Diagnosis of Diseases of the Chest

THIRD EDITION

Robert G. Fraser, M.D.
Professor Emeritus
Department of Radiology
University of Alabama at Birmingham
Birmingham, Alabama

J.A. Peter Paré, M.D.
Professor Emeritus
Department of Medicine
McGill University
Montreal, Quebec

P.D. Paré, M.D.
Professor of Medicine
University of British Columbia
Head, Respiratory Division
University of British Columbia and
    St. Paul's Hospital
Vancouver, British Columbia

Richard S. Fraser, M.D.
Associate Professor of Pathology
McGill University
Pathologist, Montreal General Hospital
Head, Department of Pathology
Montreal Chest Hospital Institute
Montreal, Quebec

George P. Genereux, M.D.
Professor of Radiology
University of Saskatchewan, Saskatoon
Radiologist, University of Saskatchewan Hospital
Saskatoon, Saskatchewan

1990
W.B. SAUNDERS COMPANY
Harcourt Brace Jovanovich, Inc.
Philadelphia   London   Toronto   Montreal   Sydney   Tokyo

W. B. SAUNDERS COMPANY
Harcourt Brace Jovanovich, Inc.

The Curtis Center
Independence Square West
Philadelphia, PA 19106

Library of Congress Cataloging-in-Publication Data
(Revised for vol. 3)

Diagnosis of diseases of the chest.

Rev. ed. of: Diagnosis of diseases of the chest /
Robert G. Fraser, J. A. Peter Paré. 2nd ed. 1977–
Includes bibliographies and indexes.

1. Chest—Diseases—Diagnosis—Collected works.
2. Thoracic Diseases—diagnosis. 3. Thoracic Radiology.
I. Fraser, Robert G., 1921–

RC941.D52   1990   87–4678

ISBN 0–7216–3879–1 (set)

ISBN 0–7216–3870–8 (v. 1)

ISBN 0–7216–3871–6 (v. 2)

ISBN 0–7216–3872–4 (v. 3)

Listed here are the latest translated editions of this book together with the language of the translation and the publisher.

Italian (2nd Edition)—Editrice Ambrosiana, Milan, Italy
Spanish (2nd Edition)—Salvat Editores S.A., Barcelona, Spain
Portuguese (2nd Edition)—Editora Manole Ltda., Sao Paulo, Brazil
German (2nd Edition, Vol. IV)—F. K. Schattauer Verlag, Stuttgart, West Germany

Editor: Lisette Bralow
Designer: W. B. Saunders Staff
Production Manager: Carolyn Naylor
Manuscript Editor: Carol Robins
Illustration Coordinator: Walt Verbitski
Indexer: Julie Schwager/Kathy Garcia

Volume I ISBN 0-7216-3870-8
Volume II ISBN 0-7216-3871-6
Volume III ISBN 0-7216-3872-4
Set ISBN 0-7216-3879-1

Diagnosis of Diseases of the Chest

Printed in the United States of America

Last digit is the print number: 9   8   7   6   5   4   3   2   1

DEDICATION

This volume is dedicated to the memory of Dr. George Genereux, whose untimely death ended the distinguished career of a dear friend and co-author.

PREFACE TO THE THIRD EDITION

—vanity of vanities; all is vanity.
What profit hath a man of all his labour which
he taketh under the sun?
One generation passeth away, and another
generation cometh.

—ECCLESIASTES 1:2

It has been 20 years since the two senior authors began writing the first edition of this book, and during the preliminary stages of planning for the third edition, we grudgingly acknowledged a mild but inescapable attrition in the motivation and initiative we possessed formerly. More importantly, we recognized the need to prepare to hand over the reins for the writing of future editions to dependable and tested hands. As a result, we felt obliged to augment the authorship of this edition with young, fertile minds, and we didn't have far to look: our two sons, RSF and PP, were devoting much of their professional lives to the pathologic and physiologic manifestations of chest disease, respectively, and it was logical that they should take up the cudgel to prevent their fathers from wallowing in their own misconceptions. We also felt the need for the addition of a third creative mind, this time a radiologist, to bring about renewed vigor and enthusiasm to the description and illustration of roentgenologic pathology; again we had to look no further than our own back yard to find GG, an internationally renowned radiologist with a vast clinical experience in chest disease. As the first volume of this third edition has evolved, it has become abundantly clear that we possessed much wisdom in seeking the collaboration of these three. The new authors have reorganized many chapters and have greatly improved the text by preparing a much more accurate description and illustration of the pathologic manifestations of thoracic disease, a more thorough discussion of normal and pathologic physiology, and fresh new material on the roentgenologic manifestations of many conditions.

It was stated in the Preface to the First Edition that the book was written with the aim of emphasizing the value of the roentgenogram as the *first* rather than the *major* step in the diagnosis of chest disease. In the subsequent 15 year interval, we have not seen cause to alter this opinion. However, despite the usefulness of this approach from a practical day-to-day viewpoint, we have come to realize more fully that the ultimate foundation upon which diagnosis must be based is a knowledge of chest disease itself. In addition to a thorough familiarity with normal structure and function, this includes a detailed knowledge of physiologic and pathologic alterations as well as the etiologies and pathogenetic mechanisms behind them. Although intimated in the first two editions, this belief has reached full fruition in the present text in which all aspects of the normal and diseased chest have been given roughly equal coverage. Whatever emphasis was formerly placed on roentgenology is now of necessity less evident. This should not be interpreted as a diminution in our belief of the importance of the roentgenogram in diagnosis but rather as an extension of the previously unstated but implied importance of the broader view. This approach has necessarily involved the inclusion of a vast amount of new information and has resulted unavoidably in a comprehensive reference work rather than a textbook. The scope of the text is such that it will find its greatest use in the hands of specialists such as respirologists, thoracic surgeons, and radiologists and pathologists whose particular interest lies in diseases of the chest. However, those with a more general outlook, such as internists and house officers, will also find the book useful as an occasional reference source.

What will the reader find new? In addition to the more extensive coverage of pathology and physiology and the addition of new knowledge that has appeared in the literature over the 7 or 8 year span, fresh material has appeared on the control of breathing, the respiratory muscles in health and disease, breathing during sleep, the development of the lung, host defense mechanisms, opportunistic infections, pulmonary vasculitides, the acquired immunodeficiency syndrome, the lung in transplantation, and drug-induced pulmonary disease. In addition, there is a complete reorganization of the chapter on neoplasms based on the 1982 WHO classification, and there are extensive additions to the discussion of the obstructive airway diseases, particularly with regard to pathophysiology and bronchial reactivity. A number of illustrations have been replaced and many new ones added, with emphasis on computed tomography and, to a lesser extent, magnetic resonance imaging. Virtually all illustrations of gross and microscopic pathology are new, and it is hoped that they will provide new insights into pathologic/radiologic correlation.

Since the publication of the Second Edition, a spectacular expansion of knowledge has occurred concerning the structure and function of the lung in health and disease; as a result, it has proved impossible to carry out a simple revision, and in most areas the book has been almost completely rewritten. However, all attempts have been made not to increase its length: the addition of new material, particularly in sections dealing with pathology and pathophysiology, has been balanced by the removal of out-of-date-text. To achieve a roughly equal size of the new volumes, it has been necessary to alter the order of chapters somewhat from that in the first two editions. The tables of differential diagnosis and decision trees have been incorporated into Volume IV rather than occupying a separate volume as in the second edition. The rapidity with which new knowledge is appearing has also made it necessary to publish the four volumes sequentially rather than simultaneously. We regret the necessity for this, but were we to await completion of the later volumes, the first volume would be long out of date, requiring thorough revision; the inevitable result would be a vicious cycle whereby none of the volumes would ever be published!

As anticipated, the writing style of each of the five authors has varied considerably, requiring considerable subediting in an attempt to unify syntax and nomenclature. In this regard, we and others have been concerned with the variable terminology employed by physicians in the description of the normal and diseased thorax. In an attempt to obviate this variability, in 1975 a joint committee of the American College of Chest Physicians and the American Thoracic Society published a glossary of pulmonary terms and symbols pertinent to the medical and physiologic aspects of the normal and diseased chest (Chest 67:538, 1975). At about the same time, the Fleischner Society formed a committee on nomenclature that designed and subsequently published a glossary of words and terms that they recommended for roentgenologic terminology (AJR *143*:509, 1984). Since several of the terms recommended by the ACCP/ATS Committee for use in the classification of diseases, in physical examination, and in respiratory therapy are at variance with those used in this book, we have chosen to include only the terms and symbols used in respiratory physiology and pathophysiology. Both the modified ACCP/ATS and the Fleischner glossaries are printed before Chapter 1, and the reader is urged to review them and use them regularly.

The burgeoning knowledge in the field of chest disease continues unabated. The 20-odd journals that the two senior authors reviewed in the preparation of the first and second editions have been expanded not only by the proliferation of new biomedical publications and the inclusion of a number of recognized journals in other specialized clinical disciplines, but also by the many physiology and pathology journals that were not included in the original review. As a consequence, the near-10,000 references cited in the second edition will certainly be exceeded in the third. Bibliographies have been placed at the end of each chapter and their position indicated by a black slash on page edges, thus facilitating their identification.

Once again, we invite our readers to inform us of differences of opinion they may have with the contents of this book or to offer their advice as to how future editions may be improved. It is only through such interchange of information and opinion that we can hope to establish on a firm basis the knowlege necessary for a full understanding of respiratory disease.

RGF
JAPP
PDP
RSF
GPG

ACKNOWLEDGMENTS

Coordination of the contributions of two authors in the preparation of the first two editions of this book proved to be a formidable undertaking, but in fact was relatively simple compared with the enormous problems created by attempts to assimilate material from five separate sources. The writing of the manuscript and the choice and preparation of new illustrations were the most formidable part of the undertaking, but the many steps necessary to the final product required the unselfish and enthusiastic contributions of many hands and minds, and the support and encouragement we received from many of our friends are greatly appreciated and duly acknowledged.

It is not possible to overstate our gratitude to our secretaries, who handled magnificently the tedious and necessarily exacting task of listing and filing references, transcribing manuscript from tape, typing the several drafts up to and including the final, and cheerfully coping with the innumerable problems encountered. Anne Paré of Val Morin, Quebec; Peggy Stewart of St. Paul's Hospital, Vancouver; Donna O'Connor and Wendy Segall of the Montreal General Hospital; Joan Matlock of the University of Saskatchewan Hospital; and Marianne Constantine of the Montreal Chest Hospital exhibited exemplary patience and devotion in accomplishing these thorny chores. Although these individuals have earned our heartfelt thanks, the efforts by Lynn Hogan and Susan Ullery-Lynch of the Hospital of the University of Alabama at Birmingham deserve special praise, since it was their lot to type not only the contributions from their boss but also the edited manuscript from the other four authors. Joanne Fraser carried out the tedious job of recording, filing, and checking the innumerable references, an extremely frustrating chore that she performed with meticulous accuracy. The devotion and diligence with which all these people carried out their tasks are deeply appreciated.

The majority of the case histories and roentgenograms reproduced here are of patients of staff members of the Royal Victoria Hospital, the Montreal General Hospital, the Montreal Chest Hospital Institute, the Hospital of the University of Alabama at Birmingham, and the Medical Center of the University of Saskatchewan. All illustrations of pathology derived from patients in the Montreal General Hospital and the Montreal Chest Hospital Institute. Our indebtedness to our colleagues who were caring for these patients cannot be overemphasized, not only for their generosity in permitting us to publish these case reports but also for the benefit of their experience and guidance over the years.

The superb photographic work throughout these volumes was the accomplishment of the Department of Visual Aids of the Royal Victoria Hospital; Susie Gray and Tony Zagar of the Department of Radiology, the University of Alabama at Birmingham; David Mandeville of the University of Saskatchewan Hospital; and Joseph Donohue and Anthony Graham of Montreal. Their craftsmanship and rich experience in photography are readily apparent in these pages. Caroline Lutz, Adriana Torrisi, and Maria Masluck provided expert assistance in the preparation of the pathologic material. We would also like to thank Dr. John Fleetham of the University Hospital, University of British Columbia, for his help in the preparation of the section on obstructive sleep apnea and Dr. Margot Becklake for her able assistance in revising the material on asbestos-related disease.

Throughout our labors, we received much support and cooperation from the publishers, notably Lisette Bralow, who effectively and sympathetically minimized the many obstacles we encountered.

Finally, and with immense gratitude, we recall the patience and understanding displayed by our wives and children throughout our labors. Without their continuous encouragement, this book surely would not have been completed, and we acknowledge their many virtues with much love.

RGF
JAPP
PDP
RSF
GPG

PREFACE TO
THE FIRST EDITION

This book was written with the aim of defining an approach to the diagnosis of diseases of the chest based on the abnormal roentgenogram. Experience over the years has led the authors to the conclusion that the chest roentgenogram represents the focal point or sheet anchor in the diagnosis of the majority of pulmonary diseases, many patients presenting with either no symptoms and signs or entirely nonspecific ones. This emphasis on the roentgenogram as the first step in reaching a diagnosis does not represent an attempt to relegate history and physical examination to a position of no importance, but merely an effort to place them in proper perspective. In no other medical field is diagnosis so dependent upon the intelligent integration of information from roentgenologic, clinical, laboratory, and pathologic sources as in diseases of the chest. We submit that the roentgenogram is the starting point in this investigation; the knowledge of structural change thus obtained, when integrated with pertinent clinical findings and results of pulmonary function tests and other ancillary diagnostic procedures, enables one to arrive at a confident diagnosis. Some patients manifest symptoms and signs that themselves are virtually diagnostic of some chest disorders, but even in such cases the confirmation of diagnosis requires the presence of an appropriate roentgenographic pattern.

A glance through the pages will reveal an abundance of roentgenographic illustrations that might create the illusion that this book is written primarily for the roentgenologist, but this is not our intention. In fact, the clinical, morphologic, and laboratory aspects of many diseases are described at greater length than the roentgenologic, a fact pointing up the broad interest we hope the book will engender among internists, surgeons, and family practitioners interested in chest disease. The numerous illustrations reflect the aim of the book—to emphasize the value of the roentgenogram as the *first* rather than the *major* step in diagnosis.

During the writing of the book, our original plan was considerably modified as the format unfolded and we became even more aware of the complexities of design and organization. Originally, our approach to differential diagnosis suggested a division of chapters on the basis of specific roentgenographic patterns. It soon became apparent, however, that since many diseases give rise to various different roentgenographic patterns, this method of presentation would require tedious repetition of clinical and laboratory details in several chapters. To obviate this, we planned tables of differential diagnosis, listing etiologic classifications of diseases that produce specific roentgenographic patterns and describing briefly the clinical and laboratory characteristics of each disease, thus facilitating recognition of disease states. The tables are designed to be used with the text in the following manner. When a specific pattern of disease is recognized, the appropriate table should be scanned and those conditions selected that correspond most closely with the clinical picture presented by the patient. Additional information about the likeliest diagnostic possibilities can be obtained by referring to the detailed discussions in the relevant sections of the text (page numbers are cited after each diagnosis). The tables relate to 17 basic patterns of bronchopulmonary, pleural, and mediastinal disease; they are grouped together in Chapter 5 in Volume I and may be located with ease from the black marks found on the upper corners of their pages. Each table is preceded by a detailed description and representative illustrations of the specific roentgenographic pattern. An attempt has been made to indicate the relative incidence of the diseases.

Although our original plan called for a one volume presentation, it soon became apparent that the length of the text and the number and size of illustrations necessary for full coverage of the subject required two volumes. Volume I includes descriptions of the normal chest, methods and techniques of investigation, clinical features, and roentgenologic signs of chest diseases, the tables of differential diagnosis, and chapters devoted to diseases of developmental origin and the infectious diseases; in Volume II appear detailed discussions of the morphologic, roentgenologic, and clinical aspects of all other diseases of the thorax arranged in chapters according to etiology.

The roentgenograms have been reproduced by two different techniques, the majority in Volume I by the logEtronic method and those in Volume II by direct photography. The publishers have been generous in allotting sufficient space for the reproduction of the roentgenograms in a size adequate for good detail recognition.

Much of the material in the book has been based on our personal experience gained in the past almost two decades, during which we have had a predominant interest in pulmonary disease. Obviously, this experience has been greatly enhanced by the extensive literature that has accumulated during these years, and we are mindful of the tremendous help we have received from the contributions of others. Our free use of the literature is reflected in the extensive bibliography.

Certain differences from the contents of other books on respiratory disease will be noted. First, this text contains no reference to treatment. Since drug therapies and surgical techniques are constantly changing, any attempt to include them would make the book out of date almost before it was published. Second, we have intentionally made only passing reference to pulmonary disease peculiar to children, a full description of which would require a complete separate text.

The relative incidence of respiratory diseases has changed considerably over the last quarter century. In some diseases, such as tuberculosis and bronchiectasis, a decreased frequency reflects improved public health measures and therapeutic innovations; in others, man's therapeutic triumphs have proved a mixed blessing, enabling patients with disabling chronic respiratory disease to live longer despite formerly fatal pneumonias. Perhaps even more important, man himself is responsible for varying the spectrum of respiratory disease as a result of his irresponsible insistence upon increasing the amount and variety of atmospheric pollutants. Inhaled contaminated air not only is regarded as the major etiologic factor in chronic obstructive pulmonary disease and the inorganic dust pneumoconioses, but also has been incriminated in the etiology of several hypersensitivity diseases of the lungs. This last group comprises the "extrinsic" form of allergic alveolitis. The number of conditions involved, when added to the better known "intrinsic" counterpart—the collagen diseases—is largely responsible for the length of the chapter devoted to immunologic diseases. Other changes that have contributed to the "new face" of pulmonary disease include increasing knowledge of the hormonal effects of neoplasms; the discovery that various immunologic defects may reduce host resistance to infection; and finally the appearance in the western world of parasitic infestations and bacterial infections formerly considered so rare in those areas as to warrant little consideration in differential diagnosis, but now of some importance because of the modern day ease of intercontinental travel. Although the novelty of these recent changes may have led the authors to consider them in greater detail and length than is their due, the emphasis may serve to bring them into proper perspective.

Finally, we recognize our fallibility. It is inevitable that some observations in a text of this magnitude will prove erroneous in time or will find disagreement among our knowledgeable readers. This we expect and accept. We sincerely hope that such differences of opinion will be made known to us, so that they may be weighed and, where appropriate, introduced into subsequent editions or revisions. It is only through such interchange of information and opinion that we can hope to establish on a firm basis the knowledge necessary to a full understanding of respiratory disease.

R.G.F.
J.A.P.P.

CONTENTS

VOLUME III

Glossary of Words, Terms and Symbols in Chest Medicine and Roentgenology

"Then you should say what you mean," the March Hare went on.
"I do," Alice hastily replied; "at least— at least, I mean what I say—that's the same thing, you know."
"Not the same thing a bit!" said the Hatter. "Why, you might just as well say that 'I see what I eat' is the same thing as 'I eat what I see!' "

This well-known excerpt from Lewis Carroll's *Alice's Adventures in Wonderland* points out a problem that confronts many physicians in today's constantly expanding scientific literature—the use of words and terms that mean different things to different people. The frequency with which imprecise or frankly erroneous words are employed to describe roentgenographic images (for example) is astonishing; common usage has created a jargon that has led to confusion if not to actual communication breakdown. In 1975, a joint committee of the American College of Chest Physicians and the American Thoracic Society published a glossary of pulmonary terms and symbols* pertinent to the medical and physiologic aspects of chest disease, but it omitted words that specifically related to chest roentgenology. As a consequence, the Fleischner Society formed a Committee on Nomenclature several years ago to draw up a glossary of roentgenologic words and terms and this task now has been completed and the glossary published.† We list herewith a number of words, terms, and symbols selected from the two publications that we hope our readers will refer to and use. The precise definition of some words has been altered slightly to coincide with usage in this book.

---

*Pulmonary Terms and Symbols; A report of the ACCP/ATS Joints Committee on Pulmonary Nomenclature. Chest 67:583, 1975.
†Glossary of Terms for Thoracic Radiology: Recommendations of the Nomenclature Committee of the Fleischner Society. Am J Roentgenol *143*:509, 1984.

WORDS OR TERMS USED IN ROENTGENOLOGY

Word or Term	Comments
abscess *n., pl.* -es. 1. (pathol.) An inflammatory mass, the central part of which has undergone purulent liquefaction necrosis. It may communicate with the bronchial tree. 2. (radiol.) Within the lung, a mass presumed to be caused by infection. The presence of gas within the mass, with or without a fluid level, represents a cavity (q.v.) and implies a communication with the bronchial tree. Otherwise, a pulmonary mass can be considered to represent an abscess in the morpholgic sense only by inference. *Qualifiers:* Expressing clinical course: acute, chronic. Expressing etiology: bacterial, fungal, etc. Expressing site of involvement: lung, mediastinum, etc.	Should be used only with reference to masses of presumed infectious etiology. The word is not synonymous with cavity (*q.v.*).

WORDS OR TERMS USED IN ROENTGENOLOGY *Continued*

Word or Term	Comments
acinar pattern *n.* (radiol.) A collection of round or elliptic, ill-defined, discrete or partly confluent opacities in the lung, each measuring 4 to 8 mm in diameter and together producing an extended, inhomogeneous shadow. *Synonyms:* Rosette pattern; acinonodose pattern (used specifically with reference to endobronchial spread of tuberculosis); alveolar pattern.	An inferred conclusion usually used as a descriptor. An acceptable term, preferred to cited synonyms (especially "alveolar pattern," which is an inaccurate descriptor).
acinar shadow *n.* (radiol.) A round or slightly elliptic pulmonary opacity 4 to 8 mm in diameter presumed to represent an anatomic acinus rendered opaque by consolidation. Usually employed in the presence of many such opacities (*see* acinar pattern).	An inferred conclusion sometimes applicable as a roentgenologic descriptor.
acinus *n.* (anat.) The portion of lung parenchyma distal to the terminal bronchiole and consisting of respiratory bronchioles, alveolar ducts, alveolar sacs, and alveoli (*see* acinar shadow, acinar pattern).	A specific feature of pulmonary anatomy.
aeration *n.* (physiol./radiol.) 1. The state of containing air. 2. The state or process of being filled or inflated with air. *Qualifiers:* overaeration (preferred) or hyperaeration; underaeration (preferred) or hypoaeration. *Synonym:* Inflation.	An acceptable term with reference to the inspiratory phase of respiration. Inflation is preferred in sense 2.
air, *n.* (radiol.) Inspired atmospheric gas. The word is sometimes used to describe gas within the body regardless of its composition or site.	With reference to pneumothorax, subcutaneous emphysema, or the content of the stomach, colon, etc., gas is the more accurate term and is preferred.
air bronchiologram *n.* (radiol.) The equivalent of air bronchogram but in airways assumed to be bronchioles because of their peripheral location and diameter.	An acceptable term.
air bronchogram *n.* (radiol.) The roentgenographic shadow of an air-containing bronchus peripheral to the hilum and surrounded by airless lung (whether by virtue of absorption of air, replacement of air, or both), a finding generally regarded as evidence of the patency of the more proximal airway. Hence, any bandlike tapering and/or branching lucency within opacified lung corresponding in size and distribution to a bronchus or bronchi and presumed to represent an air-containing segment of the bronchial tree.	A specific feature of roentgenologic anatomy whose identify is often inferred. A useful and recommended term.
air-fluid level *n.* (radiol.) A local collection of gas and liquid that, when traversed by a horizontal x-ray beam, creates a shadow characterized by a sharp horizontal interface between gas density above and liquid density below.	A useful roentgenologic descriptor. Since with rare exception (*e.g.,* fat-fluid level) the upper of the two absorbant media is "air" (gas), it is sufficient to describe such an appearance as a "fluid level."
air space *n.* (*adj.* air-space) (anat./radiol.) The gas-containing portion of lung parenchyma, including the acini and excluding the interstitium and purely conductive portions of the lung. *Synonyms:* Acinar consolidation, alveolar consolidation (when used as an adjective in relation to air-space consolidation).	An inferred conclusion usually used as a roentgenologic descriptor. An acceptable term whose use as an adjective is also appropriate.

WORDS OR TERMS USED IN ROENTGENOLOGY *Continued*

Word or Term	Comments
air-trapping *n.* (pathophysiol./radiol.) The retention of excess gas in all or part of the lung at any stage of expiration.	A specific roentgenologic sign to be employed only if excess air retention is demonstrated by a dynamic study, *e.g.*, inspiration-expiration roentgenography or fluoroscopy. *Not* to be used with reference to overinflation of the lung at full inspiration (total lung capacity).
airway *n., adj.* (anat./radiol.) A collective term for the air-conducting passages from the larynx to and including the respiratory bronchioles. *Synonyms:* Conducting airway; tracheobronchial tree.	A useful anatomic term. May be used as an adjective in relation to disease or abnormality. Note that the respiratory bronchioles are both conducting and gas-exchanging airways and thus constitute the transitory zone.
alveolarization *n.* (radiol.) The opacification of groups of alveoli by a contrast medium.	A misnomer whose use is to be deplored. Excessive filling of peripheral lung structure by contrast media usually employed for bronchography may opacify respiratory bronchioles but not alveoli. Thus, the correct term is "bronchiolar filling or opacification."
anterior junction line *n.* (radiol.) A vertically oriented linear or curvilinear opacity approximately 1 to 2 mm wide, commonly projected on the tracheal air shadow. It is produced by the shadows of the right and left pleurae in intimate contact between the aerated lungs anterior to the great vessels (and sometimes the heart); hence, it never extends above the suprasternal notch (*cf.* posterior junction line). *Synonyms:* Anterior mediastinal septum, line, or stripe.	A specific feature of roentgenologic anatomy; to be preferred to cited synonyms.
aortopulmonary window *n.* 1. (anat.) A mediastinal space bounded anteriorly by the posterior surface of the ascending aorta; posteriorly by the anterior surface of the descending aorta; superiorly by the inferior surface of the aortic arch; inferiorly by the superior surface of the left pulmonary artery; medially by the left side of the trachea, left main bronchus, and esophagus; and laterally by the left lung. Within it are situated fat, the ductus ligament, the left recurrent laryngeal nerve, and lymph nodes. 2. (radiol.) A zone of relative lucency in the mediastinal shadow that is seen to best advantage in the left anterior oblique or lateral projection and that corresponds to the anatomic space defined above. On a posteroanterior roentgenogram of the chest, the lateral margin of the space constitutes the aortopulmonary window interface. *Synonym:* Aortic-pulmonic window.	A specific feature of roentgenologic anatomy.
atelectasis *n.* (pathophysiol./radiol.) Less than normal inflation of all or a portion of the lung with corresponding diminution in volume. *Qualifiers* may be employed to indicate severity (mild, moderate, severe), mechanism (resorption, relaxation, cicatrization, adhesive), or distribution (*e.g.*, lobar, platelike [*q.v.*], discoid). *Synonyms:* Collapse, loss of volume, anectasis.	Generally this term is preferable to "collapse" in describing loss of volume. The word "collapse" connotes total atelectasis in which lung tissue has been reduced to its smallest volume. Anectasis is usually used in reference to failure of lung expansion in the neonate.

WORDS OR TERMS USED IN ROENTGENOLOGY *Continued*

Word or Term	Comments

azygoesophageal recess *n.* 1. (anat.) A space or recess in the right side of the mediastinum into which the medial edge of the right lower lobe (crista pulmonis) extends. It is limited superiorly by the arch of the azygos vein, inferiorly by the diaphragm, posteriorly by the azygos vein in front of the vertebral column, and medially by the esophagus and its adjacent structures. (The exact relationship between the medial edge of the lung and the mediastinal structures is variable.) 2. (radiol.) In a frontal chest roentgenogram, a vertically oriented interface between air in the right lower lobe and the adjacent mediastinum that represents the medial limit of the anatomic azygoesophageal recess.

> *Synonyms:* Infraazygos recess; right pleuroesophageal line or stripe; right paraesophageal line or stripe.

A specific feature of roentgenologic anatomy. The use of the term "recess" to identify an interface is inappropriate; thus, azygoesophageal recess interface is preferred.

bat's-wing distribution *n.* (radiol.) A spatial arrangement of roentgenographic opacities in a frontal roentgenogram that bears a vague resemblance to the shape of a bat in flight; said of coalescent, ill-defined opacities that are approximately bilaterally symmetric and that are confined to the medulla of the lungs (*q.v.*).

> *Synonym:* Butterfly distribution.

A roentgenologic descriptor of limited usefulness.

bleb *n.* 1. (pathol.) A gas-containing space within or contiguous to the visceral pleura of the lung. 2. (radiol.) A local, thin-walled lucency contiguous with the pleura, usually at the lung apex.

> *Synonyms:* Type I bulla (pathol.); bulla; a form of pulmonary air cyst (radiol.)

An inferred conclusion seldom justifiable by roentgenogram alone. Bulla or air cyst is preferred.

bronchiole *n.* (anat./radiol.) An airway that contains no cartilage in its wall. A bronchiole may be purely conducting (up to and including the terminal bronchiole) or transitory (the respiratory bronchioles that carry out both conduction and gas exchange).

A specific feature of pulmonary anatomy.

bronchocele *n. See* mucoid impaction.

bronchus *n.* (anat./radiol.) A conducting airway distal to the tracheal bifurcation that contains cartilage in its wall.

A specific feature of pulmonary anatomy.

bulla *n., pl.* -lae. 1. (pathol.) A sharply demarcated region of emphysema; a gas-containing space that may contain nothing but gas or may contain overdistended and ruptured alveolar septa and blood vessels. 2. (radiol.) Sharply demarcated hyperlucent area of avascularity within the lung, measuring 1 cm or more in diameter and possessing a wall less than 1 mm in thickness. *Qualifiers:* small, medium, large.

The preferred term to describe all thin-walled air-containing spaces in the lung with the exception of pneumatocele (*q.v.*).

butterfly distribution *n.* (radiol.) *See* bat's-wing distribution.

To be distinguished from the use of this term in general medicine to describe the distribution of certain cutaneous lesions.

WORDS OR TERMS USED IN ROENTGENOLOGY *Continued*

Word or Term	Comments
calcification *n.* 1. (pathophysiol.) (a) The process by which one or more deposits of calcium salts are formed within lung tissue or within a pulmonary lesion. (b) Such a deposit of calcium salts. 2. (radiol.) A calcific opacity within the lung that may be organized (*e.g.*, concentric lamination), but which does not display the trabecular organization of true bone. *Qualifiers:* "eggshell," "popcorn," target, laminated, flocculent, nodular, etc.	An explicit conclusion; may be used as a descriptor. To be distinguished from ossification (*q.v.*).
carina *n.* (anat./radiol.) The keel-shaped ridge that separates the right and left main bronchi at the tracheal bifurcation.	A specific feature of pulmonary anatomy.
carinal angle *n.* (anat./radiol.) The angle formed by the right and left main bronchi at the tracheal bifurcation. *Synonyms:* Bifurcation angle; angle of tracheal bifurcation.	A definitive anatomic and roentgenologic measurement.
cavity *n.* 1. (pathol.) A mass within lung parenchyma, the central portion of which has undergone liquefaction necrosis and has been expelled via the bronchial tree, leaving a gas-containing space, with or without associated fluid. 2. (radiol.) A gas-containing space within the lung surrounded by a wall whose thickness is greater than 1 mm and usually irregular in contour.	A useful descriptor without etiologic connotation. The word must not be used interchangeably with abscess (*q.v.*), which may exist without bronchial communication and therefore without cavitation.
circumscribed *adj.* (radiol.) Possessing a complete or nearly complete visible border.	An acceptable descriptor.
clot *n.* (pathol.) A semisolidified mass of blood elements.	*Cf.* thrombus.
coalescence *n.* (radiol.) The joining together of a number of opacities into a single opacity; confluence (*q.v.*).	An acceptable descriptor.
coin lesion *n.* (radiol.) A sharply defined, circular opacity within the lung suggestive of the appearance of a coin and usually representing a spherical or nodular lesion. *Synonyms:* Pulmonary nodule, pulmonary mass.	A roentgenologic descriptor, the use of which is to be condemned. The term "coin" may be descriptive of the shadow, but certainly not of the lesion producing it.
collapse *n.* (radiol.) A state in which lung tissue has undergone complete atelectasis.	The term is acceptable when employed strictly as defined, but "atelectasis" is preferred, since the degree of loss of lung volume can be qualified by mild, moderate, or severe.
collateral ventilation *n.* (physiol./radiol.) The process by which gas passes from one lung unit (acinus, lobule, segment, or lobe) to a contiguous unit via alveolar pores (pores of Kohn), canals of Lambert, or direct airway anastomoses. *Synonym:* Collateral air drift.	An inferred conclusion usually based on fairly reliable signs. A useful term. The channels of peripheral airway communication also function as a mechanism for transmission of liquid from one unit to another (*e.g.*, in acute airspace pneumonia).
confluence *n.* (radiol.) The nature of opacities that are contiguous with or adjacent to one another. *Antonym:* Discrete (*q.v.*).	A useful descriptor; confluence is to be distinguished from coalescence (*q.v.*), which is the act of becoming confluent.

WORDS OR TERMS USED IN ROENTGENOLOGY *Continued*

Word or Term

Comments

consolidation *n.* 1. (pathophysiol.) The process by which air in the lung is replaced by the products of disease, rendering the lung solid (as in pneumonia). 2. (radiol.) An essentially homogeneous opacity in the lung characterized by little or no loss of volume, by effacement of pulmonary blood vessels, and sometimes by the presence of an air bronchogram (*q.v.*).

An inferred conclusion, applicable only in an appropriate clinical setting when the opacity can with reasonable certainty be attributed to replacement of alveolar air by exudate, transudate, or tissue. Not to be used with reference to all homogeneous opacities.

corona radiata *n.* (radiol.) A circumferential pattern of fine linear spicules, approximately 5 mm long, extending outward from the margin of a solitary pulmonary nodule through a zone of relative lucency.

A sign of limited usefulness in the differentiation of benign and malignant nodules.

cor pulmonale *n.* 1. (pathol./clin.) Right ventricular hypertrophy and/or dilatation occurring as a result of an abnormality of lung structure or function. 2. (radiol.) The combination of pulmonary arterial hypertension and chronic lung disease, with or without evidence of enlargement of right heart chambers. *Qualifiers:* acute, chronic.

An inferred roentgenologic conclusion based on usually reliable signs. An acceptable descriptor. Despite the pathologic definition, roentgenologic evidence of cardiomegaly need not be present.

cortex *n.* (radiol.) The peripheral 2 to 3 cm of lung parenchyma adjacent to the visceral pleura, either over the convexity of the thorax or in the interlobar fissures. (*See* medulla and hilum.)

The peripheral part of an arbitrary subdivision of the lung into three zones from the hilum to the visceral pleura. Of limited usefulness.

CT number *n.* (radiol./physics) In computed tomography, a quantitative numerical statement of the relative attenuation of the x-ray beam at a specified point; loosely, the relative attenuation of a specified tissue absorber, usually expressed in Hounsfield units (HU).

cyst *n.* 1. (pathol.) A circumscribed space whose contents may be liquid or gaseous and whose wall is generally thin and well defined and lined by epithelium. 2. (radiol.) A gas-containing space of any size possessing a thin wall. *Qualifiers:* foregut (bronchogenic, esophageal duplication); postinfectious.

This term is entirely nonspecific and should not possess inferred conclusion as to etiology. It is the preferred term to describe any thin-walled gas-containing space in the lung possessing a wall thickness greater than 1 mm.

defined *adj.* (radiol.) The character of the border of a shadow. *Qualifiers:* well, sharply, poorly, distinctly.

An acceptable descriptor.

demarcated *adj.* (radiol.) Distinct from adjacent structures. *Qualifiers:* well, sharply, poorly.

An acceptable descriptor. (*Cf.* defined.)

dense *adj.* (radiol.) Possessing density (*q.v.*). Usually used in describing or comparing roentgenographic shadows with respect to their light transmission.

A recommended term in the context defined. Should not be used in referring to the opacity of an absorber of x-radiation. (*See* opaque, opacity.)

density *n.* 1. (physics) The mass of a substance per unit volume. 2. (photometry/radiol.) The opacity of a roentgenographic shadow to visible light; film blackening. 3. (radiol.) The shadow of an absorber more opaque to x-rays than its surround; an opacity or radiopacity. 4. The degree of opacity of an absorber to x-rays, usually expressed in terms of the nature of the absorber (*e.g.*, bone, water, or fat density).

In sense 2, the term refers to a fundamental characteristic of the roentgenogram, and its use is recommended. In senses 3 and 4, it refers to the character of the absorber and has an exactly opposite connotation with respect to film blackening. Because of this potential confusion, the term should *never* be used to mean an "opacity" or "radiopacity."

WORDS OR TERMS USED IN ROENTGENOLOGY *Continued*

Word or Term	Comments
diffuse *adj.* 1. (pathophysiol.) Widely distributed through an organ or type of tissue. 2. (radiol.) Widespread and continuous (said of shadows and by inference of the states or processes producing them). *Synonyms:* Disseminated, generalized, systemic, widespread.	A useful and acceptable term. In the context of chest radiology, "diffuse" connotes widespread, anatomically continuous but not necessarily complete involvement of the lung or other thoracic structure or tissue; "disseminated" connotes widespread but anatomically discontinuous involvement; and "generalized" connotes complete or nearly complete involvement whereas "systemic" connotes involvement of a thoracic structure or tissue as part of a process involving the entire body.
discrete *adj.* (radiol.) Separate, individually distinct; hence, with respect to opacities, usually circumscribed. *Antonyms:* Confluent, coalescent.	An acceptable descriptor.
disseminated *adj.* 1. (pathophysiol.) Widely but discontinuously distributed through an organ or type of tissue. 2. (radiol.) Widespread but anatomically discontinuous (said of shadows and by inference of the states or processes producing them). *Synonyms:* Diffuse (*q.v.*), generalized, systemic.	A useful and acceptable term.
doubling time *n.* (radiol.) The time span over which a pulmonary nodule or mass doubles in volume (increases its diameter by a factor of 1.25).	An acceptable term. The concept should be used with caution as a criterion for distinguishing benign from malignant nodules.
embolus *n.* 1. (pathol.) A clot or mass of foreign material that has been carried by the bloodstream to occlude partly or completely the lumen of a blood vessel. 2. (radiol.) (a) A lucent defect or obstruction within an opacified blood vessel presumed to represent an embolus in the pathologic sense. (b) An acutely dilated pulmonary artery presumed to represent the presence of blood clot or other embolic material. *Qualifiers:* acute, chronic; air, fat, amniotic fluid, parasitic, neoplastic, tissue, foreign material (*e.g.*, iodized oil, mercury, talc); septic, therapeutic, paradoxic.	In sense 2(a), an inferred conclusion based on reliable evidence (arteriography); in sense 2(b), based on highly suggestive evidence (conventional roentgenography) in the appropriate clinical setting. A useful descriptor, particularly in arteriography.
emphysema *n.* 1. (pathol.) (a) A morbid condition of the lung characterized by abnormally expanded air spaces distal to the terminal bronchiole, with or without destruction of the air-space walls (per Ciba Conference, 1959). (b) As above, but "with destruction of the walls of involved air spaces" specified (per World Health Organization, 1961, and American Thoracic Society, 1962). 2. (radiol.) Overinflation of all or a portion of one or both lungs, with or without associated oligemia (*q.v.*), presumed to represent morphologic emphysema.	In radiology, an inferred conclusion based on usually reliable signs (if the disease is moderate or advanced). Applicable only in an appropriate clinical setting and, in the sense of the ATS definition, not applicable to spasmodic asthma or compensatory overinflation.
fibrocalcific *adj.* (radiol.) Of or pertaining to sharply defined, linear, and/or nodular opacities containing calcification(s) (*q.v.*), usually occurring in the upper lobes and presumed to represent old granulomatous lesions.	A widely used and acceptable roentgenologic descriptor.

WORDS OR TERMS USED IN ROENTGENOLOGY *Continued*

Word or Term	Comments
fibronodular *adj.* (radiol.) Of or pertaining to sharply defined, approximately circular opacities occurring singly or in clusters, usually in the upper lobes, and associated with linear opacities and distortion (retraction) of adjacent structures. A finding usually presumed to represent old granulomatous disease.	An inferred conclusion usually employed as a roentgenologic descriptor. Its use is not recommended.
fibrosis *n.* 1. (pathol.) (a) Cellular fibrous tissue or dense acellular collagenous tissue. (b) The process of proliferation of fibroblasts leading to the formation of fibrous or collagenous tissue. 2. (radiol.) Any opacity presumed to represent fibrous or collagenous tissue; applicable to linear, nodular, or stellate opacities that are sharply defined, that are associated with evidence of loss of volume in the affected portion of the lung and/or with deformity of adjacent structures, and that show no change over a period of months or years. Also applicable with caution to a diffuse pattern of opacity if there is evidence of progressive loss of lung volume or if the pattern of opacity is unchanged over time.	In radiology, an inferred conclusion often used as a descriptor. An acceptable term if used in strict accordance with the criteria cited.
fissure *n.* 1. (anat.) The infolding of visceral pleura that separates one lobe or a portion of a lobe from another. 2. (radiol.) A linear opacity normally 1 mm or less in width that corresponds in position and extent to the anatomic separation of pulmonary lobes or portions of lobes. *Qualifiers:* minor, major, horizontal, oblique, accessory, anomalous, azygos, inferior accessory. *Synonym:* Interlobar septum.	A specific feature of anatomy.
Fleischner's line(s) *n.* (radiol.) A straight, curved, or irregular linear opacity that is visible in multiple projections; is usually situated in the lower half of the lung; is usually approximately horizontal but may be oriented in any direction; and may or may not appear to extend to the pleural surface. Such lines vary markedly in length and width; their exact pathologic significance is unknown.	An acceptable term. However, the term "linear opacity," properly qualified with respect to location, dimensions, and orientation, is preferred. There are no synonyms ("platelike," "discoid," and "platter" atelectasis should *not* be employed as synonyms; in the absence of clear histologic evidence of the significance of Fleischner's lines, the inferred identification of such lines with a form of atelectasis is unwarranted).
fluffy *adj.* (radiol.) In describing opacities: ill-defined, lacking clear-cut margins; resembling down. *Synonyms:* Shaggy, poorly defined.	An imprecise descriptor of limited usefulness.
ground-glass pattern *n.* (radiol.) Any extended, finely granular pattern of pulmonary opacity within which normal anatomic details are partly obscured. Term derived from a fancied resemblance to etched or abraded glass. *Synonym:* Granular pattern.	A nonspecific roentgenologic descriptor of limited usefulness; the synonym is preferred.
hernia *n.* (clin./morphol./radiol.) The protrusion of all or part of an organ or tissue through an abnormal opening.	An inferred conclusion to be used only within the precise terms of the definition. Thus, in the thorax the word is appropriate in relation to the diaphragm but should not be used with reference to pulmonary overinflation and mediastinal displacement.

WORDS OR TERMS USED IN ROENTGENOLOGY *Continued*

Word or Term	Comments
hilum, *n., pl.* -la. 1. (anat.) A depression or pit in that part of an organ where the vessels and nerves enter. 2. (radiol.) The composite shadow at the root of each lung composed of bronchi, pulmonary arteries and veins, lymph nodes, nerves, bronchial vessels, and associated areolar tissue. *Synonyms:* Lung root; hilus (hili).	A specific element of pulmonary anatomy. Hilum (hila) is preferred to hilus (hili).
homogeneous *adj.* (radiol.) Of uniform opacity or texture throughout. *Antonyms:* Inhomogeneous, nonhomogeneous, heterogeneous.	A useful roentgenologic descriptor. Inhomogeneous is the preferred antonym.
honeycomb pattern *n.* 1. (pathol.) A multitude of irregular cystic spaces in pulmonary tissue that are generally lined with bronchiolar epithelium and have markedly thickened walls composed of dense fibrous tissue, with or without associated chronic inflammation. 2. (radiol.) A number of closely approximated ring shadows representing air spaces 5 to 10 mm in diameter with walls 2 to 3 mm thick that resemble a true honeycomb; a finding whose occurrence implies "end-stage" lung.	It is recommended that the term be used strictly in accordance with the dimensional limits cited, in which case it possesses specific connotation.
hyperemia *n.* 1. (pathol./physiol.) An excess of blood in a part of the body; engorgement. 2. (radiol.) Increased blood flow. *Synonym:* Pleonemia (*q.v.*).	While semantically correct, this word has come through common usage to mean the increased blood flow that is part of the inflammatory response. We recommend that it be used as a descriptor only in arteriography. The synonym is preferred when indicating increased blood flow to the lungs.
hypertension *n.* (clin./radiol.) Elevation above normal levels of systolic and/or diastolic pressure within the systemic or pulmonary vascular bed. Generally accepted empiric levels of pressure for systemic arterial hypertension are 140 systolic, 90 diastolic; systemic venous hypertension, 12 mm Hg; pulmonary arterial hypertension, 30 mm Hg systolic; 15 diastolic; pulmonary venous hypertension, 12 mm Hg. *Synonym:* High blood pressure.	With the exception of systemic arterial hypertension, roentgenologic assessment of hypertension in each of the four vascular compartments constitutes an inferred conclusion, although based on usually reliable signs.
infarct *n.* (Literally, a portion of tissue stuffed with extravasated blood or serum.) 1. (pathol.) A zone of ischemic necrosis surrounded by hyperemic lung resulting from occlusion of the region's feeding vessel, usually by an embolus. 2. (radiol.) A pulmonary opacity that, by virtue of its temporal development and in the appropriate clinical setting, is considered to result from thromboembolic occlusion of a feeding vessel. The opacity is commonly but not exclusively hump-shaped and pleura-based when viewed in profile and poorly defined and round when viewed *en face.*	An inferred roentgenologic conclusion acceptable in the proper clinical setting and with appropriate signs. Subsequent events may establish that the opacity was the result of either hemorrhage or tissue necrosis. The word should not be used in the absence of an opacity (*e.g.,* with oligemia).

WORDS OR TERMS USED IN ROENTGENOLOGY *Continued*

Word or Term	Comments
infiltrate *n.* 1. (pathophysiol.) Any substance or type of cell that occurs within or spreads through the interstices (interstitium and/or alveoli) of the lung, which is foreign to the lung or which accumulates in greater than normal quantity within it. 2. (radiol.) (a) An ill-defined opacity in the lung that neither destroys nor displaces the gross morphology of the lung and is presumed to represent an infiltrate in the pathophysiologic sense. (b) Any ill-defined opacity in the lung.	An inferred and often unwarranted conclusion used as a descriptor. The term is almost invariably used in sense 2(b), in which it serves no useful purpose, and, lacking a specific connotation, is so variably used as to cause great confusion. The term's use as a descriptor is to be condemned. The preferred word is "opacity," properly qualified with respect to location, dimensions, and definition.
inflation *n.* (physiol./radiol.) The state or process of being expanded or filled with gas; used specifically with reference to the expansion of the lungs with air. *Qualifiers:* overinflation (preferred) or hyperinflation; underinflation (preferred) or hypoinflation. *Synonyms:* Aeration, inhalation, inspiration.	"Inflation" connotes expansion with gas or air. "Aeration" connotes the admission of air, exposure to air. "Inhalation" refers specifically to the act of drawing air into the lungs in the process of breathing (as opposed to exhalation); "inspiration," with reference to breathing, is similar in connotation. The word "inflation" is the preferred term, since it avoids the confusion that surrounds the meaning of aeration as a result of common misusage.
interface *n.* (radiol.) The common boundary between the shadows of two juxtaposed structures or tissues of different texture or opacity (*e.g.,* lung and heart). *Synonyms:* Edge, border.	A useful roentgenologic descriptor.
interstitium *n.* (anat./radiol.) A continuum of loose connective tissue throughout the lung consisting of three subdivisions: (a) bronchoarterial (axial), surrounding the bronchoarterial bundles from the hila to the point at which bronchiolar walls become intimately related to lung parenchyma; (b) parenchymal (acinar), situated between alveolar and capillary basement membranes; and (c) subpleural, situated between the pleura and lung parenchyma and continuous with the interlobular septa and perivenous interstitial space that extends from the lung periphery to the hila. *Synonym:* Interstitial space.	A useful anatomic term. The interstitium of the lung is not normally visible roentgenographically and only becomes visible when disease (*e.g.,* edema) increases its volume and attenuation.
Kerley line *n.* (radiol.) A linear opacity, which, depending on its location, extent, and orientation, may be further classified as follows: Kerley A line—an essentially straight linear opacity 2 to 6 cm in length and 1 to 3 mm in width, usually situated in an upper lung zone, that points toward the hilum centrally and is directed toward but does not extend to the pleural surface peripherally. Kerley B line—a straight linear opacity 1.5 to 2 cm in length and 1 to 2 mm in width, usually situated at the lung base, and oriented at right angles to the pleural surface with which it is usually in contact. Kerley C lines—a group of branching, linear opacities producing the appearance of a fine net, situated at the lung base and representing Kerley B lines seen *en face*. *Synonym:* Septal line(s).	A specific feature of pathologic/roentgenologic anatomy. Except when it is essential to distinguish A, B, and C lines, the term "septal line" is preferred. "Lymphatic line" is anatomically inaccurate and should never be used.

WORDS OR TERMS USED IN ROENTGENOLOGY *Continued*

Word or Term	Comments
line *n*. (radiol.) A longitudinal opacity no greater than 2 mm in width (*cf*. stripe).	A useful word appropriately employed in the description of roentgenographic shadows within the mediastinum (*e.g.,* anterior junction line) or lung (interlobar fissures).
linear opacity *n*. (radiol.) A shadow resembling a line; hence, any elongated opacity of approximately uniform width. *Synonyms:* Line, line shadow, linear shadow, band shadow.	A generic roentgenologic descriptor of great usefulness. "Band shadow" and "line shadow" have been employed by some to identify elongated shadows more than 2 mm wide and less than 2 mm wide, respectively; "linear opacity," qualified by a statement of specific dimensions, is the preferred term. The length, width, anatomic location, and orientation of such a shadow should be specified.
lobe *n*. (anat./radiol.) One of the principal divisions of the lungs (usually three on the right, two on the left), each of which is enveloped by the visceral pleura except at the hilum and in areas of developmental deficiency where fissures are incomplete. The lobes are separated in whole or in part by pleural fissures.	A specific feature of pulmonary anatomy.
lobule *n*. (anat./radiol.) A unit of lung structure. A subdivision of lung parenchyma that is of two types: (a) primary, arising from the last respiratory bronchiole and consisting of a series of alveolar ducts, atria, alveolar sacs, and alveoli, together with their accompanying blood vessels and nerves; (b) secondary, composed of a variable number of acini (usually 3 to 5) and bounded in most cases by connective tissue septa.	Acinus is the preferred anatomic/physiologic unit of lung structure. Since a primary lobule is not visible roentgenographically, the use of the term has been largely abandoned. When unmodified, the word "lobule" refers to a secondary lobule. A secondary pulmonary lobule occasionally becomes visible when it is either selectively consolidated or its surrounding connective tissue septa become visible from a process such as edema.
lucency *n*. (radiol.) The shadow of an absorber that attenuates the primary x-ray beam less effectively than do surrounding absorbers. Hence, in a roentgenogram, any circumscribed area that appears more nearly black (of greater photometric density) than its surround. Usually applied to local shadows of air density whose attenuation is less than that of surrounding lung (*e.g.,* a bulla) or of fat density when surrounded by a more effective absorber such as muscle. *Synonyms:* Radiolucency, translucency, transradiancy.	This term employed by analogy with "opacity," is acceptable in American usage, although it is etymologically indefensible. In British usage, "transradiancy" is preferred.
lymphadenopathy *n*. (clin./pathol./radiol.) Any abnormality of lymph nodes; by common usage usually restricted to enlargement of lymph nodes. *Synonym:* Lymph node enlargement.	Since "adeno-" specifically relates to a glandular structure and since lymph nodes are not glands, the term is a misnomer and its use is to be condemned in favor of its synonym.
marking(s) *n*. (radiol.) A descriptor variously used with reference to the shadows produced by a combination of normal pulmonary structures (blood vessels, bronchi, etc.). Usually used in the plural and following "lung" or "bronchovascular." *Synonym:* Linear opacity.	When used alone, a vague descriptor of little value and not recommended. With proper qualification, the term is acceptable.

WORDS OR TERMS USED IN ROENTGENOLOGY *Continued*

Word or Term	Comments
mass *n.* (radiol.) Any pulmonary or pleural lesion represented in a roentgenogram by a discrete opacity greater than 30 mm in diameter (without regard to contour, border characteristics, or homogeneity), but explicitly shown or presumed to be extended in all three dimensions. *Synonym:* Tumor *(q.v.).*	A useful and recommended descriptor. Should always be qualified with respect to size, location, contour, definition, homogeneity, opacity, and number. Its use as a qualifier of "lesion" is to be deplored.
medulla *n.* (radiol.) That portion of the lung situated between the hilum and cortex *(q.v.).*	A term and concept of limited usefulness.
miliary pattern *n.* (radiol.) A collection of tiny discrete opacities in the lungs, each measuring 2 mm or less in diameter, and generally uniform in size and widespread in distribution. *Synonym:* Micronodular pattern.	An acceptable descriptor without etiologic connotation.
mucoid impaction *n.* (radiol.) A broad I-, Y-, or V-shaped roentgenographic opacity caused by the presence within a proximal airway (lobar, segmental, or subsegmental bronchus) of thick, tenaceous mucus, usually associated with airway dilatation. The shape of the opacity depends upon the branching pattern of airway involved. *Synonym:* Bronchocele *(q.v.).*	An inferred conclusion based on usually reliable signs. A useful descriptor preferred to its synonym.
Mueller maneuver *n.* (physiol.) Inspiration against a closed glottis, usually but not necessarily from a position of residual volume.	A useful technique for producing transient decrease in intrathoracic pressure.
nodular pattern *n.* (radiol.) A collection of innumerable, small discrete opacities ranging in diameter from 2 to 10 mm, generally uniform in size and widespread in distribution, and without marginal spiculation *(cf.* reticulonodular pattern).	An acceptable roentgenologic discriptor without specific pathologic or etiologic implications. The size of the nodules should be specified, either as a range or as an average.
nodule *n.* (radiol.) Any pulmonary or pleural lesion represented in a roentgenogram by a sharply defined, discrete, approximately circular opacity 2 to 30 mm in diameter *(cf.* mass). *Synonym:* Coin lesion *(q.v.).*	A useful and recommended descriptor to be used in preference to its synonym, which is a colloquial abomination. Should always be qualified with respect to size, location, border characteristics, number, and opacity.
oligemia *n.* 1. (pathol./physiol.) Reduced blood flow to the lungs or a portion thereof. 2. (radiol.) General or local decrease in the apparent width of visible pulmonary vessels, suggesting less than normal blood flow. *Qualifiers:* acute, chronic; local, general. *Synonym:* Reduced blood flow.	An inferred conclusion usually used as descriptor and appropriately based on reliable signs. An acceptable term.
opacity *n.* (radiol.) The shadow of an absorber that attenuates the x-ray beam more effectively than do surrounding absorbers. Hence, in a roentgenogram, any circumscribed area that appears more nearly white (of lesser photometric density) than its surround. Usually applied to the shadows of nonspecific pulmonary collections of fluid, tissue, etc., whose attenuation exceeds that of the surrounding aerated lung. *Synonym:* Radiopacity *(cf.* density).	An essential and recommended roentgenologic descriptor. In the context of roentgenologic reporting, "radiopaque" is acceptable but seems redundant; however, it is preferred in British usage. "Density" *(q.v.)* should *never* be used in this context.

WORDS OR TERMS USED IN ROENTGENOLOGY *Continued*

Word or Term	Comments
opaque *adj.* (radiol.) Impervious to x-rays. *Synonym:* Radiopaque.	Opaque and radiopaque are both acceptable terms, although the former is preferred (*see* opacity).
ossification *n.* (radiol.) Calcific opacities within the lung that represent trabecular bone; applicable to calcific opacities that either display morphologic characteristics of trabecular bone (trabeculation and a defined cortex) or occur in association with a lesion known histologically to produce trabecular bone within lung (*e.g.,* mitral stenosis). *Synonyms:* Ossific nodulation, ossific nodule(s).	A useful roentgenologic term, although usually an inferred conclusion. To be distinguished from "calcification" (*q.v.*).
paraspinal line *n.* (radiol.) A vertically oriented interface usually seen in a frontal chest roentgenogram to the left (rarely to the right) of the thoracic vertebral column. It extends from the aortic arch to the diaphragm and represents contact between aerated lower lobe and adjacent mediastinal tissues. The anatomic interface is situated posterior to the descending aorta and is seen between the left lateral margin of the aorta and the spine. *Synonyms:* Left paraspinal pleural reflection; left paraspinal interface.	A specific feature of roentgenologic anatomy. Either of the synonyms cited is preferred inasmuch as the shadow represents an interface, not a line.
parenchyma *n.* 1. (anat.) The gas-exchanging portion of the lung consisting of the alveoli and their capillaries, estimated to comprise approximately 90 per cent of total lung volume. 2. (radiol.) All lung tissue exclusive of visible pulmonary vessels and airways.	A useful anatomic concept and an acceptable roentgenologic descriptor.
perfusion *n.* (physiol./radiol.) The passage of blood into and out of the lung. *Synonym:* Pulmonary blood flow.	A useful and recommended term.
phantom tumor *n.* (radiol.) A shadow produced by a local collection of fluid in one of the interlobar fissures (most often the minor fissure), usually possessing an elliptic configuration in one roentgenographic projection and a rounded configuration in the other, thus resembling a tumor. It is commonly caused by cardiac decompensation and usually disappears with appropriate therapy. *Synonyms:* Vanishing tumor, pseudotumor.	An explicit diagnostic conclusion from serial roentgenograms but only an inferred conclusion from a single examination. An acceptable descriptor.
platelike atelectasis *n.* (radiol.) A linear or planar opacity presumed to represent diminished volume in a portion of the lung; usually situated in lower lung zones. *Synonyms:* Platter, linear, or discoid atelectasis.	An inferred conclusion usually not subject to proof and often unwarranted. Its use as a descriptor is not recommended. "Linear opacity" is preferred.
pleonemia *n.* (pathol./physiol./radiol.) Increased blood flow to the lungs or a portion thereof, manifested roentgenologically by a general or local increase in the width of visible pulmonary vessels. *Synonyms:* Increased blood flow, hyperemia.	An inferred conclusion often used as a descriptor and based on usually reliable signs. An acceptable term preferrable to hyperemia (*q.v.*).
pneumatocele *n.* (pathol./radiol.) A thin-walled, gas-filled space within the lung usually occurring in association with acute pneumonia (most commonly of staphylococcal etiology) and almost invariably transient.	An inferred conclusion. An acceptable descriptor if used in accordance with the precise definition.

WORDS OR TERMS USED IN ROENTGENOLOGY *Continued*

Word or Term	Comments
pneumomediastinum *n.* (pathol./radiol.) A state characterized by the presence of gas in mediastinal tissues outside the esophagus, tracheobronchial tree, or pericardium. *Qualifiers:* spontaneous, traumatic, diagnostic. *Synonym:* Mediastinal emphysema.	An appropriate descriptor based on roentgenologic signs alone; preferred to its synonym.
pneumonia *n.* (pathol./radiol.) Infection (or noninfectious inflammation) of the air spaces and/or interstitium of the lung. *Qualifiers* may be employed to indicate temporal course (acute, chronic), predominant anatomic involvement (air-space or lobar, interstitial, bronchial), or etiology (bacterial, viral, fungal). *Synonym:* Pneumonitis.	An inferred conclusion, based on usually reliable signs. Generally preferred to its synonym, although the latter is sometimes used to designate infection caused by viruses or *Mycoplasma pneumoniae.*
pneumothorax *n.* (pathol./radiol.) A state characterized by the presence of gas within the pleural space. *Qualifiers:* spontaneous, traumatic, diagnostic, tension (*q.v.*).	A diagnostic conclusion appropriately based on roentgenologic evidence alone.
popcorn calcification *n.* (radiol.) A cluster of sharply defined, irregularly lobulated, calcific opacities, usually within a pulmonary nodule, suggesting the appearance of popcorn.	An acceptable descriptor.
posterior junction line *n.* (radiol.) A vertically oriented, linear or curvilinear opacity approximately 2 mm wide, commonly projected on the tracheal air shadow, and usually slightly concave to the right. It is produced by the shadows of the right and left pleurae in intimate contact between the aerated lungs. It represents the plane of contact between the lungs posterior to the trachea and esophagus and anterior to the spine; hence, in contrast to the anterior junction line, it may project both above and below the suprasternal notch. *Synonyms:* Posterior mediastinal septum; posterior mediastinal line; supraaortic posterior junction line or stripe; mesentery of the esophagus.	A specific feature of roentgenologic anatomy; to be preferred to cited synonyms.
posterior tracheal stripe *n.* (radiol.) A vertically oriented linear opacity ranging in width from 2 to 5 mm, extending from the thoracic inlet to the bifurcation of the trachea, and visible only on lateral roentgenograms of the chest. It is situated between the air shadow of the trachea and the right lung and is formed by the posterior tracheal wall and contiguous mediastinal interstitial tissue. *Synonym:* Posterior tracheal band.	A specific feature of radiologic anatomy; to be preferred to its synonym.
primary complex *n.* 1. (pathol.) The combination of a focus of pneumonia due to a primary infection (*e.g.,* tuberculosis or histoplasmosis) with granulomas in the draining hilar or mediastinal lymph nodes. 2. (radiol.) (a) One or more irregular opacities of variable extent and location assumed to represent consolidation of lung parenchyma, associated with enlargement of hilar or mediastinal lymph nodes, an appearance presumed to represent active infection. (b) One or more small, sharply defined parenchymal opacities (often calcified) associated with calcification of hilar or mediastinal lymph nodes, an appearance usually regarded as evidence of an inactive process.	A useful inferred conclusion. "Primary complex" is to be preferred to "Ranke complex," which is acceptable but rarely used. "Ghon complex" represents an inappropriate use of the eponym and is unacceptable (Ghon described the pulmonary abnormality alone, which thus becomes a Ghon focus or Ghon lesion).

WORDS OR TERMS USED IN ROENTGENOLOGY *Continued*

Word or Term	Comments
profusion *n.* (radiol.) The number of small opacities per unit area or zone of lung. In the ILO classification of radiographs of the pneumoconioses, the qualifiers 0 through 3 subdivide the profusion into 4 categories. The profusion categories may be further subdivided by employing a 12-point scale.	A useful word to describe the number of opacities in any diffuse disease, including the pneumoconioses.
pseudocavity *n.* (radiol.) A state in which a pulmonary nodule or mass possesses a central portion that is more lucent than its periphery (thus suggesting cavitation) but in which subsequent computed tomography or pathologic examination reveals only the presence of necrotic tissue high in lipid content, with no true cavity. *Synonym:* Simulated cavity.	An inferred conclusion sometimes used as a descriptor. The term is without etiologic connotation.
pulmonary edema *n.* 1. (pathophysiol.) The accumulation of liquid in the interstitial compartment of the lung with or without associated alveolar filling. Specifically, the accumulation of water, protein, and solutes (transudate), usually due to one or a combination of the following: (a) increased pressure in the microvascular bed, (b) increased microvascular permeability, or (c) impaired lymphatic drainage. Also, the accumulation of water, protein, solutes, and inflammatory cells (exudate) in response to inflammation of any type (*e.g.,* infection, allergy, trauma, or circulating toxins). 2. (radiol.) A pattern of opacity (usually bilaterally symmetrical) believed to represent interstitial thickening or alveolar filling when associated findings and/or history suggest one of the processes enumerated above. *Qualifiers:* interstitial, air-space, alveolar. *Synonyms:* Wet, boggy, or moist lung.	An inferred conclusion often employed as a descriptor, based on usually reliable signs. A useful and acceptable term when used in an appropriate clinical setting. The synonyms are colloquialisms to be avoided.
respiratory failure *n.* (physiol.) A state characterized by an arterial P_{O_2} below 60 mm Hg or an arterial P_{CO_2} above 49 mm Hg, at rest at sea level, resulting from impaired respiratory function. *Synonym:* Pulmonary insufficiency.	A useful term that should be restricted to clinical and physiologic usage. It is preferred to its synonym.
reticular pattern *n.* (radiol.) A collection of innumerable small linear opacities that together produce an appearance resembling a net. *Qualifiers:* fine, medium, coarse. *Synonym:* Small irregular opacities (in the ILO classification of radiographs of the pneumoconioses).	A recommended descriptor that usually indicates predominant abnormality of the pulmonary interstitium. The synonym should be restricted to the roentgenographic characterization of pneumoconiosis.
reticulonodular pattern *n.* (radiol.) A collection of innumerable small, linear, and nodular opacities that together produce a composite appearance resembling a net with small superimposed nodules. In common usage, the reticular and nodular elements are dimensionally of similar magnitude. *Qualifiers:* fine, medium, coarse.	An acceptable roentgenologic descriptor that usually indicates predominant abnormality of the pulmonary interstitium.
right tracheal stripe *n.* (radiol.) A vertically oriented linear opacity approximately 2 to 3 mm wide extending from the thoracic inlet to the right tracheobronchial angle. It is situated between the air shadow of the trachea and the right lung and is formed by the right tracheal wall and contiguous mediastinal interstitial tissue and pleura. *Synonym:* Right paratracheal stripe or band.	A specific feature of radiologic anatomy; to be preferred to the cited synonym since the opacity is caused chiefly by the tracheal wall itself.

WORDS OR TERMS USED IN ROENTGENOLOGY *Continued*

Word or Term	Comments
segment *n.* (anat./radiol.) One of the principal anatomic subdivisions of the pulmonary lobes served by a major branch of a lobar bronchus. *Qualifier:* bronchopulmonary.	A useful anatomic and roentgenologic descriptor.
septal line(s) *n.* (radiol.) Usually used in the plural, a generic term for linear opacities of varied distribution produced when the interstitium between pulmonary lobules is thickened (*e.g.*, by fluid, dust deposition, cellular material). *Synonym:* Kerley line (*q.v.*).	A specific feature of roentgenologic pathology, sometimes inferred. A recommended term. "Kerley line" is acceptable, particularly when seeking to identify a particular type of septal line (*e.g.*, Kerley B line).
shadow *n.* (radiol.) In clinical roentgenography, any perceptible discontinuity in film blackening (or fluoroscopic image or CRT display) attributed to the attenuation of the x-ray beam by a specific anatomic absorber or lesion on or within the body of the patient; an opacity or lucency. The word should always be qualified as precisely as possible with respect to size, contour, location, opacity, lucency, and so on.	A useful and recommended descriptor to be employed only when more specific identification is not possible.
silhouette sign *n.* (radiol.) 1. The effacement of an anatomic soft tissue border by either a normal anatomic structure (*e.g.*, the inferior border of the heart and left hemidiaphragm) or a pathologic state such as airlessness of adjacent lung or accumulation of fluid in the contiguous pleural space. 2. A sign of conformity, and hence, of the probable adjacency of a pathologic opacity to a known structure.	Useful in detecting and localizing an opacity along the axis of the x-ray beam. Although the physical basis underlying the production of this sign is contentious, the term is a widely accepted and useful descriptor. Despite the fact that the definition implies *loss* of silhouette, the term has acquired such common popularity that its continued use is recommended.
small irregular opacities *n.* (radiol.) A collection of innumerable small linear opacities that together produce an appearance resembling a net. In the ILO/1980 classification of radiographs of the pneumoconioses, the qualifiers s, t, and u subdivide the dimensions of the opacities into three diameter ranges—up to 1.5 mm, 1.5 to 3 mm, and 3 to 10 mm, respectively. *Synonym:* Reticular pattern (*q.v.*).	A term to be employed specifically to describe roentgenographic manifestations of the pneumoconioses; the synonym is preferred for nonpneumoconiotic disease.
small rounded opacities *n.* (radiol.) A collection of innumerable pulmonary nodules ranging in diameter from bare visibility up to 10 mm, usually widespread in distribution. In the ILO/1980 classification of radiographs of the pneumoconioses, the qualifiers p, q, and r subdivide the dimensions of the opacities into three diameter ranges—up to 1.5 mm, 1.5 to 3 mm, and 3 to 10 mm, respectively. *Synonym:* Nodular pattern (*q.v.*).	A term to be employed specifically to describe roentgenographic manifestations of the pneumoconioses; the synonym is preferred for nonpneumoconiotic disease.

WORDS OR TERMS USED IN ROENTGENOLOGY *Continued*

Word or Term

Comments

stripe *n.* (radiol.) A longitudinal composite opacity measuring 2 to 5 mm in width (*cf.* line).

An acceptable descriptor when limited to anatomic structures within the mediastinum (*e.g.*, right tracheal stripe).

subsegment *n.* (anat./radiol.) A unit of pulmonary tissue supplied by a bronchus of lesser order than a segmental bronchus.

A useful anatomic and roentgenologic descriptor.

tension *adj.* 1. (physiol./clin.) When used with reference to pneumo- or hydrothorax, a state characterized by cardiorespiratory functional impairment. 2. (radiol.) The accumulation of gas or fluid in a pleural space in an amount sufficient to cause airlessness of the ipsilateral lung, marked depression of the ipsilateral hemidiaphragm, and displacement of the mediastinum to the opposite side.

An inferred conclusion to be used only in the presence of clinical cardiorespiratory embarrassment. In fact, "tension" in relation to pneumothorax exists only during the expiratory phase of the respiratory cycle, since pleural pressure on inspiration is usually subatmospheric. The word should not be employed as in the term "tension cyst," which does not satisfy the criteria cited.

thromboembolism *n.* (pathol./clin./radiol.) Partial or complete occlusion of the lumen of a blood vessel by a thrombus (*q.v.*).

An inferred conclusion sometimes based on reliable signs (in conventional roentgenography) or a diagnostic conclusion based on roentgenologic evidence alone (in angiography).

thrombosis *n.* (pathol./radiol.) The state or process of thrombus formation within a blood vessel or heart chamber.

Cf. clot.

thrombus *n.* (pathol./radiol.) A mass of semisolidified blood, composed chiefly of platelets and fibrin with entrapped cellular elements, at the site of its formation in a blood vessel or heart chamber.

A useful descriptor to be employed only in the precise sense of the definition. (*Cf.* embolus.)

tramline shadow *n.* (radiol.) Parallel or slightly convergent linear opacities that suggest the planar projection of tubular structures and that correspond in location and orientation to elements of the bronchial tree. They are generally assumed to represent thickened bronchial walls.

Synonyms: Thickened bronchial wall, tubular shadow (*q.v.*).

A roentgenologic descriptor which is not recommended in deference to either of the synonyms. Such shadows are of possible pathologic significance only when they occur outside the limits of the hilar shadows where bronchial walls may be seen normally.

tubular shadow *n.* (radiol.) 1. Paired, parallel, or slightly convergent linear opacities presumed to represent the walls of a tubular structure seen *en face* (*e.g.*, a bronchus). 2. An approximately circular opacity presumed to represent the wall of a tubular structure seen end-on.

Synonyms: Tramline shadow (*q.v.*), thickened bronchial wall.

Acceptable if the anatomic nature of a shadow is obscure; otherwise the more precise "thickened bronchial wall" is to be preferred.

tumor *n.* 1. (general) A swelling or morbid enlargement. 2. (pathol./radiol.) Literally, a mass (*q.v.*), not differentiated as to its neoplastic or non-neoplastic nature.

Synonym: Mass.

A useful descriptor, although "mass" is preferred. The use of the word as a synonym for neoplasm is to be condemned.

WORDS OR TERMS USED IN ROENTGENOLOGY *Continued*

Word or Term	Comments
Valsalva maneuver *n.* (physiol.) Forced expiration against a closed glottis, usually but not necessarily from a position of total lung capacity.	A useful technique to produce transient increase in intrathoracic pressure.
vasoconstriction *n.* 1. (physiol.) Narrowing of muscular blood vessels by contraction of their muscle layer. 2. (radiol.) Local or general reduction in the caliber of visible pulmonary vessels (oligemia [*q.v.*]), presumed to result from decreased flow occasioned by contraction of muscular pulmonary arteries. *Qualifiers:* hypoxic, reflex.	An inferred conclusion based on usually reliable signs. The word is not synonymous with oligemia; although the latter is a *sign* of vasoconstriction, it may also occur when vessel narrowing is organic (as in emphysema) rather than functional and potentially reversible.
vasodilation *n.* (radiol.) The local or general increase in the width of visible pulmonary vessels resulting from increased pulmonary blood flow. *Synonym:* Vasodilatation.	An inferred conclusion based on usually reliable signs.
ventilation *n.* (physiol./radiol.) The movement of air into and out of the lungs; inspiration and expiration. *Qualifiers:* hyperventilation (preferred), or overventilation; hypoventilation (preferred), or underventilation.	The term always implies a biphasic dynamic process of admission and expulsion; hence, it cannot be assessed from a single static image (*see* inflation).

V_T/T_I Mean inspiratory flow

V_T/T_E Mean expiratory flow

V_E $\dfrac{V_t \times T_i}{T_i \times T_{Tot}}$

DIFFUSING CAPACITY TESTS AND SYMBOLS

Dx Diffusing capacity of the lung expressed as volume (STPD) of gas (x) uptake per unit alveolar-capillary pressure difference for the gas used. Unless otherwise stated, carbon monoxide is assumed to be the test gas: i.e., D is D_{CO}. A modifier can be used to designate the technique: e.g., Dsb is single breath carbon monoxide diffusing capacity and Dss is steady state CO diffusing capacity

D_M Diffusing capacity of the alveolar capillary membrane (STPD)

θx Reaction rate coefficient for red cells; the volume STPD of gas (x) which will combine per minute with 1 unit volume of blood per unit gas tension. If the specific gas is not stated, θ is assumed to refer to CO and is a function of existing O_2 tension

Qc Capillary blood volume (usually expressed as Vc in the literature, a symbol inconsistent with those recommended for blood volumes). When determined from the following equation, Qc represents the effective pulmonary capillary blood volume, i.e., capillary blood volume in intimate association with alveolar gas:

$$\frac{1}{D} = \frac{1}{D_M} + \frac{1}{\theta \cdot Qc}$$

D/V_A Diffusion per unit of alveolar volume with D expressed STPD and V_A expressed as liters BTPS. This method is preferred to the occasional practice of expressing both values STPD

BLOOD GAS MEASUREMENTS*

Pa_{CO_2} Arterial carbon dioxide tension

Sa_{O_2} Arterial oxygen saturation

Cc_{O_2} Oxygen content of pulmonary end-capillary blood

---

*Symbols for these measurements are readily composed by combining the general symbols recommended earlier.

$P(A-a)O_2$ Alveolar-arterial oxygen pressure difference. The previously used symbol, A-aDO_2 is not recommended.

$C(a-\bar{v})O_2$ Arteriovenous oxygen content difference

PULMONARY SHUNTS

$\dot{Q}sp$ Physiologic shunt flow (total venous admixture) defined by the following equation when gas and blood gas data are collected during ambient air breathing:

$$\dot{Q}sp = \frac{Cc_{O_2} - Ca_{O_2}}{Cc_{O_2} - C\bar{v}_{O_2}} \cdot \dot{Q}$$

$\dot{Q}san$ A special case of $\dot{Q}sp$ (often called anatomic shunt flow) defined by the above equation when blood and gas data are collected after sufficiently prolonged breathing of 100% O_2 to assure an alveolar N_2 less than 1%

$\dot{Q}s/\dot{Q}t$ The ratio $\dot{Q}sp$ or $\dot{Q}_{SAN}$ to total cardiac output

BRONCHIAL REACTIVITY

PC_{20} Provocative concentration of an inhaled agonist producing a 20% decrease in FEV_1

PD_{20} Provocative dose of an inhaled agonist producing a 20% decrease in FEV_1

$PD_{40}SGaw$ Provocative dose of an inhaled agonist producing a 40% decrease in SGaw

Isocapnic hyperventilation (eucapnic hyperventilation) = "hyperventilation" with addition of CO_2 to the inspired air to keep end tidal P_{CO_2} constant (Iso) and/or normal (Eu-). Used to assess bronchoconstrictive response to cold and/or dry air

SLEEP STUDIES

Polysomnography   The evaluation during sleep of vital functions and a quantitative evaluation of sleep parameters overnight

NREM   Nonrapid eye movement sleep

REM   Rapid eye movement sleep

Apnea   Cessation of air flow for greater than 10 seconds

Sleep apnea   The presence of 30 or greater apneas in an overnight, 7 hour sleep study. (Apnea frequency >4/hr)

V_DA The alveolar dead space volume defined as V_DA/f

$\dot{V}_DA$ Ventilation of the alveolar dead space (BTPS), defined by the following equation: $V_DA = V_D - V_{DAN}$

MEASUREMENTS OF MECHANICS OF BREATHING*

PRESSURE TERMS

Paw   Pressure in the airway, level to be specified

Pao   Pressure at the airway opening

Ppl   Intrapleural pressure

P_A Alveolar pressure

P_L Transpulmonary pressure

Pbs   Pressure at the body surface

P(A-ao)   Pressure gradient from alveolus to airway opening

Pw   Transthoracic pressure

Ptm   Transmural pressure pertaining to an airway or blood vessel

Pes   Esophageal pressure used to estimate Ppl

Pga   Gastric pressure; used to estimate abdominal pressure

Pdi   Transdiaphragmatic pressure; used to estimate the tension across the diaphragm

Pdi Max   Maximal transdiaphragmatic pressure; used to measure the strength of diaphragmatic muscle contraction

PI Max (also MIP)   Maximal inspiratory pressure; measured at the mouth, used to assess the strength of inspiratory muscles

PE Max (also MEP)   Maximal expiratory pressure; measured at the mouth, used to assess the strength of the expiratory muscles

FLOW-PRESSURE RELATIONSHIPS†

R   A general symbol for resistance, pressure per unit flow

Raw   Airway resistance

Rti   Tissue resistance

R_L Total pulmonary resistance, measured by relating flow-dependent transpulmonary pressure to airflow at the mouth

Rus   Resistance of the airways on the alveolar side (upstream) of the point in the airways where intraluminal pressure equals Ppl, measured under conditions of maximal expiratory flow

Rds   Resistance of the airways on the oral side (downstream) of the point in the airways where intraluminal pressure equals Ppl, measured under conditions of maximal expiratory flow

Gaw   Airway conductance, the reciprocal of Raw

Gaw/V_L Specific conductance, expressed per liter of lung volume at which G is measured (also SGaw)

VOLUME-PRESSURE RELATIONSHIPS

C   A general symbol for compliance, volume change per unit of applied pressure

Cdyn   Dynamic compliance, compliance measured at points of zero gas flow at the mouth during active breathing. The respiratory frequency should be designated; e.g., Cdyn40

Cst   Static compliance, compliance determined from measurements made during conditions of interruption of air flow

C/V_L Specific compliance

E   Elastance, pressure per unit of volume change, the reciprocal of compliance

Pst   Static transpulmonary pressure at a specified lung volume; e.g., PstTLC is static recoil pressure measured at TLC (maximal recoil pressure)

PstTLC/ TLC   Coefficient of lung reaction expressed per liter of TLC

W   A general symbol for mechanical work of breathing, which requires use of appropriate qualifying symbols and description of specific conditions

BREATHING PATTERN

T_I Inspiratory time

T_E Expiratory time

T_{Tot} Total respiratory cycle time

T_I/T_{Tot} Ratio of inspiratory to total respiratory cycle time—Duty cycle

V_T Tidal volume

---

*All pressures are expressed relative to ambient pressure and gases are at BTPS unless otherwise specified.

†Unless otherwise specified, the lung volume at which all resistance measurements are made is assumed to be FRC.

TERMS AND SYMBOLS USED IN RESPIRATORY PHYSIOLOGY AND PATHOPHYSIOLOGY

GENERAL SYMBOLS

P	Pressure, blood, or gas
$\dot{X}$	A time derivative indicated by a dot above the symbol (rate). This symbol is used for both instantaneous flow and volume per unit time
%X	Per cent sign *preceding* a symbol indicates percentage of the predicted normal value
X/Y%	Per cent sign *following* a symbol indicates a ratio function with the ratio expressed as a percentage. Both components of the ratio must be designated; e.g., $FEV_1/FVC\% = 100 \times FEV_1/FVC$
X_A or Xa	A small capital letter or lower case letter on the same line following a primary symbol is a qualifier to further define the primary symbol. When small capital letters are not available on typewriters or to printers, large capital letters may be used as subscripts; e.g., $X_A = XA$

GAS PHASE SYMBOLS

PRIMARY SYMBOLS (LARGE CAPITAL LETTERS)

V	Gas volume. The particular gas as well as its pressure, water vapor conditions, and other special conditions must be specified in text or indicated by appropriate qualifying symbols
F	Fractional concentration of gas

COMMON QUALIFYING SYMBOLS

I	Inspired
E	Expired
A	Alveolar
T	Tidal
D	Dead space or wasted ventilation
B	Barometric
L	Lung
STPD	Standard conditions: Temperature 0 degrees Centigrade, pressure 760 mm Hg, and dry (0 water vapor)
BTPS	Body conditions: Body temperature, ambient pressure, and saturated with water vapor at these conditions

ATPD	Ambient temperature and pressure, dry
ATPS	Ambient temperature and pressure, saturated with water vapor at these conditions
an	Anatomic
p	Physiologic
rb	Rebreathing
f	Respiratory frequency per minute
max	Maximal
t	Time

BLOOD PHASE SYMBOLS

PRIMARY SYMBOLS (LARGE CAPITAL LETTERS)

Q	Blood volume
$\dot{Q}$	Blood flow, volume units and time must be specified
C	Concentration in the blood phase
S	Saturation in the blood phase

QUALIFYING SYMBOLS (LOWER CASE LETTERS)

b	Blood in general
a	Arterial
c	Capillary
ć	Pulmonary end-capillary
v	Venous
v̄	Mixed venous

VENTILATION AND LUNG MECHANICS TESTS AND SYMBOLS

LUNG VOLUME COMPARTMENTS*

RV	Residual volume; that volume of air remaining in the lungs after maximal exhalation. The method of measurement should be indicated in the text or, when necessary, by appropriate qualifying symbols
ERV	Expiratory reserve volume; the maximal volume of air exhaled from the end-expiratory level

---

*Primary components are designated as volumes. When volumes are combined they are designated as capacities. All are considered to be at BTPS unless otherwise specified.

V_T Tidal volume; that volume of air inhaled or exhaled with each breath during quiet breathing, used only to indicate a subdivision of lung volume

IRV   Inspiratory reserve volume; the maximal volume of air inhaled from the end-inspiratory level

IC   Inspiratory capacity; the sum of IRV and V_T

IVC   Inspiratory vital capacity; the maximal volume of air inhaled from the point of maximal expiration

VC   Vital capacity; the maximal volume of air exhaled from the point of maximal inspiration

FRC   Functional residual capacity; the sum of RV and ERV (the volume of air remaining in the lungs at the end-expiratory position). The method of measurement should be indicated, as with RV

TLC   Total lung capacity; the sum of all volume compartments or the volume of air in the lungs after maximal inspiration. The method of measurement should be indicated, as with RV

RV / TLC%   Residual volume to total lung capacity ratio, expressed as a per cent

CV   Closing volume; the volume exhaled after the expired gas concentration is inflected from an alveolar plateau during a controlled breathing maneuver. Since the value obtained is dependent on the specific test technique, the method used must be designated in the text and, when necessary, specified by a qualifying symbol. Closing volume is often expressed as a ratio of the VC, i.e., (CV/VC%)

CC   Closing capacity; closing volume plus residual volume, often expressed as a ratio of TLC, i.e., (CC/TLC%)

VL   Actual volume of the lung, including the volume of the conducting airways

V_A Alveolar gas volume

FORCED SPIROMETRY MEASUREMENTS*

FVC   Forced vital capacity; vital capacity performed with a maximally forced expiratory effort

FIVC   Forced inspiratory vital capacity; the maximal volume of air inspired with a maximally forced effort from a position of maximal expiration

---

*All values are BTPS unless otherwise specified.

FEVt   Forced expiratory volume (timed). The volume of air exhaled in the specified time during the performance of the forced vital capacity; e.g., FEV_1 for the volume of air exhaled during the first second of the FVC

FEVt / FVC%   Forced expiratory volume (timed) to forced vital capacity ratio, expressed as a percentage

FEF25–75%   Mean forced expiratory flow during the middle of the FVC (formerly called the maximal mid-expiratory flow rate)

PEF   The highest forced expiratory flow measured with a peak flow meter

$\dot{V}maxX$ Forced expiratory flow, related to the total lung capacity or the vital capacity of the lung at which the measurement is made. *Modifiers refer to the amount of lung volume remaining when the measurement is made.* For example: $\dot{V}max75\%$ = Instantaneous forced expiratory flow when the lung is at 75% of its TLC

$\dot{V}max50$ Instantaneous forced expiratory flow when 50% of the vital capacity remains to be exhaled

$\dot{V}maxXp$ Forced expiratory flow at "X" percentage of vital capacity on a partial flow volume curve, initiated from a volume below TLC

MVVx   Maximal voluntary ventilation. The volume of air expired in a specified period during repetitive maximal respiratory effort

MEASUREMENTS OF VENTILATION

$\dot{V}_E$ Expired volume per minute (BTPS)

$\dot{V}_I$ Inspired volume per minute (BTPS)

$\dot{V}_{CO_2}$ Carbon dioxide production per minute (STPD)

$\dot{V}_{O_2}$ Oxygen consumption per minute (STPD)

$\dot{V}_A$ Alveolar ventilation per minute (BTPS)

V_D The physiologic dead space volume defined as V_D/f

$\dot{V}_D$ Ventilation per minute of the physiologic dead space (wasted ventilation), BTPS, defined by the following equation:
$$\dot{V}_D = \dot{V}_E(Pa_{CO_2} - P_{E_{CO_2}})/Pa_{CO_2}$$

V_{DAN} Volume of the anatomic dead space (BTPS)

$\dot{V}_{DAN}$ Ventilation per minute of the anatomic dead space, that portion of conducting airway in which no significant gas exchange occurs (BTPS)

Obstructive apnea	Apnea with respiratory effort
Central apnea	Apnea without respiratory effort
Mixed apnea	Apnea initially without, but later with, respiratory effort
Hypopnea	Reduced respiratory effort with associated decrease in arterial saturation
Apnea index	Number of apneas divided by the total sleep time in hours
Arousal	Short neurologic awakening

PULMONARY DYSFUNCTION

TERMS RELATED TO ALTERED BREATHING

Many terms are in use, such as tachypnea, hyperpnea, hypopnea, and so on. Simple descriptive terms, such as rapid, deep, or shallow breathing, should be used instead.

Dyspnea	A subjective sensation of difficult or labored breathing
Overventilation	A general term indicating excessive ventilation. When unqualified, it refers to *alveolar overventilation*, excessive ventilation of the gas-exchanging areas of the lung manifested by a fall in arterial CO_2 tension. The term *total overventilation* may be used when the minute volume is increased regardless of the alveolar ventilation. (When there is increased wasted ventilation, total overventilation may occur when alveolar ventilation is normal or decreased)
Underventilation	A general term indicating reduced ventilation. When otherwise unqualified, it refers to alveolar underventilation, decreased effective alveolar ventilation manifested by an increase in arterial CO_2 tension. (Over- and underventilation are recommended in place of hyper- and hypoventilation to avoid confusion when the words are spoken)

TERMS DESCRIBING BLOOD GAS FINDINGS

Hypoxia	A term for reduced oxygenation
Hypoxemia	A reduced blood oxygen content or tension
Hypocarbia	(hypocapnia) A reduced arterial carbon dioxide tension
Hypercarbia	(hypercapnia) An increased arterial carbon dioxide tension

TERMS DESCRIBING ACID-BASE FINDINGS

Acidemia	A pH less than normal; the value should always be given
Alkalemia	A pH greater than normal; the value should always be given
Hypobasemia	Blood bicarbonate level below normal
Hyperbasemia	Blood bicarbonate level above normal
Acidosis	A clinical term indicating a disturbance that can lead to acidemia. It usually is indicated by hypobasemia when metabolic (nonrespiratory) in origin and by hypercarbia when respiratory in origin. There may or may not be accompanying acidemia. The term should always be qualified as metabolic (nonrespiratory) or respiratory
Alkalosis	A clinical term indicating a disturbance that can lead to alkalemia. It usually is indicated by hyperbasemia when metabolic (nonrespiratory) in origin and by hypocarbia when respiratory in origin. There may or may not be accompanying alkalemia. The term should always be qualified as metabolic (nonrespiratory) or respiratory

OTHER TERMS

Pulmonary insufficiency	Altered function of the lungs that produces clinical symptoms, usually including dyspnea
Acute respiratory failure	Rapidly occurring hypoxemia or hypercarbia due to a disorder of the respiratory system. The duration of the illness and the values of arterial oxygen tension and arterial carbon dioxide tension used as criteria for this term should be given. The term *acute ventilatory failure* should be used only when the arterial carbon dioxide tension is increased. The term *pulmonary failure* has been used to indicate respiratory failure due specifically to disorders of the lungs
Chronic respiratory failure	Chronic hypoxemia or hypercarbia due to a disorder of the respiratory system. The duration of the condition and the values of arterial oxygen tension and arterial carbon dioxide tension used as criteria for this term should be given
Obstructive pattern	(Obstructive ventilatory defect) Slowing of air flow during forced ventilatory maneuvers

Restrictive pattern — (Restrictive ventilatory defect) Reduction of vital capacity not explainable by airways obstruction

Impairment — A measurable degree of anatomic or functional abnormality which may or may not have clinical significance. *Permanent impairment* is that which persists after maximal medical rehabilitation has been achieved

Disability — A legally determined state in which a patient's ability to engage in a specific activity under a particular circumstance is reduced or absent because of physical or mental impairment. *Permanent disability* exists when no substantial improvement of the patient's ability to engage in the specific activity can be expected

C H A P T E R

Embolic and Thrombotic Diseases of the Lungs

PULMONARY THROMBOSIS

Although embolization is undoubtedly the most frequent mechanism involved to explain the presence of intrapulmonary thrombus, *in situ* thrombosis of pulmonary vessels is probably more common than is generally appreciated. However, because of the difficulty in distinguishing thromboembolus from *in situ* thrombus both radiologically and pathologically, and because the predisposing conditions for pulmonary thrombosis are frequently the same as those for systemic venous thrombosis, it can be difficult to state with certainty which of the two processes is operative. The pathogenesis and effects of pulmonary vascular thrombosis are related to some extent to the site and can be conveniently discussed under three categories: (1) arteries, (2) arterioles and capillaries, and (3) veins.

Pulmonary Arteries

It is in the pulmonary arteries that the distinction between *in situ* thrombosis and embolism can be particularly difficult; in fact, in some cases, differentiation is not possible. Probably the most common underlying cause of *in situ* arterial thrombosis is *infectious pneumonia*, in which vascular damage occurs in relation to abscesses and foci of active granulomatous inflammation. Thrombosis related to primary or metastatic neoplasm is also relatively common; it can result from either invasion of the vessel by the neoplasm or vascular compression by expanding tumor. Less common causes include immune-mediated vasculitis,[1] trauma,[2] aneurysms,[3] indwelling catheters,[4] congenital heart anomalies associated with decreased pulmonary blood flow such as tetralogy of Fallot,[5] and sickle-cell trait or disease;[6-8] in the last named condition, thrombosis is sometimes associated with sudden death.[9] Other pulmonary and cardiac diseases, such as emphysema,[10] pneumoconiosis, mitral stenosis, and primary pulmonary hypertension,[11] have also been associated; however, pulmonary thromboemboli occur with such frequency in these conditions that it is difficult, if not impossible, to estimate with any degree of accuracy the true incidence of thrombosis.

Pathologically, *in situ* arterial thrombosis should be suspected grossly if there is adjacent parenchymal disease or if there is extensive and continuous thrombus in multiple vessels; the formation of a cast of the arterial tree would not be possible with the multiple fragments of thrombus characteristic of emboli. In one literature review of 100 cases considered to represent *in situ* thrombosis, the site of thrombus formation was the right lung in 49 per cent, the left in 6 per cent, and both lungs in 45 per cent;[11] the author suggested that the longer course of the right pulmonary artery and its association with other mediastinal structures were responsible for the higher incidence in this lung. Histologically, *in situ* thrombosis should be considered when there is associated vasculitis or if the thrombus is eccentrically located on the side of the vessel wall adjacent to a focus of parenchymal inflammation (Fig. 9–1). The genesis of isolated thrombi unassociated with pneumonia or other active inflammatory pulmonary disease cannot be determined histologically in most instances; although such *in situ* thrombi undoubtedly occur, they are usually considered thromboemboli.

Thrombosis is found most often in small elastic or muscular arteries supplying lung that is already the site of disease; as a result, the effects of the thrombus are often difficult to evaluate in determining roentgenographic or clinical manifestations. An exception is the necrosis and cavitation that occur in some cases of pneumonia (lung "gangrene") or vasculitis, the pathogenesis being related at least in part to the thrombosis and resulting ischemia. In addition, thrombus can occasionally extend proximally from a focus of active parenchymal inflammation, especially in tuberculosis;[11] such extension can sometimes occur as far as the pulmonary trunk and opposite main pulmonary artery, resulting in severe obstruction of pulmonary blood flow and cor pulmonale.

Pulmonary Arterioles and Capillaries

Thrombosis of small pulmonary vessels occurs in immunologically mediated leukocytoclastic vasculitis (*see* page 1264); in these cases, it is usually associated with other evidence of vascular damage, particularly parenchymal hemorrhage. Fibrin thrombi, believed to be the product of an acute hypercoagulability state, are also found in the lungs of animals and humans who have died of "shock"[12] and disseminated intravascular coagulation[13] related to such conditions as septicemia and amniotic fluid

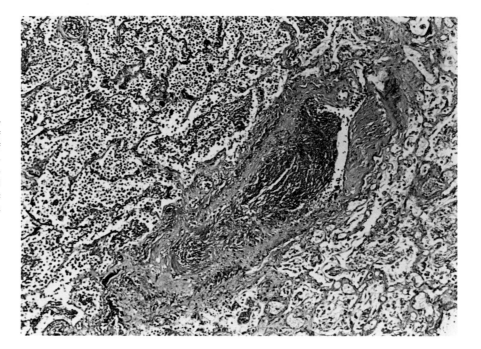

Figure 9–1. Pulmonary Artery Thrombosis *in Situ*. The left portion of the figure shows alveolar airspaces full of polymorphonuclear leukocytes, representing an acute bacterial pneumonia. A pulmonary artery at the junction of affected and unaffected lung reveals eccentric thrombosis in relation to the pneumonia (× 80).

embolism. *In situ* thrombosis of small as well as large pulmonary vessels can occur in sickle cell disease.[6]

PULMONARY VEINS

As in the arterial circulation, pulmonary venous thrombosis commonly develops secondary to an infectious process or neoplasm. Other related conditions include those in which there is decreased blood flow, such as tetralogy of Fallot,[5] sclerosing mediastinitis,[14, 15, 718] and veno-occlusive disease; in fact, venous thrombosis has been considered by some to be intimately involved in the pathogenesis of the last-named disorder.

PULMONARY THROMBOEMBOLISM

INCIDENCE

Estimates of the incidence of pulmonary thromboembolism vary considerably in different series, largely as a result of differences in the character of the population under study and the techniques and criteria used in diagnosis. In general, thromboemboli are an infrequent cause of hospital admission, ranging in incidence from 0.49 to 2.5 per cent of medical patients and 0.09 to 0.6 per cent of surgical patients in three series.[16] As a *diagnosed* complication of hospitalization, they are also relatively uncommon; in one retrospective study of patients discharged from the hospital over a 10-year period, the incidence was only 0.21 per cent.[16] The incidence of fatal pulmonary embolism after routine surgery is also very low, estimated at only two to three per 1,000 procedures.[17] Despite these figures, however, it is well recognized that the true incidence

of thromboembolism is much higher, a belief that is based on three observations:

1. Signs and symptoms are lacking in many patients; it has been estimated that about 80 per cent of pulmonary thromboembolic episodes are unrecognized as a result of the absence of clinical findings.[18, 19]

2. A definitive diagnosis is difficult to make during life, even when symptoms and signs are present.[20]

3. Thromboemboli are frequently identified at autopsy; in retrospective necropsy studies, the incidence in most series ranges from 5 to 20 per cent.[16, 22, 23] If lung specimens are examined in detail prospectively, the incidence is even higher: in one series of 61 consecutive necropsies, 64 per cent were found to contain organized or recent thromboemboli.[24] In another investigation of 263 right lungs,[25] emboli were found in 51.7 per cent, and, as the authors admitted, the true incidence must have been even higher, since only one lung was examined. Even when the pulmonary embolism is of major degree, the correct diagnosis is often not made before death: of 54 autopsies performed at the Peter Bent Brigham Hospital on patients with this finding, the correct diagnosis was made ante mortem in only 16 (30 per cent); misdiagnosis was most frequent in the elderly and in patients with established pneumonia.[26] Misdiagnosis is not invariably related to underdiagnosis; in one study, 61.9 per cent of all clinical diagnoses of pulmonary embolism were false positives.[21]

Although the precise incidence of pulmonary thromboembolism is not known, it appears to be increasing,[27] particularly in previously healthy young adults.[28, 29] Some of this increase can be attributed to a higher index of clinical suspicion and improved, readily accessible diagnostic facilities.[27] However, there appears to be a real increase for which not all the causal factors are known, although the increasing complexity of surgical procedures and the vast increase in the use of oral contraceptives (see further on) are at least partly responsible.

An accurate estimate of the frequency of pulmonary thromboembolism as a major or significant contributory cause of death is difficult to establish because of the subjectivity involved in such estimates. Nevertheless, the condition is clearly of great importance; for example, it has been estimated that pulmonary thromboembolism is responsible for 50,000 deaths per year in the United States.[30] In their study of 263 right lungs, Morrell and Dunnill[25] considered that death was attributable to thromboembolism in 56 (43 per cent) of the 136 patients in whom these were found and in 21 per cent of the total number of patients. These high figures are in sharp contrast to the 2.7 to 8.8 per cent in the three series quoted by Morrell,[16] figures that are more in keeping with our experience and with that of others.[16, 23]

ETIOLOGY AND PATHOGENESIS

The pathogenesis of pulmonary thromboembolism can be conveniently considered under (1) the development of venous and cardiac thrombosis and (2) the effects on the lungs of the thromboemboli themselves.

Venous and Cardiac Thrombosis

Since by definition pulmonary thromboembolism is characterized by the transport to and impaction within the lung of a fragment of thrombus, the process must be preceded by the development of thrombus elsewhere in the circulatory system. In the great majority of cases, this occurs in the veins of the legs, particularly the thighs. Other relatively common sites are the pelvic veins (including the periprostatic veins in men), the inferior vena cava, and the right atrium. The right ventricle[31] (rarely in association with a right ventricular myxoma),[32, 33] right-sided heart valves, superior vena cava,[34] and the veins of the neck and arms are infrequent sources. The incidence of deep venous thrombosis in the arms[35] is estimated to be less than 2 per cent of all cases;[36] however, complicating pulmonary embolism is not proportionately rare, being reported in three of 25 patients in one series[37] and in five of 16 in another.[38] Foci of peripheral thrombosis are sometimes multiple, making detection of the precise source of an embolus difficult; for example, in one necropsy study of 78 patients known to have had pulmonary embolism,[39] peripheral thrombi were found in 62, at multiple sites in more than a third; the leg veins were involved in 46 per

cent, the right atrium in 23 per cent, the inferior vena cava in 19 per cent, and the pelvic veins in 16 per cent. It should be emphasized that the source of thrombus is not found during life in up to 50 per cent of cases of fatal embolism[40, 41] and may not be identifiable even at autopsy.[40]

The pathogenesis of cardiac and venous thrombosis is complex and is related to one or more of three major factors: (1) an alteration in blood flow, caused by either stasis or local turbulence; (2) endothelial damage, usually the result of trauma or inflammation; and (3) a change in the coagulability of blood, caused by either substances or processes that increase the clotting tendency or a deficiency of substances inhibiting clot formation. A thorough discussion of the pathogenesis and effects of these three factors is essential for an understanding of pulmonary thromboembolism.

ALTERED BLOOD FLOW

The rate of blood flow through the systemic veins to the heart depends upon the input from the arterial side of the circulation, the resistance to venous flow, the milking action of the local musculature, and, in those veins in which they are present, intraluminal valves. An alteration in any of these can lead to a decrease in blood flow that may predispose to thrombus formation. Many of the clinical conditions associated with venous thrombosis, particularly in the legs, are in turn associated with an abnormality of one or more of these factors. Such conditions include left-sided heart failure and shock (decreased arterial input),[27, 42] obesity, pregnancy, intra-abdominal tumors, right-sided heart failure, external pressure from leg casts or bandages (increased resistance to flow),[43] strokes[42, 44] and the postsurgical or paraplegic state (immobility with loss or decrease of muscle activity), and varicose veins.[17, 27, 42, 45, 46] Slowing of blood flow that is caused by intrinsic abnormality of the blood itself, such as in multiple myeloma[47, 48] and sickle-cell anemia,[49] also predisposes to thrombosis.

Because of their distance from the heart and the effects of gravity and immobility, the legs are the most vulnerable site for an alteration in venous blood flow, and the frequency of pulmonary thromboembolism directly parallels thrombosis in this site. In high-risk patients, deep venous thrombosis in the legs is common, being found in 27 to 60 per cent of patients in large autopsy series.[23, 50, 51] When detected by phlebography and scanning techniques, thrombosis associated with immobility or surgery is equally frequent; in their study of 160 patients undergoing total hip replacement, Stamatakis and colleagues[52] found evidence of deep venous thrombosis in the legs in 81 (50 per cent). In another series of 132 consecutive patients undergoing elective surgery (not on the legs), 40 (30 per cent) showed evidence of thrombosis by ^{125}I fibrinogen test and phlebography;[53] only 20 of these had clinical signs, only four had detectable pulmonary emboli, and in 14 there was evidence of lysis of the thrombus within 72 hours. Isotopic scanning techniques and radiographic phlebography have shown deep venous thrombosis (DVT) in up to 60 per cent of patients with strokes,[44] and in 34 to 37 per cent of patients with myocardial infarction;[54, 55] in the latter group, the incidence of DVT appears to be closely associated with the severity of myocardial damage and does not occur in the majority of cases of uncomplicated myocardial infarction.[56]

In the legs, most thrombi appear to be initiated by local fibrin–platelet–red blood cell aggregates, often in the region of a valve pocket.[51, 57, 719] Although many initially form in the calf, it is clear from postmortem anatomic studies[50, 51, 57] and in vivo phlebographic investigations[52, 58] that a substantial proportion arise in the veins of the thigh. It is widely believed that it is from this site rather than the calf where the majority of clinically significant pulmonary thromboemboli arise,[23, 59–61] although occasional well-documented cases have been described in which the calf was the site of origin.[62]

Localized areas of blood turbulence are probably responsible, at least in part, for the thrombus related to foreign objects, such as indwelling Swan-Ganz arterial catheters,[63, 64] pacing catheters,[65] and cerebrospinal fluid shunt[66] or inferior vena cava plication[67] devices.

ENDOTHELIAL INJURY

The role of endothelial injury in the genesis of deep venous thrombosis is currently believed to be of little importance in most situations.[51, 68, 719] In his study of 50 small thrombi in the pockets of femoral vein valves, Sevitt[57] generally identified no evidence of antecedent intimal damage; however, he did find within apparently normal valves microscopic foci of fibrin thrombi, which he speculated were the precursors of future macroscopic thrombi. In addition, although experimental venous trauma is associated with limited platelet adherence to exposed subendothelial tissue, it has been found to be a weak promoter of fibrin thrombus formation.[719] Thus, venous thrombosis secondary to injury or inflammation of the vessel wall (thrombophlebitis) is probably uncommon compared to the typical bland thrombosis unassociated with these events. Despite these observations, endothelial injury can be a significant factor in some situations in which there is localized venous trauma, such as total hip replacement.[52] It may also be important in the thrombosis associated with bacterial endocarditis and immunologically mediated vasculitis.

Paradoxically, the contrast medium used to detect venous thrombosis can itself initiate thrombosis, presumably as a result of endothelial damage;[69, 70] it has been estimated that this complication occurs in 3 to 5 per cent of patients undergoing this procedure.[70] A follow-up study of a group of

patients 5 to 10 years after proven venous thrombosis in a lower limb revealed a surprising incidence of filling defects, presumably representing organized thrombi in vessels initially found to be patent; the authors suggested that the diagnostic venography might have been responsible.[71]

COAGULATION ABNORMALITIES

Most instances of venous thrombosis and pulmonary thromboembolism, particularly those that are acute and massive, are associated with medical, surgical, or obstetric conditions with well-defined risk factors.[72] However, some patients in whom peripheral venous thrombosis develops, with or without associated embolization, are otherwise healthy. In many such cases, questioning will reveal other potential pathogenetic factors for the thrombosis, such as sitting for long periods in a cramped position while traveling (as has been reported in active duty servicemen[73, 74]) or standing for long periods at work in occupations such as nursing.[75, 76] In such circumstances and in those in which no other pathogenetic factors are evident, the possibility of a hypercoagulable state should be considered. Although the existence of such a condition has long been suspected and there is abundant indirect evidence for its presence, its precise nature has been documented only rarely. Thus, a familial deficiency of antithrombin III, an alpha-2-globulin capable of inactivating thrombin and factor Xa, is associated with a substantially increased incidence of deep venous thrombosis and occasionally pulmonary emboli,[77] usually in association with a second risk factor, such as pregnancy or surgery, but in one instance following venography.[69] Similarly, deficiencies of either of the coagulation inhibition proteins C or S may be associated with recurrent venous thrombosis and pulmonary thromboembolism.[720, 721]

Patients with myeloproliferative disorders manifesting thrombocytosis (such as polycythemia vera and essential thrombocythemia)[78] are prone to thrombotic and hemorrhagic complications, whereas those with reactive thrombocytosis tend not to be.[79] Platelet aggregate formation has been proposed as a factor in the pathogenesis of recurring venous thrombosis, and in such patients treatment with dipyridamole and aspirin has been shown to increase platelet survival time[80, 81] and prevent venous thrombosis.[81] Physical conditioning, pedalling devices, and such physical methods as elastic or pneumatic compression and electrical stimulation of the muscles of the extremities have been shown to prevent thrombosis, possibly by increasing fibrinolytic activity[82–84] in addition to increasing flow. In addition, some disease entities, including hypertension and hyperlipidemia,[85] predispose to thrombosis because of an apparent alteration in the noncellular elements of the coagulation system. As in other conditions which have been associated with a tendency to increased coagulation, such as the postoperative and posttraumatic states, the precise alteration in blood components leading to this has not been clearly defined and is likely multifactorial and complex.

Two other factors that predispose to thrombus formation—neoplasms and oral contraceptives—deserve more detailed discussion. Patients with certain neoplasms, particularly those of the lung, gastrointestinal tract, and genitourinary tract,[86] show a propensity for the development of venous thrombosis, and affected patients have an increased incidence (approximately four-fold) of pulmonary thromboembolism. In some cases, the thrombus has been associated with intravascular mucus, suggesting that this might be the initiator of thrombosis; in others, alteration in the normal level of coagulation factors such as fibrinogen, antithrombin, and thromboplastin has been identified.[722]

Since the late 1960s, it has become evident that there is an increased risk of venous thrombosis and pulmonary thromboembolism in women taking oral contraceptives.[87–92] The risk is dose-related[90] and is believed to be especially serious in patients with congenital left-to-right intracardiac shunts.[93] The culpable ingredient in the hormone pill is thought to be estrogen,[94] which both augments clotting and impairs fibrinolysis;[95] lowering the estrogen content of such medication has resulted in a decrease in morbidity but not mortality caused by venous thromboembolic disease.[96]

Several epidemiologic studies support the association. The incidence of postoperative thromboembolism is increased three to four times in women taking oral contraceptives,[97] and it has been estimated that healthy women between the ages of 20 and 34 taking oral contraceptives run a risk of death from pulmonary or cerebral embolism that is seven to eight times that in nonusers.[88] Stated another way, one of every 2,000 women taking oral contraceptives in one study required inpatient treatment for venous thrombosis in contrast to only one of 20,000 not taking these drugs.[89] Since thromboembolism is an uncommon cause of death in healthy women in this age group, these figures are statistically equivalent to eight deaths per half-million users of the contraceptive pill compared to one death per half-million nonusers. However, the risk of thromboembolism due to pregnancy itself should be balanced against these figures when contraceptive therapy is being considered.

MISCELLANEOUS FACTORS

A number of other conditions that are associated with venous thrombosis and pulmonary thromboembolism are characterized by a pathogenesis that is even less well understood:

1. It has been shown in many studies that the incidence of thromboembolism increases with age.[16, 25] It is not known to what extent this is a feature of the aging process itself or simply a reflection of the increased incidence of the other known risk factors in this group.

2. Blood group O has been shown to be the least likely to be associated with venous thrombosis, particularly in postoperative and pregnant or puerperal women.[98, 99]

3. Cigarette smoking has been claimed to increase the risk of venous thromboembolism,[100] although evidence for this association is not at all convincing.[92] For example, two studies of patients with recent myocardial infarction[101, 102] found a significantly greater incidence of deep venous thrombosis in nonsmokers than in smokers; isotopic scanning revealed deep venous thrombosis in 42 of 74 (56 per cent) nonsmokers but in only 24 of 126 (19 per cent) smokers (whose smoking had been stopped on hospital admission).

4. Strangely, thromboembolism appears to be an infrequent cause of mortality in patients with chronic renal failure. In a series of 2,255 autopsies on adults, the overall incidence of pulmonary embolism was 32.3 per cent (18.4 per cent microscopic, 4.4 per cent macroscopic, and 9.9 per cent both); by contrast, in the 95 patients with chronic renal failure (serum creatinine level over 5.0 mg/dl), the incidence was only 9.47 per cent (all microscopic).[103]

This brief discussion of the pathogenesis of venous and cardiac thrombosis has separated predisposing factors into three groups. However, it is important to realize that in many clinical conditions two and sometimes all three of these are involved in the increased risk and that assessment of the relative importance of each can be exceedingly difficult.[104, 105] The multifactorial pathogenesis of thromboembolism is well illustrated by pregnancy, in which the incidence is clearly increased; in addition to increased venous pressure in the legs and the risk of varicosities in the pelvic and leg veins, there is an increase in the concentration of several components of the clotting mechanism.[108] An additional hazard in pregnancy is thrombophlebitis of the ovarian veins, especially in the presence of sepsis.[108, 109] Most studies indicate that thromboembolic disease is not common ante partum;[108] for example, in one study, measurement of the uptake of ^{125}I-labeled fibrinogen[104] revealed puerperal deep vein thrombosis in only one of 100 women considered to be at high risk. Instead, embolism tends to occur during the postpartum period, most often after difficult or traumatic delivery and especially if there has been hemorrhage.[110] However, others have shown an increased incidence of thrombosis and pulmonary embolism in pregnancy, even during the first trimester;[109, 111] for example, in one investigation of women over the age of 35 who required assisted delivery and were taking estrogen therapy to inhibit lactation, the incidence of peripheral thrombosis was increased tenfold.[105]

Because of the risk and expense of administering prophylactic low-dose heparin to all patients considered to be susceptible to thromboembolic disease, attempts have been made to identify those patients who should receive such medication based on a predictive index calculated from euglobulin lysis time, concentration of fibrin-related antigen, percentage overweight for height, and presence or absence of varicose veins.[106, 107]

Thromboembolism

A fragment of embolized thrombus lodged within a pulmonary artery has two immediate consequences—an increase in pressure proximal to the thrombus and a decrease or cessation of flow distal to it. The effects of thromboemboli are largely a result of these two consequences, the final clinical, roentgenographic, and pathologic manifestations being modified by a number of factors, including the size of the embolus, the presence of bacteria within the thrombus (septic embolism), the presence and extent of underlying lung abnormality (including previous thromboemboli), and the presence of extrapulmonary disease, particularly of the cardiovascular system. These manifestations can be discussed under four headings: (1) hemorrhage and infarction, (2) atelectasis, (3) hypertension, and (4) edema.

HEMORRHAGE AND INFARCTION

Parenchymal consolidation secondary to sudden occlusion of a pulmonary artery is due to one or more of three processes: (1) hemorrhage alone, (2) hemorrhage with necrosis of lung parenchyma (infarction), or (3) pneumonia. The last-named occurs in association with septic thromboemboli (*see* later) or with infection superimposed on infarcted lung. The first two are a direct consequence of a deficiency of pulmonary arterial blood flow and may represent in part different manifestations of the severity of the vascular occlusion. It should be noted that because clinical and roentgenographic findings seldom permit reliable differentiation between hemorrhage and infarction, at least in their early stages, the two are usually referred to under the single term infarction; in addition, pure pulmonary hemorrhage has sometimes been referred to as "incipient" or "incomplete" infarction.[112] Although it is likely that some of these latter cases do in fact represent true tissue necrosis as well as hemorrhage at a stage before pathologic or roentgenographic identification is possible, it is clear that others are simply a reflection of reversible ischemic damage to the alveolocapillary membrane.

Despite this fundamental pathogenetic distinction, we feel it proper to use the word "infarct" roentgenographically *in all situations in which a pulmonary opacity develops within one or more bronchopulmonary segments or subsegments distal to an occluded pulmonary artery.* Should follow-up examinations show rapid clearing, it would be reasonable to consider the lesion to be caused by hemorrhage alone. Should the opacity clear more slowly, over several weeks, the reasonable inference can be made that the vascular insult resulted in tissue death. On the other hand, from a pathologic point of view, a precise distinction between hemorrhage and infarction is usually possible, and in the following pathologic descriptions these terms are used according to their specific connotation.

Although the precise pathogenesis of pulmonary hemorrhage following thromboembolism has not been clearly established, the probable mechanism is ischemic damage to endothelial and alveolar epithelial cells, permitting the passage of red blood cells and edema into the airspaces. The hemorrhage has been considered to be derived from the bronchial arteries via bronchopulmonary anastomoses[116] but theoretically can also come from the pulmonary artery itself when the vessel is only partly occluded or after clot retraction or fibrinolysis has partly reopened the vessel.

It is not known precisely what proportion of emboli result in infarction, although some necropsy reviews have suggested that the incidence is as low as 10 to 15 per cent.[24, 113] From both clinical and experimental findings, however, it is well known that pulmonary vascular occlusion, particularly of one of the main pulmonary arteries, usually results in no permanent tissue damage unless other factors coexist.[114] The most common underlying condition predisposing to infarction is congestive heart failure,[112] an association believed to be explained by increased pulmonary venous pressure and resulting decreased bronchial artery blood flow.

Experimentally, ligation of the pulmonary veins in the presence of thromboembolism has been shown to cause pulmonary infarction, supporting this hypothesis.[114] Shock, possibly by decreasing blood flow through the bronchial arteries, is also frequently accompanied by infarction.[22] Other conditions associated with an increased incidence of infarction include malignancy (especially of the lung in one series),[115] multiple emboli, the number of lobes containing emboli, the presence of peripheral as opposed to central emboli,[22, 116] and, experimentally, chest wall compression and pleural effusion.[114] In one recent study in which the factors associated with pulmonary infarction were examined, the major determinants were the functional status of the patient, the number of lobes containing emboli, the presence of left ventricular failure, and the coexistence of lung cancer.[115] Using discriminant analysis on a group of 21 patients, the combination of these four variables predicted the presence of infarction with 70 per cent accuracy; the size of the infarct was correlated most strongly with the use of vasodilators and the embolic burden.[115]

ATELECTASIS

Pathophysiologic consequences of sudden occlusion of a pulmonary vessel include local decrease in compliance and in ventilation, caused at least partly by bronchoconstriction resulting from decreased Pco_2 within the bronchus supplying the occluded segment.[117-119] Loss of lung volume follows and is attributable at least in part to surfactant depletion;[120-123] this manifestation of pulmonary embolism is a common roentgenographic finding and is usually more striking when accompanied by infarction.[124]

After induction of pulmonary embolism in dogs,[125] airway resistance increased but bronchography showed no change in caliber of the large bronchi. If this takes place in humans, the airway obstruction must occur in small bronchi, bronchioles, or alveolar ducts.[126] In fact, experiments in dogs have implicated airways of 0.5 to 3.5 mm in diameter as being responsible for this response;[127] roentgenographic opacification with powdered tantalum of airways as small as 0.5 mm in diameter showed that all outlined intrapulmonary airways constricted equally after either ipsilateral or contralateral vascular occlusion by embolus. Airways whose initial caliber was 0.5 to 3.0 mm were the site of maximal narrowing, which occurred 80 to 120 seconds after embolization; the caliber became normal again in 4 to 40 minutes. Subsequently, it was shown[128] that autologous thrombi injected into the pulmonary artery of the left diaphragmatic lobe of dogs resulted in narrowing of right-sided airways of 0.4 to 15 mm in inner diameter, indicating reflex bronchoconstriction. Prior section of the left cervical vagus nerve significantly reduced contralateral bronchoconstriction, indicating that the parasympathetic nervous system partially controls airway narrowing after acute pulmonary thromboembolism. Using a similar technique plus bronchial pressure measurements, another group[129] injected aged, fresh, and inert (agarose) clots as emboli, to assess mechanical and humoral factors in the pathogenesis of bronchoconstriction. Bronchoconstriction of airways 0.3 to 3.0 mm in diameter occurred in all three groups. Since humoral effects derived from the thrombus could be discounted or minimized in the inert agarose and aged clots, it was concluded that mechanical factors were the common denominator. Bronchoconstriction was usually transient, the airways returning to normal dimensions within 5 minutes; the time of bronchoconstriction correlated with a drop in pulmonary compliance and an increase in airway resistance. This transient bronchoconstriction in response to pulmonary embolism in dogs has been demonstrated by radionuclide imaging,[130] unilateral pulmonary artery occlusion resulting in immediate diminution in ventilation of the ischemic lung and return to normal in 4 to 6 hours. Inhalation of 8 per cent CO_2 improved ventilation in some dogs.

Humoral effects of thrombi may be involved in the pathogenesis of bronchoconstriction. Experiments with animals showed that thrombi passing through the bloodstream to the lungs collect platelets which, when exposed to fresh thrombin, release serotonin and histamine, giving rise to bronchoconstriction.[131] In animals[131] and in humans,[132] this response can be prevented with heparin. In animals, postembolic bronchoconstriction is evidenced functionally by decreased lung compliance and increased resistance.[133]

Clinical and physiologic studies in humans also have indicated that pulmonary emboli induce the release of vasoactive and bronchoconstrictive substances such as serotonin, prostaglandins, and histamine, leading to bronchoconstriction, vasoconstriction, and perhaps altered pulmonary microcirculatory permeability.[134] Physiologic evidence of bronchoconstriction was found in 61 of 72 patients with pulmonary emboli, and only some had rhonchi.[135] In another study,[136] only 12 of 250 patients with acute pulmonary embolism (proved by angiography) had sufficient wheezing to justify a diagnosis of bronchial asthma; six of the 12 had an allergic diathesis, bronchial asthma having been diagnosed several years before embolism developed.

HYPERTENSION

The effects of pulmonary embolism on the pulmonary vasculature are somewhat similar to its effects on the airways. Small pulmonary emboli increase pulmonary arterial pressure and arterial hypoxemia, the pressure rise depending on both mechanical blockage and vasoconstriction.[137] Angiography after induction of pulmonary air embolism in dogs[138, 139] showed that air injected into the main pulmonary artery resulted in a 140 per cent increase in pulmonary arterial pressure, no change in pulmonary wedge or left atrial pressures, and a 28 per cent decrease in cardiac output; all these changes disappeared within 13 minutes. Proximal branches of the pulmonary artery became wide and tortuous, and peripheral branches tapered rapidly with both unilateral and bilateral embolization. With the former, peripheral vasoconstriction occurred in the nonembolized lung, indicating a reflex origin. The angiograms also revealed faster passage of contrast material from pulmonary arteries to pulmonary veins, indicating that the increased pressure had opened arteriovenous anastomoses, creating a right-to-left shunt and explaining at least partly the arterial hypoxemia. Additional evidence for vasoconstriction in humans with thromboembolic disease lies in the partial reversibility of chronic pulmonary hypertension following the administration of vasodilating agents.[141]

Multiple small pulmonary emboli rarely cause sudden death and do so only when there is severe underlying lung disease. These patients may have no symptoms indicative of an embolic episode, but occlusion of the major portion of the pulmonary vascular tree almost inevitably results in acute pulmonary hypertension, cor pulmonale, and right-sided heart failure (a small atrial or ventricular septal defect may be sufficient to relieve the right-sided hypertension and is the rare exception to this general rule). Even if there are multiple pulmonary emboli, pulmonary hypertension is not sustained until at least 50 per cent (probably closer to 70 per cent) of the pulmonary vascular tree is occluded.[142–147] However, transient pulmonary hypertension may result from vasoconstriction, particularly when smaller vessels are occluded;[142, 148–152] this may depend on a reflex or humoral mechanism.[145, 153]

When an increase in pulmonary artery pressure is discovered in patients with recent pulmonary embolism, it is usually necessary to exclude previous embolic occlusions or underlying disease, such as chronic obstructive pulmonary disease (COPD), as being responsible for the pulmonary hypertension. In such patients, the ratio of the mean pulmonary arterial pressure to the severity of vascular occlusion observed angiographically may effectively distinguish those patients in whom recent pulmonary embolism is the primary determinant of the postembolic hemodynamic abnormality from those in whom the pre-embolic hemodynamic abnormalities play the dominant role.[154] The presence of pulmonary hypertension in patients with COPD is an indication of advanced disease; a simple measurement of the FEV_1 as an indicator of the severity of disease may be useful in distinguishing underlying disease from embolic disease as the cause of the rise in pulmonary artery pressure.[155]

PULMONARY EDEMA

Diffuse pulmonary edema sometimes develops after pulmonary embolism.[140] Many patients are in heart failure at the time of the embolic episode,[159, 160] in which case the edema is readily explained on this basis alone. In experiments on animals, however, embolization of only one lung sometimes resulted in bilateral pulmonary edema, suggesting the possibility of a neurogenic mechanism.[161, 162] Another possible pathogenetic mechanism of pulmonary edema, applicable only in patients suffering massive embolism, is the pulmonary arterial hypertension that accompanies obstruction of a large cross section of the pulmonary vascular bed. Since right ventricular output must pass through a markedly reduced vascular bed, the pulmonary hypertension that inevitably ensues can conceivably cause high capillary hydrostatic pressures with resultant edema, analogous to that which occurs in some individuals at high altitudes; as might be expected, this is particularly true of patients with congenital absence of the right or left pulmonary artery.[163] Pulmonary edema localized to the left upper lobe has been well documented in a patient with massive embolism affecting the vasculature of the left lower lobe and right lung.[164] Sparing of the nonperfused areas of lung in both acute and chronic pulmonary embolization has been reported in patients who develop noncardiogenic pulmonary edema.[165, 166]

PATHOLOGIC CHARACTERISTICS

Lung Parenchyma

In the majority of instances, lung parenchyma distal to a pulmonary thromboembolus is either normal or shows only mild atelectasis and minimal intra-alveolar hemorrhage or edema. When changes are more marked, they consist of either hemorrhage alone or a combination of hemorrhage and necrosis. In the early stages, the two may be difficult to distinguish grossly, possessing a typical appearance of a more or less wedge-shaped area of deep red consolidation whose base abuts the pleura.

In the absence of tissue death, parenchymal hemorrhage usually disappears fairly rapidly and its residue may not be grossly detectable if the lung is examined a week or more after the embolic episode. Occasionally, deposition of hemoglobin-derived pigment on parenchymal and vascular interstitial tissue imparts a distinct yellow appearance to the previously affected lung for weeks after the initial event. In the early stages, histologic examination shows only intra-alveolar hemorrhage and

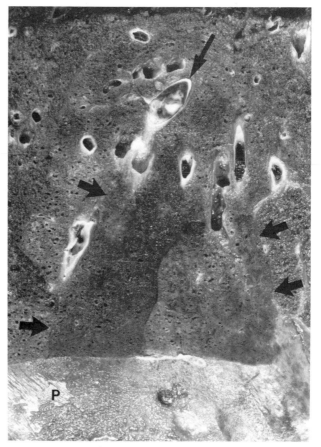

Figure 9–2. Recent Pulmonary Infarct. A wedge-shaped focus of hemorrhagic lung parenchyma is present adjacent to the pleura (*small arrows*). The lobule at the left is somewhat more hemorrhagic, although the entire area is necrotic. The lung architecture is easily identified in the necrotic regions. Note the thrombus in the feeding pulmonary artery (*large arrow*) and the fibrinous pleuritis (P).

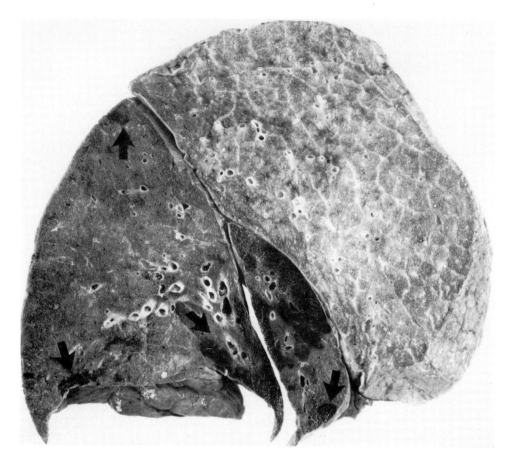

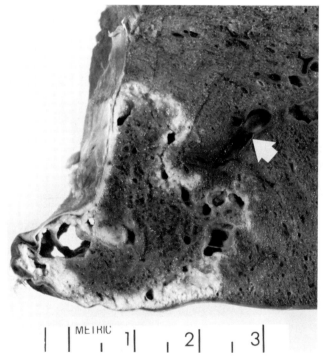

Figure 9–3. Thromboembolism with Multiple Pulmonary Infarcts. A slice of right lung shows multiple recent pleural-based infarcts in the middle and lower lobes (*arrows*).

edema, with intact alveolar walls. Later on, hemosiderin-laden macrophages usually are the only evidence of prior damage.

Within 1 or 2 days of the thromboembolic event, an infarct becomes more easily recognizable as a firm, more or less wedge-shaped area of hemorrhagic consolidation typically abutting the pleura (Fig. 9–2). Although it is usually well demarcated, patchy areas of parenchymal hemorrhage may be present adjacent to it; it is this zone that can cause the poor definition of infarcts roentgenographically. Overlying fibrinous pleuritis is often present at this stage (Fig. 9–2). Multiple foci of infarction are not infrequent (Fig. 9–3). With time, the necrotic parenchyma becomes clearly demarcated from adjacent lung by a zone of organization tissue that may be red in appearance (reflecting the vascularity of the organization tissue) or distinctly white as a result of the influx of a large number of polymorphonuclear leukocytes (Fig. 9–4). Eventually, the infarcted parenchyma is completely replaced by fibrous tissue, resulting in a contracted, somewhat elongated scar associated with pleural puckering. Cavitation within the infarct usually but not invariably[167, 168] indicates the presence of superimposed infection, although it may be difficult to distinguish this from primary pneumonia with secondary vascular thrombosis. Whatever the etiology, cavitation is typically associated with a prominent leukocytic infiltrate, the enzymes from the latter presumably causing liquefaction of necrotic tissue as a precursor to drainage

Figure 9–4. Organizing Pulmonary Infarct. A well-demarcated infarct is present in the basal aspect of the lower lobe. At the junction of necrotic and viable parenchyma, there is a distinct zone of white tissue representing a prominent polymorphonuclear leukocytic reaction. In relation to this, there is focal liquefaction and cavitation. Note that the underlying lung architecture in the necrotic zone is preserved; note also the pulmonary artery thrombus (*arrow*) and the residual pleuritis.

and cavity formation. Occasionally, the hemorrhagic appearance of a partly organized infarct is lacking, the affected parenchyma appearing white and granular; such a lesion can be mistaken grossly for neoplasm.

Histologically, infarcted lung parenchyma shows coagulative necrosis, which in the early stages may be somewhat obscured by alveolar hemorrhage and edema. Organization by granulation tissue is identifiable at the periphery after several days (Fig. 9–5). Reactive epithelial changes, particularly of type 2 pneumocytes, are often present at the margin of the infarct; when expectorated, these cells occasionally give rise to a false-positive cytologic diagnosis of malignancy.[169] Long-standing infarcts show dense parenchymal fibrosis in which the underlying lung architecture often can still be recognized. Airways within the fibrotic region may remain patent and viable, reflecting the preservation of the bronchial circulation; recanalized thrombus may be identifiable in pulmonary arteries (Fig. 9–6). The pleura in the vicinity of the infarct typically shows a prominent increase in vascularity as well as fibrosis and retraction into the lung itself (Fig. 9–6).

Experimental investigations in dogs and observations on humans with protracted pulmonary artery occlusion reveal a gradual increase in the bronchial circulation, which anastomoses freely with pulmonary vessels until the normal pulmonary arterial blood flow is equaled.[170, 171] Systemic-pulmo-

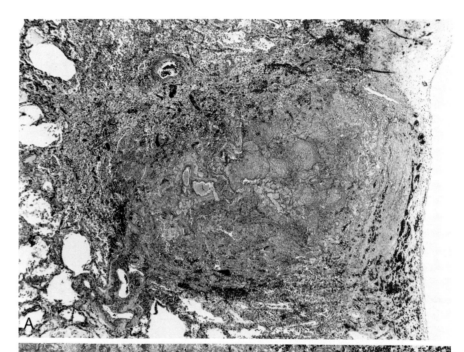

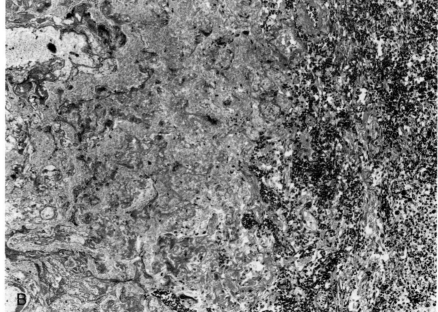

Figure 9–5. Organizing Pulmonary Infarct. A histologic section at low power (*A*) reveals a fairly well demarcated focus of necrotic lung parenchyma surrounded by a zone of organization tissue. Note the prominent vascularity in the adjacent pleura. A magnified view (*B*) shows coagulative necrosis of lung tissue on the left and granulation tissue on the right. (*A*, × 25; *B*, × 100.)

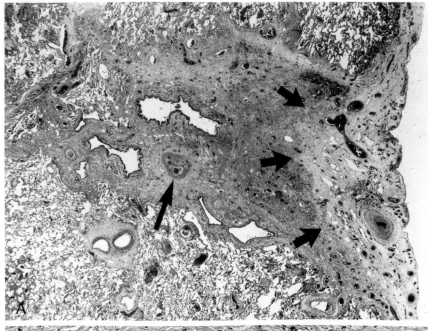

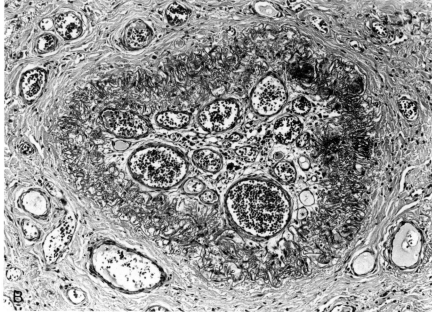

Figure 9–6. Remote Pulmonary Infarct. A histologic section (*A*) reveals a well-demarcated area of parenchymal fibrosis that abuts the pleura; the pleura itself is fibrotic and retracted into the lung (*short arrows* denote the pleura-lung interface). Note the histologically viable bronchi within the infarct and the partly occluded pulmonary artery (*large arrow*) containing recanalized thrombus. A magnified view (*B*) shows the pulmonary artery to better advantage. (*A*, × 10; *B*, × 120.)

nary arterial anastomoses are usually inapparent on postmortem aortography 3 to 7 days after embolization, but are well formed by 3 to 4 weeks; these anastomoses presumably play a major role in the lung's response to later emboli.[39]

Thromboembolus and Pulmonary Vessels

The fate of pulmonary thromboemboli depends on multiple factors, including the status of the patient's fibrinolytic system, the degree of organization of the thrombus before its embolization, and the amount of new thrombus added *in situ*. Although emboli occasionally change little in size, thereby causing chronic vascular obstruction,[172] the vast majority are largely degraded by one or more of three mechanisms—lysis, fragmentation and peripheral embolization, and organization and recanalization.

LYSIS

Both roentgenographic[173] and perfusion scanning[174] studies have established that, in many cases, flow through obstructed arteries returns relatively rapidly in the first few days after embolization. These clinical observations have been substantiated experimentally by several workers. In one investigation in which serial roentgenograms were obtained of dogs following administration of thromboemboli labeled with powdered tantalum, Austin and his coworkers[175] found a gradual decrease in the breadth of the radiopaque labels in the individual clots, particularly during the first 2 to 4 days after embolization. In another study of fresh clot emboli in dogs,[176] the volume of the embolized clot was seen to diminish by 50 per cent in 3 hours. Such rapid and extensive dissolution suggests the effect of fibrinolysis. This subject is discussed in greater detail on page 1773.

FRAGMENTATION AND PERIPHERAL EMBOLIZATION

In the study by Austin and colleagues,[175] the clots were observed to fragment into multiple small pieces which embolized further towards the periph-

ery of the lung; this change was observed somewhat later than lysis and was most prominent after the first week following embolization. The pathogenesis of this fragmentation may be related to splitting of the thrombus into smaller and smaller pieces as a result of ingrowth of endothelial cells and macrophages from the vessel wall.[177]

ORGANIZATION AND RECANALIZATION

Ingrowth of fibroblasts, capillaries, and endothelial cells from the vessel wall into the peripheral portion of a thrombus can also result in its organization and eventual incorporation into the wall as a fibrous plaque, typically in an eccentric location (Fig. 9–7). Alternatively, some thrombi undergo lysis and

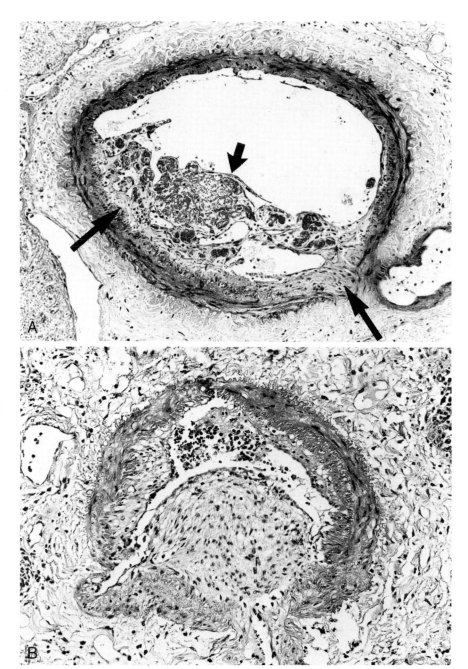

Figure 9–7. Organizing Thromboembolus. A histologic section of a muscular artery of medium size (*A*) shows a small amount of thrombus (*short arrow*) in the lower aspect. Its luminal surface is smooth and covered by endothelial cells; the thrombus was originally in direct contact with the vessel wall but has been partly replaced by fibrous tissue (*long arrows*). A section of another vessel (*B*) shows a more advanced stage of organization, the thrombus being completely replaced by fibrous tissue. Such eccentric intimal thickening is highly suggestive of remote thromboembolism.

Illustration continued on following page

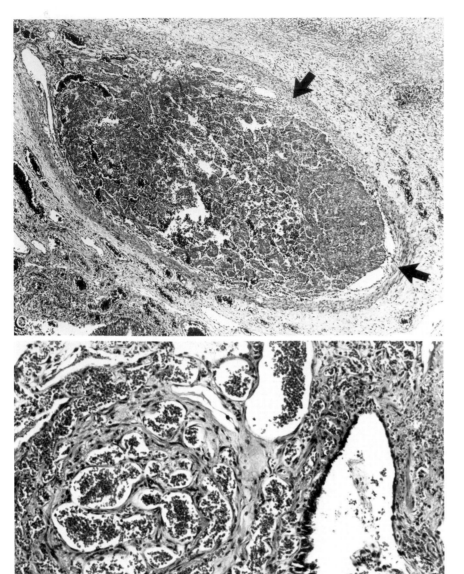

Figure 9–7 *Continued* In another section (*C*), a large muscular pulmonary artery is almost completely occluded by thrombus. Adherence of the thrombus to the vessel wall by fibroplastic ingrowth is evident in several foci (*arrows*). Note also that the central portion of the thrombus is divided into numerous small fragments as a result of simultaneous lysis and organization; such a process typically causes multiple small intraluminal channels rather than focal eccentric intimal thickening. *D*, An advanced stage of this process is illustrated in a small muscular artery. (*A*, × 130; *B*, × 140; *C*, × 40; *D*, × 150.)

organization in their central portion at the same time as they undergo peripheral organization, resulting in the formation of multiple small vascular channels within the original lumen (recanalization) (Fig. 9–7). Although the lumens of such embolized vessels are inevitably diminished in cross-sectional area, these processes undoubtedly result in a much greater flow than would have been possible without organization.

In addition to changes attributable to organization of the thromboembolus, the pulmonary artery wall itself can undergo several alterations in the acute stage of embolization. Occasionally, necrosis and inflammation may be seen (Fig. 9–8),[178, 179] possibly caused by local ischemia induced by the impacted thrombus. Splits in the intimal and medial elastic laminae, focal areas of medial fibrosis, and both true and false saccular aneurysms have also been attributed to thromboemboli.[178, 180] Sevitt[180] has speculated that at least some of these changes might be caused by mechanical stretching at the time of embolic impaction.

Despite the angiographic evidence of rapid dissolution in some cases, many recent thromboemboli remain intact and can be recognized grossly at necropsy by one or more of three characteristics: (1) the presence of distinct laminations (Fig. 9–9) (corresponding to alternating bands of platelet-fibrin deposition during the initial stages of venous thrombosis), (2) adherence to the vessel wall (indi-

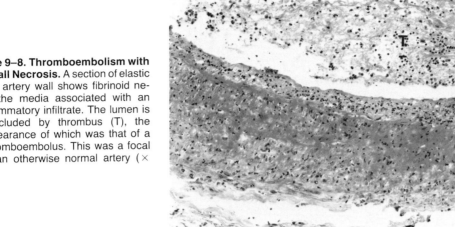

Figure 9–8. Thromboembolism with Arterial Wall Necrosis. A section of elastic pulmonary artery wall shows fibrinoid necrosis of the media associated with an acute inflammatory infiltrate. The lumen is mostly occluded by thrombus (T), the gross appearance of which was that of a typical thromboembolus. This was a focal lesion in an otherwise normal artery (× 120).

cating organization), or (3) in larger vessels, the presence of a coiled appearance (due to imperfect fit and folding of the thrombus as it lodges in the artery). If these features are lacking, it may be difficult to distinguish with certainty a recent thromboembolus from a postmortem clot. Organizing and organized thromboemboli can also be recognized in many cases as areas of intraluminal fibrosis containing small hemorrhagic spaces (representing areas of recanalization) and as fibrous bands or webs traversing the lumen (Fig. 9–10).[156–158, 181, 182]

Histologic sections show thrombi in various stages of organization, depending both on the extent of pulmonary arterial reaction and on the degree of organization that occurred at the initial venous site of thrombosis. Medium- to large-sized muscular arteries are most commonly affected; in one necropsy study of 54 patients,[39] the muscular arteries were involved in all cases, elastic arteries in only 20, and the arterioles in 22. Determining the precise time at which a particular thromboembolic episode occurred is extremely difficult in most cases; however, evidence of organization in the vessel and contiguous thrombus indicates a duration of at least 1 or 2 days and is sufficient to exclude embolus as the immediate cause of death. The absence of this reaction, however, does not necessarily imply a more recent event, since organization may not proceed at the same rate in all parts of the thrombus. Remote, organized thromboemboli can be recognized by eccentric areas of intimal fibrosis and by fibrous bands traversing the lumen (Figs. 9–7 and 9–10).[181, 182] Intimal thickening originating from pulmonary emboli can undergo transformation to atherosclerotic plaques.[183]

ROENTGENOGRAPHIC MANIFESTATIONS

Consideration of the manifestations of pulmonary thromboembolic disease should be prefaced by a further reminder that most episodes are asymptomatic and produce no detectable changes on plain chest roentgenograms. Even if the diagnosis is suspected clinically and confirmed angiographically, in many cases no abnormalities are seen on plain films (*see* page 1756).[181, 187] Roentgenologically apparent changes usually occur only when a fairly large segmental artery is occluded or when obstruction of many small vessels has impaired pulmonary hemodynamics.[188] The statement made by Figley and associates[189] in discussing life-threatening embolism is appropriate: "The principal evidence of embolism on the chest roentgenogram is often the paucity of abnormalities for a patient in such dire straits."

An excellent review of techniques and results of imaging of pulmonary embolism, including diagnostic criteria of value, has been published by Sostman and his colleagues[723] and by Alderson and Martin.[724]

Anatomic Distribution

Most embolic occlusions occur in the lower lobes, probably as a result of hemodynamic flow patterns. The right lung is involved more frequently than the left, especially the posterior basal segment.[39, 114, 188, 190, 191] One report of pulmonary infarction[192] stated that it was in the upper lobes in nine of the 60 patients studied, but this figure probably is too high for all thromboembolic episodes (that is, including those in which infarction

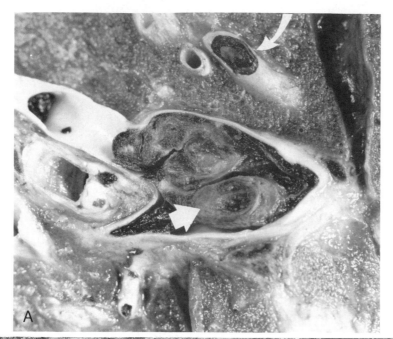

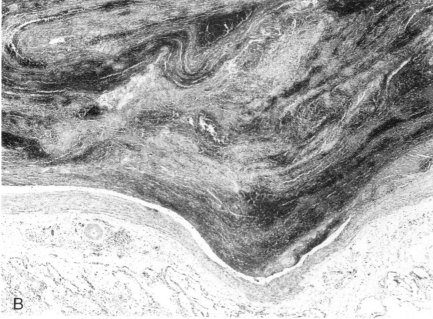

Figure 9–9. Recent Thromboembolus. A gross specimen of a lobar pulmonary artery (*A*) shows a recent thromboembolus, focally with prominent lamination (*short arrow*). Occlusion of a small segmental branch is also apparent (*curved arrow*). In a histologic section (*B*), dark and light bands alternate in a pattern characteristic of recent thrombus, the former caused by red blood cells and the latter by platelet-fibrin aggregates. Note the absence of reaction in the adjacent arterial wall (× 25).

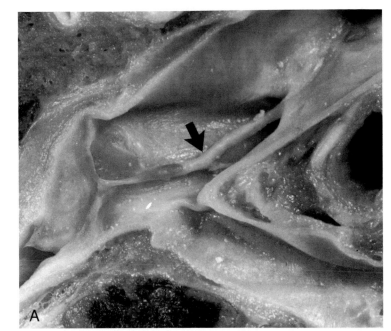

Figure 9–10. Remote Thromboembolus: Intraluminal Fibrous Bands. A gross specimen of a lobar pulmonary artery and its proximal branches (A) shows a cord-like fibrous band traversing the vessel lumen (*arrow*). This appearance is diagnostic of organized thrombus, most often caused by embolism. A histologic section through a medium-sized elastic artery (B) reveals several broad fibrous bands separating the lumen into multiple compartments. There is no evidence of residual thrombus (× 25).

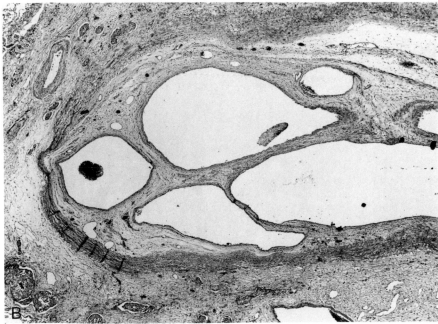

does not occur). Fleischner[190] believed that up to 10 per cent of upper lobe embolism may be acceptable in necropsy studies, but probably is too high for experience based on clinical material. Since people spend approximately one third of their lives recumbent in bed, when the disparity of blood flow to upper and lower lung zones almost disappears, the marked predilection of thromboembolism for lower lobes appears surprising—particularly since most embolic episodes occur in hospitalized patients, many of them in bed postoperatively. Thus the roentgenologist must bear in mind the possibility of infarction as a cause of upper lobe opacities.[193]

The roentgenographic manifestations of thromboembolism can be divided into those with and those without increase in roentgenographic density—that is, with and without infarction.

Thromboembolism Without Infarction

When changes relating to thromboembolism without infarction are visible on plain roentgenograms of the chest—and it must be stressed again that this is uncommon except when embolism is massive—they may be distinctive and should strongly suggest the diagnosis. There are four changes: oligemia, change in vessel size, alteration in size and configuration of the heart, and loss of lung volume.

OLIGEMIA

Peripheral oligemia may be local, caused· by occlusion of a fairly large lobar or segmental pulmonary artery (Fig. 9–11), or general, the result of widespread small vessel thromboembolism. The first description of local oligemia resulting from embolism was by Westermark in 1938,[194] and although some authors[146, 189, 195] regard the sign as seldom convincing, others have confirmed it as a valid sign of embolism.[124, 190, 196–198] In a study of 25 patients with massive pulmonary embolism in whom plain film and angiographic abnormalities were correlated,[124] local oligemia was observed in *all*—in fact, 79 per cent of such zones apparent on the arteriogram were recognizable on the plain roentgenogram. It was concluded that changes in vascularity were the principal diagnostic changes on the plain roentgenogram. In another series,[119] local oligemia was reported in eight of ten cases. Further, induction of pulmonary embolism (confirmed by angiography) in ten dogs[197] resulted in roentgenographic evidence of local oligemia in five animals during the first day, mainly as increased radiolucency of affected lung zones; it disappeared within 24 to 36 hours.

Even more impressive were the results of the experimental study carried out on dogs by Grossman and his colleagues:[201] employing a fourth-generation computed tomography (CT) scanner

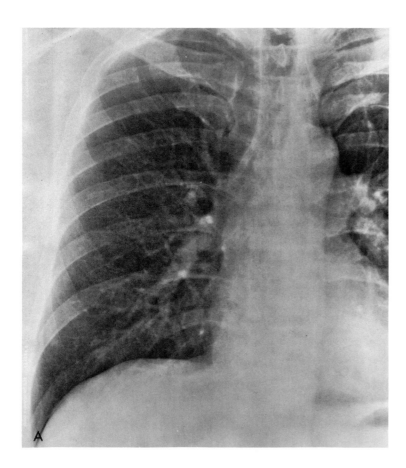

Figure 9–11. Pulmonary Embolism Without Infarction: The Westermark Sign. On admission of a 52-year-old man to the hospital, a posteroanterior roentgenogram (*A*) revealed no significant abnormalities. Several days following abdominal surgery, he experienced abrupt onset of right chest pain and dyspnea.

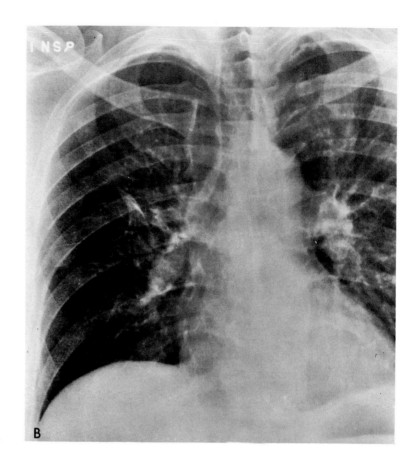

Figure 9–11 *Continued* A roentgenogram at this time (*B*) showed an obvious increase in diameter and a change in configuration of the right interlobar artery (*arrowheads*); also, the distal end of this artery appeared "knuckled" and the vessels peripheral to it diminutive. The overall density of the right lower zone was considerably less than that of the left, indicating diminished perfusion (the Westermark sign). A lung scan (*C*) revealed absence of perfusion of the lower half of the right lung.

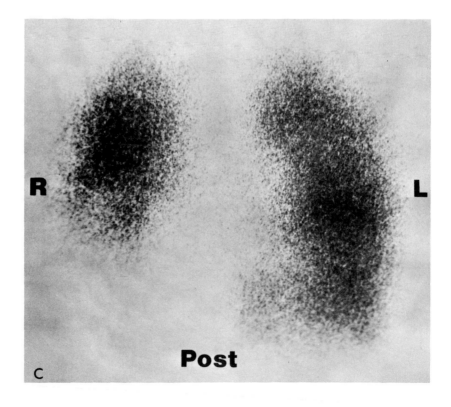

with a 2-second scan time and a 512-by-512 matrix, these authors scanned the thorax of 17 dogs following balloon occlusion of a major lower lobe pulmonary artery. In *all* dogs, lung parenchyma distal to the occluded vessel revealed an appreciable reduction in Hounsfield units compared to identical anatomic zones of the contralateral lung, reflecting oligemia; contrast medium was not used. The time between vessel occlusion and the CT examination ranged from 1 minute to 9 hours, and there appeared to be little relationship between the time interval after occlusion and the degree of hypoperfusion. In no case was an abnormality identifiable on conventional roentgenograms obtained at the same time as the CT scan, although in 16 of the 17 animals a perfusion deficit corresponding to the zone of oligemia identified by CT was observed on radionuclide scanning with ^{99m}Tc macroaggregated albumin (MAA). The fact that the oligemia was caused by a reduction in blood volume was confirmed by carrying out a computer analysis of the labeled erythrocyte mass: in all cases there was a decline in the mass distal to the occluded vessel. For reasons that the authors were unable to explain, the oligemia was consistently identified in all animals in the prone position but seldom in the supine position; in fact, the density of affected zones of animals in the latter position was the same as contralateral normal lung. On the basis of such studies and assuming that the results of animal experimentation can be transposed to humans, it appears that CT possesses considerable promise in the identification of oligemia in acute pulmonary embolism in man (*see* Fig. 9–25, page 1739); however, since prompt radionuclide scanning can be expected to yield similar information at much lower cost, the routine employment of CT in this clinical setting is unlikely to achieve widespread use.

The value of full lung tomography in the appreciation of local oligemia after embolism[199] was emphasized in studies with the technique described by Fraser and Bates[200] in the study of emphysema; characteristic abnormalities were detected on full lung tomograms in all 23 cases of pulmonary embolism. If tomographic findings are equivocal, Beamish[196] recommends combining tomography with the rapid intravenous infusion of contrast medium to visualize local oligemia.

Oligemia is more often detected when a whole lung or a major part of it is deprived of its pulmonary artery circulation (Fig. 9–12), the unilateral oligemia contrasting markedly with the pleonemia of the other lung.[202–206]

General pulmonary oligemia in thromboembolic disease is almost invariably the result of widespread occlusion of smaller arteries (the rare exception is the case in which thromboembolism of large pulmonary arteries is the predominant morphologic abnormality; see Fig. 4–146, page 655). The diffuse oligemia is nearly always accompanied by signs of pulmonary artery hypertension (Fig. 9–13)—enlargement of the central pulmonary arteries, cor pulmonale, cardiac decompensation, and dilation of the superior vena cava and azygos vein (Fig. 9–14).[198] Absence of pulmonary overinflation differentiates diffuse thromboembolism from diffuse emphysema.

CHANGES IN THE PULMONARY ARTERY

Enlargement of a major hilar pulmonary artery is a leading sign of pulmonary embolism (*see* Fig. 9–11),[146, 205–209] and is of particular value when serial roentgenograms reveal progressive enlargement of the affected vessel.[205] In a study of 25 patients with massive pulmonary embolism (defined arteriographically as involvement of at least half the major pulmonary arterial branches),[124] Kerr and colleagues described "plump" hilar shadows in 14, 13 of which were on the right. These authors experienced difficulty (as have we) in appreciating dilatation of the left interlobar artery on a posteroanterior chest roentgenogram, probably because of overlap by the heart; however, this vessel is often clearly seen posterior to the left upper lobe bronchus on a lateral roentgenogram, and a diameter greater than 18 mm can be regarded as reasonable evidence of dilatation. In the right hilum, the presence of a thrombus can be assessed by measurement of the diameter of the descending branch of the pulmonary artery where it relates to the intermediate stem bronchus. The normal maximal diameter of this artery at total lung capacity (TLC) is 16 mm in adult men and 15 mm in adult women; when values are exceeded, it may be reasonably concluded that the vessel is enlarged.[211] Perhaps more reliable than this absolute measurement, however, is increase in size of the affected vessel in serial examinations, which is strong evidence of thromboembolism, especially if peripheral oligemia is present (*see* Fig. 9–11). Widening of the pulmonary artery usually diminishes rapidly, and the artery reverts to normal size within a few days after lysis and fragmentation of the thrombus.[189]

A more recent study by Palla and coworkers achieved impressive results.[210] In a conventional roentgenographic study of 73 patients with confirmed pulmonary embolism and of 85 age-matched patients in whom an original suspicion of embolism was not confirmed, these authors found a significant dilatation of the proximal portion of the right interlobar artery in the former group (p<0.01). The transverse diameter of the vessel was measured at four points, namely, the junction of the right superior pulmonary vein with the interlobar artery and at three 1-cm intervals distally; only at the proximal two points did increased diameters reach statistical significance. In the patients with emboli, the mean diameter of the vessel at the venoarterial junction was 17.8 mm (SD 3.94 mm) compared with a mean diameter in the nonembolic patients of 15.7 mm (SD 3.14 mm); this difference was highly sig-

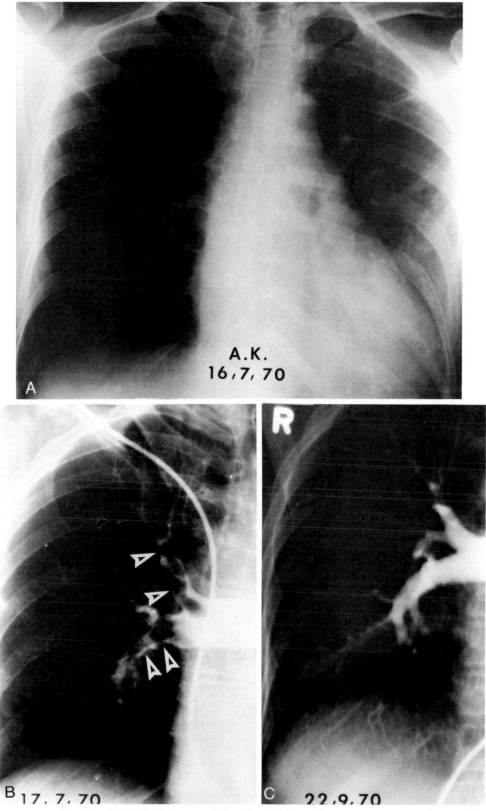

Figure 9–12. Westermark's Sign in Acute Pulmonary Thromboembolism. An overpenetrated anteroposterior roentgenogram of the chest (A) discloses a hypertranslucent right lung, its vessels being diminutive compared with faintly visible vessels in the left lung. Cardiac size is moderately increased. The combined features strongly suggest massive pulmonary thromboembolism in the right lung. A view of the right lung (B) from a pulmonary angiogram reveals intraluminal filling defects (*arrowheads*) that severely compromise blood flow through the ascending and descending branches of the right pulmonary artery, accounting for the oligemia in A. Two months later, a repeat pulmonary angiogram (C) shows complete resolution of the emboli.

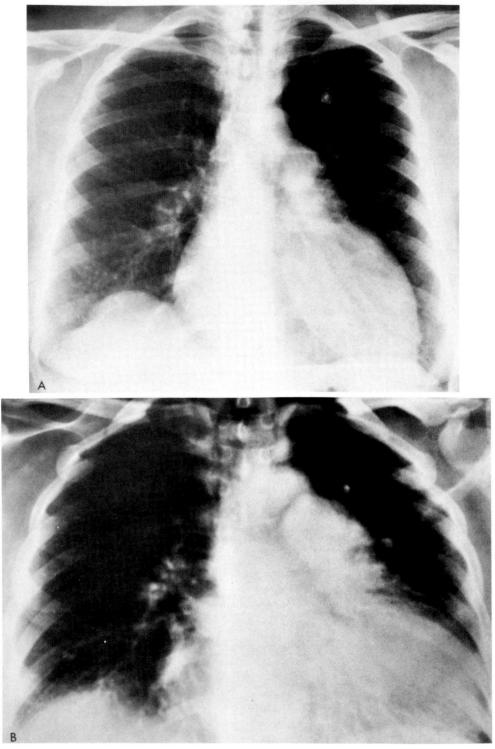

Figure 9–13. Multiple Peripheral Embolization. A posteroanterior roentgenogram (*A*) of a 41-year-old woman reveals generalized, symmetric oligemia of both lungs. The hilar pulmonary arteries are enlarged and taper rapidly as they proceed distally; the heart is moderately enlarged, and its contour is typical of right ventricular dilatation and cor pulmonale; the lungs are not overinflated. A pulmonary angiogram exposed 10 seconds following the rapid intravenous injection of contrast medium (*B*) reveals persistent opacification of the chambers on the right side of the heart at a time when all contrast media should have passed through the lungs into the systemic circulation, indicating severe pulmonary arterial hypertension.

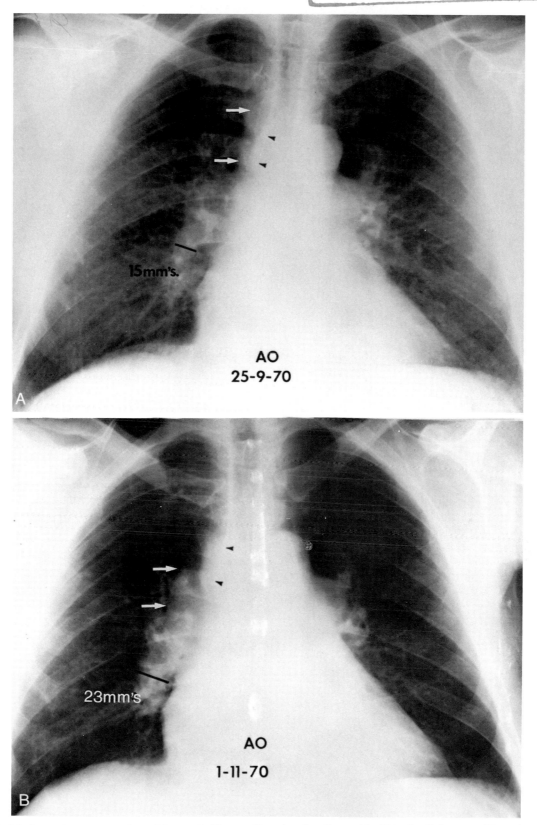

Figure 9–14. Acute Cor Pulmonale and Systemic Venous Hypertension Caused by Massive Pulmonary Thromboembolism. A posteroanterior roentgenogram (*A*) is normal; note the appearance of the superior vena cava (*arrows*), azygos vein (*arrowheads*), and right interlobar artery (measuring 15 mm in transverse diameter). Two months later, this elderly man suffered the sudden onset of retrosternal pain and dyspnea 10 days after prostatic surgery; a repeat chest roentgenogram (*B*) discloses marked enlargement of the vena cava (*arrows*), azygos vein (*arrowheads*), and the cardiac shadow; the hilar arterial vasculature is distinctly dilated, the right interlobar artery now measuring 23 mm. The combined features are highly suggestive, if not diagnostic, of cor pulmonale associated with massive thromboembolism. A perfusion lung scan (not shown) disclosed an absence of perfusion in the right lung and large deficits in the left mid and lower lung zones.

nificant (p = 0.004). At a point 1 cm distal to the venoarterial junction, comparable figures for the patients with emboli were 16.3 mm (SD 4.10) and for the patients without emboli 14.0 mm (SD 3.05); this difference was also highly significant (p = 0.001). In about one fourth of the patients with pulmonary embolism, enlargement was so marked that the artery assumed a "sausage" configuration, corresponding to the "knuckle sign" described below; this feature was regarded by the authors as particularly suggestive of the diagnosis. In all cases, the presence or absence of an acute embolic episode was confirmed by perfusion lung scanning.

It is almost certain that the increase in size of the right interlobar artery is the result of distention of the vessel by the thrombus itself, *not* of increased vascular pressure. In the latter case, the increase in resistance due to local embolization causes immediate redistribution of blood flow to lung areas of normal vascular resistance; in fact, this redistribution of blood flow may be evidenced on plain roentgenograms by an increase in the size of the vessels (*see* Fig. 9–25, page 1739). Such local "hyperemia" was observed in at least one zone in ten of 25 patients with massive pulmonary embolism studied by Kerr and coworkers.[124] Only when there is widespread involvement in both lungs (70 per cent of the cross-sectional area of the vascular bed) does the increased resistance increase the size of the hilar artery, and then this is bilateral and symmetric (*see* Fig. 9–13). Diminished pulsation in enlarged thrombosed hilar vessels may be apparent fluoroscopically,[202, 203, 206] but this sign is seldom convincing, pulsation usually being relatively inapparent even in normal pulmonary arteries.

Of equal importance to increase in size of an interlobar artery is the abrupt tapering of the occluded vessel distally; the vessel may terminate suddenly, creating the so-called "knuckle sign" (Figs. 9–15 and 9–16).[119, 184, 202] Also, occluded vessels may be more sharply delineated than normal, a sign probably relating to diminished pulsation.

CARDIAC CHANGES (COR PULMONALE)

Acute cor pulmonale is not a common roentgenologic accompaniment of thromboembolism, being observed in only 10 per cent of 126 patients.[212] It occurs most often with widespread multiple peripheral emboli (*see* Fig. 9–13) and sometimes—when a large enough area of the arterial system is occluded—with massive central embolization (*see* Fig. 4–146, page 655). The signs are those of cardiac enlargement due to dilation of the right ventricle, increase in size of the main pulmonary artery, and, usually, increase in size and rapidity of tapering of the hilar pulmonary vessels.[184, 205] Dilation of the azygos vein and superior vena cava may be apparent, reflecting right-sided cardiac decompensation (Fig. 9–14). It may be very difficult to recognize any of these signs, particularly cardiac

enlargement, in a patient with restricted ventilation whose chest roentgenogram was exposed at the bedside, most likely in the supine position.[189] Cardiac enlargement may not occur in the rare case of multiple pulmonary emboli in which an atrial or ventricular septal defect relieves pressure on the right cardiac chambers through a right-to-left shunt (Fig. 9–17).

LOSS OF LUNG VOLUME

Loss of volume of a lower lobe in pulmonary embolism without infarction may be manifested roentgenographically by elevation of the hemidiaphragm (Fig. 9–18), or downward displacement of the major fissure, or both. The mechanism probably relates to a deficit of surfactant resulting from loss of pulmonary artery perfusion as well as to bronchoconstriction. Loss of lung volume is a more frequent finding when infarction is present (*see* farther on). Studies of 25 patients with massive pulmonary embolism[124] showed loss of volume in eight, seven of whom had infarction.

Thromboembolism with Infarction

Thromboembolism may increase roentgenographic density by consolidating lung parenchyma, regardless of whether the infarction is associated with tissue necrosis or with simple hemorrhage and edema. Parenchymal consolidation is nearly always the result of embolism rather than thrombosis *in situ*—although, in a small percentage of patients, thrombi may arise *in situ* without any previous embolic episode, particularly in those with chronic cardiorespiratory disease or degenerative changes in the pulmonary arteries.[202, 203, 206]

The roentgenologic changes in embolism with and without infarction are basically the same, except that in the former instance the oligemia is replaced by parenchymal consolidation. Increased size and abrupt tapering of the feeder artery are common to both conditions, but loss of lung volume occurs most often and is more severe with infarction (Fig. 9–19). Of 25 cases of massive pulmonary embolism studied by Kerr and colleagues,[124] eight (including seven with pulmonary infarction) had elevation of the ipsilateral hemidiaphragm. In a retrospective study of 66 necropsy-proven cases of pulmonary embolism with infarction, Talbot and associates[213] found elevation of the hemidiaphragm in 26 (40 per cent) and regarded this as the single most useful roentgenographic sign of infarction. In a study of 50 patients with angiographically documented acute pulmonary embolism, Szucs and associates[187] found relatively nonspecific abnormalities on the plain roentgenogram in 71 per cent, consisting of pulmonary opacity, pleural effusion, or elevated hemidiaphragm; in the remaining 29 per cent, the roentgenogram was normal. Of interest in this series was the incidence of different roentgenographic

Text continued on page 1733

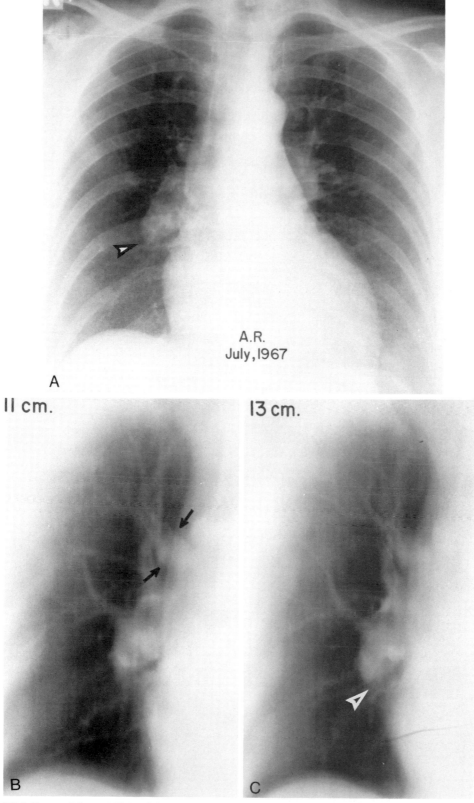

Figure 9–15. Dilatation and Amputation of the Right Interlobar Artery (Knuckle Sign) As Evidence of Pulmonary Thromboembolism. A conventional posteroanterior chest roentgenogram (*A*) reveals an enlarged cardiac shadow. The lungs are normal except for a suggestion of oligemia in the right upper and left lower lung zones. The hilar arteries are dilated, and the right interlobar artery tapers rapidly and appears to terminate abruptly (*arrowhead*), an appearance that is confirmed on detail views of the right lung (*B, C*) from conventional linear tomograms (*arrowhead*). This constitutes a positive knuckle sign. The proximal part of the ascending right pulmonary artery is also dilated (*arrows*).

Illustration continued on following page

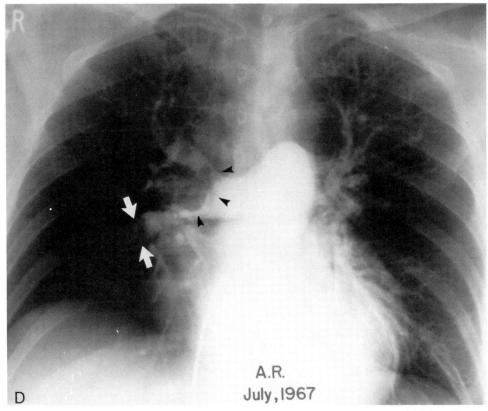

Figure 9–15 *Continued* A pulmonary angiogram in anteroposterior projection (*D*) discloses a large saddle embolus (*arrowheads*) partly obstructing the bifurcation of the ascending and descending branches of the right pulmonary artery. The right interlobar artery is completely occluded (*arrows*), accounting for the features illustrated in *A* to *C*. Several segmental arterial branches in the left upper lobe and lingula are also obstructed. The patient is a middle-aged woman with a history of progressive dyspnea.

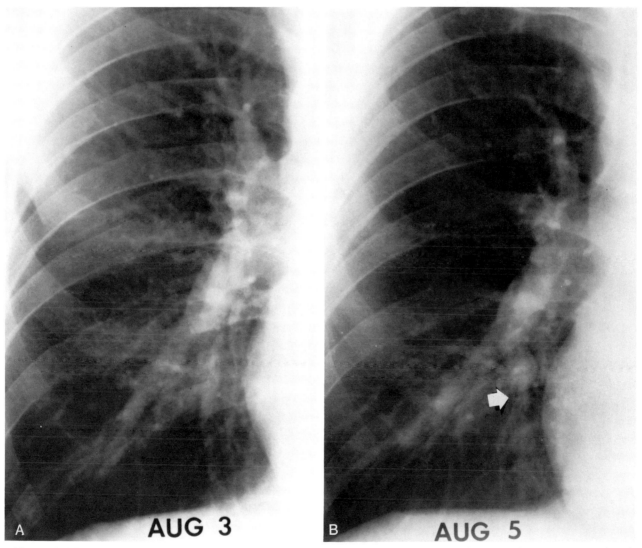

Figure 9–16. Thromboembolism, Infarction, and Healing. *A*, Sequential views of the right lung from posteroanterior chest roentgenograms reveal no abnormality. Two days later (*B*), however, a segmental branch in the lower lobe is focally enlarged and abruptly tapered (*arrow*). This feature is highly suggestive of an impacted thromboembolism in a segmental artery, creating a "knuckle sign."

Illustration continued on following page

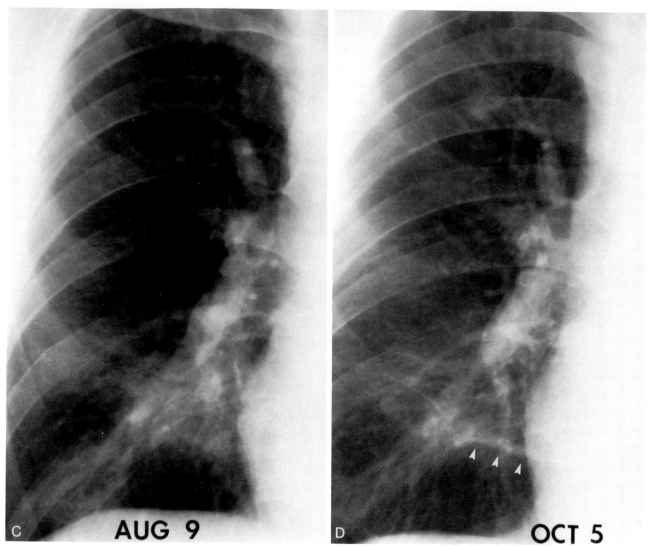

Figure 9–16 *Continued* Four days later (*C*), an ill-defined parenchymal opacity had appeared in the posterior basal segment of the lower lobe, representing an infarct. Approximately 2 months later (*D*), the only residuum is a linear opacity (*arrowheads*) at the site of the previous area of consolidation, consistent with a scar. The patient is a 35-year-old renal transplant recipient who complained of the acute onset of mild dyspnea the day before the roentgenogram in *B*.

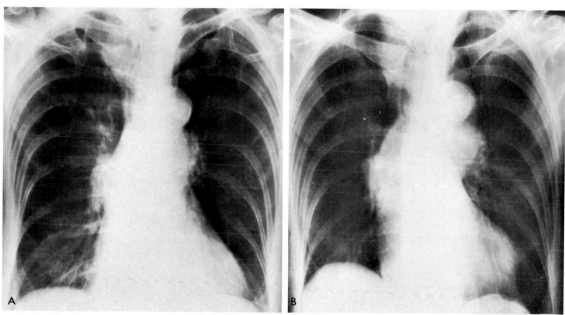

Figure 9–17. Massive Central and Peripheral Pulmonary Emboli Without Cardiac Enlargement (Atrial Septal Defect). A posteroanterior roentgenogram (*A*) of a 76-year-old woman reveals no convincing evidence of significant abnormality in the lungs; the pulmonary vasculature and cardiovascular silhouette are within normal limits except for moderate atherosclerosis of the aorta. One month later, following the abrupt onset of severe dyspnea, an anteroposterior roentgenogram (*B*) reveals a considerable change in the appearance of the chest: the hilar pulmonary arteries are increased in size, and their peripheral branches are thin and attenuated; there is severe bilateral pulmonary oligemia. This appearance strongly suggested multiple pulmonary emboli, but the absence of cardiac enlargement with such extensive arterial obstruction was difficult to explain. At necropsy, the reason for the absence of significant cardiac enlargement was readily explained by the demonstration of an atrial septal defect which permitted partial relief of hypertension in the right heart chambers through a right-to-left shunt. Huge saddle emboli were present in the right and left main pulmonary arteries and extended into and expanded the main hilar vessels bilaterally; multiple peripheral emboli were also present. Note that in contrast to the situation depicted in Figure 9–13, the enlargement of the hilar pulmonary arteries in this patient related to the physical presence of thrombus rather than to the development of pulmonary arterial hypertension.

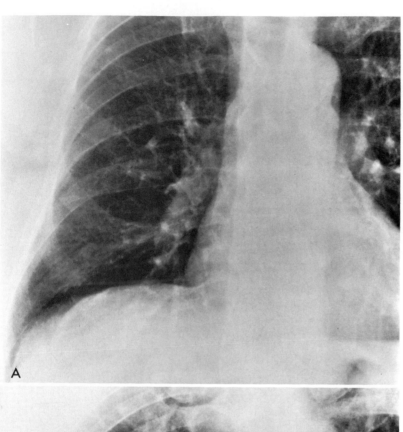

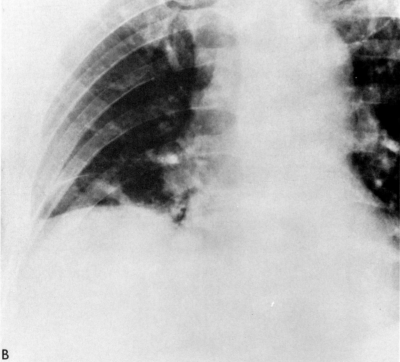

Figure 9–18. Atelectasis Associated with Pulmonary Embolism. When this 72-year-old man was admitted to the hospital, his chest roentgenogram (A) was normal. Several days following laparotomy, he suffered a typical clinical episode of pulmonary embolism. An anteroposterior roentgenogram (B) showed moderate elevation of the right hemidiaphragm associated with a fat, bulging right interlobar artery. The only opacity in the right lower lobe is an obliquely oriented line shadow. This loss of volume is presumably the result of reduced perfusion and surfactant deficit.

Figure 9–19. Pulmonary Infarction with Rapid Resolution. A view of the right lung from a conventional posteroanterior chest roentgenogram (*A*) reveals a homogeneous opacity occupying the lower half of the right lower lobe. The right hemidiaphragm is moderately elevated and the right interlobar artery is plump. The findings are highly suggestive of pulmonary infarction. Eight days later (*B*), the lower-lobe consolidation has resolved and the hemidiaphragm has descended to its normal position. The patient is an afebrile elderly woman with the acute onset of dyspnea and hemoptysis. The rapidity of resolution is compatible with pulmonary hemorrhage secondary to thromboembolism.

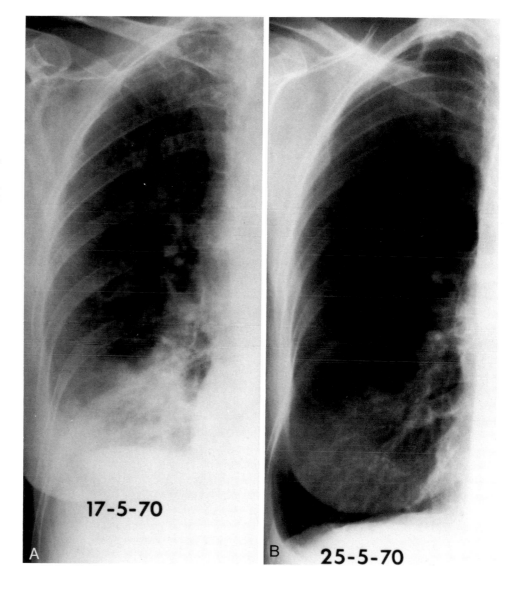

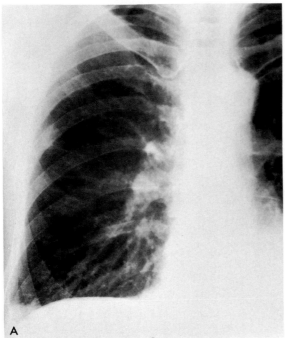

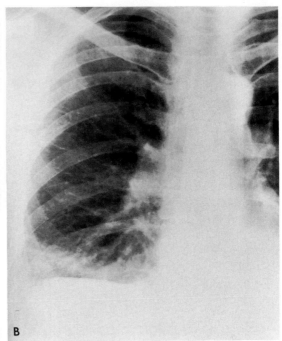

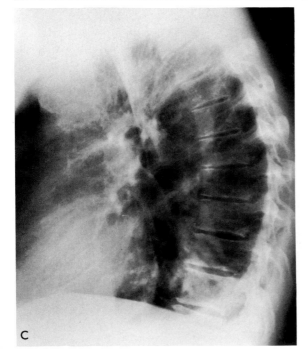

Figure 9–20. Pulmonary Infarct, Right Lower Lobe. Three days after laparotomy, this 57-year-old man suffered abrupt onset of right-sided chest pain. A view of the right hemithorax from a posteroanterior roentgenogram exposed 24 hours later (*A*) reveals a rather poorly defined shadow of homogeneous density nestled in the costophrenic sulcus; there is a small pleural effusion. Three days later, posteroanterior (*B*) and lateral (*C*) roentgenograms demonstrate considerable increase in the extent of parenchymal consolidation. The right hemidiaphragm has risen since the previous examination. Although the shadow is poorly visualized in lateral projection, the presence of disease is indicated by obliteration of the posterior portion of the hemidiaphragm. Roentgenographic resolution was incomplete 3 weeks later, indicating that the process was one of necrosis rather than hemorrhage alone.

abnormalities in relation to time after the acute episode. For example, loss of lung volume, as evidenced by elevation of a hemidiaphragm, was observed in 50 per cent of patients within 24 hours of onset of symptoms but in only 15 per cent when symptoms had been present longer. However, the incidence of pulmonary opacities was reversed, these being found in 37 and 57 per cent of patients, respectively. Elevation of the ipsilateral hemidiaphragm occurs with roughly equal frequency in cases resulting in lung necrosis and in those with simple hemorrhage and edema.[146, 188] Since tissue necrosis is most common in patients with cardiorespiratory disease, concomitant roentgenographic signs of cor pulmonale, pulmonary venous hypertension, and edema increase the likelihood that an opacity represents tissue necrosis rather than simple hemorrhage.

The roentgenographic patterns of pulmonary infarction are specific only insofar as the shadows are segmental in distribution and homogeneous in density. In the early stages, particularly, any increase in density is ill defined; it is commonest in the base of the right lower lobe, often nestled in the costophrenic sinus (Fig. 9–20). The majority of cases of pulmonary infarction involve one or perhaps two bronchopulmonary segments, thus affecting a relatively small volume of lung parenchyma. However, as emphasized by Jacoby and Mindell,[221] infarction occasionally may involve the whole or a major portion of a lobe. In fact, of 49 cases of pulmonary embolism with infarction studied by Talbot and associates,[213] massive lobar consolidation was found in seven. Since the majority of patients in both these reports were subsequently studied at necropsy, their illness was obviously much more severe and the incidence of lobar consolidation much greater than would be expected in the general population of patients with pulmonary embolism. The oft-repeated observation that infarction invariably relates to a visceral pleural surface[188, 190] is of little value in differential diagnosis, since the majority of pneumonias do also. The interval between the embolic episode and any increase in roentgenographic density ranges from 10 to 12 hours[190, 195] to several days after occlusion,[190] and in one series density increased in equal numbers of cases within 24 hours and later.[192] Experiments in dogs[119, 725] and necropsy studies on human lungs[726] have shown that ischemic areas usually become atelectatic and congested within 24 hours.

The so-called "classic" configuration of an infarct as a "truncated cone" is fairly common. This "typical" configuration consists of homogeneous wedge-shaped consolidation in the lung periphery, with its base contiguous to a visceral pleural surface and its rounded, convex apex toward the hilum (Figs. 9–21 and 9–22).[188, 190, 195] Originally described by Hampton and Castleman[112] in 1940, this configuration has come to bear the euphonious eponym

of "Hampton's hump"; it is highly suggestive of pulmonary infarction (Fig. 9–23). The size of the consolidated area varies from patient to patient and, in the case of multiple infarctions, from one area to another (Fig. 9–24). They are usually 3 to 5 cm in diameter,[190] in a range extending from bare visibility up to 10 cm. An air bronchogram is rarely seen in a pulmonary infarct;[222] this absence, combined with peripheral homogeneous consolidation, should strongly suggest infarction rather than acute airspace pneumonia. However, an air bronchogram does not completely rule out infarction: in three of our patients with pulmonary embolism, an air bronchogram was apparent within 24 hours of appearance of a pulmonary opacity, presumably reflecting delayed filling of the airways with blood and edema fluid. Cavitation in pulmonary infarction is rare,[184] being found in only 2.7 per cent of cases at necropsy.[223] It usually—but not invariably[167, 168, 224]—indicates septic pulmonary emboli (see farther on), lesions often misdiagnosed.[225]

Just as CT appears to be capable of revealing zones of oligemia with greater accuracy than conventional roentgenography (Fig. 9–25), it is possible that it should be able to demonstrate pulmonary infarcts with greater precision, and such appears to be the case, in both experimental animals and in man (Fig. 9–26). In an experimental study of 15 dogs in which pulmonary infarcts were created by transcatheter electrocoagulation of the pulmonary artery, Lourie and his colleagues[226] observed areas of increased opacity on CT scans in 13 dogs immediately after electrocoagulation, whereas only nine dogs manifested patchy opacities on conventional roentgenograms. At the end of 1 week, CT scans were abnormal in 13 of the 15 dogs compared with seven with abnormal roentgenograms. At the end of 2 weeks, CT scans were abnormal in seven of 12 dogs and chest roentgenograms were abnormal in two of eleven dogs. Clearly, in this experimental study, CT more accurately identified the earlier phases of infarction (81 per cent of dogs during the immediate post-occlusion period and 87 per cent by the end of 1 week). According to Sinner,[227] the superiority of CT over conventional roentgenography applies in humans as well: this investigator studied 16 patients with clinical evidence of pulmonary thromboembolism (corroborated in most by perfusion lung scans) and observed areas of increased attenuation in all; CT evidence of pulmonary infarction was often identified during the first 48 hours following the acute clinical episode, at a time when chest roentgenograms were normal in six of the 16 patients. In seven of the 16 patients, a distinct wedge-shaped opacity was observed. By and large, the single or multiple defects observed on perfusion lung scans matched well with attenuation changes observed on CT (Fig. 9–27). Although the results of this study are perhaps not surprising, it is again clear that since radionuclide

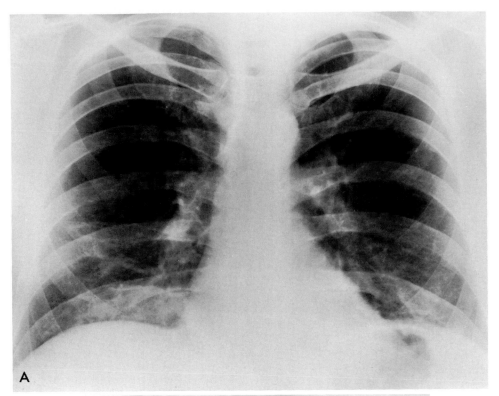

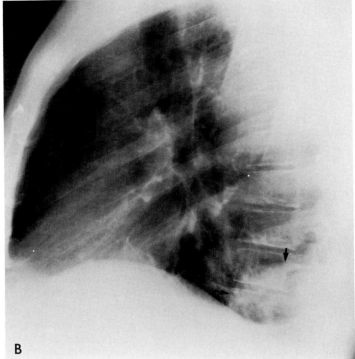

Figure 9–21. Pulmonary Infarct, Right Lower Lobe. Posteroanterior (A) and lateral (B) roentgenograms of a 40-year-old man reveal a fairly well-circumscribed shadow of homogeneous density occupying the posterior basal segment of the right lower lobe. In lateral projection, the shadow has the shape of a truncated cone with its apex directed toward the hilum (Hampton's hump) (arrows). A small effusion can be identified in lateral projection. This combination of changes is highly suggestive of pulmonary infarction; the history and biochemical findings were compatible with the diagnosis.

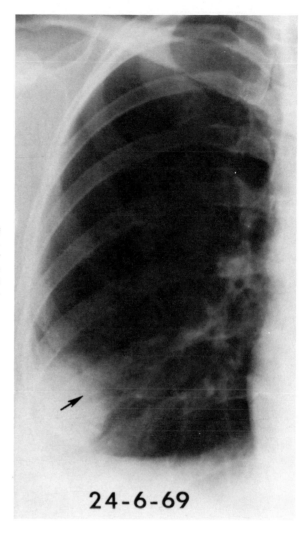

Figure 9–22. Hampton's Hump in Pulmonary Infarction. A view of the right lung from a posteroanterior chest roentgenogram reveals a homogeneous opacity in the right costophrenic angle possessing a convex contour (*arrow*) towards the hilum. This constitutes the typical features of a Hampton's hump and is highly suggestive of a pulmonary infarct. The patient is a young man with a history of acute chest pain associated with thrombophlebitis of the right leg.

scans detected lobar or segmental defects with no less accuracy than CT, and since the cost of this procedure is much less, it appears unlikely that CT will gain much support as a cost-effective procedure.

Similarly, magnetic resonance imaging (MRI) appears to hold considerable promise in the study of pulmonary thromboembolism, both in the experimental animal[727–729] and in patients.[730–733] Pope and his colleagues[729] studied the influence of gating, cardiac cycle, and timing of rephasing gradients upon the detection of pulmonary emboli by MRI in dogs, and found that cardiac gating in systole and late magnetization rephasing yielded the best diagnostic accuracy. Gated images were clearly superior to ungated; with combined cardiac and respiratory gating, sensitivity was 82 per cent and specificity 88 per cent. Although these results are encouraging, it is probable that because of cost and the comparable efficiency of ventilation-perfusion ($\dot{V}/\dot{Q}$) scintigraphy, MRI is unlikely to gain wide acceptance as a diagnostic technique in pulmonary thromboembolism.

Patterns of Resolution of Pulmonary Infarction

The time course of resolution of infarction varies widely and is a reliable indicator of the nature of the consolidative process. If embolism results only in parenchymal hemorrhage and edema, clearing may occur within 4 to 7 days,[228] often without residua; in fact, we have seen one patient in whom it cleared in 3 days. When embolism leads to necrosis, however, resolution averages 20 days[189]—and according to Fleischner may take as long as 5 weeks.[229]

A valuable sign differentiating pulmonary infarction from acute pneumonia is the pattern of resolution, which was described by Woesner and associates.[230] The shadow of acute pneumonia appears to break up, rendering an originally homogeneous opacity inhomogeneous as scattered areas of radiolucency appear within it, whereas the shadow of a pulmonary infarct gradually diminishes but maintains its homogeneity and roughly its original shape. These authors likened a resolving infarct

Text continued on page 1745

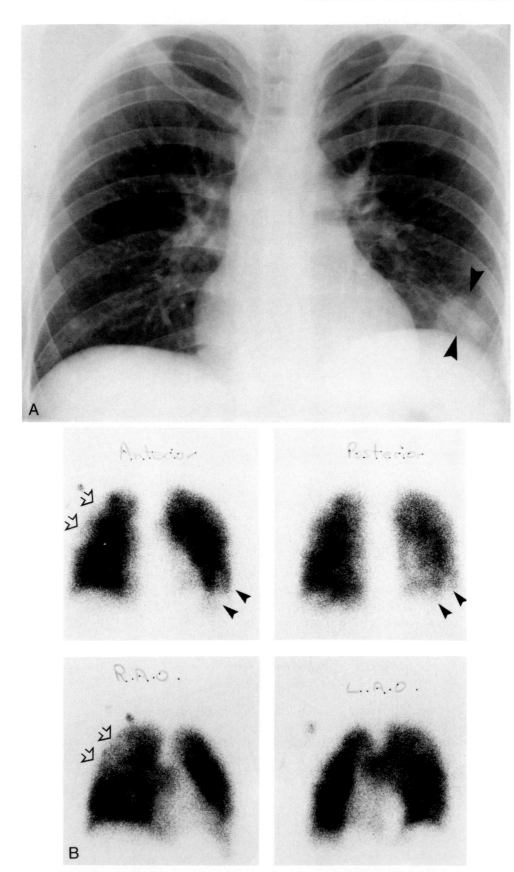

Figure 9–23. CT Depiction of Acute Pulmonary Thromboembolism and Infarction (Hampton's Hump). A conventional posteroanterior chest roentgenogram (*A*) discloses a round homogeneous opacity (*arrowheads*) in the left lower lobe; the left hemidiaphragm is slightly elevated. The right lung is normal. Perfusion lung scintigrams in anterior, posterior, and shallow right and left anterior oblique projections (*B*) reveal perfusion deficits in both lungs, the most notable being situated in the right upper (*open arrows*) and left lower lobes (*arrowheads*). Ventilation scans (not shown) were normal.

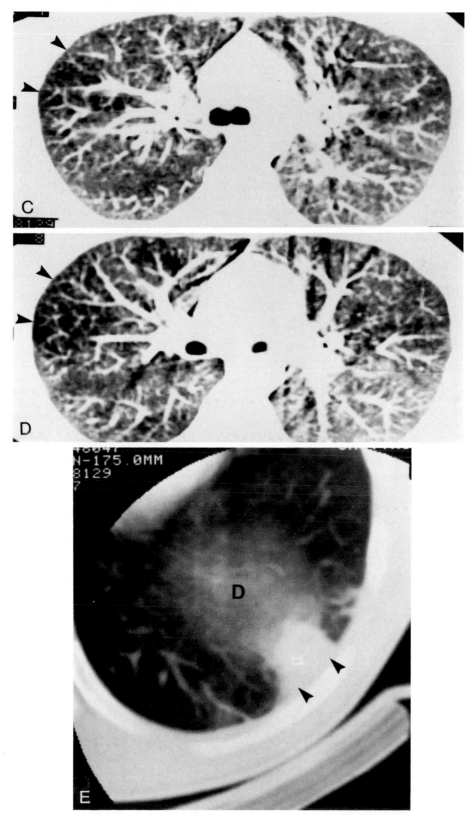

Figure 9–23 *Continued* CT scans through the carina (*C*) (above) and 1 cm caudad (*D*) (below) reveal areas of decreased attenuation (*arrowheads*) in the anterior and lateral aspect of the right upper lobe. Note that these areas, representing diminished perfusion, correspond with those identified on the perfusion scintigrams in *B*. A detail view of the left lower lobe from a transverse CT scan (*E*) shows a pleural-based truncated opacity (*arrowheads*) in the posterolateral costophrenic recess. The blunted medial contour is typical of a Hampton's hump. The top of the left hemidiaphragm (D) can be identified anterior to the infarct. The patient is a young man with an acute onset of left chest and shoulder pain.

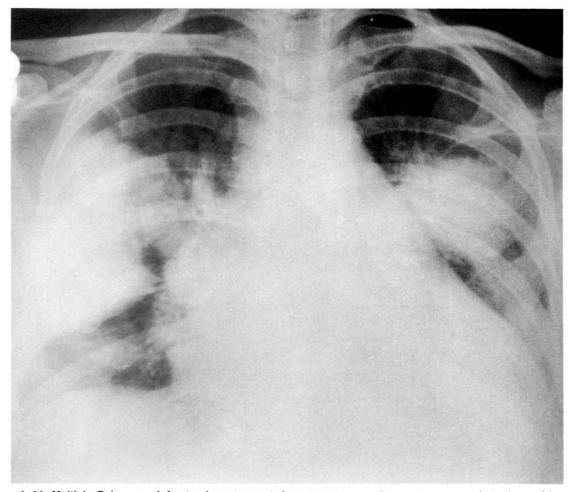

Figure 9–24. Multiple Pulmonary Infarcts. An anteroposterior roentgenogram demonstrates several shadows of homogeneous density in both lungs. Those on the right possess a configuration suggesting a truncated cone (Hampton's hump) with their apices directed toward the hilum. The main shadow in the left lung is roughly circular in shape, suggesting that its base may be contiguous to the anterior or posterior chest wall. At necropsy, multiple infarcts were present in both lungs, the major lesion on the left being in the superior segment of the lower lobe.

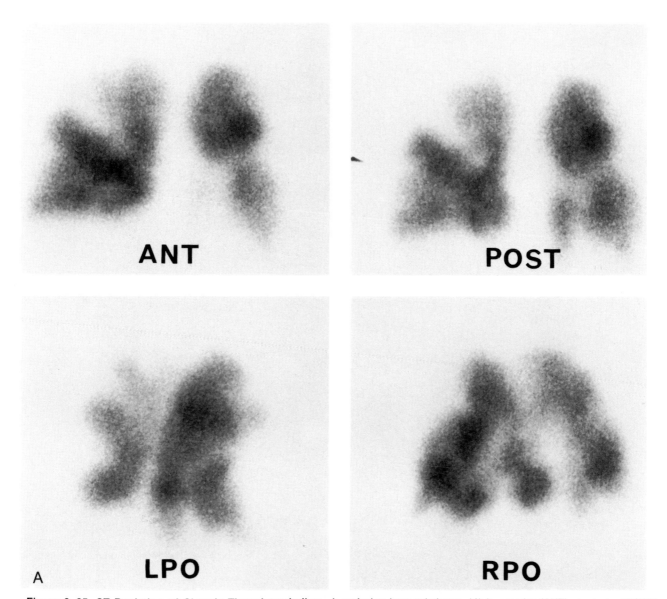

Figure 9–25. CT Depiction of Chronic Thromboembolism. A perfusion lung scintigram (*A*) in anterior (ANT), posterior (POST), right posterior oblique (RPO) and left posterior oblique (LPO) projections show multiple segmental deficits in both lungs: a ventilation scan (not shown) was normal.

Illustration continued on following page

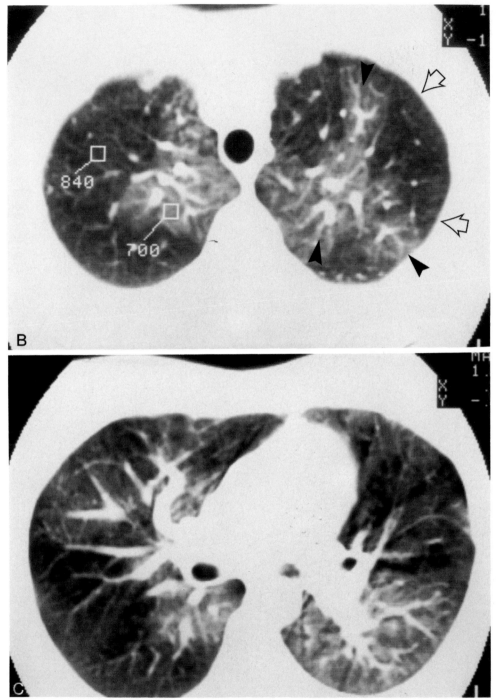

Figure 9–25 *Continued* The combined scintigraphic findings are highly suggestive of thromboembolic disease. CT scans through the upper (*B*) and lower (*C*) lobes reveal sharply contrasting, contiguous areas of high (*arrowheads*) and low (*open arrows*) CT attenuation that represent zones of increased perfusion and oligemia, respectively (note values in Hounsfield units in cursor boxes in the upper lobes). In those areas with increased perfusion, the vessels are larger than normal, contrasting with the smaller size of those in the hyperlucent lung. The patient is a 47-year-old woman with chronic and progressive dyspnea.

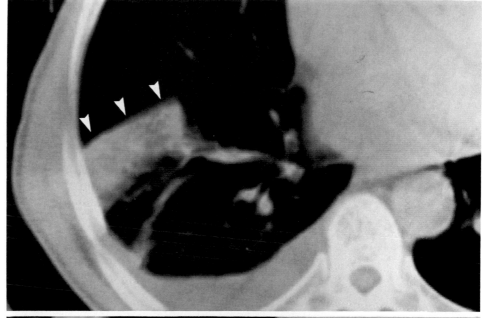
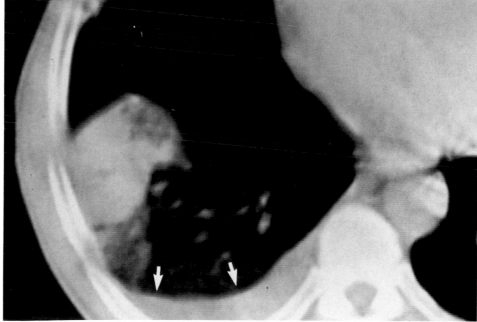

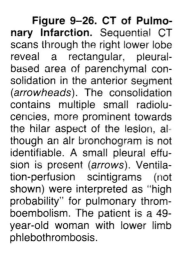

Figure 9–26. CT of Pulmonary Infarction. Sequential CT scans through the right lower lobe reveal a rectangular, pleural-based area of parenchymal consolidation in the anterior segment (*arrowheads*). The consolidation contains multiple small radiolucencies, more prominent towards the hilar aspect of the lesion, although an air bronchogram is not identifiable. A small pleural effusion is present (*arrows*). Ventilation-perfusion scintigrams (not shown) were interpreted as "high probability" for pulmonary thromboembolism. The patient is a 49-year-old woman with lower limb phlebothrombosis.

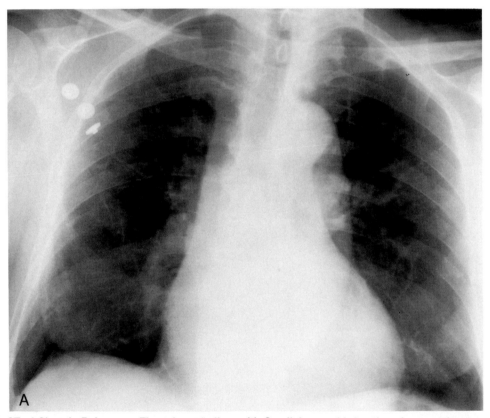

Figure 9–27. CT of Chronic Pulmonary Thromboembolism with Small Areas of Infarction. A conventional posteroanterior chest roentgenogram (A) reveals moderate cardiomegaly. Scattered areas of oligemia are present in both lungs.

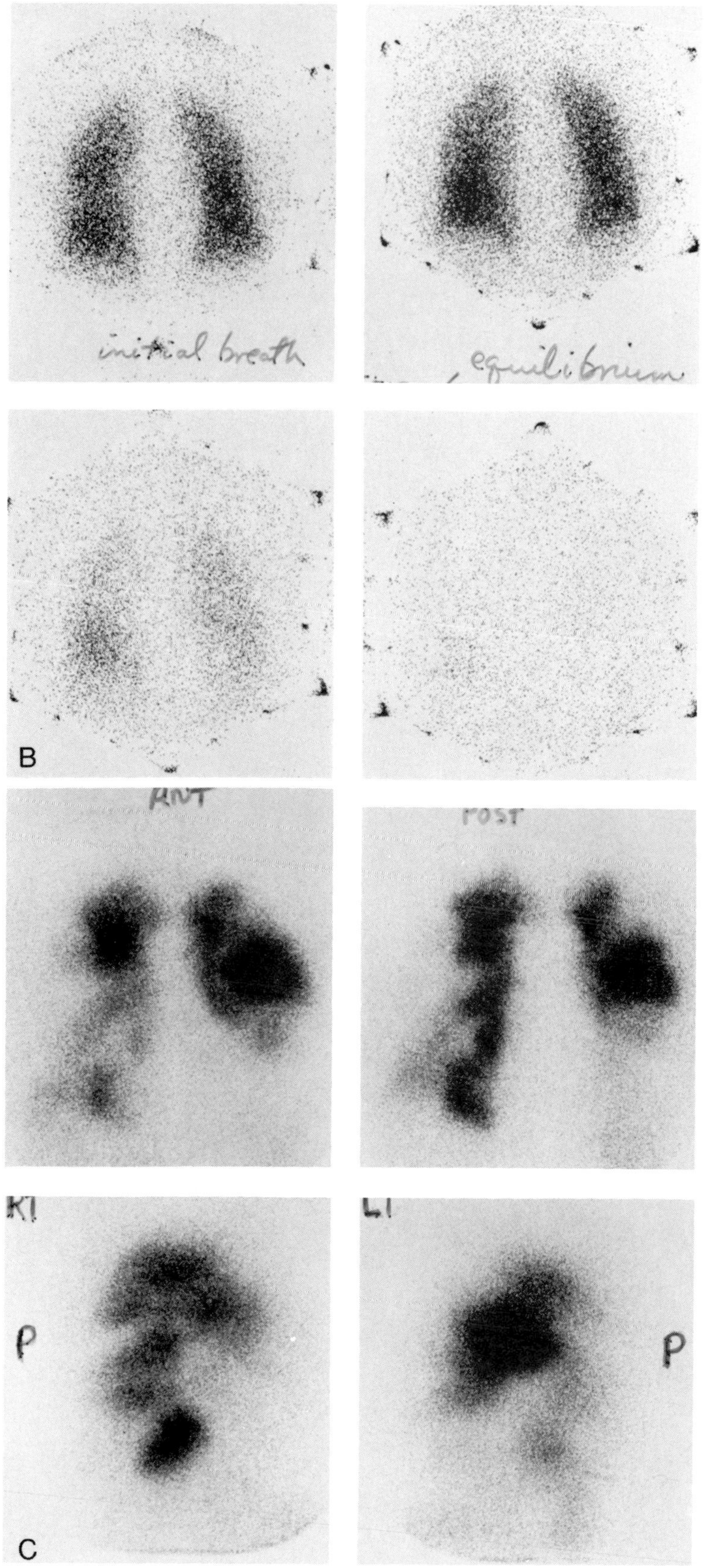

Figure 9–27 *Continued* A ventilation scintigram (*B*) is normal, whereas a perfusion scan (*C*) shows multiple deficits in both lungs, the largest being located in the left lower and the right middle and lower lobes. The scan pattern is strongly suggestive of pulmonary thromboembolism.

Illustration continued on following page

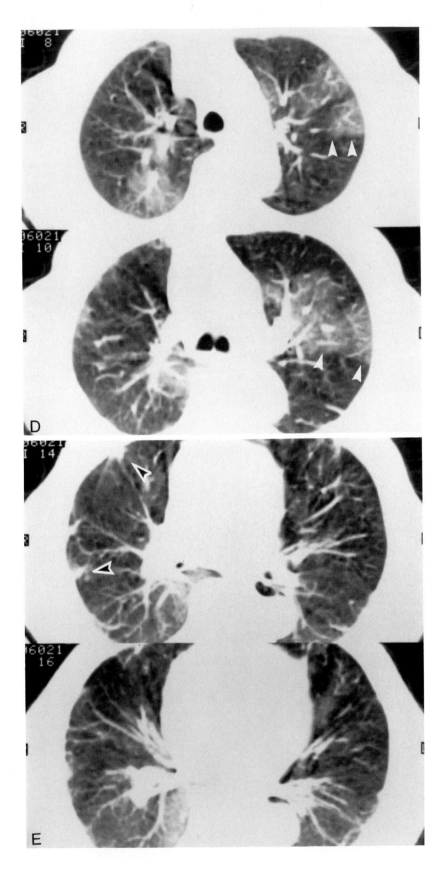

Figure 9–27 *Continued* Sequential CT scans through the upper (*D*) and lower (*E*) lobes reveal triangular areas of increased attenuation (*small arrowheads* in *D*) alternating with contiguous regions of diminished attenuation. The vessels in the former zones are larger than are those in the latter, indicating redistribution of blood flow from the oligemic lung. Several subpleural opacities (*large arrowheads* in *E*) are visible in the lower lobes, suggesting healed (fibrotic) or healing infarcts. The patient is a 72-year-old man.

to a melting ice cube, thus the term "the melting sign." We concur with their observation, but consider this sign applicable only in the resolving stages of either lesion and, therefore, of no value at a time when the institution of appropriate therapy is vital.

The short-term and long-term patterns of resolution of pulmonary infarction vary considerably. The long-term effects have been clarified by Goldrick and his colleagues[231] in a follow-up study of 32 patients with 58 angiographically proven pulmonary infarcts; serial chest roentgenograms were obtained on all patients over a period of 3 months or longer. Complete roentgenographic resolution occurred in 29 (50 per cent) of the 58 infarcts; of the remainder, residual findings included linear scars (14), pleurodiaphragmatic adhesions (nine), and localized pleural thickening (six). In all cases, the residual features were diminutive when compared with the original abnormality. Follow-up perfusion lung images performed at time intervals similar to those of the chest roentgenograms were available for 44 infarcts: seven of these showed complete resolution, and the remaining 37 showed a residual but much smaller perfusion defect.

LINE SHADOWS

During the period of resolution, the major roentgenographic abnormalities consist of linear opacities caused by a variety of different mechanisms. Line shadows probably constitute one of the most frequent roentgenographic manifestations of pulmonary embolism and infarction; in one series they were observed at some stage in 21.6 per cent of cases.[192] Their pathogenesis in pulmonary embolism is discussed in Chapter 4 (*see* page 633) and is only summarized here. Four types may occur: "platelike atelectasis," parenchymal scarring, thrombosed arteries and veins, and line shadows of pleural origin.

Platelike Atelectasis. These linear opacities, almost always in the lung bases 1 to 3 cm above the hemidiaphragm, are usually roughly horizontal. They are 1 to 3 mm thick and usually several centimeters long; at least one extremity abuts the pleural surface (Fig. 9–28). Westcott and Cole[734] carried out a detailed roentgenologic/pathologic correlative study of ten patients in whom a linear opacity characteristic of plate atelectasis was present on their last antemortem roentgenogram and on whom autopsy was subsequently performed. All ten revealed pathologic evidence of peripheral subpleural linear collapse combined with invagination of overlying pleura. The atelectasis was either deep to incomplete fissures or extended to pre-existing pleural clefts; however, in both situations, the surface of the lung appeared folded in at the sight of linear atelectasis. This frequent association with

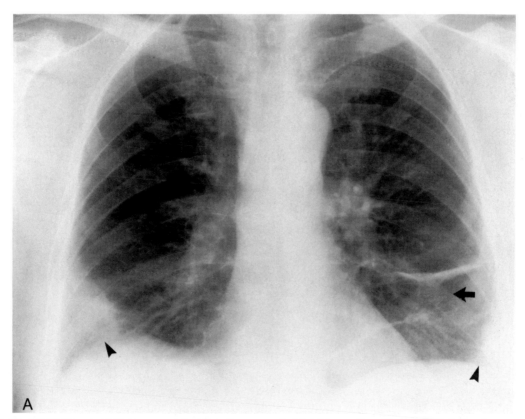

Figure 9–28. CT Features of Pulmonary Infarction Accompanied by Linear Opacities. A conventional posteroanterior chest roentgenogram (*A*) discloses hemispheric, homogeneous opacities in both costophrenic angles (*arrowheads*), highly suggestive of pulmonary infarcts. Two linear opacities are present in the left lower lobe, the cephalad lesion being horizontal and somewhat wider and longer than the obliquely oriented caudad lesion. Note the round opacity (*arrow*) contiguous with the inferior part of the broader line.

Illustration continued on following page

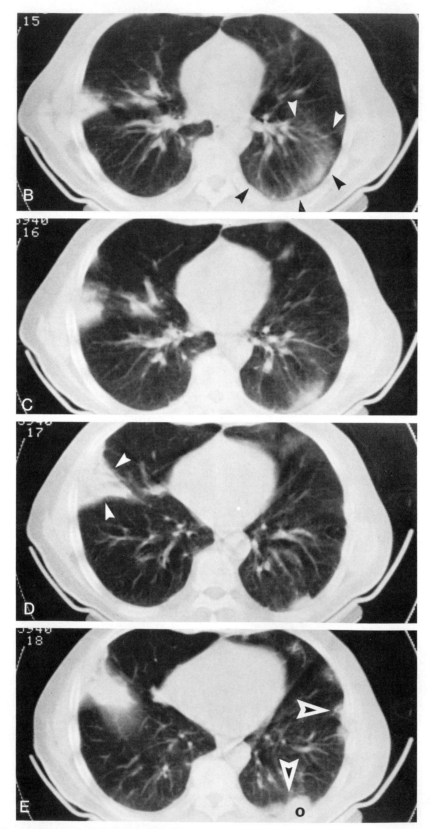

Figure 9–28 *Continued B* and *C,* Sequential CT scans through the middle lobe, lingula, and lower lobes (*B, C*) reveal an inhomogeneous wedge-shaped area of consolidation in the lateral segment of the middle lobe (*small arrowheads*), and multiple truncated or hemispheric pleura-based opacities (*large arrowheads*) in the left upper lobe. These features are characteristic of the varied CT appearance of pulmonary infarction. CT scans through the lower lobes (*D* and *E*) demonstrate a vague ground-glass opacity (*between arrowheads*) that extends from the posterior chest wall forward to the level of the inferior hilum; this appearance is analogous to that produced by a thickened minor fissure (obviously not the case in this instance) and suggests that the linear shadow in *A* represents a thin sheet of infolded pleura and contiguous, central plate-like atelectasis. The contiguous hemispheric opacity (O) that relates to the linear opacity in *A* is shown on the more caudad scans (*B* and *C*). The patient is a 60-year-old man with a history of recent prostate surgery.

congenital pleural clefts, indentations, scars, and incomplete fissures suggested to these investigators that plate atelectasis may develop preferentially at sites of pre-existing pleural invagination. Although six of the ten patients manifested pathologic evidence of acute pulmonary embolism, these authors[734] contended that there was no evidence that the atelectasis directly represented thrombosed vessels or infarcts. The linear opacities were caused by atelectasis alone in six patients, atelectasis associated with edema in three, and atelectasis combined with "alveolitis" in one. In addition to the theories proposed by these researchers, we suspect that in patients with thromboembolic disease, the pathogenesis of these linear opacities probably relates at least in part to altered alveolar surface tension resulting from decreased surfactant production.[120-123]

Parenchymal Scarring. As with platelike atelectasis, linear shadows caused by scarring secondary to lung necrosis extend to a pleural surface (see Fig. 4–130, page 637). Fleischner and his colleagues[232] stated that these opacities often terminate in a nodular rounded extremity at the pleural surface, a finding not observed in atelectasis. Contrary to what might be expected from the segmental distribution of pulmonary infarction, these line shadows lie in any plane and run in almost any direction, apparently without regard to segmental distribution. They may be up to 10 cm long but most are shorter than the shadows of platelike atelectasis. An important differential feature is that the line shadows of platelike atelectasis disappear within a few days, whereas those of healed infarction are permanent.

The long line shadows of healed infarction may have a sizable pleural component. In pathologic studies, Reid found that as the necrotic tissue of infarction shrinks through scarring, it causes inward retraction of contiguous visceral pleura, and she suggested that this infolded pleura may contribute to the formation of line shadows (see Fig. 4–126, page 635).[233]

Thrombosed Arteries and Veins. Simon[234] described line shadows, usually horizontal in the lung bases, in middle-aged and elderly subjects whose history did not suggest thromboembolism and who had no abnormalities that might suggest a cause for platelike atelectasis. Although the pathologic basis of many of these lines is elusive, some have been shown to represent a thrombosed artery, with or without fibrosis in contiguous lung parenchyma (Fig. 9–29). In some instances, simultaneous bronchography and tomography failed to show any relation between the lines and the bronchial tree. More recently, Simon and Reid[235] and Simon[236] suggested that horizontal or inclined long line shadows represent thrombosed veins more often than arteries (Fig. 9–30). Their evidence was both inferential and direct: inferential in that the direction of the line shadow was identical to that followed by a pulmonary vein, particularly the relationship of its medial extremity to the left atrium; and direct in that the position of the line shadow was related to that of the vein in subsequent angiography. We have seen many cases in which the distribution of line shadows was similar to that described by Simon and Reid. The major clues to their nature lie in their orientation (not conforming to bronchovascular distribution) and the relationship of their medial extremity to the left atrium. The shadows are 2 to 10 mm thick, and in our cases followed the distribution of a major upper lobe vein just as frequently as veins draining the middle and lower zones. In at least one of our patients, angiography performed when a line was clearly visible on plain roentgenograms showed rough correspondence, anatomically, to a pulmonary vein; in fact, the shadow became opacified during the capillary and venous phases of filling, suggesting either recanalization within the thrombosed vein or marked vascularity of pathologic tissue around the vein. (However, opacification of a line shadow during the venous phase of an angiogram does not positively identify it as a vein: platelike atelectasis could opacify in the same fashion.) These opacities cannot be caused purely by blood clot within the vein itself: the density of clot is identical to that of blood and thus should not produce a different roentgenographic shadow.

A roentgenologic clue to the identity of these oblique line shadows is their usual visualization in posteroanterior but not lateral projection (the shadow of platelike atelectasis should be visible in both planes). However, fluoroscopy with rotation of the patient into various positions usually reveals the shadow 10 to 15 degrees from the lateral plane, extending from within the body of a lobe toward the left atrium and terminating at the major fissure. At its junction with the major fissure, the shadow usually expands into a small triangle with its base on the fissure, suggesting pleural infolding.

Despite the lack of more precise pathologic confirmation, the evidence that has accumulated over the past few years lends considerable support to the thesis that these opacities represent thrombosed veins (or occasionally arteries) associated with edema and hemorrhage in the surrounding parenchyma. Current knowledge dictates that visualization of such shadows on a chest roentgenogram, particularly if the clinical setting is such that a thromboembolic episode might be anticipated, should alert physicians to the possibility of thromboembolism.

Line Shadows of Pleural Origin. As indicated in Chapter 4, these line shadows are seen frequently and are caused either by thickening of an interlobar fissure (often the accessory fissure on the right side) or by fibrous pleural thickening over the anterior or posterior lung surfaces, resulting from the pleuritis that frequently accompanies pulmonary infarction (see Fig. 4–127, page 635). These rather stringy

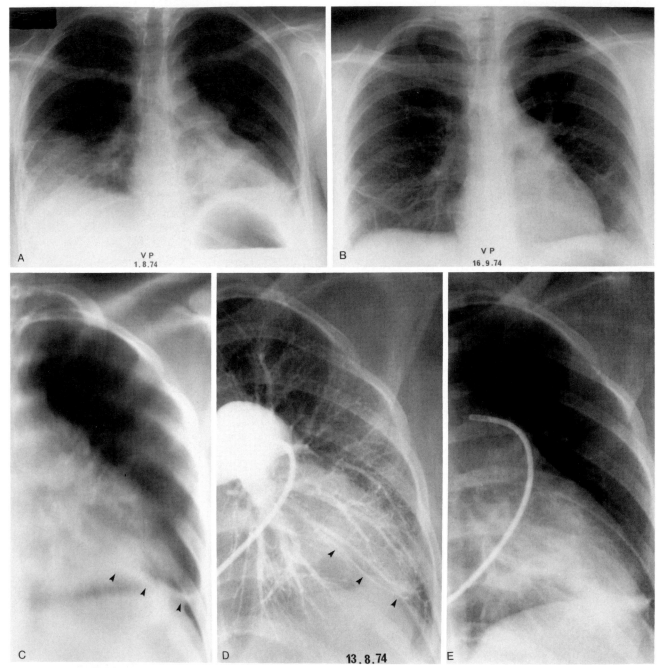

Figure 9–29. Vascularized Linear Opacity As a Sign of Pulmonary Thromboembolism: Query Recanalization of a Thrombosed Pulmonary Artery. A conventional posteroanterior chest roentgenogram (*A*) shows large homogeneous opacities in the middle lobe and both lower lobes consistent with pulmonary infarcts. Approximately 6 weeks later, a repeat study (*B*) reveals almost complete resolution of the infarcts although several curvilinear opacities persist. A detail view of the left lung from an anteroposterior linear tomogram (*C*) demonstrates one curvilinear opacity (*arrowheads*) in the lower lobe. A pulmonary angiogram during the arterial (*D*) and late venous (*E*) phases shows a patent but obviously enlarged central arterial system. Note that the linear shadow that was identified in *C* relates most closely to a nontapering, essentially branchless lateral segmental artery (*arrowheads*). The patient is a young woman with multiple recurrent pulmonary thromboemboli and cor pulmonale.

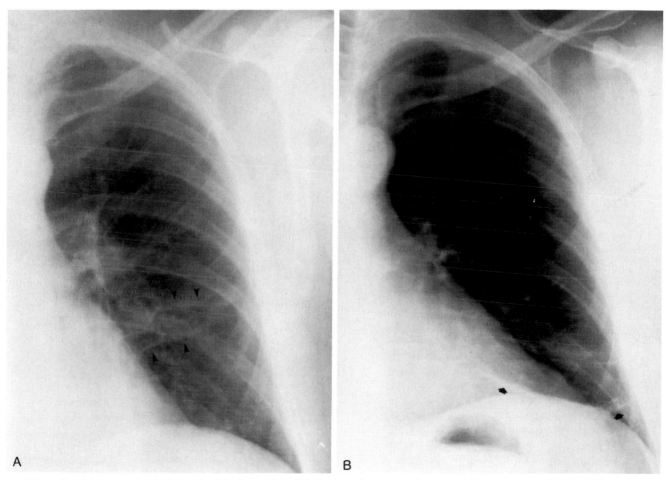

Figure 9–30. Vascularized Linear Opacity As a Sign of Pulmonary Thromboembolism: Query Recanalization of a Thrombosed Pulmonary Vein. A view of the left lung from a conventional posteroanterior chest roentgenogram (*A*) shows two faint curvilinear opacities (*arrowheads*) in the lower third of the lung contiguous with the hilum. Clinically, the patient presented with acute dyspnea and left chest discomfort. Nine months later, a repeat chest roentgenogram (*B*) reveals a curvilinear supradiaphragmatic opacity (*arrows*) that extends proximally in a fashion suggesting a relationship to the venous system.

Illustration continued on following page

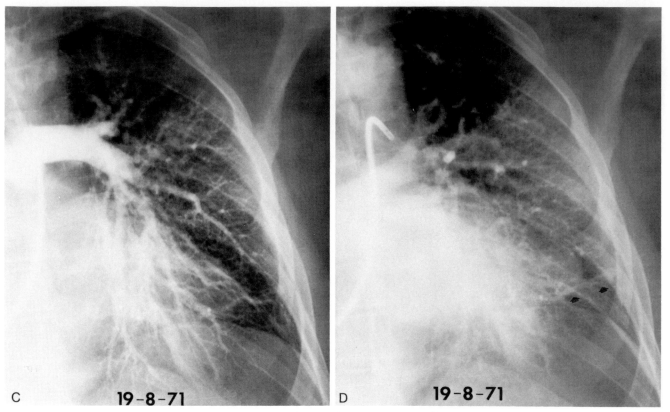

Figure 9–30 *Continued* A selective left pulmonary angiogram during the arterial (*C*) and venous (*D*) phases reveals normal hilar arteries; however, major perfusion deficits are present in the left upper lobe and costophrenic angle, particularly evident during the venous phase. Note that the linear opacity that was identified in *B* is maximally opacified during the late venous phase of the study (*arrows*). The faint central radiolucency that extends along the opacity is consistent with venous thrombosis with recanalization.

shadows are usually horizontal or oblique, not unlike scars of old pulmonary infarction.

Pleural Effusion

As a roentgenographic manifestation of thromboembolic disease, pleural effusion is as common as, if not commoner than, parenchymal consolidation:[146, 184, 192, 238] it nearly always indicates infarction. The parenchymal shadow may be diminutive or hidden by the fluid,[188, 207] so confusing the diagnostic possibilities that an embolic episode will be suggested only if there is a high index of suspicion. The amount of pleural fluid is frequently small but may be abundant. It is more often unilateral.[190, 205] When predominantly infrapulmonary, it may be mistaken for hemidiaphragmatic elevation.[190] Pleural fluid usually develops and absorbs synchronously with the infarction, but sometimes appears later and clears sooner.[189]

Pneumothorax

Pneumothorax, a rare complication,[188] is thought to develop most often during intermittent positive pressure breathing or when an infarct has become infected.[239] In the latter circumstances, the clinical and roentgenologic course is fairly charac-

teristic:[240] (1) all such patients have an underlying condition, often rheumatic heart disease; (2) the infarcted area is large; (3) after the infarction, the patient feels better for a while but then produces copious amounts of blood-tinged, purulent sputum and has fever, leukocytosis, and acute cardiac failure. This third phase, which lasts several days to weeks and reflects excavation of the infarcted area, is followed by a second brief period of quiescence; finally, 2 to 3 weeks after the infarction bronchopleural fistula develops, and this is often fatal.

MICROTHROMBOEMBOLISM

Microscopic emboli of fibrin-platelet thrombus occur in association with all recognized sites of extrapulmonary thrombosis, including the deep veins, prosthetic heart valves, and arteriovenous cannulas.[12] The process is essentially identical to emboli of larger fragments of thrombus, but because of their small size, the clinical and roentgenographic manifestations are generally absent or minimal.[214] Rarely, the number of aggregates may be sufficient to cause significant effects, typically in situations in which blood has been present outside the vascular system for some period of time, such as in hemodialysis,[215] plasmapheresis,[216] and massive transfusions of stored blood.[215, 217–219] Identical emboli can be seen in the systemic vessels in patients in whom extracorporeal circulation is employed during cardiac surgery;[219] filters can dramatically decrease the number of such emboli.[218]

Pathologic examination of the lungs in such cases[216, 219] shows platelet-fibrin aggregates within capillaries and precapillary arterioles, apparently occluding their lumens. Since many of these patients are critically ill from their primary disease, the role of the microemboli in morbidity and mortality is seldom clear. Occasional cases of rapid death have occurred, associated with dyspnea, bronchospasm, and hypotension. In addition to a mechanical occlusive effect, it has been speculated that platelet-derived chemical mediators may also play a role in the pathogenesis of pulmonary disease.[216] In 22 patients who died from extensive burns, there was a significant correlation in lung sections between numbers of megakaryocytes and fibrin microthrombi, supporting a relationship between disseminated intravascular coagulation (DIC) and numbers of pulmonary megakaryocytes.[220]

SEPTIC EMBOLISM

The pulmonary manifestations of septic emboli may be the only indication of serious underlying infection, and since the roentgenographic changes are often distinctive, their recognition early in the disease should permit diagnosis and prompt institution of therapy.[241]

Septic pulmonary embolism occurs most often in younger people, the majority of the 17 patients described by Jaffe and Koschmann being under 40 years of age.[242] Emboli originate from two major sites—the heart (in association with bacterial endocarditis of the tricuspid valve or a ventricular septal defect) and the peripheral veins (septic thrombophlebitis). The tricuspid valve may have been normal before infection, or may have been congenitally malformed, or the site of rheumatic endocarditis. Since tricuspid endocarditis may not give rise to signs implicating this valve,[243] septic pulmonary emboli may be the first clue to this diagnosis.

In 13 of Jaffe and Koschmann's 17 cases, the emboli were thought to arise from lesions in the right side of the heart (two of the 13 had septic thrombophlebitis also). A predisposing factor is nearly always present, most often drug addiction, alcoholism, general infections in patients with immunologic deficiencies (particularly lymphoma), congenital heart disease, and dermal infections.[248] A single case has been described of candidiasis and septic emboli in a patient who swallowed a toothpick that traversed the duodenum, penetrated the inferior vena cava, and became impacted in the right ventricle.[249] When host defenses are deficient opportunistic infections must be considered, and blood samples should be cultured for fungi as well as bacteria.

Septic pulmonary emboli can occasionally originate from the pharynx, infection extending to the parapharyngeal space and internal jugular venous system. This clinical presentation has been referred to as Lemierre's syndrome or postanginal sepsis.[244–246] The oral anaerobes, particularly Bacteroides and Fusobacterium species, are the most common pathogens associated with this syndrome. Staphylococcal osteomyelitis may also be the primary site of origin, ten such cases having been reported by Felman and Shulman.[247] In this report it was emphasized that in many cases the osteomyelitis is overlooked and that primary therapy directed toward the pulmonary complications may be unsuccessful until the osteomyelitis is recognized and treated directly.

Additional uncommon sites of septic thrombophlebitis include arm veins in patients with a history of intravenous drug abuse, pelvic veins in association with pelvic infection,[241] and veins near infected indwelling catheters and arteriovenous shunts such as those used for hemodialysis.[250, 251] There has been one report of septic emboli in association with a transvenous pacemaker.[252]

In Jaffe and Koschmann's series,[242] the organism most often grown on blood cultures was coagulase-positive Staphylococcus aureus and, second, streptococci. In four of the 17 patients, blood cultures were negative. Cultures of sputum from many of these patients grew organisms different from those on their blood cultures.

Although many cases of pulmonary infection associated with thromboembolism are the result of the presence of organisms within the thrombus itself (true septic emboli), it should be appreciated that secondary bacterial infection of initially sterile infarcts can result in a similar pathologic and roentgenographic appearance (Fig. 9–31).

Pulmonary disease secondary to septic emboli is usually manifested by multiple, rather ill-defined, round or wedge-shaped opacities in the periphery of the lungs. They may be uniform in size or vary widely, reflecting recurrent showers of emboli. Jaffe and Koschmann noted their apparently migratory nature; they appear first in one area and then in another as older lesions resolve and new ones appear. Cavitation is frequent (Fig. 9–32) and may occur rapidly; the cavities are usually thin-walled, and many have no fluid level. Occasionally, there develops within one or more cavities a central loose body simulating a fungus ball,[253, 254] termed the "target sign" by Zelefsky and Lutzker;[253] these represent pieces of necrotic lung that have been sequestered within the cavity and roentgenographically simulate the intracavitary loose bodies that develop in some patients with invasive aspergillosis (see page 991). Since both septic embolism and invasive aspergillosis tend to occur in compromised hosts and since the etiology and therapy of the two conditions differ substantially, it is obviously essential to establish the etiologic diagnosis as early as possible. It is also important to realize that such

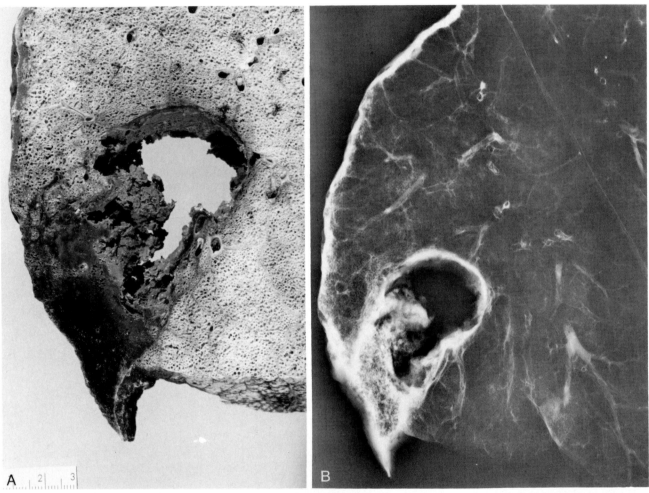

Figure 9–31. Pulmonary Infarct with Cavitation Secondary to Bacterial Superinfection. A magnified view of a slice of left lower lobe (*A*) shows a well-defined recent infarct with proximal cavitation. Note the focus of shaggy necrotic lung projecting into the cavity. A roentgenogram of the specimen (*B*) shows an appearance that simulates an intracavitary fungus ball. The patient had multiple foci of bronchopneumonia and bland infarction but no evidence of extrathoracic infection; thus, the cavitation was considered to represent secondary infection of a previously sterile infarct rather than septic embolization.

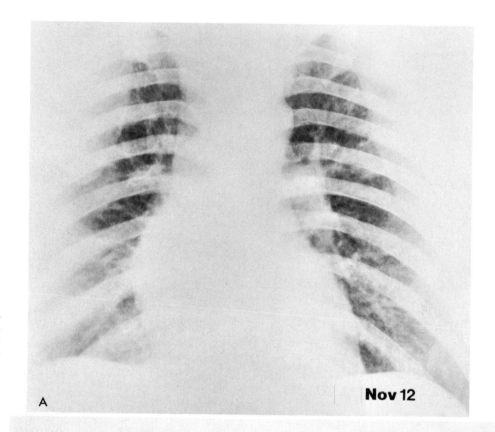

Figure 9–32. Massive Septic Embolism. Shortly before the roentgenogram illustrated in *A*, a 31-year-old man suffered a massive right pulmonary embolism related to severe thrombophlebitis of one leg. This film reveals relatively clear lungs, a normal left hilum, and an almost absent right hilum. A lung scan performed shortly thereafter (*B*) reveals a total lack of perfusion of the right lung and a segmental defect in the midportion of the left lung.

Illustration continued on following page

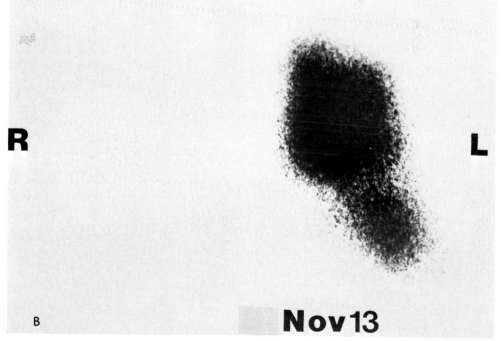

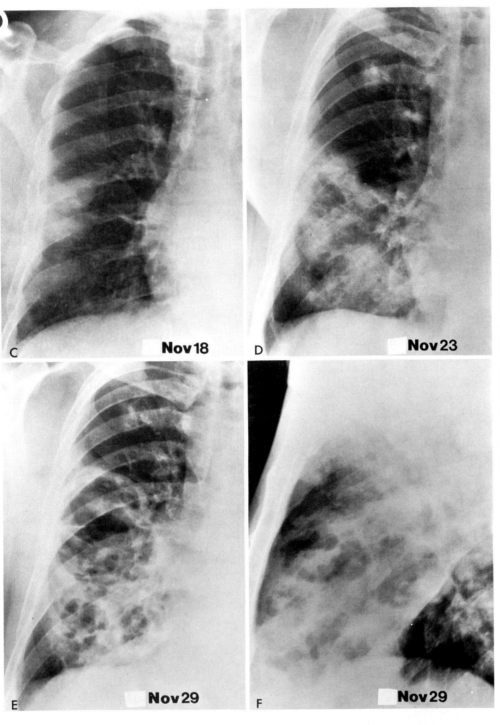

Figure 9–32 *Continued* Five days after the acute episode (*C*), a poorly defined opacity has appeared in the axillary portion of the right lung in a configuration compatible with a pulmonary infarct; there is a small right pleural effusion. Five days later (*D*), much of the lower half of the right lung has become consolidated, several areas of radiolucency scattered throughout the consolidated lobe suggesting cavitation. After another 5 days (*E* and *F*), numerous shaggy cavities have appeared in the consolidation, representing multiple abscesses as a result of septic infarction. The disease is situated predominantly in the right middle and upper lobes.

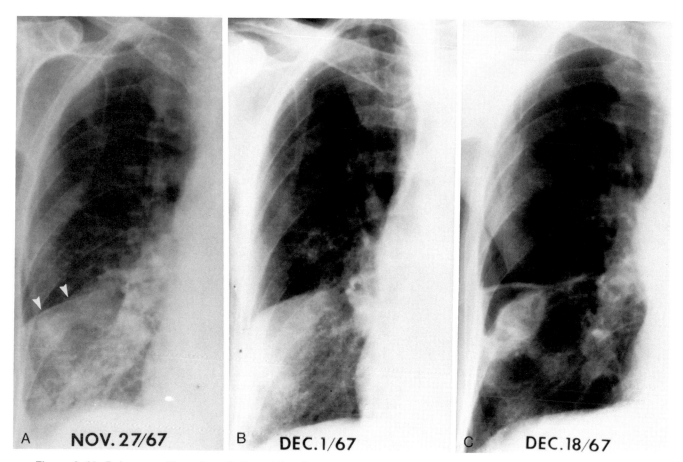

Figure 9–33. Pulmonary Thromboembolism, Infarction, and Cavitation. A view of the right lung from a posteroanterior chest roentgenogram (*A*) reveals extensive consolidation in the lateral segment of the middle lobe. Note the absence of an air bronchogram. The minor fissure (*arrowheads*) is slightly thickened and depressed. Four days later (*B*), the consolidation has partly resolved on its hilar aspect, suggesting that it represents hemorrhagic edema. However, 18 days later (*C*), a cavity had appeared that contained an eccentrically situated lung slough or hematoma. At autopsy several days later, these features were shown to be caused by a bland infarct associated with tissue necrosis and cavitation. The intracavitary mass consisted of sloughed noninfected lung parenchyma. The patient is a 72-year-old bedridden man who initially complained of cough, chest pain, and hemoptysis.

intracavitary loose bodies can be associated with secondary bacterial infection of a bland infarct (*see* Fig. 9–31) and, rarely, with bland infarcts themselves (Fig. 9–33). Acute septic embolism may be associated with hilar and mediastinal lymph node enlargement that may be massive as in the four patients described by Gumbs and McCauley,[255] in all of whom the etiology was *S. aureus*. Pleural effusion, in the form of empyema, is an infrequent complication.

Roentgenograms sometimes show multiple, small, poorly defined opacities that simulate diffuse bronchopneumonia and therefore require extreme alertness to detect the diagnosis, particularly if the emboli stem from bacterial endocarditis. In questionable cases, the diagnosis can be confirmed by pulmonary arteriography with or without lung scanning.

Affected patients are often young and many have a history of drug addiction. Some present with a sore throat, although the initial pharyngitis may have cleared by the time the infection reaches the retropharyngeal space.[245] Fever, cough (with or without expectoration of purulent material), and hemoptysis are the most common symptoms. Hemoptysis may be massive—in one report of three addicts with this complication, two died from asphyxia.[256] The presence of fever in drug addicts should always raise the suspicion of infective endocarditis: in a series of 87 consecutive admissions of drug abusers with a temperature of 38.1°C or more, 13 per cent were proven to have infected heart valves.[257] Infection originating from a right heart valve may give rise to a murmur, but in many cases this is soft and atypically located and its significance may be overlooked.[248]

The source of infection must be identified, since antibotic therapy alone may not control the infection. Additional therapeutic procedures may be required, including removal of catheters, arteriovenous shunts or prosthetic valves, ligation of the inferior vena cava or ovarian veins,[241, 258] or surgical drainage. The tricuspid valve may need to be replaced if infection cannot be controlled.[259] Early surgical resection of a lobe may be indicated.[259]

THE ACCURACY OF CHEST ROENTGENOGRAPHY IN THE DIAGNOSIS OF PULMONARY EMBOLISM

Possibly the most definitive study that has been carried out to date to test the accuracy of the chest roentgenogram in the diagnosis of pulmonary embolism was carried out by Greenspan and his colleagues[260] and published in 1982, and the results of this study, while perhaps not surprising, are surely not encouraging. These authors garnered the chest roentgenograms of 152 patients who were all suspected at one time of having pulmonary embolism but in whom only 108 proved to have embolism on the basis of a positive pulmonary angiogram (the remaining 44 patients were assumed not to have embolism on the basis of either a normal perfusion scintiscan or a pulmonary angiogram). The roentgenograms were randomized and presented for interpretation to nine readers (seven of whom were radiologists specializing in pulmonary disease). The question "Does this patient have pulmonary embolism?" required a "yes," "no," or "don't know" answer. The results were as follows: the average true-positive ratio (sensitivity) was 0.33 (range 0.52 to 0.88) (sic); the average true-negative ratio (sensitivity) was 0.59 (range 0.31 to 0.80); the false-positive and false-negative ratios, respectively, were 0.21 (range 0.05 to 0.39) and 0.41 (range 0.15 to 0.70). A predictive index, reflecting the overall accuracy of diagnosis, was 0.40 (range 0.17 to 0.57) for the entire group.

On the basis of this study, the authors concluded that although the chest roentgenogram may provide additional information in the evaluation of patients suspected of having pulmonary embolism, it cannot be considered a definitive examination, in and of itself. Its major importance lies in the exclusion of other disease processes that can mimic acute pulmonary embolism and in providing correlation with $\dot{V}/\dot{Q}$ lung scans.

PULMONARY ANGIOGRAPHY

Pulmonary arteriography is the single most definitive technique for investigating suspected pulmonary thromboembolic disease,[261–263] and even extremely ill patients usually tolerate the procedure well.[189] However, it carries a risk of morbidity and mortality.

Techniques

Best results are obtained if the contrast medium is injected through a catheter whose tip is in the right or left pulmonary artery (Fig. 9–34). This permits not only a clear view of the ipsilateral pulmonary arterial tree but also the measurement of pulmonary artery pressure. The study may reveal partial or complete occlusion of lobar or segmental vessels, but is seldom useful when the obstructed vessels are subsegmental or smaller.[146, 261, 264] Small pulmonary vessels may be inadequately seen because (1) the contrast medium is diluted during cardiac systole; (2) vessel detail may be obscured by overlap of many opacified vessels; and (3) blood flow tends to be diverted away from embolized vessels. In such cases, it may be necessary to perform subsegmental arteriography, first in anteroposterior (AP) projection[265] and then in other projections if the AP study is inconclusive. In a review of 57 positive pulmonary arteriograms, it was found that additional views were necessary in 26 cases[266]—the right posterior oblique projection for the right lung and the left posterior oblique or lateral projection for the left lung. In a study of the reliability of selective pulmonary arteriography in the diagnosis of pulmonary embolism, Quinn and his colleagues[735] concluded that this procedure carried out in the conventional manner is reliable in the detection of emboli in segmental or larger pulmonary arteries but that observer disagreement becomes considerable for emboli situated in subsegmental pulmonary arteries; they suggested that emboli of this size are at the resolution limit of the technique. However, wedge arteriography (which is seldom indicated) permits identification of vessels 2 mm or smaller in diameter,[267] an ability that is enhanced by magnification;[268] only a small amount of contrast medium should be injected, probably not more than 1 ml.

Some interest has been expressed in the performance of bedside, flow-directed, wedge pulmonary angiography in the diagnosis of pulmonary embolic disease, but Le Page and Gracia[269] concluded that this procedure is characterized by a low sensitivity and specificity and is of little value as either a screening procedure or a diagnostic tool: in a predictive study involving 74 unequivocally positive conventional pulmonary angiograms, these authors concluded that flow-directed, wedge arteriography would have detected the embolism in only 48 per cent of the cases in which the right lower lobe alone was embolized, in 10 per cent of the cases in which the left lower lobe alone was embolized, and in 30 per cent of the cases in which both lower lobes were embolized.

The development of intravenous digital subtraction angiography (DSA) has stimulated interest in the accuracy with which this technique can provide diagnostic information in patients with suspected pulmonary embolism. To test this accuracy, Reilley and her colleagues[270] carried out an experimental study on eight canines in which perfusion lung scanning, magnification pulmonary arteriography, and DSA were performed prior to and

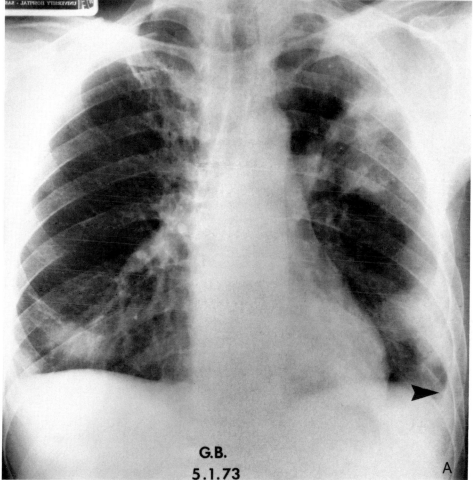

Figure 9–34. Value of Oblique Arteriography in the Demonstration of Pulmonary Thromboembolism. A conventional postero-anterior chest roentgenogram (*A*) shows multiple well defined and poorly defined homogeneous opacities in both lungs, involving predominantly the lower lobes. The lesions relate intimately to visceral pleura and on the left are associated with a small pleural effusion (*arrowhead*). Cardiac size and configuration are normal.

Illustration continued on following page

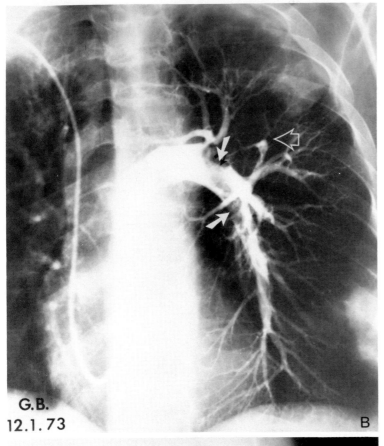

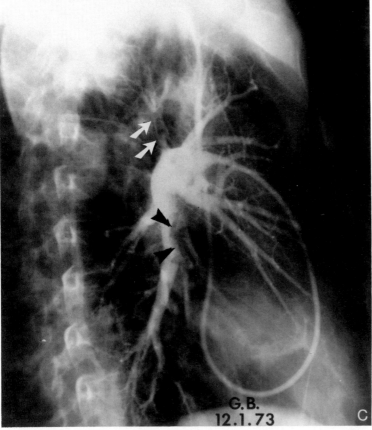

Figure 9–34 *Continued* A selective left pulmonary arteriogram in left anterior oblique (*B*) and steep right anterior oblique projections (*C*) reveals multiple intraluminal filling defects, both central (*arrows*) and eccentric (*arrowheads*). A segmental artery (*open arrow*) in the upper lobe in *B* is amputated. These features are diagnostic of multiple pulmonary thromboemboli.

following absorbable gelatin sponge (Gelfoam) embolization of selected pulmonary arteries. The DSA study was performed in two stages, one in which contrast medium was injected into an iliac vein and the other an arterial phase injection in which the tip of the catheter was placed in a selected pulmonary artery. Two parameters were evaluated on the DSA images: (1) *arterial cut-off*, representing the effect of occluded vessels, and (2) a *parenchymal phase*, representing a reduction in peripheral perfusion analogous to the wedge-shaped defects seen on scintigraphic perfusion images. The results were as follows: the sites of embolization were identified in six (75 per cent) of eight animals on perfusion lung scans, in seven (93 per cent) of eight animals by magnification arteriography, in six of eight in the arterial phase DSA study, and in all eight dogs in the parenchymal phase DSA examinations.

The accuracy of DSA has also been tested in humans by Pond and his colleagues,[271] who carried out a prospective study of 33 patients with suspected embolism: they performed intravenous DSA as the initial examination followed immediately by conventional pulmonary arteriography with selective right or left main pulmonary artery injections. Intravenous studies of diagnostic quality were obtained in 31 (93.9 per cent) of the 33 patients; the remaining two were technically unsatisfactory. Of the satisfactory intravenous studies, pulmonary embolism was correctly diagnosed in 12 cases and excluded in 18; emboli were detected in major and second-order branches and occasionally in third-order branches. There was one false-positive intravenous study, but the overall accuracy was 90.9 per cent (considering all studies) and 96.8 per cent (excluding the two inadequate intravenous examinations).

Despite the excellent results obtained by Pond and his colleagues,[271] other investigators have not been as fortunate: of 54 patients suspected of having pulmonary embolism studied by DSA, Musset and his associates[770] found 13 (24 per cent) to be technically unsatisfactory; of the interpretable angiograms, there were 27 per cent false-positive results. The authors concluded that although the diagnosis of pulmonary embolism cannot be excluded on the basis of normal DSA findings, this may be the technique of choice in the screening of life-threatening pulmonary embolism for which curative emergency treatment with thrombolytic agents or embolectomy may be indicated.

Although there is little argument that DSA is less expensive, safer, faster, and easier to perform than conventional pulmonary arteriography, the success rate in the limited studies reported to date leaves some doubt regarding its reliability as an acceptable substitute for routine angiography. Perhaps the technological advances that can be expected in future years will improve the outlook.

Known allergy to contrast medium is an absolute contraindication to pulmonary angiography, and recent myocardial infarction and ventricular irritability are relative contraindications. A report of 367 consecutive studies[263] recorded complications in 13 patients (4 per cent) relating to catheterization (cardiac perforation, pyrogenic reaction, and arrhythmias) and contrast medium (bronchospasm, angioneurotic edema, and anaphylaxis) in roughly equal numbers. There was one death from cardiac shock immediately after injection of the medium. Two perforations occurred early in the study when a relatively stiff catheter was being used, and all three patients in whom acute bronchospasm developed had a history of asthma. In another series of 298 patients,[273] two patients who died had severe underlying embolic disease and pulmonary hypertension. In the urokinase pulmonary embolism trial reported in 1973,[274] 310 pulmonary angiograms were performed on 160 patients without a fatality; complications included one cardiac perforation and five instances of ventricular arrhythmias, all of which responded to therapy. In an earlier study[275] of previously healthy patients who suffered massive pulmonary embolism, cardiac arrest requiring brief external cardiac massage followed the injection of contrast medium in several cases. It has been suggested that if the pulmonary arterial pressure exceeds 80 mm Hg and pulmonary embolectomy appears indicated, the patient should be placed on right heart bypass before angiography is performed.[276, 277]

In patients in whom pulmonary arteriography is contraindicated for one reason or another, both MRI[730-733] and CT can provide noninvasive alternatives in selective circumstances. Although experience is rather limited to date, Godwin and his colleagues[278] effectively employed CT in three patients to demonstrate emboli and thrombi within central pulmonary arteries; the technique established the diagnosis in one patient and in another served as a follow-up of central thromboembolism, thus avoiding repeat angiography. A more recent experimental study by Ovenfors and his colleagues[279] suggested that CT scanning with contrast enhancement may permit identification of emboli in lobar and segmental arteries (Fig. 9–35).

Angiographic Abnormalities

The multifarious angiographic criteria reported for the diagnosis of pulmonary embolism were summarized by Sagel and Greenspan[262] and are listed in Table 9–1. They pointed out that although the importance of secondary signs has been stressed, these signs reflect nothing more than diminished pulmonary arterial perfusion, a common manifestation of several pulmonary and cardiac diseases from which pulmonary embolism must be differentiated. In fact, there is only one established angiographic criterion for the definitive diagnosis of pulmonary embolism—direct observation of an intraluminal filling defect.[119, 146, 149, 280-283] However, the secondary signs listed in Table 9–1 may

Text continued on page 1764

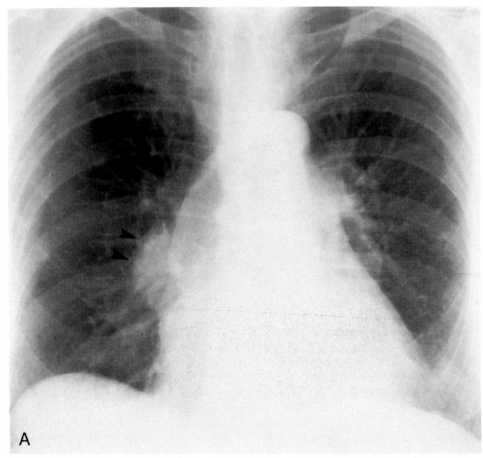

Figure 9–35. Chronic Pulmonary Thromboembolism: Scintigraphic, Arteriographic, and CT Manifestations. A conventional posteroanterior chest roentgenogram (*A*) reveals an enlarged heart whose configuration is compatible with enlargement of the right ventricle. The hilar arteries, particularly the right interlobar artery (*arrowheads*), are prominent. No abnormality is seen in the lungs.

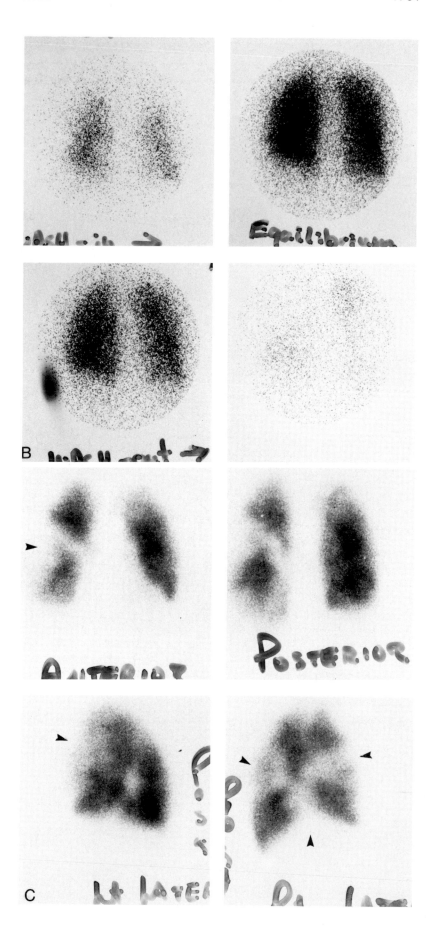

Figure 9–35 *Continued* A ventilation lung scintigram (*B*) is normal, whereas a perfusion scan (*C*) reveals multiple segmental defects in both lungs (*arrowheads*). These studies indicate a high probability of pulmonary thromboembolism.

Illustration continued on following page

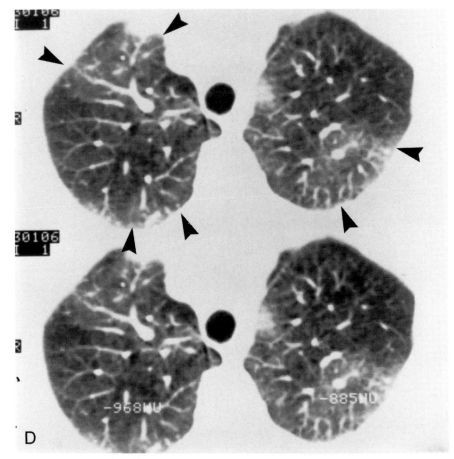

Figure 9–35 *Continued* A CT scan through the upper lobes (*D*) discloses geographic areas of maintained perfusion (*arrowheads*) in the anterior portion of the left upper lobe that contrast sharply with contiguous areas of diminished CT density (compare the CT attenuation values in the two zones). Note that the vessels are larger in the well-perfused areas than in the oligemic zones.

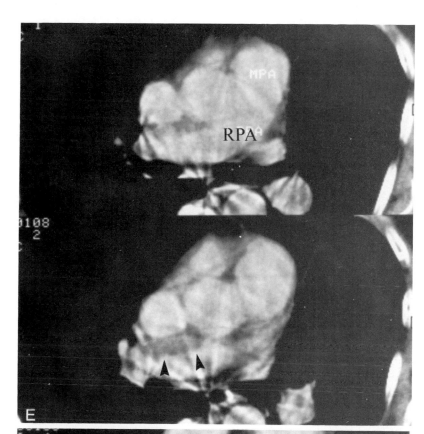

Figure 9–35 *Continued* Contrast-enhanced CT scans through the right pulmonary artery (RPA) (*E*) and its descending branches (*F*) reveal an elongated filling defect (*arrowheads*) adjacent to the anterior wall of the right pulmonary artery, and a number of smaller, eccentric defects on the anterior part of the descending arteries (*arrows*).

Illustration continued on following page

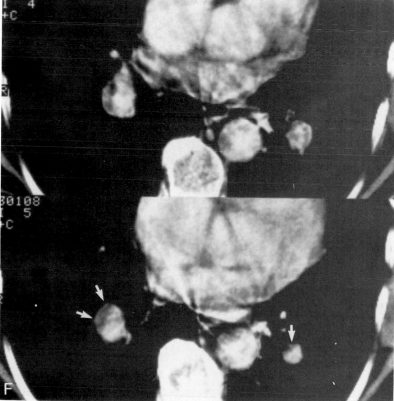

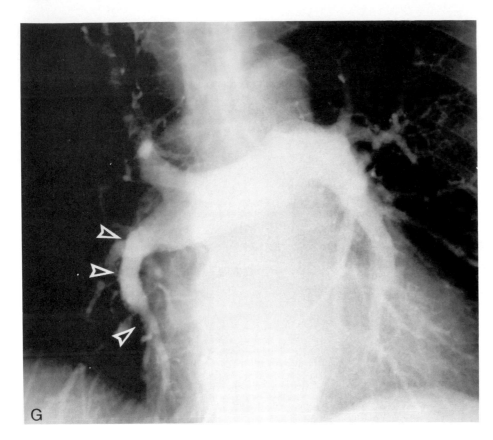

Figure 9–35 *Continued* A pulmonary arteriogram in anteroposterior projection (*G*) demonstrates the anterolateral plaque-like defects (*arrowheads*) in the descending branches, although the anteriorly positioned thrombus in the right artery is hidden from view. The patient is a 63-year-old man with a long history of exertional dyspnea.

be useful by directing attention to areas in which manifestations of embolism may be subtle; in such cases, segmental or wedge arteriography, especially with magnification, should reveal intraluminal defects in smaller vessels.

Care must be taken not to misinterpret an opacified artery seen end-on as a blunt obstruction.

Table 9–1. Angiographic Criteria Reported for the Diagnosis of Pulmonary Embolism*

PRIMARY SIGN

A. Filling defect
  1. Persistent intraluminal radiolucency, central or marginal, without complete obstruction of blood flow
  2. Trailing edge of an intraluminal radiolucency when there is complete obstruction of distal blood flow

SECONDARY SIGNS

A. Abrupt occlusion ("cutoff") of a pulmonary artery without visualization of an intraluminal filling defect
B. Perfusion defect (asymmetric filling)
  1. Areas of oligemia or avascularity
  2. Focal areas in which the arterial phase is prolonged (especially when localized to the lower lung fields); this is usually accompanied by slow filling and emptying of the pulmonary veins.
  3. Tortuous, abruptly tapering peripheral vessels, with a paucity of branching vessels ("pruning")

*Reprinted from Sagel SS, Greenspan RH: Radiology *99*:541, 1971, with permission of the authors and editor.

Tapering of vessels usually connotes circumferential organization and recanalization and, therefore, an old thromboembolic episode.[280] In follow-up angiographic studies,[284] weblike deformities of vessels identified *in vivo* at the precise sites of intra-arterial filling defects previously shown angiographically (Fig. 9–36) were assumed to be remnants of emboli as has been shown pathologically (*see* Fig. 9–10).[156, 157] In fact, in some patients pulmonary emboli may fail to resolve normally, resulting in chronic pulmonary thromboembolism, pulmonary hypertension, respiratory insufficiency, cor pulmonale, and death. In such cases, Mills and his colleagues[293] advocate combined pulmonary and bronchial arteriography, the former to delineate the location of obstructions within the pulmonary vascular tree and the latter to establish whether the peripheral branches of the obstructed pulmonary arteries are patent. Peripheral patency of the pulmonary circulation is necessary if surgical removal of chronic thromboemboli is to be successful; back bleeding of arterial blood from the bronchial circulation can establish peripheral patency at the time of surgery, but preoperative bronchial arteriography can predict the potential success of embolectomy. Of nine patients with chronic pulmonary embolism studied by Mills and his colleagues,[293] embolectomy resulted in clinical improvement in seven.

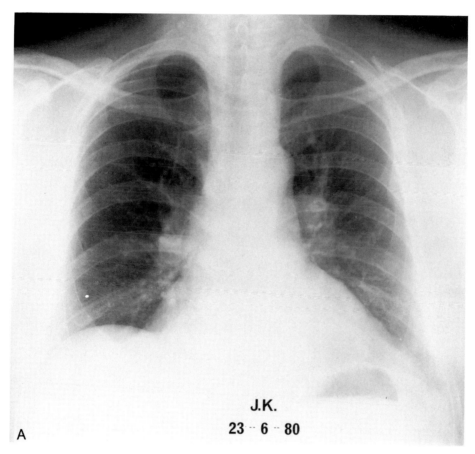

Figure 9–36. Pulmonary Thromboembolism and Cor Pulmonale: Scintigraphic Features. A posteroanterior chest roentgenogram (*A*) shows enlargement and increased rapidity of tapering of the hilar pulmonary arteries indicating precapillary pulmonary hypertension. The lungs are otherwise normal. The heart is slightly enlarged.

Illustration continued on following page

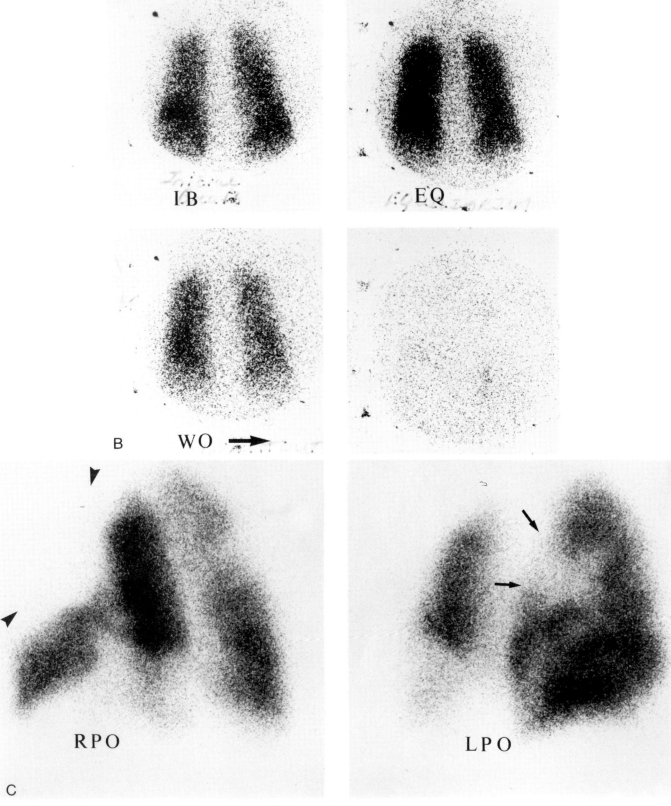

Figure 9–36 *Continued* A ventilation scintigram (*B*) is normal, whereas perfusion scans in left posterior oblique (LPO) and right posterior oblique positions (*C*) reveal a total lack of activity in the right upper lobe (*arrowheads*) and segmental defects in the right lower and left upper lobes (*arrows*).

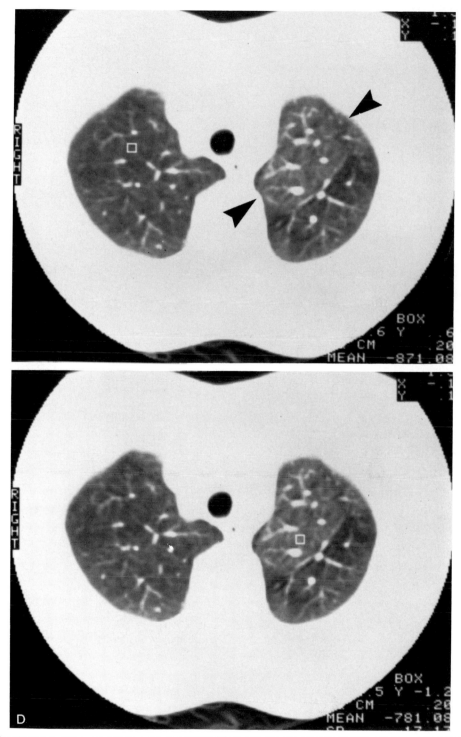

Figure 9–36 *Continued* A CT scan (*D*) through the upper lobes reveals an opacity in the anterior segment of the left upper lobe (*arrowheads*) possessing a sharply defined "geographic" quality strongly suggestive of a segmental boundary. The opaque area corresponds to the zone of maintained perfusion identified on the perfusion scintigram. The posterior part of the left upper lobe and the whole right upper lobe are oligemic, the vessels generally being smaller than in areas of maintained perfusion. CT attenuation values in the oligemic areas (−871 Hounsfield units) and plethoric area (−781 Hounsfield units) are slightly lower and higher, respectively, than normal.

Illustration continued on following page

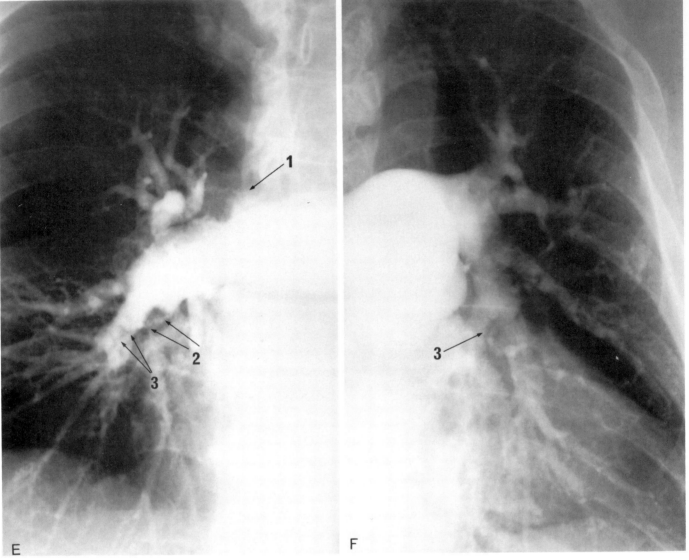

Figure 9–36 *Continued* Detail views of the right (*E*) and left (*F*) lungs from a pulmonary arteriogram reveal occlusion of the ascending branch of the right pulmonary artery (*1*), plaque-like defects in the right interlobar artery (*2*), and intraluminal curvilinear defects (*3*) consistent with organized thrombi (webs). These features are indicative of chronic thromboemboli.

Occasionally, a variety of clinical entities can mimic pulmonary embolism both clinically and scintigraphically, leading to pulmonary angiography for confirmation of an embolic episode. Five such instances have been reported by Cassling and his colleagues,[736] including examples of Takayasu arteritis, angiopathy of unknown etiology, angiosarcoma, and sarcoidosis. We have seen a single patient who presented with a history highly suggestive of acute pulmonary embolism but who was shown angiographically to have a severe narrowing of a segmental artery subsequently proven to be caused by small cell carcinoma (Fig. 9–37).

Many workers[262, 285–287] have emphasized the importance of assessing concomitant disease that might affect the pulmonary vasculature and alter the angiographic pattern, and Sagel and Greenspan[262] tabulated conditions associated with nonuniform pulmonary arterial perfusion (Table 9–2).

Techniques have been developed for quantifying the angiographic severity of major pulmonary embolism,[288–290] but from a practical point of view these are useful only in epidemiologic studies.

Pulmonary Artery Pressures

Measurement of the right ventricular and pulmonary arterial pressures is often very helpful in the evaluation of patients with thromboembolic disease,[291] and these pressures should always be carefully recorded before pulmonary angiography. Even if the angiogram reveals no evidence of major vessel occlusion, the pulmonary arterial pressure may be raised, suggesting multiple microemboli throughout the lungs. On the basis of their own experience and a review of the literature, however, Haegelin and Murray[292] believe that this combina-

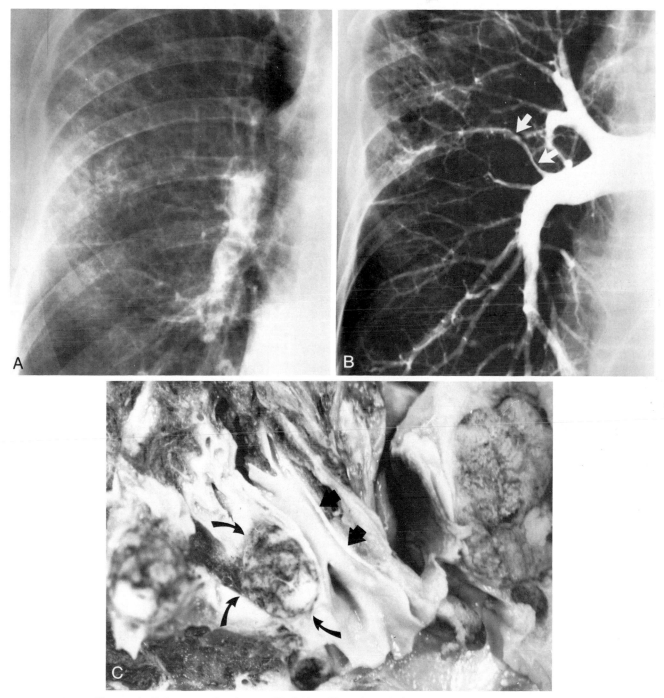

Figure 9–37. Metastatic Pulmonary Carcinoma Mimicking Thromboembolism. A view of the right lung from a posteroanterior roentgenogram (*A*) reveals a number of poorly defined opacities in the axillary portion of the right upper lobe. This 60-year-old man presented with a history of abrupt onset of right-sided chest pain, and a provisional diagnosis of acute pulmonary thromboembolism was made. A selective right pulmonary arteriogram (*B*) revealed no evidence of embolism but showed diffuse concentric narrowing of a branch of the right interlobar artery (*arrows*) extending towards the axillary opacity. At autopsy a few days later, the arterial narrowing was shown to be caused by compression by enlarged lymph nodes containing metastatic small cell carcinoma. A magnified view of the medial portion of the right lung (*C*) shows the narrowed artery (*arrows*) and the contiguous enlarged nodes (*curved arrows*). The peripheral opacities were caused by the carcinoma.

Table 9–2. Conditions Associated with Nonuniform Pulmonary Arterial Perfusion*

I. *Emphysema (focal or diffuse)*
II. *Inflammatory diseases*
    Pneumonia (including tuberculosis)
    Lung abscess
    Bronchiectasis
    Pulmonary fibrosis:
        Interstitial fibrosis
        Fibrothorax
III. *Congenital*
    Absence or hypoplasia of a pulmonary artery
    Peripheral pulmonary stenosis
    Bronchopulmonary sequestration
IV. *Extrinsic obstruction of a pulmonary artery or vein by compression or actual invasion*
    Neoplasms:
        Benign
        Malignant
    Inflammatory:
        Fibrosing mediastinitis
    Aortic aneurysms
V. *Intrinsic obstruction of a pulmonary artery*
    Thromboembolic disease:
        Blood clot
        Tumor
        Fat
    The Eisenmenger reaction: superimposed obliterative arteriolitis develops in large left-to-right intracardiac and extracardiac shunts
    Arteritis
VI. *Postcapillary pulmonary (venous) hypertension*
    Left ventricular failure
    Mitral valvular disease
    Pulmonary veno-occlusive disease
VII. *Focal hypoventilation (frequently associated with atelectasis or air trapping)*
    Bronchial obstruction:
        Inflammatory processes
        Neoplasm
        Reflex bronchoconstriction
          Asthma
          Pulmonary embolism
    Splinting from pleural irritation:
        Inflammation ("pleuritis")
        Rib fractures

*Reprinted from Sagel, SS, Greenspan, RH.: Radiology, *99*:541, 1971, with permission of the authors and editor.

tion of findings is more characteristic of primary pulmonary hypertension, since the hypertension that accompanies multiple pulmonary emboli almost invariably connotes embolization of vessels large enough to be seen angiographically. The pulmonary arterial pressure probably is raised in most patients with positive angiographic findings, and those with a mean right ventricular pressure exceeding 22 mm Hg (30 cm saline) are likely to die.[294] When the main pulmonary arterial pressure is raised and the differential diagnosis is between acute pulmonary embolism and myocardial infarction with shock, capillary wedge pressure can be obtained with much less risk than an angiogram and usually distinguishes the two conditions, being normal in embolism and raised in myocardial infarction.[295]

Occlusion of a pulmonary artery with a balloon has been recommended[146] when the pulmonary arterial pressure is normal and thromboembolism is strongly suspected clinically. With this procedure, the pulmonary vascular resistance falls when thromboembolism is absent and rises when pulmonary vessels are occluded by thrombus.

SCINTIGRAPHY

Despite the hundreds of studies that have been performed over the past two or three decades, it is still safe to say that the optimal approach to the diagnosis of pulmonary embolism remains controversial. As has been shown, the chest roentgenogram provides a low discovery rate and a high incidence of false negatives; similarly, as we see later, clinical symptoms and signs and the results of laboratory investigation are of limited value for diagnosis because of low specificity and sensitivity. Although it is well recognized that pulmonary angiography is the definitive method of establishing the diagnosis and of demonstrating the extent of embolism, this invasive procedure is expensive, time-consuming, and possessive of potential morbidity. As a result of these considerations, it is now well accepted that ventilation-perfusion scintigraphy is the technique of choice as the initial screening procedure in the diagnosis of pulmonary embolism.

Techniques

PERFUSION

This procedure consists of the intravenous injection of macroaggregates of albumin (MAA) tagged with ^{99m}Tc (and sometimes with ^{131}I, ^{51}Cr, or ^{113M}In). The number of particles administered ranges from 250,000 to 500,000 containing 2 to 4 millicuries (mCi) of isotope. Imaging is performed with a scintillation camera in anterior, posterior, both lateral, and both posterior oblique projections. The macroaggregates are small enough that they become thoroughly mixed with the blood and are distributed throughout the lung in proportion to regional blood flow; however, the majority are large enough to become trapped within the pulmonary capillaries so that their detection provides a "static" image of regional flow at an instant in time.

VENTILATION

Ventilation images are obtained by inhaling ^{133}Xe, or Krypton 81m (^{81m}Kr). Images are created on a scintillation camera, if at all possible with the patient erect. Generally, an "equilibrium" image is obtained at the end of the wash-in phase while the patient rebreaths 10 mCi of ^{133}Xe through a closed system containing oxygen. Images are obtained in posterior projection, sometimes with sequential wash-out images at regular intervals until the ^{133}Xe clears the lungs. Although single-breath ^{133}Xe is sometimes employed, Alderson and his associates[296] have shown that these are not suitable as the sole determinant of $\dot{V}/\dot{Q}$ match or mismatch, especially when subsegmental perfusion defects are present, and that prolonged wash-out imaging improves the specificity of $\dot{V}/\dot{Q}$ studies in patients with suspected pulmonary embolism. An alternative gas for ventilation imaging is [81m]Kr, a gas that is eluted from a generator delivered on-site each day and therefore of somewhat limited availability. In several respects, this agent is regarded by some as a virtually ideal agent for ventilation imaging in patients with suspected pulmonary embolism.[724, 737] Its 190-keV primary photon energy permits ventilation imaging to be performed after the ^{99m}Tc–labeled perfusion agent has been injected. Its short physical half-life (13 seconds) and related low-radiation dose permit many ventilation views to be obtained. In addition, [81m]Kr is the easiest agent to employ in critically ill patients, even when ventilation is being assisted by a mechanical respirator. The advantages of this gas over ^{133}Xe have been discussed in detail by Alderson and Martin.[724]

An alternative to the ^{133}Xe or [81m]Kr inhalation method is aerosol inhalation lung imaging in which a labeled aerosolized liquid rather than a gas is inhaled, particularly with incorporation of the demand valve technique developed by Taplin and his colleagues.[297] Small plastic nebulizers that allow convenient production of submicronic radioaerosols from self-contained, inexpensive nebulization systems have become commercially available, permitting the production of particles of sufficiently small size to reach the lung periphery, thus obviating excess central deposition. In a study of 107 patients who were referred for evaluation of suspected pulmonary embolism, Alderson and his colleagues[738] compared ^{99m}Tc–diethylenetrianine penta-acetic acid (DTPA) aerosol with radioactive gases as adjuncts to perfusion scintigraphy and found that the radioaerosol inhalation studies, performed with improved nebulizers, were diagnostically equivalent to ventilation imaging. It is probable that this is now the most widely used technique in the study of ventilation in patients with suspected pulmonary thromboembolism; it possesses the advantage of providing static images in multiple projections; further, any expired radioactivity can be trapped in a filter.

At the time of writing, it is too early to determine the impact of either single-photon emission computed tomography (SPECT) or ^{111}In–labeled platelets in the diagnosis of pulmonary embolism. SPECT permits separation of radionuclide activity in front of and behind the area of interest whereas the scintillation camera provides single planar images with overlap of normal and abnormal lung regions. In an experimental study in which the lower lobe segmental pulmonary arteries of six dogs were embolized and pulmonary perfusion evaluated with SPECT, conventional gamma camera imaging, and angiography, Osborne and his colleagues[298] determined that although selective segmental arteriography was the most sensitive method of detecting the emboli, SPECT was much more sensitive than the scintillation camera in evaluating the presence of emboli at 2 hours and at 1, 2, and 8 weeks after embolization. Similar beneficial results were obtained by Kahn and associates in a study of four patients with thromboembolic disease.[299] It would thus appear that this technique holds considerable promise.

Scintigraphic Abnormalities and Criteria for Diagnosis

Ventilation-perfusion studies of the lung are widely used to screen patients with suspected pulmonary embolism and to select those requiring pulmonary angiography. Pulmonary emboli are rarely, if ever, identified angiographically in patients with normal perfusion images, so that when scintigraphy is normal arteriography is not indicated.[307–309] By contrast, when $\dot{V}/\dot{Q}$ studies demonstrate sizable perfusion defects in the absence of ventilatory impairment ($\dot{V}/\dot{Q}$ mismatch) or of associated roentgenographic abnormalities, the probability of embolism is high (see Figs. 9–35 and 9–36). As pointed out by Biello and his colleagues,[310] arteriography is generally unnecessary in these patients unless the diagnosis is still uncertain, unless anticoagulant therapy is contraindicated, or unless surgical intervention is proposed. Conversely, when $\dot{V}/\dot{Q}$ studies demonstrate perfusion defects that correspond in size and location to zones of decreased ventilation ($\dot{V}/\dot{Q}$ match), embolism is unlikely and no further evaluation is usually required.[310]

As pointed out by Biello and his colleagues,[310] there are certain well-defined situations in which abnormalities observed on conventional roentgenograms and $\dot{V}/\dot{Q}$ scans are such that a positive statement regarding the presence or absence of embolism cannot be made, the findings thus becoming indeterminate. The most frequent of these is one in which the scintigraphic abnormalities correspond in anatomic distribution to opacities identified on chest roentgenograms. On the basis of their experience with 146 patients with abnormal $\dot{V}/\dot{Q}$ studies, these authors[311] proposed a scheme by which the probability of pulmonary embolism can be estimated on the strength of three combinations of $\dot{V}/\dot{Q}$ patterns and roentgenographic abnormalities:

1. When the perfusion defect was substantially smaller than the corresponding roentgenographic abnormality, pulmonary embolism was present infrequently.

2. When the perfusion defect was substantially larger than the corresponding roentgenographic opacity, pulmonary embolism was present in a high percentage of patients.

3. When the perfusion defect and radiographic opacity were of about equal size, the frequency of pulmonary embolism was approximately 25 per cent. On the basis of these and the foregoing observations, a scheme for the interpretation of $\dot{V}/\dot{Q}$ images was designed (Table 9–3). For comparison purposes, another scheme for the scintigraphic diagnosis of pulmonary embolism has been selected by the multi-institutional committee currently involved in the prospective National Institutes of Health (NIH)-sponsored PIOPED trial (Prospective Investigation of Pulmonary Embolism Diagnosis). These criteria are listed in Table 9–3 alongside those proposed by Biello and his colleagues.

Subsequently, Carter and his associates[312] carried out a study in which the relative accuracy of the Biello scheme was compared with a somewhat simpler scheme that had been developed and was in use over a period of years at the University of Michigan; the latter scheme had been synthesized from the results from several groups published in the literature prior to 1978. In a study of 70 $\dot{V}/\dot{Q}$ scintiscans, the results of this comparison were rather impressive: observers employing the Biello scheme had a significantly smaller average number of "indeterminate" interpretations (41 per cent) than did the observers using the Michigan scheme (55 per cent); in addition, the Biello group showed a slight improvement in positive predictive value without a deterioration in the negative predictive value compared with the Michigan group. It was concluded that the diagnostic scheme introduced by Biello and his colleagues[310] represents a useful improvement for the diagnosis of pulmonary embolism by $\dot{V}/\dot{Q}$ imaging.

Hypoperfusion due to embolic arterial occlusion is unaccompanied by significant regional hypoventilation, thus resulting in increased dead space ventilation and a high $\dot{V}/\dot{Q}$ ratio, a fact originally reported by Bass and his colleagues.[313] Using the same ^{133}Xe method to study patients with COPD,[314] they showed that regional hypoventilation was accompanied by regional hypoperfusion; however, the decrease in ventilation was greater than that in perfusion resulting in venous admixture and a low $\dot{V}/\dot{Q}$ ratio. Although several studies[315–318] have confirmed these findings and have established the value of combined ventilation and perfusion scanning, there is both experimental and clinical[130, 319, 320] evidence that soon after embolization there is reduction in ventilation to the embolized region that, in humans, may last up to 48 hours.

Patients with COPD who are suspected of having acute pulmonary embolism comprise a difficult group, although Alderson and his coworkers[321] have clarified the problems to some extent. In a combined ventilation-perfusion-angiographic study of 83 patients with COPD and suspected pulmonary embolism,[321] these authors found that the overall sensitivity of $\dot{V}/\dot{Q}$ imaging for pulmonary embolism in their population was 0.83 and its specificity 0.92.

Table 9–3. Two Schemes for Interpretation of $\dot{V}/\dot{Q}$ Images

PROBABILITY OF PULMONARY EMBOLISM	A*	B†
None	Normal perfusion	Normal perfusion
Low	Small $\dot{V}/\dot{Q}$ mismatches	Small $\dot{Q}$ defects regardless of number, ventilation or chest X-ray findings
	Focal $\dot{V}/\dot{Q}$ matches with no corresponding radiographic abnormalities	$\dot{Q}$ defect substantially smaller than chest X-ray
	Perfusion defects substantially smaller than radiographic abnormalities	$\dot{V}/\dot{Q}$ match in 50% one lung or 75% of one lung zone; chest X-ray normal or nearly normal
		Single moderate $\dot{Q}$ with normal chest X-ray ($\dot{V}$ irrelevent)
		Nonsegmental $\dot{Q}$ defects
Intermediate	Diffuse, severe airway obstruction	Abnormality that is not defined by either "high" or "low"
	Matched perfusion defects and radiographic abnormalities	
	Single moderate $\dot{V}/\dot{Q}$ mismatch without corresponding radiographic abnormality	
High	Perfusion defects substantially larger than radiographic abnormalities	Two or more large $\dot{Q}$ defects; $\dot{V}$ and chest X-ray normal
	One or more large or two or more moderate-sized $\dot{V}/\dot{Q}$ mismatches with no corresponding radiographic abnormalities	Two or more large $\dot{Q}$ defects in which $\dot{Q}$ is substantially larger than either matching $\dot{V}$ or chest X-ray
		Two or more moderate $\dot{Q}$ and one large $\dot{Q}$; $\dot{V}$ and chest X-ray normal
		Four or more moderate $\dot{Q}$; $\dot{V}$ and chest X-ray normal

*Proposed by Biello et al[311] (slightly modified).
†Proposed by PIOPED.[739, 740]

False-negative interpretations occurred in three of the 16 patients who showed ventilation abnormalities in more than 50 per cent of their lungs, whereas in the 67 patients with ventilation abnormalities affecting 50 per cent or less of their lungs, the sensitivity (0.95) and specificity (0.94) for detecting pulmonary embolism were high. The authors concluded that $\dot{V}/\dot{Q}$ imaging is a reliable method for detecting pulmonary embolism in patients with regions of $\dot{V}/\dot{Q}$ match as long as ventilation abnormalities are limited in extent.

In a later study aimed at assessing the accuracy of chest roentgenograms in predicting the extent of airway disease in patients with suspected pulmonary embolism, Smith and associates[322] found that $\dot{V}/\dot{Q}$ scans were indeterminate in all 21 patients who had roentgenographic evidence of widespread COPD, in 35 per cent of those with focal obstructive disease, and in only 18 per cent of those whose chest roentgenograms revealed no evidence of COPD. The authors concluded that ventilation imaging is probably not warranted in patients with roentgenographic evidence of widespread COPD. When an attempt is made to distinguish $\dot{V}/\dot{Q}$ matching that is compatible with pulmonary embolism from that caused by COPD, a computation of the actual $\dot{V}/\dot{Q}$ ratio may be useful: in one study[323] in which a $\dot{V}/\dot{Q}$ ratio of 1.25 or higher was used to define an area of mismatch, the percentage of patients classified correctly as having either pulmonary embolism or COPD increased from 56 to 88 per cent, based simply on a consideration of the matched or mismatched character of perfusion.

Although $\dot{V}/\dot{Q}$ mismatch constitutes highly suggestive evidence of acute pulmonary embolism, especially if the chest roentgenogram is normal, a similar $\dot{V}/\dot{Q}$ abnormality can be produced by other conditions, including compression or partial occlusion of a vascular lumen by pulmonary carcinoma, lymphangitic carcinomatosis, and vascular occlusive lesions such as pulmonary artery sarcoma.[324] A rare case has been described in which a traumatic pseudoaneurysm of the right pulmonary artery resulted in a $\dot{V}/\dot{Q}$ mismatch.[324]

Serial scanning may provide information not available from a single scan.[741] Changing patterns of perfusion defects indicate multiple emboli, some areas regaining normal activity and other previously normal zones becoming unperfused.[191, 325] In one study, new perfusion defects, probably caused by further emboli, developed in 22 of 63 patients under treatment of pulmonary embolism;[174] most appeared within 2 weeks after the initial episode. This frequency suggests that anticoagulants are not very effective in preventing embolism, although the incidence of new defects was even higher in untreated patients.

Serial scans are also useful in following patients with known pulmonary embolism to assess resolution. Of 74 patients with a clinical diagnosis of pulmonary embolism,[174] one third showed almost complete recovery, one third improved 25 per cent or more, and the others remained the same or worsened. Perfusion was restored most rapidly in the first few days, and more slowly during the next 2 to 3 weeks. The degree of recovery in individual patients varied greatly but tended to be most rapid initially and slower later; it was almost nil after 3 to 4 months. Patients who had large perfusion defects (>30 per cent of one lung) showed considerable improvement but, on average, recovered less completely than those with small defects.

In another study of 70 such patients,[326] the scan became normal in one third of 34 patients with small emboli (on average, 10 days after onset of symptoms), in three of 14 with medium-sized defects (average, 18 days), and in only four of 22 patients with large defects (average, 23 days). Correlation of recovery with age showed the return to normal perfusion in 57 per cent of patients less than 40 years old but in none over 60 years; in fact, less than half of the latter group had significant scan improvement. A similar follow-up of 40 patients with pulmonary embolism[191] showed that, within 4 months, blood flow had returned to normal in 27 (67 per cent) and had improved in three others; of the 31 patients with an embolism of "intermediate" severity, 13 had normal scans later and 16 showed improvement, whereas only two of the nine patients with "severe" embolism had normal scans later and six improved.

It should be borne in mind that in other diseases (e.g., pneumonia, congestive heart failure, and atelectasis) sequential scanning can also show rapid improvement in regional perfusion. Asthma in particular is easily confused with pulmonary embolism (without infarction) because of its characteristic fleeting areas of reduced ventilation and perfusion even in patients with few symptoms and normal chest roentgenograms.[327]

Errors can be made in assuming that all new areas of hypoperfusion represent new emboli in patients with pulmonary hypertension.[328] A region of lung whose feeding artery is partly occluded by an embolus may be well perfused on an initial scan at a time when neighboring branches are completely occluded, but fragmentation and peripheral embolization of the thrombus in the completely occluded vessel may render a previously "normal" segment relatively underperfused and engender an erroneous interpretation of recurrent embolism.

METHODS FOR DIAGNOSIS OF DEEP VEIN THROMBOSIS

Phlebography (Venography)

Phlebography is used to outline the deep veins extending from the calf to the inferior vena cava in order to determine the presence and site of thrombus formation. In one prospective study,[329] 70 per cent of patients with pulmonary embolism proven by angiography showed evidence of thrombosis of the deep veins of the legs; it must be assumed that either the remaining 30 per cent had other sources for embolism (e.g., the deep pelvic veins, renal veins, inferior vena cava, or right atrium) or that all or most of the thrombi in the legs had embolized.[329, 330] Usually, the veins are opacified by injecting contrast medium into a foot vein; the iliac veins can be displayed by femoral vein or intraosseous injection.[331] The procedure is recommended in patients with recurrent pulmonary embolism for whom thrombectomy and venous ligation are being contemplated,[332, 333] particularly if anticoagulant therapy has apparently been unsuccessful.[60] If fibrinolytic plus anticoagulant therapy does not control the embolic episodes and the patient is too ill to tolerate bilateral ascending phlebography, Dow[334] has recommended that retrograde phlebography be performed (after pulmonary angiography) before inferior vena cava or venous ligation, both through one catheter in an antecubital vein. Rudikoff and his colleagues[335] extended this technique by recommending a sequence of angiography beginning with right iliac and vena caval opacification, proceeding to pulmonary arteriography, and terminating with retrograde left iliac vein opacification. Of 137 patients with pulmonary embolism studied by this technique, 15 (11 per cent) were found to have thrombus in the iliocaval system.

In a prospective study of patients clinically suspected of having pulmonary embolism, Hull and his coworkers[329] performed pulmonary angiography and venography in those in whom the perfusion lung scan was abnormal; they found that some of the patients with abnormal perfusion scans and normal pulmonary angiograms had proximal vein thrombosis, suggesting that such thrombosis could have been associated with pulmonary emboli that were undetected by selective angiography, either for technical reasons or because of lysis of the thrombi and migration distally into the pulmonary microcirculation. It seems to us reasonable to conclude from these findings that patients with positive lung scans (even if indeterminate) should undergo a diagnostic procedure to detect the presence of proximal vein thrombosis before a decision is made to administer anticoagulant therapy.

Venography has at least three disadvantages: (1) it is painful; (2) it can itself induce thrombosis in 3 to 4 per cent of patients; and (3) when standard techniques are employed, the external and common iliac veins are inadequately opacified in up to 18 per cent of patients. As a result, Hull and his colleagues[336, 337] have recommended that the technique be replaced in the investigation of suspected venous thrombosis by impedance plethysmography and ^{125}I-fibrinogen leg scanning.

An interesting prospective study was carried out by Dorfman and his coworkers[771] in which $\dot{V}/\dot{Q}$ scans were employed to determine the incidence of occult pulmonary emboli in patients with proven deep venous thrombosis. Fifty-eight patients without symptoms of pulmonary embolism but with venographically proven venous thrombosis were subjected to chest roentgenography, ^{99m}Tc perfusion scans, and ^{133}Xe ventilation scans: of the 49 patients with deep venous thrombosis proximal to the calf veins, 17 (35 per cent) had high probability scans; of all 58 patients, only 12 (21 per cent) had normal scans. The authors concluded that baseline $\dot{V}/\dot{Q}$ lung scanning can be a valuable procedure in patients with proven above-knee deep venous thrombosis.

Scintigraphy

The intravenous injection of ^{125}I-labeled fibrinogen (along with daily doses of oral iodine), followed by scanning of the legs, can aid in the detection of thrombosis and thus the prevention of pulmonary embolism.[332] The technique is inaccurate in the veins of the upper thigh and pelvis, where a Doppler ultrasonic flow detector or impedance plethysmography may provide more information (see farther on).[338] It is also said to be unreliable as a diagnostic test for deep vein thrombosis in patients who have recently been heparinized. A ^{125}I-labeled fibrinogen uptake study, with or without an ultrasound flow detector test or impedance plethysmography, can be used to monitor deep vein thrombosis postoperatively, to detect extension of thrombosis from the leg into the thigh, and to decide whether anticoagulant therapy is needed.[17, 332] The test has also been used to assess the potential benefits of such methods of prophylaxis as electrical stimulation of the calf muscles, pneumatic compression of the calves, passive flexion of the foot during surgery, and small doses of heparin injected subcutaneously.[332, 339–343] However, there is no convincing evidence that techniques that reduce the frequency of small calf thrombi detectable by the ^{125}I-fibrinogen technique will lower the incidence of pulmonary embolism.[17] In fact, as discussed earlier, it seems probable that most thrombi reaching the lungs originate in the iliofemoral axis rather than in the calf.

Scintigraphic detection of venous thrombi in man by ^{111}In-labeled autologous platelets was first reported by Davis and associates.[300] It has been shown in animals[301] and in humans[302] that such platelets can adhere to venous thrombi, target-to-background ratios being sufficient to permit external "hot spot" imaging with a scintillation camera. The correlation between venography and scintigraphy in the diagnosis of deep venous thrombosis has been excellent.[303] Whereas ^{125}I-labeled fibrinogen has been found to be useful in the detection of calf vein thrombosis as it forms, ^{111}In-labeled platelets will reveal already established thrombi high in the iliofemoral segment.[304] Tissue confirmation of a pulmonary embolus was obtained in a patient who continued to incorporate labeled platelets into a suspected pulmonary embolus after 5 weeks of heparin therapy; reluctance to accept the evidence provided by an unproven technique precipitated the thoracotomy, even in the presence of a positive angiogram.[305] This technique was also used successfully to detect deep venous thrombosis in 13 of 29 patients with acute exacerbations of COPD, nine of the 13 being in the calf; pulmonary emboli were found at autopsy in the one patient who died.[306]

Future developments of this scintigraphic method will be awaited with interest.

Ultrasonography

A noninvasive procedure showing a high degree of accuracy in the detection of fresh thrombi in popliteal and proximal veins is the Doppler ultrasound flow detection method.[343, 338] Normal venous sound is recognized by its cyclic nature, coincident with the respiratory cycle, and by its modification with the Valsalva and Mueller maneuvers. Thrombosis in the iliofemoral veins is readily recognizable by alteration in audible sounds or flow-velocity patterns recorded over the common femoral vein. This method is said to correlate well with iliac phlebography[344] and has been recommended for screening high-risk patients, phlebography being reserved to confirm the diagnosis before starting therapy. However, others[345] have reported a low percentage of positive findings in patients with pulmonary emboli; as a result, this method of assessing flow variation has largely been replaced by impedance plethysmography.

Impedance Plethysmography

This technique, originally described by Mullick and Wheeler and their colleagues in the 1970s,[346, 347] is based on variations in blood flow measured by a change in electrical resistance between electrodes fastened to the calf. Since blood is an excellent conductor of electricity, the change in limb venous blood volume when a thigh cuff is inflated normally results in decreased resistance; when the cuff pressure is released, a prompt increase in resistance follows. Constant dilatation of the deep venous system caused by thrombotic occlusion results in little or no change in resistance with this maneuver.

As previously noted, lower limb venography induces deep venous thrombosis in 3 to 4 per cent of patients,[336] and therefore a safe and reliable noninvasive method of determining deep vein patency is highly desirable; it appears that impedance plethysmography achieves this purpose, especially when combined with fibrinogen scanning.[336, 348, 349–352] With venography used as a standard, the sensitivity of this method in the identification of thrombi above the knee has been estimated to be 95 per cent.[350, 353] One group of investigators[351] has obtained similar results using impedance plethysmography in combination with quantitative analysis of fibrin degradation products. Radiofibrinogen leg scanning and impedance plethysmography are now generally recommended as screening procedures in all patients at risk for,[354] or suspected of having, pulmonary embolism.[350, 355]

Thermography

Conventional infrared telethermography has been successfully employed for the diagnosis of deep vein thrombosis since the early 1970s.[356, 357]

Henderson and associates[358] showed that thermograms performed after exercise of the lower limbs were positive in patients who developed thrombosis detected by the fibrinogen-uptake test after abdominal surgery. However, a later study,[359] in which similar methods were employed postoperatively with exercise, failed to detect a significant difference in the incidence of thrombosis in patients whose thermograms were positive and in those whose thermograms were negative.

In recent years, a new thermographic technique, liquid crystal contact color thermography, has been developed and appears to show considerable promise as a noninvasive screening study for the diagnosis of deep venous thrombosis in high-risk patients.[360] As pointed out by Pochaczevsky and associates,[360] cholesteric crystals possess the property of changing colors in consistent, predictable patterns in response to local temperature changes. The technique consists of imbedding liquid crystals in elastic, flexible sheets, which are then inflated and adapted to the contour of extremities of various sizes and shapes. Preliminary results have shown excellent correlation with ascending phlebography, the two methods being in agreement in 90 per cent of cases.[360]

Magnetic Resonance Imaging

A prospective study of 16 patients was recently carried out by Spritzer and his colleagues[742] in which limited flip-angle, gradient-refocused MRI was compared with venography for the presence or absence of deep venous thrombosis. They showed that thrombosed vessels possessed decreased-to-absent signal intensity whereas patent vessels were characterized by high signal intensity. In 16 of 17 extremities, MRI allowed accurate detection and localization of the thrombi that had been identified by venography, permitting the authors to conclude that MRI with limited flip-angle, gradient-refocused pulse sequences appears to be a sensitive, noninvasive means of detecting deep venous thrombosis.

Comparison of Angiography and Isotopic Scanning

In several studies, pulmonary scintigraphy and angiography have been correlated in the evaluation of patients with pulmonary embolism.[283, 361 366, 743–745] By and large, all studies agree on two basic principles.

1. Pulmonary $\dot{V}/\dot{Q}$ scans and angiograms are complementary—not competitive—techniques in the evaluation of pulmonary embolic disease.

2. Each method has diagnostic limitations.

A study of 14 patients with pulmonary embolism established by both lung scanning and selective pulmonary angiography, and in whom other cardiopulmonary disease had been excluded,[363] showed that the lung scan better depicted capillary flow and the angiogram better detected embolic material in large vessels but that the findings with both correlated reasonably well overall in the assessment of embolic involvement. When embolization involved less than 40 per cent of the lung, it was better demonstrated by the perfusion scan, whereas more extensive involvement was more reliably recorded by angiogram. Agreement was closest when a massive clot completely obstructed either a part of the main pulmonary artery or a junction of the main and lobar pulmonary arteries. It was concluded that although overall correlation was good, either technique could result in significantly underestimating the extent of embolism and both might be necessary to determine this reasonably accurately.

Using subselective, scintigraphically guided, magnification arteriography and eight-view perfusion scintigraphy in a study of experimental canine emboli, Bookstein and associates found excellent angiographic-scintigraphic correlation both immediately after embolization and during the entire course of lysis.[367] In a study of 71 patients with findings indicative of pulmonary embolism who underwent lung scanning and then pulmonary angiography,[364] the scan predicted specific arteriographic evidence of pulmonary embolism in 75 per cent of those in whom the scan defects were characteristic of embolism (i.e., the perfusion defects corresponded to specific anatomic segments and the chest roentgenograms were normal or suggested pulmonary embolism). This study confirmed previous observations that in patients with COPD, congestive cardiac failure, or bronchial asthma, only pulmonary arteriography can establish the diagnosis of embolism with certainty. A remarkably high degree of correlation of results of scanning and arteriography was found in a study[365] of 48 patients in whom these were performed because of the clinical possibility of pulmonary embolism. There was 94 per cent agreement between the scan and both arteriogram and plain roentgenogram, and in all cases a negative scan correlated with a negative arteriogram. All correlative studies have shown that although scanning is not as reliable as angiography in assessing oligemia at the lung bases, it has the theoretic advantage of depicting the circulation in the lung periphery, an area poorly visualized by angiography.[261, 368] The volume of lung parenchyma is 20 to 30 times the size of a supply vessel 1 to 2 mm in diameter and is easily visualized by scanning when the vessel is occluded; by contrast, vessels of this size are seldom well depicted angiographically.[369]

A study by Gilday and associates[361] of 101 patients thought clinically to have pulmonary embolism who were subjected to both lung scanning and angiography sums up the position of these two procedures in the investigation of a suspected embolic episode. In all 44 patients with pulmonary emboli shown by angiography, scans were abnormal, and none of the 21 patients with normal lung scans had emboli on angiography. Correlation between scan and angiogram was good (85 per cent) when the distribution of focal scan defects was lobar but was less (64 per cent) when this was segmental. In 77 per cent of the 53 patients judged on pulmonary scanning to have a high probability of pulmonary embolism, emboli were demonstrated angiographically.

As might be anticipated from the foregoing, the findings on $\dot{V}/\dot{Q}$ scintigraphy exert a considerable influence on whether pulmonary angiography is to be performed. In a prospective-retrospective study of 600 patients clinically suspected of having pulmonary embolism, Sostman and his colleagues[370] assessed the use of pulmonary angiography in relation to $\dot{V}/\dot{Q}$ scintigraphy at two teaching hospitals. Of the 60 patients who underwent angiography (30 in each institution), the scintigraphic diagnosis was shown to have a major impact on the frequency of requests for angiography, inconclusive scintigraphy being the principal reason for such requests; however, nearly half the patients for whom scintigraphic assessment was indecisive were managed without further diagnostic measures. Few patients in the low-probability and high-probability scintigraphic categories received angiography. It has also been shown that regardless of the findings on $\dot{V}/\dot{Q}$ scintigraphy, pulmonary angiography (including selective injection and magnification) can effectively rule out clinically significant pulmonary thromboembolism: of a group of 180 consecutive patients with suspected pulmonary embolism and negative pulmonary arteriograms, not one of the 167 untreated patients died as a result of thromboembolic disease during the acute illness;[371] of the 147 patients who survived (20 died from unrelated causes), none suffered episodes of recurrent embolism during a minimum 6-month follow-up.

Follow-up studies of patients with normal scintigraphic findings have shown similar results: of 68 patients with suspected pulmonary embolism and normal lung scans in one study, thromboembolic disease developed in only one.[307] Similarly, McNeil and associates[372] followed 42 young patients ranging in age from 18 to 40 who presented with pleural pain and who had normal findings on perfusion scanning; all remained in good health, and none had a recurrence of chest pain over a period of 6 to 18 months.

We conclude that $\dot{V}/\dot{Q}$ scintigraphy should be the initial screening procedure in patients suspected of having acute pulmonary embolism. If the findings are abnormal but inconclusive and if the suspicion of embolism is high on the basis of clinical and roentgenographic findings, angiography should be performed. If angiographic results are negative, impedance plethysmography and fibrinogen lower limb scanning (or venography) may reveal the site of thrombosis for peripherally located pulmonary emboli.[329] Gilday and his associates[361] also recommend pulmonary angiography to confirm a scan diagnosis before pulmonary embolectomy, inferior vena caval interruption, or thrombolytic therapy. We are in general agreement with the requirement for angiography before the institution of thrombolytic therapy or any form of surgery, but do not favor its invariable use before starting anticoagulant therapy. If a pulmonary scan is positive and there is strong clinical evidence of an acute embolic episode but the chest roentgenogram is normal, we hold that anticoagulant therapy should be started without further diagnostic intervention. In fact, if the chest roentgenogram reveals an abnormality consistent with embolism and infarction and the patient has symptoms and signs of peripheral venous thrombosis, there seems to be little indication for a scan. In such cases, the results of this procedure should not influence the decision to institute anticoagulant therapy.

CLINICAL MANIFESTATIONS

The clinical manifestations of pulmonary thromboembolic disease depend on several factors that, individually or in combination, influence the effect of vascular occlusion on the lung parenchyma: (1) the presence or absence of cardiopulmonary disease; (2) the size, number, and location of emboli; (3) whether vessel occlusion is complete or partial; and (4) the time interval between embolic episodes.[143] Most pulmonary thromboemboli produce no symptoms or cause such minimal distress that they may be recognized only in retrospect, regardless of whether the occlusion has occurred in the smaller vessels, the segmental arteries, or even the lobar arteries. In fact, even though supposedly normal persons may die suddenly as a result of pulmonary embolism,[373, 374] a large embolus obstructing a major vessel may give rise to only minor disturbance in circulatory dynamics and minimal clinical and roentgenographic findings.[149] In such cases, serial angiograms show disappearance of the clot within a few days as a result of lysis, or fragmentation and dispersal to smaller vessels, or a combination of both.[144, 150, 375–377] In a patient with cardiovascular disease, however, a similar episode is much more likely to lead to infarction, cardiac arrhythmia, systemic hypotension, and death. Symptoms and signs are also often absent during individual episodes of multiple pulmonary emboli that are of sufficient severity to cause chronic cor pulmonale over time.[144, 172, 380] The major clue to the diagnosis of pulmonary embolism is a well-defined predisposing condition.[45, 72]

When present, the most common symptoms of angiographically proven thromboembolism are dyspnea (over 80 per cent of patients), cough (70 per cent), and pleural pain (58 to 70 per cent).[72, 381] Hemoptysis is comparatively uncommon (20 to 33 per cent of cases),[72, 146, 207, 382–384] but is obviously important to recognize because it implies hemorrhage or infarction. The onset of dyspnea or pain is usually abrupt, an observation that aids in differentiation from pneumonia, in which the onset is usually more gradual and is accompanied by cough productive of purulent material. Rarely, dyspnea is sporadic and is associated with wheezing, simulating bronchial asthma.[132, 136, 385, 386] In about 50 per cent of cases, close questioning will elicit a history of one or more transitory episodes of dyspnea in the past, harbingers of later, more distressing embolism and infarction.[113, 144, 369, 382, 387] In fact, it has been estimated[378, 379] that any patient who has had a pulmonary embolism has a 30 per cent chance of a further embolic episode, an incidence much greater than that occurring in a general hospital population. Chest pain can be of two types: *retrosternal,* similar to that of of angina pectoris,[114, 145] or *pleuritic,* a consequence of pulmonary infarction.

Physical findings of thromboembolism are usually nonspecific—tachypnea, rales, tachycardia (with or without arrhythmias), and manifestations of pulmonary arterial hypertension.[381] Fever is fairly common and should not be regarded as a useful sign in distinguishing infarction from pneumonia.

The presence of signs and symptoms of deep venous thrombosis, particularly in the legs, is supportive evidence of pulmonary thromboembolism and must be carefully assessed in all patients in whom the latter diagnosis is entertained. Localized pain or tenderness in the calf, popliteal fossa, or thigh, especially if associated with a discrepancy in the diameter of the legs, suggests venous thrombosis. In some cases, pain may be elicited by dorsiflexion of the foot (Homans' sign). Although these findings are helpful when present, their absence does not in any way militate against a diagnosis of thromboembolism: since approximately 50 per cent of patients who suffer a fatal embolism show no clinical evidence of deep thrombosis during life,[40, 41] it is not unusual for persons who recover from pulmonary embolism to have no symptoms or signs of peripheral thrombosis. When it is recognized, pulmonary embolism usually occurs within weeks of the detection of peripheral venous thrombosis,[388] although in some cases it may precede such evidence.[389] For example, in one study of 93 patients who were referred to surgeons after medical therapy had failed to control pulmonary emboli,[60] 46 showed no clinical evidence of venous thrombosis; however, leg signs later developed in 36 and venography confirmed thrombosis in all (thrombosis never became clinically evident in the others).

Although the clinical manifestations of pulmonary thromboembolism and infarction are chiefly respiratory or cardiac,[390, 391] they can also mimic acute abdominal or cerebral disease.[205, 207, 382, 390, 392] Diaphragmatic pleuritis, ileus, and a rise in serum bilirubin may suggest a diagnosis of acute cholecystitis. Neurologic signs include restlessness, anxiety, syncope, convulsions, irrational behavior, hemiparesis or monoparesis, confusion, and coma.[114, 390, 392, 393] They appear mainly in elderly, bedridden, or cardiac patients and almost certainly are caused by a combination of previous cerebrovascular disease, hypoxemia, and acute cerebral vasospasm resulting from hypocarbia.

In general, pulmonary thromboembolic disease consists of the following three fairly well-defined syndromes that reflect the size and numbers of thrombi: (1) massive pulmonary embolism, (2) pulmonary infarction, and (3) pulmonary hypertension.

MASSIVE PULMONARY EMBOLISM

Massive pulmonary embolism results when a thrombus lodges in the bifurcation of main branches of the pulmonary artery, obstructing at least 50 per cent of the pulmonary vascular bed. As a result of acute cor pulmonale, central venous pressure rises and cardiac output falls. Peripheral venous vasoconstriction may prevent systemic hypotension, but with very high resistance in the lesser circulation the blood pressure falls, and the clinical presentation is that of circulatory collapse or shock.[295] Patients complain of severe dyspnea and retrosternal pain, and tachycardia, tachypnea, and—in some—cyanosis develop. Auscultation may reveal bronchial breathing but rarely rales or a friction rub. The jugular veins are distended, and gallop rhythm is invariably audible. There may be a diffuse systolic lift at the left sternal edge, with accentuation of the pulmonic component of the second heart sound. If the right ventricle fails acutely, a finding often associated with severe systemic hypotension, these signs of pulmonary hypertension may be absent.[72, 275, 295, 331, 394]

Although characteristic, this dramatic clinical presentation is absent in some cases.[395, 396] Rare reported findings include pulsus alternans and intensification of cyanosis caused by development of a right-to-left shunt through a patent foramen ovale. This latter development is an uncommon sequel to pulmonary hypertension, which in one instance was shown to be dramatically reversed with thrombolytic therapy of an intraventricular thrombus and pulmonary emboli.[397] Massive pulmonary embolism must be distinguished from myocardial infarction[398] and, when neurologic manifestations predominate,[392] from a cerebrovascular accident.

PULMONARY INFARCTION

Occasionally, pulmonary infarction may be caused by fragmentation and peripheral embolization of a central pulmonary thromboembolus, in which case the clinical picture may be the same as in massive embolism. More commonly, however, infarction is seen in relation to occlusion of segmental or subsegmental arteries.[22] In these cases, the patient complains of dyspnea of acute onset, pain on breathing, and possibly hemoptysis. Tachycardia and fever are often present; the latter is usually low

grade (37.2 to 37.7° C), but temperature may go as high as 39.5° C. Fever occurs in 18 per cent[146] to 50 per cent of cases.[399] Findings include locally decreased breath sounds, rales, rhonchi, friction rub, and signs of pleural effusion.[119, 207, 374] Rarely, pulmonary emboli of this size traverse a congenital septal defect or a patent foramen ovale, causing paradoxical embolism.[400, 401] The differential diagnosis includes pneumonia, atelectasis, and primary pleural effusion. However, pneumonia usually causes higher fever and purulent expectoration and the onset is more insidious. It may be difficult to rule out atelectasis, since both complications are common postoperatively. The pleural effusion of pulmonary infarction is usually grossly bloody, unless diluted with the transudate of heart failure. If an infarct cavitates (which is rare), confusion may arise with acute lung abscess.[224, 240] Since patients with sickle-cell disease are prone to both pneumonia and infarction, the difficulty in differentiation is increased in these patients.[49, 402, 403]

Thromboembolic disease is particularly difficult to diagnose in patients with COPD, largely because of abnormal perfusion scans. However, this has been shown not to be a problem in young smokers: in a study of 40 smokers (at least one pack/year) aged 18 to 29 years, perfusion scans were completely normal in all.[404] When perfusion scans mismatch with ventilation scans and the defects are segmental or lobar in size and few in number, emboli are almost certainly the cause, even in patients who manifest some roentgenographic evidence of obstructive pulmonary disease. When COPD is roentgenographically widespread, perfusion scans are invariably indeterminate and angiography is required for confirming a definitive diagnosis of pulmonary embolic disease.[322] In one study of three COPD patients with angiographically proven pulmonary embolism, the Pa_{CO_2} dropped immediately in all, a finding that may suggest the diagnosis.[405] It is difficult to assess the frequency with which acute exacerbations of COPD are precipitated by pulmonary embolism, although our own experience would suggest that this is uncommon. In two separate studies, the incidence of proximal lower limb thrombosis was documented in 6 per cent[352] and 30 per cent[306] of patients whose symptoms of COPD underwent acute clinical deterioration.

PULMONARY HYPERTENSION

When a multitude of thromboemboli, usually of small size, impact in arteries and arterioles and cause vascular obstruction, arterial hypertension is almost inevitable. If only a small cross section of the vascular bed is occluded, most patients are asymptomatic. If more than 50 per cent of the vascular bed is affected, progressive dyspnea on exertion and, in some patients, right ventricular failure develop. Some complain of episodic transient dyspnea, presumably a result of intermittent microembolism. Recurrent attacks of cardiac arrhythmia, particularly atrial flutter, may occur.[406] Unusual clinical findings reported in association with pulmonary hypertension include a continuous murmur (believed to be caused by pulmonary artery stenosis[407]) and paralysis of the left vocal cord (caused by compression of the recurrent laryngeal nerve between the aorta and pulmonary artery).[408] The latter condition has been reported more often in association with primary hypertension,[409, 410] a disease difficult to differentiate from multiple pulmonary embolization and considered further in Chapter 10.

Laboratory Findings

Laboratory tests, including serum enzyme levels of lactate dehydrogenase (LDH) and serum glutamic-oxalo-acetic transaminase (SGOT) and the measurement of fibrin and fibrinogen degradation products, have been largely abandoned as useful criteria of thromboembolic disease. Wacker's triad—an increased level of LDH, a normal level of SGOT, and a slightly increased level of serum bilirubin[411, 412]—occurs in approximately 12 per cent of cases of pulmonary embolism,[187] and has not been found to be useful in distinguishing embolism from myocardial infarction or pneumonia.[187, 413, 414] On the other hand, levels of creatinine phosphokinase (CPK) may distinguish myocardial infarction from massive pulmonary embolism.[415]

The body reacts to thrombus formation by increasing serum fibrinolytic activity. This response is effective in the microcirculation, where capillary endothelial cells contain large amounts of plasminogen activator, the enzyme that converts plasminogen to plasmin, which in turn acts on fibrinogen and fibrin. Fibrinolysis leads to the formation of substances known as fibrinogen-fibrin degradation products (FDP-fdp) or fibrin split products (FSP); these can be measured by several methods, including radioimmunoassay,[416] a staphylococcal clumping test,[417] and tanned red cell hemagglutination inhibition immunoassay.[418, 419] In patients with deep vein thrombosis in the leg, the serum levels of FDP-fdp may be significantly increased, although there is overlap in patients with and without proved deep vein thrombosis.[413, 420–422] When deep vein thrombosis is extensive, levels are considerably higher and hence of greater diagnostic value.[421, 423] Since many of these studies were carried out postoperatively, any FDP-fdp increases produced by the lysis of thrombi at the operative site would have tended to mask increases due to deep vein thrombosis.[420] FDP-fdp levels are higher with pulmonary thromboembolism than with deep vein thrombosis alone and, although false-positive and false-negative results occur, the technique helps substantiate a clinical diagnosis.[413, 420, 421, 424, 425–427]

In one study, a quantitative determination of FDP was found to be a practical and reliable screening test for deep venous thrombosis and, when used in conjunction with impedance plethysmography, was shown to improve both sensitivity and specificity of the latter.[351] The high levels of fibrin-fibrinogen split products in pulmonary embolism reflect the abundance of plasminogen activator in capillary endothelial cells. This rise may be very transient,[428] which may explain why some authors[413] have been unable to confirm this finding. Levels of FDP-fdp are highest in patients with acute symptoms and those in whom cardiac catheterization shows increased total pulmonary resistance.[427]

Although potentially helpful in the diagnosis of pulmonary thromboembolism, fibrin split products are also considerably increased and hypofibrinogenemia and thrombocytopenia also are present in patients with disseminated intravascular coagulation (DIC),[429] during normal labor (and particularly in complicated pregnancy at term), and in liver disease, recent myocardial infarction,[427] malignancy, immunologically mediated connective tissue disease, infection, vasculitis, renal disease, and leukemia.[429] The suggestion that plasma and serum concentration of deoxyribonucleic acid (DNA) can be useful diagnostic measurements in the diagnosis of pulmonary embolism[430] was not confirmed in a later study in which patients who did not show abnormalities on angiography or scintigraphy were used as controls.[431]

The leukocyte count seldom exceeds 15,000/mm³. Forty-four of 47 patients with angiographically proven pulmonary embolism had counts below this, and in almost half the count was less than 10,000/mm³.[399] Any increase in neutrophils is usually associated with fever and symptoms and signs of pulmonary infarction.

Sanguineous pleural fluid strongly suggests pulmonary infarction, particularly if malignancy has been excluded. Serous effusion is probably caused by cardiac failure.[432]

Pulmonary function studies reveal restrictive disease. The resting lung volume is decreased and airway resistance is increased, and lung compliance and diffusing capacity are reduced. Most of the patients hyperventilate.[119, 433] Arterial blood gas analysis reveals low PO_2 values and respiratory alkalosis.[119, 433–435] The arterial PO_2 was ≤ 80 mm Hg in 36 patients with angiographically proven acute pulmonary embolism,[187] and it was concluded that this is a sensitive and useful test for screening patients suspected of having this disorder. Despite this, the urokinase study group reported arterial PO_2 values of 80 mm Hg or greater in 13 of 113 similar patients, including three of 70 with massive pulmonary embolism.[72, 436] Furthermore, pulmonary embolism is commoner in older patients, in whom PaO_2 is normally 80 mm Hg or less. The value of blood gas studies in this disorder is limited by the occurrence of similar changes in heart failure, atelectasis, and pneumonia, the main conditions to be differentiated. This hypoxemia cannot always be corrected by the patient's breathing 100 per cent oxygen, suggesting intrapulmonary venous shunting that may be due to pulmonary edema.[151, 399, 437] In most cases, however, the hypoxemia is probably caused chiefly by $\dot{V}/\dot{Q}$ abnormality. Several authors[433, 438–440] stress the value of determining the difference between end tidal and arterial P_{CO_2} as a measurement of large areas of ventilated but unperfused lung. This procedure was introduced by Severinghaus and Stupfel[441] on an experimental basis and was adapted by Robin and associates for clinical use.[438, 439] It is estimated that at least 20 to 30 per cent of lung parenchyma must be unperfused before the P_{CO_2} difference exceeds 6 mm Hg, and compensatory measures that restrict ventilation of the unperfused lung develop rapidly after embolism and render this test almost valueless by 48 hours after the event.[399]

In a review of the subject of gas exchange following pulmonary thromboembolism, it was concluded that the severity and mechanism of abnormalities are likely to depend upon the size and location of emboli, the presence or absence of preexisting cardiopulmonary disease, and the time elapsed since embolization. Arterial blood gas alterations, changes in the Bohr dead space, and arterial-to-end tidal CO_2 gradient are neither sufficiently sensitive nor specific to be of great use in the differential diagnosis of pulmonary embolism.[442]

Interpretation of the results of pulmonary function studies in thromboembolic disease requires consideration of many factors. Many of these patients are extremely ill and cannot cooperate. A predisposing condition, such as heart failure, obesity, recent major surgery, or pregnancy, may influence lung function. Pleural pain may prevent full expansion of the thoracic cage, creating a degree of functional impairment that does not truly reflect the state of the lung parenchyma. The very nature of thromboembolic disease as a dynamic process renders comparison difficult between the results in two series or even between two patients. The most striking finding during pulmonary function assessment 7 to 30 days after onset of the latest embolic episode[443] was the minimal disturbance occasioned by even recurrent emboli in elderly, apparently very ill patients. However, these studies are valuable aids to the diagnosis of pulmonary vascular occlusive disease caused by multiple emboli before pulmonary hypertension develops.[444, 674]

Electrocardiographic Changes

Electrocardiographic (ECG) changes appear early and are often transient; they are caused by acute pulmonary hypertension and hypoxemia and therefore are commonest after massive pulmonary embolism.[187, 275, 445–448] When recurrent embolism results in occlusion of approximately 70 per cent of the pulmonary vascular bed, ECG changes reflect cor pulmonale. Reports of positive ECG changes in

70 per cent or more of patients[390, 445, 448, 449] probably reflect both early recording and moderate-sized emboli; those indicating little or no value of the ECG[380, 383, 399, 450] probably include delayed recordings and smaller emboli.

Certain ECG patterns are considered diagnostic of acute pulmonary embolism; these include an S wave in lead I and an inverted Q wave or T wave or both in lead III, with inversion of the T waves recorded over the right side of the heart. Other less reliable changes are those of right axis deviation and a pattern of right bundle branch block or right ventricular hypertrophy. A leftward shift of the frontal plane electrical axis, attributed to myocardial ischemia from hypoxemia, has been reported.[451] Atrial arrhythmias are frequent,[452] particularly in patients with established heart disease.[187] Early and frequent tracings may be necessary to detect these changes.[114, 449] In contrast to the low diagnostic specificity of the ECG in acute pulmonary embolism, there is no question of the value of the ECG in right ventricular hypertrophy secondary to recurrent thromboembolism; transient T wave inversion in leads V1 to V3 superimposed on the chronic changes may indicate acute pulmonary embolic episodes.[382]

PROGNOSIS

As discussed previously, it is very likely that most thromboembolic episodes are unrecognized clinically:[21, 391, 453] careful search of the pulmonary vascular tree at necropsy has revealed organized thrombi in more than 50 per cent of unselected patients, most of whom had neither a clinical history suggestive of thromboembolic episodes nor pathologic evidence that the emboli had caused morbidity or mortality.[24, 25, 158] It thus must be concluded that the prognosis in the majority of thromboembolic events is good.

In most of these cases, however, the emboli are small and lodge in subsegmental or segmental vessels. By contrast, the outcome of massive thromboembolism (affecting the pulmonary trunk or large portions of one or both main pulmonary arteries) is substantially less favorable: although this event is rarely fatal in adolescents,[746] it is probable that the majority of adult patients so affected die within 30 minutes[154] to 2 hours.[145] On the other hand, the prognosis is much more favorable for those who survive the acute event, partial or complete resolution of the thromboembolism being the rule. Follow-up studies of 15 patients who survived major or massive embolism[173] showed earliest complete resolution at 14 days, and in two others at 15 and 34 days. Serial photoscanning of 69 patients[191] revealed that most of them had complete or nearly complete return of pulmonary blood flow by 4 months. Similarly, follow-up of 33 patients at 30 months[453] showed residual angiographic abnormalities in four and chronic cor pulmonale in none.

In nearly all patients, the resolution of pulmonary embolism is complete clinically and hemodynamically within 4 to 6 weeks of the acute event and is also complete or almost complete roentgenographically and angiographically.[455–457] A minority of patients will complain of dyspnea on exertion or will manifest clinical findings suggesting recurrent embolic episodes; when studied at the time of the initial embolic episode, such patients will have shown significant pulmonary hypertension greater than a mean of 30 mm Hg.[456] Invariably, follow-up studies will be abnormal; pulmonary hypertension tends to persist but an exercise study may be required for it to become apparent.[455, 458]

Patients with pulmonary hypertension caused by chronic thrombotic obstruction of major pulmonary arteries may benefit from embolectomy.[172, 455, 459, 460] In such cases, Moser and his group[461, 462] have accomplished direct visualization of emboli through an angioscope to confirm the diagnosis; the distal tip of this fiberoptic instrument is covered by an inflatable balloon and is inserted through a jugular vein or directly into a pulmonary artery at thoracotomy. Although they and others[172, 455] have had surprising success with thromboendarterectomy, the immediate postoperative course can be stormy as a result of reperfusion pulmonary edema in anatomic locations distal to sites of thrombus removal.[460]

The prognosis of acute pulmonary thromboembolic disease is improved by thrombolytic and anticoagulant therapy. Seriously ill patients should receive either streptokinase or urokinase unless there are anatomic lesions elsewhere that may bleed excessively.[330, 457, 463–465] In contrast to anticoagulants, these agents actually dissolve thrombi and thus prevent long-term disability;[466–468] we suspect that they are underused. Natural fibrinolytic activity of blood can be augmented by strenuous exercise and by physical methods such as elastic compression, electrical stimulation of lower limb muscles, pedaling devices, and pneumatic compression; the use of such methods can reduce the incidence of thrombus formation.[82–84]

In the original controlled trial of heparin in the treatment of pulmonary embolism by Barritt and Jordan in 1960,[469] when five of the 19 controls died and five developed recurrent emboli, it was deemed unethical to withhold heparin from then on; since that time, anticoagulation for thromboembolic disease has been accepted as mandatory for both treatment and prophylaxis.[470–476] Heparin is not equally effective preoperatively for all types of surgery; similarly, it is less effective in the prophylaxis of medical conditions and is not useful at all in the prophylaxis or treatment of thromboembolic disease associated with malignancy. Oral anticoagulants are probably of benefit[477] but are contraindicated during pregnancy in which they should be replaced by heparin.[478] They are also of no value in the rare devastating coagulopathy known as Trousseau's syndrome[479] in which recurring arterial and venous thrombotic events, amputation of limbs, and death eventually occur in the absence of continuous intravenous heparin therapy.

The prognosis of patients with thromboembolic disease may be altered by ligation of or insertion of an umbrella into the inferior vena cava, procedures that are recommended in the presence of septic pulmonary emboli or recurrent small emboli associated with pulmonary hypertension, congestive heart failure, or contraindications to anticoagulant therapy.[457] However, they are accompanied by a high mortality rate in very sick patients, especially those with heart failure.[457] The subsequent development of inadequate venous blood return can result in cardiac limitation to exercise.[766] The prognosis associated with the surgical removal of thromboemboli in chronic vessel obstruction is improved, but whether pulmonary embolectomy can salvage patients with acute massive pulmonary embolism who would not otherwise have survived is controversial;[157] however, apparent successes have been reported.[480, 481]

The major complication associated with the treatment of thromboembolic disease is hemorrhage that occurs with about equal frequency with anticoagulant and fibrinolytic therapy. During 3,862 courses of anticoagulant treatment in one study,[182] 163 (6.8 per cent) hemorrhagic episodes were identified. Some authorities consider that the risk of angiography is less than that of anticoagulant therapy and recommend that patients who show nonspecific or inconclusive abnormalities on lung scan undergo an angiogram before being subjected to anticoagulant therapy.[483] Even those receiving low-dose heparin are not without risk of hemorrhage.[330] Hemorrhage is rarely fatal and occurs most frequently in the brain or gastrointestinal tract.[482] Massive hemothorax consequent upon heparin therapy for pulmonary infarction is extremely uncommon.[484] Sources of error that result in hemorrhage during anticoagulant therapy have been reviewed.[457, 485–487]

The incidence of symptoms originating in the legs—pain, swelling, eczema, pigmentation, varices, induration, and even ulceration—is similar after inferior vena cava ligation and following therapy with anticoagulants alone.[488] Thrombolytic treatment has been reported to be ineffective in preventing the post-thrombotic syndrome.[466] Venography at the time of acute thromboembolic disease has been suspected as being one cause of the post-phlebitic leg.[71]

SUMMARY

Pulmonary thromboembolism, with or without infarction, is a common disease that is often undiagnosed or misdiagnosed. Diagnosis frequently depends upon the physician's alertness to complaints of the sudden onset of dyspnea or pleuritic pain, particularly if this is followed by hemoptysis. Suspicion should be heightened if there are predisposing conditions such as recent fracture, surgical procedures, heart disease, obesity, pregnancy, or estrogen therapy. The diagnosis is virtually certain if the pulmonary symptoms develop in patients with evidence of peripheral venous thrombosis, although the latter is apparent in less than 50 per cent of cases.

If there is even the slightest clinical evidence of pulmonary thromboembolism, a chest roentgenogram, ECG, radioisotopic lung scan, and blood gases should be carried out promptly. Radioisotopic scanning, ultrasonography, impedance plethysmography, and phlebography of the legs are useful to provide circumstantial evidence of pulmonary embolism, to document progression of peripheral thrombus formation, and to decide whether thrombectomy or ligation of peripheral veins or of the inferior vena cava should be done.

A normal chest roentgenogram does not exclude the diagnosis. Positive findings include local oligemia (Westermark's sign), increased caliber and abrupt tapering of the descending branch of the pulmonary artery, hemidiaphragmatic elevation, basal line shadows, and parenchymal consolidation. Parenchymal consolidation varies widely but is nearly always basal and abutting against a visceral pleural surface and often is associated with a small pleural effusion. Although CT appears to be capable of revealing zones of oligemia with greater accuracy than conventional roentgenography and can even demonstrate thrombi within central pulmonary arteries, it appears unlikely that it will gain much support as a cost-effective diagnostic procedure, since radionuclide scans detect lobar or segmental defects with an equivalent accuracy.

Local "cold" zones on a radioisotopic scan without corresponding roentgenographic opacities are virtually pathognomonic of thromboembolism if the scan defect is segmental and chronic lung disease can be reasonably excluded on the basis of history, plain roentgenographic findings, and/or a normal ventilation scan.

Pulmonary angiography is the most definitive technique for diagnosing thromboembolism. Since DSA is less expensive, safer, faster, and easier to perform than conventional pulmonary arteriography, it appears probable that this procedure will become the examination of choice for the evaluation of patients suspected of having pulmonary emboli. Indications for the use of arteriography in the investigation of possible thromboembolic disease are in dispute. Whereas it is generally agreed that it must be performed to confirm a scan diagnosis before pulmonary embolectomy, inferior vena cava interruption, or thrombolytic therapy, some dispute its requirement before starting anticoagulant therapy. While recognizing the views of those who insist upon angiographic proof before instituting this therapy, we subscribe to the position that if a pulmonary scan is positive in a patient with strong clinical evidence of a recent embolic episode, and the chest roentgenogram is normal or reveals abnormalities compatible with the diagnosis, angiography should be avoided and anticoagulant therapy started at once. Possible exceptions are patients with COPD, in whom perfusion defects are likely without embolism. Although the diagnosis sometimes cannot be established short of pulmonary angiography, the administration of anticoagulant therapy on suspicion alone is preferable to confirmation of the diagnosis at necropsy.

EMBOLI OF EXTRAVASCULAR TISSUES AND SECRETIONS

Fragments of virtually any organ, normal tissue, or body secretion can theoretically gain access to the systemic circulation and be transported to the lungs. Some, such as megakaryocytes and trophoblast cells, do this with such frequency that the process can be considered a normal phenomenon. Other fragments are found only in pathologic conditions, in which circumstances tissue disruption with venous laceration is a necessary precondition; thus, the underlying pathogenesis is frequently trauma, most often associated with labor, accidental or battlefield injuries, or procedures such as venipuncture or surgery. Occasionally, a necrotizing inflammatory process can release small tissue fragments into the bloodstream with similar results. As a result of their inherent invasive properties, neoplastic cells can gain access to the systemic circulation without the aid of trauma; although in these circumstances emboli are usually microscopic and of no consequence from a vascular point of view, occasional large fragments or numerous small ones can cause significant vascular obstruction.

With the exception of neoplastic tissue, amniotic fluid, and possibly fat, the vast majority of these emboli are discovered incidentally at autopsy and are of little or no clinical or roentgenographic importance.

FAT EMBOLISM

Although intact fragments of adipose tissue are occasionally found in the pulmonary arteries following severe trauma, the term fat embolism traditionally refers to the presence of globules of free fat within the vasculature. Exogenous fatty material, such as ethiodized oil used as roentgenographic contrast media, is also usually excluded from the definition and is discussed further on (see page 1803). The subject was extensively reviewed in a 1962 monograph by Sevitt.[489]

Etiology and Pathogenesis

The commonest source of fat emboli is the bone marrow. Arguments in favor of this site are summarized by Sevitt:[489] (1) the presence of free marrow fat in the vicinity of recent fractures; (2) the presence of pulmonary fat emboli in experimental animals after fracture or marrow disruption; (3) the presence of fat globules in the blood of humans after fractures and a variety of orthopedic procedures; (4) the frequency with which bone marrow fragments are present in association with fat emboli; (5) a positive correlation between the extent of pulmonary fat embolism and the severity of bone injury; (6) the prevention in experimental animals of fat embolism after fracture by prior venous ligation or application of a tourniquet; and (7) experiments in which marrow fat stained with a dye was traced into the lung.

Pulmonary fat embolism has also been reported in patients and in experimental animals that have suffered crush injury,[489] suggesting an origin from nonosseous fat; however, as Sevitt has noted,[489] such emboli are unlikely to be of importance unless extensive areas of the body are involved, in which circumstance it would be difficult to exclude concomitant bone trauma. In patients in whom the lesser circulation is already compromised, however, an origin of fat from soft tissues may be of considerable significance; for example, there has been a report of two patients with emphysema and one with kyphoscoliosis who had a history of falls and bruises but no fractures; all three died 3 to 5 hours after admission and were found at autopsy to have extensive fat embolism.[490] Additional potential sources of fat emboli include fatty liver (induced by a variety of drugs such as steroids[491, 492] and alcohol[493]), poisons (including carbon tetrachloride, phosphorus, and methyl alcohol[489]), intravenously infused lipid emulsions utilized in long-term hyperalimentation,[747] and following liposuction.[717] The possibility that intravascular fat can be derived from altered blood lipoproteins or chylomicrons or from stress-induced lipemia has also been considered,[489, 494, 495] but there is no conclusive evidence that these mechanisms are of any importance.[489]

Accidental or battlefield trauma is by far the most common antecedent of pulmonary fat embolism; autopsy series on patients who have died after injury show an incidence ranging from 67 to 97 per cent.[494, 496, 497] In addition to trauma, however, any condition or procedure that disrupts the marrow has the potential of causing this complication. Examples include sickle-cell disease with bone marrow infarction, intraosseous venography,[498, 499] epileptic[500, 501] and other convulsive states,[489] replacement arthroplasty,[502, 503] acute osteomyelitis,[506] and external cardiac massage.[504] The widespread use of the last-named procedure probably makes it the commonest cause of fat embolism after accidental fractures; in one necropsy study of 57 patients who had had external cardiac massage, pulmonary fat emboli were identified in 46 (80 per cent).[504] Pulmonary fat embolism has also been associated occasionally with a variety of nontraumatic conditions such as diabetes mellitus,[494, 498–500, 502, 503, 505, 506] pancreatitis, severe burns, extracorporeal circulation, and corticosteroid therapy.[492] It has even been suggested that fat may contribute to the roentgenographically apparent and often undiagnosed diffuse interstitial disease following bone marrow transfusion.[507]

Although it is well accepted that the vast majority of fat emboli to the lungs and systemic organs are derived from traumatized bone marrow, the effects of the fat and possible pathogenetic mechanisms of these effects are controversial. The presence of roentgenographic changes and of signs and symptoms of pulmonary disease shortly after trauma has understandably led to the belief that the intravascular fat itself is responsible. However, in some autopsy studies,[508, 509] little correlation has been found between the presence of intravascular fat and clinical manifestations, leaving the pathogenetic relationship of the two open to question. In addition, although there is some indication that early surgical stabilization of extensive long bone fractures can decrease the incidence and severity of post-traumatic pulmonary insufficiency,[748, 749] when pelvic or long bone fractures are unaccompanied by sepsis or by severe injuries to the brain, chest, or abdomen, the severity of adult respiratory distress syndrome (ARDS) appears to be relatively mild and recovery is common.[750] Sevitt[489] has stated that pulmonary fat emboli are unlikely to be of clinical significance in previously healthy individuals and that pulmonary manifestations are more likely to be secondary to the complications of systemic emboli, particularly to the brain, or to conditions such as ARDS that result from the initial injury or its nonembolic complications.

Even if fat emboli are accepted as an important cause of pulmonary disease, the pathogenetic mechanisms are unclear. Fat appears to be transported to the lungs as neutral triglycerides,[510] and it has been proposed[511] that these are converted by intrapulmonary lipases into free fatty acids that can exert a direct toxic effect on the pulmonary endothelium. Such damage could result in the release of chemotoxins from leukocytes, further exaggerating the injury.[751] Supporting this hypothesis are experimental studies in which severe pulmonary edema and hemorrhage have resulted from the injection of free fatty acids into the pulmonary arteries.[512, 513] However, experimental studies in which neutral fat has been injected have not found evidence for conversion to free fatty acids;[513–516] in addition, it has been suggested that severe trauma itself can result in complement activation.[752]

It is also possible that fat emboli, if sufficient in number, can cause vascular obstruction; in support of this is the observation that pulmonary arterial pressure can rise transiently in experimental animals soon after embolization.[514] Mechanical vascular obstruction accompanied by unexplained sludging of erythrocytes has also been proposed as the cause of hemorrhagic necrosis in the skin and brain.[516] However, in most cases the typical 1- to 3-day delay of symptoms and the usual absence of acute right heart failure suggest that these are not important mechanisms of clinical pulmonary disease in most cases. Finally, it has been suggested that intravascular coagulation, possibly instituted by thromboplastin released from the fat itself, may be important in the pathogenesis.[516, 517]

Typically, the full clinical syndrome of fat embolism develops 1 to 3 days after trauma. The reasons for this delay are unclear, but it has been suggested that they can be explained by (1) continuing embolization from the site of injury, (2) the conversion of neutral triglycerides to unsaturated fatty acids, and (3) imbalance between coagulation and fibrinolysis, leading to deposition of fibrin in pulmonary vessels. From the pulmonary circulation, small fat droplets pass into the general systemic circulation and form emboli in many organs, notably the brain, kidneys, and skin.[518]

Pathologic Characteristics

Pathologically,[489, 508] the lungs of patients who have died with fat emboli are frequently heavy, ranging from 871 to 1404 gm in Scully's series of 102 cases,[508] and show patchy areas of hemorrhage and edema. Fat is most easily identified in frozen sections with fat-soluble dyes, but can also be recognized within arterioles and capillaries as round-to-oval spaces, 20 to 40 μm in diameter, apparently compressing red blood cells to one side (Fig. 9–38).

It can also be seen within alveolar airspaces, where it is ingested by macrophages and eventually carried up the mucociliary escalator or transported to regional lymphatics. Fat can appear within pulmonary capillaries very rapidly after trauma;[489, 519] however, histologic evidence of its presence is rare if the interval between injury and death is more than 4 weeks.[503, 505]

Roentgenographic Manifestations

Pulmonary fat embolism is unrecognized in many cases if it is not severe, partly because symptoms are mild or absent but especially because the chest roentgenogram is often normal—as, for example, in 87.5 per cent of patients in one series in whom the diagnosis of fat embolism was based on the presence of lipiduria.[520] When present, roentgenographic appearances in the lungs are those of ARDS of any cause, consisting of widespread airspace consolidation due to alveolar hemorrhage and edema, often with discrete acinar shadows (Fig. 9–39). The distribution is predominantly peripheral rather than central,[521, 522] usually involving the basal regions to a greater degree than does pulmonary edema of cardiac origin. Further differentiation from cardiogenic edema is provided by the absence of cardiac enlargement and of signs of pulmonary venous hypertension; however, in the series reported by Curtis and associates,[523] diffuse linear opacities resembling interstitial edema were just as common as airspace opacities. The time lapse between trauma and roentgenographic signs is usually 1 to 2 days.[518, 521] This delay in the appearance of signs differentiates fat embolism from traumatic lung contusion. In the latter, roentgenographic opacity invariably appears immediately after injury,

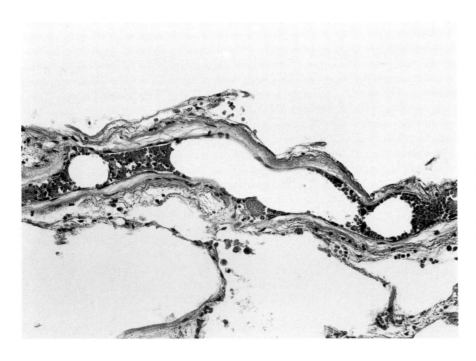

Figure 9–38. Fat Emboli. The lumen of this pulmonary arteriole shows one elongated and two circular spaces that are devoid of blood cells. Such an appearance is suggestive of fat and was confirmed by lipid stains. This histologic section is from a young man who died several hours after a motor vehicle accident; there was no clinical or pathologic evidence of acute lung damage (× 190).

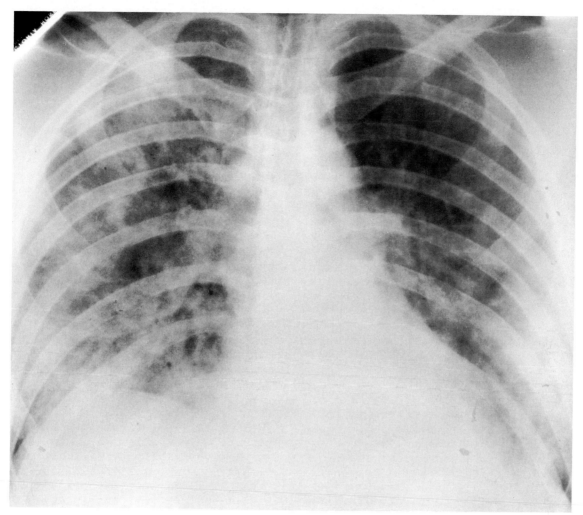

Figure 9–39. Traumatic Fat Embolism. An anteroposterior roentgenogram of a 21-year-old man 3 days after a severe automobile accident reveals extensive involvement of both lungs by patchy shadows of unit density. In many areas the shadows are confluent, but in some they are relatively discrete, permitting identification of individual acinar shadows. For some unknown reason, the left upper lung is less severely involved. Complete roentgenographic resolution occurred 7 days later.

and whereas the opacity usually clears rapidly (in 24 to 26 hours), the roentgenographic resolution of fat embolism takes 7 to 10 days or even up to 4 weeks.[524] Further differentiation lies in the extent of lung involvement: lung contusion seldom affects both lungs diffusely and symmetrically; and when both lungs are involved, the roentgenographic changes are usually more severe in the lung deep to the site of maximal trauma.

Clinical Manifestations

Fat embolism is commonest in young people with leg fractures sustained in vehicular accidents[494, 525, 526] and elderly people with hip fractures or after arthroplasty.[502, 503, 527] Of the 45 cases reported by Ross,[528, 529] 42 had fractures of the femur or tibia and three had pelvic fractures. Despite this, it should be emphasized that the amount of embolized fat in these circumstances is usually insufficient to cause symptoms: in a review of 670 patients with fractures of the femur or tibia,[494] only eight (1.2 per cent) had clinical evidence of fat embolism.

Symptoms usually appear 1 to 2 days after injury.[504, 518, 521] In a review of 15 cases,[526] the mean time of onset was 40 hours, but symptoms may appear almost immediately[499, 522] or within 12 hours.[522, 530] The clinical manifestations can be divided into those arising from the lungs and those originating in other viscera. Symptoms from involvement of the lungs are cough, dyspnea, hemoptysis, and pleural pain; signs include pyrexia, tachypnea, tachycardia, rales, rhonchi, and friction rub.[494, 526] Acute cor pulmonale with cardiac failure, cyanosis, and circulatory shock may occur.[505, 526] Manifestations of fat embolism elsewhere are chiefly caused by involvement of the central nervous system and skin; they include confusion, restlessness, stupor, delirium, and coma,[526, 531, 532] the last-named signifying a poor prognosis. Petechiae are common,[526, 533] particularly along the anterior axillary folds[534] and in the conjunctiva[526] and retina,[526] a distribution which has been attributed to fat floating on the bloodstream and thus affecting vessels that are uppermost.[535] Hypocalcemia usually develops because of the affinity of calcium ions for free fatty acids released by the hydrolysis of fat emboli; the serum calcium level may be of prognostic value.[505, 526] Hemolytic anemia[526, 532, 533] and thrombocytopenia[505, 534] have been reported. Fat droplets may be detected in the urine or sputum,[526] but this is not a reliable indication of the diagnosis;[505] fat droplets are found rarely in cerebrospinal fluid.[536] The triad of petechial rash, cerebral manifestations, and typical pulmonary changes 1 to 2 days after trauma is virtually pathognomonic of fat embolism.

Using these criteria for diagnosis in 30 patients, Curtis and associates[523] recognized three fairly distinct syndromes:

1. Eighteen patients had the classic syndrome consisting of tachypnea, tachycardia, petechiae, and cerebral symptoms. In three of these, the chest roentgenogram revealed localized patchy opacities; in six, bilateral linear opacities simulating interstitial edema; in six, a pattern of alveolar edema; and in only three, normal findings—two patients died of massive pulmonary thromboembolism.

2. Ten patients developed ARDS, all with DIC and very high A-a gradients for oxygen; six died.

3. Two patients died within 24 hours as a result of shunting of fat to the systemic circulation; one had pulmonary hypertension and the shunt occurred through an atrial septal defect, and in the other the shunt was presumably within the lungs.

By contrast, in a review of their experience from 1968 to 1977 using similar criteria, Guenter and Braun[543] recognized 54 patients with the fat embolism syndrome; there were no deaths. An autopsy survey covering the same period identified only one additional case of fat embolism.

In a prospective, randomized, double-blind evaluation of the efficacy of corticosteroid therapy in the prophylaxis of the fat embolism syndrome in high-risk patients, a significant improvement was observed in corticosteroid-treated patients (zero of 21) compared with those who were placebo-treated (nine of 41).[544]

Pulmonary function tests reveal stiffness of the lungs, a diffusion defect, increase in the A-a O_2 gradient, and $\dot{V}/\dot{Q}$ inequality.[526, 532, 537] Severe hypoxemia may persist despite inhalation of 100 per cent oxygen.[537] Decreased diffusing capacity[538] and Pao_2[542] have been observed in patients with fractures of the long bones who have no chest symptoms, indicating subclinical fat embolism to the lungs. Follow-up shows a return to normal pulmonary function.[494]

BONE MARROW EMBOLISM

Pulmonary bone marrow emboli are seen not uncommonly at necropsy in individuals who have sustained fractures or experienced external cardiac massage. In one necropsy study of 51 adult patients who had undergone the latter procedure, eight (15 per cent) showed pulmonary bone marrow emboli.[574] In another review of 203 consecutive necropsies of patients who had sustained multiple fractures, bone marrow emboli were identified in 13 (6 per cent).[575] The true incidence is probably influenced by both the severity of the trauma and the number of lung sections examined; for example, in a study of lungs from 205 victims of an airplane crash in which injury was undoubtedly severe, emboli were found in 60 (29 per cent).[519] Although fractures and external cardiac massage are the most commonly recognized antecedents, a number of other conditions in which bone disruption may occur have been associated, including convulsions (caused by electroconvulsive therapy, epilepsy, eclampsia, or tetanus[575]), bone biopsy,[576] and even vertebral compression fractures related to osteoporosis.[577] It is likely that emboli are also frequent but unrecognized in individuals who sustain solitary and nonlethal fractures or who undergo certain orthopedic procedures such as total hip replacement. Fragments of infarcted marrow, in the absence of known trauma, can also be found in patients with sickle-cell disease.[6]

As in fat embolism, in the vast majority of cases the pathogenesis is related to traumatic fragmentation of marrow and its entry under pressure into disrupted marrow sinusoids or veins. Free fat emboli are probably also present in the majority of cases; in fact, in their study of plane crash victims, Bierre and Koelmeyer[519] found a positive correlation between the extent of fat and bone marrow embolization.

The embolized fragments usually are identified histologically as incidental findings within small muscular arteries or arterioles. Tissue may fill the lumen completely or partly; in the latter case, thrombus may develop at its periphery. Experimental studies have documented periarterial interstitial edema in vessels distal to the emboli;[753] the adjacent pulmonary parenchyma shows no consistent abnormality. When emboli are recent, the histologic appearance is that of normal marrow; occasionally, spicules of bone can be identified (Fig. 9–40).[575, 578] With time, the hematopoietic cells degenerate and disappear and the residual fat and necrotic cells become incorporated into the vessel wall as a fibrous plaque.[578, 754] Infarction of lung parenchyma has not been documented.

The vast majority of bone marrow emboli are of no clinical significance, being discovered incidentally at autopsy or in surgically excised lungs. Although they have been implicated as a major or contributory cause of death in some patients,[577] a true pathogenetic relationship is questionable; in these cases, clinical effects are more likely related to associated free fat embolism or to other systemic disease. Despite this, experimental studies in rabbits have suggested the possibility of the development of chronic hypertension.[754]

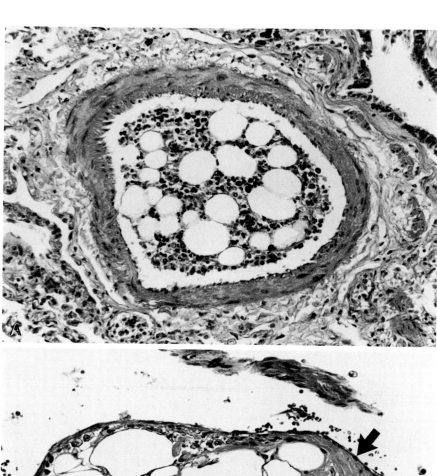

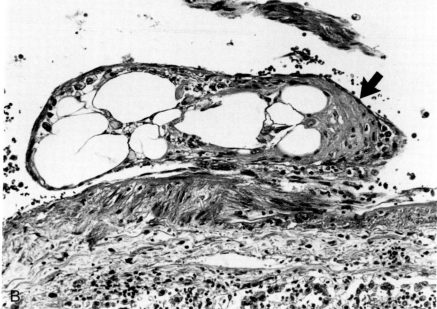

Figure 9–40. Bone Marrow Emboli.
A histologic section of a muscular pulmonary artery (*A*) contains a recent bone marrow embolus; the section is from a patient with myocardial infarction who underwent unsuccessful resuscitation. In a section from another patient who had successful resuscitation but died 10 days later (*B*), the embolus is partly organized; note the loss of marrow cells, focal fibrosis (*arrow*), and adherence of the embolus to the vessel wall. (*A* and *B*, × 180.)

AMNIOTIC FLUID EMBOLISM

Amniotic fluid embolism is a rare but highly lethal complication of pregnancy in which amniotic fluid enters the bloodstream through tears in the uterine veins and is carried to the lungs. Although first recognized in 1926, the entity was not clearly defined until the publication in 1941 of Steiner and Lushbaugh's review,[541] and their description still stands:

> Profound shock coming on suddenly and unexpectedly in a woman who is in unusually severe labor or has just finished such a labor, especially if she is an elderly multipara with an excessively large, perhaps dead, fetus and with meconium in the amniotic fluid, should lead to a suspicion of this possibility. If, also, the shock is introduced by a chill which is followed by dyspnea, cyanosis, vomiting, restlessness and the like and is accompanied by a pronounced fall in blood pressure and a rapid, weak pulse, the picture is more complete. If pulmonary edema now develops quickly in the known absence of previously existing heart disease the diagnosis is reasonably certain.

The incidence of the condition is difficult to establish. Courtney[545] stated that it results in a maternal mortality rate of one in 20,000 to 30,000 deliveries and accounts for 4 to 6 per cent of maternal deaths; another study estimated that about 10 per cent of 1,400 maternal deaths in the United States in 1967 were attributable to the disease.[546] However, because of the difficulty in making the diagnosis at autopsy unless special stains are employed and because of the undoubted presence of nonlethal but unsubstantiated disease in an unspecified number of women,[547, 548] the true incidence is likely to be somewhat higher. Perhaps the most meaningful statement concerning its significance is from a 1961 report from the Sloan Hospital for Women[549] that it was the commonest cause of maternal death during labor or immediately post partum. The subject has been review by Aguillon and his colleagues,[550] by Courtney,[545] and by Morgan.[551]

Pathogenesis

Virtually no amniotic fluid escapes into the maternal circulation during normal pregnancy, labor, or delivery.[552] Only when there is disruption of the uterine wall in association with rupture of the placental membranes can embolization take place. Such disruption can occur in three regions:

1. Through small tears in the veins of the endocervix or lower uterine segment. Such tears can occur during normal labor but are of no significance if covered by fetal membranes; if these have separated, however, uterine contractions against a head impacted in the birth canal can repeatedly pump amniotic fluid into the maternal venous circulation. These circumstances are said to be those most likely to be associated with a lethal outcome.[547]

2. Through the placental site, usually in cases of uterine rupture, placenta previa, premature separation, or cesarean section when the incision involves the placental implantation site.

3. Less commonly, elsewhere in the uterine wall in association with some form of myometrial trauma.

Amniotic fluid is composed of fetal urine, secretions from the amniotic membrane, and a variety of particulate material derived from the fetus, including squames and lanugo hairs from the skin, fat from the vernix caseosa, and mucin and bile from the meconium. It is these particulates that are believed to be responsible for the clinical and pathologic manifestations of disease, meconium being particularly important in this regard.[541, 547] In support of the importance of particulates in pathogenesis are experiments in which no significant harmful effects resulted from the injection of filtered amniotic fluid into the peripheral and pulmonary circulation.[547, 553, 547]

The pathophysiologic consequences of intravascular amniotic fluid can be discussed under four headings: pulmonary vascular obstruction, anaphylaxis, infection and septic shock, and coagulation disturbances.

Pulmonary Vascular Obstruction. Once amniotic fluid enters the maternal circulation, particulate matter is quickly filtered out in the pulmonary vascular bed. Pulmonary artery pressure rises abruptly as a result of a combination of mechanical obstruction and (probably) reflex vasoconstriction.[547] Blood flow to the left side of the heart decreases and cardiac output falls, followed by systemic hypotension and peripheral vascular collapse; permeability pulmonary edema develops rapidly. The severe pulmonary hypertension induces acute right ventricular failure, and hypoxemia causes cerebral manifestations, including restlessness, convulsions, and coma.

Anaphylaxis. The reaction of rabbits to the intravenous injection of meconium was thought by Steiner and Lushbaugh to simulate anaphylactic shock.[541] Although Attwood[547] speculated that substances such as blood group antigens normally present in amniotic fluid might act as agents that can trigger a Type I immunologic reaction, he concluded that in fact no good evidence for such a mechanism exists.

Infection and Septic Shock. Some cases of amniotic fluid embolism are associated with prolonged rupture of membranes and the presence of infected amniotic fluid,[547] in which circumstance systemic hypotension might be related in part to endotoxemia. In the appropriate clinical setting, the presence of positive blood cultures and histologic evidence of chorioamnionitis should suggest this mechanism.

Coagulation Disturbances. Amniotic fluid is a powerful coagulant, 1 ml of a thrombokinase-like constituent within it capable of coagulating 10 liters of blood.[554] Because of this property and because it constitutes a volume equivalent to one quarter of the total maternal blood volume at term, it represents the body's largest reservoir of active coagulant, and its introduction into the systemic circulation can cause profound disturbances in blood coagulation. Such disturbances can occur in up to 40 per cent of patients who survive the first hour after the initial embolic event,[550] and are probably related chiefly to a decrease in circulating fibrinogen, in turn the result of several factors:

1. A direct effect due to the thromboplastic activity of the cellular components of the amniotic fluid, with resultant formation of fibrin and consumption of fibrinogen.

2. An enhancement of this process by activation of the fibrinolytic system, both directly by tissue activator released from the amniotic cells and indirectly by a reaction to the excess fibrin.

3. Plasmin activation, leading to proteolysis of fibrin and fibrinogen, further depleting these hemostatic factors.[555]

4. Possibly, platelet aggregation around particulate material in pulmonary arterioles and capillaries, with further enhancement of the activity of the coagulation system.

The combination of some or all of these processes results in severe fibrin depletion and the clinical and pathologic picture of DIC.[555, 556] However, in a report of an apparent successful response to cryoprecipitate therapy in a patient with proven amniotic fluid embolism, the fibrinogen level was within normal limits at the time of treatment and the authors attributed the response to plasma fibronectin, which is also a component of the cryoprecipitate.[557] Fibronectin is believed to play a role in maintaining the integrity of the reticuloendothelial system, and it has been suggested that the beneficial results that are observed in patients with ARDS in response to cryoprecipitate therapy may be due to this substance rather than to its fibrinogen content.[557]

Pathologic Characteristics

Pathologic findings have been described in detail by Attwood[547] and by Peterson and Taylor.[558] Grossly, the lungs may be edematous and may show focal areas of hemorrhage, but frequently they are unremarkable; in Peterson and Taylor's 40 cases, the average combined lung weight was only 748 gm, the upper limit of normal being 600 to 700 gm. Although focal areas of interstitial or airspace edema may be seen, the most striking histologic finding is the presence of foreign material within medium- to small-sized pulmonary arteries and arterioles. This consists of squames, fragments of hair (which are refractile and well demonstrated by polarized microscopy), and somewhat amorphous basophilic material (sometimes containing greenish-yellow pigment) that is considered to represent mucin and bile derived from meconium. Similar material can be seen in the systemic circulation, particularly in the brain and kidney, but in these

sites is generally considered to be without clinical or pathologic importance.[547, 558–561] In experimental animals,[562] epithelial squames can be identified up to 3 weeks and lanugo hairs and mucin up to 7 months after the intravenous injection of human amniotic fluid; in most instances, little histologic reaction is present.[562] In one patient who survived, a lung biopsy performed one month after the embolic episode confirmed the suspected diagnosis.[563]

Although much intravascular foreign material can be recognized with hematoxylin and eosin (H & E) stain, it is more easily demonstrated with special techniques, which should always be performed before excluding a diagnosis of amniotic fluid embolism histologically. Several techniques can be employed, the most useful being those to demonstrate acid mucopolysaccharides;[564] others have suggested using immunohistochemical staining for keratin (to identify squames)[565] or fetal isoantigen (in cases where it differs from that of the mother).[755]

Pathologic evidence of uterine trauma is present in many cases; of the 30 patients on whom adequate material was available, Peterson and Taylor[558] identified amniotic fluid within uterine vessels in the myometrium or broad ligament in 15.

Roentgenographic Manifestations

Roentgenographic changes in the lungs are poorly documented; in most cases, the condition is so rapidly fatal that roentgenograms are not obtained and few of the rare nonfatal cases are diagnosed. In line with the pathologic characteristics, the major roentgenologic sign is airspace pulmonary edema indistinguishable from acute pulmonary edema of other cause; in fact, this was the sole change described in the cases we could locate in the literature.[557, 563, 566–568] Whether cardiac enlargement accompanies the edema depends on the severity of pulmonary arterial hypertension and consequent cor pulmonale, but almost certainly vascular occlusion severe enough to cause roentgenographically demonstrable cardiomegaly will be fatal.

Since the predominant roentgenographic manifestation is widespread airspace consolidation, the chief differential diagnoses are massive pulmonary hemorrhage and aspiration of liquid gastric contents (Mendelson's syndrome).

Clinical Manifestations

Typically, the clinical manifestations of amniotic fluid embolism are abrupt in onset and rapidly progressive. In Peterson and Taylor's series of 40 cases,[558] disease was heralded by dyspnea and cyanosis in 20 patients, sudden profound shock disproportionate to blood loss in 12, and signs of CNS irritability (convulsions, hyperreflexia, and other signs) in eight. Thirty patients died as a direct result of the embolic episode, 29 within 6 hours of the clinical onset and one after 31 hours; excessive bleeding was a contributory cause in eight. In the other ten cases, death was attributed to uncontrollable uterine hemorrhage. Fibrinogen levels were low in all four patients in whom they were measured.

Manifestations in Anderson's 32 patients[569] included dyspnea and cyanosis (developing late) in 23, shock in 18, apparent cardiac arrest in 19, and grand mal convulsions in 13; 11 became semicomatose or comatose before death. The time interval from onset of symptoms to death ranged from 10 minutes to 32 hours; death occurred within 1 hour in 11 patients.

Because of the frequently rapid clinical course and of the necessity in most cases for histologic examination of lung tissue for definitive diagnosis, almost all recognized cases of amniotic fluid embolism end fatally. However, the disease is occasionally nonfatal,[547] the diagnosis being made in some cases by cytologic examination of blood aspirated from a Swan-Ganz catheter.[548, 756] In addition, there are six reports in the literature in which amniotic fluid "contents" have been recovered from the lungs ante mortem.[548, 557, 563, 568]

Predisposing factors to amniotic fluid embolism include tumultuous labor, uterine stimulants, meconium in the amniotic fluid, intrauterine fetal distress and death, older age of the mother, and multiparity. The first two are important because of the attendant increase in uterine pressure, but it is important to recognize that tumultuous labor is not an absolute prerequisite for embolization, being described in less than 30 per cent of patients in one series[558] and in only 28 per cent of reported cases in a review of the literature.[551] Analysis of 40 cases by Peterson and Taylor[558] revealed an older age of the mother (average 32 years), premature placental separation (in 18 patients), intrauterine death (in 16), meconium staining of amniotic fluid (in 14), and clinically hypertonic labor (in 11). Prolonged gestation, large infants, and the type of delivery were not factors; none of the babies was considered premature or postmature, and only four women were nulliparous. In all reported series, patients have been in the 35th to 42nd week of pregnancy at the time of embolization.

Despite the fact that intrauterine death increases the permeability of fetal membranes and diminishes their strength, the increased permeability can hardly be envisioned as an acute phenomenon; thus, it is most improbable that fetal death *per se* is the cause of amniotic fluid embolism.[551] The high correlation between intrauterine death and fetal distress is probably related to contamination of the amniotic fluid with meconium, rendering the effects of embolization more damaging. Full-term pregnancy in the presence of an intrauterine contraceptive device is uncommon, but four proven cases of amniotic fluid embolism have been reported in such circumstances.[551]

EMBOLIC MANIFESTATIONS OF PARASITIC INFESTATION

Immature forms of many human metazoan parasites travel through the systemic circulation to the lungs, where they lodge within pulmonary arterioles and capillaries. Although, strictly speaking, this represents embolization, in most cases the clinical and pathologic effects are not related to vascular obstruction or damage; instead, pulmonary disease typically occurs in the adjacent lung parenchyma and represents a host reaction to the migrating organism during part of its life cycle. Examples of parasites that cause this form of disease include *Ascaris lumbricoides*, *Strongyloides stercoralis*, *Ancylostoma duodenale*, *Necator americanus*, *Toxicara canis* and *cati*, *Paragonimus* species, and probably *Wucheria bancrofti* and *Brugia malayi*.

In some instances, however, parasites cause disease that is related directly to pulmonary vascular obstruction. Undoubtedly, the most important of these organisms are *Schistosoma* species in which eggs released into the systemic or portal venous circulation lodge within pulmonary arteries and arterioles and cause endarteritis obliterans and pulmonary arterial hypertension. Embolized *Ascaris suum* eggs can sometimes lead to the same process;[772] although there are no clinical manifestations of this process, ingestion of *A. suum* larvae can result in massive pulmonary edema, presumably on a hypersensitivity basis.[570] Occasionally, whole mature organisms can be transported to the lung and become lodged within larger pulmonary vessels; the commonest of these is *Dirofilaria immitis* (the heart worm of the dog),[773] which is typically associated with adjacent parenchymal necrosis that is roentgenographically manifested by a solitary pulmonary nodule. Rarely, other adult worms such as *Schistosoma* species can behave similarly.[774] An unusual complication of hepatic hydatid disease occurs when a cyst ruptures into the hepatic veins and its contents are embolized to the lungs.[775] A thorough discussion of these parasites and the diseases they cause is given in Chapter 6.

EMBOLISM OF NEOPLASTIC TISSUE

Since all cases of hematogenous pulmonary metastases must be derived from tumor fragments lodged within pulmonary vessels, it is evident that these are one of the most common forms of emboli. Because of the small size of most tumor fragments, however, effects related to vascular obstruction are seldom apparent. When tumor emboli are of sufficient size or number to mimic thromboemboli, the clinical, pathologic, and roentgenographic manifestations can be identical, including pulmonary infarction, acute cor pulmonale, and sudden death, or a slowly progressive syndrome of dyspnea and pulmonary hypertension;[571, 572] a scintigram, considered to be typical, has been described in the latter syndrome.[573, 776] The subject is considered in greater detail in Chapter 8.

EMBOLISM OF TROPHOBLAST OR MEGAKARYOCYTIC CELLS

Embolism to the lungs by trophoblast cells is virtually a normal finding in pregnancy; in one autopsy study of 220 pregnant or puerperal women in which a number of lung sections were examined, they were found in 43.6 per cent.[757] The greatest number are seen in the peripartum period, a finding probably related to the trauma of labor. In rare cases, the extent of embolism has been such as to suggest a cause of death;[757] in the vast majority of patients, however, the presence of trophoblast cells is of no clinical or pathologic significance and they disappear mostly by *in situ* degeneration shortly after their appearance in the lungs.[579]

Megakaryocytes are so frequently identified within pulmonary vessels in autopsy and surgically excised lung tissue that their presence is in all likelihood a normal finding. In fact, it has been suggested that a substantial proportion of platelet production occurs within the lungs.[758] This subject is considered more fully on page 145.

MISCELLANEOUS CAUSES OF EXTRAVASCULAR TISSUE EMBOLISM

Rarely, the following tissues or secretions have been reported as embolizing to the lungs:
1. *Skin*,[580] possibly derived from venipuncture.
2. *Liver*, secondary to massive hepatic necrosis or trauma.[582]
3. *Bone*, following bone marrow transplantation.[583]
4. *Gastrointestinal contents*, in a patient with Budd-Chiari syndrome and ileal diverticulitis.[584]
5. *Transitional epithelium*, apparently secondary to severe urethritis.[581]
6. *Myocardium*, after surgical correction of pulmonary atresia.[759]
7. In some pregnant women, minute clusters of large, eosinophilic cells that have been considered by several authors to be derived from emboli of *endometrial decidua*.[585, 586]
8. *Neural tissue*, invariably secondary to severe trauma, either during birth or as a result of accidental or battlefield injury.[587, 588]
9. *Bile*, usually in patients with a combination of biliary tract obstruction and liver trauma, the latter secondary to accidental injury, percutaneous cholangiography, or needle biopsy.[589] Only ten cases of bile embolism had been documented by 1984;[589] since intrahepatic biliary duct pressure is higher than venous pressure in the presence of duct obstruction,[589] any form of hepatic damage that causes communication between veins and ducts can result in bile embolization. Although these emboli have been implicated in the cause of death in some cases,[590] it is likely that most are of no clinical significance.

EMBOLI OF FOREIGN MATERIAL

AIR EMBOLISM

Air may enter either the greater or lesser circulation, and although the terminology applied to these two routes varies considerably in the literature, we prefer the following nomenclature:
Pulmonary air embolism. Most commonly, air enters the systemic venous circulation and passes to the right side of the heart and then to the lungs; very occasionally, air can enter a pulmonary artery and embolize to lung parenchyma distally.
Systemic air embolism. Air enters the pulmonary venous circulation and passes to the left side of the heart and then to the systemic arterial network.

Just as these routes are different, so are the pathologic and clinical manifestations of the emboli. In pulmonary air embolism, the effects derive from obstruction of the pulmonary circulation and thus are felt *by* the lungs; in systemic air embolism, the effects derive from an abnormality *within* the lung and are felt chiefly by the two vital organs, the heart and the brain.

Pathogenesis

SYSTEMIC AIR EMBOLISM

The most common site of air entry in systemic air embolism is the pulmonary veins. This can occur only when (1) there is an opening in a vessel exposed to air, and (2) the pressure of the air exceeds the pressure in the vessel. These two criteria are met in a variety of circumstances. The easiest to comprehend, and possibly the most common, occurs with the insertion of a needle into the thoracic cavity for thoracentesis or needle biopsy.[760–762] In these situations, air can enter a pulmonary vein in three situations:[591] (1) when a needle, accidentally inserted into the lung during attempted induction of pneumothorax, enters a pulmonary vein, injection of air will obviously result in embolism; (2) when a needle containing no stylet or stopcock is introduced into the lung for biopsy and enters a pulmonary vein, air may enter the vein if atmospheric pressure exceeds venous pressure, as during deep inspiration; and (3) when a needle introduced into the lung for biopsy pierces a bronchus or pulmonary cyst and a contiguous vein, air can enter the vein if the bronchial or cyst pressure exceeds venous pressure, as during a cough. In these circumstances, air embolism can thus be prevented by ensuring that suction on a syringe does not produce blood, that the needle hole is occluded by a stylet or stopcock, and that patients undergoing lung biopsy are cautioned against coughing or straining after the needle point has entered the lung.

Systemic air embolism can also occur in several situations in which the thorax is intact. One of the most common is during scuba diving, in which the pathogenesis is related to poor ventilation of a bulla because of partial or complete obstruction of its feeding airway. Smith[592] calculated that the volume of air in a space distal to a partly or completely occluded bronchus doubles every 33 feet of a diver's ascent, producing sufficient distention to explode the airspace. He stated that lethal air embolism can result from breath-holding during ascent from depths as little as 10 feet; in fact, a case has been described of a 21-year-old man who died during an attempt to swim across a 25-yard pool at a depth of 6 feet.[593] Death in these situations is caused by the excess pulmonary pressure and volume forcing air into the pulmonary circulation and sending a stream of bubbles to the left side of the heart. Such episodes can be prevented by exhaling during ascent so that poorly ventilated spaces do not overdistend as pressure within them diminishes.

Similar circumstances are possible during assisted positive pressure breathing, perhaps particularly in neonates: Kogutt[594] has reported six cases of systemic air embolism as a complication of respiratory therapy in neonates; in the only infant who survived, there was no clinical symptomatology, the diagnosis being made by roentgenographic findings alone. Although positive pressure breathing increases both pulmonary venous and airspace pressures, a gradient favorable to the occurrence of air embolism may develop if excessively high pressures are used for hyperinflation.

A similar pathophysiologic process undoubtedly underlies the air embolism that occurs in status asthmaticus[595] and hyaline membrane disease of the newborn:[596–598] in both situations, the sequence of events probably consists of alveolar rupture, interstitial emphysema, and pneumomediastinum (and sometimes pneumothorax); as air is forced through the subadventitial plane of the pulmonary veins, it may enter the lumen and cause systemic embolism. In circumstances of diffuse interstitial emphysema associated with hyaline membrane disease, death may also result from compression of pulmonary veins and other mediastinal structures by gas—the "airblock syndrome" first described by Macklin and Macklin in 1944.[599] Massive air embolism may also occur via communication of a major pulmonary artery and a contiguous airspace within the lung: an example has been reported in a 14-year-old boy who developed a side-to-side perforation of a left pulmonary artery branch to the superior branch of the left lower lobe bronchus secondary to an adjacent lung abscess;[600] intermittent positive pressure

ventilation caused increased intrabronchial pressure and direct passage of air into the left lower lobe pulmonary artery resulting in fatal systemic air embolism. Cerebral air embolism has followed laser resection of an endobronchial carcinoid tumor.[777]

PULMONARY AIR EMBOLISM

Pulmonary air embolism occurs as a result of air entering the systemic venous circulation and passing to the right side of the heart and the lungs; rarely it is caused by air entering the pulmonary arteries directly and passing into the distal pulmonary circulation. The former is usually iatrogenic and occurs most often in a surgical setting; any surgical procedure in which the wound is above the level of the heart—for example, during craniotomy in the sitting (Fowler's) position[602]—places the patient at risk for this complication. Air can also enter systemic veins and pass to the right heart and pulmonary circulation by a variety of other mechanisms—through an intravenous apparatus, during diagnostic and therapeutic air insufflation procedures (e.g., into joints, urinary bladder, vagina, fallopian tubes, and uterus, or into the peritoneal or retroperitoneal space), and occasionally during operative obstetrics and at delivery of patients with placenta previa.[603] A patient has also been described who died from air embolism to the right side of the heart during pneumonectomy for carcinoma;[604] air entered the systemic venous system through a communication between a bronchus and the azygos vein while the patient was receiving positive pressure ventilation. In the case of infusion catheters, the usual mode of entry is direct injection. However, in a case reported by Tuddenham and Paskin,[605] air passed spontaneously through a fibrous tract that had formed around a catheter inserted into a central vein for prolonged hyperalimentation; air was apparent roentgenologically in the pulmonary outflow tract. The authors emphasized this potential hazard of centrally placed catheters for recording central venous pressure and for hyperalimentation. A recent report[763] documented 23 cases of air embolism in a series of 100 patients undergoing contrast-enhanced CT; the amount of embolism was minimal in 20 patients and moderate in three. The locations of the emboli were the subclavian or axillary vein in nine patients, a brachiocephalic vein in three, the internal jugular vein in two, the superior vena cava in two, the right ventricle in two, and the main pulmonary artery in 12. There were no immediate or delayed complications.

The occurrence of air embolism in operative obstetrics has been related to manual vaginal manipulations, which tend to produce a piston effect, forcing air into an open placental sinus. Of similar pathogenesis were eight cases[606] in which fatal air embolism occurred during late stages of pregnancy. Air forced into the vagina during orogenital sex play had separated the amniotic membranes from the uterine wall and entered the uterine veins.

At first glance, the cause of death in pulmonary air embolism might be assumed to be the formation of an air block in the outflow tract of the right ventricle and pulmonary arteries, preventing peripheral pulmonary blood flow. However, experimental studies by Hartveit and Warren and their coworkers[607, 608] have clearly shown that the ill effects of air embolism cannot be attributed solely to vascular obstruction by air bubbles; a highly complex series of events is involved, chief of which is probably the formation of fibrin plugs and their impaction in terminal branches of the pulmonary arteries. The interested reader is directed to these two reports for detailed discussion of these complex forces. Briefly, when blood and air are whipped together in the right chambers of the heart, blood is altered and liberates fibrin. (As whipping is the classic laboratory method of defibrinating blood, this finding is not surprising.) Probably, fibrin formation results from platelet damage produced by whipping—a significant decrease in platelets in the peripheral blood is usual with pulmonary air embolism. The sequence of events after the formation of fibrin is readily apparent: contraction of the right ventricle forces the changed blood into the pulmonary circulation, where the fibrin mesh impacts in terminal branches of the pulmonary arteries. The fibrin plugs block the passage of air bubbles caught in the mesh behind them, arresting the pulmonary circulation. The major pathogenetic role of clotting has been supported by experiments on mice[607] in which animals pretreated with heparin showed better survival rates, particularly with lower doses of air. In addition to fibrin thrombus formation, there is also an increase in the number of fat droplets in the blood, probably derived from plasma lipids and formed by the mechanical churning of air, blood, and fibrin.

Although this description refers specifically to pulmonary air embolism, cerebral and cardiac effects of systemic air embolism are probably of the same nature. It is important to note that a much smaller quantity of air is needed to cause death from air originating in the lesser circulation and going to the heart and brain than from air entering the systemic venous system and being trapped in the lungs.

Air that enters the pulmonary circulation in large quantity can also result in permeability pulmonary edema,[778] a fact that was well illustrated by the case of a young man who blew air into tubing connected to a catheter in his arm;[764] the edema peaked in intensity after 12 hours and protein content was very high; the patient recovered within 48 hours of the air infusion.

Pathologic Characteristics

The gross morphologic changes in those who die from pulmonary air embolism are well documented, both in humans[609] and experimental animals.[607] Bloody froth formed by the whipping action of the right atrium and ventricle fills these chambers and extends into the central and peripheral branches of the pulmonary artery and sometimes the superior and inferior vena cava. The pulmonary veins are virtually empty of blood; so also are the left atrium and left ventricle, which are contracted upon themselves and contain only a very small quantity of black blood. The systemic arterial system contains no air bubbles. Repeated sublethal intravenous injections of air in rabbits has been shown to produce pulmonary arterial intimal fibrosis.[610, 765]

Roentgenographic Manifestations

The roentgenologic manifestations of air embolism in living patients have been fairly well documented in the small number of reports that have appeared in the literature.[594, 600, 605, 611] As expected, the principal sign is the presence of visible gas in cardiac chambers, major pulmonary arteries or veins, or systemic arteries in many sites throughout the body. In pulmonary air embolism, gas is present in right heart chambers and central pulmonary arteries; in systemic air embolism, gas will be identified in the left heart chambers, aorta, or more peripheral branches of the systemic arterial tree such as in the neck, shoulder girdles, or upper abdomen. In the two cases reported by Siegle and his colleagues,[598] intracardiac air was identified roentgenographically ante mortem. Vinstein and associates[597] emphasized the importance of the identification of gas within the vascular system, especially within hepatic veins. Taylor,[601] who described the postmortem diagnosis of air embolism by roentgenography, emphasized both the difficulty of demonstrating intravascular gas with standard necropsy techniques and the importance of its roentgenographic demonstration at necropsy.

Kizer and Goodman[612] list the following radiographic manifestations of pulmonary air embolism: (1) air in the main pulmonary artery, (2) pulmonary edema, (3) focal oligemia, (4) enlarged central pulmonary arteries, (5) atelectasis, (6) intracardiac air, (7) air in the hepatic venous circulation, and (8) no abnormality.

Clinical Manifestations

Air embolism originating systemically and involving the lungs is undoubtedly, in most instances, a benign occurrence not recognized by any clinical findings. If the amount of air entering the lung is considerable, there may be pulmonary edema[764, 778] or even systemic hypotension as a consequence of the obstruction to outflow from the pulmonary circulation; such circumstances can occasionally prove fatal.[601] A precordial murmur resembling the sound of a "mill wheel" has been described in some patients.[613] Occasionally, the intrusion of air into the pulmonary circulation is followed by its migration to systemic vessels supplying vital organs, particularly the heart and brain; this in turn results in an abrupt onset of hypotension, convulsions, coma and death. If coronary vessels are obstructed, ECG changes may indicate myocardial ischemia or ventricular dysrhythmia.[602]

EMBOLISM OF TALC, STARCH, AND CELLULOSE (DRUG ADDICT'S LUNG)

Emboli of talc, starch, and cellulose are seen in individuals who have chronically engaged in intravenous drug abuse. In most instances, the complication occurs with medications intended solely for oral use; pills are crushed in a spoon or bottle top, water is added, and the mixture heated and drawn into a syringe, sometimes using absorbent cotton as a filter. The habit is usually a result of a shortage of available heroin, although some addicts use the drugs in this manner to counteract the sedative effect of the narcotic drugs themselves.[614-617] Oral medication misused in this way includes amphetamines[616] and closely related drugs such as methylphenidate hydrochloride (Ritalin) and tripelennamine,[615, 618-624] methadone hydrochloride,[614, 617, 625, 626] hydromorphone hydrochloride (Dilaudid),[628] phenyltoloxamine,[629] propoxyphene (Darvon), secobarbital, pentazocine (Talwin),[630, 631] meperidine,[632-635] and propylhexedrine.[636] A particularly popular combination of these drugs, intended for nonparenteral use, consists of pentazocine (Talwin) and tripelennamine (pyribenzamine).[637] All these oral medications have in common the addition of an insoluble filler to bind the medicinal particles together and to act as a lubricant to prevent the tablets from sticking to punches and dyes during manufacture.[618] The most widely used filler is talc (magnesium silicate). Cornstarch is used in secobarbital and pentazocine and is also occasionally mixed with heroin and other drugs by addicts. Microcrystalline cellulose is a prominent component of pentazocine.[466, 638]

Illegally acquired "street" heroin also contains diluents such as maltose, lactose, and quinine. Most of these are water-soluble[639] and induce no pulmonary damage. Occasionally, however, talc is used as a filler; in this case, the pathologic effects are identical to those of abused oral medications. However, since the use of such contaminated drug is likely to be intermittent, the quantity of embolized talc is usually small and the clinical and roentgenographic effects minimal or nil.

Pathogenesis

When injected intravenously, the fillers become trapped within pulmonary arterioles and capillaries and cause vascular occlusion, sometimes associated with thrombosis. Presumably related to this, tran-

sient pulmonary hypertension has been reported following the intravenous injection of 450-mg pentazocine tablets;[643] rare cases of sudden death have also been attributed to acute occlusion of the pulmonary vasculature after the intravenous injection of talc.[629, 644] A more common event is the development of chronic pulmonary hypertension. Although this may be caused in part by vascular alterations directly caused by the talc emboli, it is likely that parenchymal interstitial fibrosis and emphysema are also involved (see farther on). In time, the foreign particles emigrate through the vessel wall and come to lie in the adjacent perivascular and parenchymal interstitial tissue where they engender a foreign body giant cell reaction and fibrosis. The pathogenesis of the long-term complications of panacinar emphysema and confluent parenchymal disease is unclear.[617]

The most hazardous fillers are talc and cellulose; cornstarch alone, although causing a histiocytic and foreign body giant cell reaction, appears to be relatively innocuous.[640, 641] Animal studies have shown that 90 per cent of maize starch emboli are removed within 24 hours, providing an explanation for the diminished inflammatory changes.[642] As might be predicted, the severity of roentgenographic and pulmonary function abnormalities is related to the quantity of drug injected.[617]

Pathologic Characteristics

In the early stages of disease, the lungs of intravenous drug abusers with foreign body emboli show variable numbers of more or less discrete parenchymal nodules measuring up to 1 mm in diameter.[631, 645] In long-standing disease, there is a tendency for the nodules to become confluent, especially in the upper lobes, producing large areas of consolidation resembling the progressive massive fibrosis (PMF) seen in the pneumoconioses.[617, 627, 646, 647] Panacinar emphysema, sometimes with bulla formation, may also be evident.[617, 648]

Histologically, the small nodules consist of loosely formed granulomas containing many large multinucleated giant cells and surrounded by a small amount of fibrous tissue (Fig. 9–41). Although some involve the lumens and walls of smaller muscular arteries and arterioles, in most instances they are present entirely in the parenchymal interstitium. Intervening panacinar emphysema is common in long-standing cases (Fig. 9–41). Evidence of recent, organizing, or organized thrombus can be seen[640] but is uncommon. Focal vascular dilatation ("angiomatoid" lesions) and medial muscular hypertrophy have occasionally been observed.[640, 644] Sections of the large foci of upper lobe consolidation seen in long-standing disease show sheets of multinucleated giant cells, usually not organized in discrete granulomas (Fig. 9–42); a variable degree of fibrosis is also present.

Foreign material is readily identifiable within

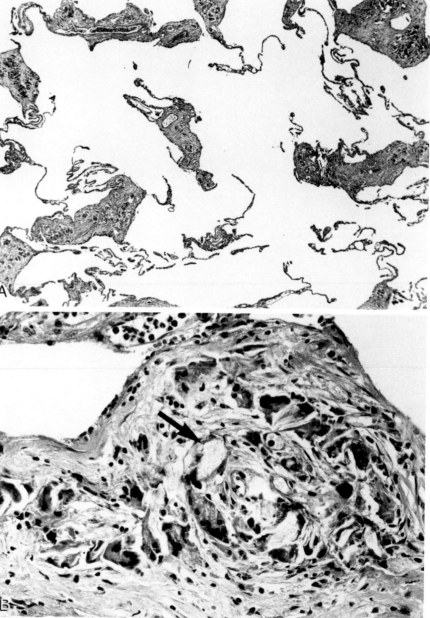

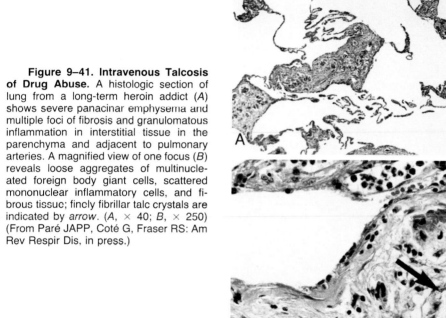

Figure 9–41. Intravenous Talcosis of Drug Abuse. A histologic section of lung from a long-term heroin addict (*A*) shows severe panacinar emphysema and multiple foci of fibrosis and granulomatous inflammation in interstitial tissue in the parenchyma and adjacent to pulmonary arteries. A magnified view of one focus (*B*) reveals loose aggregates of multinucleated foreign body giant cells, scattered mononuclear inflammatory cells, and fibrous tissue; finely fibrillar talc crystals are indicated by *arrow*. (*A*, × 40; *B*, × 250) (From Paré JAPP, Coté G, Fraser RS: Am Rev Respir Dis, in press.)

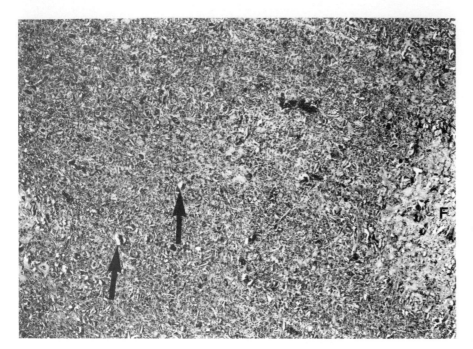

Figure 9–42. Intravenous Talcosis of Drug Abuse. A histologic section from a large focus of consolidated upper lobe parenchyma shows complete effacement of normal lung architecture by a mononuclear inflammatory infiltrate and innumerable multinucleated foreign body giant cells; there is also focal fibrosis (F). Even at this magnification, talc is visible as small white areas (*arrows*) (× 40). (From Paré JAPP, Coté G, Fraser RS: Am Rev Respir Dis, in press.)

the histiocytic and giant cells and is particularly well seen in polarized light. Talc can be identified as irregular, birefringent aggregates of plate-like crystals ranging from 5 to 15 μm in length. Cellulose crystals tend to be larger (10 to 40 μm in length) and show characteristic reactions with Congo red and methenamine silver stains.[630, 640] Starch crystals are characteristically round and contain a central maltese cross.[640, 641] All particles may be recognized in material obtained by fine needle aspiration[649] or bronchoalveolar lavage.[650] Smaller particles can pass through the lesser circulation and have been found in the lungs, liver, bone marrow, spleen, lymph nodes, and fundi;[651] in the last location they may be identified clinically on ophthalmoscopic examination. Because of the association of intravenous drug abuse with acquired immunodeficiency syndrome (AIDS), clinical and pathologic findings characteristic of this disorder may be seen in addition to those of talc emboli.[767, 779]

Roentgenographic Manifestations

In our experience based on a 10-year follow-up of a group of affected patients,[617, 652] the intravenous abuse of drugs containing talc or cellulose and intended for oral use may result in a sequence of changes that are likely dose-related and that can progress following cessation of the intravenous abuse. The earliest finding is of a widespread micronodulation, the diameter of individual nodules ranging from bare visibility to about 1 mm (Fig. 9–43); the pattern does not have a reticular component, the opacities being distinct and "pinpoint" in character, simulating alveolar microlithiasis. Although some authors have described a midzonal predominance of these micronodules,[614, 653] the dis-

tribution we have observed has been diffuse and uniform throughout the lungs. In our cases, profusion of nodules did not vary from patient to patient, severity of involvement being evidenced by size alone. Roentgenograms revealing the earliest discernible changes and those of advanced disease seemed to show the same number of nodules, the only difference being that the older ones were larger and therefore more clearly visible. This rather unusual finding is different from the pattern of progression usually associated with the pneumoconioses. In some patients, the widespread nodularity is associated with loss of volume, sometimes severe.

In the later stages of the disease, the opacities in the upper lobes may coalesce to form an almost homogeneous opacity that closely resembles the progressive massive fibrosis of silicosis or coalworker's pneumoconiosis except for the presence of an air bronchogram (Fig. 9–44).[627, 646, 647, 654] Pulmonary arterial hypertension and cor pulmonale may develop (Fig. 9–45).[623, 653, 655, 656] In the very late stages of the disease, increasing disability and deteriorating function are associated with roentgenographic evidence of emphysema and bullae;[645, 652] the chest roentgenogram may be diagnostic at this stage, revealing a combination of micronodular opacities, coalescent upper lobe lesions resembling progressive massive fibrosis, and lower lobe emphysema or bullae (Fig. 9–46).[647] The lungs may be massively consolidated, as in one case reported by Feigin.[768] Pneumothorax, sometimes recurrent, has been described.[617] Mediastinal lymph node enlargement has been reported in two cases.[614, 617] Gallium 67 scans have been found to be positive.[650, 657]

It is important to realize that some patients may complain of dyspnea and may even have evidence

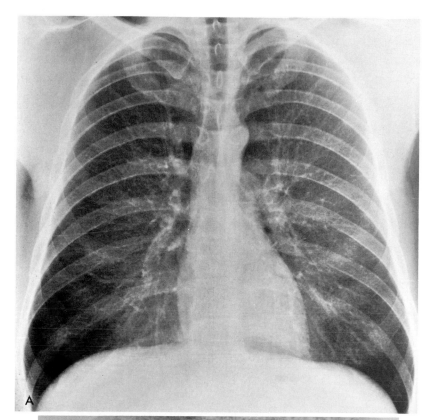

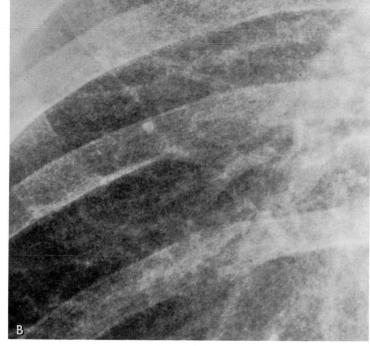

Figure 9–43. Pulmonary Talcosis in Intravenous Drug Abuse. This asymptomatic 22-year-old man had been "shooting" heroin and methadone for 4 years at the time these roentgenograms were obtained. There is widespread involvement of both lungs by tiny micronodular opacities (*A*), seen to better advantage on a roentgenographically magnified image (2:1) of the right lower zone (*B*). There is no anatomic predominance. The pattern is similar to the discrete opacities of alveolar microlithiasis (*see* Figure 2–2, page 320).

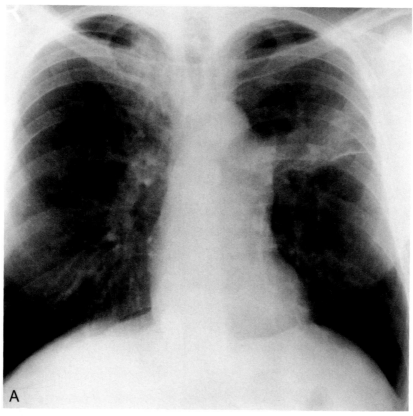

Figure 9–44. Progressive Massive Fibrosis in Intravenous Talcosis of Drug Abuse. A conventional posteroanterior chest roentgenogram (*A*) shows a homogeneous opacity in the anterior segment of the left upper lobe and a somewhat smaller area of consolidation in the right upper lobe partly hidden behind the clavicle and first rib. Innumerable micronodular opacities could be identified throughout the lungs on the original roentgenogram (as in Fig. 9–43). The hila are elevated and the central arteries slightly enlarged.

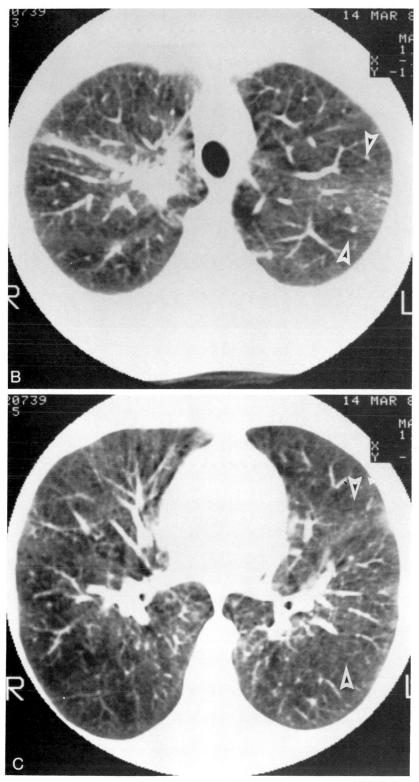

Figure 9–44 *Continued* CT scans through the upper (*B*) and lower (*C*) lobes reveal a patchy ground-glass increase in CT attenuation within both lungs (*between arrowheads*).

Illustration continued on following page

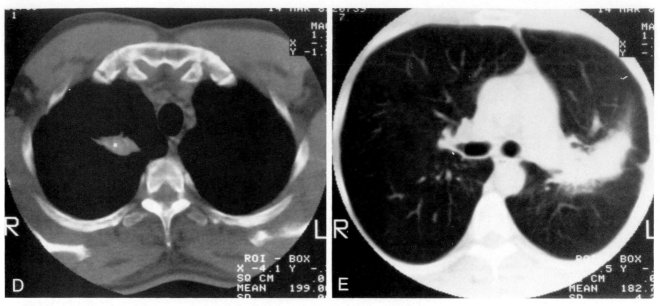

Figure 9–44 *Continued* CT scans in *D* and *E* with narrow and wide window settings, respectively, show focal areas of homogeneous consolidation in the upper lobes. Note that the CT attenuation in these focal lesions is much higher than soft tissue (+180 to +199 Hounsfield units), a point of possible diagnostic importance in distinguishing such opacities from malignancy; this CT feature is possibly caused by the talc content of the lesions. The patient is a 38-year-old man with a long history of intravenous drug abuse.

of talc deposits in their retina and yet have a normal chest roentgenogram.[617]

Clinical Manifestations

Most addicts who inject oral medications or heroin doctored with insoluble fillers are asymptomatic, granulomas being found incidentally at necropsy in those who die from other causes.[616–618, 639, 658] Symptoms usually develop in very heavy users and consist of dyspnea and occasionally persistent cough.[614, 617] Rhonchi are heard in some but are not necessarily related to the foreign body reaction, since most of these individuals are also heavy cigarette smokers. Cor pulmonale may be manifest as a result of extensive vascular and parenchymal disease. As in the pneumoconioses that result from inhalation of silica and silicates, the reaction to intravenously injected talc progresses and disability increases after cessation of exposure.[617]

Organized thrombi and scars are visible in the forearms of nearly all addicts who inject drugs intravenously. Glistening particles can be seen in the fundi, principally at the posterior pole surrounding the foveal area; these may be the earliest clue to illicit use of such drugs, since they have been detected in addicts whose chest roentgenograms and pulmonary function are normal.[617, 659] These minute particles are usually of no clinical consequence; however, occasional cases have been reported in which retinal detachment, vitreous hemorrhage, and retinal neovascularization have been identified.[660–662]

Pulmonary Function Tests

There are a number of studies in which pulmonary function has been assessed in intravenous drug users, but in most cases there has not been a clear indication of the inclusion of patients who have abused oral medications. Overland and associates[663] studied 512 intravenous drug abusers, 96 per cent of whom were cigarette smokers, but did not specify the number who were abusing drugs intended for oral use: in 247 (48 per cent), pulmonary function tests were normal; in 190 (38 per cent), the diffusing capacity was less than 75 per cent of normal, and in the remainder there was obstructive or restrictive impairment with or without some reduction in diffusion. In another evaluation of 12 asymptomatic addicts, most of whom admitted to injecting oral drugs intravenously,[664] the only significant abnormality was a decreased diffusing capacity. Itkonen and associates[637] compared pulmonary function tests in 20 intravenous abusers of pentazocine and tripelennamine with an equal number of "pure" heroin users, and in the former group found a higher percentage of respiratory symptoms, a greater reduction in the mean diffusing capacity, and abnormal responses to submaximal steady-state exercise testing. This lowering of diffusing capacity of the lungs for carbon monoxide (DL_{CO}) correlates with decreased perfusion determined by radionuclide scanning[614, 625, 628, 664] and undoubtedly reflects vascular obstruction by talc particles.

Our studies of addicts who admitted intravenous abuse of oral medications[617] also indicated a

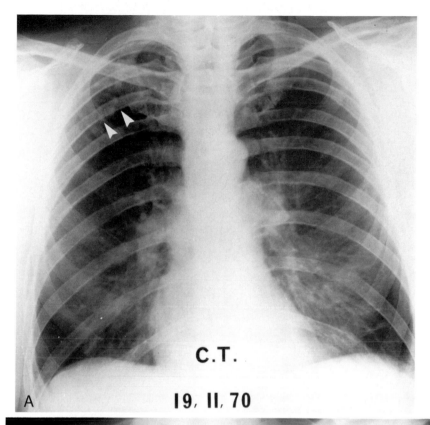

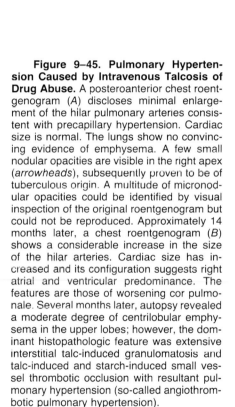

Figure 9–45. Pulmonary Hypertension Caused by Intravenous Talcosis of Drug Abuse. A posteroanterior chest roentgenogram (*A*) discloses minimal enlargement of the hilar pulmonary arteries consistent with precapillary hypertension. Cardiac size is normal. The lungs show no convincing evidence of emphysema. A few small nodular opacities are visible in the right apex (*arrowheads*), subsequently proven to be of tuberculous origin. A multitude of micronodular opacities could be identified by visual inspection of the original roentgenogram but could not be reproduced. Approximately 14 months later, a chest roentgenogram (*B*) shows a considerable increase in the size of the hilar arteries. Cardiac size has increased and its configuration suggests right atrial and ventricular predominance. The features are those of worsening cor pulmonale. Several months later, autopsy revealed a moderate degree of centrilobular emphysema in the upper lobes; however, the dominant histopathologic feature was extensive interstitial talc-induced granulomatosis and talc-induced and starch-induced small vessel thrombotic occlusion with resultant pulmonary hypertension (so-called angiothrombotic pulmonary hypertension).

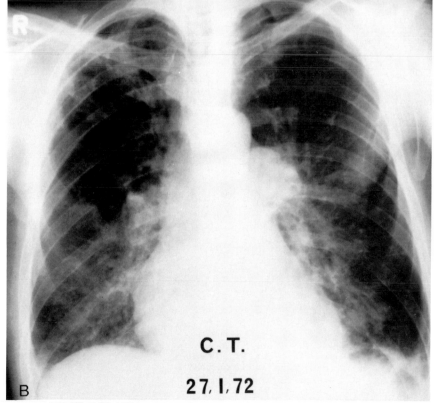

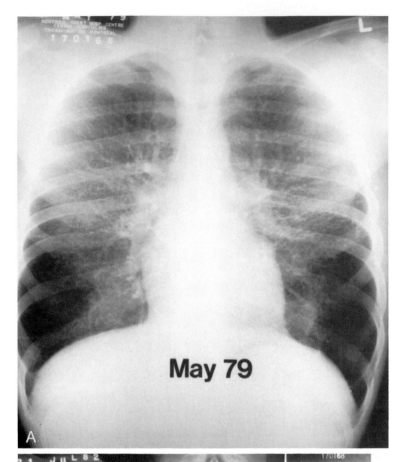

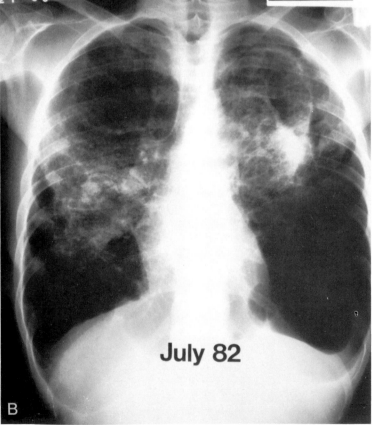

Figure 9–46. Progressive Massive Fibrosis As a Long-Term Effect of Intravenous Talcosis of Drug Abuse. A conventional chest roentgenogram (*A*) reveals a diffuse micronodular pattern throughout both lungs with considerable upper and midzonal predominance. The patient was a chronic intravenous drug abuser, and the pattern is characteristic of intravenous talcosis. Three years later (*B*), large irregular opacities had appeared in both midlung zones, simulating the progressive massive fibrosis seen in silicosis. A pneumothorax is present on the left.

significant impairment of gas transfer, accompanied by a strange combination of obstructive and restrictive insufficiency but little or no hyperinflation or air trapping, at least in the early stages. However, in a follow-up of some of our original patients and in two others we have seen with a remote history of intravenous abuse of oral medications,[652] we found severe reduction of flow rates and diffusion accompanied by hyperinflation and air trapping. These patients were hypoxemic and very disabled by dyspnea; in addition to talcosis, there was roentgenographic and pathologic evidence of emphysema, bullae, and complicating pneumothorax (Fig. 9–46).

IODIZED OIL EMBOLISM

Iatrogenic pulmonary oil embolism is almost invariably a complication of lymphangiography with ethiodized poppy seed oil (Ethiodol) and only occasionally after procedures such as hysterosalpingography, urethrography, and myelography.[665–668] In one case it followed iophendylate (Pantopaque) ventriculography in a young patient with a ventriculoatrial shunt.[669] Pathologic findings have been infrequently described. In one study, lung biopsy performed within 12 hours after the lymphatic injection of ethiodized oil[670] showed lipid droplets widely distributed throughout the pulmonary capillary bed, corresponding to fine granular stippling observed throughout both lungs roentgenologically. Biopsy specimens obtained the next day revealed less lipid in the parenchymal interstitial space, and it was no longer exclusively in the capillary bed, much having passed into the extravascular interstitial tissue and some into the alveoli. At this stage, roentgenography usually shows a fine reticular pattern,[671] which may persist for up to 11 days.[667] In fact, oil embolism produces a reticular pattern in relatively pure form (see Figure 4–64, page 558). In some cases, necropsy reveals reactive changes in pulmonary endothelial cells and an interstitial histiocytic and giant cell reaction indicating passage of lipid outside the vascular space.[673] A staining technique has been described for distinguishing neutral fat from lipiodol.[676]

Roentgenographic evidence of oil embolism was found in 44 of 80 patients,[671] most of whom had pelvic or abdominal lymphatic obstruction. It is postulated that such obstruction permits uptake of the contrast medium by systemic veins, so that the oil arrives in the lungs earlier and in greater concentration than it would otherwise. The small peripheral vessels may be so filled with lipid contrast material as to present an arborizing pattern similar to that seen on pulmonary arteriography (see Fig. 4–64, page 558).[672]

Not all patients subjected to lymphangiography show roentgenographic evidence of this abnormality in their lungs. However, both postmortem studies shortly after the procedure[673, 672] and photoscans of sputum after lymphangiography with ^{131}I-labeled oil[675] showed conclusively that a considerable quantity of oil may be present in the lungs without roentgenographically demonstrable signs.

In a study of five patients after lymphangiography with ^{131}I-labeled ethiodized oil,[677] deposition in the lungs was maximal in the first 24 hours; in three patients, more than 40 per cent of the total dose was found in the lungs. Mean biologic half-life in the lung was 8 days (range, 5.2 to 12.6 days). Clearance was slower from the upper zones, seemingly correlating with blood flow. Interestingly, clearance was most rapid in the two active ambulant outpatients, who remained in a relatively upright semi-Fowler's position for 48 hours after lymphangiography.

Few patients have symptoms. Mild fever may develop within 48 hours after lymphangiography. Very rarely, cough, chills, dyspnea, cyanosis, or hypotension develop, and the ECG shows evidence of right ventricular strain.[671] In some patients lymphangiography may provoke severe reactions and prolonged expectoration of oil.[678] Six deaths consequent upon lymphangiography have been reported, the majority in patients known to have had pulmonary insufficiency previously.[679]

Several investigators have documented decreased diffusing capacity after lymphangiography.[670, 677, 679–681] In a study of 20 patients, Fraimow and colleagues[670] found a fall in average diffusing capacity from 21.2 to 15.9 ml CO/min/mm Hg; others have found a 16 to 34 per cent and 8 to 40 per cent (mean, 22 per cent) decrease from control levels.[677, 681] Decrease is maximal at 24 to 48 hours,[670, 681] an early fall in gas transfer being attributed to reduced pulmonary capillary blood flow and a later drop to interference with the membrane component of diffusion when the oil moves into the interstitial tissue.[679, 681] The reduction in diffusing capacity may persist even after most of the oil has cleared,[677, 681] possibly caused by an inflammatory effect on the alveolar wall as the oil is metabolized to cytotoxic fatty acid. In one study of nine patients, serial measurements of diffusing capacity showed a return to normal levels in 1 month or less.[681] There is also reduction in lung compliance[680] and in arterial PO_2, particularly after a high dose of a contrast agent.[670, 682, 683] As might be expected, ventilatory ability is not altered despite impairment of gas exchange and decreased pulmonary compliance.[670, 681]

METALLIC MERCURY EMBOLISM

Like air, mercury may be introduced into either the arterial or the venous circulation. In the former case, it originates from syringes used for arterial blood gas sampling[684] that contain the liquid as an anaerobic sealant, or it may come from arterial pressure monitors incorporating a liquid mercury manometer connected directly to an intra-arterial needle. Since it is the systemic arterial circulation that is involved, the thorax is not affected.

Pulmonary embolization may be accidental or intentional—accidentally from injury from a broken thermometer or from venous blood sampling with a mercury-sealed syringe, and intentionally from injection by drug abusers or patients attempting suicide.[685, 686] The metal reaches the right ventricle and is disseminated throughout the pulmonary arterial tree: the result is a distinctive, almost alarming, roentgenographic appearance (Fig. 9–47). Although mercury is moderately viscous, it will flow readily through a 22-gauge needle, permitting accidental leakage or self-injection into the vascular system. The incidence of pulmonary mercury embolism is low but not insignificant—it developed in nine (0.9 per cent) of 1,063 patients who had cardiac catheterizations or blood gas determinations,[687] and the incidence seems to be increasing with the use of such injections by drug abusers "for kicks."

Pathologically, the inflammatory reaction in the lungs is relatively mild.[688] The mercury may remain within the pulmonary arteries, eventually becoming encased in thrombus. It can also emigrate into the adjacent interstitium and alveolar airspaces, where it causes a foreign body giant cell reaction.

Roentgenographically, the appearance is distinctive because of the very high density of mercury. The presentation may be in the form of spherules or of short tubular structures representing mercury-filled arterial segments. The distribution is usually bilateral and fairly symmetric. Being denser than plasma, mercury flows to dependent portions of the lung, so that the predominant distribution depends on the body position at the moment of injection. A local collection of mercury may be apparent in the heart, usually near the apex of the right ventricle, distinguishing it from aspirated mercury in the bronchi (Fig. 9–47). Roentgenograms of the abdomen may reveal scattered mercury deposits in the liver, spleen, or kidney as a result of passage through the pulmonary capillary bed and into the systemic circulation. In patients in whom the mercury has been self-administered, roentgenograms of the forearms may reveal aggregations of mercury droplets within the soft tissues at the site of injection.[689]

Clinically, the body's reaction to pulmonary mercury embolism varies but appears to be predominantly systemic. Toxicity is manifested by a metallic taste, excessive salivation, gingivitis, stomatitis, diarrhea, nephrosis, tremor (Hatter's shakes), and erethism.[688] Symptoms are believed to occur when sufficient metallic mercury is oxidized to the soluble mercuric ion Hg^{++}, which has a selective affinity for sulfhydryl groups and acts by inhibiting enzymes containing them.[688] This effect does not occur in everyone with pulmonary mercury embolism; for example, of nine patients in whom embolism oc-

curred as a complication of catheterization,[687] six had symptoms of chronic mercurialism but three suffered no ill effects.

Metallic mercury can reach the lungs by either embolization or aspiration, and since to the best of our knowledge the latter does not cause mercurialism, the two should be distinguished whenever possible. We know of no roentgenographic method that distinguishes the intrabronchial from the intravascular location, especially when the metal is in the lung periphery, although its presence within the heart chambers (Fig. 9–47) proves its vascular location. Aspiration usually occurs after accidental breakage of a thermometer or indwelling intestinal tube[690] or during a suicide attempt.[691] In contrast to embolized mercury, aspirated mercury does not appear to initiate an inflammatory reaction[691] and is slowly removed by the ciliary escalator and cough.[690]

COTTON FIBER EMBOLISM

It is probable that in the majority of cases, fragments of cotton fibers are introduced into the pulmonary circulation by contamination of needles or intravenous catheters from clothing, bedding, or gauze used to wipe the needle. Rare examples secondary to cardiac catheterization[692] and angiography[693] have also been described, and it has been suggested that the material can occasionally be derived from intravenous fluid itself.[694] In one necropsy study of 74 children who had received intravenous fluid strained through a cotton filter, intrapulmonary fibers were demonstrated in 61; there was a direct correlation between the amount of fluid administered and the number of cotton fibers per unit area of lung.[695] These emboli result in no clinical or roentgenographic findings and are invariably discovered incidentally at autopsy or in a lung biopsy specimen.

Histologically, the fibers can be recognized as elongated, refractile foreign material associated with a variable inflammatory reaction. In the early stages,[692, 696] this consists simply of platelet thrombus within an acute inflammatory cellular exudate; later, the inflammation becomes granulomatous and is associated with large, multinucleated foreign body–type giant cells (Fig. 9–48). Although the granulomatous focus containing the cotton is initially located within the lumen and wall of small arteries and arterioles, it can eventually emigrate outside the vessel wall into the alveolar interstitium or airspaces;[692, 696] in the latter location, it can be confused with inhaled foreign material, suggesting a diagnosis of allergic alveolitis.

BARIUM EMBOLISM

Rarely, barium embolization to the lungs has been observed as a complication of routine barium

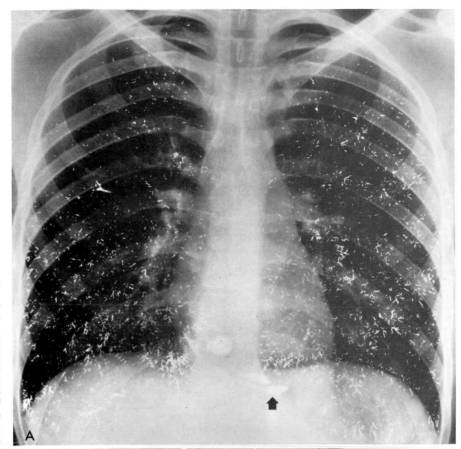

Figure 9–47. Metallic Mercury Embolization. A posteroanterior roentgenogram (A) reveals a multitude of short linear and branching opacities of metallic density distributed widely throughout both lungs, seen to better advantage in a magnified view of the lower portion of the right lung (B). It would be difficult to be certain whether this metallic mercury was within the vascular or airway system of the lungs if it were not for the presence of a pool of mercury lying in the inferior aspect of the right ventricular chamber (arrows in A). This young male drug addict injected metallic mercury into an antecubital vein for a special "kick." (Courtesy of Dr. William Beamish, University Hospital, Edmonton, Alberta.)

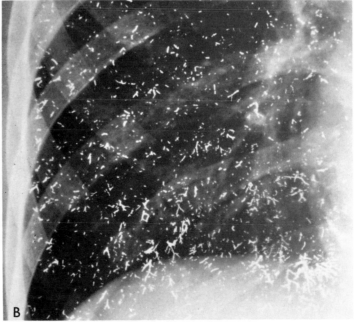

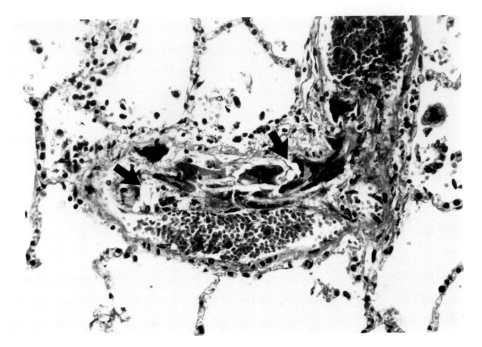

Figure 9–48. Cotton Fiber Embolism. A histologic section of a small pulmonary artery shows several multinucleated foreign body giant cells adjacent to one wall. In their midst are multiple irregularly shaped spaces (*arrows*) that showed the presence of refractile material on polarization microscopy. The appearance is characteristic of cotton fiber embolism (× 250).

enema[697, 698] and of barium "enema" performed inadvertently via the vagina.[699] Mucosal lacerations can usually be identified,[699] enabling entry of injected barium into the venous system. Pathologically, the barium can be seen within pulmonary arterioles and capillaries as refractile and often angulated crystalline material. In one case, it was present within pulmonary endothelial cells that were enlarged and showed a finely vacuolated appearance.[699] The condition is serious, and the majority of reported patients have died, either immediately or within 24 hours of the event.

MISCELLANEOUS FOREIGN BODY EMBOLISM

Macroscopic Foreign Bodies

Bullets or bullet fragments can enter the extrathoracic systemic veins or the right side of the heart and be carried to the lungs to lodge within pulmonary arteries (Fig. 9–49).[700–702] Thrombus can form around the metal with resultant infarction.[700] However, both clinical observations and experimental studies[703] have shown that metallic foreign bodies can remain within the pulmonary vasculature for prolonged periods without untoward effects.

Radiopaque foreign material, such as wire loops, balloons filled with contrast medium, and silicone-tantalum mixtures are used therapeutically in both the pulmonary and systemic circulations to obliterate arteriovenous malformations or to control intractable hemorrhage;[704, 705] in the systemic circulation, escape of material to the venous side will result in opacities of metallic density within the lungs.

Plastic intravenous catheters, whole or in fragments, may be carried in the systemic venous circulation to the right heart chambers and pulmonary circulation, a complication that usually occurs when a polyethylene catheter is cut by the sharp bevel of the needle housing it. The catheter may break or be cut during dressing changes or be detached from the connector.[706] Occasionally, the catheter can fracture spontaneously.[769] Embolized catheters *must* be removed surgically, or, if they have not advanced too far, by ureteric stonecatcher.[707, 708] A review of the literature[706] showed that 17 of 28 patients who received no treatment died of directly related cardiopulmonary complications, whereas all 34 patients from whom catheters were removed survived and were asymptomatic. This iatrogenic error can be avoided by the use of a needle-in-catheter rather than a catheter-in-needle.[706, 709] In the former type, the needle is discarded; in the latter, it is withdrawn over the catheter and left in place, a potential source of shearing of the polyethylene tubing.[710]

Microscopic Foreign Bodies

A variety of particulate materials, including glass, rubber, plastic, and cellulose, have been found in fluid destined for intravenous injection.[694, 711, 712] In one study, between 100 and 1,500 particles greater than 5 μm in diameter per liter of fluid were identified from four different manufacturers.[712] A number of these particles are undoubtedly retained within the lungs after infusion, and those that pass through the pulmonary capillary sieve must inevitably end up somewhere in the systemic circulation. Although there are no known clinical

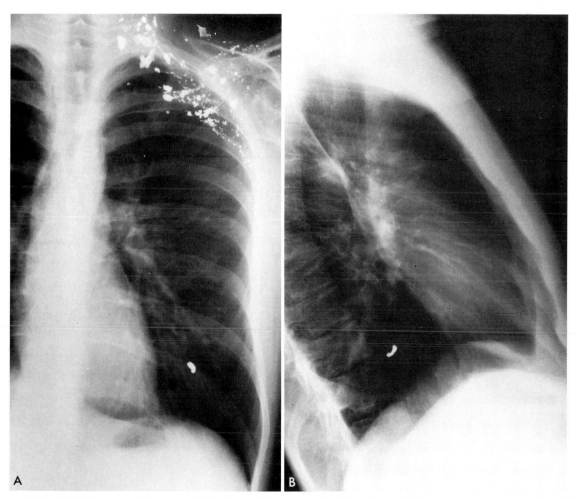

Figure 9–49. Bullet Fragment Embolus to the Lung. Posteroanterior (*A*) and lateral (*B*) roentgenograms reveal multiple metallic foreign bodies in the soft tissues of the left shoulder. In addition, a solitary metallic fragment is situated in the midportion of the left lower lobe. It is assumed that this fragment gained entry to a vein in the shoulder and embolized to the lung by way of the right heart chambers.

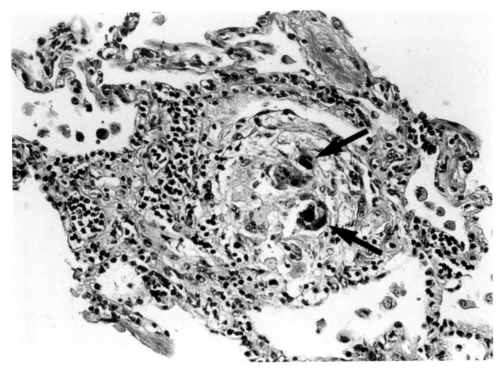

Figure 9–50. Chronic Hemodialysis with Granulomatous Pneumonitis. A magnified view of lung parenchyma shows an interstitial lymphocytic infiltrate and a single well-circumscribed granuloma containing several ill-defined, non-refractile foreign particles (*arrows*). Similar granulomas and patchy interstitial pneumonitis were present throughout both lungs and were considered to represent a reaction to microemboli related to long-term hemodialysis. The patient was a 65-year-old woman with no respiratory symptoms; the chest roentgenogram was normal (× 250).

or roentgenographic manifestations of these emboli, their long-term effects, if any, are unknown. However, of importance to the pathologist is the granulomatous reaction that may develop in relation to some of the foreign material and that may be a source of confusion in the interpretation of biopsy specimens.

Foreign material resembling a silicone antifoaming agent was detected within the pulmonary vasculature in seven of 11 patients who had undergone extracorporeal circulation;[713] although there was no histologic reaction, the longest postoperative survival was only 90 hours. Pulmonary granulomas and isolated interstitial giant cells containing foreign material have been detected in patients on long-term hemodialysis (Fig. 9–50);[714, 715] although the nature of the foreign material has not been identified in all cases, in some it has been shown to be silicone, apparently derived from the dialysis tubing. In one patient, minute fragments of embolized polytef (Teflon) from a tricuspid Beall prosthesis has resulted in a similar pulmonary granulomatous reaction.[716] Clinical and roentgenographic manifestations have been absent in these patients.

BRONCHIAL ARTERY THROMBOSIS AND EMBOLISM

Although bronchial artery *thrombosis* is seldom recognized, it probably occurs fairly frequently in association with infections or neoplasms. The clinical, roentgenographic, and pathologic effects, if any, tend to be minimal, although in some cases partial thrombosis associated with injury to the vessel wall may result in interstitial or parenchymal hemorrhage. It is probable that hemorrhage can also occur in some cases of systemic vasculitis affecting the bronchial arteries (*see* Fig. 7–31, page 1256).

The vast majority of bronchial artery *emboli* consist of foreign material introduced therapeutically in an attempt to control recurrent or massive hemoptysis.[780] The embolic material is varied and includes absorbable gelatinous sponge (Gelfoam), polyvinyl alcohol (Ivalon), isobutyl-2-cyanoacrylate (Bucrylate), and Gianturco coils.[781] Such substances either can completely obstruct the lumen of the vessel following injection or can partly obstruct it and subsequently induce thrombosis that causes complete luminal obliteration.

Pathologic examination of bronchial arteries recently embolized with foreign material shows thrombus related to the material; in one experimental study on the effects of polyvinyl alcohol (PVA),[782] vasculitis was also observed. Tomashefski and his colleagues[781] have described the long-term reaction to injected PVA in three patients with cystic fibrosis: fibrosis and mild chronic inflammation, including a foreign body giant cell reaction, were observed in relation to the PVA (Fig. 9–51); focal arterial wall damage and occasional spicules of PVA

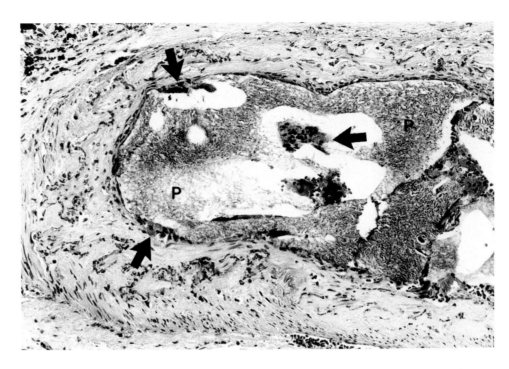

Figure 9–51. Bronchial Artery Polyvinyl Alcohol Embolus. A portion of bronchial artery shows complete luminal occlusion by clumps of polyvinyl alcohol (P) rimmed by occasional multinucleated foreign body giant cells (*arrows*). The specimen was from an autopsy 6 weeks after embolization for massive hemoptysis (× 160).

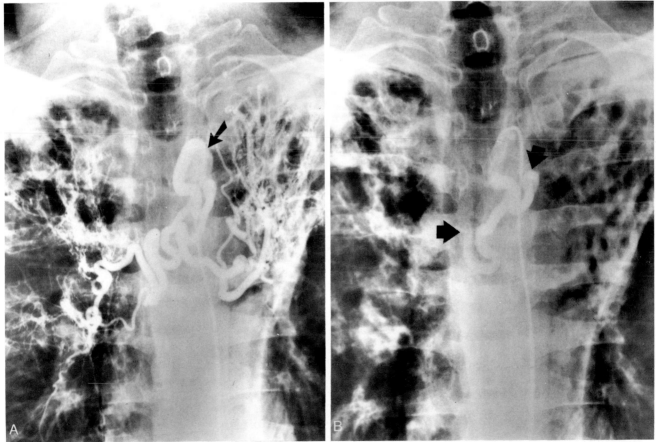

Figure 9–52. Bronchial Artery Embolization for Life-Threatening Pulmonary Hemorrhage. A bronchial artery angiogram (*A*) reveals marked dilatation of the vessel within the mediastinum and a remarkable increase in flow to a partly atelectatic left upper lobe; note the origin of the bronchial artery from the top of the aortic arch (*arrow*). The left upper lobe is the site of severe bronchiectasis and scarring. This 40-year-old man had cystic fibrosis and presented with hemoptysis amounting to 600 ml during the previous 24 hours. Bronchoscopy revealed a great deal of blood in the left upper lobe bronchus. Following the injection of polyvinyl alcohol foam (Ivalon) particles, a repeat injection of contrast medium (*B*) reveals total obstruction of both left and right branches of the bronchial artery (*arrows*) and an absence of flow to the left upper lobe. The embolization resulted in cessation of the hemoptysis.

were identified in the perivascular connective tissue, indicating transmural migration of the foreign material, presumably by a process similar to that seen with embolized talc and cotton. Experimentally, bronchial wall necrosis has been produced after bronchial artery occlusion by glass microspheres.[783] Despite the foregoing, the effects of therapeutic emboli on the bronchial wall itself and on tissues supplied by the bronchial arteries are usually not evident and appear to be minimal.

Roentgenographically, the appearances are as might be anticipated: initial opacification of the bronchial artery and its peripheral arborization usually reveals a markedly dilated, hypertrophied vascular tree (Fig. 9–52); following embolization, the artery can be seen to be completely blocked at a variable distance from its origin, peripheral flow being nonexistent.

REFERENCES

1. Slavin RE, de Groot WJ: Pathology of the lung in Behçet's disease. Am J Surg Pathol 5:779, 1981.
2. Dimond EG, Jones TR: Pulmonary artery thrombosis simulating pulmonic valve stenosis with patent foramen ovale. Am Heart J 47:105, 1954.
3. Chiu B, Magil A: Idiopathic pulmonary arterial trunk aneurysm presenting as cor pulmonale: Report of a case. Hum Pathol 16:947, 1985.
4. Connors AF, Castele RJ, Farhat NZ, et al: Complications of right heart catheterization. Chest 88:567, 1985.
5. Ferencz C: The pulmonary vascular bed in tetralogy of Fallot. I. Changes associated with pulmonic stenosis. Bull Johns Hopkins Hosp 106:81, 1960.
6. Haupt HM, Moore GW, Bauer TW, et al: The lung in sickle cell disease. Chest 81:332, 1982.
7. Israel RH, Salipante JS: Pulmonary infarction in sickle cell trait. Am J Med 66:867, 1979.
8. Nussbaum RL, Rice L: Morbidity of sickle cell trait at high altitude. South Med J 77:1049, 1984.
9. Heath D, Thompson IM: Bronchopulmonary anastomoses in sickle-cell anaemia. Thorax 24:232, 1969.
10. Ryan SF: Pulmonary embolism and thrombosis in chronic obstructive emphysema. Am J Pathol 43:767, 1963.
11. Savacool JW, Charr R: Thrombosis of the pulmonary artery. Am Rev Tuberc 44:42, 1941.
12. Editorial: Pulmonary microembolism. Lancet, 1:429, 1967.
13. Robboy SJ, Colman RW, Minna JD: Pathology of disseminated intravascular coagulation. Hum Pathol 3:327, 1972.
14. Nasser WK, Feigenbaum H, Fisch C: Clinical and hemodynamic diagnosis of pulmonary venous obstruction due to sclerosing mediastinitis. Am J Cardiol 20:725, 1967.
15. Katzenstein A-LA, Mazur MT: Pulmonary infarct: an unusual manifestation of fibrosing mediastinitis. Chest 77:521, 1980.
16. Morrell MT: The incidence of pulmonary embolism in the elderly. Geriatrics 25:138, 1970.
17. Browse NL: Prevention of venous thromboembolism. N Engl J Med 287:145, 1972.
18. Coon WW, Coller FA: Clinicopathologic correlation in thromboembolism. Surg Gynecol Obstet 109:259, 1959.
19. Spittell JA Jr: Pulmonary thromboembolism—some editorial comments. Dis Chest 54:401, 1968.
20. Mercer J, Talbot IC: Clinical diagnosis: a post-mortem assessment of accuracy in the 1980s. Postgrad Med J 61:713, 1985.
21. Modan B, Sharon E, Jelin N: Factors contributing to the incorrect diagnosis of pulmonary embolic disease. Chest 62:388, 1972.
22. Tsao M, Schraufnagel D, Wang N: Pathogenesis of pulmonary infarction. Am J Med 72:599, 1982.
23. Beckering RE Jr, Titus JL: Femoral-popliteal venous thrombosis and pulmonary embolism. Am J Clin Pathol 52:530, 1969.
24. Freiman DG, Suyemoto J, Wessler S: Frequency of pulmonary thromboembolism in man. N Engl J Med 272:1278, 1965.
25. Morrell MT, Dunnill MS: The post-mortem incidence of pulmonary embolism in a hospital population. Br J Surg 55:347, 1968.
26. Goldhaber SZ, Hennekens CH, Evans DA, et al: Factors associated with correct antemortem diagnosis of major pulmonary embolism. Am J Med 73:822, 1982.
27. Silver D, Helfrich LR, Woodard WT: Management of pulmonary embolism. Med Clin North Am 54:361, 1970.
28. Morrell MT, Truelove SC, Barr A: Pulmonary embolism. Br Med J 2:830, 1963.
29. Loehry CA: Pulmonary emboli in young adults. Br Med J 1:1327, 1966.
30. Moser KM: Pulmonary embolism. Am Rev Respir Dis 115:829, 1977.
31. Waller BF, Dean PJ, Mann O, et al: Right ventricular outflow obstruction from thrombus with small peripheral pulmonary emboli. Chest 79:224, 1981.
32. Gonzalez A, Altieri PI, Marquez E, et al: Massive pulmonary embolism associated with a right ventricular myxoma. Am J Med 69:795, 1980.
33. Bortolotti U, Mazzucco A, Valfre C, et al: Right ventricular myxoma: review of the literature and report of 2 patients. Ann Thorac Surg 33:277, 1982.
34. Goldstein MF, Nestico P, Olshan AR, et al: Superior vena cava thrombosis and pulmonary embolus: association with right atrial mural thrombus. Arch Intern Med 142:1726, 1982.
35. Sundqvist S-B, Hedner U, Kullenberg HKE, et al: Deep venous thrombosis of the arm: a study of coagulation and fibrinolysis. Br Med J 283:265, 1981.
36. Coon WW, Willis PW III: Thrombosis of axillary and subclavian veins. Arch Surg 94:657, 1967.
37. Adams JT, McEvoy RK, deWeese JA: Primary deep venous thrombosis of upper extremity. Arch Surg 91:29, 1965.
38. Tomlin CE: Pulmonary infarction complicating thrombophlebitis of the upper extremity. Am J Med 12:411, 1952.
39. Smith George T, Dexter L, Dammin GJ: Postmortem quantitative studies in pulmonary embolism. In Sasahara AA, Stein M (eds): Pulmonary Embolic Disease. New York, Grune & Stratton, 1965, pp 120–130.
40. Greenberg H: Refractory dyspnea and orthopnea. Evidence of recurrent pulmonary embolism and infarction. Am Rev Respir Dis 92:215, 1965.
41. Sevitt S: Venous thrombosis and pulmonary embolism. Their prevention by oral anticoagulation. Am J Med 33:703, 1962.
42. Clagett GP, Salzman EW: Prevention of venous thromboembolism in surgical patients. N Engl J Med 290:93, 1974.
43. Starkie CM, Harding LK, Fletcher DJ, et al: (The Birmingham eclampsia study group): Intravascular coagulation and abnormal lung-scans in pre-eclampsia and eclampsia. Lancet 2:889, 1971.
44. Warlow C, Ogston D, Douglas AS: Venous thrombosis following strokes. Lancet 1:1305, 1972.
45. Fred HL: Bacterial pneumonia or pulmonary infarction? Dis Chest 55:422, 1969.
46. Youssef AH, Barkhan P: Inhibition by aspirin of release of antiheparin activity from human platelets. Br Med J 3:394, 1969.
47. Catovsky D, Ikoku NB, Pitney WR, et al: Thromboembolic complications in myelomatosis. Br Med J 3:438, 1970.
48. Monta LE, Ramanan SV: Recurrent pulmonary embolism. A sign of multiple myeloma. JAMA 233:1192, 1975.
49. Barrett-Connor E: Pneumonia and pulmonary infarction in sickle cell anemia. JAMA 224:997, 1973.
50. Gibbs NM: Venous thrombosis of the lower limbs with particular reference to bed-rest. Br J Surg 45:209, 1957.
51. McLachlin J, Paterson JC: Some basic observations on venous thrombosis and pulmonary embolism. Surgery 93:1, 1951.
52. Stamatakis D, Kakkar VV, Sagar S, et al: Femoral vein thrombosis and total hip replacement. Br Med J 2:223, 1977.
53. Kakkar VV, Flanc C, Howe CT, et al: Natural history of postoperative deep-vein thrombosis. Lancet 2:230, 1969.
54. Murray TS, Lorimer AR, Cox FC, et al: Leg-vein thrombosis following myocardial infarction. Lancet 2:792, 1970.
55. Maurer BJ, Wray R, Shillingford JP: Frequency of venous thrombosis after myocardial infarction. Lancet 2:1385, 1971.
56. Cristal N, Stern J, Ronen M, et al: Identifying patients at risk for thromboembolism: use of 125 I-labeled fibrinogen in patients with acute myocardial infarction. JAMA 236:2755, 1976.
57. Sevitt S: The structure and growth of valve-pocket thrombi in femoral veins. J Clin Pathol 27:517, 1974.
58. Browse NL, Thomas ML: Source of non-lethal pulmonary emboli. Lancet 1:258, 1974.
59. Le Quesne LP: Relation between deep vein thrombosis and pulmonary embolism in surgical patients. N Engl J Med 291:1292, 1974.
60. Mavor GE, Galloway JMD: The iliofemoral venous segment as a source of pulmonary emboli. Lancet 1:871, 1967.
61. Kakkar VV, Howe CT, Flanc C, et al: Natural history of postoperative deep-vein thrombosis. Lancet 2:230, 1969.
62. Bartter T, Hollingsworth HM, Irwin RS, et al: Pulmonary embolism from a venous thrombus located below the knee. Arch Intern Med 147:373, 1987.
63. Yorra FH, Oblath R, Jaffe H, et al: Massive thrombosis associated with use of the Swan-Ganz catheter. Chest 65:682, 1974.
64. Goodman DJ, Rider AK, Billingham ME, et al: Thromboembolic complications with the indwelling balloon-tipped pulmonary arterial catheter. N Engl J Med 291:777, 1974.
65. Prozan GB, Shipley RE, Madding GF, et al: Pulmonary thromboembolism in the presence of an endocardiac pacing catheter. JAMA 206:1564, 1968.

66. Gibney RTN, Donovan F, Fitzgerald MX: Recurrent symptomatic pulmonary embolism caused by an infected Pudenz cerebrospinal fluid shunt device. Thorax 33:662, 1978.
67. Braun TI, Goldberg SK: An unusual thromboembolic complication of a Greenfield vena caval filter. Chest 87:127, 1985.
68. Sevitt S: Pathology and pathogenesis of deep vein thrombosis. In: Poller L (ed): Recent Advances in Thrombosis. London, Churchill Livingstone, 1973, p 17.
69. Winter JH, Fenech A, Bennett B, et al: Thrombosis after venography in familial antithrombin III deficiency. Br Med J 283:1436, 1981.
70. Hull R, Hirsh J, Sackett DL, et al: Cost effectiveness of clinical diagnosis, venography, and noninvasive testing in patients with symptomatic deep-vein thrombosis. N Engl J Med 304:1561, 1981.
71. Browse NL, Clemenson G, Thomas ML: Is the postphlebitic leg always postphlebitic? Relation between phlebographic appearances of deep-vein thrombosis and late sequelae. Br Med J 281:1167, 1980.
72. Wenger NK, Stein PD, Willis PW III: Massive acute pulmonary embolism: the deceivingly nonspecific manifestations. JAMA 220:843, 1972.
73. Kent DC, Reid D: Pulmonary embolism in active duty servicemen. Arch Environ Health 12:509, 1966.
74. Editorial: Pulmonary embolism in active-duty servicemen. JAMA 196:360, 1966.
75. Ramsay LE, MacLeod MA: Incidence of idiopathic venous thromboembolism in nurses. Br Med J 4:446, 1973.
76. Sartwell PE, Masi AT, Arthes FG, et al: Thromboembolism and oral contraceptives: An epidemiologic case-control study. Am J Epidemiol 90:365, 1969.
77. Marciniak E, Farley CH, DeSimone PA: Familial thrombosis due to antithrombin III deficiency. Blood 43:219, 1974.
78. Davis RB: Acute thrombotic complications of myeloproliferative disorders in young adults. Am J Clin Pathol 84:180, 1985.
79. Wu KK: Platelet hyperaggregability and thrombosis in patients with thrombocythemia. Ann Intern Med 88:7, 1978.
80. Davis JW, Davis RF: Prevention of cigarette smoking-induced platelet aggregate formation by aspirin. Arch Intern Med 141:206, 1981.
81. Steele P: Trial of dipyridamole-aspirin in recurring venous thrombosis. Lancet 2:1328, 1980.
82. Williams RS, Logue EE, Lewis JL, et al: Physical conditioning augments the fibrinolytic response to venous occlusion in healthy adults. N Engl J Med 302:987, 1980.
83. Leading article: Physical methods of prophylaxis against venous thrombosis. Br Med J 282:1341, 1981.
84. Editorial: Natural fibrinolysis and its stimulation. Lancet 1:1401, 1981.
85. Editorial: Predisposition to thrombosis. Lancet 2:1430, 1974.
86. Greenspan RH, Steiner RE: The radiologic diagnosis of pulmonary thromboembolism. In Simon M, Potchen EJ, LeMay M (eds): Frontiers of Pulmonary Radiology. New York, Grune & Stratton, 1969.
87. Royal College of General Practitioners Report by Records Unit and Research Advisory Service of RCGP: Oral contraception and thrombo-embolic disease. J Coll Gen Pract 13:267, 1967.
88. Inman WHW, Vessey MP: Investigation of deaths from pulmonary, coronary, and cerebral thrombosis and embolism in women of childbearing age. Br Med J 2:193, 1968.
89. Vessey MP, Doll R: Investigation of relation between use of oral contraceptives and thromboembolic disease. Br Med J 2:199, 1968.
90. Inman WHW, Vessey MP, Westerholm B, et al: Thromboembolic disease and the steroidal content of oral contraceptives. A report to the Committee on safety of drugs. Br Med J 2:203, 1970.
91. Report from the Boston Collaborative Drug Surveillance Programme: Oral contraceptives and venous thromboembolic disease, surgically confirmed gallbladder disease, and breast tumours. Lancet 1:1399, 1973.
92. Vessey MP, Doll R: Investigation of relation between use of oral contraceptives and thromboembolic disease. A further report. Br Med J 2:651, 1969.
93. Oakley Celia, Somerville J: Oral contraceptives and progressive pulmonary vascular disease. Lancet 1:890, 1968.
94. Leading Article: Oral contraceptives and thromboembolism. Br Med J 2:187, 1968.
95. Leading Article: Blood clotting and the pill. Br Med J 4:378, 1972.
96. Bottiger LE, Boman G, Eklund G, et al: Oral contraceptives and thromboembolic disease: effects of lowering oestrogen content. Lancet 1:1097, 1980.
97. Vessey MP, Doll R, Fairbairn AS, et al: Postoperative thromboembolism and the use of oral contraceptives. Br Med J 3:123, 1970.
98. Jick H, Westerholm B, Vessey MP, et al: Venous thromboembolic disease and ABO blood type: A cooperative study. Lancet 1:539, 1969.
99. Talbot S, Wakley EJ, Ryrie D, et al: ABO blood-groups and venous thromboembolic disease. Lancet 1:1257, 1970.

100. Frederiksen H, Ravenholt RT: Thromboembolism, oral contraceptives, and cigarettes. Public Health Rep 85:197, 1970.
101. Marks P, Emerson PA: Increased incidence of deep vein thrombosis after myocardial infarction in non-smokers. Br Med J 3:232, 1974.
102. Handley AJ, Teather D: Influence of smoking on deep vein thrombosis after myocardial infarction. Br Med J 3:230, 1974.
103. Mossey RT, Kasabian AA, Wilkes BM, et al: Pulmonary embolism: low incidence in chronic renal failure. Arch Intern Med 142:1646, 1982.
104. Jewett JF: Pulmonary embolism and renal vein thrombosis. N Engl J Med 291:529, 1974.
105. Jeffcoate TNA, Miller J, Roos RF, et al: Puerperal thromboembolism in relation to the inhibition of lactation by oestrogen therapy. Br Med J 4:19, 1968.
106. Crandon AJ, Peel KR, Anderson JA, et al: Postoperative deep vein thrombosis: identifying high-risk patients. Br Med J 281:343, 1980.
107. Crandon AJ, Peel KR, Anderson JA, et al: Prophylaxis of postoperative deep vein thrombosis: selective use of low-dose heparin in high-risk patients. Br Med J 281:345, 1980.
108. Evans GL, Dalen JE, Dexter L: Pulmonary embolism during pregnancy. JAMA 206:320, 1968.
109. Leading Article: Antepartum pulmonary embolism. Br Med J 3:307, 1972.
110. Aaro LA, Juergens JL: Thrombophlebitis and pulmonary embolism as complications of pregnancy. Med Clin North Am 58:4829, 1974.
111. Henderson SR, Lund CJ, Creasman WT: Antepartum pulmonary embolism. Am J Obstet Gynecol 112:476, 1972.
112. Hampton AO, Castleman B: Correlation of postmortem chest teleroentgenograms with autopsy findings. With special reference to pulmonary embolism and infarction. Am J Roentgenol 43:305, 1940.
113. Smith GT, Dammin GJ, Dexter L: Postmortem arteriographic studies of the human lung in pulmonary embolization. JAMA 188:143, 1964.
114. Parker BM, Smith JR: Pulmonary embolism and infarction. A review of the physiologic consequences of pulmonary arterial obstruction. Am J Med 24:402, 1958.
115. Schraufnagel DE, Tsao M, Yao YT, et al: Factors associated with pulmonary infarction. Am J Clin Pathol 84:15, 1985.
116. Dalen JE, Haffajee CI, Alpert JS, et al: Pulmonary embolism, pulmonary hemorrhage and pulmonary infarction. N Engl J Med 296:1431, 1977.
117. Comroe JH Jr: Pulmonary arterial blood flow: Effects of brief and permanent arrest. Am Rev Resp Dis 85:179, 1962.
118. Newhouse MT, Becklake MR, Macklem PT, et al: Effect of alterations in end-tidal CO_2 tension on flow resistance. J Appl Physiol 19:745, 1964.
119. Llamas R, Swenson EW: Diagnostic clues in pulmonary thromboembolism evaluated by angiographic and ventilation-blood flow studies. Thorax 20:327, 1965.
120. Tierney DF: Pulmonary surfactant in health and disease. Dis Chest 47:247, 1965.
121. Pattle RE: The lining layer of the lung alveoli. Br Med Bull 19:41, 1963.
122. Mead J: Mechanical properties of lungs. Physiol Rev 41:281, 1961.
123. Clements JA: Surfactant in pulmonary disease. N Engl J Med 272:1336, 1965.
124. Kerr IH, Simon G, Sutton GC: The value of the plain radiograph in acute massive pulmonary embolism. Br J Radiol 44:751, 1971.
125. Jaffe RB, Figley MM: Roentgenographic evaluation of bronchial size following pulmonary embolization. Radiology 88:425, 1967.
126. Nadel JA, Colebatch HJH, Olsen CR: Location and mechanism of airway constriction after barium sulfate microembolism. J Appl Physiol 19:387, 1964.
127. Austin JHM, Sagel SS: Alterations of airway caliber after pulmonary embolization in the dog. Invest Radiol 7:135, 1972.
128. Austin JHM: Intrapulmonary airway narrowing after pulmonary thromboembolism in dogs: Partial control by the parasympathetic nervous system. Invest Radiology 8:315, 1973.
129. Robinson AE, Puckett CL, Green JD, et al: In vivo demonstration of small-airway bronchoconstriction following pulmonary embolism. Radiology 109:283, 1973.
130. Isawa T, Taplin GV, Beazell J, Criley JM: Experimental unilateral pulmonary artery occlusion: Acute and chronic effects on relative inhalation and perfusion. Radiology 102:101, 1972.
131. Thomas DP, Tanabe G, Khan M, et al: Humoral factors mediated by platelets in experimental pulmonary embolism. In Sasahara AA, Stein M (eds): Pulmonary Embolic Disease. New York, Grune & Stratton, 1965, pp 59–64.
132. Gurewich V, Sasahara AA, Stein M: Pulmonary embolism, bronchoconstriction and response to heparin. In Sashara AA, Stein M. (eds): Pulmonary Embolic Disease. New York, Grune & Stratton, 1965, pp 162–169.
133. Stein M, Tanabe G, Khan M, et al: Pulmonary response to macro-

and micro-thromboembolism. *In* Sasahara AA, Stein M (eds): Pulmonary Embolic Disease. New York, Grune & Stratton, 1965, pp 141–148.

134. Meth RF, Tashkin DP, Hansen KS, et al: Pulmonary edema and wheezing after pulmonary embolism. Am Rev Respir Dis *111*:693, 1975.

135. Sasahara AA, Cannilla JE, Morse RL, et al: Clinical and physiologic studies in pulmonary thromboembolism. Am J Cardiol *20*:10, 1967.

136. Windebank WJ, Boyd G, Moran F: Pulmonary thromboembolism presenting as asthma. Br Med J *1*:90, 1973.

137. Soloff LA, Rodman T: Acute pulmonary embolism: I. Review. Am Heart J *74*:710, 1967.

138. Josephson S, Ovenfors C-O: Experimental pulmonary air embolism: Angiographic study in dogs. Invest Radiol *5*:220, 1970.

139. Josephson S: Pulmonary hemodynamics during experimental air embolism: Evidence of vasoconstriction. Scand J Clin Lab Invest *26*(Suppl 115):37, 1970.

140. Dombert MC, Rouby JJ, Smiejan JM, et al: Pulmonary oedema during pulmonary embolism. Br J Dis Chest *81*:407, 1987.

141. Dantzker DR, Bower JS: Partial reversibility of chronic pulmonary hypertension caused by pulmonary thromboembolic disease. Am Rev Respir Dis *124*:129, 1981.

142. Dexter L, Smith GT: Quantitative studies of pulmonary embolism. Am J Med Sci *247*:641, 1964.

143. Davison P: Functional aspects of the cor pulmonale syndrome. Br J Dis Chest *54*:186, 1960.

144. Baker RR, Wagner HN Jr: Pulmonary embolectomy in the treatment of massive pulmonary embolism. Surg Gynecol Obstet *122*:513, 1966.

145. Gorham LW: A study of pulmonary embolism: Part II. The mechanism of death; based on a clinicopathological investigation of 100 cases of massive and 285 cases of minor embolism of the pulmonary artery. Arch Intern Med *108*:189, 1961.

146. Wiener SN, Edelstein J, Charms BL: Observations on pulmonary embolism and the pulmonary angiogram. Am J Roentgenol *98*:859, 1966.

147. Wood P: Pulmonary hypertension with special reference to the vasoconstrictive factor. Br Heart J *20*:557, 1958.

148. Fouche RF, D'Silva JL: Hypertransradiancy of one lung field and its experimental production by unilateral miliary embolisation of pulmonary arteries in cats. Clin Radiol *11*:100, 1960.

149. Cooley RN: Pulmonary thromboembolism—the case for the pulmonary angiogram. Am J Roentgenol *92*:693, 1964.

150. Mounts R, Molnar W, Marable SA, et al: Angiography in recent pulmonary embolism with follow-up studies: Preliminary report. Radiology *87*:713, 1966.

151. Dexter L: Cardiovascular responses to experimental pulmonary embolism. *In* Sasahara AA, Stein M, (eds): Pulmonary Embolic Disease. New York, NY, Grune & Stratton, 1965, pp 101–109.

152. Parmley LF Jr, North RL, Ott BS: Hemodynamic alterations of acute pulmonary thromboembolism. Circ Res *12*:450, 1962.

153. Thomas DP, Gurewich V, Ashford TP: Platelet adherence to thromboemboli in relation to the pathogenesis and treatment of pulmonary embolism. N Engl J Med *274*:953, 1966.

154. McIntyre KM, Sasahara AA: The ratio of pulmonary arterial pressure to pulmonary vascular obstruction: index of preembolic cardiopulmonary status. Chest *71*:692, 1977.

155. Fanta CH, Wright TC, McFadden ER: Differentiation of recurrent pulmonary emboli from chronic obstructive lung disease as a cause of cor pulmonale. Chest *79*:92, 1981.

156. Freiman DG: Pathologic observations on experimental and human thromboembolism. *In* Sasahara AA, Stein M (eds): Pulmonary Embolic Disease. New York, Grune & Stratton, 1965, pp 81–85.

157. Korn D, Gore I, Blenke A, Collins DP: Pulmonary arterial bands and webs: An unrecognized manifestation of organized pulmonary emboli. Am J Pathol *40*:129, 1962.

158. Morrell MT, Dunnill MS: The post-mortem incidence of pulmonary embolism in a hospital population. Br J Surg *55*:347, 1968.

159. Short DS: A survey of pulmonary embolism in a general hospital. Br Med J *1*:790, 1952.

160. Yuceoglu YZ, Rubler S, Eshwar KP, et al: Pulmonary edema associated with pulmonary embolism: A clinicopathological study. Angiology *22*:501, 1971.

161. Swenson EW, Llamas R, Ring GC: Hypoxemia and edema of the lungs in experimental pulmonary thromboembolism. *In* Sasahara AA, Stein M (eds): Pulmonary Embolic Disease. New York, Grune & Stratton, 1965, pp 170–180.

162. Singer D, Hesser C, Pick R, Katz LN: Diffuse bilateral pulmonary edema associated with unilobar miliary pulmonary embolization in the dog. Circ Res *6*:4, 1958.

163. Hackett PH, Creagh CE, Grover RF, et al: High-altitude pulmonary edema in persons without the right pulmonary artery. N Engl J Med *302*:1070, 1980.

164. Hyers TM, Fowler AA, Wicks AB: Focal pulmonary edema after massive pulmonary embolism. Am Rev Resp Dis *123*:232, 1981.

165. Jackson J, Thompson N, Miller YE: Chronic pulmonary emboli: sparing of affected regions of lung from noncardiogenic pulmonary edema. Chest *89*:463, 1986.

166. Bedard CK, Bone RC: Westermark's sign in the diagnosis of pulmonary emboli in patients with the adult respiratory distress syndrome. Crit Care Med *5*:137, 1977.

167. Redline S, Tomashefski JF Jr, Altose MD: Cavitating lung infarction after bland pulmonary thromboembolism in patients with the adult respiratory distress syndrome. Thorax *40*:915, 1985.

168. Libby LS, King TE, LaForce FM, et al: Pulmonary cavitation following pulmonary infarction. Medicine *64*:342, 1985.

169. Bewtra C, Dewan N, O'Donahue WJ Jr: Exfoliative sputum cytology in pulmonary embolism. Acta Cytol *27*:489, 1983.

170. Gahagan T, Manzor A, Isaac B, Mathur AN: Reestablishment of pulmonary-artery flow after prolonged complete occlusion: Studies in dogs. JAMA *198*:639, 1966.

171. Liebow AA, Hales MR, Bloomer W, et al: Studies on the lung after ligation of the pulmonary artery: II. Anatomical changes. Am J Pathol *26*:177, 1950.

172. Moser KM, Spragg RG, Utley J, et al: Chronic thrombotic obstruction of major pulmonary arteries: results of thromboendarterectomy in 15 patients. Ann Intern Med *99*:299, 1983.

173. Dalen JE, Banas JS Jr, Brooks HL, et al: Resolution rate of acute pulmonary embolism in man. N Engl J Med *280*:1194, 1969.

174. Secker-Walker RH, Jackson JA, Goodwin J: Resolution of pulmonary embolism. Br Med J *4*:135, 1970.

175. Austin JHM, Wilner GD, Dominguez C: Natural history of pulmonary thromboemboli in dogs: Serial radiographic observation of clots labeled with powdered tantalum. Radiology *116*:519, 1975.

176. Moser KM, Guisan M, Bartimmo EE, et al: *In vivo* and post mortem dissolution rates of pulmonary emboli and venous thrombi in the dog. Circulation *48*:170, 1973.

177. Sevitt S: Organic fragmentation in pulmonary thrombo-emboli. J Pathol *122*:95, 1977.

178. Salyer WR, Salyer DC, Hutchins GM: Local arterial wall injury caused by thromboemboli. Am J Pathol *75*:285, 1974.

179. Meyer JS: Thromboembolic pulmonary arterial necrosis and arteritis in man. Arch Pathol *70*:63, 1960.

180. Sevitt S: Arterial wall lesions after pulmonary embolism, especially ruptures and aneurysms. J Clin Pathol *29*:665, 1976.

181. Korn D, Gore I, Blenke A, et al: Pulmonary arterial bands and webs: An unrecognized manifestation of organized pulmonary emboli. Am J Pathol *40*:129, 1962.

182. Vanek J: Fibrous bands and networks of postembolic origin in the pulmonary arteries. J Pathol Bacteriol *81*:537, 1961.

183. Sevitt S, Walton KW: Atherosclerotic lesions from the reduction of pulmonary emboli. Atherosclerosis *59*:173, 1986.

184. Williams John R, Wilcox WC: Pulmonary embolism: Roentgenographic and angiographic considerations. Am J Roentgenol *89*:333, 1963.

185. Maddison FE, Wright RR, Tooley WH: Chest radiography following unilateral pulmonary artery occlusion. An experimental study. Radiology *88*:435, 1967.

186. Williams JR, Wilcox C, Andrews GJ, et al: Angiography in pulmonary embolism. JAMA *184*:473, 1963.

187. Szucs MM Jr, Brooks HL, Grossman W, et al: Diagnostic sensitivity of laboratory findings in acute pulmonary embolism. Ann Intern Med *74*:161, 1971.

188. Torrance DJ Jr: Roentgenographic signs of pulmonary artery occlusion. Am J Med Sci *237*:651, 1959.

189. Figley MM, Gerdes AJ, Ricketts HJ: Radiographic aspects of pulmonary embolism. Semin Roentgenol *2*:389, 1967.

190. Fleischner FG: Roentgenology of the pulmonary infarct. Semin Roentgenol *2*:61, 1967.

191. Tow DE, Wagner HN Jr: Recovery of pulmonary arterial blood flow in patients with pulmonary embolism. N Engl J Med *276*:1053, 1967.

192. Stein GN, Chen JT, Goldstein F, et al: The importance of chest roentgenography in the diagnosis of pulmonary embolism. Am J Roentgenol *81*:255, 1959.

193. Starr DC: Apical pulmonary infarction—an unusual manifestation of thromboembolic disease. J Can Assoc Radiol *24*:272, 1973.

194. Westermark N: On the roentgen diagnosis of lung embolism. Acta Radiol *19*:357, 1938.

195. Beilin DS, Fink JP, Leslie LW: Correlation of postmortem pathological observations with chest roentgenograms. Radiology *57*:361, 1951.

196. Beamish WE: Radiologic diagnosis of pulmonary embolism including the application of full-chest tomography. J Can Assoc Radiol *21*:217, 1970.

197. Wolfe WG, Sabiston DC Jr: A study of changes in the roentgenogram of the chest in experimental pulmonary embolism. Surg Gynecol Obstet *127*:492, 1968.

198. Fleischner FG: Recurrent pulmonary embolism and cor pulmonale. N Engl J Med *276*:1213, 1967.

199. Fletcher BD, Donner MW: The use of full-chest tomography in the roentgenographic evaluation of pulmonary embolism. Dis Chest 54:13, 1968.
200. Fraser RG, Bates DV: Body section roentgenography in the evaluation and differentiation of chronic hypertrophic emphysema and asthma. Am J Roentgenol 82:39, 1959.
201. Grossman D, Ritter CA, Tarner RJ, et al: Successful identification of oligemic lung by transmission computed tomography after experimentally produced acute pulmonary arterial occlusion in the dog. Invest Radiol 16:275, 1981.
202. Keating DR: Thrombosis of pulmonary arteries. Am J Surg 90:447, 1955.
203. Ball KP, Goodwin JF, Harrison CV: Massive thrombotic occlusion of the large pulmonary arteries. Circulation 14:766, 1956.
204. Fleischner FG: Unilateral pulmonary embolism with increased compensatory circulation through the unoccluded lung: Roentgen observations. Radiology 73:591, 1959.
205. Fleischner FG: Pulmonary embolism. Clin Radiol 13:169, 1962.
206. Ring Alfred, Bakke JR: Chronic massive pulmonary artery thrombosis. Ann Intern Med 43:781, 1955.
207. Fleischner FG: Pulmonary embolism. Can Med Assoc J 78:653, 1958.
208. Chrispin AR, Goodwin JF, Steiner R: The radiology of obliterative pulmonary hypertension and thrombo-embolism. Br J Radiol 36:705, 1963.
209. Teplick JG, Haskin ME, Steinberg SB: Changes in the main pulmonary artery segment following pulmonary embolism. Am J Roentgenol 92:557, 1964.
210. Palla A, Donnamaria V, Petruzzelli S, et al: Enlargement of the right descending pulmonary artery in pulmonary embolism. Am J Roentgenol 141:513, 1983.
211. Chang CH, Davis WC: A roentgen sign of pulmonary infarction. Clin Radiol 16:141, 1965.
212. Laur A: Roentgen diagnosis of pulmonary embolism and its differentiation from myocardial infarction. Am J Roentgenol 90:632, 1963.
213. Talbot S, Worthington BS, Roebuck EJ: Radiographic signs of pulmonary embolism and pulmonary infarction. Thorax 28:198, 1973.
214. Harker LA, Slichter SJ: Studies of platelet and fibrinogen kinetics in patients with prosthetic heart valves. N Engl J Med 283:1302, 1970.
215. Bischel MD, Scoles BG, Mohler JG: Evidence for pulmonary microembolization during hemodialysis. Chest 67:335, 1975.
216. Rubenstein MD, Wall RT, Wood GS, et al: Complications of therapeutic apheresis, including a fatal case with pulmonary vascular occlusion. Am J Med 75:171, 1983.
217. Reul GJ Jr, Beall AC Jr, Greenberg SD: Protection of the pulmonary microvasculature by fine screen blood filtration. Chest 66:4, 1974.
218. Patterson RH Jr, Twichell JB: Disposable filter for microemboli: Use in cardiopulmonary bypass and massive transfusion. JAMA 215:76, 1971.
219. Jenevein EP, Weiss DL: Platelet microemboli associated with massive blood transfusion. Am J Pathol 45:313, 1964.
220. Wells S, Sissons M, Hasleton PS: Quantitation of pulmonary megakaryocytes and fibrin thrombi in patients dying from burns. Histopathology 8:517, 1984.
221. Jacoby CG, Mindell HJ: Lobar consolidation in pulmonary embolism. Radiology 118:287, 1976.
222. Bachynski JE: Absence of the air bronchogram sign: A reliable finding in pulmonary embolism with infarction or hemorrhage. Radiology 100:547, 1971.
223. Coke LR, Dundee JC: Cavitation in bland infarcts of the lung. Can Med Assoc J 72:907, 1955.
224. Grieco MH, Ryan SF: Aseptic cavitary pulmonary infarction. Am J Med 45:811, 1968.
225. Arora YC, Lyons HA, Cantor PA: Unusual clinical and roentgenographic features of pulmonary infarction. Am Rev Respir Dis 82:232, 1960.
226. Lourie GL, Pizzo SV, Ravin C, et al: Experimental pulmonary infarction in dogs: A comparison of chest radiography and computed tomography. Invest Radiol 17:224, 1982.
227. Sinner WN: Computed tomographic patterns of pulmonary thromboembolism and infarction. J Computr Assist Tomogr 2:395, 1978.
228. Castleman B: Pathologic observations on pulmonary infarction in man. In Sasahara AA, Stein M, (eds): Pulmonary Embolic Disease. New York, Grune & Stratton, 1965, pp 86–92.
229. Fleischner FG: Observations on the radiologic changes in pulmonary embolism. In Sasahara AA, Stein M (eds): Pulmonary Embolic Disease, New York, Grune & Stratton, 1965, pp 206–213.
230. Woesner ME, Sanders I, White GW: The melting sign in resolving transient pulmonary infarction. Am J Roentgenol 111:782, 1971.
231. McGoldrick PJ, Rudd TG, Figley MM, et al: What becomes of pulmonary infarcts? Am J Roentgenol 133:1039, 1979.
232. Fleischner F, Hampton AO, Castleman B: Linear shadows in the lung (interlobar pleuritis atelectasis and healed infarction). Am J Roentgenol 46:610, 1941.
233. Reid L: Personal communication (through Dr. George Simon), 1968.
234. Simon G: The cause and significance of some long line shadows in the chest radiograph. Proc R Soc Med 58:861, 1965.
235. Simon G, Reid L: Personal communication, 1968.
236. Simon G: Further observations on the long line shadow across a lower zone of the lung. Br J Radiol 43:327, 1970.
237. Tudor J, Maurer BJ, Wray R, et al: Lung shadows after acute myocardial infarction. Clin Radiol 24:365, 1973.
238. Kaye Josse, Cohen G, Sandler A, et al: Massive pulmonary embolism without infarction. Br J Radiol 31:326, 1958.
239. Blundell JE: Pneumothorax complicating pulmonary infarction. Br J Radiol 40:226, 1967.
240. McFadden ER Jr, Luparello F: Bronchopleural fistula complicating massive pulmonary infarction. Thorax 24:500, 1969.
241. Fred HL, Harle TS: Septic pulmonary embolism. Dis Chest 55:483, 1969.
242. Jaffe RB, Koschmann EB: Septic pulmonary emboli. Radiology 96:527, 1970.
243. Bain RC, Edwards JE, Scheifley CH, et al: Right-sided bacterial endocarditis and endarteritis. A clinical and pathologic study. Am J Med 24:98, 1958.
244. Hadlock FP, Wallace RJ, Rivera M: Pulmonary septic emboli secondary to parapharyngeal abscess: postanginal sepsis. Radiology 130:29, 1979.
245. Hadlock FP, Wallace RJ Jr, Rivera M: Pulmonary septic emboli secondary to parapharyngeal abscess: postanginal sepsis. Radiology, 130:29, 1979.
246. Celikel TH, Muthuswamy PP: Septic pulmonary emboli secondary to internal jugular vein phlebitis (postanginal sepsis) caused by Eikenella corrodens. Am Rev Respir Dis 130:510, 1984.
247. Felman AH, Shulman ST: Staphylococcal osteomyelitis, sepsis, and pulmonary disease: Observations of 10 patients with combined osseous and pulmonary infections. Radiology 117:649, 1975.
248. Roberts WC, Buchbinder NA: Right-sided valvular infective endocarditis. A clinicopathologic study of twelve necropsy patients. Am J Med 53:7, 1972.
249. Noble J Jr, Cohen RB: Candida septicemia and pulmonary lesions. N Engl J Med 286:1309, 1972.
250. Goodwin NJ, Castronuovo JJ, Friedman EA: Recurrent septic pulmonary embolization complicating maintenance hemodialysis. Ann Intern Med 71:29, 1969.
251. Levi J, Robson M, Rosenfeld JB: Septicaemia and pulmonary embolism complicating use of arteriovenous fistula in maintenance haemodialysis. Lancet 2:288, 1970.
252. Waisser E, Kuo C-S, Kabins SA: Septic pulmonary emboli arising from a permanent transvenous cardiac pacemaker. Chest 61:503, 1972.
253. Zelefsky MN, Lutzker LG: The target sign: a new radiologic sign of septic pulmonary emboli. Am J Roentgenol 129:453, 1977.
254. Silingardi V, Canossi GC, Torelli G, et al: The radiology "target sign" of septic pulmonary embolism in a case of acute myelogenous leukemia. Respiration 42:61, 1981.
255. Gumbs RV, McCauley DI: Hilar and mediastinal adenopathy in septic pulmonary embolic disease. Radiology 142:313, 1982.
256. Webb DW, Thadepalli H: Hemoptysis in patients with septic pulmonary infarcts from tricuspid endocarditis. Chest 76:99, 1979.
257. Marantz PR, Linzer M, Feiner CJ, et al: Inability to predict diagnosis in febrile intravenous drug abusers. Ann Intern Med 106:823, 1987.
258. Hussey HH: Pulmonary embolism. JAMA 226:1351, 1973.
259. MacMillan JC, Milstein SH, Samson PC: Clinical spectrum of septic pulmonary embolism and infarction. J Thorac Cardiovasc Surg 75:670, 1978.
260. Greenspan RH, Ravin CE, Polansky SM, et al: Accuracy of the chest radiograph in diagnosis of pulmonary embolism. Invest Radiol 17:539, 1982.
261. Weidner W, Swanson L, Wilson G: Roentgen techniques in the diagnosis of pulmonary thromboembolism. Am J Roentgenol 100:397, 1967.
262. Sagel SS, Greenspan RH: Nonuniform pulmonary arterial perfusion: Pulmonary embolism? Radiology 99:541, 1971.
263. Dalen JE, Brooks HL, Johnson LW, et al: Pulmonary angiography in acute pulmonary embolism: Indications, techniques, and results in 367 patients. Am Heart J 81:175, 1971.
264. Ormond RS, Gale HH, Drake EH, et al: Pulmonary angiography and pulmonary embolism. Radiology 86:658, 1966.
265. Bookstein JJ: Segmental arteriography in pulmonary embolism. Radiology 93:1007, 1969.

9

266. Gomes AS, Grollman JH, Mink J: Pulmonary angiography for pulmonary emboli: rational selection of oblique views. Am J Roentgenol 129:1019, 1977.
267. Stein PD: Wedge arteriography for the identification of pulmonary emboli in small vessels. Am Heart J 82:618, 1971.
268. Greenspan RH, Simon AL, Ricketts HJ, et al: In vivo magnification angiography. Invest Radiol 2:419, 1967.
269. Le Page JR, Gracia RM: The value of bedside wedge pulmonary angiography in the detection of pulmonary emboli: a predictive and prospective evaluation. Radiology 144:67, 1982.
270. Reilley RF, Smith CW, Price RR, et al: Digital subtraction angiography: limitations for the detection of pulmonary embolism. Radiology 149:379, 1983.
271. Pond GD, Ovitt TW, Capp MP: Comparison of conventional pulmonary angiography with intravenous digital subtraction angiography for pulmonary embolic disease. Radiology 147:345, 1983.
272. Ludwig JW, Verhoeven LAJ, Kersbergen JJ, et al: Digital subtraction angiography of the pulmonary arteries for the diagnosis of pulmonary embolism. Radiology 147:639, 1983.
273. Moses DC, Silver TM, Bookstein JJ: The complementary roles of chest radiography, lung scanning, and selective pulmonary angiography in the diagnosis of pulmonary embolism. Circulation 49:179, 1974.
274. Urokinase pulmonary embolism trial: Pulmonary angiography. Circulation 47(Suppl 2):38, 1973.
275. Sutton GC, Honey M, Gibson RV: Clinical diagnosis of acute massive pulmonary embolism. Lancet 1:271, 1969.
276. Sautter RD, Fletcher FW, Emanuel DA, et al: Pulmonary arteriography in the operating room. Chest 57:423, 1970.
277. Bookstein JJ: Segmental arteriography in pulmonary embolism. Radiology 93:1007, 1969.
278. Godwin JD, Webb WR, Gamsu G, et al: Computed tomography of pulmonary embolism. Am J Roentgenol 135:691, 1980.
279. Ovenfors C-O, Goodwin JD, Brito AC: Diagnosis of peripheral pulmonary emboli by computed tomography in the living dog. Radiology 141:519, 1981.
280. Williams JR, Wilcox WC: Pulmonary embolism: Roentgenographic and angiographic considerations. Am J Roentgenol 89:333, 1963.
281. Ferris EJ, Stanzler RM, Rourke JA, et al: Pulmonary angiography in pulmonary embolic disease. Am J Roentgenol 100:355, 1967.
282. Simon M, Sasahara AA: Observations on the angiographic changes in pulmonary thromboembolism. In Sasahara AA, Stein M (eds): Pulmonary Embolic Disease. New York, Grune & Stratton, 1965, pp 214–224.
283. Alexander JK, Gonzalez DA, Fred HL: Angiographic studies in cardiorespiratory diseases. Special reference to thromboembolism. JAMA 198:575, 1966.
284. Peterson KL, Fred HL, Alexander JK: Pulmonary arterial webs. A new angiographic sign of previous thromboembolism. N Engl J Med 277:33, 1967.
285. Stein PD, O'Connor JF, Dalen JE, et al: The angiographic diagnosis of acute pulmonary embolism: Evaluation of criteria. Am Heart J 73:730, 1967.
286. Bookstein JJ, Silver TM: The angiographic differential diagnosis of acute pulmonary embolism. Radiology 110:25, 1974.
287. Cassling RJ, Lois JF, Gomes AS: Unusual pulmonary angiographic findings in suspected pulmonary embolism. Am J Roentgenol 145:995, 1985.
288. Miller GAH, Sutton GC, Kerr IH, et al: Comparison of streptokinase and heparin in treatment of isolated acute massive pulmonary embolism. Br Med J 2:681, 1971.
289. Walsh PN, Greenspan RH, Simon M, et al: An angiographic severity index for pulmonary embolism. Circulation 47(Suppl 2):101, 1973.
290. Tibbutt DA, Fletcher EWL, Thomas ML, et al: Evaluation of a method for quantifying the angiographic severity of major pulmonary embolism. Am J Roentgenol 125:895, 1975.
291. MacLean LD, Shibata HR, McLean APH, et al: Pulmonary embolism: The value of bedside scanning, angiography and pulmonary embolectomy. Can Med Assoc J 97:991, 1967.
292. Haegelin HF, Murray JF: Means of distinguishing pulmonary emboli and other causes of pulmonary hypertension. Dis Chest 53:138, 1968.
293. Mills SR, Jackson DC, Sullivan DC, et al: Angiographic evaluation of chronic pulmonary embolism. Radiology 136:301, 1980.
294. Del Guercio LRM, Cohn JD, Feins NR, et al: Pulmonary embolism shock: Physiologic basis of a bedside screening test. JAMA 196:751, 1966.
295. Oakley CM: Diagnosis of pulmonary embolism. Br Med J 2:773, 1970.
296. Alderson PO, Biello DR, Khan AR, et al: Comparison of 133Xe single-breath and washout imaging in the scintigraphic diagnosis of pulmonary embolism. Radiology 137:481, 1980.
297. Taplin GV, Elam D, Griswold ML, et al: Aerosol inhalation in lung imaging. Radiology 112:431, 1974.
298. Osborne DR, Jaszczak RJ, Greer K, et al: Detection of pulmonary emboli in dogs: comparison of single photon emission computed tomography, gamma camera imaging and angiography. Radiology 146:493, 1983.
299. Khan BO, Jarritt PH, Cullum I, et al: Radionuclide section scanning of the lungs in pulmonary embolism. Br J Radiol 54:586, 1981.
300. Davis HH, Heaton WA, Siegel BA, et al: Scintigraphic detection of atherosclerotic lesions and venous thrombi in man by indium-111 labelled autologous platelets. Lancet 1:1185, 1978.
301. Sostman HD, Neumann RD, Zoghbi SS, et al: Experimental studies with 111Indium-labeled platelets in pulmonary embolism. Invest Radiol 17:367, 1982.
302. Sostman HD, Neumann RD, Loke J, et al: Detection of pulmonary embolism in man with 111In-labeled autologous platelets. Am J Roentgenol 138:945, 1982.
303. Fenech A, Hussey JK, Smith FW, et al: Diagnosis of deep vein thrombosis using autologous indium111-labelled platelets. Br Med J 282:1020, 1981.
304. Fenech A, Dendy PP, Hussey JK, et al: Indium-III labelled platelets in diagnosis of leg-vein thrombosis: preliminary findings. Br Med J 280:1571, 1980.
305. Ezekowitz MD, Eichner ER, Scatterday R, et al: Diagnosis of a persistent pulmonary embolus by indium-111 platelet scintigraphy with angiographic and tissue confirmation. Am J Med 72:839, 1982.
306. Winter JH, Buckler PW, Bautista AP, et al: Frequency of venous thrombosis in patients with an exacerbation of chronic obstructive lung disease. Thorax 38:605, 1983.
307. Kipper MS, Moser KM, Kortman KE, et al: Longterm follow-up of patients with suspected pulmonary embolism and a normal lung scan. Chest 82:411, 1982.
308. Rosenow EC III, Osmundson PJ, Brown ML: Pulmonary embolism. Mayo Clin Proc 56:161, 1981.
309. Robin ED: Overdiagnosis and overtreatment of pulmonary embolism: The emperor may have no clothes. Ann Intern Med 87:775, 1977.
310. Biello DR, Mattar AG, Osei-Wusu A, et al: Interpretation of indeterminate lung scintigrams. Radiology 133:189, 1979.
311. Biello DR, Mattar AG, McKnight RC, et al: Ventilation-perfusion studies in suspected pulmonary embolism. Am J Roentgenol 133:1033, 1979.
312. Carter WD, Brady TM, Keyes JW Jr, et al: Relative accuracy of two diagnostic schemes for detection of pulmonary embolism by ventilation-perfusion scintigraphy. Radiology 145:447, 1982.
313. Bass H, Heckscher T, Anthonisen NR: Regional pulmonary gas exchange in patients with pulmonary embolism. Clin Sci 33:355, 1967.
314. Anthonisen NR, Bass H, Heckscher T, et al: Recent observation on the measurement of regional V/Q ratios in chronic lung disease. J Nucl Biol Med 11:73, 1967.
315. McNeil BJ, Holman BL, Adelstein SJ: The scintigraphic definition of pulmonary embolism. JAMA 227:753, 1974.
316. DeNardo GL, Goodwin DA, Ravasini R, et al: The ventilatory lung scan in the diagnosis of pulmonary embolism. N Engl J Med 282:1334, 1970.
317. Williams O, Lyall J, Vernon M, et al: Ventilation-perfusion lung scanning for pulmonary emboli. Br Med J 1:600, 1974.
318. Farmelant MH, Trainor JC: Evaluation of a 133Xe ventilation technique for diagnosis of pulmonary disorders. J Nucl Med 12:586, 1971.
319. Wolfe WC, Pircher FJ, Sabiston DC Jr: Diagnosis of pulmonary embolism by radioactive ventilation scanning. Surg Forum 17:119, 1966.
320. Kessler RM, McNeil BJ: Impaired ventilation in a patient with angiographically demonstrated pulmonary emboli. Radiology 114:111, 1975.
321. Alderson PO, Biello DR, Sachariah KG, et al: Scintigraphic detection of pulmonary embolism in patients with obstructive pulmonary disease. Radiology 138:661, 1981.
322. Smith R, Ellis K, Alderson PO: Role of chest radiography in predicting the extent of airway disease in patients with suspected pulmonary embolism. Radiology 159:391, 1986.
323. Meignan M, Simonneau G, Oliveira L, et al: Computation of ventilation-perfusion ratio with Kr-81m in pulmonary embolism. J Nucl Med 25:149, 1984.
324. Dillon WP, Taylor AT, Mineau DE, et al: Traumatic pulmonary artery pseudoaneurysm simulating pulmonary embolism. Am J Roentgenol 139:818, 1982.
325. Moser KM, Miale A Jr: Interpretive pitfalls in lung photoscanning. Am J Med 44:366, 1968.
326. Winebright JW, Gerdes AJ, Nelp WB: Restoration of blood flow after pulmonary embolism. Arch Intern Med 125:241, 1970.
327. Vernon P, Burton GH, Seed WA: Lung scan abnormalities in asthma and their correlation with lung function. Eur J Nucl Med 12:16, 1986.

328. Moser KM, Longo AM, Ashburn WL, et al: Spurious scintiphoto-graphic recurrence of pulmonary emboli. Am J Med 55:434, 1973.

329. Hull RD, Hirsh J, Carter CJ, et al: Pulmonary angiography, ventilation lung scanning, and venography for clinically suspected pulmonary embolism with abnormal perfusion lung scan. Ann Intern Med 98:891, 1983.

330. Bell WR: Pulmonary embolism: progress and problems. Am J Med 72:181, 1982.

331. Leading Article: Managment of pulmonary embolism. Br Med J 4:133, 1968.

332. Browse NL: Prophylaxis of pulmonary embolism. Br Med J 2:780, 1970.

333. Browse NL, Thomas ML, Solan MJ, et al: Prevention of recurrent pulmonary embolism. Br Med J 3:382, 1969.

334. Dow JD: Retrograde phlebography in major pulmonary embolism. Lancet 2:407, 1973.

335. Rudikoff JC, Clapp PR, Ferris EJ: Iliocaval thrombi in pulmonary thromboembolic disease. Am J Roentgenol 126:1019, 1976.

336. Hull R, Hirsh J, Sackett DL, et al: Replacement of venography in suspected venous thrombosis by impedance plethysmography and ^{125}I-fibrogen leg scanning: A less invasive approach. Ann Intern Med 94:12, 1981.

337. Hull R, Hirsh J, Sackett DL, et al: Combined use of leg scanning and impedance plethysmography in suspected venous thrombosis: an alternative to venography. N Engl J Med 296:1497, 1977.

338. Little JM, Binns M: Spontaneous change in frequency of deep-vein thrombosis detected by ultrasound. Lancet 2:1229, 1972.

339. Clark WB, MacGregor AB, Prescott RJ, et al: Pneumatic compression of the calf and postoperative deep-vein thrombosis. Lancet 2:5, 1974.

340. Roberts VC, Cotton LT: Prevention of postoperative deep-vein thrombosis in patients with malignant disease. Br Med J 1:358, 1974.

341. Lahnborg G, Bergstöm K, Friman L, et al: Effect of low-dose heparin on incidence of postoperative pulmonary embolism detected by photoscanning. Lancet 1:329, 1974.

342. Roberts VC: Fibrinogen uptake scanning for diagnosis of deep vein thrombosis: A plea for standardization. Br Med J 3:455, 1975.

343. O'Brien JR: Detection of thrombosis with iodine-125 fibrinogen. Data reassessed. Lancet 2:396, 1970.

344. Yao ST, Gourmos C, Hobbs JT: Detection of proximal-vein thrombosis by Doppler ultrasound flow-detection method. Lancet 1:1, 1972.

345. Cheely R, McCartney WH, Perry JR, et al: The role of noninvasive tests versus pulmonary angiography in the diagnosis of pulmonary embolism. Am J Med 70:17, 1981.

346. Mullick SC, Wheeler HB, Songster GF: Diagnosis of deep venous thrombosis by measurement of electrical impedance. Am J Surg 119:417, 1970.

347. Wheeler HB, Mullick SC, Anderson JN, et al: Diagnosis of occult deep vein thrombosis by a noninvasive bedside technique. Surgery 70:20, 1971.

348. Simon G: Further observations on the long line shadow across a lower zone of the lung. Br J Radiol 43:327, 1970.

349. Moser KM, Brach BB, Dolan GF: Clinically suspected deep venous thrombosis of the lower extremities: A comparison of venography, impedance plethysmography and radio-labeled fibrinogen. JAMA 237:2195, 1977.

350. Sasahara AA, Sharma GVRK, Paris AF: New developments in the detection and prevention of venous thromboembolism. Am J Cardiol 43:1214, 1979.

351. Foti MEG, Gurewich V: Fibrin degradation products and impedance plethysmography: measurements in the diagnosis of acute deep vein thrombosis. Arch Intern Med 140:903, 1980.

352. Prescott SM, Richards KL, Tikoff G, et al: Venous thromboembolism in decompensted chronic obstructive pulmonary disease: a prospective study. Am Rev Respir Dis 123:32, 1981.

353. Wilson JE: Diagnostic methods for deep venous thrombosis. Arch Intern Med 140:893, 1980.

354. Moser KM, Lemoine JR, Nachtwey FJ, et al: Deep venous thrombosis and pulmonary embolism. JAMA 246:1422, 1981.

355. Moser KM, Le Moine JR: Is embolic risk conditioned by location of deep venous thrombosis? Ann Intern Med 94(Part I):439, 1981.

356. Ritchie WGM, Soulen RL, Lapayowker MS: Thermographic diagnosis of deep venous thrombosis. Radiology 131:341, 1979.

357. Aronen HJ, Suoranta HT, Taavitsainen MJ: Thermography in deep venous thrombosis of the leg. Am J Roentgenol 136:1179, 1981.

358. Henderson HP, Cooke ED, Bowcock SA, et al: After-exercise thermography for predicting postoperative deep vein thrombosis. Br Med J 1:1020, 1978.

359. Lindhagen A, Berggvist D, Hallbook T, et al: After-exercise thermography and prediction of deep vein thrombosis. Br Med J 284:1825, 1982.

360. Pochaczevsky R, Pillari G, Feldman F: Liquid crystal contact thermography of deep venous thrombosis. Am J Roentgenol 138:717, 1982.

361. Gilday DL, Poulose KP, DeLand FH: Accuracy of detection of pulmonary embolism by lung scanning correlated with pulmonary angiography. Am J Roentgenol 115:732, 1972.

362. Moser KM, Harsanyi P, Rius-Garriga G, et al: Assessment of pulmonary photoscanning and angiography in experimental pulmonary embolism. Circulation 39:663, 1969.

363. McIntyre KM, Sasahara AA: Correlation of pulmonary photoscan and angiogram as measures of the severity of pulmonary embolic involvement. J Nucl Med 12:732, 1971.

364. Poulose KP, Reba RC, Gilday DL, et al: Diagnosis of pulmonary embolism: A correlative study of the clinical, scan, and angiographic findings. Br Med J 3:67, 1970.

365. Linton DS Jr, Bellon EM, Bodie JF, et al: Comparison of results of pulmonary arteriography and radioisotope lung scanning in the diagnosis of pulmonary emboli. Am J Roentgenol 112:745, 1971.

366. Urokinase pulmonary embolism trial: Interrelationships of pulmonary angiograms, lung scans, hemodynamic measurements and fibrinolytic findings. Circulation 47(Suppl 2):73, 1973.

367. Bookstein JJ, Feigin DS, Seo KW, et al: Diagnosis of pulmonary embolism. Radiology 136:15, 1980.

368. Fred HL, Burdine JA Jr, Gonzalez DA, et al: Arteriographic assessment of lung scanning in the diagnosis of pulmonary thromboembolism. N Engl J Med 275:1025, 1966.

369. UCLA Interdepartmental Conference (Moderator: Webber MM: Discussants: Bloomer WE, Crandell PH, Drinkard J, et al): The use of radioisotope scanning in medical diagnosis: Applications in diseases of brain, lung, liver, and heart. Ann Intern Med 67:1059, 1967.

370. Sostman HD, Ravin CE, Sullivan DC, et al: Use of pulmonary angiography for suspected pulmonary embolism: influence of scintigraphic diagnosis. Am J Roentgenol 139:673, 1982.

371. Novelline RA, Baltarowich OH, Athanasoulis CA, et al: The clinical course of patients with suspected pulmonary embolism and a negative pulmonary arteriogram. Radiology 126:561, 1978.

372. McNeil BJ, Hessel SJ, Branch WT: The value of the lung scan in the evaluation of young patients with pleuritic chest pain. J Nucl Med 17:163, 1976.

373. Breckenridge RT, Ratnoff OD: Pulmonary embolism and unexpected death in supposedly normal persons. N Engl J Med 270:298, 1964.

374. Cohen H, Daly JJ: Unheralded pulmonary embolism. Br Med J 2:1209, 1957.

375. Sautter RD, Fletcher FW, Emanuel DA, et al: Complete resolution of massive pulmonary thromboembolism. JAMA 189:948, 1964.

376. Chait A, Summers D, Krasnow N, et al: Observations on the fate of large pulmonary emboli. Am J Roentgenol 100:364, 1967.

377. Fred HL, Axelrad MA, Lewis JM, et al: Rapid resolution of pulmonary thromboemboli in man. An angiographic study. JAMA 196:1137, 1966.

378. Barker NW, Nygaard KK, Walters W, et al: A statistical study of post-operative venous thrombosis and pulmonary embolism. II. Predisposing factors. Mayo Clin Proc 16:1, 1941.

379. Barker NW, Nygaard KK, Walters W, et al: A statistical study of post-operative venous thrombosis and pulmonary embolism. III. Time of occurrence during the postoperative period. Mayo Clin Proc 16:17, 1941.

380. Amos JAS: Thrombosis of the major pulmonary arteries. Br Med J 2:659, 1958.

381. Sasahara AA, McIntyre KM, Criss AJ, et al: Aggressive approach to the management of pulmonary embolism. Cardiovasc Clin 1:262, 1970.

382. Goodwin John F: The clinical diagnosis of pulmonary thromboembolism. In Sasahara AA, Stein M (eds), Pulmonary Embolic Disease. New York, Grune & Stratton, 1965, pp 239–255.

383. Spittell JA Jr: Thrombophlebitis and pulmonary embolism. Circulation 27:976, 1963.

384. Rosenberg DML, Pearce C, McNulty J: Surgical treatment of pulmonary embolism. J Thorac Cardiovasc Surg 47:1, 1964.

385. Webster JR Jr, Saadeh GB, Eggum PR, et al: Wheezing due to pulmonary embolism: Treatment with heparin. N Engl J Med 274:931, 1966.

386. Olazábal F Jr, Román-Irizarry LA, Oms JD, et al: Pulmonary emboli masquerading as asthma. N Engl J Med 278:999, 1968.

387. Leading Article: Prevention of pulmonary embolism. Br Med J 2:1, 1973.

388. Gore I, Tanaka K: Phlebothrombosis, pulmonary embolization and pulmonary hypertension. Am J Med Sci 244:351, 1962.

389. Stevens AE: The late appearance of leg symptoms in pulmonary embolus. Lancet 2:1005, 1961.

390. Israel HL, Goldstein F: The varied clinical manifestations of pulmonary embolism. Ann Intern Med 47:202, 1957.

391. Hildner FJ, Ormond RS: Accuracy of the clinical diagnosis of pulmonary embolism. JAMA 202:567, 1967.

392. Fred HL, Willerson JT, Alexander JK: Neurological manifestations of pulmonary thromboembolism. Arch Intern Med 120:33, 1967.

393. Bang AN, Iversen K, Schmidt H: Thromboemboliske lungesyg-

9

domme. Belyst ved klinik og sektionsfund på et større hospitalsmateriale. (Thromboembolic lung lesions.) Nord Med 60:1413, 1958.

394. Dalen JE, Dexter L: Pulmonary embolism. JAMA 207:1505, 1969.

395. Parmley LF Jr, Senior RM, McKenna DH, et al: Clinically deceptive massive pulmonary embolism. Chest 58:15, 1970.

396. McDonald IG, Hirsh J, Hale GS, et al: Saddle pulmonary embolism: A surgical emergency. Lancet 1:269, 1970.

397. Shenoy MM, Friedman SA, Dhar S, et al: Streptokinase lysis of intraventricular thrombus and pulmonary emboli with resolution of acquired intracardiac shunt. Ann Intern Med 103:65, 1985.

398. Shaw RA, Schonfeld SA, Whitcomb ME: Pulmonary embolism presenting as coronary insufficiency. Arch Intern Med 141:651, 1981.

399. Sasahara AA: Clinical studies in pulmonary thromboembolism. In Sasahara AA, Stein M (eds): Pulmonary Embolic Disease. New York, Grune & Stratton, 1965, pp 256–264.

400. Meister SG, Grossman W, Dexter L, et al: Paradoxical embolism: Diagnosis during life. Am J Med 53:292, 1972.

401. Loscalzo J: Paradoxical embolism: clinical presentation, diagnostic strategies, and therapeutic options. Am Heart J 112:141, 1986.

402. Bromberg PA: Pulmonary aspects of sickle cell disease. Arch Intern Med 133:652, 1974.

403. Petch MC, Sargent GR: Clinical features of pulmonary lesions in sickle-cell anemia. Br Med J 3:31, 1970.

404. Wallace JM, Moser KM, Hartman MT, et al: Patterns of pulmonary perfusion scans in normal subjects. 2: the prevalence of abnormal scans in young smokers. Am Rev Respir Dis 125:465, 1982.

405. Lippmann M, Fein A: Pulmonary embolism in the patient with chronic obstructive pulmonary disease: a diagnostic dilemma. Chest 79:39, 1981.

406. Johnson JC, Flowers NC, Horan LG: Unexplained atrial flutter: A frequent herald of pulmonary embolism. Chest 60:29, 1971.

407. Fraser RS, Lynne-Davies P: Continuous chest murmur acquired following pulmonary thromboembolism. Chest 65:562, 1974.

408. Albertini RE: Vocal cord paralysis associated with pulmonary emboli. Chest 62:508, 1972.

409. Brinton WD: Primary pulmonary hypertension. Br Heart J 12:305, 1950.

410. Soothill JF: A case of primary pulmonary hypertension with paralysed left vocal cord. Guys Hosp Rep 100:232, 1951.

411. Wacker Warren EC, Snodgrass PJ: Serum LDH activity in pulmonary embolism diagnosis. JAMA 174:2142, 1960.

412. Wacker WEC, Rosenthal M, Snodgrass PJ, et al: A triad for the diagnosis of pulmonary embolism and infarction. JAMA 178:8, 1961.

413. Ruckley CV, Das PC, Leitch AG, et al: Serum fibrin/fibrinogen degradation products associated with postoperative pulmonary embolus and venous thrombosis. Br Med J 4:395, 1970.

414. Snodgrass PJ, Amador E, Wacker WEC: Serum enzymes in the diagnosis of pulmonary embolism. In Sasahara AA, Stein M (eds): Pulmonary Embolic Disease. New York, Grune & Stratton, 1965, pp 93–100.

415. Coodley EL: Enzyme profiles in the evaluation of pulmonary infarction. JAMA 207:1307, 1969.

416. Allington MJ: Detection of fibrin(ogen) degradation products by a latex dumping method. Scand J Haematol (Suppl) 13:115, 1971.

417. Hawiger J, Niewiarowski S, Gurewich V, et al: Measurement of fibrinogen and fibrin degradation products in serum by staphylococcal clumping test. J Lab Clin Med 75:93, 1970.

418. Merskey C, Johnson AJ, Pert JH, et al: Pathogenesis of fibrinolysis in defibrination syndrome: Effect of heparin administration. Blood 24:701, 1964.

419. Merskey C, Kleiner GJ, Johnson AJ: Quantitative estimation of split products of fibrinogen in human serum, relation to diagnosis and treatment. Blood 28:1, 1966.

420. Cooke ED, Gordon YB, Bowcock SA, et al: Serum fibrin (fibrinogen) degradation products in diagnosis of deep vein thrombosis and pulmonary embolism after hip surgery. Lancet 2:31, 1975.

421. Gurewich V, Hume M, Patrick M: The laboratory diagnosis of venous thromboembolic disease by measurement of fibrinogen/fibrin degradation products and fibrin monomer. Chest 64:585, 1973.

422. Gallus AS, Hirsh J, Gent M: Relevance of preoperative and postoperative blood tests to postoperative leg-vein thrombosis. Lancet 2:805, 1973.

423. Tibbutt DA, Chesterman CN, Allington MJ, et al: Measurement of fibrinogen-fibrin-related antigen in serum as aid to diagnosis of deep vein thrombosis in outpatients. Br Med J 1:367, 1975.

424. Wilson JE III, Frenkel EP, Pierce AK, et al: Spontaneous fibrinolysis in pulmonary embolism. J Clin Invest 50:474, 1971.

425. Sonnabend D, Cooper D, Fiddes P, et al: Fibrin degradation products in thrombo-embolic disease. Pathology 4:47, 1972.

426. Cash JD, Woodfield DG, Das PC, et al: Diagnosis of suspected or occult pulmonary embolus. Br Med J 2:576, 1969.

427. Rickman FD, Handin R, Howe JP, et al: Fibrin split products in acute pulmonary embolism. Ann Intern Med 79:664, 1973.

428. Light RW, Bell WR: LDH and fibrinogen-fibrin degradation products in pulmonary embolism. Arch Intern Med 133:372, 1974.

429. Cooper HA, Bowie EJW, Owen CA Jr: Evaluation of patients with increased fibrinolytic split products (FSP) in their serum. Mayo Clin Proc 49:654, 1974.

430. Sipes JN, Suratt PM, Teates CD, et al: A prospective study of plasma DNA in the diagnosis of pulmonary embolism. Am Rev Respir Dis 118:475, 1978.

431. Lippmann ML, Morgan L, Fein A, et al: Plasma and serum concentrations of DNA in pulmonary thromboembolism. Am Rev Respir Dis 125:416, 1982.

432. Griner Paul F: Bloody pleural fluid in pulmonary infarction. JAMA 202:947, 1967.

433. Sasahara Arthur A, Stein M, Simon M, et al: Pulmonary angiography in the diagnosis of thromboembolic disease. N Engl J Med 270:1075, 1964.

434. Wilhelmsen Lars, Selander S, Söderholm B, et al: Recurrent pulmonary embolism. Medicine 42:335, 1963.

435. Just-Viera JO, Yeager GH: Massive pulmonary embolism. II. Predictable mortality and cardiopulmonary changes in dogs breathing room air. Ann Surg 159:636, 1964.

436. Urokinase pulmonary embolism trial: Phase I results. A cooperative study. JAMA 214:2163, 1970.

437. Leland O, Stevens Jr, Sasahara AA: Hemodynamic observations in patients with pulmonary thromboembolism. In Sasahara AA, Stein M (eds): Pulmonary Embolic Disease. New York, Grune & Stratton, 1965, pp 110–119.

438. Robin ED, Julian DG, Travis DM, et al: A physiologic approach to the diagnosis of acute pulmonary embolism. N Engl J Med 260:586, 1959.

439. Robin ED, Forkner CE Jr, Bromberg PA, et al: Alveolar gas exchange in clinical pulmonary embolism. N Engl J Med 262:283, 1960.

440. MacKeen AD, Landrigan PL, Dickson RC: Early diagnosis of acute pulmonary embolism. Can Med Assoc J 85:233, 1961.

441. Severinghaus JW, Stupfel M: Alveolar dead space as an index of distribution of blood flow in pulmonary capillaries. J Appl Physiol 10:335, 1957.

442. Dantzker DR, Bower JS: Alterations in gas exchange following pulmonary thromboembolism. Chest 81:495, 1982.

443. Colp CR, Williams MH Jr: Pulmonary function following pulmonary embolization. Am Rev Respir Dis 85:799, 1962.

444. Nadel JA, Gold WM, Jennings DB, et al: Unusual disease of pulmonary arteries with dyspnea. Structure-function relationships. Am J Med 41:440, 1966.

445. Lichstein E, Seckler SG: Evaluation of acute chest pain. Med Clin North Am 57:1481, 1973.

446. Winsor T: Electrocardiogram and pulmonary infarction (acute cor pulmonale). JAMA 204:807, 1971.

447. Schwaber JR: The diagnosis of pulmonary embolism. Med Clin North Am 53:365, 1969.

448. Smith M, Ray CT: Electrocardiographic signs of early right ventricular enlargement in acute pulmonary embolism. Chest 58:205, 1970.

449. Cutforth RH, Oram S: The electrocardiogram in pulmonary embolism. Br Heart J 20:41, 1958.

450. Littmann D: Observations on the electrocardiographic changes in pulmonary embolism. In Sasahara AA, Stein M (eds): Pulmonary Embolic Disease. New York, Grune & Stratton, 1965, pp 186–198.

451. Lynch RE, Stein PD, Bruce TA: Leftward shift of frontal plane QRS axis as a frequent manifestation of acute pulmonary embolism. Chest 61:443, 1972.

452. Webber DM, Phillips JH Jr: A re-evaluation of electrocardiographic changes accompanying acute pulmonary embolism. Am J Med Sci 251:381, 1966.

453. Paraskos JA, Adelstein SJ, Smith RE, et al: Late prognosis of acute pulmonary embolism. N Engl J Med 289:55, 1973.

454. Donaldson GA, Williams C, Scannell JG, et al: A reappraisal of the application of the Trendelenburg operation to massive fatal embolism. Report of a successful pulmonary-artery thrombectomy using a cardiopulmonary bypass. N Engl J Med 268:171, 1963.

455. Benotti JR, Ockene IS, Alpert JS, et al: The clinical profile of unresolved pulmonary embolism. Chest 84:669, 1983.

456. Riedel M, Stanek V, Widimsky J, et al: Longterm follow-up of patients with pulmonary thromboembolism: late prognosis and evolution of hemodynamic and respiratory data. Chest 81:151, 1982.

457. Wilson JE III: Pulmonary embolism: diagnosis and treatment. Clin Notes Respir Dis 20:3, 1981.

458. Shuck JW, Walder JS, Kam TH, et al: Chronic persistent pulmonary embolism: report of 3 cases. Am J Med 69:790, 1980.

459. Daily PO, Johnston GG, Simmons CJ, et al: Surgical management of chronic pulmonary embolism: surgical treatment and late results. J Thorac Cardiovasc Surg 79:523, 1980.

460. Levinson RM, Shure D, Moser KM: Reperfusion pulmonary edema after pulmonary artery thromboendarterectomy. Am Rev Respir Dis 134:1241, 1986.

461. Moser KM, Shure D, Harrell JH, et al: Angioscopic visualization of pulmonary emboli. Chest 77:198, 1980.
462. Shure D, Gregoratos G, Moser KM: Fiberoptic angioscopy: role in the diagnosis of chronic pulmonary arterial obstruction. Ann Intern Med 103:844, 1985.
463. Marder VJ: The use of thrombolytic agents: choice of patient, drug administration, laboratory monitoring. Ann Intern Med 90:802, 1979.
464. Sasahara AA, Sharma GVRK, Tow DE, et al: Clinical use of thrombolytic agents in venous thromboembolism. Arch Intern Med 142:684, 1982.
465. Bell WR, Meek AG: Current concepts: guidelines for the use of thrombolytic agents. N Engl J Med 301:1266, 1979.
466. Editorial: Streptokinase and deep venous thrombosis. Lancet 1:1035, 1981.
467. Editorial: Pulmonary embolism: therapeutic dilemma? Lancet 2:1396, 1981.
468. Sharma GVRK, Burleson VA, Sasahara AA: Effect of thrombolytic therapy on pulmonary-capillary blood volume in patients with pulmonary embolism. N Engl J Med 303:842, 1980.
469. Barritt DW, Jordan SC: Anticoagulant drugs in the treatment of pulmonary embolism: a controlled trial. Lancet 1:1309, 1960.
470. Sasahara AA, Sharma GVRK, Paris AF: New developments in the detection and prevention of venous thromboembolism. Am J Cardiol 43:1214, 1979.
471. Robbins SL: Pathology, 3rd ed., Vol. II. Philadelphia, WB Saunders Co, 1967.
472. Urokinase pulmonary embolism trial: Phase I results. A cooperative study. JAMA 214:2163, 1970.
473. Jaffe RB, Koschmann EB: Septic pulmonary emboli. Radiology 96:527, 1970.
474. Roberts WC, Buchbinder NA: Right-sided valvular infective endocarditis. A clinicopathologic study of twelve necropsy patients. Am J Med 53:7, 1972.
475. Silingardi V, Canossi GC, Torelli G, et al: The radiologic 'target sign' of septic pulmonary embolism in a case of acute myelogenous leukemia. Respiration 42:61, 1981.
476. Gumbs RV, McCauley DI: Hilar and mediastinal adenopathy in septic pulmonary embolic disease. Radiology 142:313, 1982.
477. Poller L: Oral anticoagulants reassessed. Br Med J 284:1425, 1982.
478. Gray JD: Cardiovascular and respiratory agents during pregnancy: implications for fetal development. Clin Invest Med 8:339, 1985.
479. Bell WR, Starksen NF, Tong S, et al: Trousseau's syndrome: devastating coagulopathy in the absence of heparin. Am J Med 79:423, 1985.
480. Hall RJC, Sutton GC, Kerr IH: Long-term prognosis of treated acute massive pulmonary embolism. Br Heart J 39:1128, 1977.
481. Glassford DM Jr, Alford WC Jr, Burrus GR, et al: Pulmonary embolectomy. Ann Thorac Surg 32:28, 1981.
482. Coon WW, Willis PW III: Hemorrhagic complications of anticoagulant therapy. Arch Intern Med 133:386, 1974.
483. Cheely R, McCartney WH, Perry JR, et al: The role of noninvasive tests versus pulmonary angiography in the diagnosis of pulmonary embolism. Am J Med 70:17, 1981.
484. Millard CE: Massive hemothorax complicating heparin therapy for pulmonary infarction. Chest 59:235, 1971.
485. Hattersley PG, Mitsuoka JC, King JH: Sources of error in heparin therapy of thromboembolic disease. Arch Intern Med 140:1173, 1980.
486. Walker AM, Jick H: Predictors of bleeding during heparin therpy. JAMA 244:1209, 1980.
487. Van Renterghem D, Bogaerts Y, Tasson J, et al: Intrabronchial bleeding and life-threatening atelectasis in pulmonary embolism. Eur J Respir Dis 65:144, 1984.
488. Young AE, Thomas ML, Browse NL: Comparison between sequelae of surgical and medical treatment of venous thromboembolism. Br Med J 4:127, 1974.
489. Sevitt S: Fat Embolism. London, Butterworths, 1962.
490. Lessells AM: Fatal fat embolism after minor trauma. Br Med J 282:1586, 1981.
491. Hill RB Jr: Fatal fat embolism from steroid-induced fatty liver. N Engl J Med 265:318, 1961.
492. Pastore L, Kessler S: Pulmonary fat embolization in the immunocompromised patient. Am J Surg Pathol 6:315, 1982.
493. Durlacher SH, Meier JR, Fisher RS, et al: Sudden death due to pulmonary fat embolism in chronic alcoholics with fatty livers. J Forensic Sci 4:215, 1959.
494. Benatar SR, Ferguson AD, Goldschmidt RB: Fat embolism—some clinical observations and a review of controversial aspects. Q J Med 41:85, 1972.
495. Weisz GM, Steiner E: The cause of death in fat embolism. Chest 59:511, 1971.
496. Sevitt S: The significance and classification of fat-embolism. Lancet 2:825, 1960.
497. Vance BM: Significance of fat embolism. Arch Surg 23:426, 1931.
498. Young AE, Evans IL, Irving D, et al: Fat embolism after pertrochanteric venography. Br Med J 4:592, 1973.
499. Thomas ML, Tighe JR: Death from fat embolism as a complication of intraosseous phlebography. Lancet 2:1415, 1973.
500. Kaufman HD, Finn R, Bourdillon RE: Fat embolism following an epileptic seizure. Br Med J 1:1089, 1966.
501. Todd N: Fatal fat embolism during ritual initiation. Can Med Assoc J 113:133, 1975.
502. Gresham GA, Kuczynski A, Rosborough D: Fatal fat embolism following replacement arthroplasty for transcervical fractures of femur. Br Med J 2:617, 1971.
503. Sevitt S: Fat embolism in patients with fractured hips. Br Med J 2:257, 1972.
504. Jackson CT, Greendyke RM: Pulmonary and cerebral fat embolism after closed-chest cardiac massage. Surg Gynecol Obstet 120:25, 1965.
505. Editorial: Fat embolism. Lancet 1:672, 1972.
506. Broder G, Ruzumna L: Systemic fat embolism following acute primary osteomyelitis. JAMA 199:1004, 1967.
507. Lipton JH, Russell JA, Burgess KR, et al: Fat embolization and pulmonary infiltrates after bone marrow transplantation. Med Pediatr Oncol 15:24, 1987.
508. Scully RE: Fat embolism in Korean battle casualties: Its incidence, clinical significance, and pathologic aspects. Am J Pathol 32:379, 1956.
509. Dines DE, Burgher LW, Okazaki H: The clinical and pathologic correlation of fat embolism syndrome. Mayo Clin Proc 50:407, 1975.
510. Hallgren B, Kerstall J, Rudenstam C-M, et al: A method for the isolation and chemical analysis of pulmonary fat embolism. Acta Chir Scand 132:613, 1966.
511. Peltier LF: Fat embolism. III. The toxic properties of neutral fat and free fatty acids. Surgery 40:665, 1956.
512. Derks CM, Jacobovitz-Derks D: Embolic pneumopathy induced by oleic acid. Am J Pathol 87:143, 1977.
513. Jones JG, Minty BD, Beeley JM, et al: Pulmonary epithelial permeability is immediately increased after embolisation with oleic acid but not with neutral fat. Thorax 37:169, 1982.
514. Jacobovitz-Derks D, Derks CM: Pulmonary neutral fat embolism in dogs. Am J Pathol 95:29, 1979.
515. Reidbord HE: Pulmonary fat embolism. Arch Pathol 98:122, 1974.
516. Thompson PL, Williams KE, Walters MN-I: Fat embolism in the microcirculation: an in-vivo study. J Pathol 97:23, 1969.
517. Saldeen T: Fat embolism and signs of intravascular coagulation in a posttraumatic autopsy material. J Trauma 10:273, 1970.
518. Maruyama Y, Little JB: Roentgen manifestations of traumatic pulmonary fat embolism. Radiology 79:945, 1962.
519. Bierre AR, Koelmeyer TD: Pulmonary fat and bone marrow embolism in aircraft accident victims. Pathology 15:131, 1983.
520. Glas WW, Grekin TD, Musselman MM: Fat embolism. Am J Surg 85:363, 1953.
521. Berrigan TJ Jr, Carsky EW, Heitzman ER: Fat embolism. Roentgenographic pathologic correlation in 3 cases. Am J Roentgenol 96:967, 1966.
522. Heitzman ER: The Lung: Radiologic-Pathologic Correlations. St. Louis, The CV Mosby Co, 1973, pp 127, 137.
523. Curtis A McB, Knowles GD, Putnam CE, et al: The three syndromes of fat embolism: pulmonary manifestations. Yale J Biol Med 52:149, 1979.
524. Williams JR, Bonte FJ: Pulmonary damage in nonpenetrating chest injuries. Radiol Clin North Am 1:439, 1963.
525. Dines DE, Linscheid RL, Didier EP: Fat embolism syndrome. Mayo Clin Proc 47:237, 1972.
526. Burgher LW, Dines DE, Linscheid RL: Fat embolism and the adult respiratory distress syndrome. Mayo Clin Proc 49:107, 1974.
527. Hagley SR, Lee FC, Blumbergs PC: Fat embolism syndrome with total hip replacement. Med J Aust 145:541, 1986.
528. Ross AP: The effect of heparin in experimental fat embolism. Surgery 66:765, 1969.
529. Ross AP: The fat embolism syndrome: With special reference to the importance of hypoxia in the syndrome. J Ann R Coll Surg Engl 46:159, 1970.
530. Aufranc OE, Jones WN, Butler JE: Fat embolism. A complication of fractures of the femur and tibia. JAMA 213:2249, 1970.
531. Tscherne H, Schreyer H, Magerl F: Pulmonale and kardiale röntgenbefunde bei traumatischer fettembolie. (Pulmonary and cardiac roentgen findings due to traumatic fat embolism.) Fortschr Roentgenstr 106:703, 1967.
532. Sproule Brian J, Brady JL, Gilbert JAL: Studies on the syndrome of fat embolization. Can Med Assoc J 90:1243, 1964.
533. Evarts Charles M: Diagnosis and treatment of fat embolism. JAMA 194:899, 1965.
534. Hoare EM: Platelet response in fat embolism and its relationship to petechiae. Br Med J 2:689, 1971.

535. Tachakra SS: Distribution of skin petechiae in fat embolism rash. Lancet 1:284, 1976.
536. Cross HE: Examination of CSF in fat embolism. Report of a case. Arch Intern Med 115:470, 1965.
537. Wiener L, Forsyth D: Pulmonary pathophysiology of fat embolism. Am Rev Respir Dis 92:113, 1965.
538. Davidson FF, Murray JF: Use of pulmonary diffusing capacity measurements to detect unsuspected fat embolism. Am Rev Respir Dis 106:715, 1972.
539. Editorial: Fat embolism and hypoxaemia. Lancet 2:1360, 1974.
540. Gurd AR, Wilson RI: The fat embolism syndrome. J Bone Joint Surg (Br) 56:408, 1974.
541. Steiner PE, Lushbaugh CC: Maternal pulmonary embolism by amniotic fluid as a cause of obstetric shock and unexpected deaths in obstetrics. JAMA 117:1245, 1941.
542. Hutchins PM, Macnicol MF: Pulmonary insufficiency after long bone fractures: absence of circulating fat or significant immunodepression. J Bone Joint Surg 67:835, 1985.
543. Guenter CA, Braun TE: Fat embolism syndrome: changing prognosis. Chest 79:143, 1981.
544. Schonfeld SA, Ploysongsang Y, DiLisio R, et al: Fat embolism prophylaxis with corticosteroids: prospective study in high-risk patients. Ann Intern Med 99:438, 1983.
545. Courtney LD: Amniotic fluid embolism. Obstet Gynecol Surv 29:169, 1974.
546. Philip RS: Amniotic fluid embolism. NY State J Med 67:2085, 1967.
547. Attwood HD: Amniotic fluid embolism. Pathol Ann 7:145, 1972.
548. Masson RG, Ruggieri J, Siddiqui MM: Amniotic fluid embolism: definitive diagnosis in a survivor. Am Rev Respir Dis 120:187, 1979.
549. Shnider SM, Moya F: Amniotic fluid embolism. Review article. Anesthesiology 22:108, 1961.
550. Aguillon A, Andjus T, Grayson A, Race GJ: Amniotic fluid embolism: A review. Obstet Gynecol Surv 17:619, 1962.
551. Morgan M: Amniotic fluid embolism. Anaesthesia 34:20, 1979.
552. Sparr RA, Pritchard JA: Studies to detect the escape of amniotic fluid into the maternal circulation during parturition. Surg Gynecol Obstet 107:560, 1958.
553. Attwood HD, Downing SE: Experimental amniotic fluid and meconium embolism. Surg Gynecol Obstet 120:255, 1965.
554. Weiner AE, Reid DE, Roby CC: The hemostatic activity of amniotic fluid. Science 110:190, 1949.
555. Woodfield DG, Galloway RK, Smart GE: Coagulation defect associated with presumed amniotic fluid embolism in the mid-trimester of pregnancy. J Obstet Gynecol Br Commonwealth 78:423, 1971.
556. Ratnoff OD, Vosburgh GJ: Observations on the clotting defect in amniotic-fluid embolism. N Engl J Med 247:970, 1952.
557. Rodgers GP, Heymach GJ III: Cryoprecipitate therapy in amniotic fluid embolization. Am J Med 76:916, 1984.
558. Peterson EP, Taylor HB: Amniotic fluid embolism: An analysis of 40 cases. Obstet Gynecol 35:787, 1970.
559. Liban E, Raz S: A clinicopathologic study of fourteen cases of amniotic fluid embolism. Am J Clin Pathol 31:477, 1969.
560. Turner R, Gisack M: Massive amniotic fluid embolism. Ann Emerg Med 13:359, 1984.
561. Mulder JI: Amniotic fluid embolism: an overview and case report. Am J Obstet Gynecol 152:430, 1985.
562. Attwood HD: A histological study of experimental amniotic-fluid and meconium embolism in dogs. J Pathol Bacteriol 88:285, 1964.
563. Wasser WG, Tessler S, Kamath CP, et al: Nonfatal amniotic fluid embolism: a case report of postpartum respiratory distress with histopathologic studies. Mount Sinai J Med 46:388, 1979.
564. Roche WD Jr, Norris HJ: Detection and significance of maternal pulmonary amniotic fluid embolism. Obstet Gynecol 43:729, 1974.
565. Garland IWC, Thompson WD: Diagnosis of amniotic fluid embolism using an antiserum to human keratin. J Clin Pathol 36:625, 1983.
566. Arnold HR, Gardner JE, Goodman PH: Amniotic pulmonary embolism. Radiology 77:629, 1961.
567. Cornell SH: Amniotic pulmonary embolism. Am J Roentgenol 89:1084, 1963.
568. Lumley J, Owen R, Morgan M: Amniotic fluid embolism: a report of three cases. Anaesthesia 34:33, 1979.
569. Anderson DG: Amniotic fluid embolism: A re-evaluation. Am J Obstet Gynecol 98:336, 1967.
570. Phills JA, Harold AJ, Whiteman GV, et al: Pulmonary infiltrates, asthma, and eosinophilia due to Ascaris suum infestation in man. N Engl J Med 286:965, 1972.
571. Hadfield JW, Sterling JC, Wraight EP: Multiple tumour emboli simulating a massive pulmonary embolus. Postgrad Med J 58:792, 1982.
572. Margolis ML, Jarrell BE: Pulmonary tumor microembolism. South Med J 78:757, 1985.
573. Crane R, Rudd TG, Dail D: Tumor microembolism: pulmonary perfusion pattern. J Nucl Med 25:877, 1984.
574. Carstens PHB: Pulmonary bone marrow embolism following external cardiac massage. Acta Pathol Microbiol Scand 76:510, 1969.
575. Rappaport H, Raum M, Horrell JB: Bone marrow embolism. Am J Pathol 27:407, 1951.
576. Yoell JH: Bone marrow embolism to lung following sternal puncture. AMA Arch Pathol 67:373, 1959.
577. Pyun KS, Katzenstein RE: Widespread bone marrow embolism with myocardial involvement. Arch Pathol 89:378, 1970.
578. Schinella RA: Bone marrow emboli: Their fate in the vasculature of the human lung. Arch Pathol 95:386, 1973.
579. Park WW: Experimental trophoblastic embolism of the lungs. J Pathol Bacteriol 75:257, 1958.
580. Nosanchuk JS, Littler ER: Skin embolus to lung. Arch Pathol 87:542, 1969.
581. Becker SN, Seo IS, Cornog J: Atypical transitional epithelial cells in a pulmonary embolus. Chest 61:198, 1972.
582. Straus R: Pulmonary embolism caused by liver tissue. Arch Pathol 33:69, 1942.
583. Abrahams C, Catchatourian R: Bone fragment emboli in the lungs of patients undergoing bone marrow transplantation. Am J Clin Pathol 79:360, 1983.
584. Smith RRL, Hutchins GM: Pulmonary fecal embolization complicating the Budd-Chiari syndrome. N Engl J Med 298:1069, 1978.
585. Hartz PH: Occurrence of decidua-like tissue in the lung. Am J Clin Pathol 26:48, 1956.
586. Park WW: The occurrence of decidual tissue within the lung: report of a case. J Pathol Bacteriol 67:503, 1954.
587. Bohm N, Keller KM, Kloke WD: Pulmonary and systemic cerebellar tissue embolism due to birth injury. Virchows Arch 398:229, 1982.
588. Valdes-Dapena MA, Arey JB: Pulmonary emboli of cerebral origin in the newborn. Arch Pathol 84:643, 1967.
589. Balogh K: Pulmonary bile emboli: Sequelae of iatrogenic trauma. Arch Pathol Lab Med 108:814, 1984.
590. Armellin GM, Smith RC, Faithfull GR: Pulmonary bile emboli following percutaneous cholangiography and biliary drainage. Pathology 13:615, 1981.
591. Wescott JL: Air embolism complicating percutaneous needle biopsy of the lung. Chest 63:108, 1973.
592. Smith FR: Air embolism as a cause of death in scuba diving in the Pacific Northwest. Dis Chest 52:15, 1967.
593. Bayne CG, Wurzbacher T: Can pulmonary barotrauma cause cerebral air embolism in a non-diver? Chest 81:648, 1982.
594. Kogutt MS: Systemic air embolism secondary to respiratory therapy in the neonate: six cases including one survivor. Am J Roentgenol 131:425, 1978.
595. Segal AJ, Wasserman M: Arterial air embolism: A cause of sudden death in status asthmaticus. Radiology 99:271, 1971.
596. Bowen FW Jr, Chandra R, Avery GB: Pulmonary interstitial emphysema with gas embolism in hyaline membrane disease. Am J Dis Child 126:117, 1973.
597. Vinstein AL, Gresham EL, Lim MO, et al: Pulmonary venous air embolism in hyaline membrane disease. Radiology 105:627, 1972.
598. Siegle RL, Eyal FG, Rabinowitz JG: Air embolus following pulmonary interstitial emphysema in hyaline membrane disease. Clin Radiol 27:77, 1976.
599. Macklin MT, Macklin CC: Malignant interstitial emphysema of the lungs and mediastinum as an important occult complication in many respiratory diseases and other conditions: An interpretation of the clinical literature in the light of laboratory experiment. Medicine 23:281, 1944.
600. Cholankeril JV, Joshi RR, Cenizal JS, et al: Massive air embolism from the pulmonary artery. Case report. Radiology 142:33, 1982.
601. Taylor JD: Post-mortem diagnosis of air embolism by radiography. Br Med J 1:890, 1952.
602. Campkin TV, Perks JS: Venous air embolism. Lancet 1:235, 1973.
603. O'Quin RJ, Lakshminarayan S: Venous air embolism. Arch Intern Med 142:2173, 1982.
604. Cleveland JC: Fatal air embolism to the right side of the heart during pneumonectomy for carcinoma: result of broncho-azygous vein communication and positive-pressure ventilation. Chest 71:556, 1977.
605. Tuddenham WJ, Paskin DL: Radiographic demonstration of air embolism. Medical Radiogr Photogr 50:16, 1974.
606. Fatteh A, Leach WB, Wilkinson CA: Fatal air embolism in pregnancy resulting from orogenital sex play. Forensic Sci 2:247, 1973.
607. Hartveit F, Lystad H, Minken A: The pathology of venous air embolism. Br J Exp Pathol 49:81, 1968.
608. Warren BA, Philp RB, Inwood MJ: The ultrastructural morphology of air embolism: Platelet adhesion to the interface and endothelial damage. Br J Exp Pathol 54:163, 1973.
609. Gottlieb JD, Ericsson JA, Sweet RB: Venous air embolism: A review. Anesth Analg 44:773, 1965.
610. Boerema B: Appearance and regression of pulmonary arterial

lesions after repeated intravenous injection of gas. J Pathol Bacteriol 89:741, 1965.

611. Faer JM, Messerschmidt GL: Nonfatal pulmonary air embolism: radiolgraphic demonstration. Am J Roentgenol 131:705, 1978.

612. Kizer KW, Goodman PC: Radiographic manifestations of venous air embolism. Radiology 144:35, 1982.

613. Ericsson JA, Gottlieb JD, Sweet RB: Closed-chest cardiac massage in the treatment of venous air embolism. N Engl J Med 270:1353, 1964.

614. Douglas FG, Kafilmout KJ, Patt NL: Foreign particle embolism in drug addicts: Respiratory pathophysiology. Ann Intern Med 75:865, 1971.

615. Hopkins GP, Taylor DG: Pulmonary talc granulomatosis. A complication of drug abuse. Am Rev Respir Dis 101:101, 1970.

616. Kalant H, Kalant OJ: Death in amphetamine users: Causes and rates. Can Med Assoc J 112:299, 1975.

617. Paré JA, Peter, Fraser RG, Hogg JC, et al: Pulmonary "mainline" granulomatosis: Talcosis of intravenous methadone abuse. Medicine 58:229, 1979.

618. Hopkins GB: Pulmonary angiothrombotic granulomatosis in drug offenders. JAMA 221:909, 1972.

619. Lewman LV: Fatal pulmonary hypertension from intravenous injection of methylphenidate (Ritalin) tablets. Hum Pathol 3:67, 1972.

620. Hahn HH, Schweid AI, Beaty HN: Complications of injecting dissolved methylphenidate tablets. Arch Intern Med 123:656, 1969.

621. Willey RF: Abuse of methylphenidate (Ritalin). N Engl J Med 285:464, 1971.

622. O'Driscoll WG, Lindley GR: Self-administration of tripelennamine by a narcotic addict. N Engl J Med 257:376, 1957.

623. Wendt VW, Puro HE, Shapiro J, et al: Angiothrombotic pulmonary hypertension in addicts. "Blue velvet" addiction. JAMA 188:755, 1964.

624. Lerner AM, Oerther FJ: Characteristics and sequelae of paregoric abuse. Ann Intern Med 65:1019, 1966.

625. Soin JS, Wagner HN, Thomashaw D, et al: Increased sensitivity of regional measurements in early detection of narcotic lung disease. Chest 67:325, 1975.

626. Zientara M, Moore S: Fatal talc embolism in a drug addict. Hum Pathol 1:324, 1970.

627. Stern WZ, Subbarao K: Pulmonary complications of drug addiction. Semin Roentgenol 18:183, 1983.

628. Camargo G, Colp C: Pulmonary function studies in ex-heroin users. Chest 67:331, 1975.

629. Gross EM: Talc embolism: Sudden death following intravenous injection of phenyltoloxamine. Forensic Sci 2:475, 1973.

630. Tomashefski JF Jr, Hirsch CS, Jolly PN: Microcrystalline cellulose pulmonary embolism and granulomatosis. Arch Pathol Lab Med 105:89, 1981.

631. Zeltner TB, Nussbaumer U, Rudin O, et al: Unusual pulmonary vascular lesions after intravenous injections of microcrystalline cellulose. Virchows Arch 395:207, 1982.

632. Krainer L, Berman E, Wishnick SD: Parenteral talcum granulomatosis: A complication of narcotic addiction. Lab Invest 11:671, 1962.

633. Marschke G, Haber L, Feinberg M: Pulmonary talc embolization. Chest 68:824, 1975.

634. Smith RH, Graf MS, Silverman JF: Successful management of drug-induced talc granulomatosis with corticosteroids. Chest 73:552, 1978.

635. Schwartz IS, Bosken C: Pulmonary vascular talc granulomatosis. JAMA 256:2584, 1986.

636. Sturner WO, Spruill FG, Garriott JC: The propylhederine-associated fatalities: Benzedrine revisited. J Forensic Sci 19:372, 1974.

637. Itkonen J, Schnoll S, Daghestani A, et al: Accelerated development of pulmonary complications due to illicit intravenous use of pentazocine and tripelennamine. Am J Med 76:617, 1984.

638. Houck RJ, Bailey GL, Daroca PJ Jr, et al: Pentazocine abuse: report of a case with pulmonary arterial cellulose granulomas and pulmonary hypertension. Chest 77:227, 1980.

639. Siegel H, Bloustein P: Continuing studies in the diagnosis and pathology of death from intravenous narcotism. J Forensic Sci 15:179, 1970.

640. Tomashefski JF Jr, Hirsch CS: The pulmonary vascular lesions of intravenous drug abuse. Human Pathol 11:133, 1980.

641. Johnston WH, Waisman J: Pulmonary corn starch granulomas in a drug user. Arch Pathol 92:196, 1971.

642. Clark MC, Flick MR: Permeability pulmonary edema caused by venous air embolism. Am Rev Respir Dis 129:633, 1984.

643. Farber HW, Falls R, Glauser FL: Transient pulmonary hypertension from the intravenous injection of crushed, suspended pentazocine tablets. Chest 80:178, 1981.

644. Waller BF, Brownlee WJ, Roberts WC: Self-induced pulmonary granulomatosis: a consequence of intravenous injection of drugs intended for oral use. Chest 78:90, 1980.

645. Groth DH, Mackay GR, Crable JV, et al: Intravenous injection of talc in a narcotics addict. Arch Pathol 94:171, 1972.

646. Feigin DS: Talc: understanding its manifestations in the chest. Am J Roentgenol 146:295, 1986.

647. Crouch E, Churg A: Progressive massive fibrosis of the lung secondary to intravenous injection of talc: a pathologic and mineralogic analysis. Am J Clin Pathol 80:520, 1983.

648. Pingleton SK, Bone RC, Pingleton WW, et al: Prevention of pulmonary emboli in a respiratory intensive care unit: efficacy of low-dose heparin. Chest 79:647, 1981.

649. Tao L, Morgan RC, Donat EE: Cytologic diagnosis of intravenous talc granulomatosis by fine needle aspiration biopsy. Acta Cytol 28:737, 1984.

650. Farber HW, Fairman RP, Glauser FL: Talc granulomatosis: laboratory findings similar to sarcoidosis. Am Rev Respir Dis 125:258, 1982.

651. Mariani-Costantini R, Jannotta FS, Johnson FB: Systemic visceral talc granulomatosis associated with miliary tuberculosis in a drug addict. Am J Clin Pathol 78:785, 1982.

652. Paré JAP, Coté G, Fraser RS: Long-term follow-up of drug addicts with pulmonary intravenous talcosis. In press.

653. Genereux GP, Emson HE: Talc granulomatosis and angiothrombotic pulmonary hypertension in drug addicts. J Can Assoc Radiol 25:87, 1974.

654. Sieniewicz DJ, Nidecker AC: Conglomerate pulmonary disease: a form of talcosis in intravenous methadone abusers. Am J Roentgenol 135:697, 1980.

655. Robertson CH Jr, Reynolds RC, Wilson JE: Pulmonary hypertension and foreign-body granulomas in intravenous drug abusers: documentation by cardiac catheterization and lung biopsy. Am J Med 61:657, 1976.

656. Arnett EN, Battle WE, Russo JV, et al: Intravenous injection of talc-containing drugs intended for oral use: a cause of pulmonary granulomatosis and pulmonary hypertension. Am J Med 60:711, 1976.

657. Brown DG, Aguirre A, Weaver A: Gallium-67 scanning in talc-induced pulmonary granulomatosis. Chest 77:561, 1980.

658. Johnston EH, Goldbaum LR, Whelton RL: Investigation of sudden death in addicts. With emphasis on the toxicologic findings in thirty cases. Med Ann DC 38:375, 1969.

659. Murphy SB, Jackson WB, Paré JAP: Talc retinopathy. Can J Opthalmol 13:152, 1978.

660. Bluth LL, Hanscom TA: Retinal detachment and vitreous hemorrhage due to talc emboli. JAMA 246:980, 1981.

661. Brucker AJ: Disk and peripheral retinal neovascularization secondary to talc and cornstarch emboli. Am J Opthalmol 88:864, 1979.

662. Kresca LJ, Goldberg MF, Jampol LM: Talc emboli and retinal neovascularization in a drug abuser. Am J Opthamol 87:334, 1979.

663. Overland ES, Nolan AJ, Hopewell PC: Alteration of pulmonary function in intravenous drug abusers: prevalence, severity, and characterization of gas exchange abnormalities. Am J Med 68:231, 1980.

664. Thomashow D, Summer WR, Soin J, et al: Lung disease in reformed drug addicts: diagnostic and physiologic correlations. Johns Hopkins Med J 141:1, 1977.

665. Ulm AH, Wagshul EC: Pulmonary embolization following urethrography with an oily medium. N Engl J Med 263:137, 1960.

666. Clouse ME, Hallgrimsson J, Wenlund DE: Complications following lymphography with particular reference to pulmonary oil embolization. Am J Roentgenol 96:972, 1966.

667. Gough JH, Gough MH, Thomas ML: Pulmonary complications following lymphography with a note on technique. Br J Radiol 37:416, 1964.

668. Keats TE: Pantopaque pulmonary embolism. Radiology 67:748, 1956.

669. Allen WE, D'Angelo CM: Pulmonary oil embolization following pantopaque ventriculography in a patient with a ventriculovenous shunt. Case report. J Neurosurg 35:623, 1971.

670. Fraimow W, Wallace S, Lewis P, et al: Changes in pulmonary function due to lymphangiography. Radiology 85:231, 1965.

671. Bron Klaus M, Baum S, Abrams HL: Oil embolism in lymphangiography; Incidence, manifestations, and mechanism. Radiology 80:194, 1963.

672. Takahashi M, Abrams HL: Arborizing pulmonary embolization following lymphangiography: Report of three cases and an experimental study. Radiology 89:633, 1967.

673. Hallgrimsson J, Clouse ME: Pulmonary oil emboli after lymphography. Arch Pathol 80:426, 1965.

674. Helmers RA, Zavala DC: Serial exercise testing in pulmonary embolism. Chest 94:517, 1988.

675. Richardson P, Crosby EH, Bean HA, et al: Pulmonary oil deposition in patients subjected to lymphography: Detection by thoracic photoscan and sputum examination. Can Med Assoc J 94:1086, 1966.

676. Felton WL II: A method for the identification of lipiodol in tissue sections. Lab Invest 1:364, 1952.

677. Fallat RJ, Powell MR, Youker JE, et al: Pulmonary deposition and

clearance of ^{131}I-labeled oil after lymphography in man: Correlation with lung function. Radiology 97:511, 1970.

678. Belin RP, Shea MA, Stone NH, et al: Iodoliposputosis following lymphangiography. Report of a case. Dis Chest 48:543, 1965.

679. Weg JG, Harkleroad LE: Aberrations in pulmonary function due to lymphangiography. Dis Chest 53:534, 1968.

680. Gold WM, Youker J, Anderson S, et al: Pulmonary-function abnormalities after lymphangiography. N Engl J Med 273:519, 1965.

681. White RJ, Webb JAW, Tucker AK, et al: Pulmonary function after lymphography. Br Med J 4:775, 1973.

682. Fabel H, Kunitsch G, St Stender H: Störungen der Lungenfunktion nach Lymphographie. (Disturbances of pulmonary function following lymphangiography.) Fortschr Roentgenstr 107:609, 1967.

683. LaMonte CS, Lacher MJ: Lymphangiography in patients with pulmonary dysfunction. Arch Intern Med 132:365, 1973.

684. Devlin HB, Sudlow M: Peripheral mercury embolization occurring during arterial blood sampling. Br Med J 1:347, 1967.

685. Johnson HRM, Koumides O: Unusual case of mercury poisoning. Br Med J 1:340, 1967.

686. Hill DM: Self-administration of mercury by subcutaneous injection. Br Med J 1:342, 1967.

687. Buxton JT Jr, Hewitt JC, Gadsden RH, et al: Metallic mercury embolism. Report of cases. JAMA 193:573, 1965.

688. Naidich TP, Bartelt D, Wheeler PS, et al: Metallic mercury emboli. Am Roentgenol 117:886, 1973.

689. Vas W, Tuttle RJ, Zylak CJ: Intravenous self-administration of metallic mercury. Radiology 137:313, 1980.

690. Tsuji HK, Tyler GC, Reddington JV, et al: Intrabronchial metallic mercury. Chest 57:322, 1970.

691. Schulze W: Röntgenologische studien nach aspiration von metallischen quecksilber. (Roentgenographic studies of metallic mercury aspiration.) Fortschr Roentgenstr 89:24, 1958.

692. Johnston B, Smith P, Heath D: Experimental cotton-fibre pulmonary embolism in the rat. Thorax 36:910, 1981.

693. Adams DF, Olin TB, Kosek J: Cotton fiber embolization during angiography. Radiology 84:678, 1965.

694. Garvan JM, Gunner BW: The harmful effects of particles in intravenous fluids. Med J Aust 2:1, 1964.

695. Jaques WE, Mariscal GG: A study of the incidence of cotton emboli. Bull Int Assoc Med Museums 32:63, 1951.

696. von Glahn WC, Hall JW: The reaction produced in the pulmonary arteries by emboli of cotton fibers. Am J Pathol 25:575, 1949.

697. Truemner KM, White S, Vanlandingham H: Fatal embolization of pulmonary capillaries. JAMA 173:119, 1960.

698. Roman PW, Wagner JH, Steinbach SH: Massive fatal embolism during barium enema study. Radiology 59:190, 1952.

699. David R, Berezesky IK, Bohlman M, et al: Fatal barium embolization due to incorrect vaginal rather than colonic insertion. Arch Pathol Lab Med 107:548, 1983.

700. Collins DH: Bullet embolism: A case of pulmonary embolism following the entry of a bullet into the right ventricle of the heart. J Pathol Bacteriol 60:205, 1948.

701. Straus R: Pulmonary embolism caused by a lead bullet following a gunshot wound of the abdomen. Arch Pathol 33:63, 1942.

702. Hafez A, Dartevelle P, Lafont D, et al: Pulmonary arterial embolus by an unusual wandering bullet. Thorac Cardiovasc Surg 31:392, 1983.

703. Brewer LA III, Bai AF, King EL, et al: The pathologic effects of metallic foreign bodies in the pulmonary circulation. J Thorac Cardiovasc Surg 38:670, 1959.

704. Terry PB, Barth KH, Kaufman SL, et al: Balloon embolization for treatment of pulmonary arteriovenous fistulas. N Engl J Med 302:1189, 1980.

705. Leitman BS, McCauley DI, Firooznia H: Multiple metallic pulmonary densities after therapeutic embolization. JAMA 248:2155, 1982.

706. Bernhardt LC, Wegner GP, Mendenhall JT: Intravenous catheter embolization to the pulmonary artery. Chest 57:329, 1970.

707. Edelstein J: Atraumatic removal of a polyethylene catheter from the superior vena cava. Chest 57:381, 1970.

708. Soni J, Osatinsky M, Smith T, et al: Nonsurgical removal of polyethylene catheter from the right cardiac cavities. Chest 57:398, 1970.

709. Doering RB, Stemmer EA, Connolly JE: Complications of indwelling venous catheters. Am J Surg 114:259, 1967.

710. Ross AM: Polyethylene emboli: How many more? Chest 57:307, 1970.

711. Editorial: Glass embolism. Lancet 2:1300, 1972.

712. Turco SJ, Davis NM: Detrimental effects of particulate matter on the pulmonary circulation. JAMA 217:81, 1971.

713. Thomassen RW, Houbert JP, Winn DF Jr, et al: The occurrence and characterization of emboli associated with the use of a silicone antifoaming agent. J Cardiovasc Thorac Surg 41:611, 1961.

714. Leong AS-Y, Disney APS, Gove DW: Spallation and migration of silicone from blood-pump tubing in patients on hemodialysis. N Engl J Med 306:135, 1982.

715. Krempien B, Bommer J, Ritz E: Foreign body giant cell reaction in lungs, liver and spleen. Virchows Arch (Pathol Anat) 392:73, 1981.

716. Robinson MJ, Nestor M, Rywlin AM: Pulmonary granulomas secondary to embolic prosthetic valve material. Hum Pathol 12:759, 1981.

717. Ross RM, Johnson GW: Fat embolism after liposuction. Chest 93:1294, 1988.

718. Berry DF, Buccigrossi D, Peabody J, et al: Pulmonary vascular occlusion and fibrosing mediastinitis. Chest 89:296, 1986.

719. Thomas DP: Venous thrombogenesis. Ann Rev Med 36:39, 1985.

720. Comp PC, Esmon CT: Recurrent venous thromboembolism in patients with a partial deficiency of proteins. N Engl J Med 311:1525, 1984.

721. Griffin JH, Evatt B, Zimmerman TS, et al: Deficiency of protein C in congenital thrombotic disease. J Clin Invest 68:1370, 1981.

722. Min K-W, Gyorkey F, Sato C: Mucin-producing adenocarcinomas and nonbacterial thrombotic endocarditis. Pathogenetic role of tumor mucin. Cancer 45:2374, 1980.

723. Sostman HD, Rapoport S, Gottschalk A, et al: Imaging of pulmonary embolism. Invest Radiol 21:443, 1986.

724. Alderson PO, Martin EC: Pulmonary embolism: diagnosis with multiple imaging modalities. Radiology 164:297, 1987.

725. Sutnick AI, Soloff LA: Pulmonary arterial occlusion and surfactant production in humans. Ann Intern Med 67:549, 1967.

726. Comroe JH Jr: Pulmonary arterial blood flow: Effects of brief and permanent arrest. Am Rev Respir Dis 85:179, 1962.

727. Gamsu G, Hirji M, Moore EH, et al: Experimental pulmonary emboli detected using magnetic resonance. Radiology 153:467, 1984.

728. Stein MG, Crues JV III, Bradley WG Jr, et al: MR imaging of pulmonary emboli: an experimental study in dogs. AJR 147:1133, 1986.

729. Pope CF, Sostman D, Carbo P, et al: The detection of pulmonary emboli by magnetic resonance imaging. Evaluation of imaging parameters. Invest Radiol 22:937, 1987.

730. Thickman D, Kressel HY, Axel L: Demonstration of pulmonary embolism by magnetic resonance imaging. AJR 142:921, 1984.

731. Moore EH, Gamsu G, Webb VR, et al: Pulmonary embolus: detection and follow-up using magnetic resonance. Radiology 153:471, 1984.

732. Fisher MR, Higgins CB: Central thrombi in pulmonary arterial hypertension detected by MR imaging. Radiology 158:223, 1986.

733. White RD, Winkler ML, Higgins CB: MR imaging of pulmonary arterial hypertension and pulmonary emboli. AJR 149:15, 1987.

734. Westcott JL, Cole S: Plate atelectasis. Radiology 155:1, 1985.

735. Quinn MF, Lundell CJ, Klotz TA, et al: Reliability of selective pulmonary arteriography in the diagnosis of pulmonary embolism. AJR 149:469, 1987.

736. Cassling RJ, Lois JF, Gomes AS: Unusual pulmonary angiographic findings in suspected pulmonary embolism. AJR 145:995, 1985.

737. Rosen JM, Biello DR, Siegel BA, et al: Kr-81m ventilation imaging: clinical utility in suspected pulmonary embolism. Radiology 154:787, 1985.

738. Alderson PO, Biello DR, Gottschalk A, et al: Tc-99m-DTPA aerosol and radioactive gases compared as adjuncts to perfusion scintigraphy in patients with suspected pulmonary embolism. Radiology 153:515, 1984.

739. Sostman HD, Rapoport S, Gottschalk A, et al: Imaging of pulmonary embolism. Invest Radiol 21:443, 1986.

740. Wellman HM: Pulmonary thromboembolism: current status report on the role of nuclear medicine. Semin Nucl Med 16:236, 1986.

741. Alderson PO, Dzebolo NN, Biello DR, et al: Serial lung scintigraphy: utility in diagnosis of pulmonary embolism. Radiology 149:797, 1983.

742. Spritzer CE, Sussman SK, Blinder RA, et al: Deep venous thrombosis evaluation with limited-flip-angle, gradient-refocused MR imaging: preliminary experience. Radiology 166:371, 1988.

743. Spies WG, Burstein SP, Dillehay GL, et al: Ventilation-perfusion scintigraphy in suspected pulmonary embolism: correlation with pulmonary angiography and refinement of criteria for interpretation. Radiology 159:383, 1986.

744. Braun SD, Newman GE, Ford K, et al: Ventilation-perfusion scanning and pulmonary angiography: correlation in clinical high-probability pulmonary embolism. AJR 143:977, 1984.

745. Bogren HG, Berman DS, Vismara LA, et al: Lung ventilation-perfusion scintigraphy in pulmonary embolism. Diagnostic specificity compared to pulmonary angiography. Acta Radiolo [Diagn] 19:933, 1978.

746. Bernstein D, Coupey S, Schonberg SK: Pulmonary embolism in adolescents. Am J Dis Child 140:667, 1986.

747. Kitchell CC, Balogh K: Pulmonary lipid emboli in association with long-term hyperalimentation. Hum Pathol 17:83, 1986.

748. Gustilo RB, Corpuz V, Sherman RE: Epidemiology, mortality and morbidity in multiple trauma patients. Orthopedics 8:1523, 1985.

749. Johnson KD, Cadambi A, Seibert GB: Incidence of adult respiratory distress syndrome in patients with multiple musculoskeletal injuries:

effect of early operative stabilization of fractures. J Trauma 25:375, 1985.

750. Modig J, Hedstrand U, Wegenius G: Determinants of early adult respiratory distress syndrome. A retrospective study of 220 patients with major fractures. Acta Chir Scand 151:413, 1985.

751. Oryarzun M, Doerschuck C: Personal communication.

752. Kapur MM, Jain P, Gidh M: The effect of trauma on serum C3 activation and its correlation with injury severity score in man. J Trauma 26:464, 1986.

753. Yamamoto M: Pathology of experimental pulmonary bone marrow embolism. I. Initial lesions of the rabbit lung after intravenous infusion of allogeneic bone marrow with special reference to its pathogenesis. Acta Pathol Jpn 35(1):45, 1985.

754. Yamamoto M: Pathology of experimental pulmonary bone marrow embolism. II. Post-embolic pulmonary arteriosclerosis and pulmonary hypertension in rabbits receiving an intravenous infusion of allogeneic bone marrow. Acta Pathol Jpn 37(5):705, 1987.

755. Ishiyama I, Mukaida M, Komuro E, et al: Analysis of a case of generalized amniotic fluid embolism by demonstrating the fetal isoantigen (A blood type) in maternal tissues of B blood type, using immunoperoxidase staining. Am J Clin Pathol 85:239, 1986.

756. Lee KR, Catalano PM, Ortiz-Giroux S: Cytologic diagnosis of amniotic fluid embolism. Report of a case with a unique cytologic feature and emphasis on the difficulty of eliminating squamous contamination. Acta Cytol 30:177, 1986.

757. Attwood HD, Park WW: Embolism to the lungs by trophoblast. J Obstet Gynaecol Br Comm 68:611, 1961.

758. Aabo K, Hansen KB: Megakaryocytes in pulmonary blood vessels. I: Incidence at autopsy; clinicopathologicical relations especially to disseminated intravascualar coagulation. Acta Pathol Microbial Scand 86:285, 1978.

759. Lie JT: Myocardium as emboli in the systemic and pulmonary circulation. Arch Pathol Lab Med 111:261, 1987.

760. Cianci P, Posin JP, Shimshak RR, et al: Air embolism complicating percutaneous thin needle biopsy of lung. Chest 92:749, 1987.

761. Aberle DR, Gamsu G, Golden JA: Fatal systemic arterial air embolism following lung needle aspiration. Radiology 165:351, 1987.

762. Tolly TL, Feldmeier JE, Czarnecki D: Air embolism complicating percutaneous lung biopsy. AJR 150:555, 1988.

763. Woodring JH, Fried AM: Nonfatal venous air embolism after contrast-enhanced CT. Radiology 167:405, 1988.

764. Clark MC, Flick MR: Permeability pulmonary edema caused by venous air embolism. Am Rev Respir Dis 129:633, 1984.

765. Balk AG, Mooi WJ, Dingemans KP, et al: Development and regression of pulmonary arterial lesions after experimental air embolism. A light and electronmicroscopic study. Virchows Arch (Pathol Anat) 406:203, 1985.

766. Miller TD, Staats BA: Impaired exercise tolerance after inferior vena caval interruption. Chest 93:776, 1988.

767. Lewis JH, Sundeen JT, Simon GL, et al: Disseminated talc granulomatosis. An unusual finding in a patient with acquired immunodeficiency syndrome and fatal cytomegalovirus infection. Arch Pathol Lab Med 109:147, 1985.

768. Feigin DS: Talc: understanding its manifestations in the chest. AJR 146:295, 1986.

769. Prager D, Hertzberg RW: Spontaneous intravenous catheter fracture and embolization from an implanted venous access port and analysis by scanning electron microscopy. Cancer 60:270, 1987.

770. Musset D, Rosso J, Petitpretz P, et al: Acute pulmonary embolism: diagnostic value of digital subtraction angiography. Radiology 166:455, 1988.

771. Dorfman GS, Cronan JJ, Tupper TB, et al: Occult pulmonary embolism: a common occurrence in deep venous thrombosis. AJR 148:263, 1987.

772. Piggott J, Hansbarger EA Jr, Neafie RC: Human ascariasis. Am J Clin Pathol 53:223, 1970.

773. Neafie RC, Piggott J: Human pulmonary dirofilariasis. Arch Pathol 92:342, 1971.

774. Shaw AFB, Ghareeb AA: The pathogenesis of pulmonary schistosomiasis in Egypt with special reference to Ayerza's disease. J Pathol Bacteriol 146:401, 1938.

775. Richmond DR, Bernstein L: Hydatid pulmonary embolism. Case report. Aust Ann Med 17:270, 1968.

776. Chan CK, Hutcheon MA, Hyland RH, et al: Pulmonary tumor embolism: a critical review of clinical, imaging, and hemodynamic features. J Thorac Imaging 2:4, 1987.

777. Ross DJ, Mohsenifar Z, Potkin RT, et al: Pathogenesis of cerebral air embolism during neodymium-YAG kaser photoresection. Chest 94:660, 1988.

778. Smelt WL, Baerts WD, de Langhe JJ, et al: Pulmonary edema following air embolism. Acta Anaesthesiol Belg 38:201, 1987.

779. Ben-Haim SA, Ben-Ami H, Edoute Y, et al: Talcosis presenting as pulmonary infiltrates in an HIV-positive heroin addict. Chest 94:656, 1988.

780. Uflacker R, Kaemmerer A, Picon PD, et al: Bronchial artery embolization in the management of hemoptysis: technical aspects and long-term results. Radiology 157:637, 1985.

781. Tomashefski JF Jr, Cohen AM, Doershuk CF: Longterm histopathologic follow-up of bronchial arteries after therapeutic embolization with polyvinyl alcohol (Ivalon) in patients with cystic fibrosis. Hum Pathol 19:555, 1988.

782. Castaneda-Zuniga WR, Sanchez R, Amplatz K: Experimental observations on short- and long-term effects of arterial occlusion with Ivalon. Radiology 126:783, 1978.

783. Boushy SF, Helgason AH, North LB: Occlusion of the bronchial arteries by glass microspheres. Am Rev Respir Dis 103:249, 1971.

10

Pulmonary Hypertension and Edema

GENERAL CONSIDERATIONS OF PULMONARY BLOOD FLOW AND PRESSURE

The anatomy of the pulmonary circulation and the principles that govern blood flow through the pulmonary vascular tree are discussed in detail in Chapter 1 (*see* page 71). Only a brief overview is given here.

The pulmonary vasculature consists of a highly branched system of arteries, arterioles, capillaries, venules, and veins that can accommodate the entire cardiac output at low driving pressures. The pulmonary arteries and arterioles accompany the bronchi, bronchioles, and alveolar ducts. There are approximately 17 generations of arterial vessels between the main pulmonary artery and arterioles measuring 10 to 15 μm in diameter.[1, 2] Unlike the tracheobronchial tree, in which most of the resistance to airflow is in the large airways, the majority of the resistance in the pulmonary arterial tree is in the smaller blood vessels (muscular arteries and arterioles).

The total cross-sectional areas of the tracheobronchial tree and the pulmonary arterial tree versus distance from the alveolar surface have been calculated by Culver and Butler (Fig. 10–1).[3] It is apparent that the two trees begin with similar-sized "trunks" but that the total cross-sectional area of the airways greatly exceeds that of the blood vessels in the periphery of the lung. These small vessels are also the site of the majority of vascular smooth muscle, and it is the modulation of the caliber of these vessels that distributes arterial blood flow to cause the best match of ventilation and perfusion. Pulmonary capillaries arise from the arterioles and form an extensive, almost "sheet-like" layer of blood that is situated in the alveolar walls in intimate contact with the alveolar gas. The pulmonary venules begin at the distal end of the capillary bed and run in the intralobular septa back to the hilum; they

do not run in association with the pulmonary arteries and airways. Anastomoses between the bronchial and pulmonary arterial systems occur at the capillary and postcapillary levels.

The pulmonary vascular circuit is a low-pressure system, the mean arterial pressure being only about one sixth of the systemic arterial pressure; the circuit has a remarkable capacity to compensate for a large physiologic increase in blood flow (e.g., during exercise) without a corresponding increase in pressure. This reduction in vascular resistance is

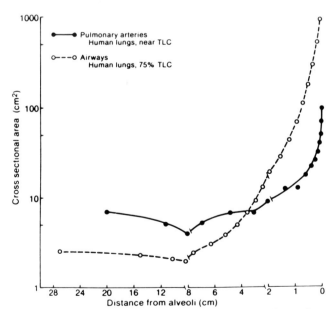

Figure 10–1. Pulmonary Arterial and Airway Cross-Sectional Area. The total cross-sectional area of the tracheobronchial tree and the pulmonary vascular tree increases greatly as they branch toward the gas-exchanging portion of the lung. These data show that the total area occupied by small airways exceeds that occupied by small pulmonary vessels. (From Culver BH, Butler J: Mechanical influences on the pulmonary microcirculation. Ann Rev Physiol 40:187, 1980. With permission of the authors and publisher.)

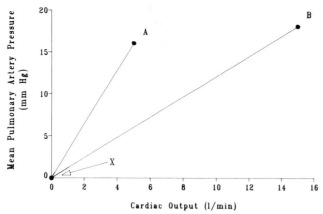

Figure 10-2. Pulmonary Vascular Pressure Flow Curves. Mean pulmonary arterial pressure is plotted against cardiac output. The slope of the line is pulmonary vascular resistance. A large increase in cardiac output is associated with only a slight increase in mean pulmonary vascular pressure. *See* text for discussion.

achieved mainly by "recruiting" pulmonary vessels that are not perfused at rest. This ability to recruit vessels with minor increases in pressure results in a pulmonary vascular pressure-flow curve, as illustrated in Figure 10-2. When the cardiac output is low (A), pulmonary vascular resistance is given by the slope A-X or

16 mm Hg/5 liters/minute = 3.2 mm Hg/liter/minute

If the cardiac output is increased to 15 liters/minute (B), pulmonary artery pressure increases only slightly to 18 mm Hg and now pulmonary vascular resistance is given by the slope B X or

18 mm Hg/15 liters/minute = 1.2 mm Hg/liter/minute

This substantial decrease in resistance occurs simply because of vascular recruitment and *not* because of relaxation of pulmonary vascular smooth muscle. The variability of vascular resistance with changing cardiac output has occasionally led to confusion in the interpretation of changes in vascular resistance. To prove the presence of pulmonary "vasodilation," it is necessary to show a decrease in pressure at a fixed flow or a shift in the position or slope of the pressure-flow curve.

Pulmonary vascular resistance (PVR) is calculated by dividing the driving flow by the cardiac output:

$$PVR = P_{Pa} - P_{La}/\dot{Q}$$

where PVR = pulmonary vascular resistance, P_{Pa} = pulmonary artery pressure, P_{La} = left atrial pressure, and $\dot{Q}$ = cardiac output. The driving pressure is the difference between mean pulmonary arterial and mean left atrial pressure. In practice, the pulmonary wedge pressure provides a reliable estimate of left atrial pressure in the absence of large vein obstruction. Pulmonary vascular resis-

tance calculated in this way represents the summed resistances of the arteries, capillaries, and veins in series. An increase in pulmonary arterial pressure can occur because of an increase in blood flow, increased resistance to flow through arteries, capillaries, or veins, or because of an increased left atrial pressure.

Alterations in the pulmonary vascular tree may be of cardiac or pulmonary origin. In either event, they can be classified into three main categories on the basis of the quantity of pulmonary blood flow—increased, normal, or decreased. In each of these categories, the changes may be general or local. Chen and his colleagues[1] have classified cardiac and pulmonary diseases according to specific pulmonary blood flow patterns, and the interested reader is directed to their article for a tabulated presentation of this rather complex subject.

The major roentgenographic effects of many intrathoracic diseases are reflected in changes in the pulmonary vascular tree. Some of these diseases are local (e.g., unilateral or lobar emphysema) and usually cause changes in roentgenographic density that can be appreciated by comparison with regions of normal lung. However, the majority of diseases, whether pulmonary or cardiac in origin, are of general distribution. Since assessment of change in lung density owing to generalized increase or decrease in blood flow can be grossly inaccurate, a change in density is much less important than an alteration in vascular pattern.

In the roentgenologic assessment of diseases of the pulmonary vascular system, signs are related to a relative change in the caliber of hilar pulmonary arteries and of lobar and segmental pulmonary arteries as they proceed distally. Attention must be directed not only to the pulmonary arteries but also to the size and contour of the heart, the size of the main pulmonary artery, and the caliber of the pulmonary veins, since each is important to the overall evaluation of any abnormality in hemodynamics. Whereas severe degrees of overvascularity (pleonemia) and undervascularity (oligemia) may be readily apparent, minor degrees may be exceedingly difficult to appreciate on standard roentgenograms. Although serial roentgenography and tomography (either conventional or computed) may aid in evaluation, only angiography can provide proof of vascular abnormality in questionable cases.

Much has been written about the reliability of the plain roentgenogram in estimating pulmonary arterial and venous pressures. That the *presence* of pulmonary hypertension can be recognized roentgenographically is undisputed, but the degree of accuracy with which its *severity* can be estimated on both the arterial and venous sides of the capillary bed is controversial. Regardless of precision, there is no doubt that much information concerning hemodynamics can be obtained from the intelligent integration of individual signs, including enlargement of cardiac chambers, increase in size of the main pulmonary artery and its hilar branches, the rapidity with which pulmonary arteries taper distally and the distribution of this narrowing, the caliber of the pulmonary veins and their discrepant size in the upper and lower lung zones, and, finally, the presence or absence of septal edema (B lines of Kerley). The interested reader is directed to the many excellent correlative studies that describe the roentgenographic signs from which pulmonary vascular pressures may be predicted.[5–16]

PULMONARY HYPERTENSION

With several exceptions, abnormalities of the pulmonary vascular tree are related to the presence of pulmonary hypertension, arterial or venous or both. Pulmonary arterial hypertension may be defined as an increase to above normally accepted values for pressure in the main pulmonary artery at rest or during exercise as measured with a catheter. Generally accepted values for these pressures are 30 mm Hg systolic and 18 mm Hg mean pulmonary arterial pressure, above which pulmonary arterial hypertension may be said to be present.[17] Pulmonary venous hypertension is present when the pressure in the pulmonary veins measured indirectly by a catheter wedged in a pulmonary artery exceeds 12 mm Hg. Slight increases in pulmonary arterial pressure generally cause no clinical, roentgenographic, or electrocardiographic signs, even with mean pulmonary arterial pressures as high as 24 mm Hg.[18] As the resistance to pulmonary blood flow increases, pulmonary arterial pressure rises, providing a greater impedance to right ventricular ejection. This increase in right ventricular afterload produces clinical and electrocardiographic signs and, eventually, roentgenologic changes indicative of strain and resultant hypertrophy of the right ventricle. With further rises in pressure, catheterization studies may show elevation not only of pulmonary arterial and right ventricular systolic pressures but also of right ventricular diastolic pressure, indicating the onset of right ventricular failure.

Pathologic Characteristics

Although there are differences in the pathologic abnormalities that occur in the pulmonary vasculature, depending on the etiology of the hypertension, in fact many of the changes are similar or identical. This is particularly true in cases of idiopathic (primary) pulmonary hypertension and of hypertension related to congenital cardiovascular disease, hepatic disease, and anorexigenic drugs, conditions that are characterized by a group of vascular changes collectively known as *plexogenic pulmonary arteriopathy*. General pathologic features that occur in these and other forms of pulmonary arterial hypertension will be described at this point;

additional information about features specific to individual etiologies is discussed in the appropriate sections. Further details of pathogenesis and morphologic features can be found in the comprehensive text by Wagenvoort and Wagenvoort.[184]

In pulmonary arterial hypertension of significant degree, the large elastic arteries, especially the main pulmonary artery, are often somewhat dilated and sometimes are larger in diameter than the aorta; the dilatation may be so severe that localized aneurysm formation is the result. If the hypertension is related to congenital cardiovascular disease and thus is present at birth, the fetal configuration of elastic laminae (consisting of fairly uniform concentric bands) tends to be preserved;[19] by contrast, if the hypertension is acquired, elastic laminae tend to possess an irregular, fragmented appearance similar to that of the normal adult vessel. An increase in acidic ground substance and a focal loss of elastic tissue in the media (so-called cystic medial necrosis) are sometimes present, and, as in the aorta, can be associated with dissecting aneurysm.[185]

Some degree of pulmonary arterial atherosclerosis is a common manifestation of aging, but in the presence of pulmonary hypertension, it increases in both severity and extent.[20] Grossly, this abnormality appears as yellow streaks or plaques similar to those seen in the systemic arteries; histologically, they consist of intimal fibrous tissue containing aggregates of lipid-laden macrophages (foam cells) (Fig. 10–3). Complicating features such as necrosis, calcification, and ulceration are rare.

Medial hypertrophy of muscular arteries is seen in almost all forms of pulmonary hypertension (Fig. 10–4). It is most often caused by a combination of muscle hypertrophy and hyperplasia, but in some cases these changes are accompanied by an increase in intermuscular connective tissue.[21] Additional smooth muscle cells are usually arranged in the same fashion as the normal circular muscle coat; however, new bundles of longitudinal muscle are also fairly common, often situated in an intimal location (Fig. 10–4). Intimal fibrosis is frequently associated with medial hypertrophy and may be so severe as to virtually obliterate the vascular lumen; in such cases, larger vessels can be identified grossly as thick, rigid pipe-like structures projecting above the surface of the lung (Fig. 10–5). Almost paradoxically, the media in such cases may be atrophic, apparently as a consequence of the intimal fibrosis (Fig. 10–5).

Muscle hypertrophy also occurs in pulmonary arterioles. In some cases, this is caused by an increase in the size and number of muscle fibers already present in the arteriolar wall, but in others it represents extension of muscle into vessels that formerly contained none (so-called arterialization of pulmonary arterioles). These new muscle cells appear to be derived from pericytes and "intermediate cells" normally present in the arteriolar wall.[22]

In addition to the changes described above,

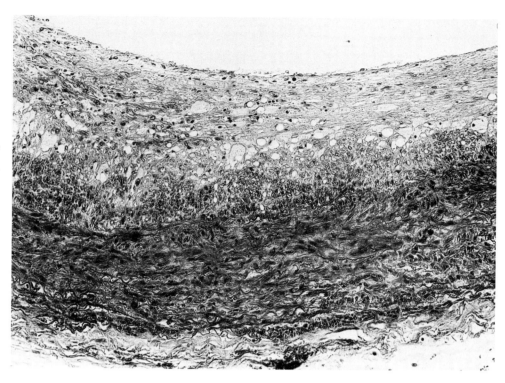

Figure 10–3. Pulmonary Artery Atherosclerosis. A histologic section of a large elastic artery shows intimal fibrosis and the presence of multiple foam cells, features representing the earliest stage of atherosclerosis (× 130).

several abnormalities are often present in small to medium-sized muscular arteries that together characterize plexogenic pulmonary arteriopathy. These include cellular intimal proliferation, plexiform and dilatation lesions, fibrinoid "necrosis," and vasculitis. *Intimal thickening* of muscular arteries in the early stages of hypertension, either primary or secondary to congenital cardiovascular disease, is typically characterized by the presence of loose connective tissue containing numerous cells; these are often elongated and arranged in more or less concentric layers, creating a distinctive "onion skin" appearance (Fig. 10–6). Ultrastructurally, the cells show features of myofibroblasts[23] and are possibly derived from the media. This cellular proliferation is often out of proportion to the degree of medial hypertrophy and can result in almost complete luminal obliteration (Fig. 10–6). Recognition of this change is important because there is evidence that its presence, at least when extensive, is associated with progressive pulmonary vascular disease despite repair of cardiovascular anomalies.[24]

A *plexiform lesion* refers to a distinctive abnormality of small muscular arteries (usually 110 to 200 μm in diameter) that often develops at a short distance beyond the origin of the vessel from its parent branch. The lesion consists of localized vascular dilatation associated with an intraluminal plexus of numerous slit-like vascular channels (Fig. 10–7); the latter are separated by a small amount of connective tissue and a variable number of plump fibroblast-like cells. The plexus itself often continues distally into a thin-walled, somewhat tortuous and dilated vascular channel. The pathogenesis of plexiform lesions has been debated; Wagenvoort and

Wagenvoort[184] have theorized that it results from organization of intraluminal thrombus, possibly secondary to fibrinoid "necrosis" and inflammation of the adjacent vessel wall. The presence of thrombus in relation to some plexiform lesions (Fig. 10–7) is consistent with this hypothesis.

Plexiform lesions are considered by some authorities[23] to represent one of several "dilatation lesions" that can be seen in plexogenic pulmonary arteriopathy. Another such lesion, which is relatively uncommon, is the *angiomatoid lesion;* as its name suggests, this consists of a cluster of tortuous, dilated, usually thin-walled vascular channels resembling an angioma (Fig. 10–8).

The term *fibrinoid necrosis* is used to describe the presence of homogeneous eosinophilic material in the wall of small pulmonary arteries and arterioles (Fig. 10–9). Although the term is commonly used, strictly speaking it is incorrect because there is usually no evidence of tissue necrosis; instead, the lesion most likely represents the accumulation of fibrin and other proteins within the media unaccompanied by true cell death. Whatever its nature, it is not an uncommon finding in plexogenic arteriopathy, particularly in the presence of high pulmonary arterial pressures. Occasionally, these foci are associated with an acute inflammatory reaction, indicating true vasculitis.

Pathogenesis

The pressure drop across any vascular bed is directly related to the blood flow through and the blood viscosity in that particular bed; an increase in flow or viscosity will cause an increase in pressure

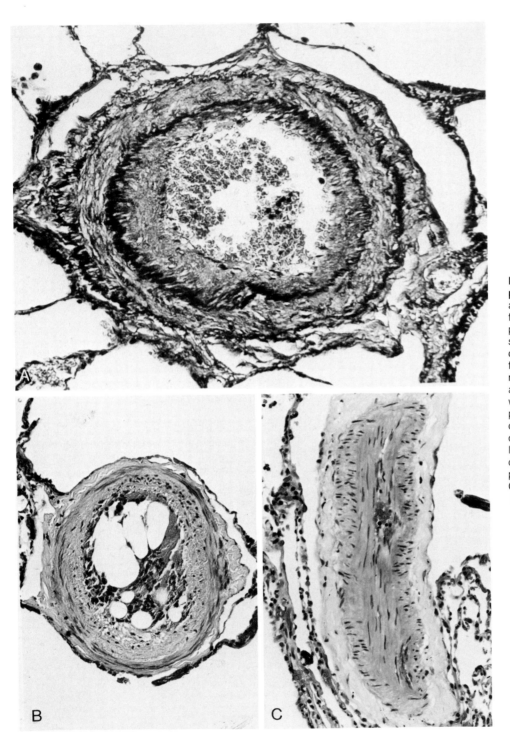

Figure 10–4. Pulmonary Hypertension: Muscular Hyperplasia. A histologic section (*A*) of a medium-sized muscular artery from a 27-year-old woman with primary pulmonary hypertension shows a moderate degree of medial thickening and mild intimal fibrosis. Cross (*B*) and longitudinal (*C*) sections through two small arteries from a 63-year-old woman with severe chronic obstructive pulmonary disease (COPD) and cor pulmonale demonstrate clearly defined outer circular and inner longitudinal muscle. (A fragment of embolized bone marrow is present in *B*.) (*A*, Verhoeff–van Gieson, × 200; *B* and *C*, H&E, × 160.)

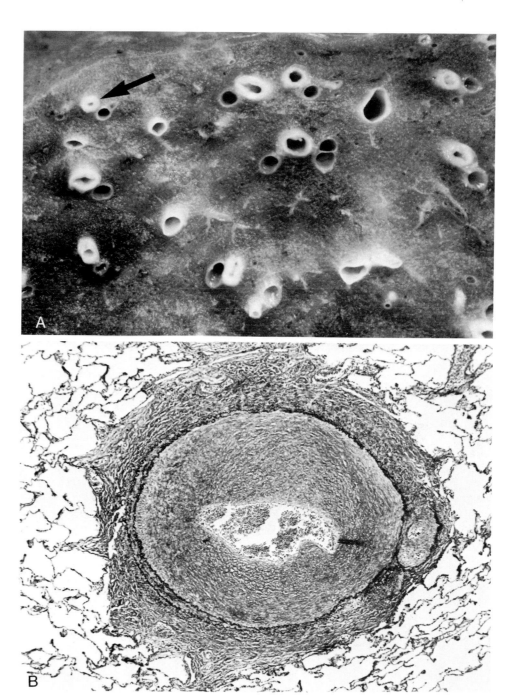

Figure 10–5. Pulmonary Hypertension: Intimal Fibrosis. A magnified view of peripheral lung parenchyma (*A*) shows marked thickening of the walls of many muscular arteries; in some (*arrow*), the lumen is almost obliterated. A corresponding histologic section demonstrates the thickening to be caused predominantly by intimal fibrosis; note also the extensive medial atrophy. (*B*, Verhoeff–van Gieson, × 52.)

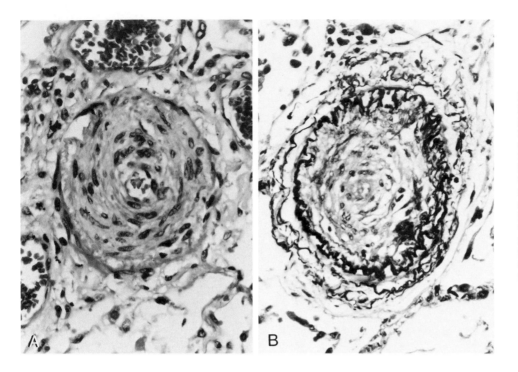

Figure 10–6. Pulmonary Hypertension: Cellular Intimal Fibrosis. A histologic section of a pulmonary artery (*A*) of a young man with an atrial septal defect shows almost complete obliteration of its lumen by cellular fibrous tissue. The cell nuclei are somewhat elongated and arranged roughly in concentric layers, resulting in a somewhat whorled appearance. A section of the same vessel stained for elastic tissue (*B*) shows the cellular proliferation to be entirely within the intima. (*A*, H&E, × 160; *B*, Verhoeff–van Gieson, × 160.)

for any given vascular geometry. The pressure across the vascular bed is indirectly related to the radius of its vessels; the total cross-sectional area of the vascular tree can decrease because of a loss of pulmonary vessels, intraluminal occlusion of a proportion of the vessels, vascular smooth muscle contraction and shortening, or vascular wall thickening. Finally, pulmonary arterial pressure can be increased as a result of an increase in the downstream or venous pressure. The pathophysiologic mechanisms that can result in pulmonary hypertension are listed in Table 10–1.

The mechanism of production of pulmonary hypertension varies from patient to patient, and multiple factors are responsible in many. In some instances, such as in the early stages of primary pulmonary hypertension, there is reason to believe that the rise in pulmonary arterial pressure is caused by vasoconstriction, and therefore is reversible.[25, 26] In other cases, obstruction of the pulmonary vascular tree is largely or completely caused by structural changes and is therefore irreversible.

Vasoconstriction may be produced by hypoxemia or acidosis, either metabolic or respiratory in origin,[27–30] and there is evidence that this type of vasoconstriction may be reversed, at least partly, by the administration of oxygen or acetylcholine or by raising the pH of the blood.[27, 28, 31] In healthy people dwelling at very high altitudes, pulmonary hypertension can develop that disappears when the person is acclimatized at sea level.[32] Angiographic studies in dogs by Harrison and his colleagues[33] showed that acetylcholine can reduce pulmonary vascular resistance and increase blood flow and that the effects were the result of active vasodilatation and at a level that is demonstrable angiographically.

These authors suggest that angiography combined with injection of vasodilators may be used to differentiate increased pulmonary vascular resistance secondary to fixed morphologic vascular alterations from vasoconstriction. Pulmonary arterial constriction can also be caused by a variety of mediators of inflammation, including serotonin, histamine, angiotensin, catecholamines, prostaglandins, and leukotrienes.[34] The release of mediators is probably the mechanism of acute pulmonary hypertension in pulmonary thromboembolic disease. The increase in pressure in the pulmonary arteries resulting from postcapillary hypertension (*see* farther on) also is initially vasospastic in origin, probably mediated through a vasovagal reflex originating from a rise in left atrial and pulmonary venous pressure. The rapid fall to normal pulmonary arterial pressure following mitral valve replacement in some cases of severe pulmonary hypertension caused by mitral stenosis can be explained only on the basis of pulmonary arterial vasoconstriction.[35]

It is useful conceptually to divide the causes of pulmonary hypertension into three general groups, each of which shows somewhat different clinical, physiologic, and roentgenologic characteristics (*see* Table 10–1): those in which the major mechanisms of production are *precapillary* in location, those in which the significant physiologic disturbance arises from disease in the *postcapillary* vessels, and a third group in which the hypertension reflects a disturbance in vessels on both sides of the capillary bed— *combined precapillary and postcapillary hypertension*. In each of these groups, the capillaries may be involved to some extent and may contribute considerably to the increase in vascular resistance. For example, in emphysema the effect occurs as a result of destruc-

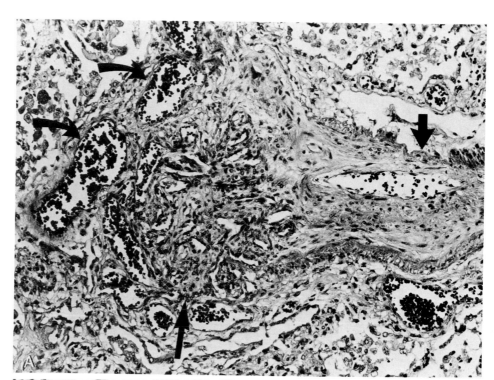

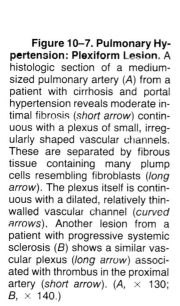

Figure 10–7. Pulmonary Hypertension: Plexiform Lesion. A histologic section of a medium-sized pulmonary artery (*A*) from a patient with cirrhosis and portal hypertension reveals moderate intimal fibrosis (*short arrow*) continuous with a plexus of small, irregularly shaped vascular channels. These are separated by fibrous tissue containing many plump cells resembling fibroblasts (*long arrow*). The plexus itself is continuous with a dilated, relatively thin-walled vascular channel (*curved arrows*). Another lesion from a patient with progressive systemic sclerosis (*B*) shows a similar vascular plexus (*long arrow*) associated with thrombus in the proximal artery (*short arrow*). (*A*, × 130; *B*, × 140.)

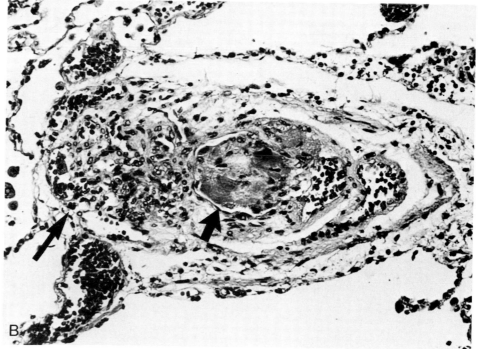

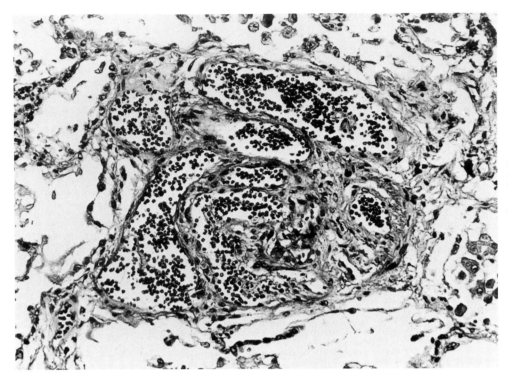

Figure 10–8. Pulmonary Hypertension: Angiomatoid Lesion. A plexus of interconnecting thin-walled dilated vascular channels resembles a small "angioma." From a patient with primary pulmonary hypertension ($\times$ 180).

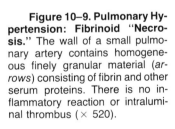

Figure 10–9. Pulmonary Hypertension: Fibrinoid "Necrosis." The wall of a small pulmonary artery contains homogeneous finely granular material (*arrows*) consisting of fibrin and other serum proteins. There is no inflammatory reaction or intraluminal thrombus ($\times$ 520).

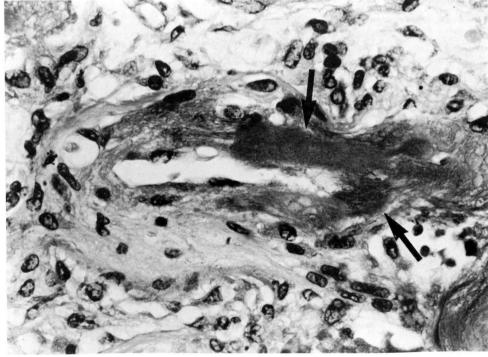

Table 10–1. Classification of Pulmonary Hypertension

PRECAPILLARY PULMONARY HYPERTENSION
Primary Vascular Disease
1. Increased flow (large left-to-right shunts)
2. Decreased flow (tetralogy of Fallot)
3. Primary pulmonary hypertension
4. Pulmonary embolic disease:
   Thrombus
   Metastatic neoplasm
   Parasites
   Miscellaneous: fat, talc, amniotic fluid
5. Immunologic abnormalities: e.g., SLE, PSS
6. High altitude
Primary Pleuropulmonary Disease
1. Emphysema
2. Diffuse interstitial or airspace disease
   Fibrosis: e.g., granulomatous disease, pneumoconiosis, connective tissue disease, fibrosing alveolitis, sarcoidosis
   Neoplasm
   Postpulmonary resection
   Miscellaneous: alveolar microlithiasis, idiopathic hemosiderosis, alveolar proteinosis, cystic fibrosis, bronchiectasis
3. Pleural disease (fibrothorax)
4. Chest wall deformity
   Thoracoplasty
   Kyphoscoliosis
Alveolar Hypoventilation
1. Neuromuscular
2. Obesity
3. Chronic upper airway obstruction in children
4. Idiopathic

POSTCAPILLARY HYPERTENSION
Cardiac
1. Left ventricular failure
2. Mitral valvular disease
3. Myxoma (or thrombus) of the left atrium
4. Cor triatriatum
Pulmonary Venous
1. Congenital stenosis of the pulmonary veins
2. Chronic sclerosing mediastinitis
3. Idiopathic veno-occlusive disease
4. Anomalous pulmonary venous return
5. Neoplasms
6. Thrombosis

Abbreviations: SLE, systemic lupus erythematosus; PSS, progressive systemic sclerosis.

tion of the capillary bed; in postcapillary venous hypertension, chronic pericapillary edema can be associated with fibrosis, thereby limiting distensibility of the capillary bed.

PRECAPILLARY PULMONARY HYPERTENSION

Primary Vascular Disease

INCREASED FLOW

Included in this category are the congenital heart defects with left-to-right shunt (atrial septal defect [ASD], ventricular septal defect [VSD], patent ductus arteriosus [PDA], aorticopulmonary window, and partial anomalous pulmonary venous

drainage) and conditions associated with an increase in total blood volume such as thyrotoxicosis and chronic renal failure. Pulmonary arterial flow may be greatly increased for a long time before increased resistance results in hypertension. It is assumed that the increase in resistance is caused by an increase in vasomotor tone and that, subsequently, the morphologic changes of increased flow hypertension develop.

In an experimental study on dogs designed to clarify the angiographic and pathophysiologic manifestations of pulmonary hypertension, Friedman[36] resected the apical and middle lobes of the left lung and anastomosed the left main pulmonary artery to the ascending aorta. One month later, he ligated all branches of the left pulmonary artery except the ventral segmental artery. Extreme pulmonary hypertension developed in the ventral segment of the remaining left diaphragmatic lobe in all animals. Direct magnification angiography revealed vascular tortuosity that was most prominent with relatively acute small vessel occlusion. Long-standing hypertension resulted in sclerotic vessels that were characterized angiographically by diminished fine branching and a poor capillary phase as well as by slow flow. Pathologic studies showed typical proliferative lesions of severe pulmonary hypertension with abundant bronchopulmonary anastomoses in the later stages.

The main roentgenographic sign in these conditions is an increase in caliber of all of the pulmonary arteries throughout the lungs (Fig. 10–10). Since the hemodynamic change is one of increased flow, the degree of enlargement of the main and hilar pulmonary arteries usually is proportional to the degree of distention of the intrapulmonary vessels. Thus, when peripheral resistance is normal, the arteries taper gradually and proportionately distally. Vascular markings that normally are invisible in the peripheral 2 cm of the lungs may become visible. Although it might be thought logical that the pulmonary veins must increase in size to the same extent as the pulmonary arteries (they carry the same volume of blood), experimental studies in dogs have produced conflicting results. For example, in a study employing an isolated dog lung preparation in which cardiac output was increased by varying stroke rate alone or stroke volume alone (or both), Milne[37] observed that increased flow resulted in an increased size of the pulmonary veins that was comparable to the increase in arterial size; this occurred in the absence of any change in left atrial pressure and thus was related purely to blood flow. However, the study by Hinchcliffe and Greenspan[38] produced results that were at variance with those of Milne: these authors "labeled" the extrapulmonary veins of dogs by injecting a suspension of tantalum particles into their adventitia, thus rendering these vessels roentgenographically visible as a ring of contrast. When blood flow through the lung was almost doubled by occlusion of the contra-

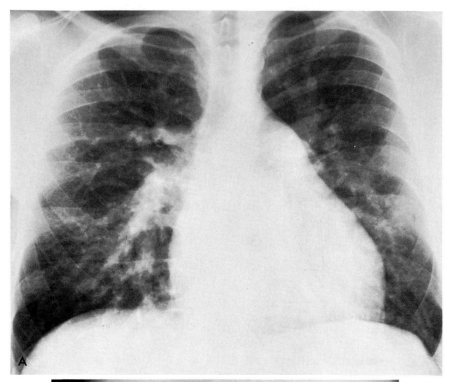

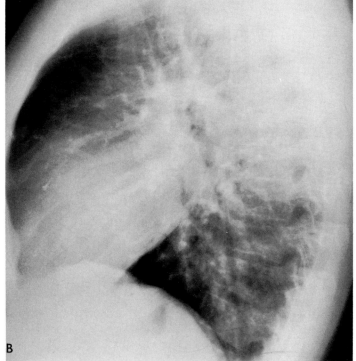

Figure 10–10. Pulmonary Pleonemia: Atrial Septal Defect. Posteroanterior (*A*) and lateral (*B*) roentgenograms of an asymptomatic 19-year-old male reveal a marked increase in the caliber of the pulmonary arteries and veins throughout both lungs; the vessels taper normally. The heart is moderately enlarged, possessing a contour consistent with enlargement of the right atrium and right ventricle. The electrocardiogram showed a right bundle branch block. An atrial septal defect was satisfactorily corrected surgically.

lateral pulmonary artery, no change was observed in the caliber of the pulmonary veins. Despite these conflicting observations, it is clear that appreciation of venous caliber is important in the assessment of shunt lesions. For example, with the development of increased vascular resistance and pulmonary hypertension, the shunt becomes balanced and eventually reversed (Eisenmenger reaction), with resultant reduction in right ventricular output and a decrease in pulmonary venous caliber.[39]

When pulmonary hypertension is long-standing and severe, the pulmonary arteries may develop calcification, presumably on an atherosclerotic basis (Fig. 10–11). This calcification usually is located in the main pulmonary artery and its major hilar branches, but occasionally it may extend into lobar branches.[40] Although such calcification is usually regarded as evidence of high pulmonary vascular resistance and irreversible vascular disease, usually in association with an Eisenmenger reaction, a case has been reported in which a large left-to-right shunt secondary to a VSD was associated with extensive pulmonary artery calcification but with near-normal pulmonary vascular resistance and no irreversible pulmonary vascular disease.[186] Very occasionally, large left-to-right shunts are not reflected in roentgenographically demonstrable enlargement of the pulmonary vascular bed or in cardiomegaly. Of 596 patients with ASDs proven by either cardiac catheterization or surgery reviewed by Baltaxe and Amplatz,[41] 14 (2.3 per cent) showed a normal heart size and a normal pulmonary vascular pattern roentgenographically; all 14 had secundum ASDs of large size, the smallest shunt amounting to 50 per cent.

It may be extremely difficult roentgenologically to recognize the presence of pulmonary arterial hypertension in cases of left-to-right shunt (Fig. 10–12). It might be assumed that increased rapidity of tapering or a disparity between proximal and peripheral pulmonary vessel size would constitute reliable evidence for the presence of hypertension. However, Doyle and associates[42] found that although the small branches of the pulmonary arterial tree are narrowed in some instances, usually they are beyond the range of visibility on plain roentgenography or angiography. These authors stated further that peripheral oligemia usually but not invariably indicates reversal of the left-to-right shunt due to increased vascular resistance, probably secondary to hypoxia. They concluded that only in very severe cases could the presence of pulmonary hypertension be determined from the chest roentgenogram. The difficulty is compounded by the fact that other signs of pulmonary arterial hypertension, such as enlargement of the main and hilar pulmonary arteries, are unreliable since these structures may be greatly enlarged when resistance is normal. It is of interest, however, that some investigators, notably Rees and Jefferson,[43, 44] regard the standard roentgenogram as being of definite value in localizing the level of the shunt. In addition, they state that the rapidity of tapering of the pulmonary vessels as they proceed distally may be a useful sign in assessing the development of hypertension, particularly in ASDs (Fig. 10–11).

Several factors operate to determine the distribution of blood flow in the lungs, both in normal subjects and in patients with cardiovascular disease. For example, in normal subjects, although the average distribution of blood flow to the right lung slightly exceeds that to the left[45] (presumably as a result of the larger volume of the right lung), blood flow to the left upper lobe is somewhat greater than that to the right (presumably as a result of the inclination of the main pulmonary artery in that direction). Patients with valvular pulmonary stenosis characteristically reverse the normal distribution pattern between right and left lungs, blood flow being greater to the left than to the right lung.[46] In cases of left-to-right shunt (Fig. 10–12) asymmetric blood flow to the two lungs has been reported by several investigators,[32, 33, 47] but the reasons for this disparity are obscure. In all studies, flow through the left lung and particularly the left upper lobe was smaller than through the right lung as assessed both roentgenologically[48, 49] and physiologically.[47] Similarly, as might be anticipated, the ratio of blood flow to upper and lower lung zones is altered in left-to-right shunts. In a radioisotopic study of regional pulmonary blood flow in patients with congenital heart disease, Friedman and colleagues[45] found that in erect normal subjects upper-lower blood flow ratios averaged 0.43, whereas in patients with left-to-right shunting this ratio was slightly but significantly raised, more so in the presence of pulmonary arterial hypertension. However, upper-lower ratios never exceeded 1.00 unless pulmonary venous hypertension was present, regardless of pulmonary arterial pressure.

According to Davies and Dow,[50] the distribution of blood flow to the right and left lungs is governed, at least in part, by the anatomic disposition of the pulmonary outflow tract. These authors found that in some cases of transposition of the great arteries, particularly when there is corrected transposition in association with a single ventricle, the pulmonary outflow tract appears to be directed toward the right hilum. This results in a prominence of the right hilar vessels roentgenographically, in earlier filling and clearing of the right lung at angiography, and in a greater flow to the right than to the left lung.

The diagnosis of left-to-right shunts may be facilitated by fluoroscopic observation of increased amplitude of pulsation of the enlarged pulmonary arteries (which tends to be of greatest magnitude in ASD and least in PDA) and enlargement of individual cardiac chambers. The character of the cardiac murmur may be distinctive, and specific signs may indicate strongly one particular anomaly (for example, incomplete right bundle branch block in

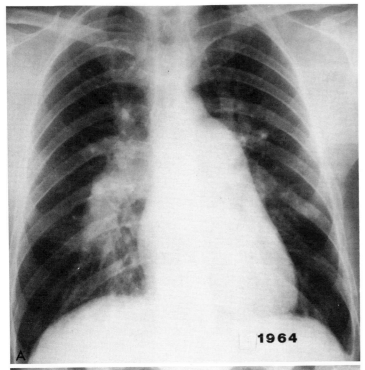

1964

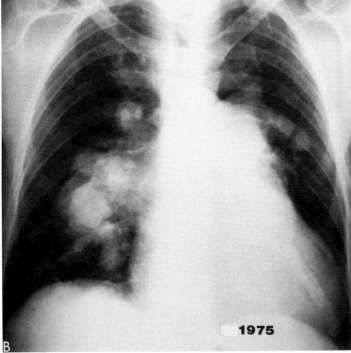

1975

Figure 10–11. Severe Eisenmenger Syndrome Caused by Atrial Septal Defect. A man presented for the first time at the age of 32 with a history of increasing shortness of breath on exertion.

A, A roentgenogram revealed marked enlargement of the hilar pulmonary arteries, which tapered rapidly as they proceeded distally. The peripheral vasculature was clearly diminished, and the size and configuration of the heart were consistent with cor pulmonale. Cardiac catheterization revealed a secundum-type atrial septal defect. Pressures in the main pulmonary artery were 113/42 mm Hg and those in the ascending aorta 99/56 mm Hg. There was a right-to-left shunt of approximately 21 per cent; pulmonary vascular resistance was equivalent to systemic levels at approximately 17 units.

B, Eleven years later the main pulmonary arteries and the heart had undergone remarkable enlargement; the peripheral oligemia was much more evident. The patient showed severe cyanosis and polycythemia. Despite supportive therapy, he died shortly after this examination. At necropsy, the lumen of the main pulmonary artery was considerably larger than that of the ascending aorta. Mural thrombi were present in the major pulmonary arteries and there was severe muscular hypertrophy and calcification of the walls of these vessels.

(Courtesy of St. Boniface Hospital, Manitoba.)

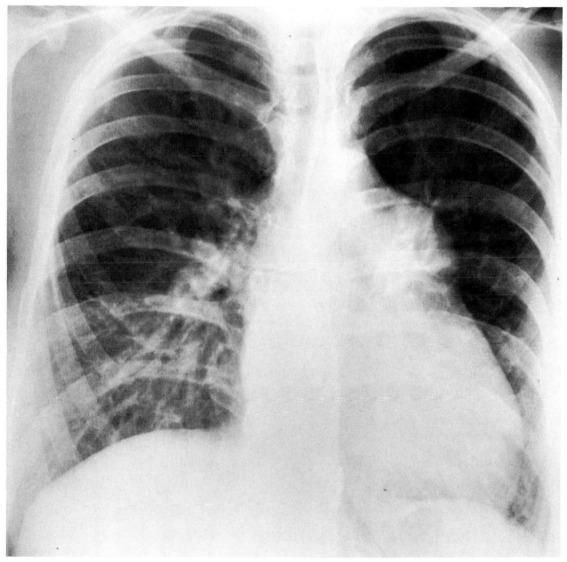

Figure 10–12. Pulmonary Pleonemia: Patent Ductus Arteriosus with Eisenmenger Reaction. A posteroanterior roentgenogram of a 20-year-old woman demonstrates an increase in caliber of the pulmonary arteries and veins throughout both lungs. Note that the left lung and particularly the left upper lobe are more radiolucent than the right, indicating less blood flow to this side. Cardiac enlargement is moderate in degree. At cardiac catheterization, the mean aortic pressure was found to be 90 mm Hg and the mean pulmonary artery pressure 100 mm Hg; the ratio of systemic to pulmonary artery flow was 3.8 to 5.0 liters per minute. The presence of a patent ductus arteriosus was established, associated with bidirectional shunt (Eisenmenger reaction). The roentgenographic signs of pulmonary arterial hypertension are unconvincing.

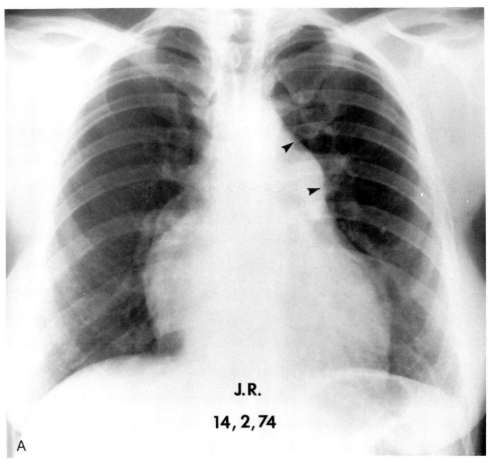

J.R.

14, 2, 74

A

Figure 10–13. Precapillary Hypertension Secondary to a Left-to-Right Intracardiac Shunt (ASD). A conventional postero-anterior chest roentgenogram (*A*) reveals moderate cardiomegaly consistent with enlargement of right heart chambers; there is no evidence of enlargement of the left atrium. The main pulmonary artery (*arrowheads*) is very prominent, although the hilar arteries appear normal. The upper-lobe vessels are roughly equal in size to those in the lower lobes, indicating the presence of increased flow to upper lobes; however, note that the lower-lobe vessels are clearly defined, thereby suggesting that postcapillary hypertension is not the cause of this phenomenon.

ASD). In many cases, however, cardiac catheterization, with or without angiocardiography, is requisite to thorough assessment, particularly in the presence of suspected pulmonary arterial hypertension. In cases in which the appearance of hilar and peripheral arteries is within normal limits, arteriography may be essential to evaluate changes in the pulmonary vasculature (Fig. 10–13). In fact, pulmonary angiography can sometimes reveal changes suggestive of angiomatoid and plexiform lesions (Fig. 10–14). To improve opacification in the angiographic demonstration of certain shunt lesions, particularly ASD and anomalous pulmonary venous drainage, Nordenstrom and colleagues[51] took advantage of the temporary changes in hemodynamics that accompany increased intra-alveolar pressure. Elevation of the intra-alveolar pressure to 40 to 50 cm H_2O, followed by right atrial or vena caval injection and sudden release of the intrapulmonary pressure, resulted in reversal of flow across ASDs and into abnormally draining pulmonary veins.

Clinically, many patients with left-to-right shunts are asymptomatic. If the shunt is large, some physical underdevelopment and a tendency to respiratory infections may occur. The patient may complain of fatigue, palpitations, and dyspnea on exertion and may exhibit signs of cardiac failure. Uncomplicated ASD is characterized by an ejection murmur, an early systolic click, and a wide splitting

of the second cardiac sound (0.05 seconds or more), which does not vary with respiration; cardiac enlargement and bulging of the precordial chest cage may develop. Ventricular septal defect produces a pansystolic murmur maximal at the third or fourth left interspace close to the sternum; the second sound is normally split or widened but, unlike its behavior in ASD, varies with respiration. The murmur of PDA before the development of pulmonary hypertension usually is long and rumbling and occupies most of systole and diastole. It is loudest in the second left interspace near the sternum and sometimes is associated with crescendo accentuation in late systole; the second pulmonic sound is increased in amplitude but normally split and changing with respiration. A widely patent left-to-right shunt caused by PDA produces systemic peripheral vascular signs of a high pulse pressure. A rare cause of left-to-right shunt is a communication between the aorta or its branches and the pulmonary artery, right heart chambers, or superior vena cava. Frequently the fistula involves the right coronary artery, the diagnosis being made in infancy by angiography following discovery of a continuous murmur on auscultation. Children are usually asymptomatic although in untreated cases symptoms may arise in later life from pulmonary hypertension, especially when the shunt volume is large.[52]

The development of pulmonary hypertension

Figure 10–13 *Continued* A right ventricular pulmonary angiogram during the arterial (*B*) and venous (*C*) phases shows the characteristic features of precapillary hypertension: the right (R) and left (L) interlobar arteries are dilated, intrapulmonary arterial branches are tortuous and sinuous (*arrowheads*), and the veins (*open arrows*) are of normal caliber. The patient is a 32-year-old woman.

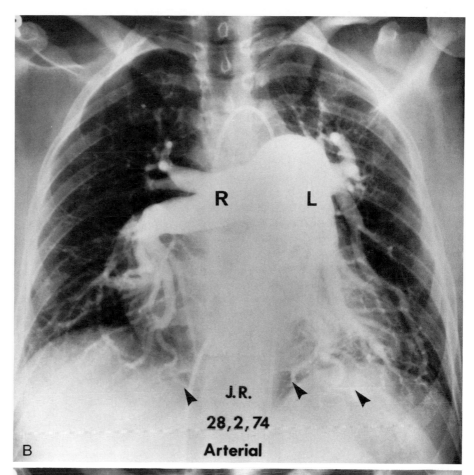

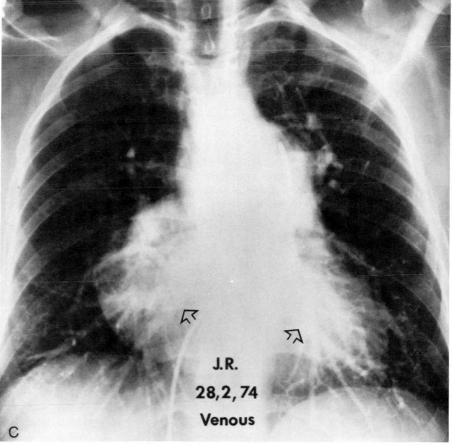

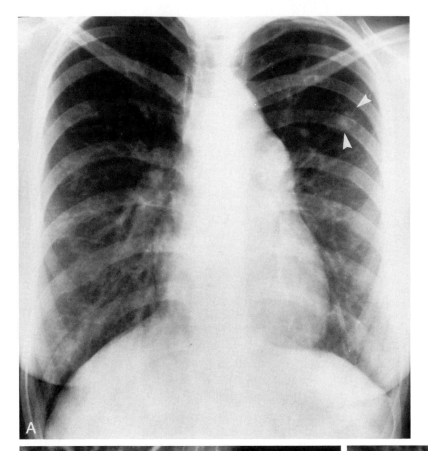

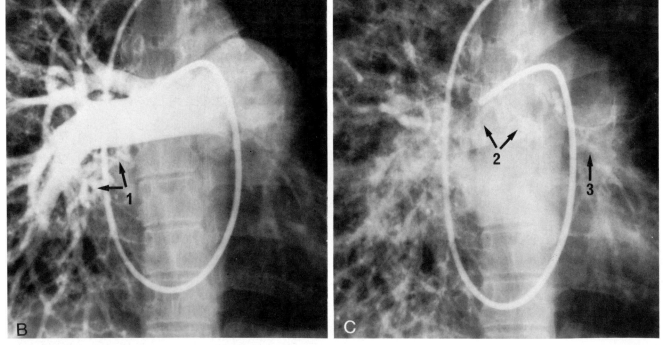

Figure 10–14. Angiographic Features of Severe Precapillary Pulmonary Hypertension Caused by a Ventricular Septal Defect. A conventional posteroanterior chest roentgenogram (A) discloses a prominent main pulmonary artery segment. The hilar arteries are increased in size and the lungs plethoric. Several poorly defined nodular opacities can be identified in the lungs, the most notable being in the left upper lobe (arrowheads). A right pulmonary arteriogram during the arterial (B) and venous (C) phases shows markedly enlarged anastomotic collateral vessels medial to the descending right pulmonary artery (1), within the mediastinum (2), and in the left hilar bronchi (3).

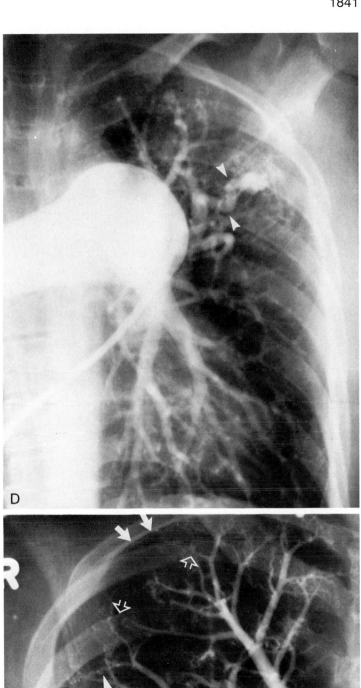

D

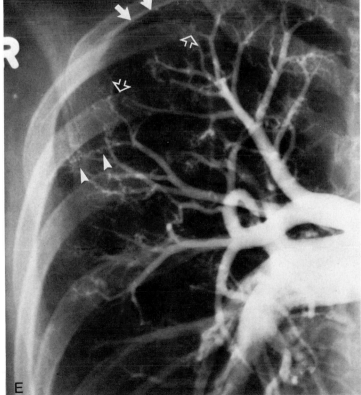

E

Figure 10–14 *Continued* A left pulmonary arteriogram (*D*) shows an enlarged, branchless, serpiginous segmental artery (*arrowheads*) that terminates in a bulbous structure distally; there is no evidence of an enlarged draining vein. A right pulmonary arteriogram (*E*) reveals multiple, small, sinuous arteries in the distal parenchyma (*arrowheads*), amputation of arteries (*open arrows*), and subpleural collaterals (*closed arrows*). The combined features are felt to be representative of severe precapillary hypertension. The patient is a young woman with a recently discovered, uncorrected ventricular septal defect. Cardiac catheterization disclosed pressures within the pulmonary artery that were almost the same as those in the systemic circulation.

in cases of left-to-right shunt gives rise to changes in the physical findings. In ASD, atrial fibrillation is a frequent occurrence and may be followed by tricuspid regurgitation and heart failure; the fixed splitting of the second heart sound becomes much narrower and the systolic murmur may become fainter. In VSD, the systolic murmur decreases in length, and an ejection systolic murmur and click may appear. In PDA, as the pressure in the pulmonary circulation rises and the shunt and shunt gradient decrease, the murmur is reduced in intensity and (as happens in many cases) the diastolic component disappears.

As indicated previously, most symptoms and signs of pulmonary hypertension are caused by cor pulmonale. Retrosternal pain, identical to angina pectoris, accompanies the very high pulmonary arterial pressures that develop in primary pulmonary hypertension and in severe hypertension with mitral stenosis. Pulmonary hypertension also causes accentuation of the second pulmonic sound and the early diastolic murmur along the left sternal border as a result of pulmonary valvular insufficiency. The parasternal thrust, tricuspid insufficiency, and liver and neck pulsations are due to cor pulmonale and failure of the right ventricle.

DECREASED FLOW (TETRALOGY OF FALLOT)

Pulmonary hypertension sometimes develops in cases of tetralogy of Fallot. Studies by Ferencz[53] indicate that the hypertension may be caused by multiple pulmonary arterial thromboses resulting from slowing of the circulation and a tendency to polycythemia. According to this author, thrombosis in the pulmonary arterial circulation is rare in patients with pulmonic stenosis without septal defects. Although creation of a systemic–pulmonary anastomosis may reverse the hypertension in some cases, this procedure can lead to rupture of small pulmonary arteries. In addition, the creation of a left-to-right shunt may result in medial hypertrophy and intimal fibrosis of the small pulmonary arteries, with consequent severe pulmonary vascular hypertension.[53] In a study of seven patients with tetralogy of Fallot who developed pulmonary arterial hypertension following subclavian–pulmonary artery anastomosis (Blalock-Taussig shunt), Puyau and Meckstroth[54] found a disproportionate increase in the size of the central pulmonary vessels compared with the peripheral vessels, a sign that was not present in a similar group of patients whose pulmonary artery pressures were normal following Blalock-Taussig shunt. These authors emphasized the importance of the early recognition of hilar enlargement in these cases, since the development of irreversible changes in pulmonary vascular resistance makes total correction impossible. Following Blalock-Taussig anastomosis severe pulmonary hypertension develops in patients over the age of 5 but not in younger children. Clinical signs suggest-

ing the presence of hypertension in such cases include an increase in cyanosis, loss of the continuous murmur, and a loud pulmonary valve closure sound. Avoidance of hypertension in this age group requires cardiac catheterization and determination of pulmonary-systemic flow and resistance ratios prior to surgery.[55] A rare but even more devastating consequence of surgical correction of tetralogy may be failure to recognize associated anomalous pulmonary venous drainage.[56] Other factors that may lead to irreversible pulmonary hypertension after surgical correction of tetralogy of Fallot include undetected agenesis of a pulmonary artery, peripheral pulmonic stenosis (coarctation), too large a shunt from a previous Blalock (or more likely Potts') anastomosis leading to heart failure, and obstruction of the pulmonary vascular bed associated with inadequate closure of the VSD and relief of the pulmonic stenosis.

In patients with tetralogy of Fallot and severe pulmonic stenosis, abnormalities in the chest roentgenograms that simulate chronic granulomatous disease can develop. Pleural and parenchymal opacities occur as a result of collateral vessels and pleuritis following multiple small hemorrhages at the lung apices, a condition that has been called "pulmonary pseudofibrosis,"[57] Other causes of opacities include varicosities of transpleural, bronchial, and other collateral vessels and possibly thromboses in small pulmonary arteries.[58, 59]

PRIMARY PULMONARY HYPERTENSION

Primary pulmonary hypertension was first described in 1951 by Dresdale and associates,[60] who reported three young women with severe exertional dyspnea and roentgenographic and clinical evidence of pulmonary hypertension and right ventricular hypertrophy. This subject has been recently reviewed.[61, 62] Primary pulmonary hypertension is a relatively uncommon condition,[63–67] the authenticity of which has been questioned by some on the basis of the demonstration at necropsy of multiple pulmonary emboli in patients considered to have had this disease during life.[68, 69] However, the dramatic response in some patients to the intravenous injection of acetylcholine[25, 70] and other vasodilating agents,[71] the presence of characteristic plexogenic arteriopathy (a pathologic state that is rarely associated with thromboemboli), and the tendency to familial occurrence[72–76] strongly support the existence of this disease as a distinct entity.

Although the majority of cases appear to occur sporadically, the disease has been reported in 52 patients from 14 North American families.[62] It has been reported in twins,[74] in five members in three generations of one family,[72] and in a father and his two children.[75] The inheritance patterns of familial primary pulmonary hypertension have been studied by Loyd and colleagues,[76] who found that although there was a widely different frequency of gene expression between families, the inheritance generally conformed to an autosomal dominant pattern.[77] These authors also pointed out that many cases considered to be sporadic could be proved to be familial if the medical records of family members who died prematurely were examined. In these familial occurrences of the disease, there is an approximate 2-to-1 female-to-male predominance. The surprising finding of a plasmin inhibitor in ten members of a kindred indicates that in some patients with familial pulmonary hypertension, pulmonary microemboli may be unable to be lysed.[78]

The relative rarity of primary pulmonary hypertension has prevented individual centers from gathering sufficiently large groups of patients to permit an adequate description of epidemiologic and clinical features. However, in 1981 the Division of Lung Disease of the National Heart, Lung, and Blood Institute of the National Institutes of Health (NIH) initiated a patient registry for the characterization of pulmonary hypertension.[67] During the next 5 years, 187 patients with presumed primary pulmonary hypertension were entered into this registry. The mean age of the patients was 36 ± 15 years with a female-to-male predominance of 1.7 to 1. The mean interval from the onset of symptoms to diagnosis was 2 years, and the most frequent presenting symptoms were dyspnea (60 per cent), fatigue (19 per cent), and syncope or near-syncope (13 per cent). Raynaud's phenomenon was observed in 10 per cent of patients, virtually all of whom were female, and a positive antinuclear antibody test was found in 29 per cent, 69 per cent of whom were female. Six per cent of patients had a familial history of pulmonary hypertension affecting a first-order relative.

The etiology and pathogenesis of primary pulmonary hypertension are unknown. The possibility that it might be drug-induced was suggested by the finding of a 20-fold increase in the incidence of the disease in Austria, Germany,[79] and Switzerland[80] during the years 1966 to 1968; in most affected patients, symptoms of rapidly progressive exertional dyspnea and syncope developed 6 to 12 months after the institution of treatment of obesity with an anorectic drug, aminorex fumarate. The pulmonary hypertension was documented by cardiac catheterization. Although it is presumed that the drug acted directly on the pulmonary vasculature, a few patients showed evidence of pulmonary and peripheral thromboembolic disease.[80] Withdrawal of the drug from the market resulted in a decline in the incidence of pulmonary hypertension.[80, 81] An attempt to reproduce the disease by administering oral aminorex to rats and dogs failed.[81] Another report has described an epidemic of pulmonary hypertension in Spain following the ingestion of toxic rapeseed oil.[82]

It is believed that the early stages of primary pulmonary hypertension are characterized by vasoconstriction of pulmonary vascular smooth muscle; with prolonged vasoconstriction there occurs vascular remodeling and eventually the changes of plexogenic pulmonary arteriopathy. A role for vasoconstriction as a predisposing factor to the development of the full-blown picture is supported by the observation that primary pulmonary hypertension is more common at altitude than at sea level.[83] In the iatrogenic variety induced by aminorex, withdrawal of the drug has resulted in symptomatic and hemodynamic improvement in some patients; similarly, spontaneous reversal has been reported,[84] suggesting that at least the early stages of primary pulmonary hypertension are caused by vasospasm unassociated with irreparable anatomic alteration in the pulmonary vasculature. Unfortunately, by the time the vast majority of patients first come to medical attention, extensive anatomic changes have already developed.

Pyrolizidine alkaloids—chemicals found in the plants *Senecio jacobaea* and *Crotalaria (C. spectabilis, C. fulva, C. laburnifolia)*—have been shown to cause pulmonary hypertension in rats.[85–88] These substances are readily available for human consumption,[85, 88] although we are not aware of convincing evidence that would implicate them in the development of pulmonary hypertension in humans. However, *C. fulva* is ingested in the West Indies as a component of bush tea and causes veno-occlusive disease of the liver.[85] The administration of the alkaloid fulvine to rats[87] results in vasoconstriction, medial hypertrophy, and necrotizing arteritis of pulmonary arteries, and thickening of the walls and proliferation of muscle fibers of pulmonary veins and venules. The experience with aminorex and *Crotalaria* suggests the possibility that pulmonary hypertension may be caused by substances which, taken by mouth, can reach the pulmonary circulation and cause obliterative vascular lesions; the route by which these metabolites of ingested foodstuffs reach the lungs may be the portal circulation, a concept supported by the rare association of portal and pulmonary hypertension. Lebrec and associates[89] have described nine patients with combined portal and pulmonary hypertension and identified 14 previously reported cases in the literature: of these 23 patients 15 had a surgical portocaval shunt established because of esophageal varices. This rare but statistically significant association[90] suggests that vasoactive or vasotoxic substances produced in the gut and normally metabolized by the liver can reach the pulmonary circulation in patients with cirrhosis, portal hypertension, and a portal-systemic shunt. McDonnell and associates[91] found a prevalence of pulmonary hypertension of 0.73 per cent in a large autopsy study of cirrhotic patients, and a prevalence of 0.61 per cent in a clinical series of 2,459 patients with biopsy-proven cirrhosis.

Another possible pathogenetic mechanism for the development of primary pulmonary hypertension is that it is part of a generalized angiopathic process;[92] for example, the incidence of Raynaud's phenomenon in patients with primary pulmonary hypertension is higher than expected. Similarly, pulmonary hypertension has been reported in association with several systemic connective tissue diseases such as polymyositis,[93] systemic lupus erythematosus,[94] and progressive systemic sclerosis (PSS).[95, 96] Deposition of amyloid in the walls of pulmonary vessels is a rare cause of pulmonary arterial hypertension.[706]

Roentgenographically, the lungs show evidence of diffuse oligemia, the peripheral pulmonary arteries being narrow and inconspicuous (Fig. 10–15).[97] The hilar pulmonary arteries are enlarged and taper rapidly distally;[97] the main pulmonary artery usually is prominent and often shows increased amplitude of pulsation fluoroscopically. Measurement of the transverse diameter of the right and left interlobar arteries provides reliable evidence of the presence or absence of dilatation and thus the likelihood of the presence of pulmonary arterial hypertension (providing conditions of increased flow such as left-to-right shunt have been excluded). As discussed in Chapter 1 (see page 83), the upper limit of the transverse diameter of the right interlobar artery from its lateral aspect to the air column of the intermediate bronchus is 16 mm in men and 15 mm in women;[98] since the transverse diameter of the left interlobar artery is often impossible to measure on a conventional posteroanterior roentgenogram, a useful alternative is to measure the vessel on a lateral roentgenogram from the circular lucency created by the left upper lobe bronchus viewed end-on to the posterior margin of the vessel as it loops over the bronchus, the accepted upper limits of normal for this measurement being 18 mm.

Although measurements in excess of these figures on conventional posteroanterior and lateral roentgenograms provide reasonably convincing evidence of the presence of pulmonary arterial hypertension, computed tomography (CT) can also allow precise noninvasive measurement of the diameter of pulmonary arteries.[99] In a study of 32 patients with cardiopulmonary disease and 26 age-and-sex-matched control subjects, Kuriyama and associates[99] found that in the normal subjects the upper limit of the diameter of the main pulmonary artery was 28.6 mm; in the patient group in which diameters were correlated with data from cardiac catheterization, a diameter of the main pulmonary artery greater than 28.6 mm readily predicted the presence of pulmonary hypertension. However, the best estimates of mean pulmonary artery pressure were obtained from the calculated cross-sectional areas of the main and interlobular pulmonary arteries (normalized for body surface area). In this study, pulmonary artery measurements not only were of value in detecting pulmonary arterial hypertension but also provided estimates of mean pulmonary artery pressure. An interesting technique has also been developed for determining serial arterial cross-sectional diameters from pulmonary wedge angiograms:[100] in a study of 11 adults comprising five normal subjects and six patients with primary pulmonary hypertension, Boxt and his colleagues[100] showed a strong correlation between arterial taper and a power function of mean pulmonary arterial pressure; the authors suggested that this technique provides a means of following the course of primary pulmonary hypertension and of studying the effects of drug therapy.

In addition to these morphologic changes in the central pulmonary arteries, patients with primary pulmonary hypertension can exhibit roentgenologic evidence of right ventricular enlargement. Overinflation does not occur, permitting ready differentiation from the diffuse pulmonary oligemia associated with emphysema. In the NIH study,[67] the chest roentgenograms were subjectively graded: prominence of the main pulmonary artery was found in 90 per cent, enlarged hilar vessels in 80 per cent, and right ventricular hypertrophy in 74 per cent. M-mode echocardiography showed right ventricular enlargement in 75 per cent of patients and paradoxical septal wall motion in 59 per cent. Lung perfusion scans were abnormal in 58 per cent of cases; the majority of the abnormalities on perfusion scintigraphy consisted of diffuse, patchy defects that were estimated to have a low probability of representing pulmonary embolism (Fig. 10–16).[67]

The main symptom in patients with primary pulmonary hypertension is dyspnea on exertion. In one series of 23 patients in whom the diagnosis was established at necropsy and in whom the clinical history did not suggest the presence of pulmonary thromboembolic disease, there was a female predominance of 5 to 1 and the median age at the time of death was 34 years; symptoms consisted of dyspnea (in 22 patients), Raynaud's phenomenon (in seven), and syncope (in six).[97] In a more recent report of 38 patients with primary pulmonary hypertension seen at the Celveland Clinic,[187] the most common symptoms in order of frequency were dyspnea on exertion (in 97 per cent), easy fatigability, chest pain, cough, dizziness, and syncope.

Signs of cor pulmonale and cardiac failure may be present, including giant jugular A waves; right atrial gallop; a loud pulmonary ejection click; an accentuated pulmonic sound; a palpable lift along the left sternal border; and, in some cases, murmurs caused by pulmonic and tricuspid insufficiency.[97] In the 187 patients from the multicenter NIH study,[67] an increase in the pulmonary component of the second heart sound was found in 93 per cent, a right-sided third or fourth heart sound in 61 per cent, tricuspid regurgitation in 40 per cent, pulmonic insufficiency in 13 per cent, cyanosis in 20 per cent, and peripheral edema in 32 per cent.

Catheterization of the right side of the heart reveals pulmonary arterial hypertension, a normal pulmonary wedge pressure, high pulmonary vas-

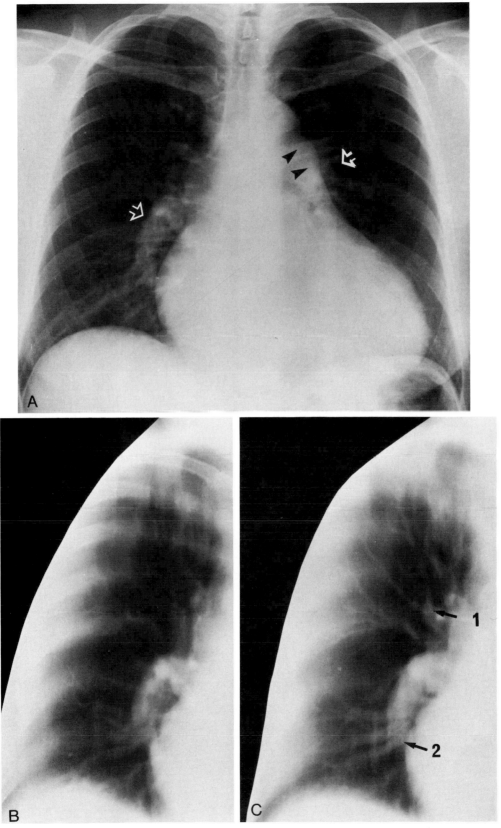

Figure 10–15. Primary Pulmonary Hypertension. A conventional posteroanterior chest roentgenogram (*A*) and detail views of the right lung from linear tomograms (*B* and *C*) reveal enlargement of the right ventricle, dilatation of the main (*arrowheads*) and hilar (*open arrows*) pulmonary arteries, and increased rapidity of tapering of pulmonary arteries as they proceed distally. The pulmonary veins in the upper (*1*) and lower (*2*) lobes in *C* are normal.

Illustration continued on following page

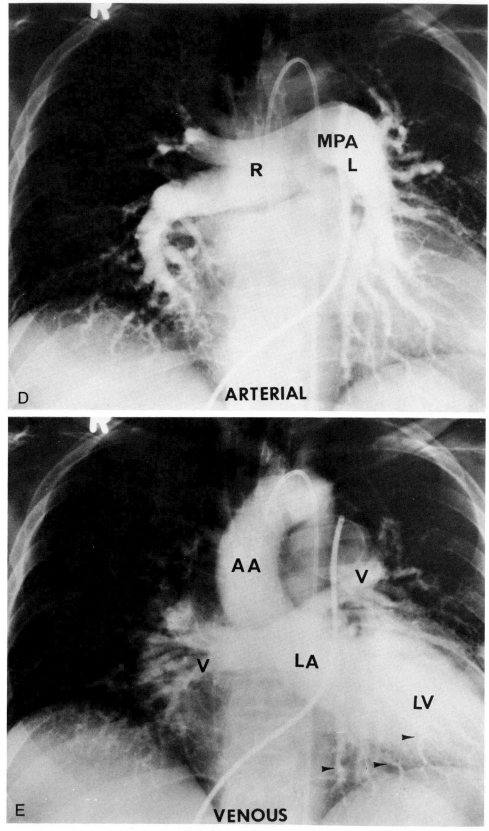

Figure 10–15 *Continued* These findings are confirmed on a pulmonary angiogram during the arterial (*D*) and venous (*E*) phases (main pulmonary artery [MPA], right [R] and left [L] pulmonary arteries); the middle and distal pulmonary arteries taper rapidly, displaying a sinuous ("corkscrew") appearance. Pulmonary veins (V) are normal. Note that some of the lower lobe arteries are persistently opacified (*arrowheads*) during the venous phase, indicative of the increased resistance to blood flow in the lower lobes. The left atrium (LA), left ventricle (LV), and ascending aorta (AA) are opacified. The patient is a young woman.

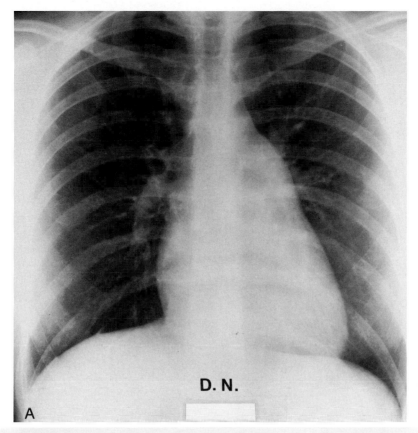

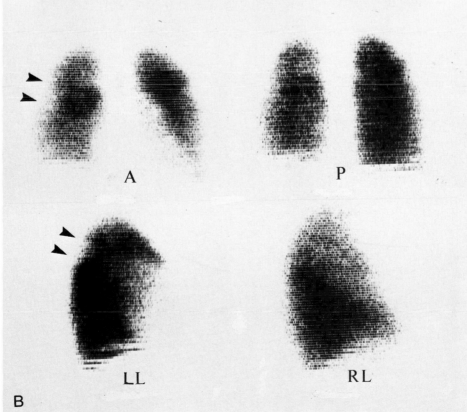

Figure 10–16. Primary Pulmonary Hypertension: Scintigraphic Findings. A posteroanterior chest roentgenogram (*A*) shows right ventricular and main pulmonary artery (*arrowheads*) enlargement; the hila, pulmonary vessels, and parenchyma are normal. Cardiac catheterization in this young woman disclosed severe precapillary hypertension; there was no evidence of a gradient across either the aortic or pulmonic valves. A four-view rectilinear pulmonary scintigraphic study (*B*) in anterior (A), posterior (P), left lateral (LL), and right lateral (RL) projections demonstrates shallow subpleural perfusion deficits (*arrowheads*) interpreted as low probability for thromboembolic disease.

cular resistance, and in patients with right ventricular failure, a low cardiac output.[63, 97] In the 187 patients from the NIH study,[67] the mean pulmonary arterial pressure was 60 ± 18 mm Hg, the pulmonary wedge pressure averaged approximately 9 mm Hg, and the cardiac index was mildly reduced at 2.27 ± 0.9 liters/minute/m^2.

Although pulmonary function may be completely normal, arterial oxygen saturation[101] and diffusing capacity are often decreased.[102] A relatively high incidence of a restrictive ventilatory defect has been observed in some studies.[103, 104] In the NIH study,[67] total lung capacity and vital capacity were mildly decreased and there was a moderate decrease in pulmonary diffusing capacity (68 per cent predicted), arterial P_{O_2} ($Pa_{O_2} = 70$ mm Hg), and arterial P_{CO_2} ($Pa_{CO_2} = 30$ mm Hg). Using the multiple inert gas technique,[105, 106] it has been shown that the gas exchange abnormalities are predominantly the result of $\dot{V}/\dot{Q}$ mismatching; significant hypoxemia occurs only when mixed venous P_{O_2} is decreased secondary to a drop in cardiac output. The fall in arterial P_{O_2} that occurs during exercise[106] is caused by a failure of cardiac output to increase sufficiently, resulting in a decrease in the mixed venous O_2 saturation; the desaturated mixed venous blood passes through shunts and low $\dot{V}/\dot{Q}$ regions, worsening the arterial P_{O_2}.

Although fatalities have been reported following lung scanning in patients with primary pulmonary hypertension,[107, 108] none of the 163 patients who had perfusion scans in the NIH study reported adverse effects. Similarly, although it has been said that patients with severe pulmonary hypertension are subject to sudden death during or following cardiac catheterization,[109] only one of the 50 patients who had pulmonary angiography in the NIH study had an adverse effect (transient hypotension). It has been suggested that adverse effects of pulmonary angiography can be diminished by performing selective left and right main pulmonary artery injections. Nicod and associates[110] carried out selective left and right main pulmonary artery injections in 67 consecutive patients with pulmonary hypertension, either primary in type or secondary to chronic thromboembolic disease, and reported no major disturbances in cardiac rhythm, no episodes of significant systemic hypotension, and no fatalities.

The majority of patients with primary pulmonary hypertension have progressive disease, and the median survival time is no more than 2 to 3 years.[62] Although the typical natural history is one of progressive dyspnea, cor pulmonale, and death, exceptions do occur; for example, repeated catheterizations may reveal no change in hemodynamics[101] or even improvement,[63] and patients have been reported to survive as long as 18 years after the onset of symptoms.[72] A reduced cardiac index and symptoms such as syncope that reflect decreased cardiac output are indicators of a poor prognosis.[111]

PULMONARY THROMBOEMBOLIC DISEASE

The majority of cases of pulmonary arterial hypertension of vascular origin probably are attributable to multiple pulmonary emboli occurring over a period of many years. Although follow-up studies on most patients who have suffered an acute pulmonary thromboembolic episode show dissolution of clots (see Chapter 9), in one series of 13 patients who years earlier had survived a severe embolic episode associated with pulmonary hypertension, nine were found to have mild degrees of persisting pulmonary hypertension (Fig. 10–17).[112] However, patients with chronic thromboembolic pulmonary hypertension usually do not give a history suggesting major pulmonary embolism or infarction.[113]

Emboli usually originate from thromboses in the systemic veins of the legs or pelvis and occasionally in the heart from myocardial or valvular disease. Less common causes of pulmonary thromboembolism are ventriculoauriculostomy, a procedure employed for relieving intracranial pressure in hydrocephalic children,[114] and pyogenic cholangitis, a not uncommon cause of pulmonary hypertension in Chinese residents of Hong Kong.[115] In some cases, pulmonary emboli can be the cause of the pulmonary hypertension that is associated with cirrhosis of the liver and portal hypertension, particularly in patients who have undergone portal-systemic shunting;[89] thrombi sometimes found in the portal venous system can be the source of the multiple pulmonary emboli, bypassing the liver through the portal-systemic anastomoses or via esophageal or gastric varices.[116] In one such case, a roentgenographic pattern of diffuse nodular opacities was considered to be caused by a fibroblastic reaction around the occluded pulmonary vessels.[117]

Rarely, pulmonary hypertension can result from chronic thrombotic occlusion of the major pulmonary arteries as in the 15 patients reported by Moser and associates[118] in whom complete or partial obstruction of a main or several lobar arteries was proven by pulmonary arteriography. These patients underwent surgical removal of the proximal pulmonary emboli and thrombi, accompanied by complete cardiac bypass and hypothermia; some degree of reperfusion pulmonary edema occurred in all patients. Primary thrombosis in the pulmonary arterial circulation is probably abetted by slowing of the circulation and the increased blood viscosity typical of polycythemia, and by the pulmonary vascular changes resulting from increased vasomotor tone, inflammation of the vessel wall, and sickling due to hemoglobin SC and hemoglobin SS disease. Because of the low mixed venous P_{O_2} and pH, the lung vessels are particularly susceptible to the increased blood viscosity caused by sickling. This unusual complication is probably more common in hemoglobin SC disease, since homozygotes for S hemoglobin tend to die at an early age.[119, 120] An

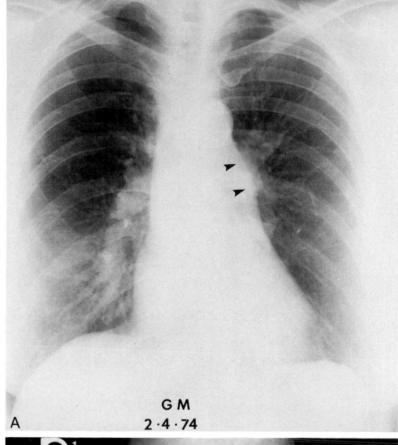

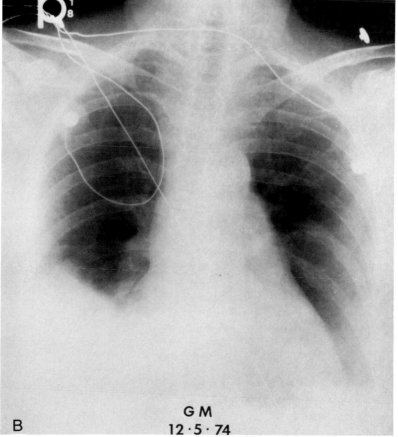

Figure 10–17. Precapillary Pulmonary Hypertension Caused by Massive Pulmonary Thromboembolism. A conventional posteroanterior chest roentgenogram (A) shows moderate enlargement of the main pulmonary artery (*arrowheads*), dilatation of hilar pulmonary arteries, and slight enlargement of the heart. There is a suggestion of oligemia in the right upper lobe. The patient, a middle-aged woman, had experienced only vague chest discomfort several days prior to this roentgenogram. Approximately 6 weeks later, following the sudden onset of severe chest pain and circulatory collapse, a chest roentgenogram (B) disclosed an increase in the size of the heart, diffuse oligemia of the right lung, and elevation of the right hemidiaphragm. These features are consistent with acute cor pulmonale caused by thromboembolism.

Illustration continued on following page

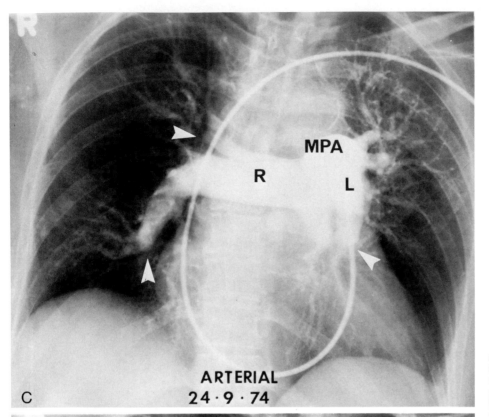

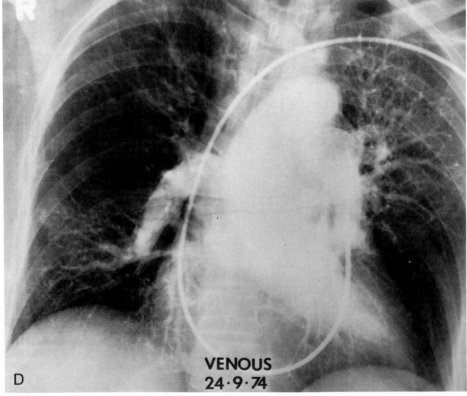

Figure 10–17 *Continued* Four and a half months later, arterial (*C*) and venous (*D*) phases of a pulmonary arteriogram reveal multiple amputated arteries (*arrowheads*) in the lower lobes and right upper lobe. The main pulmonary artery (MPA) and its right (R) and left (L) branches are dilated. During the venous phase, note the oligemia in the right mid and upper lung zones and the left lower lobe.

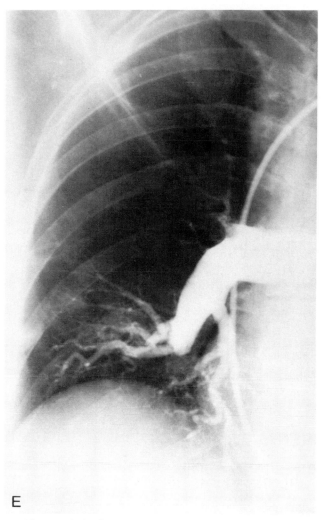

E

Figure 10–17 *Continued* The arterial vasculature is tortuous and sinuous, characteristic of chronic precapillary hypertension, a feature better shown on a detail view from a selective right pulmonary arteriogram (*E*).

even rarer cause of increased vascular resistance is seen in eclampsia, in which condition the pulmonary vessels are believed to be occluded by microthrombi from platelet-fibrin aggregates.[121, 122] When either thrombosis or embolism occurs in the major hilar pulmonary arteries, the combination of bulging hilar pulmonary arteries, severe peripheral oligemia, and cor pulmonale constitutes a virtually pathognomonic roentgenologic triad (*see* Fig. 4–146, page 655).

In the vast majority of patients, pulmonary hypertension related to thromboembolism is caused by the presence of multiple small emboli in the peripheral vasculature. The major diagnostic difficulty involves distinguishing these patients from those in whom the hypertension is primary in type and those in whom it is secondary to pulmonary veno-occlusive disease. The importance of this distinction lies in the marked differences in therapy that are appropriate in these conditions: if the hypertension is primary in type and thus caused by pulmonary vasoconstriction, vasodilator therapy is appropriate; when it is caused by thromboembolism, anticoagulants may be beneficial. Vasodilators may be contraindicated in patients with veno-occlusive disease because they can cause an increased cardiac output with a resultant rapid increase in pulmonary microvascular pressure and pulmonary edema.[123] In 19 patients with biopsy-proven plexogenic pulmonary hypertension, thromboembolic pulmonary hypertension, or veno-occlusive disease, Rich and associates[123] examined the usefulness of conventional chest roentgenography and chest scintigraphy using ^{99m}Tc-labeled albumin macroaggregates in establishing a differential diagnosis; they found that the chest roentgenogram was normal in patients with plexogenic pulmonary hypertension and thromboembolic pulmonary hypertension but that perfusion lung scanning was abnormal in seven of the eight patients with thromboembolic disease and in none of the nine patients with plexogenic pulmonary hypertension; in the former group, the scans revealed patchy, diffuse nonsegmental perfusion defects. In the two patients with veno-occlusive disease diagnosed at biopsy, the chest roentgenograms revealed evidence of pulmonary venous hypertension. The authors suggested that a combination of chest roentgenograms and perfusion scintigraphy can be useful in distinguishing these three conditions. Three studies[124–126] have confirmed the value of pulmonary scintigraphy in the differential diagnosis of thromboembolic and primary pulmonary hypertension. In our experience, CT can also be of value in the assessment of the pulmonary vasculature in patients with chronic precapillary hypertension secondary to thromboembolism (Fig. 10–18).

Morphologic features of thromboembolic pulmonary hypertension are sufficiently distinctive to enable the pathologist to suggest the cause of the hypertension in most cases.[707] Typically, multiple thrombi in various stages of organization are seen in small to medium sized muscular arteries. Eccentric intimal fibrosis and transluminal fibrous bands are common and represent completely organized thrombi. These features are discussed in greater detail on page 1712.

In addition to thrombi, many other materials can embolize to the lungs and cause pulmonary hypertension, including metastatic neoplasm (*see* page 1790), schistosomal parasites (*see* page 1790), and talc, the base in oral preparations injected intravenously by drug addicts (*see* page 1794).

The symptoms and signs of multiple pulmonary emboli are described in Chapter 9 (*see* page 1777). Nadel and his coworkers[127] described changes in size of the physiologic dead space and in arterial-alveolar gradients in patients with chronic pulmonary vascular obstruction. Exercise increased these abnormalities and in some cases resulted in pulmonary hypertension.

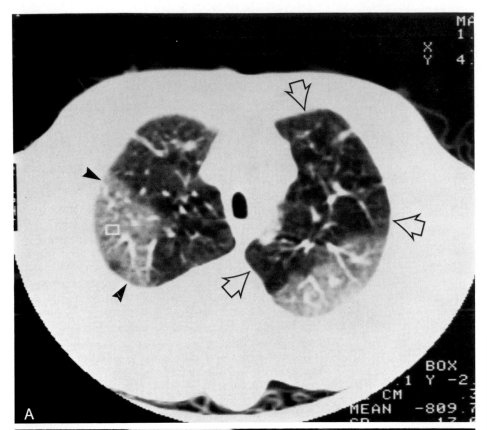

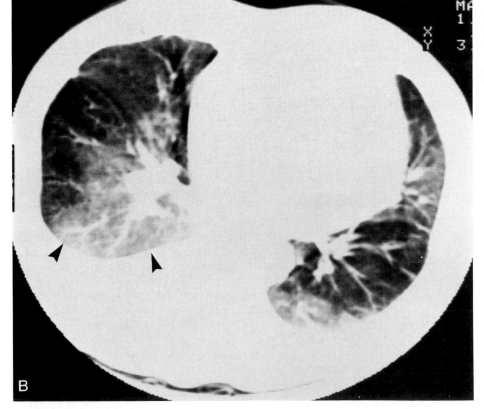

Figure 10–18. Pulmonary Hypertension: Perfusion Pattern on CT in Chronic Thromboembolism without Infarction. CT scans through the upper (*A*) and lower (*B*) lobes show sharply contrasting geographic areas of increased (*arrowheads*) and decreased (*open arrows*) attenuation, representing areas of maintained perfusion and oligemia, respectively. Note that the amorphous increase in density throughout the perfused zones is so intense that parenchymal consolidation is simulated; no such corresponding opacities were visible on a conventional roentgenogram (not depicted).

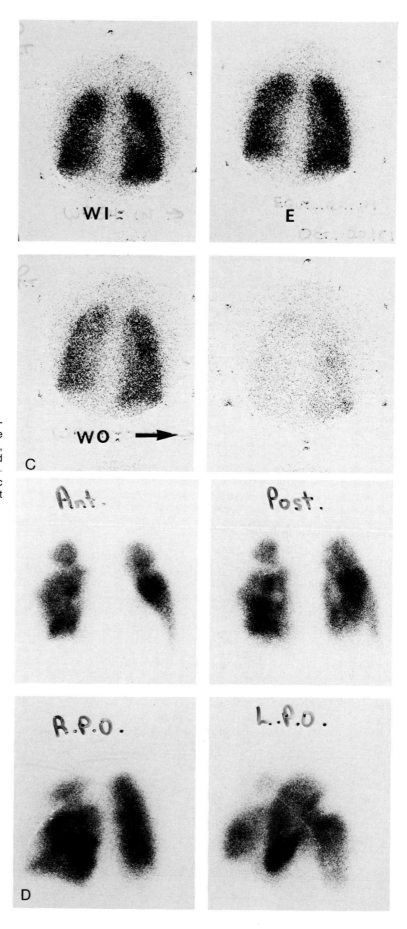

Figure 10–18 *Continued* Ventilation (*C*) and perfusion (*D*) lung scintigrams reveal features that are considered "high probability" for thromboembolism. WI, E, and WO represent the wash-in, equilibrium, and wash-out phases, respectively, of the perfusion scintigraphic study. Note the close matching of the oligemic segments on the CT and perfusion images. The patient is a 64-year-old man.

Systemic Immunologic Disorders

Isolated pulmonary hypertension, manifested pathologically by plexogenic arteriopathy, occurs occasionally in immunologically mediated connective tissue disorders, particularly PSS, mixed connective tissue disease, and SLE (Fig. 10–19). Raynaud's phenomenon is often present, suggesting that the pulmonary vasculopathy represents part of a generalized process. Pulmonary hypertension also occurs in some individuals with immunologically mediated interstitial lung disease such as rheumatoid disease and PSS; in these cases, roentgenographic and pathologic features are identical to those associated with chronic interstitial lung disease of other etiologies. Rarely, hypertension is also a complication of pulmonary vasculitis, most often Takayasu's arteritis or Behçet's disease; in these cases, the pathogenesis of the hypertension is probably related to *in situ* arterial thrombosis. This subject is considered in greater detail in relation to the specific disease entities in Chapter 7.

Pulmonary Capillary Hemangiomatosis

Pulmonary capillary hemangiomatosis, a condition first described by Wagenvoort and associates in 1978, is a rare cause of pulmonary hypertension.[128] Tron and associates reviewed the three reported cases from the literature and added four.[129] Patients are generally young adults and present with a clinical picture of pulmonary hypertension. Chest roentgenograms have been reported to show predominantly basal interstitial "shadowing" in addition to signs of pulmonary arterial hypertension. The fundamental nature of the condition is unknown; it is considered by some to represent a low-grade malignant neoplasm (*see* page 1622).

Pathologically, the most striking features are patchy areas of severe congestion which on closer examination are seen to consist of an interstitial proliferation of thin-walled blood vessels the size of capillaries (Fig. 10–20);[128] in some areas the capillaries form small nodules. They appear to invade the walls of pulmonary veins and to a lesser extent pulmonary arteries. A diagnosis of veno-occlusive disease has been made in a number of cases, even with the aid of open-lung biopsy, and this is the major differential diagnosis on histologic examination; Tron and associates[129] suggest that the use of a reticulin stain can be particularly useful in distinguishing the two. In a case reported by McGee and colleagues,[131] the chest roentgenogram was normal other than for the signs of pulmonary hypertension; pulmonary function tests showed moderate restrictive impairment with decreased lung compliance and a pressure-volume curve suggestive of increased venous pressure.

Multiple Pulmonary Artery Stenosis or Coarctation

This rare abnormality of pulmonary arteries may occur as a developmental anomaly (*see* Chapter 5, page 735) or can result from intrauterine rubella infection (*see* Chapter 6, page 1056). It may be associated with diminished vascularity in the lungs and sometimes with pulmonary arterial hypertension (Fig. 10–21).[132–137]

Compression of the Main Pulmonary Artery or Its Branches

Occasionally, an acquired disease results in diffuse pulmonary oligemia of "central" origin. For example, a mediastinal mass lying contiguous to the main pulmonary artery may compress this vessel to a degree sufficient to compromise pulmonary arterial flow.[138] In one of our patients an aneurysm of the ascending arch of the aorta compressed the pulmonary outflow tract so severely that cor pulmonale ensued; there was clear-cut roentgenographic evidence of pulmonary oligemia. Dissecting aneurysms of the pulmonary artery[139, 140] or of the aorta[141, 142] can compress the pulmonary artery. Other reported causes include primary chondrosarcoma of the sternum[138] and fibrosing mediastinitis.[143]

Primary Pleuropulmonary Disease

A wide variety of primary diseases of the lungs, pleura, chest wall, and respiratory control center (*see* Table 10–1) may cause a rise in pulmonary arterial pressure without significant change in pulmonary venous pressure. Pulmonary arterial pressures seldom reach the levels attained in cases of primary vascular disease, and the arterial and arteriolar narrowing due to intimal thickening and medial hypertrophy is less; histologic features of plexogenic arteriopathy are absent. In fact, the hypertension may be transient, reflecting episodes of pulmonary infection and its associated hypoxia. It is probable that the main cause of pulmonary arterial hypertension in this group of conditions is hypoxemia, with or without respiratory acidosis. The reduction in arterial oxygen saturation may be due to ventilation-perfusion inequality or to generalized alveolar hypoventilation. In the majority of cases the pulmonary artery pressure decreases significantly when arterial oxygen saturation is increased as a result of treatment of pulmonary infections or the administration of 100 per cent oxygen. Other probable contributory factors include hypervolemia, polycythemia, pulmonary capillary destruction, especially in cases of severe chronic obstructive pulmonary disease (COPD), and the anastomoses between the bronchial and pul-

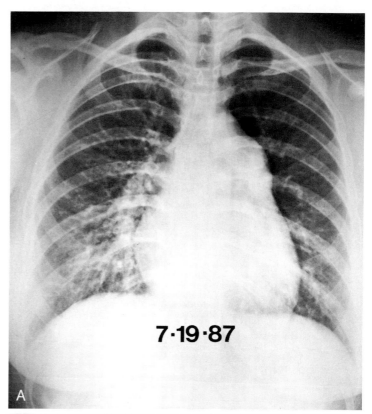

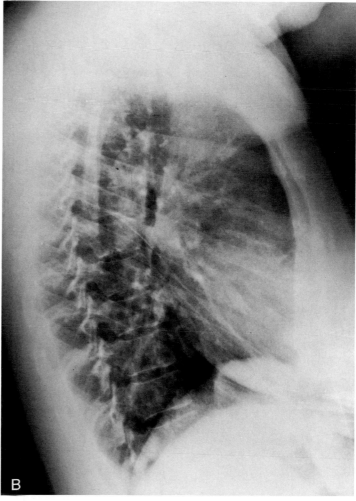

Figure 10–19. Pulmonary Arterial Hypertension Secondary to Systemic Lupus Erythematosus (SLE). The first chest roentgenograms in posteroanterior (*A*) and lateral (*B*) projection on this 32-year-old woman with SLE reveal exceptional prominence of the main pulmonary artery and mild to moderate cardiomegaly consistent with right ventricular enlargement. The pulmonary vasculature looks plethoric, but the lungs are otherwise unremarkable.

Illustration continued on following page

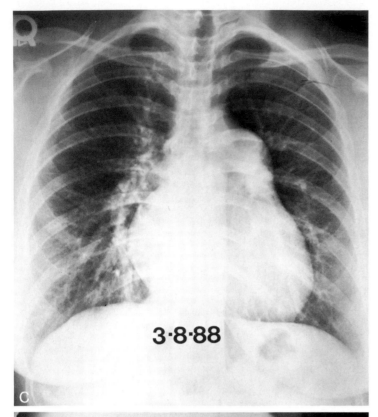

3·8·88

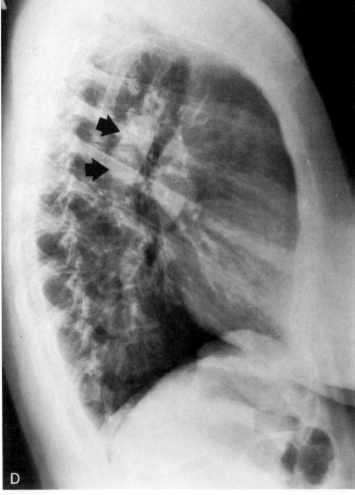

Figure 10–19 *Continued* Eight months later, repeat chest roentgenograms (*C* and *D*) showed an increase in the size of the heart and greater prominence of the main and hilar pulmonary arteries; note the markedly dilated left inter-lobar artery in *D* (*arrows*). However, a more remarkable change has occurred in the pulmonary vasculature, which now displays diffuse oligemia. These changes are characteristic of severe pulmonary arterial hypertension and cor pulmonale, attributable in this patient to vasculopathy associated with SLE. (Courtesy Dr. M. O'Donovan, Montreal General Hospital.)

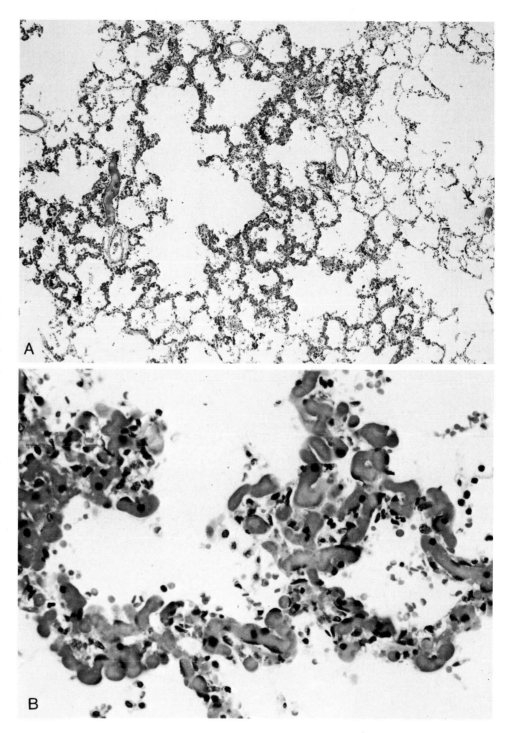

Figure 10–20. Pulmonary Capillary Hemangiomatosis. A low-power view of lung parenchyma (*A*) shows extensive "congestion" of alveolar septa (compare with normal parenchyma at right). A magnified view (*B*) shows the congestion to be caused by numerous dilated capillaries. (*A*, × 40; *B*, × 320.) (Courtesy Dr. J. Hennegan, Pathological Institute, McGill University, Montreal.)

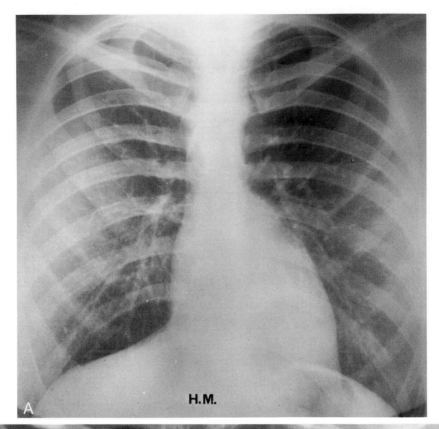

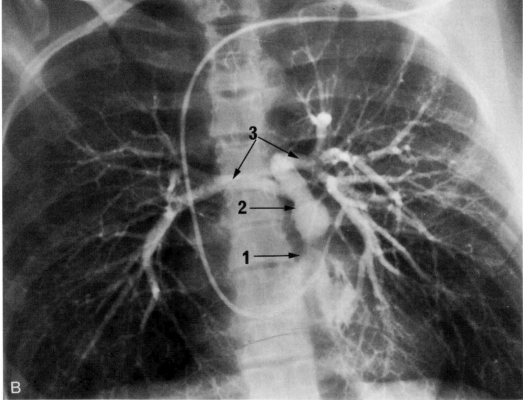

Figure 10–21. Precapillary Pulmonary Hypertension Caused by Diffuse Pulmonary Artery Stenosis. A posteroanterior chest roentgenogram (*A*) reveals cardiomegaly with a configuration consistent with right ventricular enlargement. The hila are diminutive, and the main pulmonary artery segment is barely discernible. The lungs are diffusely oligemic but are otherwise unremarkable. A right ventricular angiogram (*B*) shows multilevel pulmonary artery stenosis affecting infundibular (*1*), valvular (*2*), and supravalvular (*3*) components. The distal (intraparenchymal) arteries are small but otherwise show no abnormality. The patient is a young woman with exertional dyspnea.

monary arterial circulations, where the transmission of higher systemic pressure to the pulmonary circulation may raise pulmonary artery pressure. Many patients with pulmonary disease of sufficient severity to cause pulmonary hypertension are at risk for the development of pulmonary thromboemboli, and in some cases these may also contribute to worsening of the hypertension.[144]

CHRONIC OBSTRUCTIVE PULMONARY DISEASE

Pulmonary hypertension in chronic obstructive pulmonary disease (COPD) appears to be caused predominantly by a combination of hypoxemia and destruction of the microvasculature. Physiologic studies have shown a close correlation between pulmonary vascular resistance, oxygen saturation, and diffusing capacity during exercise.[145]

The roentgenographic manifestations of pulmonary hypertension in emphysema are identical to those of primary vascular disease; however, the invariable presence of overinflation permits ready differentiation (Fig. 10–22). Excellent correlation has been shown to exist between the diameters of the right and left interlobar arteries and the presence and severity of pulmonary arterial hypertension in patients with COPD: in a study of 61 men with COPD and 42 normal control subjects, Matthay and his colleagues[188] measured the right interlobar artery at its widest diameter on a posteroanterior roentgenogram and the left interlobar artery on the left lateral roentgenogram at its widest diameter

posterior to the circular shadow of the left upper lobe bronchus. Right-sided heart catheterization was performed on all 61 men with COPD, and in 46 the mean pulmonary artery pressure was elevated: of these 46, the right interlobar artery was dilated (>16 mm) in 43 and the left interlobar artery (>18 mm) in a similar number. When both arteries were dilated, the presence of pulmonary artery hypertension was correctly predicted in 45 of the 46 patients, including the 26 patients in whom elevation of mean pulmonary artery pressure was mild (21 to 30 mm Hg).

Even in the presence of cor pulmonale, the electrocardiogram (ECG) usually does not show the characteristic pattern of right ventricular hypertrophy that is associated with primary pulmonary vascular disease. Tall R waves in V_1 seldom are seen, and the pattern of extreme right axis deviation, with tall peaked P waves, may be due to rotation of the heart rather than right ventricular hypertrophy.

DIFFUSE INTERSTITIAL OR AIRSPACE DISEASE OF THE LUNGS

In these diseases, elevation of pulmonary artery pressure probably is related to the limited distensibility of the pulmonary vascular tree, and, therefore, hypertension becomes particularly manifest during exercise-induced increases in cardiac output. The roentgenologic changes are almost invariably dominated by the underlying pulmonary disease (Fig. 10–23), and in many cases the peripheral vascular markings are obscured.

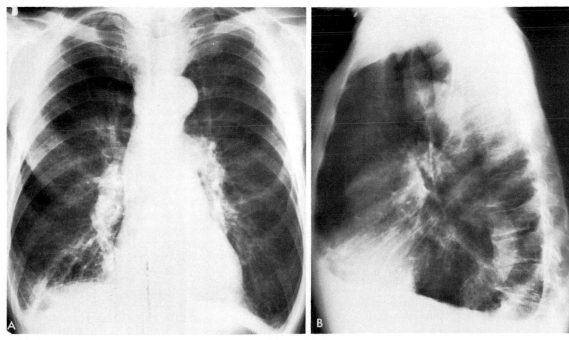

Figure 10–22. Pulmonary Arterial Hypertension Secondary to Emphysema. Posteroanterior (A) and lateral (B) roentgenograms reveal marked overinflation of both lungs, with a low flat position of the diaphragm and a marked increase in the depth of the retrosternal airspace. The lungs are diffusely oligemic, the peripheral vessels being narrow and attenuated. A discrepancy in the size of the central and peripheral pulmonary vessels is caused not only by a decrease in caliber peripherally but by an increase in size centrally; this increase in central caliber constitutes convincing evidence of pulmonary arterial hypertension. The shape of the heart suggests the presence of right ventricular hypertrophy. At necropsy, the pulmonary changes were predominantly those of panacinar emphysema.

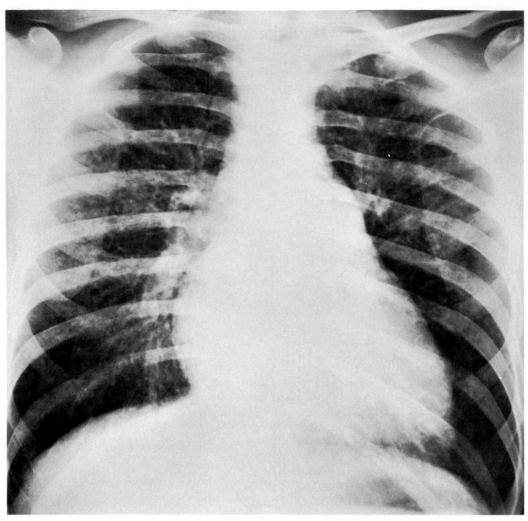

Figure 10–23. Pulmonary Arterial Hypertension in Diffuse Idiopathic Pulmonary Fibrosis. A posteroanterior roentgenogram of a 31-year-old man reveals a coarse reticular pattern throughout both lungs. The heart is moderately enlarged and possesses a contour suggesting right ventricular enlargement. The hilar pulmonary arteries are prominent, although the rapidity of tapering of these vessels as they proceed distally is difficult to assess because of the underlying interstitial disease of the lungs. Cardiac catheterization revealed a pulmonary artery pressure of 106/70 mm Hg. The necropsy diagnosis was diffuse idiopathic interstitial fibrosis.

The definitive study to date on the roentgenologic assessment of pulmonary arterial pressure in patients with diffuse interstitial pulmonary disease was performed by Austin and his colleagues from Columbia University, New York.[189] These authors carried out a roentgenographic survey of 29 patients with diffuse interstitial disease (PSS, 20; sarcoidosis, six; and miscellaneous, three) in whom cardiac catheterization had revealed pulmonary arterial hypertension and normal pulmonary wedge pressures. In general, pulmonary artery pressure was significantly related to the size of the central pulmonary arteries, and pulmonary hemodynamic abnormalities were roughly proportional to the roentgenologic severity of parenchymal disease. Perhaps because of the difficulty in objectively measuring the diameter of the right interlobar artery (mainly because of imprecise identification of the margins of the vessels as a result of contiguous disease), the transhilar-thoracic ratio proved to be

a moderately accurate predictor of pulmonary arterial pressure (the transhilar distance was defined as the sum of distances from the midsagittal line to the most lateral point of junction between each interlobar artery and upper lobe vessels). Subjective evaluation of the size of the main pulmonary artery proved to be of only moderate value as a predictor of pulmonary arterial pressure. In their estimation of pulmonary blood volume in the same patients, the authors found that three vascular signs were most useful—the transhilar-thoracic ratio, the size of the right interlobar artery, and diversion of blood flow to upper lung zones. Of these three signs, only the transhilar-thoracic ratio proved to be of value in assessing both pulmonary arterial pressure and pulmonary blood volume. Of considerable interest was the observation that diversion of blood flow to upper zones was significantly related to restriction of the pulmonary vascular bed but was not necessarily a sign of increased pulmonary arterial pressure. In another study comprising a retrospective review of 41 cases of established PSS, Steckel and his colleagues[146] found that the degree of pulmonary arterial hypertension was out of proportion to the severity of interstitial pulmonary fibrosis attributable to systemic sclerosis, suggesting the possibility of a concomitant primary vasculopathy. In this series, pulmonary arterial hypertension was evident roentgenographically or clinically in 15 patients (37 per cent).

Hilar pulmonary artery enlargement is seldom as marked as in primary vascular disease, although evidence of progressive enlargement on serial roentgenograms should suggest the diagnosis of pulmonary hypertension. The symptoms usually are attributable to the underlying disease, and the presence of pulmonary hypertension may not be clinically detectable until cor pulmonale and cardiac failure develop.

SURGICAL RESECTION

Surgical resection of diseased lung tissue can result in pulmonary arterial hypertension. Although pneumonectomy does not appear to cause a rise in pressure in a remaining normal lung in the immediate postoperative period, pathologic and physiologic evidence of hypertension can be found in patients living for 4 or more years and presumably results from small vessel sclerosis secondary to increased blood flow.[147]

FIBROTHORAX

Chronic pleural thickening rarely is associated with pulmonary arterial hypertension and cor pulmonale. We have seen two cases of unilateral calcified fibrothorax with hypoxemia, hypercapnia, secondary polycythemia, and cor pulmonale, in which physiologic studies indicated ventilation-perfusion inequality as the cause of blood gas disturbance.

CHEST DEFORMITY

Severe degrees of kyphoscoliosis and thoracoplasty may lead to pulmonary arterial hypertension and cor pulmonale, again on the basis of a poorly ventilated but relatively well-perfused lung.

ALVEOLAR HYPOVENTILATION SYNDROMES

Underventilation of normal lungs, with consequent decreased arterial blood Po_2 and increased Pco_2, may result in pulmonary hypertension. This syndrome may be primary in origin (Ondine's curse—Fig. 10–24) or due to obesity-hypoventilation syndrome, obstructive sleep apnea,[148–152] loss of altitude acclimatization,[32] or continuous depression of the respiratory center by drugs.[153]

POSTCAPILLARY PULMONARY HYPERTENSION

Postcapillary pulmonary hypertension results from any condition that increases pulmonary venous pressure above a critical level. Undoubtedly, the most common of these are diseases of the left side of the heart, usually those that cause left ventricular failure such as systemic hypertension and coronary artery disease. Less common causes include mitral stenosis, atrial myxoma, and congenital cardiac anomalies such as cor triatriatum. Pulmonary venous obstruction from a variety of causes,[154–156] including total anomalous venous drainage (see page 743) and primary veno-occlusive disease, results in similar functional effects.

When postcapillary hypertension is severe and of long standing, it induces changes within the pulmonary arterial circulation that are indistinguishable roentgenographically from those of other forms of precapillary hypertension (apart from the changes in cardiac contour, which almost always permit differentiation). Simon[5] suggests that this condition be referred to as combined precapillary and postcapillary hypertension. The roentgenographically demonstrable changes evidence superimposition of the two patterns of hypertension.

Pathologic Characteristics

Morphologic abnormalities in chronic postcapillary (venous) hypertension are present in the areries, veins, and lung parenchyma. Muscular arteries usually show medial hypertrophy, which may be marked, and muscularization of arterioles is not uncommon;[130] concomitant intimal fibrosis is usual. Although some of the medial hypertrophy may be caused by an increase in smooth muscle, there is evidence that an increase in connective tissue itself may be responsible.[21] Fibrinoid necrosis and vasculitis of small vessels have been reported[130, 157] but are rare; dilatation and plexiform lesions do not occur.

Since the primary site of hypertension is postcapillary, changes in veins and venules are almost always apparent, although they are often not as pronounced as those on the arterial side of the circulation. Medial hypertrophy and increased intimal fibrosis are common;[130, 158] in addition, the elastic laminae, which are normally irregular in distribution, may become concentrated into internal and external laminae, similar to the appearance of pulmonary arteries (so-called arterialization of pulmonary veins) (Fig. 10–25). Dilatation of the veins, especially the larger veins and those on the right side, can result in varicosities (see page 743).

The pulmonary parenchyma itself is also usually abnormal in cases of chronic postcapillary hypertension. Foci of airspace hemorrhage, either recent or old, are invariably present in individuals who have died of the disease. Remote hemorrhage

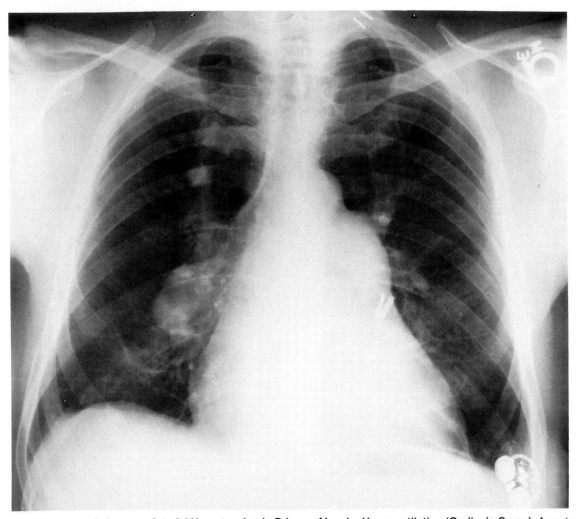

Figure 10–24. Severe Pulmonary Arterial Hypertension in Primary Alveolar Hypoventilation (Ondine's Curse). A posteroanterior roentgenogram of a 55-year-old white man reveals marked dilatation of the main pulmonary artery and its hilar branches, with rapid diminution in caliber of pulmonary arteries as they proceed distally. The heart is moderately enlarged in a configuration compatible with cor pulmonale. The lungs are not overinflated and show no evidence of primary disease. This is a case of Ondine's curse, an abnormality characterized by a failure to "remember" to breathe, with resultant alveolar hypoventilation (particularly during sleep), hypoxemia, hypercarbia, pulmonary vasoconstriction, arterial hypertension, and cor pulmonale. The pacemaker projected over the base of the left lung was pacing the left phrenic nerve in order to achieve repeated diaphragmatic contraction. (Courtesy of Dr. Richard Greenspan, Yale University, New Haven.)

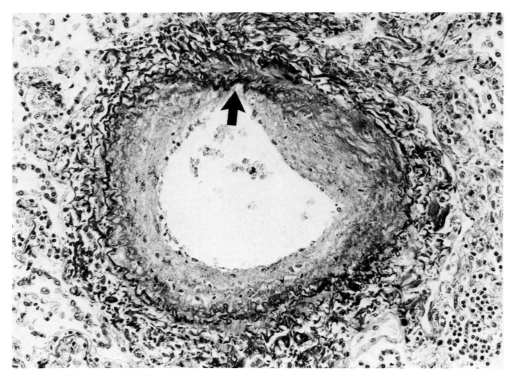

Figure 10–25. Postcapillary Hypertension in Mitral Stenosis. A histologic section of a medium-sized pulmonary vein shows intimal fibrosis and focal medial hypertrophy (*arrow*) associated with two fairly distinct elastic laminae resembling those seen in pulmonary arteries (Verhoeff–van Gieson, × 200).

appears grossly as patchy foci of red-brown discoloration 1 to 3 mm in diameter corresponding to intra-alveolar accumulation of hemosiderin-laden macrophages.[158] In severe cases, hemosiderin may also be identified lying free in the interstitial tissue. In some cases, the hemorrhage occurs as a result of leakage of red blood cells from distended pulmonary capillaries; in others, anastomoses develop between pulmonary and bronchial veins, and resulting bronchial vein varicosities can rupture and cause bright red hemoptysis.[159]

Parenchymal interstitial fibrosis and type 2 cell hyperplasia are common in postcapillary hypertension (Fig. 10–26). The pathogenesis of the fibrosis is unclear; it has been suggested that it may be caused by organization of intra-alveolar exudate,[160] but it is perhaps more likely that chronic leakage of fluid into the parenchymal interstitium is responsible. The combination of fibrosis and hemosiderin accumulation is responsible for the term "brown induration" to describe the gross appearance of these lungs. Organization of intra-alveolar fibrinous edema may be responsible for another fairly common feature of long-standing postcapillary hypertension, especially that caused by mitral stenosis—pulmonary ossification (Fig. 10–26). In this condition, irregularly shaped foci of mature bone are present within alveolar airspaces or the lumen of alveolar ducts; although usually small and visible only with the microscope, they occasionally measure up to several millimeters in diameter in which case

they are roentgenographically demonstrable (*see* farther on).

Roentgenographic Manifestations

Roentgenologically, the changes in the pulmonary vasculature are characteristic. When pulmonary vascular resistance is increased in part of the lungs and unaffected elsewhere, blood flow is redistributed from zones of high resistance to those of normal resistance. When areas of lung thus affected are sufficiently large, the discrepancy in size between normal and abnormal lung markings is readily apparent roentgenographically. This effect is observed in several primary pulmonary diseases (e.g., local obstructive emphysema [Fig. 10–27]), as well as in some affections of the cardiovascular system; we are concerned with the latter group here.

A roentgenologist made the initial empirical observation that pulmonary venous hypertension from any cause produces a distinctive alteration in the pulmonary vascular pattern. In 1958, Simon[161] observed that in mitral stenosis or left ventricular failure the lower lobe pulmonary vessels are narrowed and the upper lobe vessels distended, and he postulated that increase in pulmonary venous pressure above a critical level results in venous vasoconstriction. In erect humans, pulmonary venous pressure is higher in the lower than in the upper lobes because of a difference in hydrostatic

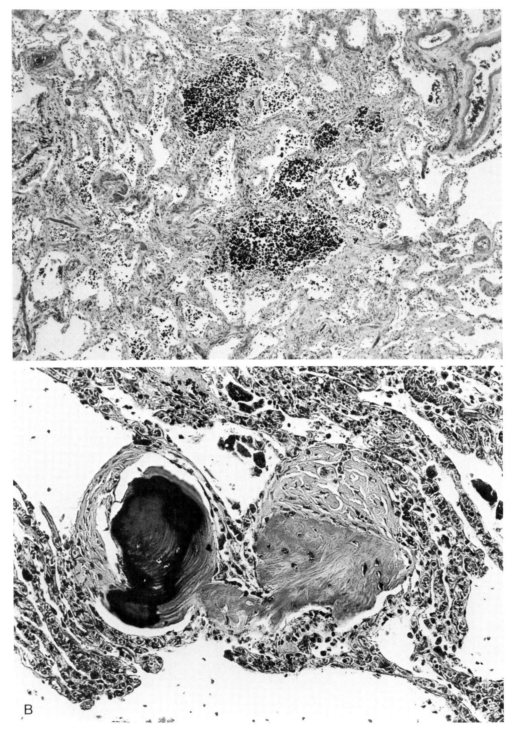

Figure 10–26. Postcapillary Hypertension in Mitral Stenosis. A histologic section of lung parenchyma from a 68-year-old woman with long-standing mitral stenosis (*A*) shows several intra-alveolar aggregates of hemosiderin-laden macrophages and a moderate degree of interstitial fibrosis. A section from another region (*B*) shows a lobulated fragment of mature bone within alveolar airspaces. (*A*, × 40; *B*, × 160.)

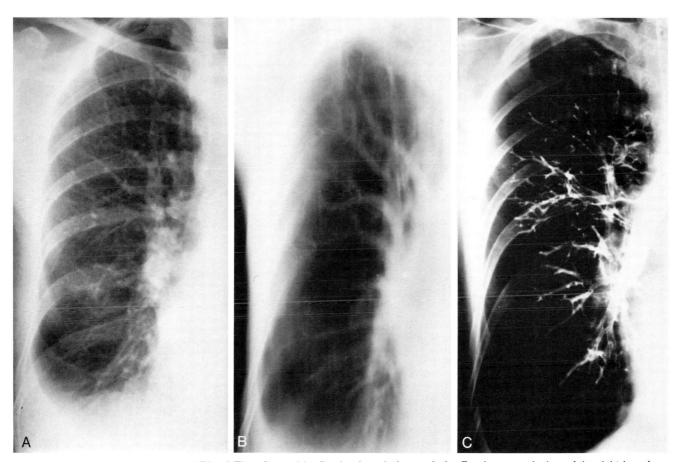

Figure 10–27. Redistribution of Blood Flow Caused by Predominantly Lower Lobe Emphysema. A view of the right lung from a conventional posteroanterior chest roentgenogram (*A*) reveals dilatation of upper lobe vessels, reduced caliber of lower-lobe vessels, and lower-zonal hyperinflation and oligemia. These findings are more clearly demonstrated on an anteroposterior linear tomogram (*B*). A right bronchogram (*C*) shows poor peripheral filling of otherwise normal lower lobe bronchi. The findings are characteristic of lower-zonal emphysema with preferential redistribution of blood flow into the upper lobes as a consequence of obliterative vascular disease. The pleural thickening at the base is caused by fibrosis, which may have contributed to the reduced perfusion.

pressure (averaging approximately 12 to 15 mm Hg in adult subjects). Therefore, the critical level is reached first in lower lung zones and resultant vasoconstriction occurs in the same order, so that peripheral vascular resistance rises in the lower zones. Since resistance in the upper lobes is unchanged initially, blood is diverted to those areas, giving a roentgenographic picture of upper lobe pleonemia and lower lobe oligemia (Figs. 10–28 and 10–29). This is in striking contrast to the normal situation, in which pulmonary perfusion increases from apex to base. With continued increase in venous pressure, the reduction in venous caliber progresses upward from the lung bases and eventually involves the upper lobes, constricting the engorged upper lobe veins and producing a pattern of diffuse alteration in the pulmonary vasculature. The inevitable result is generalized elevation of pulmonary arterial vascular resistance and pulmonary arterial hypertension (Fig. 10–30). An excellent review of the whole subject of pulmonary blood flow distribution has been published by Milne.[162]

Simon's hypothesis that reflex vasoconstriction constitutes the *mechanism* by which vascular resistance rises in the lower lobes, although never convincingly proven, was an invaluable spur to further research.[161] An alternative theory based on experimental observations in the dog was postulated by West and associates,[163] who used radioactive xenon to measure the distribution of blood flow in an isolated dog lung. These authors found greatly increased vascular resistance in the dependent lung zone when the pulmonary venous pressure was raised. Rapidly frozen sections showed accumulations of edema fluid around small arteries and veins, suggesting that resistance increases when there is interference with the tethering effect of the lung parenchyma that normally holds these vessels open. Since these important studies, however, Ritchie and his colleagues[164] showed that distribution of blood flow may remain normal when the perivascular interstitial tissues are markedly distended with fluid. In their experiments on isolated, perfused dog lungs, interstitial edema resulted in redistribution only under the specific conditions of low flow and low driving pressure. Subsequently, experiments by Muir and his coworkers[165] on anesthetized vertically suspended dogs revealed reduction in the distribution of blood flow to the base of the lungs only when *alveolar* edema was produced; the more marked the alveolar edema, the greater the reduction in flow. These authors concluded that major redistribution of blood flow occurs only with the formation of alveolar edema and that this change correlates with the associated reduction in lung volume rather than with the absolute amount of fluid present. In fact, studies with radioactive xenon[166] have shown that even in normal subjects

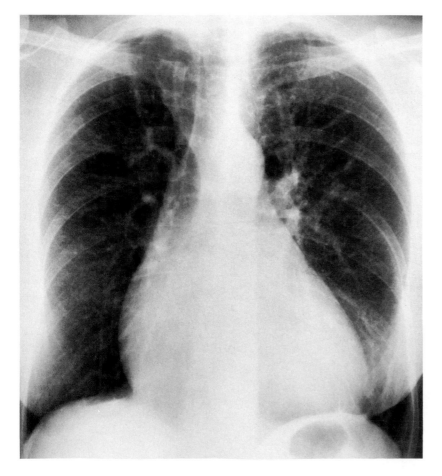

Figure 10–28. Redistribution of Blood Flow to Upper Lung Zones Caused by Pulmonary Venous Hypertension. A posteroanterior roentgenogram reveals unusually prominent vascular markings in the upper zones and rather sparse markings in the lower zones. The patient, a 42-year-old woman, had recurrent episodes of left ventricular decompensation consequent upon cardiomyopathy.

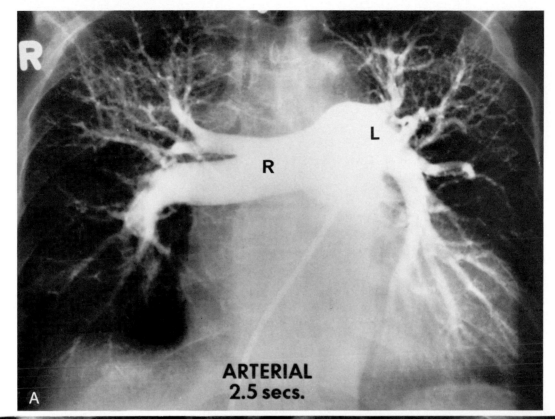

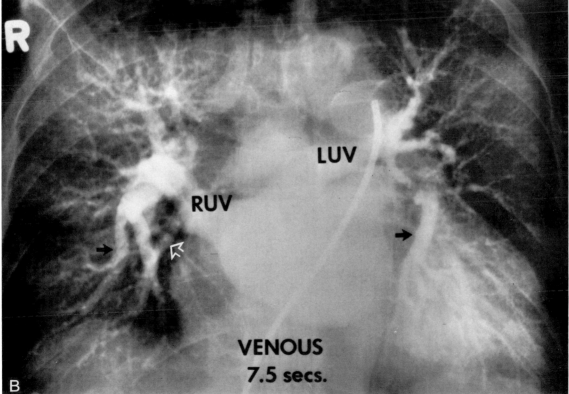

Figure 10–29. Precapillary and Postcapillary Pulmonary Hypertension: Angiographic Features. A main pulmonary artery angiogram during the arterial phase (*A*) reveals enlarged right (R) and left (L) pulmonary arteries. The middle and upper zone arteries are slightly tortuous, whereas lower lobe arteries are less well opacified and straightened, displaying few side branches. During the venous phase (*B*), the right (RUV) and left (LUV) superior veins are well opacified whereas there is only slight filling of lower lobe veins (*open arrow*). Note the persistent opacification of the lower lobe arteries (*arrows*) during the late venous phase. The findings indicate increased resistance to blood flow through the lower lobe vasculature, resulting in preferential blood flow redistribution to upper lobe vessels.

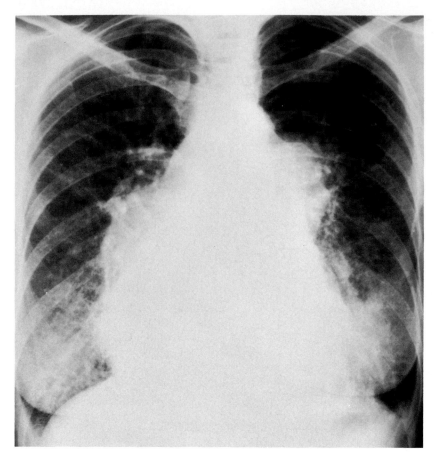

Figure 10–30. Combined Venous and Arterial Hypertension in Mitral Stenosis. A posteroanterior roentgenogram of a 40-year-old woman with a 20-year history of rheumatic heart disease reveals severe pulmonary arterial hypertension as evidenced by a moderate increase in the size of the hilar pulmonary arteries and by the rapid tapering of these vessels as they proceed distally. A slight discrepancy in the size of the upper lobe and lower lobe pulmonary vessels and well-defined Kerley B lines indicate an associated pulmonary venous hypertension. When these signs are considered in the light of the character of the cardiac enlargement, the diagnosis of chronic mitral valvular disease with pulmonary venous and arterial hypertension may be made with confidence. Following commissurotomy, several of the Kerley B lines persisted, indicating that the septal thickening was the result of fibrosis as well as edema.

the apex-to-base blood flow difference diminishes at residual volume. This phenomenon is considered to result from an increase in interstitial pressure consequent upon reduced expansion of lung parenchyma in the lower zones. The conclusions reached by Muir and associates were supported more recently in roentgenographic studies on dogs[167] that showed that the distribution of blood flow in those with interstitial edema was not significantly different from that in control animals. Not until alveolar edema was evident roentgenographically was there preferential pulmonary perfusion to upper lung zones. It is to be emphasized that the findings in these experimental studies relate only to acute left ventricular decompensation and that they should not be extrapolated to other conditions. Clinical experience with chronically elevated left atrial pressure, as in mitral stenosis, suggests that in these circumstances redistribution of flow does occur. Surette and colleagues[167] suggest that in such cases the causal mechanism for flow redistribution may be either the interstitial fibrosis that develops in the lower lung zones or the narrowing of vessels by hypertensive vascular lesions rather than a reflex as suggested by Simon[161] or perivascular interstitial edema as postulated by West and associates.[163]

Regardless of the mechanism, however, there is no doubt that a disparity between the caliber of upper and lower lobe vessels represents one of the most useful roentgenographic signs of pulmonary venous hypertension (Fig. 10–31). All too frequently, there exists an unfortunate semantic inaccuracy regarding this sign. It is common to hear the term "upper lobe venous engorgement" used to describe redistribution of blood flow from lower to upper zones; in fact, the redistribution of blood flow is *arterial* rather than venous and thus is a *flow* phenomenon caused by increased resistance to blood flow through the lower zones. Thus, *both* arteries and veins show distention, and it is conceptually preferable to employ the phrase "upper zone vascular distention" to indicate redistribution of blood flow. In fact, since distention of upper zone vessels occurs in five situations other than pulmonary venous hypertension (a supine position, predominantly lower zonal parenchymal disease, left-to-right shunts, hypervolemia, and pulmonary arterial hypertension), it is advisable *as a first approximation* to refer to the abnormality as "recruitment of upper zone vessels"; when other aspects of the roentgenographic appearance have been evaluated, it will then be possible to ascribe the recruitment to a specific etiology. The unfortunate tendency to attribute upper zonal vascular distention automatically to pulmonary venous hypertension will thus be obviated.

It is customary for roentgenologists to assess the caliber of upper zone vessels by comparing them with lower zone vessels. While it is clear that a disparity must exist in order for redistribution of flow to be present, we feel that it is often exceedingly difficult to be convinced of an increase in upper zonal vessel caliber by such a comparison. It has been our experience that subjective assessment of the caliber of vessels in the upper zones, based on experience of what constitutes the normal, is more dependable. Such an assessment is obviously facilitated by comparison with previous roentgenograms, but with few exceptions (chiefly patients with left-to-right shunts or patients whose roentgenograms have been obtained in the recumbent position), subjective assessment possesses considerable reliability even without comparison. In fact, Burko and his colleagues[168] have established objective criteria on which to base upper zonal venous distention. In a study of 100 pulmonary angiograms, 50 of which were performed in the recumbent and 50 in the sitting position, these authors found the mean pulmonary vein diameter at the level of the main pulmonary artery to be 7 mm in the supine position and 4 mm in the erect position. (Over one third of opacified pulmonary veins were too small to measure in the erect position.) From a review of the range of normal variation in the caliber of this vessel, they suggest that a pulmonary vein whose diameter is greater than 8 mm at the level of the main pulmonary artery is abnormal (Fig. 10–32). These authors also showed that upper lobe pulmonary veins are usually too small to identify on plain chest roentgenograms of normal subjects exposed in the erect position. Further, they found a considerable variation in the diameters of opacified upper lobe pulmonary veins, ranging from too small to measure to 15 mm. It is thus apparent that very occasionally a moderately distended upper lobe pulmonary vein may be identified on the chest roentgenogram of an individual who does not have pulmonary venous hypertension or redistribution of blood flow related to disease.

In a review of the chest roentgenograms of 111 patients with critical mitral stenosis (valve openings of 1.5 × 1.0 cm or less), Simon[169] found dilated upper zone vessels in all but six cases. The pulmonary artery and left atrial pressures and the degree of valve narrowing were no different in these six cases from those of the group as a whole. It is apparent, therefore, that critical mitral stenosis can be present without dilatation of the upper lobe vessels, although such an occurrence must be very uncommon. Although the presence of upper lobe vascular distention usually is evident from simple subjective assessment (or from comparison with lower lobe vascular caliber in patients in whom the severity or chronicity of venous hypertension has led to arterial hypertension), some authors have suggested that a change in contour of the right hilum may supply useful confirmatory evidence.[170, 171] Since the superior pulmonary vein forms the upper rim of the right hilar concavity, distention of this

vein flattens the concavity and may render it convex when ballooning is severe. We have seldom found this sign to be of value.

The alteration in pulmonary vascular pattern seen in mitral stenosis may be observed in mild left ventricular failure also (Fig. 10–33), but then is transient. In fact, however, the changes in the vascular pattern may be similar in all respects, including the signs of pulmonary arterial hypertension. In a study of the chest roentgenograms of 50 consecutive admissions to a coronary care unit, Tattersfield and associates[172] found the commonest abnormality to be redistribution of blood flow to upper zones (76 per cent of patients). Simon[173] suggested that such patients may be incapable of regaining complete physiologic compensation and remain in a chronic state of "incipient" decompensation.

It is of interest that signs of left ventricular failure may be apparent roentgenographically without clinical evidence of decompensation. Of 94 patients who had chest roentgenograms obtained on admission to a coronary care unit,[174] 31 (33 per cent) were found to have roentgenographic evidence of pulmonary venous hypertension (manifested most commonly by distention of upper zone vessels) without associated clinical signs. In 23 of these, however, clinically evident failure developed subsequently. In a study of 30 patients with recent myocardial infarction,[175] the severity of roentgenographic abnormality generally correlated well with levels of pulmonary capillary wedge pressure. It was found that redistribution of blood flow was the earliest manifestation of elevated wedge pressure, followed sequentially by loss of the normal sharp margins of the pulmonary vessels, the development of perihilar haze, and finally overt airspace edema.

It has been suggested[176] that the pattern of blood flow redistribution may be different in mitral insufficiency from that in other forms of pulmonary venous hypertension. Instead of symmetric dilatation of vessels in both upper zones, there occurs a more prominent dilatation of the *right* upper zone vessels, presumably as a result of reflux from the insufficient valve whose orientation posteriorly, superiorly, and to the right results in dominant flow to the right upper lobe. Of 50 cases of mitral insufficiency proved surgically or angiographically, seven showed localized dilatation of right pulmonary vessels.

In addition to the typical alteration in vascular pattern observed in pulmonary venous hypertension, particularly in mitral stenosis, other pulmonary changes occur that are worthy of note. Signs of *interstitial pulmonary edema* frequently are visible, including septal edema (Kerley A and B lines; *see* Figure 4–57, page 547) and perivascular edema (manifested by loss of definition of pulmonary vascular markings, Fig. 10–34). *Hemosiderosis*, although often visible pathologically, is not readily identifiable roentgenographically unless severe, probably be-

Text continued on page 1876

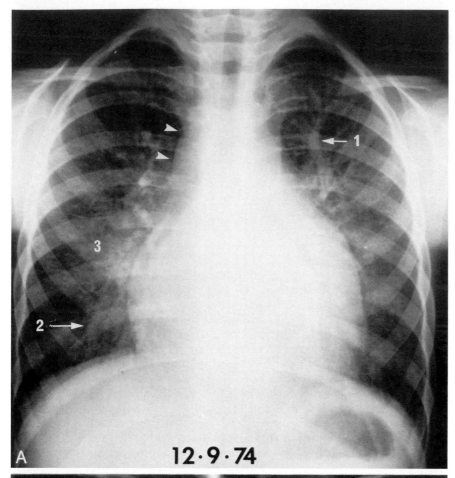

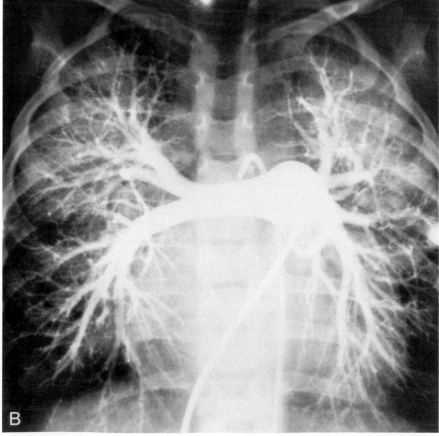

Figure 10–31. Severe Postcapillary Pulmonary Hypertension and Edema Caused by a Floppy Mitral Valve. A conventional posteroanterior chest roentgenogram (*A*) demonstrates features typical of postcapillary pulmonary hypertension—dilated upper lobe vessels (*1*), ill-defined lower lobe vessels (*2*), and diffuse interstitial edema (*3*). Cardiac size is increased in nonspecific fashion. The vascular pedicle is increased in width as a result of distention of the superior vena cava (*arrowheads*), indicating systemic venous hypertension. Anteroposterior views of the thorax from a selective main pulmonary angiogram during the arterial (*B*) and venous (*C*) phases reveal increased blood flow to the upper lobes (compare the degree of contrast-filling of the upper lobe arteries to the relatively branchless lower lobe arterial vasculature). (*See* p. 1871 for *C*.) The mid and upper zones contain a "background blush"; the lower lobes do not. Note the persistence of the lower lobe arterial pattern, the well-distended upper lobe veins (V1), and the poorly filled lower lobe veins (V2) during the venous phase.

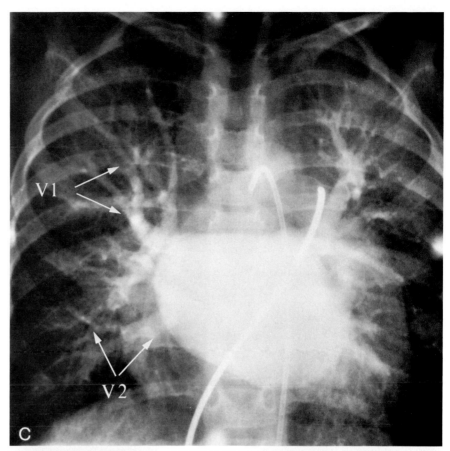

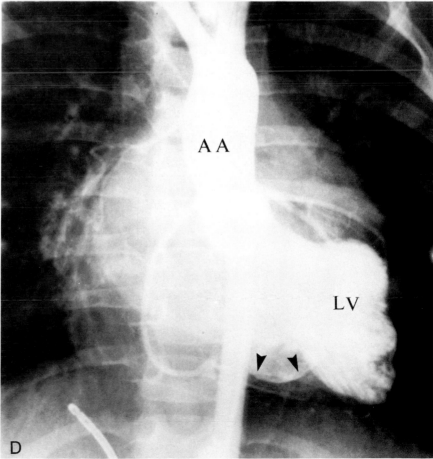

Figure 10–31 *Continued* A left ventricular angiogram (*D*) shows a prolapsed mitral valve (*arrowheads*) (floppy mitral valve syndrome) as the cause of the above-described features. LV and AA represent the left ventricle and ascending aorta, respectively. The patient is a young woman.

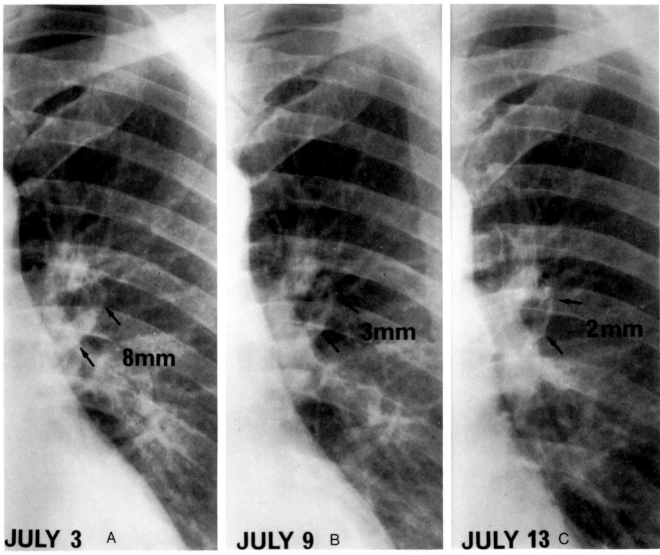

Figure 10–32. Distention of the Left Superior Pulmonary Vein As a Sign of Pulmonary Venous Hypertension. A detail view of the left hemithorax (*A*) from a conventional posteroanterior chest roentgenogram reveals a slightly dilated superior pulmonary vein (*arrows*) that measures 8 mm in transverse diameter. Six days later, following diuretic therapy (*B*), the vein (*arrows*) has diminished in size to 3 mm; subsequently, 4 days later (*C*), it has diminished to 2 mm. Note the decreasing prominence of the left heart border in the illustrative sequence. The patient is an elderly man who was admitted to hospital for a transurethral prostatectomy.

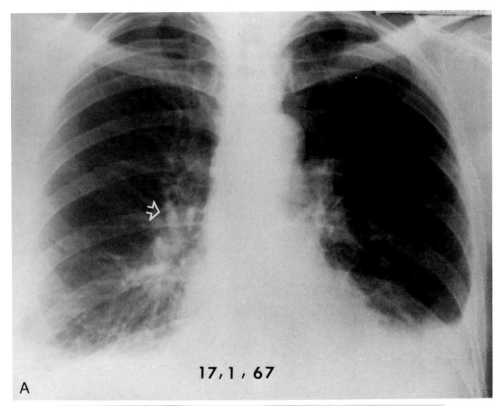

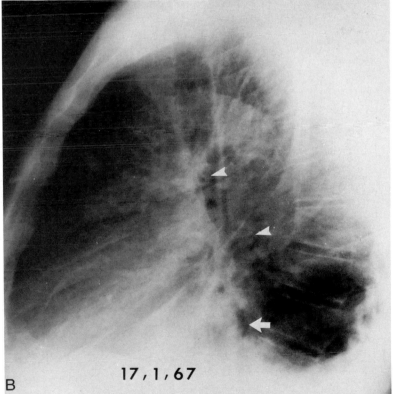

Figure 10–33. Left Ventricular Decompensation. Posteroanterior (*A*) and lateral (*B*) chest roentgenograms show mild cardiomegaly; there is redistribution of blood flow into the upper lobes, as indicated by the nearly equal size of the upper- and lower-lobe vessels; note the dilated right superior pulmonary vein (*open arrow*). The lower-lobe vessels are crowded as a result of suboptimal inspiration and bilateral pleural effusions. The anterior segment of the left lower lobe is consolidated, presumably from pneumonia (*closed arrow*). The hila are enlarged and somewhat ill defined, particularly on the left, and bronchial walls are thickened (*arrowheads*) as a result of edema.

Illustration continued on following page

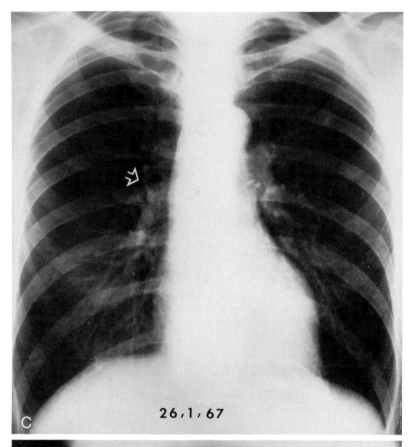

26,1,67

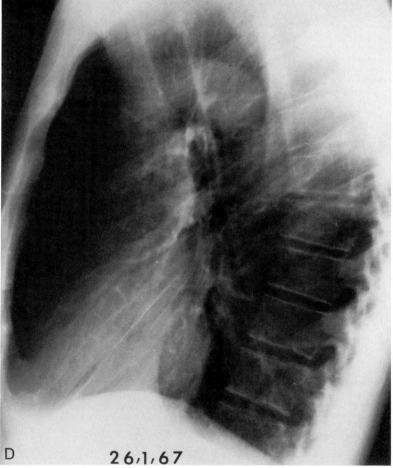

26,1,67

Figure 10–33 *Continued* Eight days later, following appropriate therapy, posteroanterior (C) and lateral (D) roentgenograms are essentially normal except for mild left ventricular enlargement. Note in particular the reduction in size and increased clarity of definition of the hila; the right superior pulmonary vein (*open arrow*) is normal. The patient is a middle-aged man with long-standing systemic hypertension.

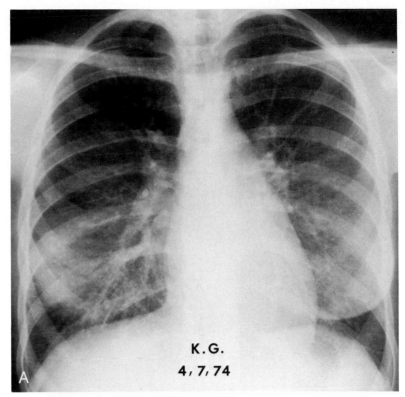

Figure 10–34. Postcapillary Hypertension Caused by a Left Atrial Myxoma. Conventional posteroanterior (*A*) and lateral (*B*) chest roentgenograms show perihilar and lower-lobe parenchymal haze, ill-defined lower-lobe bronchovascular bundles, and thickening of interlobar fissures as a result of pleural edema (*arrowheads*). On the posteroanterior projection, the heart does not appear enlarged; however, on the lateral view, there is a suggestion of left atrial (*open arrows*) and right ventricular enlargement. The findings are consistent with obstruction at or proximal to the mitral valve.

Illustration continued on following page

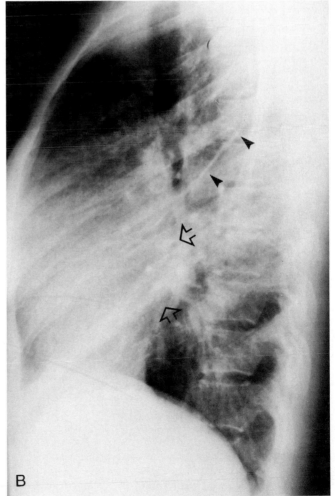

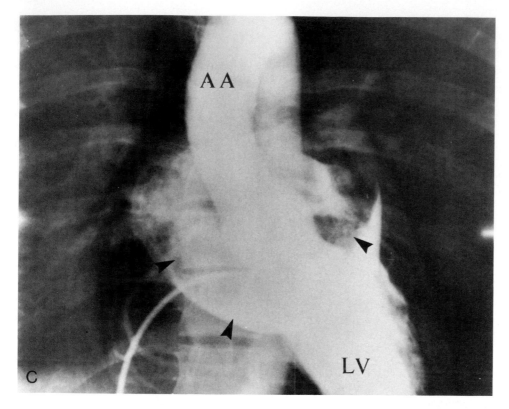

Figure 10–34 *Continued* A transseptal left atrial angiogram (*C*) discloses a large intra-atrial filling defect (*arrowheads*) consistent with a myxoma (subsequently confirmed). The left ventricle (LV) and ascending aorta (AA) are opacified with contrast medium. The patient is a young woman with intermittent episodes of exertional dyspnea.

cause of the low density of the deposits; it is manifested by tiny punctate shadows situated mainly in the midlung and lower lung zones (Fig. 10–35).

Bone formation occurs in some cases of mitral stenosis[48, 177] and is virtually pathognomonic of this entity, although it has been described in pulmonary veno-occlusive disease as well.[178] Roentgenographically, foci of parenchymal ossification appear as densely calcified nodules, 2 to 5 mm in diameter, mainly in the midlung zones and sometimes containing demonstrable trabeculae (Fig. 10–36; *see* also Fig. 4–98, page 600). They occur more commonly in males,[179, 180] are more numerous in the right lung,[181, 182] and range in incidence in reported series from 3 per cent[48] to 13 per cent.[179] Although pulmonary venous hypertension is invariably present, there is no apparent relationship between the development of ossific nodules and the degree of hypertension or associated hemosiderosis.[179]

Finally, *pulmonary fibrosis* may be apparent as a rather coarse, poorly defined reticulation, again predominantly in the middle and lower lung zones (see Fig. 10–35). A similar picture develops in some patients with malignant systemic hypertension who are kept alive with hexamethonium hydralazine, pentolinium, mecamylamine, and similar drugs.

Although it might be anticipated that roentgenographic evidence of redistribution of blood flow to upper lung zones in patients with severe mitral stenosis might disappear relatively rapidly following adequate surgical correction by closed commissurotomy or valve replacement, this is not the case. In a study of 25 patients with pure mitral stenosis designed to determine those roentgenographic criteria most helpful in the evaluation of the postoperative hemodynamic and clinical status, Seningen and his colleagues[183] employed five roentgenologic signs in an analysis of preoperative and postoperative roentgenograms:

1. Septal (Kerley B) lines.
2. Abnormal pulmonary vascular pattern (redistribution of blood flow).
3. Left atrial enlargement.
4. The ratio of the diameter of the main pulmonary artery to the diameter of the left hemithorax.
5. The diameter of the right interlobar artery.

The most useful postoperative changes were found to be left atrial size, the ratio of the width of the main pulmonary artery from the midline divided by the diameter of the left hemithorax at the diaphragm, and the diameter of the right interlobar artery distal to the right middle lobe artery. The roentgen sum of changes in these signs was 100 per cent correct in predicting significant hemodynamic change, and 86 per cent correct in predicting significant clinical improvement. A change in the abnormal vascular pattern observed preoperatively—i.e., a disappearance of signs of redistribution of blood flow—was found to be less reliable, a finding for which the authors gave two reasons: (1) hemodynamic improvement secondary to decreased pulmonary vasoconstriction may not be accompanied by a decrease in the mass of vascular wall tissue; and (2) considerable time is required for relatively fixed anatomic changes in vessels to regress.[190] This observation is of considerable importance in that the roentgenographic demonstration of persisting

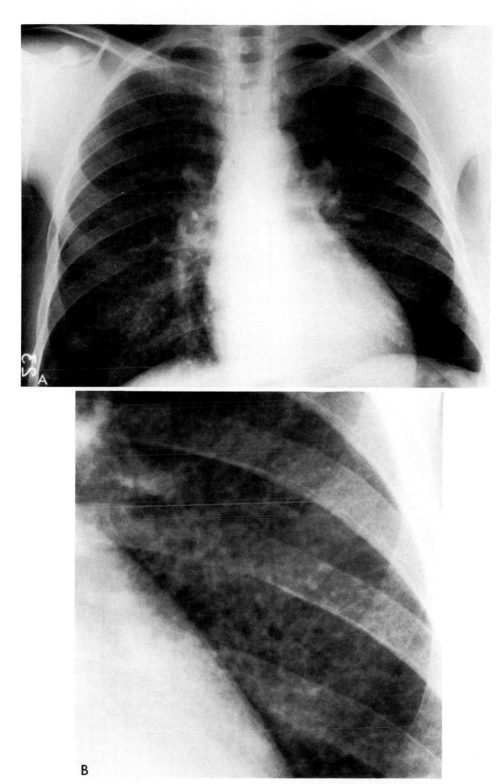

Figure 10–35. Pulmonary Hemosiderosis and Fibrosis Secondary to Recurrent Episodes of Pulmonary Edema. A posteroan-terior roentgenogram (*A*) and a magnified view of the midportion of the left lung (*B*) reveal a medium reticular pattern throughout both lungs, most evident in the mid and lower zones. This pattern did not change on sequential examinations. The patient is a 29-year-old man with severe aortic stenosis and repeated episodes of pulmonary edema.

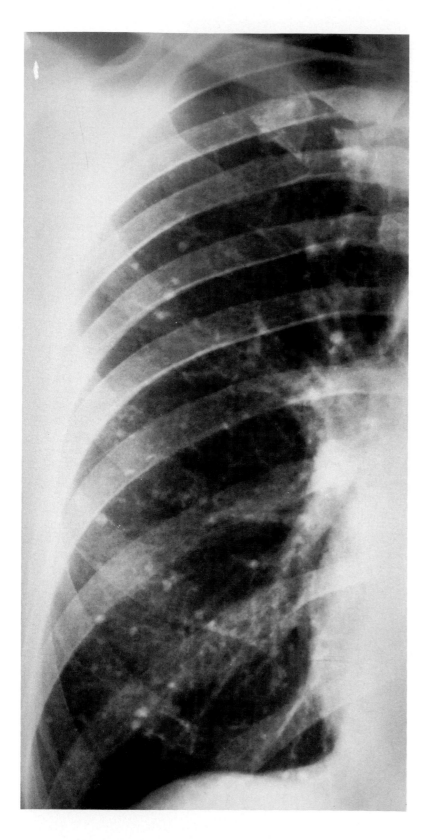

Figure 10–36. Ossific Nodules in Mitral Stenosis. A view of the right lung from a conventional posteroanterior chest roentgenogram demonstrates multiple, sharply defined 1- to 3-mm calcific (ossific) nodules most numerous in the mid and lower thirds of the lung. The patient is a middle-aged man with long-standing mitral stenosis.

upper zonal vascular distention several months following mitral commissurotomy does not necessarily indicate elevated levels of left atrial and pulmonary venous pressure. As pointed out in the next section on pulmonary edema, persistence of septal or Kerley B lines also may be a poor indicator of hemodynamic or clinical improvement, since such lines may be caused by fibrosis secondary to chronic or recurrent edema and thus will not regress or disappear despite a return to normal pulmonary hemodynamics.

Clinical Manifestations

The symptoms associated with postcapillary hypertension usually are readily differentiated from those of precapillary origin. In left ventricular failure, which is the most common cause of pulmonary venous hypertension, symptoms and signs are predominantly those arising from acute or subacute pulmonary edema. Patients typically are dyspneic and orthopneic and may be subject to paroxysmal nocturnal dyspnea—manifestations of interstitial and airspace edema. In mitral stenosis, in addition to the pink frothy expectoration typical of acute pulmonary edema, bright red blood from hemorrhaging varicosities of the bronchial veins may be expectorated. The pulmonary vascular pressure does not increase until the size of the mitral valve orifice is less than 50 per cent of normal.[191] When the orifice is very tight, a severe degree of pulmonary arterial hypertension may develop that can be differentiated from primary pulmonary hypertension only by the symptoms and signs of pulmonary edema, by the loud opening snap, and by the rumbling diastolic murmur associated with this valvular abnormality. Pulmonary venous hypertension commonly develops when a myxoma or thrombus blocks the mitral valve and the clinical course in these patients usually is punctuated by episodes of pulmonary edema or syncope that can be relieved by a change in position. In some instances left atrial myxomas give rise to systemic embolization or are associated with constitutional findings such as fever, weight loss, raised sedimentation rate, anemia, or elevation of gamma globulin levels.[192] Patients with postcapillary pulmonary hypertension due to an increased resistance between the pulmonary capillaries and the left atrium have symptoms identical to those of mitral stenosis but without the characteristic accentuation of the first heart sound, the opening snap, or the rumbling diastolic murmur. Some patients with chronic congestive heart failure[193] or pulmonary veno-occlusive disease[194] do not present with the typical clinical symptoms of orthopnea, paroxysmal nocturnal dyspnea, and pulmonary edema, and their roentgenographic findings and hemodynamic measurements may be equivocal. In such circumstances, an erroneous diagnosis of primary pulmonary arterial or interstitial disease may be made and the correct diagnosis may become apparent only when a therapeutic trial of digitalis and diuretics produces beneficial results.

The ECG findings in postcapillary hypertension reflect the cause of the hypertension and the rapidity of increase in pressure. In pure mitral stenosis, the changes may be identical to those of primary arterial hypertension with right ventricular hypertrophy. In mitral insufficiency, the ECG usually shows left ventricular hypertrophy, with or without evidence of right ventricular hypertrophy; rarely, only the latter is evident. Pulmonary function studies in patients with mitral valve disease show a progressive decrease in vital capacity and diffusing capacity and, with advancing disease, in mid-expiratory flow rates.[195] Mitral valvotomy in patients with severe disease does not result in an improvement in diffusing capacity.[196, 197] However, a considerable reduction in minute ventilation during exercise and a more nearly normal oxygen uptake may be observed after closed valvotomy.[198]

PRIMARY VENO-OCCLUSIVE DISEASE

The manifestations of pulmonary veno-occlusive disease include pulmonary arterial hypertension or pulmonary edema or both. Of the approximately 50 cases described in the literature by 1987, the diagnosis most often was made at autopsy.[199–206] However, as a result of the more widespread recognition of the variable presentations of the disease, the diagnosis is now being made more frequently ante mortem. It is a disease with no sex predilection. The age at recognition has ranged from infancy to old age, and the final histologic findings probably represent a number of different pathologic processes.[200, 207]

The pathogenesis of this disorder is unknown. A striking similarity between this entity and hepatic veno-occlusive disease (Budd-Chiari syndrome) has been noted.[208] Pulmonary veno-occlusive disease has also been reported in association with chronic active hepatitis, celiac disease,[209] and Raynaud's disease.[210] Occasional familial clusters of the disease suggest a genetic predisposition or a common environmental agent.[209, 211] We have recently observed a patient with proven pulmonary veno-occlusive disease who was taking oral contraceptive agents. In a review of the literature, Alpert found 11 cases of hepatic veno-occlusive disease associated with oral contraceptives,[212] and although the association in our patient may have been fortuitous, some studies have suggested that contraceptives may affect the pulmonary vascular prostaglandin balance, especially prostacyclin, a vasodilator and inhibitor of coagulation. Hensby and coworkers[213] measured the *in vivo* production of 6-oxo-PGF$_{1-\alpha}$ (a stable metabolite of prostacyclin) in pulmonary arterial and left ventricular blood, and found an increase in prostacyclin metabolites on the left ventricular side. They suggested that the pulmonary arterial–systemic gradient of prostacyclin may be a mechanism by which thrombosis of pulmonary veins is prevented. In their patients, the use of oral contraceptives was associated with a dramatic reduction in pulmonary endothelial prostacyclin production, leading to speculation that alteration of prostaglandin metabolism may be partly responsible for the increased risk of peripheral venous thrombosis that is observed in patients receiving oral contraceptives. The same mechanism might be responsible for the pulmonary venous obstruction and occlusion observed in patients who have hepatic and pulmonary veno-occlusive disease. Herbal "bush" teas containing *Senecio, Crotalaria,* and *Heliotropium* species may cause hepatic veno-occlusive disease in humans, and in some of these individuals pulmonary venous involvement has also been described.[214, 215] In one case report, a child is described with congenital unilateral pulmonary venous atresia in whom veno-occlusive disease subsequently developed in the contralateral lung.[216]

Pathologically, there is narrowing of the lumens of small pulmonary veins and venules by intimal fibrous tissue (Fig. 10–37), usually widespread throughout both lungs. In fact, vessel lumens may be completely obliterated by almost acellular fibrous tissue.[208] Larger pulmonary veins are usually spared. It is probable that the venous occlusions are thrombotic in origin, although the cause of the thrombosis is unknown. Histologic evidence of se-

vere pulmonary arterial hypertension is usually present in the form of medial hypertrophy of small pulmonary arteries, with or without intimal proliferation, fibrosis, and thrombi; however, the so-called plexiform lesions characteristic of primary pulmonary hypertension are absent.[207]

Roentgenographically, signs of pulmonary arterial hypertension are no different from those associated with primary or thromboembolic disease but with the important addition of signs of postcapillary hypertension, chiefly pulmonary edema (Fig. 10–38). The left atrium is not enlarged, and there is no evidence of redistribution of blood flow to upper lung zones, both important signs in distinguishing this condition from mitral stenosis.

Clinically, these patients typically have slowly progressive dyspnea and orthopnea punctuated by attacks of acute pulmonary edema; hemoptysis may occur. Rales may be heard over the lung bases, and the second pulmonic sound is accentuated in most cases. As the condition progresses, a right ventricular heave develops, together with murmurs indicative of pulmonic and tricuspid insufficiency. Pulmonary function tests reveal arterial oxygen desaturation and a reduction in diffusing capacity and lung compliance.[155] In one patient, the pressure-volume curve showed a decrease in elastic recoil at low lung volumes and an increase at high lung volumes. This pattern has also been observed

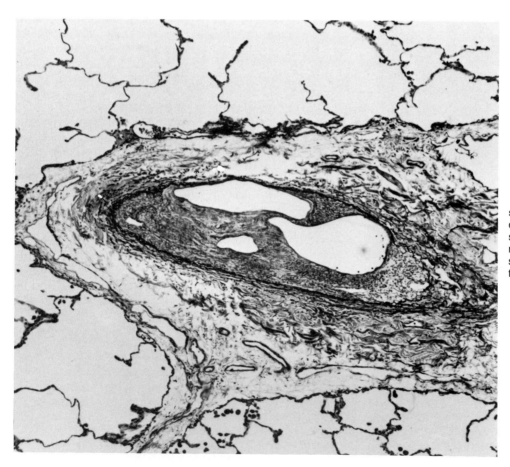

Figure 10–37. Veno-occlusive Disease. A histologic section of a medium-sized pulmonary vein shows intraluminal fibrosis and multiple variable-sized vascular spaces suggesting canalized thrombus (×40).

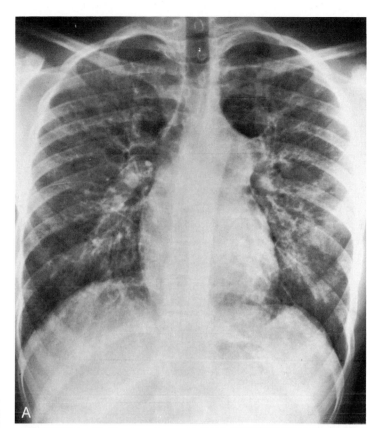

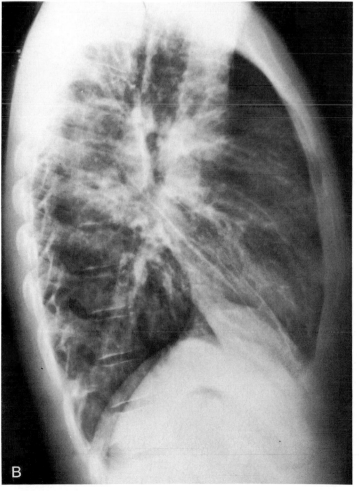

Figure 10–38. Primary Veno-occlusive Disease. Posteroanterior (*A*) and lateral (*B*) chest roentgenograms of this 16-year-old male reveal dilated main and hilar pulmonary arteries and diffuse interstitial edema (septal lines were visible on the original roentgenograms but have not reproduced). Echocardiography showed a dilated right ventricular chamber consistent with cor pulmonale but no other structural abnormality; specifically, the mitral valve and left atrium were normal in appearance. This combination of findings is virtually diagnostic of veno-occlusive disease, in a patient of this age almost certainly of the primary variety.

Illustration continued on following page

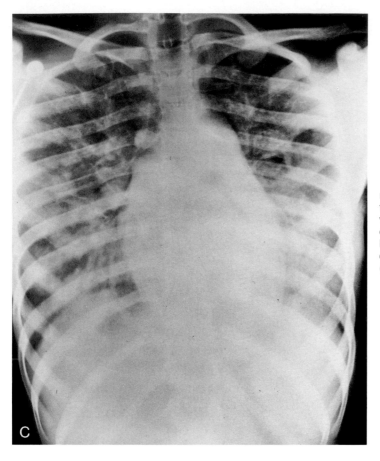

Figure 10–38 *Continued* Two weeks later, a chest roentgenogram (C) revealed massive airspace edema and the patient died shortly thereafter. At autopsy, there was widespread multifocal fibrosis of small and large intraparenchymal veins, many of which possessed numerous small lumens rather than a simple lumen. Arterioles showed abundant medial muscle and internal and external elastic laminae. (Courtesy of the Birmingham Children's Hospital.)

in patients with pulmonary venous hypertension secondary to mitral stenosis[217] and may be the result of pulmonary vascular congestion. A review[218] suggested that in pulmonary veno-occlusive disease, the pulmonary arterial wedge pressure is usually normal or low and that the combination of pulmonary venous hypertension, pulmonary arterial hypertension, and a normal pulmonary arterial wedge pressure is diagnostic of pulmonary veno-occlusive disease. The latter finding is vital to the diagnosis and is best explained on the basis that the wedged pulmonary artery catheter measures the pressure not in the small pulmonary venules, which are narrowed by the obliterative process, but in the large confluent pulmonary veins, which are usually distal to the site of obstruction; the wedge pressure therefore reflects the pressure in the large pulmonary veins and left atrium, which is normal, and not the pressure in the pulmonary capillaries, which is elevated.[207, 219] The triad of normal wedge pressure, pulmonary arterial hypertension, and pulmonary edema is virtually diagnostic of this condition. However, one other condition can cause similar findings—left atrial myxoma (*see* Fig. 10–34): the patient can present with intermittent pulmonary edema during times of mitral valve obstruction, but can have a normal pulmonary artery wedge pressure when obstruction is not present. If a careful clinical examination and investigation are done, the diagnosis of pulmonary veno-occlusive disease usu-

ally can be made ante mortem. Most patients die within 2 years of the onset of symptoms.[205]

A variation of the theme of pulmonary veno-occlusive disease is a rare condition known as *unilateral pulmonary vein atresia*. Characterized by atresia of long segments of the pulmonary veins draining one lung, the condition is believed to be congenital and to result from improper incorporation of the common pulmonary vein into the left atrium.[220] Roentgenographically, the affected lung is small, oligemic, and the site of a coarse reticular pattern caused by fibrosis secondary to chronic pulmonary edema and recurrent infection. In addition, pulmonary lymphatics and bronchial veins are dilated, probably contributing to the reticular pattern. Pulmonary arteriography reveals a marked reduction in pulmonary blood flow to the affected lung or lobe, slow circulation and stasis of contrast medium, and no evidence of pulmonary vein filling. Clinically, the condition is characterized by recurrent pulmonary infections and hemoptysis.

CHRONIC COR PULMONALE

Although the presence of pulmonary hypertension does not necessarily imply cor pulmonale, it does indicate that there is a strain on the right ventricle which, if prolonged, will inevitably lead to right ventricular hypertrophy. Strictly speaking, the term cor pulmonale should be restricted to those instances in which abnormality of lung structure or function results in right ventricular hypertrophy. Although disease of the left side of the heart and congenital cardiac disease may closely mimic true cor pulmonale, they are not generally accepted under this definition.[221] Approximately 80 per cent of cases of chronic cor pulmonale result from COPD and emphysema.[222]

Roentgenologically, cardiac enlargement is not always apparent, even when right ventricular hypertrophy is evident post mortem.[221] This failure to appreciate cardiac enlargement is particularly notable in the presence of pulmonary emphysema, when only serial roentgenography may reveal the increase.

Clinically, right ventricular thrust, usually felt along the left sternal border, may be similarly obscured by pulmonary overinflation in emphysema. A systolic thrust, sometimes a diastolic shock, and a systolic thrill may be felt over the pulmonary area. A loud P_2 sound with a pulmonary systolic ejection click, and in some cases harsh systolic and diastolic murmurs, may be heard over the same area. As right-sided heart failure develops, a systolic murmur, which is louder during inspiration, becomes audible along the left sternal border. It may be associated with a palpable pulse in the (enlarged) liver, a systolic venous pulse in the neck, and, in many cases, peripheral edema and ascites. Although this systolic murmur has been attributed to tricuspid regurgitation, catheterization studies in patients with pulmonary heart disease suggest that it more likely denotes sudden reversal of flow from the right atrium to major veins, consequent upon the large pressure variation originating in a congested right atrium.[223] Cardiac arrhythmias are rare in cor pulmonale.[224]

The ECG may be normal even in cases of known severe right ventricular hypertrophy. In one study, only two thirds of 40 patients with pathologically proven cor pulmonale had ECG tracings typical of right ventricular hypertrophy.[224] The Expert Committee Report for the World Health Organization suggested the following criteria for right ventricular hypertrophy, indicating that at least two of these signs should be present: R/S less than one in V_5 and V_6; predominant S wave in lead I or incomplete right bundle branch block; P waves taller than 2 mm in lead II; right axis deviation greater than 110 degrees; and inversion of T waves in V_1 to V_4 or V_2 and V_3.[225] This last finding is of less diagnostic value.[221]

PULMONARY ARTERY ANEURYSMS

Aneurysms of the main and lobar branches of the pulmonary artery are rare. In their 1947 review of the literature, Deterling and Clagett[226] found only eight examples in 109,571 autopsies, an incidence of one in 13,696. Only 147 pathologically proven cases had been reported in the literature to that time. If tuberculosis-related aneurysms and microscopic mycotic aneurysms associated with septic emboli or pneumonia are excluded, aneurysms of the intrapulmonary branches of the pulmonary artery are even less common; in their review of the literature in 1961, Charlton and Du Plessis[227] found only 38 examples.

Etiology and Pathogenesis

The etiology and pathogenetic mechanisms are many and diverse (Table 10–2) and are discussed only briefly here; more detailed information can be found elsewhere in the book where specific diseases are discussed.

CONGENITAL FACTORS

Congenital anomalies of the heart and great vessels are not infrequently associated with pulmonary artery aneurysm; in these circumstances, their pathogenesis can be difficult to establish precisely. In some cases, the aneurysm is related to stenosis of the pulmonary valve, right ventricular infundibulum, or a portion of the pulmonary artery itself, and represents poststenotic dilatation caused by disturbed hemodynamics.[228] In others—for example, in association with PDA—increased pulmonary blood flow and eventual arterial hypertension likely play an important role by causing distention in areas of focal vascular weakness. Although the cause of the latter is not clear in most cases, a congenital structural abnormality of the arterial wall may be important in some; however, only rarely has there been histologic evidence suggestive of such a mechanism.[229] Medial damage secondary to septic emboli from endocarditis may also be responsible in some instances.

Table 10–2. Etiology and Pathogenesis of Pulmonary Artery Aneurysms

Congenital	Deficiency of vessel wall[229]
	Postvalvular or arterial stenosis[228]
Degenerative/metabolic	Marfan's syndrome[232]
	"Cystic medial necrosis" (dissecting aneurysm)[185]
Traumatic	[233, 234]
Infectious (mycotic)	Syphilis[226]
	Tuberculosis[237]
	Pyogenic bacterial[238–240]
	Others (e.g., fungi)[241]
Immunologic	Behçet's disease (? Hughes-Stovin syndrome)[243]
	Polyarteritis nodosa (bronchial arteries)
Secondary to pulmonary disease	Hypertension (including dissecting aneurysms)[239, 240, 244, 245]
	Bronchiectasis
Idiopathic	Hughes-Stovin syndrome[243, 246, 248]

DEGENERATIVE AND METABOLIC FACTORS

Rarely, diffuse or focal dilatation of the pulmonary trunk and its main branches can occur as an isolated finding[230–231] or in association with connective tissue diseases, such as Marfan's syndrome.[232] By itself, this change is usually of little clinical consequence; however, it is very occasionally associated with dissection.[185]

TRAUMATIC FACTORS

Trauma to the chest wall can result in pulmonary arterial damage, occasionally with residual aneurysm formation.[233] Sevitt[234] has found microaneurysms (up to 1.2 mm in diameter) in association with thromboemboli and has suggested that they might be caused by physical damage resulting from impact. It is also possible that local ischemia of the arterial wall adjacent to a thromboembolus can cause necrosis and subsequent aneurysmal dilatation.[235, 236]

INFECTIOUS (MYCOTIC) FACTORS

Infection is an important pathogenetic factor in many pulmonary artery aneurysms. A variety of microorganisms can be responsible. In industrial societies, syphilis[226] and tuberculosis[237] were relatively common causes until the middle of the 20th century, but with control of these diseases in recent times, pyogenic organisms have become increasingly important.[238–240] Rarely, fungi such as *Aspergillus* species can also cause the same process.[241]

Organisms can gain access to the arterial wall by three routes:

1. By direct continuity from a focus of pulmonary parenchymal infection. Aneurysms that develop by this mechanism occur most often in chronic fibrocaseous tuberculosis, in which about 5 per cent of cases have been shown to develop them (Rasmussen's aneurysm).[237] Rupture with hemorrhage is a relatively common cause of death in these patients.[237]

2. Via the vasa vasorum derived from the bronchial arteries, a pathway that is probably the mechanism of aneurysm formation in syphilis.

3. By direct extension into a vessel wall from an intraluminal septic thromboembolus. This is probably the most common mechanism of mycotic aneurysm formation in industrialized countries today. The source of thromboemboli is usually endocarditis, particularly of the tricuspid valve in narcotic abusers,[242] and of valvular, cardiac, or vascular endothelium in patients with a variety of congenital anomalies.[239] Infectious thrombophlebitis and infected thrombi associated with intravenous catheters are occasional sources.

IMMUNOLOGIC FACTORS

Immunologically mediated vasculitis has been only rarely implicated in pulmonary artery aneu-

rysm formation, usually in the bronchial arteries in polyarteritis nodosa and in the large pulmonary arteries in Behçet's disease.[243] It has been suggested that many cases of Hughes-Stovin syndrome in fact represent the latter condition.[243]

SECONDARY FACTORS

In many cases, pulmonary arterial hypertension secondary to cardiovascular or pulmonary disease is undoubtedly an important factor in the formation of aneurysms.[227, 239, 240] The most common underlying condition is a left-to-right cardiovascular shunt, usually PDA or VSD. Occasionally, pulmonary hypertension is of the primary variety. Although dissecting aneurysms are a rare complication of pulmonary hypertension, they are invariably associated with this finding.[244, 245]

IDIOPATHIC FACTORS

Hughes-Stovin syndrome is a rare disorder characterized by aneurysms of the large and small pulmonary arteries and thrombosis of peripheral veins and dural sinuses. The syndrome was originally described in 1959 by Hughes and Stovin,[246] who reported two of their own cases and two from the literature. It is possible that there are several pathogenetic mechanisms in this syndrome, some cases being associated with congenital cardiovascular defects and others sharing similarities with Behçet's disease. An infectious basis for the aneurysms has not been substantiated by the discovery of organisms at necropsy.[247] Through 1974, eight cases of Hughes-Stovin syndrome had been reported;[248] all but one involved males, ranging in age from 14 to 37, the exception being a 25-year-old woman.[248] Pulmonary thromboembolism is a common associated finding.

Pathologic and Roentgenographic Characteristics

The pathologic and roentgenographic features of pulmonary artery aneurysms vary with the etiology and pathogenesis and are discussed in detail in the appropriate sections of the book. Aneurysms may be solitary or multiple and range in size from microscopic foci to 5 cm in diameter. Most occur in the pulmonary trunk or its major branches (Fig. 10–39), but presentation in a peripheral artery as a solitary nodule can occur.[238]

Clinical Manifestations

Clinically, signs and symptoms associated with pulmonary artery aneurysms are usually absent; in some cases, cough, dyspnea, and hemoptysis may be present.[238] Rupture into an airway can result in massive hemorrhage,[238] and thrombosis can occasionally lead to cor pulmonale.[231] Physical examination may reveal a thrill or murmur over the

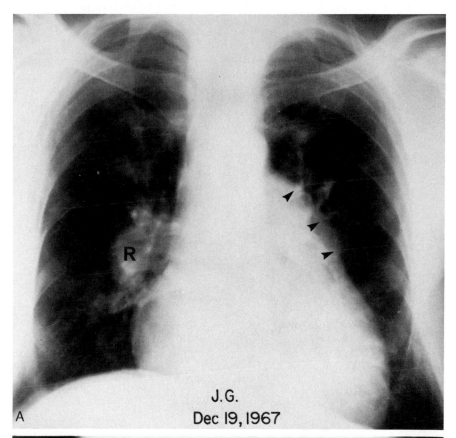

Figure 10–39. Aneurysms of the Pulmonary Arteries Secondary to Chronic Thromboembolism. Posteroanterior (*A*) and lateral (*B*) chest roentgenograms show features of severe chronic cor pulmonale — cardiomegaly with a configuration compatible with right atrial and ventricular dilatation, and marked enlargement of the main pulmonary artery (*arrowheads*) and the right (R) and left (L) interlobar arteries.

Illustration continued on following page

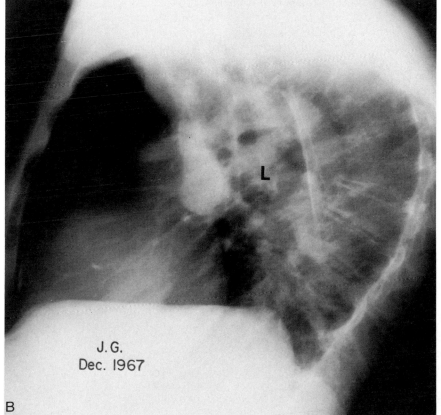

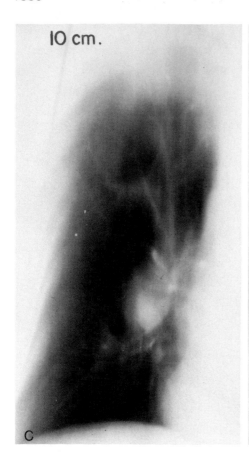

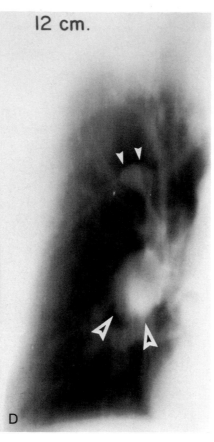

Figure 10–39 *Continued* Detail views of the right lung from conventional full lung tomograms (*C* and *D*) reveal an aneurysm in the truncus anterior (*small arrowheads*) and marked dilatation and abrupt termination of the interlobar artery (*large arrowheads*). At autopsy, these vessels were focally dilated (saccular aneurysms) proximal to totally occluded partially recanalized emboli. The patient is an elderly man.

aneurysm. In many cases, pulmonary symptoms are overshadowed by underlying cardiac or pulmonary disease. Dissecting aneurysms may present with precordial pain; proximal extension with intrapericardial hemorrhage and tamponade is a frequent cause of death.[244, 245] In Hughes-Stovin syndrome, recurrent episodes of fever, lack of response to antibiotics, hemoptysis, and respiratory symptoms resulting from recurrent pulmonary artery occlusions have been prominent clinical features. A common terminal event is massive hemoptysis.[247]

PULMONARY EDEMA

Normally, anatomic and physiologic mechanisms within the lungs keep the alveoli dry or, perhaps more correctly, ideally moist, and they maintain a constant interstitial water content. Despite the constancy of fluid content within the interstitium and alveolar airspaces, there is considerable transport of water between different tissue compartments within the lung. As in other body tissues, two physiologic factors are chiefly responsible for this fluid movement: (1) the relationship between the microvascular and perimicrovascular hydrostatic pressure and the plasma and perimicrovascular osmotic pressure, and (2) the permeability of the microvascular wall.

Normally, an ultrafiltrate of plasma moves from the pulmonary microvessels through the endothe-

lium into the interstitial compartment and from the interstitium into the pulmonary lymphatics, whence it is returned to the systemic circulation via the right lymphatic and thoracic ducts. The volume of water and protein movement are dependent on the balance of pressures across the pulmonary microvasculature and the permeability of the microvascular membrane. A disturbance of sufficient magnitude in one or both of these factors will result in an increase in the transudation or exudation of fluid from the microvessels into the interstitial tissues. Sufficient accumulation of fluid in this compartment constitutes interstitial edema; when the storage capacity of the interstitial space is exceeded, alveolar flooding and airspace edema develop. In normal circumstances, the balance of hydrostatic and osmotic forces across microvascular walls is so precise that the escape of water and protein into the interstitial tissue is exactly balanced by the removal of fluid by the intricate network of pulmonary lymphatics that absorb the fluid and return it to the systemic circulation. Additional routes for removal of lung fluid include evaporative water loss from the alveolar and bronchial surfaces, reabsorption into pulmonary and bronchial microvessels, and transport into the pleural space.

The lung is unique in the sense that edema, if sufficient in amount to flood the alveolar airspaces, results in severe disruption of the organ's primary function, the provision of adequate exchange of oxygen and carbon dioxide. With the exception of the brain, most other organs can function normally despite considerable fluid accumulation. Because of these considerations, the lung has evolved a number of anatomic and physiologic characteristics that tend to minimize the presence of excess lung liquid despite perturbations that favor its accumulation.

The most common cause of pulmonary edema is elevation of pulmonary microvascular pressure secondary to elevated pulmonary venous pressure caused by left ventricular decompensation. This form of edema is called *cardiogenic,* hemodynamic, hydrostatic, or elevated microvascular pressure pulmonary edema. A less common but nevertheless significant mechanism for the formation of pulmonary edema is an increase in the permeability of the microvascular endothelial barrier as a result of toxic injury. In its pure form, this mechanism results in the accumulation of excess water and protein in the lungs in the absence of elevated microvascular pressure and is thus termed permeability, normal microvascular pressure, or *noncardiogenic* edema. There are multiple etiologies that lead to this form of pulmonary edema and the clinical syndrome that results has been termed the adult respiratory distress syndrome (ARDS).[249, 250]

Before we begin a discussion of each of these types of pulmonary edema and diseases with which they are associated, it is desirable to review certain anatomic and physiologic considerations relating to lung fluid and solute exchange. Much of the following material has been gleaned from the excellent reviews on the subject by Fishman,[251] Robin and his colleagues,[252, 253] Staub,[254–258] Prichard,[259] Effros,[260] and others.[261, 262]

ANATOMIC CONSIDERATIONS

The Pulmonary Circulation and Microvascular Endothelium

Because of their primary role in gas exchange, a process that takes place solely by diffusion, the lungs have developed an enormous surface area for transport of oxygen and carbon dioxide. The surface area for gas exchange in the pulmonary microvessels is approximately 70 square meters,[263, 264] an area that is also potentially available for fluid exchange. The microcirculation is largely made up of an enormous interconnecting network of pulmonary capillaries, situated within alveolar walls and separated from alveolar gas by an ultrathin membrane. Although it is believed that most of the fluid exchange in the lungs takes place across the alveolocapillary endothelium, there is abundant evidence that larger precapillary and postcapillary vessels also take part, and as a result the most appropriate term for this process is *microvascular fluid exchange.*[265–267]

As discussed in Chapter 1 (*see* page 129), the pulmonary vasculature can be divided into two compartments based on the response of the blood vessels to an increase in alveolar pressure. Alveolar vessels are affected directly by such an increase by dint of compression, resulting in narrowing of the lumen. By contrast, extra-alveolar vessels are affected indirectly by alveolar pressure in that they expand during lung distention owing to the development of a more negative interstitial pressure around them. Although most of the pulmonary capillaries function as alveolar vessels, some (termed "corner vessels") behave like extra-alveolar vessels and remain patent despite an increase in alveolar pressure to values that exceed pulmonary microvascular pressure (Fig. 10–40). These corner vessels as well as small arterioles and venules contribute to fluid exchange, a fact that has been confirmed by studies that have shown that liquid exchange can occur under conditions in which alveolar pressure exceeds vascular pressure.[265, 266, 268] In fact, under Zone I conditions (*see* page 128), the rate of liquid filtration into the lung can be as much as half that in Zone III, suggesting that a considerable proportion of the lung microvessels that exchange fluid remain patent under these conditions and therefore function as extra-alveolar vessels.[257]

In any discussion of fluid exchange, the concept that the alveolocapillary wall has "thick" and "thin" sides is of considerable importance. The alveolar septum viewed in cross section by electron microscopy reveals two distinct anatomic and functional zones: a thin side for gas exchange and a thick side that serves for both structural support and fluid exchange. The difference between the two sides is the amount of interstitial tissue that separates the endothelial and epithelial cells. On the thin side, the alveolocapillary membrane measures no more than 0.3 to 0.5 μm and consists of three layers—the alveolar epithelium, the capillary endothelium, and the fused basement membranes in between. This arrangement provides the lung with an enormous area for gas exchange without the encumbrance of excessive mass. By contrast, between the basement membranes on the thick side there is a relatively wide interstitial connective tissue compartment consisting of collagen and elastic fibers, fibroblasts, contractile interstitial cells, macrophages, and ground substance. Five discrete layers separate alveolar air from capillary blood in this region—alveolar epithelium, alveolar epithelial basement membrane, the interstitial space, the capillary endothelial basement membrane, and the capillary endothelium. The thick side not only provides support for the capillary network but constitutes an essential component of the water-exchanging apparatus of the lung, operating to expedite the removal of water and proteins from the interstitial space toward the lymphatic capillaries.[251] When excess water and protein accumulate in the alveolar septa, as in interstitial pulmonary edema, they do so exclusively or predominantly on the thick side (Fig. 10–41). In a study of the ultrastructure of the alveolocapillary wall in the presence of interstitial

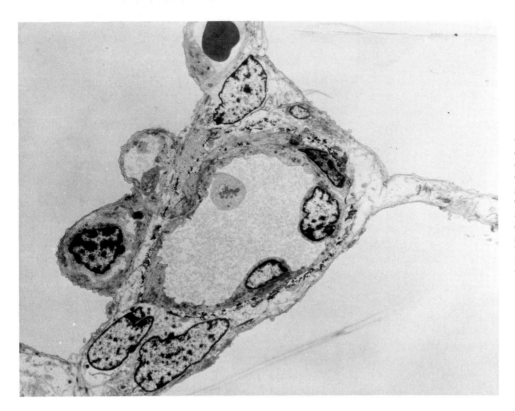

Figure 10–40. A Corner Vessel: Ultrastructure. Corner vessels are pulmonary capillaries that behave like extra-alveolar vessels. Since they are situated at the junction of three alveolar walls, lung inflation causes a dilatation of corner vessels while compressing alveolar wall vessels. (Courtesy of Dr. David Walker, Department of Pathology, University of British Columbia, Vancouver.)

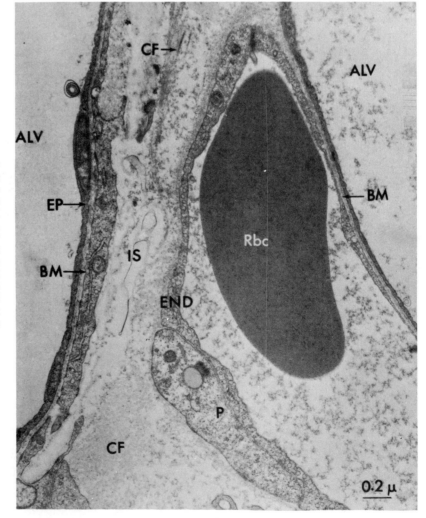

Figure 10–41. Interstitial Pulmonary Edema. The interstitial space (IS) of the thick portion of the alveolar septum has been considerably widened by edema fluid during hemodynamic pulmonary edema, whereas the opposite thin part, containing the fused basement membranes (BM), remains unchanged in thickness. ALV = alveolar space; EP = alveolar epithelium; BM = basement membrane; IS = interstitial space; CF = collagen fibers; END = capillary endothelium; Rbc = red blood cell. Transmission electron microscope (TEM) section stained with uranil acetate and lead citrate (× 12,000). (Reprinted from Fishman A: Circulation 46:389, 1972. With permission of the author and editor.)

edema, Cottrell and colleagues[269] showed that the thick side of the capillary wall was widened and the collagen fibers were separated, presumably by water; by contrast, the thin side was not expanded, thus preserving its structure for gas exchange. The pulmonary capillaries are embedded in the alveolar walls, and one alveolus may be subserved by numerous pulmonary capillaries. The alveolar wall may be made up of a multitude of thin sides and thick sides; thus, one might envisage an undulating surface created by alternating thin and thick sides.

Electron microscopic and freeze fracture studies have shown that the pulmonary capillaries are virtually indistinguishable from those found in muscle.[270] Large fenestrations between endothelial cells do not exist as they do in visceral capillaries, and the pulmonary endothelial cells are held together by tight junctions that extend, zipper-like, around the cells, thereby keeping them in close approximation (see Fig. 1–67, page 76). Strands are evident on freeze fracture through the junctional complex of endothelial cell contacts, representing protein particles within the cell membrane of opposing cells; it is these structural proteins that provide endothelial integrity. Discontinuities in these strands form the paracellular pathway or "pores" for the bulk of water transport and all of the solute transport across the endothelium. The junctional complexes of the capillary endothelium are much less well developed than those of the alveolar epithelial surface, and studies have shown that there is a correlation between the number of junctional strands and the permeability of a cellular membrane.[271] Recent studies by Walker and associates[272] suggest that large discontinuities in the tight junctions can exist at the junction between three adjacent capillary endothelial cells, such "pores" being visible on electron microscopy. Interestingly, there are relatively fewer junctional strands (and by inference, more permeable endothelium) on the venous than on the arterial end of the capillary membrane.[270]

Presumably, lipid-soluble substances can traverse the capillary endothelium by passing directly through cell membranes. By contrast, in order to cross the endothelium, water-soluble substances must be transported by pinocytosis or must pass through the paracellular pathway. It is the selective sieving of protein molecules by their molecular size that suggests that the primary pathway for protein movement across the endothelium is via the paracellular pathway. Small molecules traverse the pulmonary capillary endothelium with ease, whereas larger molecules are excluded in direct proportion to their molecular size; very large molecules do not reach the pulmonary interstitium at all. There have been a number of attempts to model and calculate the size of the "pores" between pulmonary endothelial cells by measuring transendothelial flux of different-sized tracer molecules and water, using varying microvascular pressures. No simple pore model can adequately explain the transport char-

acteristics, and it is probable that "pores" in the capillary endothelium possess a wide variety of sizes. The calculations have suggested that there are a large number of small "pores" that only allow transport of water and many fewer large "pores" that permit transport of protein.[273–276] It has been theorized that a rise in pulmonary microvascular pressure can increase the size of the gaps between endothelial cells, thus increasing protein permeability (the "stretched pore theory"). Although this theory remains controversial, it is probable that, within a range of moderately elevated microvascular pressures, lung endothelial permeability is not directly affected by pressure.[277] It should be appreciated that the "pores" through which fluid movement occurs in the pulmonary microvasculature represent a minute fraction of the total capillary surface area. The surface area occupied by "pores" may be as little as one millionth of the total endothelial surface area;[278] as a result, a doubling or tripling of the surface area occupied by "pores" might not be detected by conventional microscopic techniques, whereas it would markedly enhance fluid and solute transport.

The Bronchial Circulation and Endothelium

The bronchial circulation and the structures it supplies have been described in detail in Chapter 1 (see page 79). Briefly, in addition to providing a blood supply to the bronchial and bronchiolar walls (see below), the bronchial arteries supply the loose peribronchial and perivascular connective tissues, the visceral pleura over the mediastinal and diaphragmatic surfaces of the lungs, mediastinal and hilar lymph nodes, and the vasa vasorum of the large arteries and veins within the thorax. Within the airway walls, the bronchial vessels form two extensive plexuses, one inside the smooth muscle (the submucosal plexus) and the other outside it (the peribronchial plexus). At the level of the respiratory bronchioles, the bronchial capillary network meshes with the pulmonary capillary and venous system. The majority of the bronchial blood drains to the left side of the heart via capillary and venous anastomoses with the pulmonary circulation, although the portion that supplies the large airways returns via bronchial veins to the azygos and hemiazygos veins and ultimately reaches the right atrium. Although the total blood flow through the bronchial circulation is small relative to that through the pulmonary circulation, ranging from 1 to 5 per cent of cardiac output, the bronchial microcirculation may still play an important role in fluid exchange within the lung. The importance of the bronchial vasculature in fluid exchange could be assessed if there was accurate information concerning the total surface area for fluid exchange and the permeability of the bronchial microvascular endothelium. Unfortunately, there are few data concerning either of these variables. In some animal species,[279] the surface area of the bronchial microvessels has been calculated to be as much as one half of the corresponding airway epithelial surface area. If a similar anatomic arrangement were to exist in man, these vessels would provide a large surface area for fluid exchange.[280]

The microscopic anatomy of the bronchial microvessels is quite different from that of the pulmonary capillaries. The bronchial capillary endothelium has been described as being similar to the "visceral type" of microvessels in which many fenestrae are present between the cells.[281] Not only does the morphometry of the bronchial microvessels suggest increased permeability, but the endothelial cells also respond to pharmacologic agents in a manner that the pulmonary capillaries do not. The endothelial lining cells of the bronchial capillaries and venules contain a rich network of contractile fibers which, when stimulated, appear to be capable of widening the junctions between adjacent endothelial cells. Administration of histamine, bradykinin, or the mast cell degranulating substance 48–80 causes contraction of these intercellular fibers, enlargement of paracellular pathways, and increased permeability of the microvessels to large-molecular-weight substances and tracers such as colloidal carbon.[280] Although these anatomic and functional features make the bronchial circulation a potentially important contributor to lung fluid exchange, there is little direct evidence to implicate the bronchial circulation in the production of pulmonary edema. In one study in sheep, Nakahara and associates found a modest increase in lung lymph flow and mirovascular permeability when histamine was infused directly into the bronchial artery, but they attributed this to the effects of the drug on the pulmonary circulation via anastomotic channels.[282]

The Pulmonary Interstitium

The lung can be considered as a branching system of interstitial connective tissue that supports alveoli and airways on the one hand and the large and small vessels on the other.

Excess fluid accumulates first in the interstitium of the lung. The interstitial space can be divided into two functionally distinct compartments—an alveolar wall (parenchymal) compartment and a peribronchovascular (axial) compartment. The latter consists of an extensive and continuous network of loose connective tissue that forms a cuff around the pulmonary arteries and bronchi; it is in continuity with the interstitium surrounding the pulmonary veins and in the interlobular septa and subpleural space. The alveolar wall compartment consists of the thick side of the alveolocapillary membrane; it is bounded by the basal laminae of the pulmonary epithelium and endothelium and contains cells, interstitial ground substance, and fibers. Despite the fact that there are no qualitative differences in the connective tissue in the two "compartments," their compliance and ability to store fluid are quite different: although the parenchymal compartment constitutes a large percentage of the total interstitial space, it is very noncompliant so that interstitial edema tends to accumulate to a lesser extent in alveolar walls than in the peribronchovascular compartment. Staub and coworkers[283] have shown that not only does an interstitial phase of edema exist for a variable period before alveolar flooding occurs but edema develops in the loose connective tissue around the airways and vessels before it accumulates in the alveolar septa (*see* Fig. 4–56, page 546).

The interstitial connective tissue is a gel that contains fibers and cells. The gel itself is composed of a matrix of highly polymerized mucopolysaccharides that, in combination with proteins, form glycoproteins. In the lung, the principal mucopolysaccharides (or glycosaminoglycans, as they are also called) are chondroitin sulfate and hyaluronic acid. The glycoprotein complexes are extremely hydrophilic and can bind large amounts of water with weak hydrogen bonds; it is the association of the loosely bound water molecules and the large complex macromolecules that forms the gel. Within the gel are cells such as fibroblasts, tissue histiocytes, mast cells, and blood-derived inflammatory cells, including polymorphonuclear leukocytes and eosinophils. Collagen, elastin, and reticulin fibers run through the gel, providing a skeleton or framework for the interstitial space.

A significant portion of the water within the interstitial space forms a complex within the gel and is unavailable to large-molecular-weight solutes like serum proteins. This portion of the interstitial water volume is called the "excluded volume." The excluded volume is analogous to water contained within "capsules" which have semipermeable membranes—permeable to water and small-molecular-weight solutes but not to proteins. As a result of the excluded volume, the protein concentration (and therefore the osmotic pressure) of the interstitial fluid is greater than would be calculated from the known quantities of protein and water. It has been suggested[284] that during swelling of the interstitial space, some of the "excluded" water becomes available; by diluting interstitial protein, it lowers the interstitial osmotic pressure, thereby providing a safety factor that retards the further development of pulmonary edema. However, Bert[285] has stated that water bound to the gel glycoproteins cannot be made "available" during swelling of the gel and has suggested that only a washout of interstitial glycoprotein can decrease the excluded volume.

The size of the pulmonary interstitium is large in comparison to other organs. It is estimated that 40 per cent of the extravascular water of the lung is in the extracellular interstitial compartment. During the development of interstitial pulmonary edema, this volume can more than double before alveolar flooding occurs. The fluid storage capacity of the interstitial space increases when lung volume is increased. Gee and Williams[286] found that at a transpulmonary pressure of 5 cm H_2O, the pulmonary interstitium contained less than 1 ml of water/gm of dry lung but at a transpulmonary pressure of 15 cm H_2O the volume increased to 6 ml of water/gm of dry lung. Lung inflation in an already edematous lung can redistribute the edema fluid, shifting it from alveolar airspaces to the peribronchovascular interstitial compartment. This phenomenon has been demonstrated in animal models of both hydrostatic[287] and permeability[288] pulmonary edema and may be an explanation for the beneficial effect of positive end-expiratory pressure (PEEP); although PEEP does not decrease the amount of lung water, it can redistribute it to the interstitial space, where it has less detrimental effects on gas exchange.

The Alveolar Membrane

As described in Chapter 1 (*see* page 19), the alveolar side of the alveolocapillary membrane consists of a continuous epithelium composed of thin cytoplasmic extensions of Type 1 alveolar epithelial cells with type 2 cells interposed at irregular intervals. A continuous, well-defined basement membrane is shared with the basement membrane of the capillary endothelium on the thin side of the alveolar wall. The surface area of the alveolar membrane is approximately 70 square meters,[263] similar to the estimated surface area of the capillary bed. The intercellular junctions of the alveolar epithelium are much more highly developed than those of the capillary endothelium (*see* Fig. 1–67, page 76), and this morphologic complexity is reflected in impermeability to all lipid insoluble substances other than water.[271, 289] The permeability of the alveolar membrane can be tested by measuring the appearance of intravenously administered tracer molecules in the alveolar fluid or alternatively by measuring the appearance in the blood of tracers placed into the alveolar airspaces. Only small molecules, such as urea and sucrose, and ions, such as sodium and calcium, are able to diffuse through the alveolar epithelium, but like the capillary endothelium there appears to be a sieving that is based on molecular size.[259, 290] The size selectivity of the membrane allows the calculation of an equivalent "pore" radius that in lambs has been found to range from 0.7 to 1.4 nm; during lung inflation, however, the permeability of the membrane increases as a result of an increase in calculated "pore" radius to 3 to 4 nm.[290] This contrasts with the calculated range of "pore" sizes in the capillary endothelium in which a proportion of "pores" as large as 100 nm is required to explain the difference in lymph and plasma protein concentration.[275, 276]

The alveolar airspaces are lined by a thin layer of liquid, the total alveolar volume having been estimated to be approximately 20 ml.[259] This represents a layer averaging 0.2 to 0.3 microns in thickness spread over a surface area of 70 square meters. The liquid is not of even thickness, however; in air-filled lungs, it smooths out any irregularities in the alveolar wall and transforms the air-fluid interface into a smooth regular membrane with a constant radius of curvature.[291] This smoothing of the irregular alveolar wall is caused by the surface tension generated at the air-liquid interface.

Lymphatic Drainage

Pulmonary lymphatic capillaries are similar to those in other organs. They have a larger lumen than do blood capillaries; a discontinuous or absent basement membrane; and attenuated, irregular endothelial lining cells with many loose intercellular junctions.[292] The lymphatic endothelium is thought to offer no significant impedance to the flow of water or protein from the lung interstitium,[260] and it is generally believed that the concentration of solute in the "nonexcluded" portion of the interstitial liquid is the same as that in lymph;[255] however, it is possible that the protein concentration of lymph may be altered during its passage through regional lymph nodes.[293]

It is generally agreed that there are no lymphatic vessels in the alveolar septa,[259] although in one study in which a casting technique was employed, Pump[294] described lymphatics in some alveolar walls. The lymphatics begin as blind-ended vessels in the region of the alveolar ducts and respiratory bronchioles,[295] close to alveolar walls.[296] In 15 cases of drowning in which the lymphatics were unusually prominent, Lauweryns[297] demonstrated unequivocal histologic evidence of lymphatic capillaries in the interlobular septa, pleura, and peribronchovascular interstitium contiguous with alveolar walls. He defined these as "juxta-alveolar" lymphatic capillaries because of their topographic and probable functional relationship to the alveolar walls, without being a part of the alveolar septa themselves. The absence of lymphatic channels within the alveolar walls is easily understandable functionally. As pointed out by Staub,[254] the three-dimensional structure of the alveolar wall junction forms an interconnecting pathway through which interstitial fluid can drain to a point where it can be picked up by the lymphatic capillaries. Numerous valves, 1 to 2 mm apart, direct the flow of lymph toward the hilum in both pleural and intrapulmonary lymphatics. The pulmonary lymphatics form a superficial and a deep collecting system. The superficial system drains the pleura, interlobular septa, and "cortical" lung tissue, and reaches the hila via long lymphatic vessels that course over the surface of the lung; the vessels of the deep venous system follow the bronchovascular bundles directly to the hila and drain most of the parenchyma.[259] Most of the lymph drainage from the lungs joins lymph from the heart, mediastinum, chest wall, and diaphragm and empties into the junction of the right subclavian and jugular veins via the right lymphatic duct;[259] the remainder originates from the left lung and a portion of the right lung and empties via the main thoracic duct into the venous system. Anastomoses probably exist between the two drainage systems that allow lymph to reach the systemic circulation in the event of obstruction of one of the pathways.[259]

Tissue fluid enters the terminal lymphatics through the wide open junctions between endothelial cells. The lymphatic walls are tethered to the surrounding connective tissue by a mesh of fine filaments so that when the tissue swells there is increased traction on the lymphatics that keeps them patent and facilitates drainage.[298] Once the tissue fluid has entered the peripheral ends of the lymphatic vessels, it is pumped centrally, any bidirectional movement being prevented by the valves. The pumping is partly passive, being related to the respiratory motion of the lungs, but is also active: the larger pulmonary lymphatics are surrounded by a layer of smooth muscle that contracts rhythmically, propelling lymph centripetally.[259] Pulmonary lymphatics can generate considerable pressure when obstructed (up to 60 cm H_2O) and lymph continues to empty into the systemic circulation despite an elevation in systemic venous pressure.[259] However, it has been suggested that high venous pressure can impair lymphatic function to some extent: in one experimental study in dogs, hydrostatic pulmonary edema increased in severity when superior vena caval pressure was increased to 30 cm H_2O.[299]

PHYSIOLOGIC CONSIDERATIONS

The Starling Equation

The factors that govern the formation and removal of extravascular water within the lungs are described by the *fluid transport equation*, originally proposed by Starling (Fig. 10–42).[300] This equation describes the net flux of fluid across a membrane under steady state conditions, transport being almost entirely by bulk flow.

$$\dot{Q}f = Kf\,[(Pmv - Ppmv) = \sigma(\pi mv - \pi pmv)]$$

where $\dot{Q}f$ = the net transvascular fluid flow, a value that should be equivalent to the net lymphatic flow from the lung in the absence of edema formation; Kf = the filtration coefficient, a measure of fluid conductance; Pmv = the hydrostatic pressure in the lumen of the fluid-exchanging microvessels; Ppmv = the hydrostatic pressure in the interstitial tissue surrounding the fluid-exchanging microvessels; σ = the osmotic reflection coefficient, i.e., a number between 0 and 1 that describes the effectiveness of the membrane in preventing the flow of protein compared with the flow of water; πmv = the protein osmotic pressure in the microvascular

lumen; and πpmv = the protein osmotic pressure in the interstitial fluid surrounding the microvessels.

The factors governing the net flux of a given solute across the membrane are described separately, in the *solute transport equation*. As pointed out by Staub,[254] this equation applies only to the transport of plasma proteins because the endothelium is freely permeable to small molecules, such as nutrients and electrolytes, which flow across the membrane with water and exert no net osmotic effect.

$$\dot{Q}s = PS(\pi mv - \pi pmv) + (1 - \sigma)\,\bar{C}s\dot{Q}f$$

where $\dot{Q}s$ = the net transport of a specific protein; PS = the net permeability surface area product, a measure of the permeability of the membrane to protein; πmv and πpmv = the microvascular and perimicrovascular concentrations of the specific protein; σ = the reflection coefficient for the specific protein; and $\bar{C}s$ = the average protein concentration in the membrane.

Since the endothelial permeability and the reflection coefficient are different for protein molecules of different sizes, their net flux will be inversely related to molecular weight, and the steady state interstitial concentrations of proteins relative to their plasma concentration will also vary with molecular size. When pulmonary microvascular permeability and pressures are normal, the ratios of lymphatic (representing interstitial) to plasma protein concentrations for albumin, globulin, and fibrinogen are approximately 0.8, 0.5, and 0.2, respectively.[257] As microvascular pressure is increased, the ratios for proteins of all sizes decrease as the transport of fluid outstrips protein transport. The net result is a dilution of interstitial proteins and a decrease in the perimicrovascular interstitial osmotic pressure; this phenomenon represents one of the safety factors that limit edema formation.

Under normal steady-state conditions, there is a continual net outward flow of fluid and protein from the pulmonary microvasculature to the interstitium; these substances are then returned to the bloodstream by the lymphatics. When this balance is disrupted, edema results, initially in the interstitial space but eventually in airspaces when the imbalance of forces becomes more severe or more prolonged. Although an increase in capillary hydrostatic pressure (Pmv) or an increase in endothelial permeability (Kf) is the most common cause of edema, it is of some value to discuss each of the factors in the Starling equation individually because all are important determinants of transvascular fluid flux.

MICROVASCULAR HYDROSTATIC PRESSURE (PMV)

A gradient in intraluminal hydrostatic pressure exists in the pulmonary vasculature from the main pulmonary arteries to the large pulmonary veins and left atrium. The hydrostatic pressure in the

Figure 10–42. A Three-Compartment Model of Starling Forces. The values for microvascular and perimicrovascular hydrostatic and osmotic pressures represent rough estimates and have been chosen to illustrate the longitudinal variation of the net driving pressure (Δ P) within the exchanging vessels. The arbitrary values for Kf illustrate the relative importance of the different compartments to overall lung fluid exchange, and the values for the reflection coefficient (σ) reflect the morphometric complexity of endothelial intercellular junctions on the arterial and venous side of the microcirculation. A value of 1.0 for σ would represent a membrane that was freely permeable to water but completely impermeable to protein. The driving pressure is greatest in the precapillary vessels and least in the postcapillary venules. There is a gradient in interstitial pressure that drives fluid from the pericapillary interstitial space toward the hilum. (Modified from Staub, NC: Pathophysiology of pulmonary edema. *In* Staub NC, Taylor AE (eds): Edema. New York, Raven Press, 1984, p 719.)

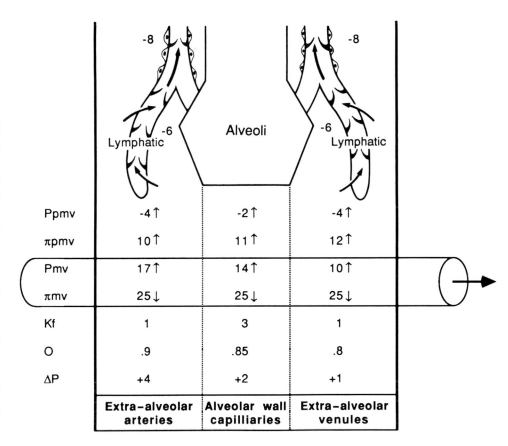

	Extra-alveolar arteries	Alveolar wall capilliaries	Extra-alveolar venules
Ppmv	-4 ↑	-2 ↑	-4 ↑
πpmv	10 ↑	11 ↑	12 ↑
Pmv	17 ↑	14 ↑	10 ↑
πmv	25 ↓	25 ↓	25 ↓
Kf	1	3	1
O	.9	.85	.8
ΔP	+4	+2	+1

fluid-exchanging vessels must be somewhere between the mean pulmonary arterial pressure (~20 cm H_2O) and the mean left atrial pressure (~5 cm H_2O). The actual value is dependent on the relative resistances of the vessels upstream and downstream from the fluid-exchanging vessels. If arterial resistance is high relative to venous resistance, a large arterial frictional pressure loss will occur and microvascular pressure will be close to venous pressure. Conversely, if venous resistance is large relative to arterial resistance and the majority of the pressure drop occurs across the venous system, pulmonary microvascular pressure will approach arterial pressure. In Zone III conditions,

$$Pmv = P_{La} + RV(P_{Pa} - P_{La})/RA + RV$$

where Pmv = microvascular pressure; P_{La} = left atrial pressure; RV and RA = venous and arterial resistances, respectively; and P_{Pa} = pulmonary arterial pressure.[255]

The results from most studies agree that venous resistance is slightly less than arterial resistance, and Staub has suggested that the value of 0.4 can be used for the normal fractional contribution of venous resistance in the calculation of Pmv.[255]

If mean pulmonary arterial pressure is 20 cm H_2O and mean left atrial pressure is 4 cm H_2O:

$$Pmv = 4 + 0.4 \times (20 - 4)$$
$$= 10.4 \text{ cm } H_2O$$

In Zone I and II conditions, the relative contributions of arterial and venous resistance will change.

Indirect measurements of the arterial and venous resistances have been made using techniques that employ a fluid bolus of low viscosity or that use rapid inflow and outflow occlusion.[301, 302] More recently, Bhattacharya and Staub[303] have made direct measurements of microvascular pressures in subpleural vessels using micropuncture techniques, and these results have allowed calculation of the serial distribution of vascular resistance within the lung. They found that approximately 40 per cent of the total pressure drop between the pulmonary artery and left atrium occurred within the alveolar wall capillaries themselves. There was very little resistance in arterial vessels larger than 50 μm in diameter or in veins larger than 20 μm in diameter. These results mean that there must be substantial variation in microvascular pressure along the relatively short length of the pulmonary capillaries and that fluid filtration may occur at the arterial end of the capillary while reabsorption from the interstitial space to the capillary lumen could occur at the venous end. As pointed out above, fluid transport across the pulmonary vascular endothelium occurs in pulmonary arterioles and venules as well as capillaries. Staub[257] has suggested a three-compartment model of lung fluid exchange in which the balance of forces and microvascular permeability vary from arterial microvessels to venous microvessels.

Although it is usual to talk of a single microvascular pressure within the pulmonary vasculature, it is obvious that there must be a large regional variation caused by the effects of gravity. Measurements of vascular pressures are normally referenced to the level of the left atrium, and in the erect position there is approximately 15 cm of lung above and 10 cm below this level. Pulmonary arterial and venous pressures decrease or increase by 1 cm H_2O pressure for each centimeter that the vessel in question is above or below the left atrium. If the pulmonary microvessels were noncompressible, the capillary pressure would also vary directly as a function of lung height. To the extent that this affects the ratios of arterial to venous resistance, capillary pressure will change. However, as pointed out by Staub,[257] the main mass of the lung is within 5 cm of the level of the left atrium in the erect as well as in the prone or supine positions. Since there is as much lung above as below this level, the integrated microvascular pressure over the height of the lung is not much different from that which would be calculated from the average P_{Pa} and P_{La} at the level of the left atrium.

PERIMICROVASCULAR INTERSTITIAL HYDROSTATIC PRESSURE (Ppmv)

Just as there is no unique value for microvascular pressure, there is also no unique value that describes the interstitial pressure of the lung. Direct measurements of pressure in the loose connective tissue near the hilum have shown it to be subatmospheric (~ -5 cm H_2O at functional residual capacity [FRC]), being more negative than pleural or alveolar pressure; it becomes progressively more negative during lung inflation (~ 12 cm H_2O at total lung capacity [TLC]).[304–306]

Using a micropuncture technique, Bhattacharya and associates[303] made direct measurements of interstitial pressure in the subpleural parenchyma in close proximity to alveolar vessels; although they were unable to obtain measurements from the alveolar septa themselves, the pressures in this location were still subatmospheric (~ -3 cm H_2O) although less so than in the perihilar region. Presumably, the pericapillary pressure is even less negative because there must be a gradient in pressure that drives fluid from the pericapillary to the perihilar (axial) interstitial compartment (see Fig. 10–42).[257]

There is probably a vertical gradient in interstitial pressure from the top to the bottom of the lung. From a study of dog lungs in which an indirect method was used to measure interstitial pressure, Parker and colleagues indicated that the vertical gradient in interstitial pressure is 0.6 cm H_2O/cm. The fact that microvascular pressure changes by 1.0 cm H_2O for each centimeter and interstitial pressure by only 0.6 cm H_2O/cm probably explains the tendency for pulmonary edema to collect preferentially in dependent lung.

PLASMA PROTEIN OSMOTIC PRESSURE (πmv)

The osmotic pressure exerted by plasma proteins is dependent on both their concentration and the permeability of the endothelial membrane to protein. It is calculated using standard equations[307, 308] or measured with osmometers[309] and represents the maximal osmotic pressure that would be produced by that concentration of protein acting across a membrane that was completely impermeable to protein (i.e., reflection coefficient of 1.0). To calculate osmotic pressure accurately, the albumin and globulin fractions of the serum protein should be known. Osmotic pressure increases alinearly with protein concentration and linearly with the albumin fraction.[308]

INTERSTITIAL PROTEIN OSMOTIC PRESSURE (πpmv)

Although plasma protein concentration (and therefore osmotic pressure) is constant throughout the microvasculature, substantial regional variations in protein concentration and osmotic pressure probably exist within the interstitium. It is assumed that the protein concentration of lung lymph represents the average protein concentration within the interstitium, although even this assumption may be invalid if there is significant sieving of protein within the interstitial space as suggested by Bert.[285] Interstitial protein concentration decreases as fluid filtration increases so that it is probable that the concentration is lowest at the base of the lung where gravity promotes the largest fluid filtration rate.[273] As discussed previously, the longitudinal variation in net filtration pressure and microvascular permeability from the arterial to the venous ends of the microvessels favors the development of differences in protein concentration between these two sites. Like the osmotic pressure of the plasma, the interstitial osmotic pressure is related to protein concentration, but because of the alinear relationship between osmotic pressure and solute concentration, a halving in protein concentration results in more than a 50 per cent decrease in osmotic pressure.

THE FILTRATION COEFFICIENT (Kf)

The filtration coefficient is a measure of endothelial permeability to water. It is analogous to the pulmonary airway conductance for air flow or diffusing capacity of the alveolocapillary membrane for a gas. The units for the filtration coefficient are ml/minute/cm H_2O/unit lung weight; the more permeable the endothelium, the larger is the value for Kf, i.e., the greater the fluid flux for a given net driving pressure. For the lung as a whole, Kf is influenced not only by the permeability of the endothelium but also by the surface area of endothelium available for fluid transport. If closed microvessels are opened (recruited) as a result of an increase in microvascular pressure, Kf will increase without an actual increase in "permeability"; for this reason, the whole organ filtration coefficient is often spoken of as the *permeability-surface area product*. It is impossible to measure Kf *in vivo,* and even in excised lung preparations the reported values simply represent the best estimates, since in order to calculate Kf precisely, it is necessary to know the four pertinent pressures (Pmv, Ppmv, πmv, and πpmv) as well as the permeability of the endothelium to protein (σ) and the net fluid flux.[257, 260]

THE OSMOTIC REFLECTION COEFFICIENT (σ)

A solute will exert a net osmotic pressure across a membrane only if the membrane is less permeable to the solute than it is to the solvent and if there is a difference in the concentration of solute on either side of the membrane. If the pulmonary capillary endothelium were impermeable to ions such as Na^+ and Cl^-, these solutes would exert an enormous osmotic pressure across the microvascular endothelium (~5000 cm H_2O at normal plasma ion concentrations).[259] Since these ions freely traverse the endothelium, there is no difference in ion concentration between plasma and interstitial fluid and thus no osmotic pressure gradient. The reflection coefficient is a numerical estimate of the permeability of the membrane to a solute and therefore is also an estimate of the effectiveness with which a given concentration of solute can exert osmotic pressure. A reflection coefficient of one means that the membrane is completely impermeable to the solute and that the osmotic pressure exerted by that solute will be equal to that measured in an osmometer; when the reflection coefficient is zero, the membrane is completely permeable to the solute and the solute exerts no osmotic pressure. A coefficient of 0.5 means that one half of the potentially available osmotic pressure is exerted by the solute.[259] Although it is often assumed that the reflection coefficient for plasma proteins is one, experimental data suggest that more appropriate values are 0.85, 0.9, and 0.98 for albumin, globulin, and fibrinogen, respectively.[257] In the presence of noncardiogenic pulmonary edema, the capillary endothelial permeability for water (Kf) and protein (σ) are altered; when the endothelium is severely damaged, the reflection coefficient approaches zero so that plasma proteins exert no effective pressure across the endothelium and the most powerful force preventing the formation of edema is lost.

Fluid Transport Across the Alveolar Epithelium

The morphologic appearance of the alveolar epithelial tight junctions suggests that the alveolar epithelium is much less permeable than the endothelium to water and solute, and physiologic studies have confirmed this.[271] The principles that govern fluid and solute transport across the endothelium are the same as those that operate across the epithelium, but the fluid conductivity is at least one order of magnitude lower; since the membrane is so restrictive, solutes that do not exert osmotic pressure across the endothelium (electrolytes) can have important effects on fluid balance across the epithelium. The protein content of the fluid lining the alveoli is unknown, but the electrolyte content is probably quite different from that in the plasma and interstitium as a result of active transport of chloride across epithelial cells into the alveolar liquid.[310, 311] The transport of fluid and solute across the alveolar epithelium can be measured accurately only when the airspaces are full of liquid; this state occurs normally only in the fetus. In the normal adult lung, the surface tension present at the interface between alveolar liquid and air exerts a pressure that tends to suck fluid from the interstitium into the airspaces. Because of the ability of a normal surfactant layer to lower surface tension, this pressure is small (~15 cm H_2O); however, when surfactant is deficient or inactivated, the increase in surface tension can play an important role in the formation of alveolar edema.[312]

Fluid Transport Across the Bronchial Endothelium

The components of the Starling equation that are necessary to calculate fluid transport across the airway endothelium are largely unknown. However, there are a number of facts that, taken together, suggest that the bronchial microvasculature may be an important site of fluid exchange: (1) the morphologic evidence of large intercellular gaps, (2) the likelihood that capillary hydrostatic pressure in these systemic microvessels is considerably higher than in the pulmonary microvasculature,[259] and (3) the probability that a more negative interstitial fluid pressure surrounds these vessels as they pass through the loose connective tissue in the peribronchovascular space.

The Safety Factors

Normally, the alveolar airspaces remain ideally moist despite substantial changes in microvascular and interstitial pressure related to posture, gravity, normal variations in the state of hydration, and changes in lung volume. The homeostasis is provided by a number of safety factors that tend to minimize accumulation of fluid in the lung.[257]

THE LYMPHATIC SYSTEM

Lung lymph flow is the first and most important safety factor. In the presence of an acute increase in microvascular pressure or permeability, lymph flow from the lung can increase tenfold or more before there is significant accumulation of pulmonary edema.[255] The rate of lung lymph flow during pulmonary edema is unknown in man. Using *Pseudomonas aeruginosa* bacteremia to induce endothelial permeability in sheep, Brigham and associates[313] obtained steady-state lymph flows of up to ten times baseline and absolute flows of up to 70 ml/hour. Scaling these results up to those of adult humans would predict that steady-state lung lymph flows of up to 200 ml/hour may be achieved.

As pointed out by Fishman,[251] it is curious that excess water should ever accumulate in the lungs in the face of such an elaborate drainage system. Whether or not a "ceiling" exists for lymphatic drainage is disputable. In their experiments on sheep subjected to *Pseudomonas* bacteremia, Brigham and associates[313] were unable to demonstrate a maximal lymph flow. However, Dumont and associates[314] suggested that the ceiling for lymphatic drainage is set by the relatively small caliber of the thoracic and right lymphatic ducts. In chronic left ventricular failure, the entire lymphatic system proliferates and the lymphatics increase in caliber.[315] For example, Uhley and colleagues[316–318] produced acute pulmonary edema in dogs by partial obstruction of the left atrium by a balloon and observed only a small absolute increase in lymph flow through the right lymphatic duct. By contrast, dogs in which chronic heart failure was induced by creation of an aortocaval anastomosis showed a major increase in pulmonary lymph flow ranging from 300 to 2800 per cent more than the normal flow of 4 ml/hour. Thus, in these experiments, at least, the lymphatics were relatively ineffectual in removing acute accumulations of lung water; however, they showed important functional expansion over a period of time and acted as a compensatory mechanism for the prevention of overt alveolar edema. These experiments were considered to be analogous to the clinical status of acute pulmonary edema (e.g., from acute myocardial infarction) on the one hand and chronic left atrial hypertension (e.g., from chronic mitral stenosis) on the other.

When lymphatic drainage is impaired because of obstruction in the lymphatic channels or the draining lymph nodes, fluid accumulates within the lungs. However, this is seldom, if ever, the sole cause of pulmonary edema. For example, partial ligation of pulmonary lymphatics causes pulmonary edema in animals in which only a mild increase in left atrial pressure has resulted from production of a mitral valve lesion.[319, 320] A clinical counterpart of this experimental work was observed in three patients in whom pulmonary edema developed in the presence of mild mitral stenosis and coexisting pneumoconiosis;[321] a discrepancy between symptoms and hemodynamic abnormalities was consistent with the contributory role of pulmonary lymphatic obliteration by interstitial pulmonary fibrosis. One might anticipate that the systemic venous hypertension that occurs in isolated right ventricular decompensation might impede lymphatic flow to a degree that would result in pulmonary edema, but this is seldom the case. As Fishman has stated,[251] the combination of tachypneic ventilatory movements and muscular contraction of the walls of the large lymphatics presumably suffices to keep the lungs free of edema. However, right ventricular decompensation alone can occasionally be responsible for the development of overt pulmonary edema;[322] for example, two patients have been described in whom pure right-sided heart failure and chronically elevated systemic venous pressure were associated with roentgenologic evidence of septal lines.[323] Both patients had clinical evidence of long-standing right ventricular outflow obstruction (longer than 12 years) and right ventricular pressures approaching systemic levels; although jugular venous pressure was markedly and chronically elevated as a result of right atrial hypertension, in neither patient was there evidence of pulmonary venous hypertension.

PROTEIN SIEVING

A second safety factor that operates in hydrostatic but not in permeability edema is dilution of the interstitial protein, resulting in a decrease in interstitial osmotic pressure during increased fluid transport. This important safety factor is dependent on the relative impermeability of the microvascular endothelium to protein. As transvascular fluid movement increases as a result of elevated microvascular hydrostatic pressure, water transport outstrips protein transport; the resulting dilution of interstitial protein decreases the osmotic pressure and attenuates the change in driving pressure that would otherwise result.[324] A corollary to the dilution of interstitial proteins is the concentration of plasma proteins that must result if the exit of water exceeds that of protein.

INTERSTITIAL COMPLIANCE

The third safety factor that tends to minimize the accumulation of edema within the lungs is the increase in tissue pressure that accompanies the swelling of the interstitium. Although the precise pressure-volume relationship of the interstitial space is unknown, there is some agreement regarding the overall shape of the relationship.[259] As fluid accumulates in the interstitial space, the structure of the tightly compacted gel resists deformation and pressure increases sharply after only a slight increase in volume. Once a certain amount of fluid has accumulated, the compliance of the gel appears to increase so that further swelling occurs despite only a slight increase in pressure. In most tissues, an additional final phase of the pressure-volume relationship exists in which the interstitial compartment again becomes stiff; in the lung, the development of alveolar flooding at this stage opens up an enormous reserve for fluid accumulation and edema can accumulate rapidly with little increase in pressure. Morphologic studies[283] suggest that the pressure-volume characteristics of the peribronchovascular interstitium are such that this space may be more compliant than that of the alveolar walls because it is in this loose connective tissue that fluid first accumulates. Montaner and coworkers[325] have suggested that the integrity of the alveolar epithelium is an important component of this safety factor; in experimental studies on dogs, they found that there was more alveolar flooding and less accumulation of interstitial lung water in pulmonary edema induced by oleic acid than in hydrostatic pulmonary edema. To the extent that the epithelium resists alveolar flooding, interstitial pressure will increase as fluid accumulates in this space. If the epithelium is damaged, as occurs in ARDS, alveolar flooding can occur at a much lower interstitial pressure. This mechanism may be important not only as a protection against the accumulation of edema but also as a protection against the impairment of gas exchange, which is a result of edema. If interstitial pressure is high in edematous lung regions, vessels in that region will be compressed and blood flow will be redistributed to less edematous regions, minimizing the mismatching of ventilation and perfusion. This increase in interstitial pressure associated with fluid accumulation may be an explanation for the redistribution of pulmonary blood "flow" evident on erect chest roentgenograms in patients with pulmonary venous hypertension; presumably, the interstitial edema is predominant in lower lung zones. When interstitial pressure fails to increase because of generalized damage to the alveolar epithelium, blood flow to the edematous regions will not decrease; as a consequence, arterial desaturation caused by pulmonary shunt will be more severe than that associated with equivalent degrees of hydrostatic edema.

THE DEVELOPMENT OF PULMONARY EDEMA

The sequence of events that occurs during the development of pulmonary edema in experimental animal models has been described by Staub and his associates,[283] and is similar for both hydrostatic and permeability edema (see Fig. 4–56, page 546).

The Interstitial Phase

The earliest manifestation of pulmonary edema, when observed through the light microscope, is the appearance of fluid in the loose connective tissue around extra-alveolar conducting vessels and airways. Excess fluid widens the peribronchovascular interstitial space and interlobular septa and distends the lymphatics (Fig. 10–43). The appearance of fluid within this compartment occurs before there is evidence of alveolar flooding and when measurements of alveolar wall thickness are virtually normal.

The Alveolar Wall Phase

As the volume of edema fluid increases, there is a progressive increase in alveolar wall thickness as fluid accumulates in the thick side of the alveolocapillary membrane. Staub and his coworkers[283] observed a transition between this phase and overt alveolar edema in which small amounts of fluid accumulated within the airspaces but were confined to the alveolar "corners."

The Alveolar Airspace Phase

Morphologic studies[283, 326, 327] have indicated that alveolar flooding is an all-or-nothing phenomenon, alveoli being either liquid-filled or air-filled. The lack of intermediate grades of filling suggests that flooding of individual alveoli occurs rapidly and completely and that some alveoli fill independently of their neighbors. The walls of fluid-filled alveoli lose their circular shape and are folded, indicating loss of volume resulting from disruption of the normal surfactant layer by the edema fluid.

In both hydrostatic and permeability edema, the protein content of the fluid in the flooded alveolar airspaces is the same as that in the interstitium,[328, 329] implying that during alveolar flooding the epithelium has lost all ability to sieve and thus permits the outpouring of pure tissue fluid. It is easy to see how this could occur in permeability edema in which the epithelium of the alveolar wall is damaged, but exactly how the epithelial barrier gives way in hydrostatic edema is unresolved. Staub has suggested that the fluid may enter the peripheral airspaces via the small airway epithelial junctions rather than the alveolar membrane;[330] if interstitial pressure becomes sufficiently positive during edema formation, fluid may breach the epithelium of the small airways and flow peripherally to the alveoli, a mechanism Staub has termed "the overflowing bathtub theory."[330]

CLASSIFICATION OF PULMONARY EDEMA

It is convenient to classify the multiple causes of pulmonary edema into two major categories on the basis of underlying pathogenetic abnormality (Table 10–3). The first category includes those conditions in which the edema results from an increase in the pulmonary microvascular pressure. Left atrial hypertension caused by left ventricular decompensation or mitral stenosis is the most common cause of high-pressure pulmonary edema (hemodynamic edema, hydrostatic edema, cardiogenic edema). A decrease in the serum osmotic pressure or in interstitial fluid pressure can contribute to the development of hydrostatic edema, although these disorders do not cause edema by themselves. The basic abnormality in hydrostatic edema is an exaggeration of the normal transvascular fluid flux and an overwhelming of the safety factors that normally

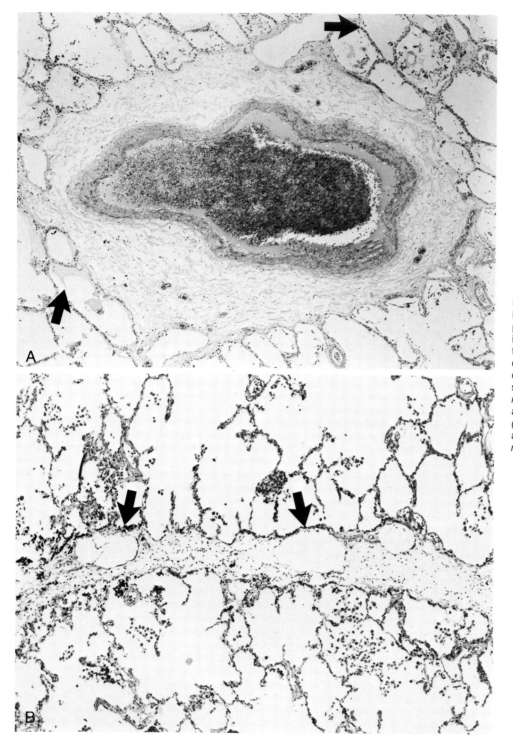

Figure 10–43. Interstitial Pulmonary Edema. *A,* A histologic section of a medium-sized pulmonary artery reveals widening of the perivascular interstitial tissue as a result of the presence of abundant fluid separating the connective tissue fibers. Mild airspace edema is also evident *(arrows)*. In the periphery of the lung, a section of an interlobular septum *(B)* shows similar widening as well as dilated lymphatic channels *(arrows)*. *(A, × 40; B, × 60.)*

Table 10–3. Classification of Pulmonary Edema

ELEVATED MICROVASCULAR PRESSURE (EMP)
Cardiogenic
    Left ventricular failure
    Mitral valvular disease
    Left atrial myxoma or thrombus
    Cor triatriatum
Affection of the pulmonary veins
    Primary (idiopathic) veno-occlusive disease
    Chronic sclerosing mediastinitis
Neurogenic
    Head trauma
    Increased intracranial pressure
    Postictal
NORMAL MICROVASCULAR PRESSURE (NMP)
(INCREASED CAPILLARY PERMEABILITY)
Inhalation of noxious fumes and soluble aerosols
    Nitrogen dioxide (silo-filler's disease)
    Sulfur dioxide
    Carbon monoxide
    Oxygen
    Ozone
    Smoke (burns)
    Ammonia
    Chlorine
    Phosgene
    Organophosphates
Aspiration of noxious fluids
    Liquid gastric contents (Mendelson's syndrome)
    Near-drowning
    Hypertonic contrast media
    Ethyl alcohol
High altitude
Transient tachypnea of the newborn
Rapid re-expansion of lung in thoracentesis
Other causes of NMP pulmonary edema
    Traumatic fat embolism
    Posttraumatic (contused lung)
    Acute radiation reaction
    Circulating toxins (alloxan, snake venom)
    Circulating vasoactive substances (histamine, kinins,
       prostaglandins, serotonin)
    Decreased capillary oncotic pressure
    Lymphatic insufficiency
COMBINED ELEVATION OF MICROVASCULAR
PRESSURE AND INCREASED CAPILLARY PERMEABILITY

control the volume of pulmonary extravascular water.

The second category includes those conditions in which the edema results from an increase in microvascular permeability (normal pressure pulmonary edema, low-pressure pulmonary edema, capillary leakage pulmonary edema, permeability pulmonary edema, noncardiogenic pulmonary edema). There are an enormous number of specific insults that can cause sufficiently widespread endothelial or epithelial damage (or both) to result in generalized pulmonary edema. Despite this variability of insults, the resulting clinical, roentgenographic, and pathologic manifestations are remarkably similar. The clinical features consist of acute respiratory failure characterized by a severe defect in the ability of the lungs to oxygenate the blood (hypoxemic respiratory failure) associated with little impairment in overall alveolar ventilation (i.e., the arterial PCO_2 is usually normal or decreased). This

clinical-pathologic-roentgenographic constellation has been termed the adult respiratory distress syndrome.[249, 250]

It is not always possible to assign individual patients with pulmonary edema to one of these major categories; in fact, a combination of permeability and cardiogenic edema is common. Coexistence of the two is particularly devastating because many of the safety factors that normally impede the accumulation of excess extravascular water are lost when the endothelium loses its selectivity for solutes.

PULMONARY EDEMA ASSOCIATED WITH ELEVATED MICROVASCULAR PRESSURE

Cardiogenic Pulmonary Edema

Undoubtedly, the most common cause of interstitial and airspace pulmonary edema is a rise in pulmonary venous pressure secondary to disease of the left side of the heart. Increased pressure within the left atrium can be transmitted to the pulmonary veins as a result of back pressure from the left ventricle (secondary to long-standing systemic hypertension, aortic valvular disease, cardiomyopathy, coronary artery disease, or myocardial infarction) or can be caused by obstruction to the left atrial outflow (as a result of mitral valve stenosis, left atrial myxoma, or cor triatriatum). Rarely, pulmonary venous hypertension can develop as a result of stenosis of the pulmonary veins themselves, either congenital (veno-occlusive disease) or acquired (sclerosing mediastinitis).

Roentgenographic Manifestations

The sequence of fluid accumulation in the lungs of dogs subjected to elevated microvascular pressure[283] is also observed in humans roentgenologically, there being two major patterns related to whether edema fluid remains relatively localized in the interstitial space or whether it occupies the airspaces of the lung also. The distinction between predominantly interstitial and predominantly airspace edema serves the useful purpose of describing two situations in which clinical and functional characteristics are different.

PREDOMINANTLY INTERSTITIAL EDEMA

Transudation of fluid into the interstitial spaces of the lung inevitably constitutes the first stage of pulmonary edema, since the capillaries are situated in this compartment. However, it must be appreciated that although this constitutes the first stage of fluid accumulation in the lungs, it is not the first sign of cardiac decompensation or pulmonary venous hypertension. As discussed previously (*see* page

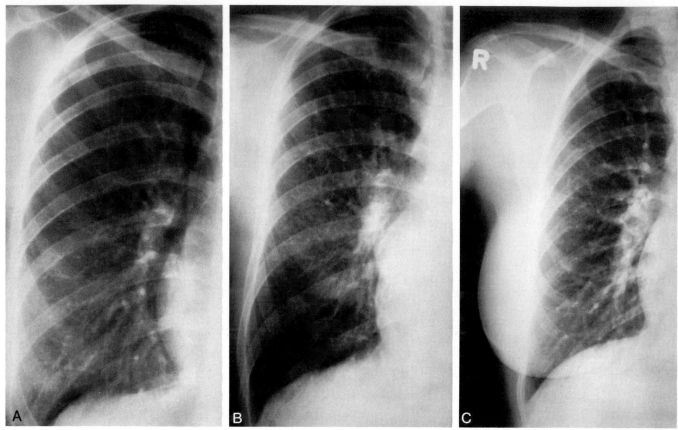

Figure 10–44. Recruitment of Upper Lobe Vessels in Postcapillary Hypertension and Left-to-Right Shunt: Roentgenographic Distinction. A view of the right lung from a conventional posteroanterior chest roentgenogram (*A*) is normal. Note that in the erect position, the upper-lobe arteries and veins are much smaller than those in the lower lobe, a reflection of the influence of gravity on blood flow. The vasculature is well defined throughout. Contrast this appearance with that in two patients with increased blood flow to the upper lobes, in *B* caused by mitral stenosis and in *C* by an atrial septal defect (ASD). *B,* Upper-lobe vessels are dilated; lower-lobe vessels are narrowed and ill-defined as a result of interstitial edema. These features are typical of postcapillary hypertension. *C,* Upper-lobe *and* lower-lobe vessels are larger than normal and are sharply defined, findings indicative of a left-to-right shunt (ASD in this instance). Note that the cause of the upper-zone vessel recruitment in *B* and *C* cannot be distinguished by the appearance of the upper-lobe vessels alone.

1863), venous hypertension usually is evidenced by redistribution of blood flow from lower to upper lung zones, so that an increase in caliber of upper zone vessels usually precedes evidence of overt edema. However, it is well to remember that upper lobe vessel "recruitment" also occurs in a number of other situations—e.g., intracardiac left-to-right shunts (Fig. 10–44). When pulmonary venous hypertension is moderate in degree or transient,[331] fluid transudation occurs into the alveolar interstitial space whence it flows rapidly centripetally and accumulates within the perivascular sheath and interlobular septa. It is this anatomic localization that produces the typical roentgenographic pattern of loss of the normal sharp definition of pulmonary vascular markings and thickening of the interlobular septa (A and B lines of Kerley—Figure 10–45). Although the presence of septal lines can be of value in confirming the diagnosis when other signs are equivocal, in our experience the frequency with which they can be identified is low compared with loss of definition of vessel markings; thus, their absence should not be construed as evidence against the diagnosis. Similarly, we have not been impressed

with the value of loss of definition of hilar pulmonary vessels as a sign of interstitial edema. Although it is frequently cited as a reliable sign of interstitial edema, in our experience the definition of hilar pulmonary arteries is seldom lost in cases of "pure" interstitial pulmonary edema, and for good reason. Since the major bronchi and arteries situated within the hila do not enter the lung until after they have divided into lobar branches, they do not possess the peribronchial and perivascular interstitium that is characteristic of intrapulmonary bronchovascular bundles. Thus, there is no reason for them to lose their definition until alveolar edema affects contiguous parenchyma and obscures their margin by a silhouetting effect. Loss of demarcation of hilar shadows should therefore be considered a sign of airspace rather than interstitial edema.

In circumstances in which edema fluid accumulates in the *parenchymal* interstitial tissues (the alveolar wall phase of Staub and associates[283]) but before the development of overt airspace edema, the accumulation usually is invisible or only faintly discernible roentgenographically as a "haze," which tends to be predominantly lower zonal or parahilar in distribution. The sequence of redistribution of blood flow, loss of the sharp marginal contour of pulmonary vessels, and, finally, perihilar haze and rosette formation was observed by McHugh and associates in 30 patients with recent myocardial infarction. Generally, the severity of roentgenographic abnormalities correlated well with pulmonary wedge pressure,[175] although it has been suggested that in acute cardiac disease states, there exists a phase lag between elevation of pulmonary wedge pressure and roentgenographic signs of pulmonary edema, possibly because of a slow transudation of fluid into the extravascular space.[332] The heart usually is enlarged, but this may not be apparent when the exciting cause is recent myocardial infarction, coronary insufficiency,[333] restrictive cardiomyopathy, left atrial myxoma, cor triatriatum, acute systemic hypertension such as that occasioned by an adrenal pheochromocytoma, or, occasionally, mitral stenosis or aortic stenosis.

If evidence for interstitial pulmonary edema is equivocal as judged from the signs described, confirmatory evidence may be provided in some cases by appreciating an increased thickness of the wall of bronchi commonly seen end-on in the parahilar zones. These bronchial walls, which we have identified in 80 per cent of a large number of normal subjects, are normally hairline in thickness (in the

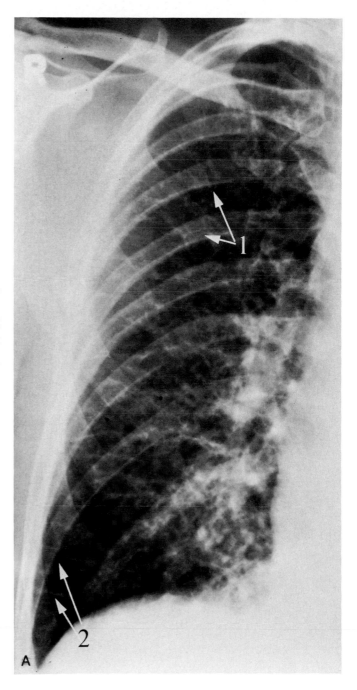

Figure 10–45. Acute Interstitial Pulmonary Edema. A view of the right lung from a posteroanterior chest roentgenogram (*A*) reveals the classic features of acute interstitial edema—septal A (*1*) and B (*2*) lines, and thickened and ill-defined bronchovascular bundles. Evidence for recruitment of upper-zone vessels is not at all convincing, a common finding in our experience in patients with *acute* interstitial edema of any etiology. The patient was an elderly man seen 4 hours after the onset of anterior chest pain caused by myocardial infarction.

Illustration continued on following page

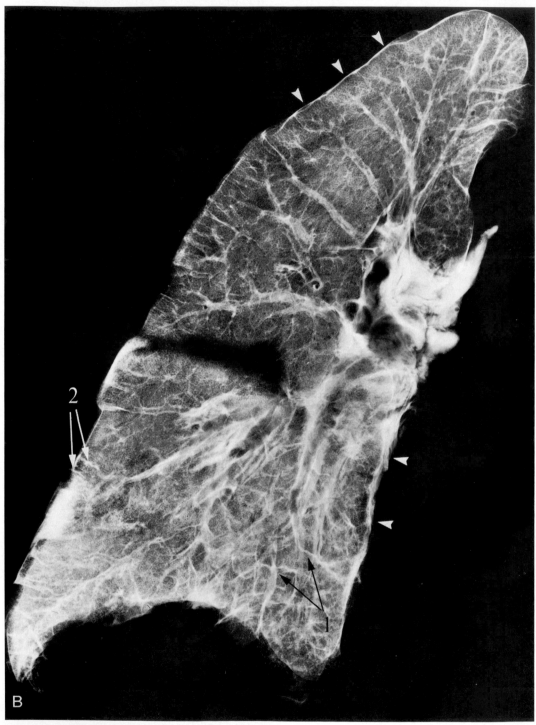

Figure 10–45 *Continued* A roentgenogram of a coronal slice through the right lung following an autopsy of a different patient (*B*) reveals similar features—septal A lines (*1*) and B lines (*2*) and thickened peribronchovascular interstitium. Note the thickened pleura (*arrowheads*), indicating the presence of pleural edema.

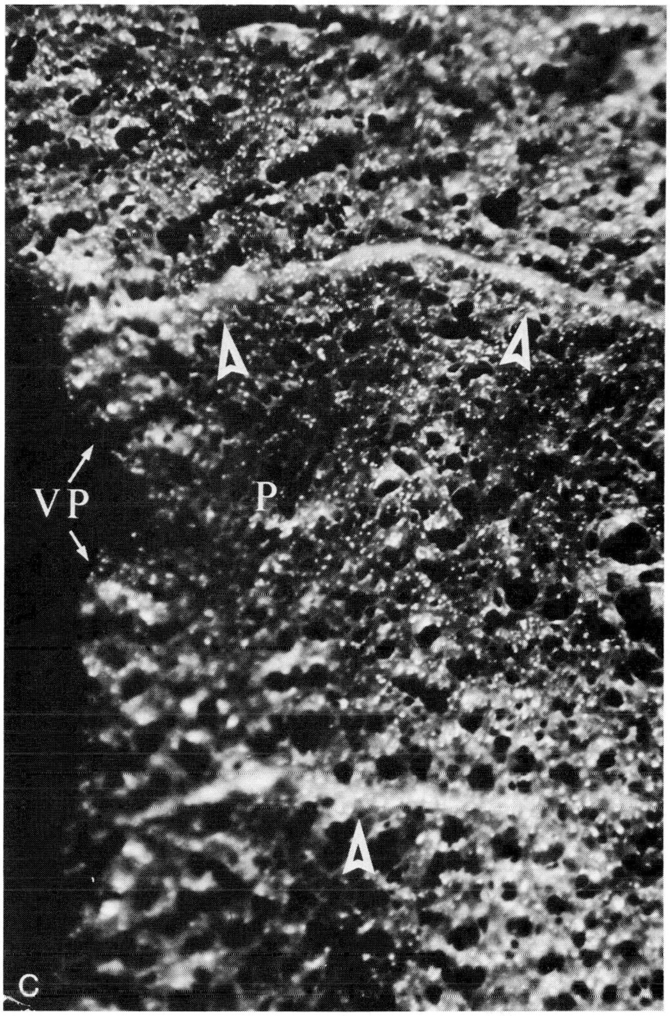

Figure 10–45 *Continued* A magnified view (*C*) of a portion of the gross specimen in *B* reveals two edematous interlobular septa (*arrowheads*) that extend perpendicular to the visceral pleura (VP, P), thus identifying them as septal B lines. (*A* and *B* from Genereux GP: Med Radiogr Photogr *61*:2, 1985.)

absence of severe chronic bronchitis). When fluid accumulates in the loose interstitial tissue surrounding them, their shadow thickens and loses its sharp definition (Fig. 10–46). Similar thickening can occur in large central airways such as the intermediate stem bronchus (Fig. 10–47). Along with Heitzman,[334] we have employed this sign to advantage in some cases in which other signs of interstitial edema have not been convincing; however, in the individual patient, it is often difficult to exclude chronic bronchitis as the cause of the bronchial wall thickening, particularly in the absence of a clinical history. In this regard, Don and Johnson[335] have suggested that peribronchial cuffing may be caused not only by an accumulation of edema fluid in the peribronchial interstitium but also by edema of the bronchial wall itself secondary to transudation from capillaries in the bronchial circulation. This should conceivably result in a narrowing of the lumen of bronchi viewed end-on, and we agree that narrowing is apparent in some cases. However, an alternative explanation for lumen narrowing is loss of pulmonary compliance: the accumulation of excess water makes the lungs stiffer than normal and reduces compliance; it is inevitable that the reduc-

tion in lung volume achieved on inspiration will be associated with a reduction in the diameter of bronchial lumens. It is possible that both mechanisms are operative; clearly, further work is necessary to clarify these issues.

Another sign of interstitial edema, but one that usually becomes evident only when the accumulation of excess water is severe, is thickening of the interlobar fissures by fluid accumulation in the pleural interstitium (Fig. 10–48).[336–338] The pleural connective tissue layer is in continuity with the interlobular septa, and it is reasonable to assume that when edema fluid accumulates in the latter sites (creating Kerley B lines), it might also collect in the pleural interstitium. In such circumstances, the excess fluid causes not only a thickening of the interlobar fissures but a widening of the pleural layer over the convexity of the lungs, particularly in the costophrenic recesses, an abnormality that is sometimes confused with pleural effusion. Small pleural effusions may be present in addition, of course.

In a hemodynamic, electrocardiographic, and roentgenographic assessment of 36 acutely ill patients with myocardial infarction or serious angina,

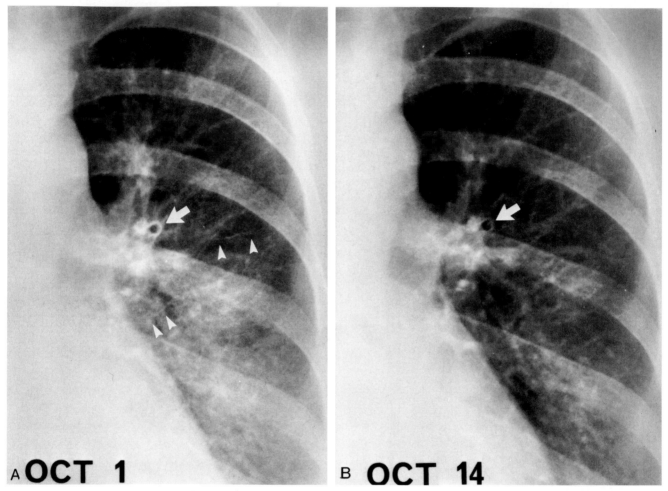

Figure 10–46. Peribronchial Cuffing in Pulmonary Edema. A detail view of the upper half of the left lung from a posteroanterior chest roentgenogram (*A*) reveals distended upper-lobe vessels, perihilar haze, septal A lines (*arrowheads*), and a thickened bronchial wall viewed end-on (*arrow*). A few days later, following diuretic therapy (*B*), signs of pulmonary edema had resolved. Note the decreased thickness of the bronchial wall (*arrow*). The patient is a middle-aged woman with renal failure.

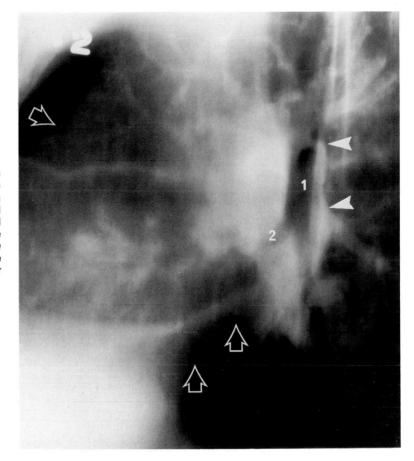

Figure 10–47. Thickening of the Intermediate Stem Line in Pulmonary Edema. A detail view of the right hilum from a conventional lateral tomogram shows a thickened posterior wall of the right main and intermediate bronchi (*arrowheads*). The abnormal bronchial wall is located posterior to the intermediate (*1*) and middle-lobe (*2*) bronchi. Septal A lines (*open arrows*) are present in the upper and lower lobes. The patient is a middle-aged man with mild left ventricular decompensation.

Heikkilä and associates[339] found a very good correlation between pulmonary arterial wedge pressure and evidence of pulmonary venous hypertension as assessed from bedside chest roentgenograms. They found that a normal chest roentgenogram was an exceptional feature of the early stages of recent myocardial infarction, since evidence for pulmonary venous hypertension presented itself immediately after mean left ventricular filling pressure rose above 10 mm Hg. Similarly, in a study of 26 patients admitted to a coronary care unit with recent myocardial infarction in whom abnormalities in bedside chest roentgenograms were correlated with pulmonary arterial diastolic pressure (assumed to reflect left ventricular end diastolic pressure), Bennett and Rees[340] found that a normal chest roentgenogram almost always correctly indicated a pulmonary arterial diastolic pressure less than 14 mm Hg. Roentgenographic evidence of pulmonary venous hypertension usually indicated a pulmonary diastolic pressure higher than 14 mm Hg, but was seen on several occasions with pressures below this level. However, both groups of investigators[339, 340] observed a time lag between the fall of pressure and roentgenologic improvement, which they considered of potential therapeutic significance. In some cases this "out of phase" delay in the disappearance of interstitial edema lasted for 12 to 22 hours after left ventricular filling pressure had returned to normal as the result of treatment. Heikkilä and colleagues found that acute sequential variation in left ventricular filling pressure was paralleled more closely by the terminal forces of the electrocardiographic P wave than by any other recorded variable. McHugh and coworkers[175] found that serious roentgenologic misinterpretation of left ventricular failure occurred occasionally in the presence of severe hypoxemia. They also observed considerable phase lags, i.e., pulmonary wedge pressure rose before roentgenographic signs became apparent and pulmonary edema persisted following successful therapy and lowering of wedge pressure to normal.

McCredie[341] has shown that measurement of pulmonary extravascular fluid volume (PEV) is an even more sensitive method for detecting abnormal quantities of fluid in the interstitial space. The PEV is the amount of fluid surrounding the perfused pulmonary vascular bed and obviously is increased in patients with pulmonary congestion and edema. Using a double isotope dilution technique, McCredie studied 45 patients with valvular heart disease and nine normal subjects and showed that there was roentgenologic evidence of interstitial pulmonary edema in only seven of the 18 patients in whom the PEV was above the normal range. The increase in PEV correlated with changes in pulmonary arterial and left atrial pressures, a relationship

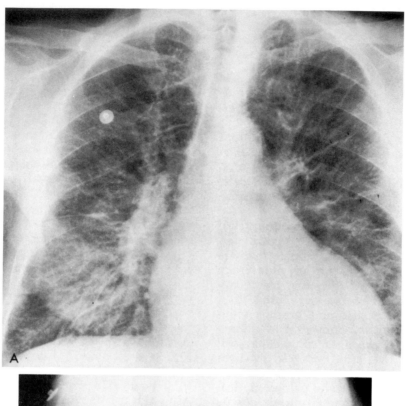

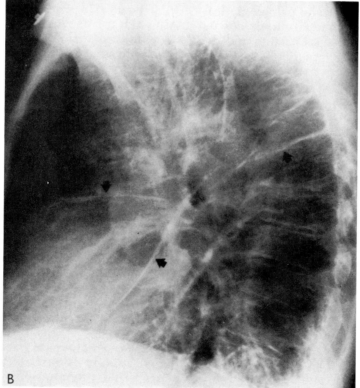

Figure 10–48. Interstitial Pulmonary Edema. Posteroanterior (*A*) and lateral (*B*) roentgenograms reveal multiple linear opacities throughout both lungs. These lines consist of a combination of long septal lines (Kerley A) and shorter peripheral septal lines (Kerley B). In lateral projection (*B*), the interlobar fissures are very prominent (*arrows*), representing pleural edema.

Illustration continued on following page

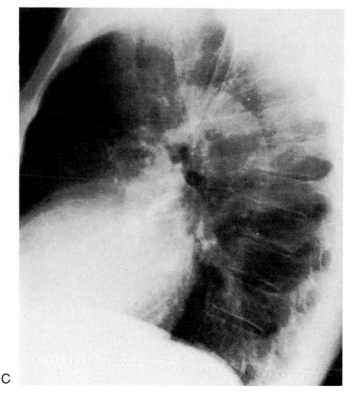

Figure 10–48 *Continued* Twenty-four hours later (*C*), the edema in the pleural interstitium had cleared completely.

C

that presumably reflected increased transudation of fluid as a result of increased intracapillary pressure.

Despite the phase lags described previously, the chest roentgenogram remains a reasonably accurate subjective method of diagnosing pulmonary edema. However, a number of imaging techniques exist that are capable of determining the quantity of excess water in the lungs objectively, including CT,[342] compton-scatter densitometry,[343] emission CT,[344, 708] and the uptake by the lungs of thallium 201. Tamaki and associates[345] showed a significantly higher uptake of thallium 201 in patients with pulmonary congestion or edema than in a group of normal controls and have recommended this technique as an extension of myocardial imaging. It also appears probable that magnetic resonance imaging (MRI) may be capable of quantifying extravascular lung water with some precision, although at the time of this writing, accumulated data are speculative and based on preliminary studies.[346-349]

With adequate treatment of the edema, the roentgenologic signs may disappear within a matter of hours (Fig. 10–48).

AIRSPACE EDEMA

Interstitial edema invariably precedes alveolar edema (Fig. 10–49), and in some patients the chest roentgenogram shows evidence of both simultaneously.[350] The sheet anchor in the roentgenologic diagnosis of airspace edema is the acinar shadow (Fig. 10–50). In the majority of cases, these shadows are confluent, creating irregular, rather poorly de-fined, patchy opacities of unit density scattered randomly throughout the lungs; in the medial third of the lungs particularly, coalescence of acinar consolidation is common. Incomplete acinar filling can result in a subacinar pattern (Fig. 10–51). The distribution varies from patient to patient but may be surprisingly similar during different episodes in one patient. In acute pulmonary edema resulting from left ventricular failure, which commonly follows myocardial infarction, patchy airspace consolidation sometimes extends to the subpleural zone or "cortex" of the lung (Fig. 10–52)—although the cortex may be completely spared, thus creating the "bat's wing" or "butterfly" pattern of edema (*see* farther on). Although the effects of gravity on the distribution of blood flow and ventilation in the normal lung have been well established, its effects on the distribution of acute pulmonary edema are not as clear. As pointed out by Fishman,[683] gravity predisposes to dependent edema both by generating higher hydrostatic pressures toward the bases and by draining interstitial fluid toward the bases via the continuous interstitial spaces. However, opposing these forces are the augmented ventilatory movements that promote the removal of fluid via the lymphatics and that are considerably more vigorous in lower than in upper lung zones. The net effect of these opposing forces is difficult to predict but, from a practical point of view, they result in maximal fluid accumulation in the lower and central lung zones.

Edema caused by cardiac disease usually is bilateral and fairly symmetric, although it may be

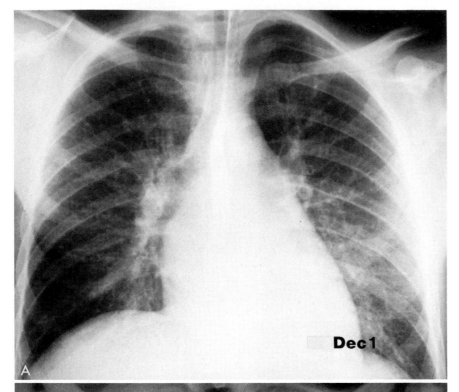

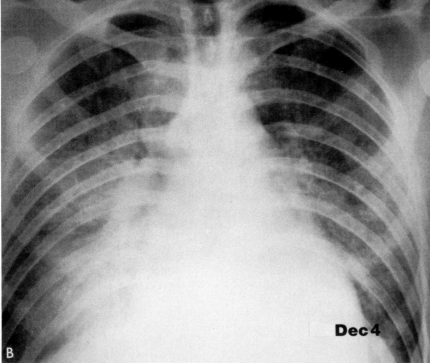

Figure 10–49. Interstitial Edema Progressing to Airspace Edema in Association with Severe Valvular Disease and Subacute Bacterial Endocarditis. The initial posteroanterior roentgenogram of this 22-year-old man (*A*) reveals diffuse interstitial edema manifested by loss of definition of vessel markings throughout both lungs and by septal lines in both costophrenic recesses. Three days later (*B*), the lungs had become massively consolidated by airspace edema. Heart size had increased considerably in this interval. Proved aortic insufficiency, mitral insufficiency, and subacute bacterial endocarditis.

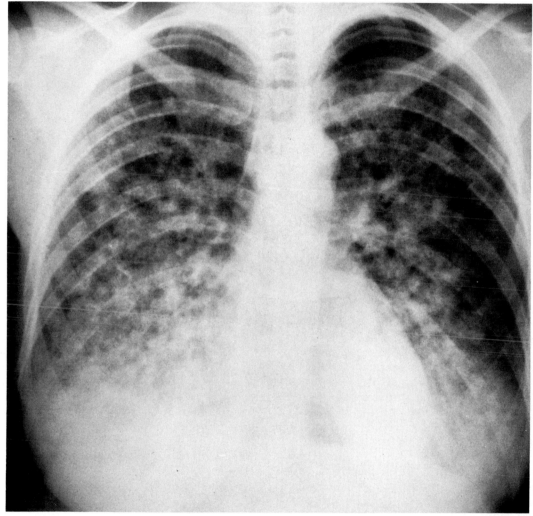

Figure 10–50. Acute Airspace Pulmonary Edema. A posteroanterior roentgenogram reveals widespread patchy airspace consolidation. Individual acinar shadows can be visualized in some areas, although generally these are coalescent, particularly in the lower lung zones. Cardiac size and configuration are normal. This 20-year-old woman had severe, periodic systemic arterial hypertension caused by a pheochromocytoma of the adrenal gland. The possibility that this represented permeability odema (ARDS) rather than cardiogenic edema was not excluded.

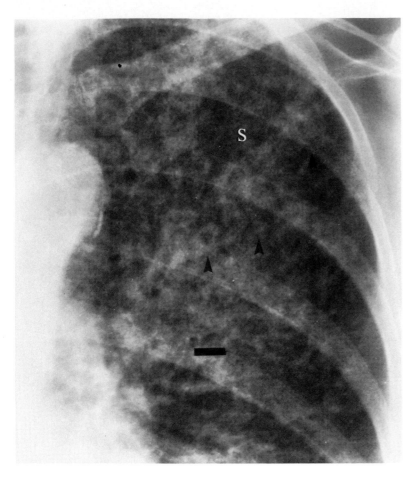

Figure 10–51. Subacinar Pattern in Acute Air-space Pulmonary Edema. A detail view of the left upper lobe from a posteroanterior chest roentgenogram shows multiple subacinar opacities (*arrowheads*) that are interspersed against a background of micro-nodules (stippling, S). These features are typical of incomplete filling of acini by pulmonary edema. The bar represents 1 cm. The patient is a middle-aged man in whom an episode of systemic hypotension developed during cardiac catheterization. (From Genereux GP: Med Radiogr Photogr 62:2, 1985.)

predominantly unilateral or in other respects "inappropriate"—that is, occupying zones of one or both lungs out of keeping with the "expected" distribution of disease arising from a central influence.[351, 352] The mechanisms underlying the development of unilateral pulmonary edema were reviewed by Azimi and associates[353] on the basis of its presence in 15 patients and have been tabulated more recently by Calenoff and his colleagues.[354] The latter authors divided the causes of unilateral pulmonary edema into two groups, ipsilateral and contralateral: *ipsilateral edema* refers to those conditions in which the pathogenetic mechanism exists on the same side as the edema and is usually associated with an alteration in the alveolocapillary membrane. Conditions listed in this category included systemic-to-pulmonary shunts in congenital heart disease, bronchial obstruction (the "drowned" lung), unilateral veno-occlusive disease, prolonged lateral decubitus position, unilateral aspiration, pulmonary contusion, and rapid thoracentesis of either air or fluid. Two cases have also been described[355] in which unilateral edema developed in the remaining lobe following lobectomy; in both cases it was caused by thrombosis of ipsilateral veins. *Contralateral edema* refers to the accumulation of excess water in a "normal" lung opposite to one with a perfusion defect. Conditions listed by Calenoff and associates[354] include proximal interruption of a pul-

monary artery, Swyer-James syndrome, acute pulmonary thromboembolism, local emphysema, lobectomy, rapid re-expansion of pneumothorax in a patient with left heart failure, systemic-to-pulmonary artery shunt, pleural disease, and unilateral sympathectomy.

In patients with cardiac decompensation, unilateral edema is probably related primarily to dependency. Leeming[356] reviewed 357 chest roentgenograms of 25 patients with pulmonary edema who were receiving intermittent positive pressure ventilation and who were often positioned on their side to promote drainage; 68 per cent of the roentgenograms showed gravity-dependent asymmetric edema and only 18 per cent showed edema predominantly in the "up" lung. Sometimes the edema was seen to shift to the contralateral lung after the patient's position was changed to the opposite side. We have seen one patient (Figure 10–53) in whom pulmonary edema was uniquely right-sided on repeated episodes of acute cardiac decompensation. When questioned, he replied that he always lay on his right side because lying on his back or left side produced marked discomfort and anxiety (a positional peculiarity apparently quite common in patients with recent myocardial infarction). It is noteworthy that predominantly unilateral edema is often right-sided, raising the question of whether the left-sided cardiac enlargement that develops in most of these patients might physically impede blood flow in the left pulmonary artery, thereby reducing capillary volume. Such a reduction certainly operates in some patients with "inappropriate" anatomic distribution of edema. We have seen examples in patients with unilateral or lobar thromboembolic disease and in others with localized pulmonary emphysema (Fig. 10–54) and unilateral fibrothorax (Fig. 10–55). Others have reported unilateral pulmonary edema in association with proximal interruption of a pulmonary artery[357] and Swyer-James syndrome.[358, 359] This theory of unequal capillary blood flow is supported by the occurrence of unilateral chronic pulmonary edema associated with pleural effusion following the surgical creation of left-to-right shunts for various congenital cardiac anomalies.[360, 361] In these cases, the pathogenesis probably is related to a combination of increased pulmonary venous pressure and capillary damage

resulting from excessive blood flow to the affected lung. Uncommon causes of unilateral pulmonary edema include raised intracranial pressure,[362] administration of 0.5 N saline through a central venous catheter inadvertently placed in a pulmonary artery,[363] and unilateral thoracic sympathectomy.[364] In the last named, one patient developed unilateral edema following contralateral sympathectomy in ARDS. The occurrence of unilateral edema in a reexpanded lung after thoracentesis of air or liquid is discussed on page 1952.

When edema is predominantly unilateral or in other ways "inappropriate," the differential diagnosis from pneumonia may be difficult[365] but may be facilitated by roentgenologic visualization of changes typical of interstitial edema. Zimmerman and his colleagues[366] have employed the "gravitational shift test" to distinguish pulmonary edema from pneumonia: by comparing bedside chest

Text continued on page 1916

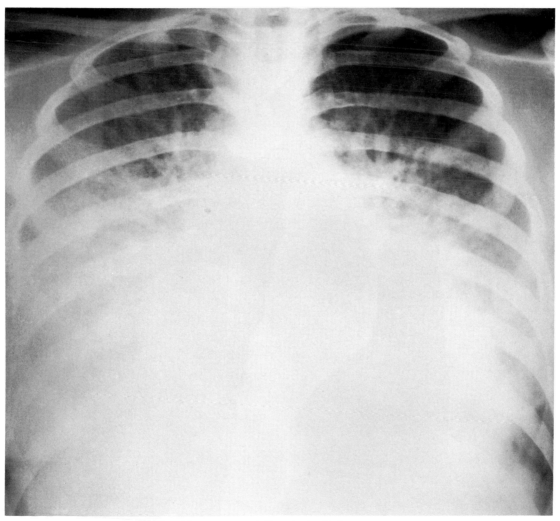

Figure 10–52. Acute Pulmonary Edema Secondary to Left Ventricular Failure. A posteroanterior roentgenogram reveals extensive consolidation of both lungs extending out to the visceral pleural surfaces. Much of the consolidation is homogeneous but individual acinar shadows can be identified in the upper lung zones. The heart is moderately enlarged. The patient, a 12-year-old girl, had had acute glomerulonephritis 2 years previously and subsequently severe systemic hypertension had developed. Six hours prior to this roentgenogram, she had the abrupt onset of severe dyspnea, pleuritic pain, and cough productive of copious frothy sputum. Both the clinical and roentgenographic pictures are typical of acute pulmonary edema secondary to left ventricular failure.

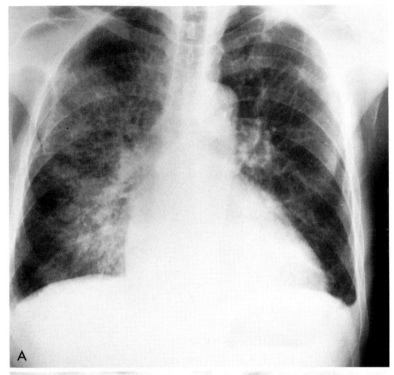

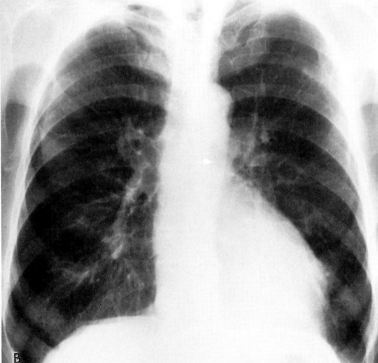

Figure 10–53. Predominantly Unilateral Pulmonary Edema: Diffuse Emphysema. A posteroanterior roentgenogram (*A*) of a 70-year-old man admitted with acute myocardial infarction reveals patchy airspace consolidation occupying the medial two thirds of the right lung characteristic of acute pulmonary edema. The left lung is unaffected, although there is a small left pleural effusion. The heart is moderately enlarged. A visit to the patient's bedside revealed the fact that he lay on his right side most of the time, since other positions seemed to intensify his shortness of breath. A roentgenogram following resolution of the edema (*B*) shows a marked increase in volume of both lungs characteristic of diffuse pulmonary emphysema. The unilaterality of the edema was clearly related to the influence of gravity. It cannot be explained on the basis of emphysema, since this disease is bilateral and symmetric.

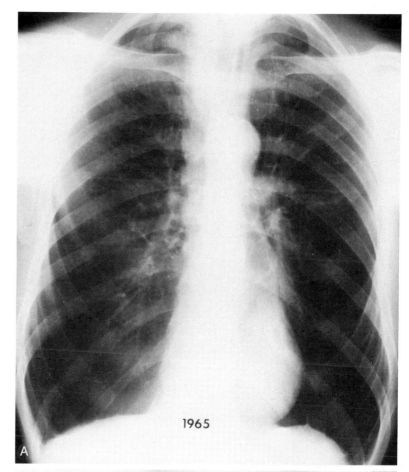

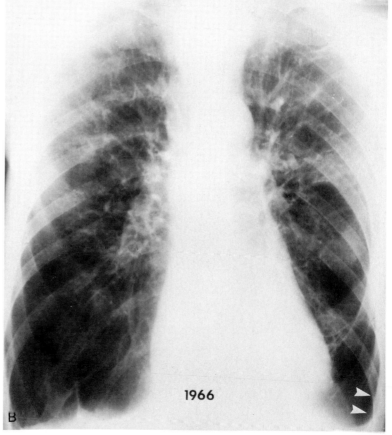

Figure 10–54. Atypical Pattern of Pulmonary Edema Associated with Predominantly Lower-Lobe Emphysema. A posteroanterior chest roentgenogram (A) shows pulmonary overinflation and striking lower-lobe oligemia indicative of advanced emphysema. Cardiac size and hilar shadows are normal. Approximately 1 year later (B), the heart had increased in size and upper-lobe vessels had become larger and poorly defined as a result of the accumulation of interstitial edema; note that lower-lobe vessels remain inconspicuous. A small pleural effusion is present on the left (arrowhead). The patient is an elderly man with a long history of chronic obstructive pulmonary disease.

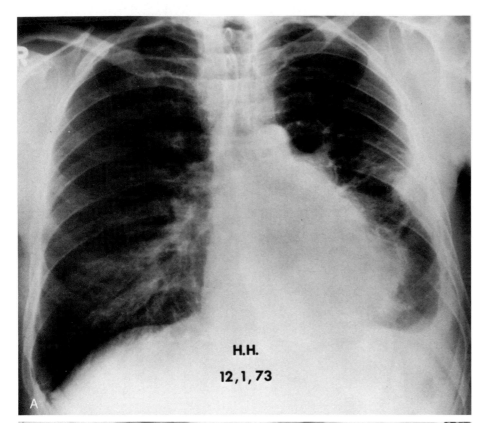

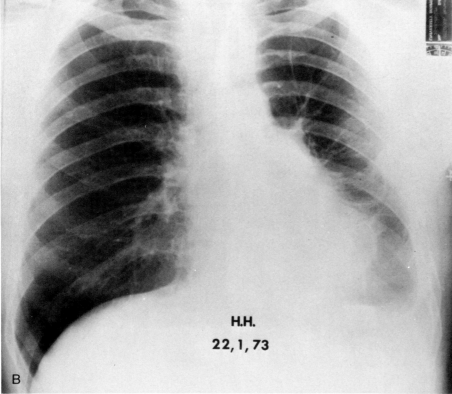

Figure 10–55. Atypical Pattern of Pulmonary Edema Caused by Unilateral Fibrothorax. A conventional posteroanterior chest roentgenogram (A) shows the typical features of left heart failure in the *right* lung as evidenced by upper-lobe redistribution of blood flow and loss of definition of bronchovascular bundles as a result of interstitial edema. However, note the absence of such findings in the left lung. The pleura is irregularly thickened over the lower half of this lung, suggesting that unilateral fibrothorax may be inhibiting ventilation with resulting hypoperfusion. Several days later, following diuretic therapy (B), signs of cardiac decompensation had resolved.

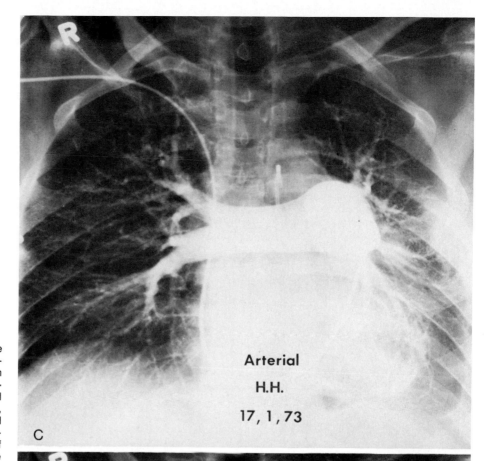

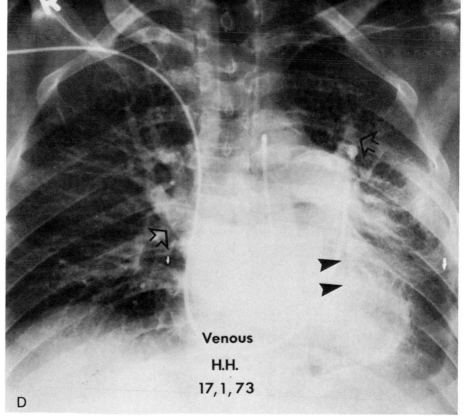

Figure 10–55 *Continued* Because of the possibility of pulmonary thromboembolism, a pulmonary angiogram was performed, revealing normal vessels in the right lung during both arterial (*C*) and venous (*D*) phases. However, note the increased resistance to blood flow through the left lower lobe as indicated by persistent opacification of the arteries (*arrowheads*) and absence of opacified veins during the venous phase of the study; the veins (*open arrows*) in the left upper lobe and right lung are normally opacified. There is no evidence of thromboembolism. The patient is an elderly man with a prior history of a traumatic hemothorax.

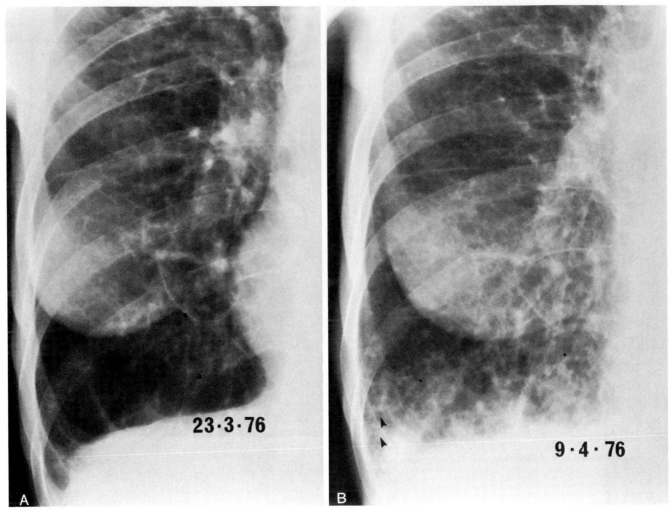

Figure 10–56. Atypical Pattern of Pulmonary Edema Associated with Bullae. A detail view of the lower half of the right lung from a posteroanterior chest roentgenogram (*A*) shows pulmonary overinflation, oligemia, and curvilinear displacement of vessels indicative of bullae. Approximately 2 weeks later, a repeat chest roentgenogram (*B*) reveals a coarse reticular pattern throughout the lower half of the right lung reminiscent of advanced interstitial lung disease. Septal B lines can be identified in the costophrenic angle (*arrowheads*). The sequence indicates that acute interstitial edema has rendered the usually invisible walls of bullae roentgenographically visible, thus forming the reticular pattern; without the prior film for comparison, it would be difficult to exclude the presence of chronic interstitial lung disease. The patient is a middle-aged woman with emphysema caused by alpha 1-antitrypsin deficiency. (From Genereux GP: Med Radiogr Photogr *61*:2, 1985.)

roentgenograms of patients examined in the supine position and after prolonged lateral decubitus positioning, these authors were able to distinguish the two conditions by observing a shift of edema fluid from one lung to the other while no change occurred in the anatomic location of pneumonia. We doubt that it is worth all the trouble; in patients in whom doubt exists, a trial of diuretic therapy with or without antibiotics would appear to be more efficacious and less time-consuming.

The roentgenologic characteristics of *septal lines* (Kerley A and B lines) are discussed in detail in Chapter 4 (*see* page 623). Several studies have indicated that Kerley B lines that are due to interstitial pulmonary edema may develop when pulmonary venous pressure (wedge pressure) is 17 to 20 mm Hg or higher.[5–12] Disappearance of the lines generally parallels that of other signs of the edema,

and their persistence after adequate therapy (such as mitral commissurotomy for mitral stenosis) usually indicates that chronic congestion and edema of the septa have led to irreversible fibrosis and hemosiderosis. Occasionally, the development of interstitial edema in patients with emphysema will make visible the walls of air sacs that cannot be seen in its absence (Fig. 10–56).

Like interstitial pulmonary edema, airspace pulmonary edema usually clears fairly rapidly in response to adequate treatment of the underlying condition, and resolution appears complete roentgenographically in not more than 3 days in most cases. It is likely that the degree of efficiency of the lymphatic system plays a major role in clearance time. Studies of lymph flow before and after experimental induction of acute heart failure showed lymph drainage to increase to 300 to 2800 per cent.[317] Pulmonary edema may clear more slowly when lymphatic drainage is hindered by factors such as systemic venous hypertension.

THE "BAT'S-WING" OR "BUTTERFLY" PATTERN OF EDEMA

These terms describe an anatomic distribution of airspace edema in which the hilum and "medulla" of the lungs are fairly uniformly consolidated and the peripheral 2 to 3 cm of lung parenchyma—the "cortex"—is relatively uninvolved (Fig. 10–57). Definition of the margin of consolidated parenchyma often is rather indistinct but may be remarkably sharp. Resolution of the edema generally begins in the periphery and spreads medially.[370] Nessa and Rigler[352] recorded an incidence of 5 per cent in 110 cases of moderate to severe edema of varying etiology. Although it has been said that this pattern of edema is seen commonly in association with uremia, Hodson[367] states that there is convincing evidence that the lesion is the result of acute left ventricular failure and that it bears no specific relationship to uremia. Localization of the edema

to the hilar and medullary portions of the lungs may be apparent in both posteroanterior and lateral roentgenographic projections,[368] and can be apparent in interstitial as well as airspace pulmonary edema, particularly on CT (Fig. 10–58). The freedom from involvement of the "cortex" usually extends along the interlobar lung fissures as well as around the convexity of the thorax, thereby creating a waist-like indentation visible in posteroanterior projection in the region of the minor fissure. Similarly, the upper and lower paramediastinal zones may be relatively free of involvement. Steckel[369] made the observation that a thin radiolucency parallel to the cardiac and aortic borders may be identified in some cases of acute pulmonary edema. He attributed this effect to contiguity of lung and heart; the active pulsation might accelerate fluid clearance from immediately adjacent parenchyma. Conversely, the absence of such a radiolucent line (which he termed the kinetic border line) may indicate a silent or akinetic heart or possibly a pericardial effusion.

Many theories have been propounded to explain the mechanism of this usual anatomic distri-

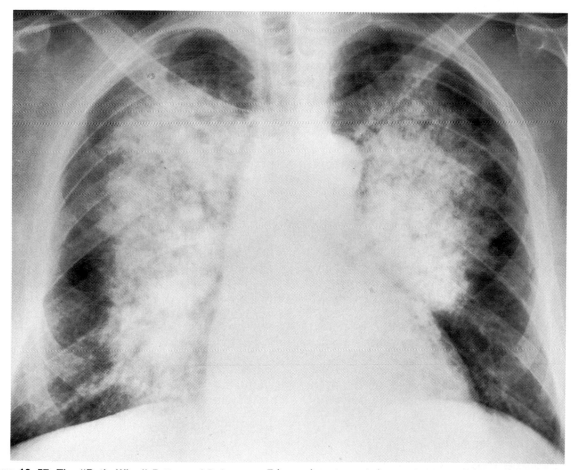

Figure 10–57. The "Bat's-Wing" Pattern of Pulmonary Edema. A posteroanterior roentgenogram demonstrates consolidation of the parahilar and "medullary" portions of both lungs, creating a bat's wing or "butterfly" appearance; the "cortex" of both lungs is relatively unaffected. The margins of the edematous lung are rather sharply defined. The consolidation is fairly homogeneous and is associated with a well-defined air bronchogram on both sides. This 59-year-old man had suffered a massive myocardial infarction 48 hours previously; he had a cough productive of pinkish sputum but was able to lie flat in bed.

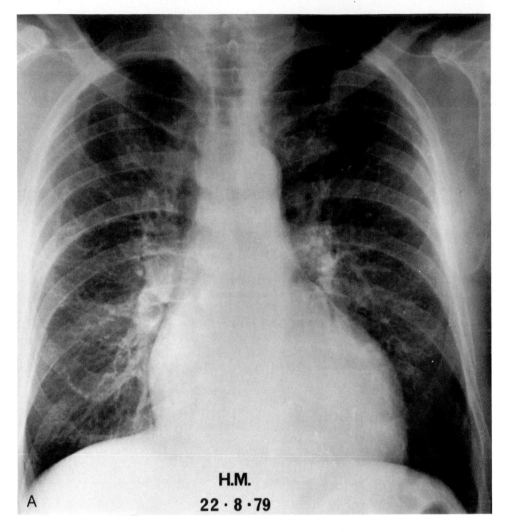

Figure 10–58. Interstitial Pulmonary Edema: CT Manifestations. A conventional posteroanterior chest roentgenogram (*A*) shows moderate left ventricular enlargement, slightly dilated upper-lobe vessels, and a loss of definition of vessels throughout both lungs indicative of diffuse interstitial edema.

bution of pulmonary edema.[371] Only three are considered here.

1. One of the more likely theories, proposed by Herrnheiser and Hinson[370] and by Prichard and her coworkers,[372] relates the distribution of the edema to peculiarities of the pulmonary vascular tree. The lungs may be divided anatomically into three portions: (a) *the hilar root area*, which contains chiefly conducting channels and little or no pulmonary parenchyma; (b) *the medullary area*, which includes the second, third, and fourth orders of bronchial and vascular divisions, with respiratory tissue intervening; and (c) *the cortex*, which measures 30 to 40 mm in thickness at the periphery of the lung and consists almost entirely of parenchyma. It has been suggested that the arterioles of the cortex may be particularly adapted for vasoconstriction or vasodilatation, much the same as in the kidney.[372] Vasoconstriction would result in the shunting of blood to the medullary zones of the lung, thus protecting the cortex from the insult of edema. In addition, the precapillary network of the medulla is disproportionately short compared with the major branches from which it arises. Because of this, high pressure within the pulmonary arteries can be readily transmitted to precapillaries and thence to the

proximal capillaries.[373] These anatomic differences in the pulmonary vasculature of the two zones may make the medulla more susceptible to transudation of fluid.

2. The experimental work on dogs by Borgström and coworkers[374] led them to the conclusion that the anatomic distribution of edema in the lungs is related to peculiarities of the pulmonary arterial and bronchial arterial circulations. They showed that when hypervolemia was present the injection of toxic material (desoxycholate) into the *pulmonary* artery resulted in *peripheral* pulmonary edema and the appearance of considerable amounts of frothy fluid in the tracheobronchial tree. By contrast, the injection of the same toxic material into the *bronchial* circulation induced *central* pulmonary edema reminiscent of the "butterfly" pattern, with sparing of the periphery; frothy sputum did not appear in the tracheobronchial tree. Thus, it was postulated that the two anatomic locations of pulmonary edema are dependent, at least partly, upon which of the two circulations suffers damage to its capillaries.

Some support for Borgström and his colleagues' conclusions was obtained clinically by Gibson,[375] who catheterized the right side of the heart in patients who had acute pulmonary edema with

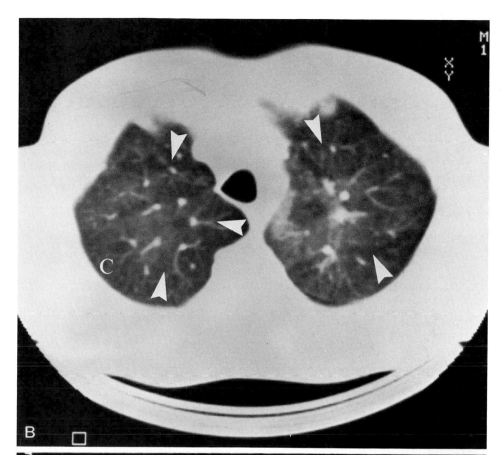

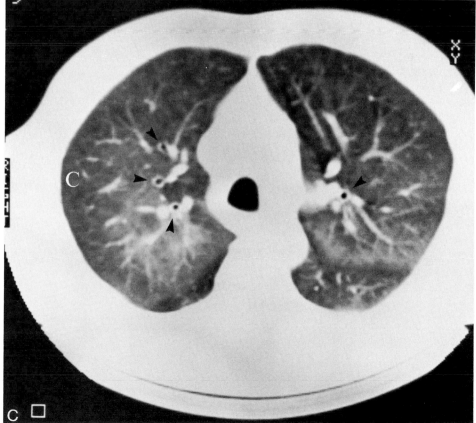

Figure 10–58 *Continued* CT scans through the apices (*B*) and the superior aspect of the hila (*C*) show a fairly symmetric increase in CT density in the medulla of each lung (*between large arrowheads* in *B*); note that the cortex (*C*) is relatively spared. Segmental bronchi are thickened (*arrowheads* in *C*) as a result of cuffs of edema. This CT pattern is typical of postcapillary hypertension. It is not certain, however, whether the increase in CT attenuation in the medulla is caused by redistributed blood flow or interstitial edema or both. The patient is a middle-aged man with hypertensive cardiovascular disease.

renal failure. Pulmonary vascular pressures were normal—or, at least, were below the colloid osmotic pressure of the plasma—suggesting an increase in capillary permeability. Additional support has been provided by Crosbie and associates,[376] who employed an isotopic technique to demonstrate increased permeability to the sodium ion in patients with renal failure. They postulated that this may be due to renin and angiotensin II, which have been shown to cause increased capillary permeability in animals.

3. A third theory, put forward by Fleischner,[377] proposes that the accumulation of fluid is dependent upon the efficiency with which the lymphatics can remove an excess. He postulated that during respiration the peripheral portion of the lungs undergoes greater volumetric change than does the medulla, and that this increased movement operates in much the same way as does muscular exercise in the extremities to stimulate increased lymphatic flow. This theory is plausible, but further experimental work is required to determine its validity. In fact, more recent studies by Wrinch and his colleagues[378] showed that between full inspiration and expiration there is little difference in the degree of lengthening and shortening of segments of the bronchial tree in the cortex as compared with the medulla.

The *clinical manifestations* of "butterfly" edema may be almost as unimpressive as the roentgenographic appearance is dramatic. Even when there is roentgenographic evidence of massive consolidation of the medial two thirds of the lungs the clinical presentation may be unremarkable, and even those patients who complain of increased dyspnea and orthopnea may have minimal or nonexistent physical signs—much the same as in diffuse interstitial edema. This dissociation of clinical and roentgenologic findings probably is attributable to the relatively mild involvement of the parenchymal compartment of the lungs (whose prime function is gas exchange) that minimizes the effect on function and physical signs.

Clinical Manifestations

The clinical manifestations of cardiogenic pulmonary edema depend on whether the onset of edema is acute or insidious. The acute form is dramatic; severe dyspnea develops over a short period (minutes to hours) and the patient is characteristically sitting bolt upright using the accessory muscles of respiration. Peripheral and central cyanosis, tachycardia, pallor, cool sweaty skin, anxiety, and an elevated blood pressure often are present. These latter findings are related to marked sympathetic stimulation. In severe cases, the patient may expectorate frothy, often blood-tinged fluid, and "air hunger" is sufficient to interfere with normal speech. In some cases, there is frank hemoptysis. Physical examination may reveal an elevated jugular

venous pressure; in the acute stages, the jugular veins may be difficult to evaluate owing to the patient's use of the cervical accessory muscles of respiration and to the considerable swings in pleural pressure. Other signs of congestive failure, such as hepatosplenomegaly and peripheral edema, may be present. Auscultation of the thorax reveals widespread crackles and expiratory wheezes. In the terminal stages there is a decrease in the patient's level of consciousness and circulatory collapse. In patients who have mitral stenosis or left ventricular failure secondary to systemic hypertension or aortic valvular disease, the episode of acute pulmonary edema may develop only following exertion or may be caused by the increase in pulmonary blood volume associated with the assumption of the supine from the erect position.

The only potentially confusing differential diagnoses are acute bronchoconstriction and upper airway obstruction. In patients with primary bronchoconstriction, evidence for sympathetic hyperreactivity is almost always lacking; examination of the chest reveals high-pitched wheezing without crackles. In acute upper airway obstruction, the chest is usually silent except for stridorous sounds confined to the central airway.

In patients in whom pulmonary edema develops less precipitously, there may be few physical findings. A history of orthopnea and paroxysmal nocturnal dyspnea is a helpful diagnostic feature in such patients, although nocturnal dyspnea and cough are also common in patients with asthma or COPD. When the edema is confined to the interstitial space, there may be no auscultatory findings, although expiratory wheezing is present in some patients at this stage. It is well to remember that the chest roentgenogram usually is more accurate than is the physical examination in identifying interstitial pulmonary edema. The quieter chest allows more careful auscultation of the heart, which may reveal a gallop rhythm or a murmur caused by valvular dysfunction. Cardiogenic pulmonary edema is not a static condition and there is usually improvement or worsening during a relatively short time course.

Physiologic Manifestations

The abnormalities of lung function that occur in pulmonary edema are caused by the effects of pulmonary vascular engorgement, interstitial fluid accumulation, and alveolar flooding.

Lung Compliance and Lung Volumes

Pulmonary vascular congestion by itself stiffens the lung,[379, 380] probably as a result of an erectile effect of vascular distention; the reduced compliance is rapidly reversed when the pulmonary microvascular pressure is decreased. During the stage of interstitial edema, compliance undergoes little further decrease but with the development of overt alveolar flooding, compliance, vital capacity, and total lung capacity all diminish as a result of both replacement of alveolar gas by fluid and a disruption of the normal surfactant-lined air-liquid interface.[381] Despite the foregoing, the relationship between changes in lung compliance and volumes and the severity of pulmonary edema is inconsistent.[382]

AIRWAY RESISTANCE AND CLOSING VOLUME

Clinical findings suggestive of airway narrowing are frequent in patients with pulmonary edema, and as discussed previously, there are anatomic reasons that may explain this finding. The pulmonary arteries and airways share a bronchovascular interstitial space, and during the development of pulmonary edema, fluid accumulates first in this space.[283] To the extent that there is competition for space within this compartment, airways can undergo narrowing. Airway resistance is increased in both acute and chronic pulmonary edema.[383, 384] In an experimental study in dogs in which pulmonary edema was induced by elevating microvascular pressure, Hogg and his colleagues[384] measured resistance of central and peripheral (< 2 mm internal diameter) airways and showed that there was a small and reversible increase in small airway resistance when pulmonary venous pressure was increased acutely; this presumably represented airway narrowing caused by vascular engorgement. However, when the venous pressure elevation was prolonged, a progressive and dramatic increase in the peripheral but not central airway resistance was observed that was thought to be secondary to peribronchovascular edema. These small airways are those that close at low lung volumes; if interstitial edema caused significant narrowing of these airways, one would predict that the closing volume test would be able to detect the change. In fact, closing volume is acutely increased in normal subjects subjected to volume overload[385] and is also increased in patients with recent myocardial infarction in whom the development of mild interstitial pulmonary edema is a distinct possibility.[386] Closing volume is also increased in patients on renal hemodialysis and decreases following removal of excess extracellular fluid.[387]

VENTILATION-PERFUSION MISMATCHING AND GAS EXCHANGE

A redistribution of blood flow to upper lung zones (recruitment of upper zone vessels) on chest roentgenograms is a time-honored sign of increased pulmonary venous pressure, although the intraobserver and interobserver error rate in its detection has not been tested to the best of our knowledge, and the accuracy of the sign in individual patients is open to some question. When redistribution is convincingly present, it predates the development of roentgenographically detectable interstitial edema.[259] In excised dog lungs, there is normally an apex-to-base gradient in regional blood flow such that flow at the base of the lung is greater. When pulmonary venous pressure is raised sufficiently to produce pulmonary edema, this pattern is altered to a point where flow to upper lung zones almost equals that to lower.[388] West[389] has suggested that perivascular edema forms first at the lung base and that edema in this location increases the regional pulmonary vascular resistance. By contrast, Muir and his colleagues[327] found a reversal in the apex-to-base flow pattern in dogs only when overt alveolar edema developed, and they suggested that alveolar wall swelling and capillary compression are required to cause flow reversal; this observation was also made roentgenographically in dogs by Surette and his colleagues.[167]

The distribution of ventilation is also affected in the presence of pulmonary edema.[390] Since the effects of edema on perfusion and ventilation distribution are inhomogeneous, $\dot{V}/\dot{Q}$ mismatching develops and arterial hypoxemia results. When edema is confined to the interstitium of the lung, arterial hypoxemia is usually mild; when airspaces are involved, true shunting of pulmonary blood combines with the $\dot{V}/\dot{Q}$ mismatching to cause more severe hypoxemia. In patients with interstitial and mild-to-moderate airspace edema, the arterial P_{CO_2} is normal or low, reflecting an overall increase in alveolar ventilation. The increase in ventilation during these stages of edema is out of proportion to the degree of hypoxemia, and it is thought that the hyperventilation may be mediated by stimulation of the "J receptors" originally described by Paintal.[391] Although most patients with acute pulmonary edema are hypocapnic or eucapnic,[392] the majority are acidemic as a result of hypoperfusion of peripheral tissues and the development of lactic acidosis.[392, 393] Approximately 10 per cent of patients in whom edema is sufficiently severe to warrant arterial blood gas analysis are hypercapnic and almost invariably manifest metabolic acidosis; that the hypercapnia cannot be attributed to pre-existing obstructive pulmonary disease has been demonstrated by subsequent assessment of pulmonary function. Although many such patients are extremely ill[394, 395] and the mortality rate high, particularly in the older age group,[396] edema in these individuals often appears to be no more severe than that in patients with normal or low arterial P_{CO_2}, and they may respond readily to appropriate therapy.[392, 397]

PULMONARY EDEMA ASSOCIATED WITH RENAL DISEASE, HYPERVOLEMIA, OR HYPOPROTEINEMIA

Both acute and chronic renal disease—with or without uremia—can be associated with acute pulmonary edema. Children with acute glomerulone-

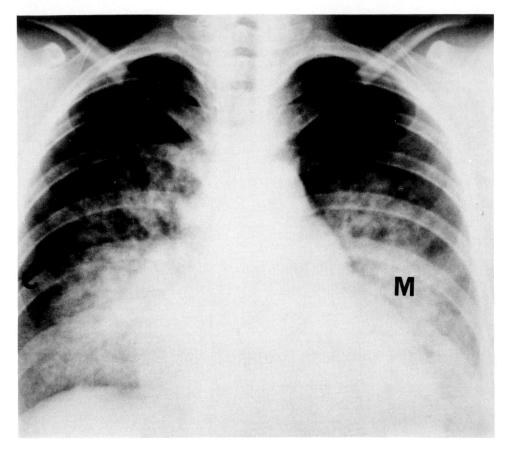

Figure 10–59. Acute Air-space Pulmonary Edema: The "Bat's-Wing" Pattern. A postero-anterior chest roentgenogram reveals a classic bat's-wing pattern of airspace consolidation consisting of a dense central core (medulla, M) surrounded by a radio-lucent peripheral zone of normal lung (cortex, C). Many characteristic features of an airspace pattern are seen, including airspace nodules, confluence of the lesions, and an air bronchogram. The heart is moderately enlarged, and it is probable that the cause of the edema in this renal transplant recipient was left ventricular failure, at least in part.

phritis may die so abruptly from cardiac failure and acute pulmonary edema that the diagnosis may be made only at autopsy.[398] In fact, the incidence of pulmonary edema in acute glomerulonephritis of infants and children is so high that MacPherson and Banerjee[399] suggested that the diagnosis of glomerulonephritis can be made with a high degree of accuracy from a plain chest roentgenogram; of 104 children ranging in age from 2 to 8 years for whom chest roentgenograms were available during the acute phase of acute glomerulonephritis, 57 (53 per cent) showed evidence of either pulmonary venous hypertension or overt pulmonary edema. From a review of all possible causes of cardiac failure in this age group, they concluded that glomerulonephritis can be implicated in approximately 75 per cent of the patients.

It is very likely that the major contributing cause to the development of pulmonary edema in renal disease is left ventricular failure, although it is probable that decreased oncotic pressure, hypervolemia, and increased capillary permeability also play a role (Fig. 10–59). In fact, in some patients with uremia, normal pulmonary capillary pressures have been recorded in the presence of pulmonary edema,[375] lending support to the influence of increased permeability.

Lung function studies on patients with severe renal failure have shown a significant reduction in diffusing capacity;[400, 401] in one study[400] this was presumed to be caused by permeability pulmonary edema, since affected patients showed no evidence of left ventricular failure. In another study,[401] hemodialysis resulted in an improvement in mid-expiratory flow rates and a reduction in gas trapping. The authors concluded that these changes could be attributed to the resolution of peribronchial edema at the lung bases.

The administration of large volumes of intravenous fluids has been shown to cause pulmonary edema in patients without underlying heart disease,[402-404] particularly during the postoperative period and in elderly patients. In many of these patients, the edema develops in the absence of known pulmonary injury and has usually been attributed to volume overload of the left ventricle with temporary high output left ventricular failure. However, it has also been shown that in some patients, fluid infusion results in pulmonary edema without functional impairment of the left ventricle and without an increase in left ventricular filling pressures or pulmonary arterial wedge pressure;[403] in these cases, the edema has been attributed at least in part to a decrease in colloid osmotic pressure. In a radiologic study of the cardiopulmonary effects of intravenous fluid overload, Westcott and Rudick[405] infused large volumes of normal saline intravenously in six dogs until obvious pulmonary edema was observed roentgenographically. Following volume overload, a statistically significant increase occurred in the size of the heart, left atrium, pulmonary arteries and veins, and systemic veins, unaccompanied by an elevation in left ventricular end-diastolic pressure or by a decrease in cardiac output or stroke volume. The authors concluded that in the absence of left ventricular failure, acute volume overload can simulate the radiographic changes produced by congestive heart failure; they suggested that the pulmonary edema may have occurred at least partly as a result of a marked decrease in serum colloid osmotic pressure. Although radiographic changes simulating congestive heart failure have also been observed in normal male volunteers whose blood volume was expanded by administration of large amounts of sodium,[406] the changes were largely those of systemic venous engorgement and pulmonary congestion in the absence of overt edema. There is little doubt that the effects on the lungs of volume overload are amplified in patients who are on the verge of cardiac or renal failure.

It is worth emphasizing that the pulmonary edema that occasionally develops in association with blood transfusion need not be the result of overloading of the circulation. Philipps and Fleischner[407] reported three cases of transient pulmonary edema in the course of blood transfusion that they attributed to incompatibility of undetermined nature. Hypervolemia was not considered the causative factor because of the small amount of transfused blood and a lack of clinical evidence of left ventricular failure. Subsequent studies[408, 409] have indicated increased capillary permeability resulting from leukoagglutinins in the pathogenesis of the edema. Increased knowledge of blood type compatibility has decreased the incidence of this complication, but the risk has not been eliminated.[410–412] These patients have an abrupt onset of chills, fever, tachycardia, nonproductive cough, and dyspnea, and sometimes they manifest blood eosinophilia.[408] Chest roentgenograms show patchy opacities affecting predominantly the parahilar and lower lung zones without associated cardiac enlargement or redistribution of blood flow. Leukoagglutinins often are demonstrable in the donors, who generally are multiparous. The antibodies develop because of incompatibility with fetal leukocytes, much in the same manner as Rhesus antibodies develop.

Pulmonary edema also occurs with increased frequency in patients with hepatic disease.[259] Tests of regional lung function suggest that pulmonary extravascular water is increased in patients with chronic hepatic failure and cirrhosis.[413] Pulmonary edema also frequently accompanies the development of acute hepatic failure.[414] It is unclear whether increased capillary pressure, increased endothelial permeability, or decreased plasma osmotic pressure is the major contributor to the development of pulmonary edema in these patients, but it is likely that a combination of these factors is responsible.

PULMONARY EDEMA SECONDARY TO AFFECTION OF THE PULMONARY VEINS

Obstructive disease of the pulmonary veins is a relatively rare cause of pulmonary venous hypertension and edema. There are at least seven etiologic factors:

1. Congenital heart disease of both high and low flow types.

2. Congenital stenosis or atresia of the pulmonary veins at their junction with the left atrium (see page 742).

3. Idiopathic veno-occlusive disease involving the small- and medium-sized veins.

4. Chronic sclerosing mediastinitis in which the pulmonary veins are involved in a cicatricial process.

5. Anomalous pulmonary venous drainage, above or below the diaphragm, in which venous compression, stenosis, or increased resistance of the hepatic sinusoids leads to a rise in pulmonary venous pressure (see page 743).

6. Rarely invasion or compression of pulmonary veins by a malignant neoplasm can cause interstitial edema and septal fibrosis; for example, these have been reported in patients who have obstructions of pulmonary veins caused by left atrial leiomyosarcoma[118] and by leukemic involvement of lymph nodes.[119]

7. Pulmonary vein thrombosis is also rare but can cause localized edema in the appropriate venous distribution (as in the cases described above of postlobectomy edema.[355]

The clinical, physiologic, and roentgenographic manifestations of pulmonary edema are usually indistinguishable from those of pulmonary venous hypertension from cardiac causes, except that in most cases the heart is of normal size. The edema is predominantly interstitial in location, although associated periodically with airspace filling. The chronic elevation of venous pressure results in pulmonary arterial hypertension indistinguishable from that associated with chronic mitral stenosis.

Primary pulmonary veno-occlusive disease is a rare and usually fatal disorder that has been described in detail previously in this chapter (see page 1879). Most patients with pulmonary veno-occlusive disease present with pulmonary arterial hypertension, but unlike primary pulmonary hypertension, there are almost invariably signs of pulmonary venous hypertension as well, with or without edema.

The etiology of pulmonary venous occlusion associated with mediastinitis is usually undetermined. A report by Stovin and Mitchinson[155] suggests that toxoplasmosis involving the pulmonary veins may be responsible for the mediastinitis in some cases, and it is well known to occur secondary to histoplasmosis (Fig. 10–60). This condition is described in detail in Chapter 19.

The possibility of anomalous pulmonary venous drainage into the hepatic veins, ductus venosus, superior vena cava, left innominate vein, azygos

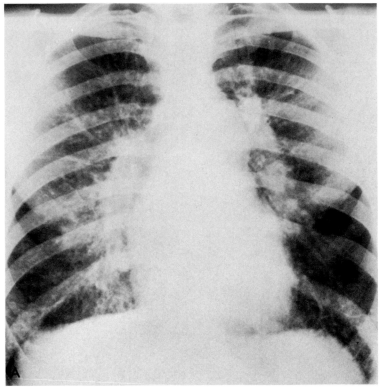

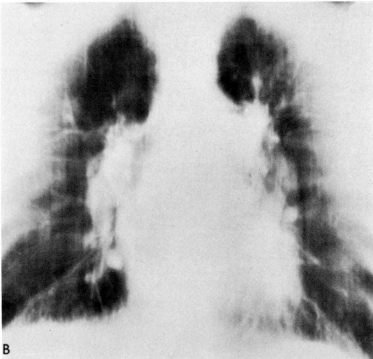

Figure 10–60. Pulmonary Edema Secondary to Pulmonary Vein Occlusion. A 36-year-old man had had progressively increasing dyspnea for 8 years, to a point of severe incapacitation at the time of admission. In addition, there was orthopnea, paroxysmal nocturnal dyspnea, a constricting substernal pain usually related to exercise, and occasional cyanosis. A posteroanterior roentgenogram (A) reveals a coarse reticular pattern throughout both lungs consistent with interstitial edema; prominent Kerley B lines are present bilaterally. The hilar pulmonary arteries are markedly enlarged and taper rapidly as they proceed distally, indicating severe pulmonary arterial hypertension. Cardiac contour is compatible with right ventricular hypertrophy. A tomogram of both lungs in anteroposterior projection (B) shows the arterial changes to better advantage; note that the vascular markings behind the heart on the left are of larger caliber than elsewhere in either lung.

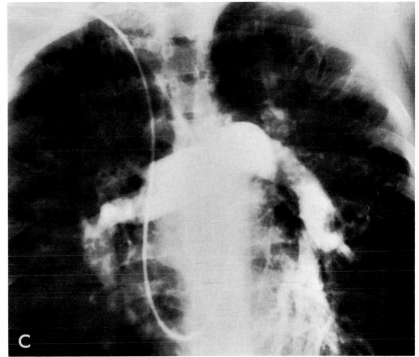

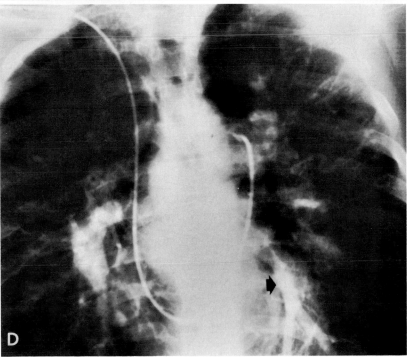

Figure 10–60 *Continued* The arterial phase of a pulmonary angiogram (*C*) shows poor opacification of all vessels except those extending into the left lower lobe; similarly, on the venous phase (*D*) the only opacified veins are those from the lower lobe (*arrow*). In *D,* although there is opacification of the left atrium as a result of flow from the left lower lobe, contrast medium is still present in the right pulmonary artery, indicating marked delay in arterial flow on this side. Cardiac catheterization revealed severe pulmonary hypertension, pressures approaching systemic levels; the wedge pressure was moderately elevated although both left atrial and right atrial pressures were normal. The final diagnosis was pulmonary venous occlusive disease affecting the veins of the right lung and left upper lobe but sparing those of the left lower lobe. The likeliest etiology was felt to be chronic granulomatous or sclerosing mediastinitis.

vein, or left superior vena cava should be borne in mind when the heart is found to be of normal size in cyanotic infants who show signs of pulmonary venous hypertension.[415–417]

NEUROGENIC AND POSTICTAL PULMONARY EDEMA

Acute pulmonary edema in association with raised intracranial pressure, head trauma, and seizures is a well-known but infrequent phenomenon. Its mechanism is poorly understood, although clinical and experimental studies suggest that both increased microvascular pressure and increased permeability may be involved. In experiments on rats and rabbits in which increased intracranial pressure was produced acutely by injection of fibrin into the cisterna magna, Sarnoff[420] interpreted the mechanism of edema as being produced by peripheral systemic vasoconstriction, bradycardia, reduced cardiac output, and consequent left atrial and pulmonary venous hypertension. Sarnoff and Kaufman[421] also observed a rise in left atrial pressure following instillation of ammonium chloride into the peritoneal cavity of cats, a phenomenon attributed to neurogenic causes.

The role of the vagus nerve in neurogenic edema is not clear. In experiments on rats and rabbits similar to those of Sarnoff, pulmonary edema did not develop when the vagus nerves were sectioned prior to the increase in intracranial pressure.[422] However, Ducker and Simmons[423] were not able to prevent neurogenic pulmonary edema by previous cervical vagotomy in dogs and monkeys subjected to increased intracranial pressure. Worthen and coworkers[424] produced pulmonary edema in dogs by introducing veratrine intracisternally; they measured left ventricular pressures before and after transection of the spinal cord at T-4, bilateral stellectomy or vagotomy (or a combination of these) and concluded that (1) systemic vasoconstriction resulted in increased venous return, which overloaded the heart and caused severe congestion of the lungs; and (2) levels of left ventricular diastolic pressure were raised chiefly because of adrenergic stimuli but also because of circulating catecholamines and the increased venous return resulting from systemic vasoconstriction. These experimental studies suggest that neurogenic pulmonary edema may be caused by transient, massive sympathetic discharge from the central nervous system (CNS), which results in generalized vasoconstriction, a shift of blood volume into the pulmonary vascular compartment, and consequent elevation of pulmonary microvascular pressure.

Clinical studies have suggested that there is also an alteration in microvascular permeability. Harari and colleagues,[425] Ducker,[427] and others[426] have reported normal microvascular pressures and protein-rich edema fluid in patients with neurogenic pulmonary edema. This combination of increased pressure and increased permeability led Theodore and Robin[428] to suggest the following scenario for the production of neurogenic pulmonary edema: an acute increase in intracranial pressure causes a generalized sympathetic discharge that results in a massive increase in pulmonary vascular pressures, barotrauma to the endothelium, and consequent increased permeability; further, by the time microvascular pressures have been measured, they may have returned to control levels, leaving barotrauma-induced changes in permeability as the major culprit. This hypothesis has been supported by individual case reports[429] in which patients with neurogenic pulmonary edema have been observed to develop episodic systemic and pulmonary vascular hypertensive crises during which pulmonary arterial wedge pressure increased to 50 mm Hg.

Despite the foregoing, there is experimental evidence that does not support the barotrauma hypothesis. Van der Zee and associates[430] and Bowers and colleagues[431] examined the effect of increased intracranial pressure in sheep on pulmonary lymphatic flow and lymphatic protein clearance. Both groups of investigators found that although there was a moderate and transient increase in pulmonary vascular pressures, there was also a prolonged and substantial increase in lung lymph flow and an increase in the ratio of lymph-plasma protein concentration, suggesting an increase in microvascular permeability. The vasoconstriction and increase in permeability were blocked by prior administration of the alpha-adrenergic blocking agent phentolamine, suggesting that both effects were mediated through the sympathetic nervous system.

Of the various causes of neurogenic edema, head trauma is one of the most frequent, and although it is often severe, it may be relatively mild and nonfatal.[362] In nontraumatized patients in whom edema develops as a consequence of raised intracranial pressure, the rise in pressure may or may not be abrupt. In three cases reported by Felman,[362] edema developed from a relatively insidious elevation of intracranial pressure caused by cerebellar astrocytoma, postmeningitic hydrocephalus, and leukemic infiltration of the meninges. The mechanism of development of postictal pulmonary edema is undoubtedly the same as that following trauma and increased intracranial pressure. It can develop immediately after an epileptic seizure or can be delayed for several hours. This type of edema occurs most often in young patients with idiopathic epilepsy and in those in whom seizures relate to expanding intracranial lesions.[432–435]

For unknown reasons, the distribution of neurogenic pulmonary edema is unpredictable and frequently asymmetric. For example, the three patients with head trauma described by Felman[362] showed predominant upper zonal distribution and the three with chronic increased intracranial pressure showed predominant right-sided localization. However, the distribution of edema was generalized in the 11 cases reported by Ducker,[427] and it is possible that positional factors and gravity effects were operative in Felman's cases.

Characteristically, the edema disappears within several days following surgical relief of increased intracranial pressure. Most patients are comatose and experience frequent periods of apnea when pulmonary edema develops. Thus, they are likely to aspirate acid gastric juice and suffer prolonged hypoxemia. It is possible that these mechanisms can be invoked as the pathogenesis in some cases. Patients who are unconscious following head trauma who do not develop overt pulmonary edema have been found to have abnormalities in gas exchange characterized by mismatching of ventilation and perfusion and an increase in shunt, and it is possible that these gas exchange problems represent subclinical pulmonary edema.[436]

PULMONARY EDEMA ASSOCIATED WITH NORMAL MICROVASCULAR PRESSURE

During the past two decades, a distinct change has occurred in the incidence and pathogenesis of acute respiratory failure. Before that time, respiratory insufficiency usually occurred in patients who had chronic lung disease, either obstructive or restrictive, and was often associated with a poor prognosis. In recent years, a new constellation of conditions has appeared in which acute respiratory failure develops in patients who do not have severe preexisting pulmonary disease, and the clinical and roentgenographic features associated with this have come to be known as the *adult respiratory distress syndrome* (ARDS). This term was coined by Petty and Ashbaugh in 1971[437] and is now in general usage to describe the noncardiogenic pulmonary edema that develops as a result of a wide variety of conditions. Since 1971, our knowledge of the roentgenographic, morphologic, and clinical nature of the entity and of the many disparate conditions that predispose to its development has accumulated in abundance. Some authorities have opposed the use of the term ARDS on the basis that it serves as a "wastebasket" that will inevitably be a repository for all the various etiologic entities regardless of their nature;[438, 439] they take the firm stance that it is desirable to prevent further confusion by applying specific etiologic connotations in the diagnoses, such as "acute pulmonary insufficiency associated with"— shock, pancreatitis, or whatever condition.[438] As Fishman asks,[439]

. . . would it not be reasonable to encourage the dissection of the "adult respiratory distress syndrome" according to etiologic entities, each with its own pathogenesis and natural history, so that clinicians will find it easier to compare bedside observations, physiologists will be encouraged to produce meaningful experimental rep-

licas of the human disorders, and pathologists will be abetted in their efforts to relate structural abnormalities to antecedent functional derangements?

The major advocates for the preservation of the term point out that "ARDS is a fact" and that it serves as a useful description of a group of pulmonary insults that have similar clinical, pathologic, physiologic, and roentgenographic features.[437] There is merit to both approaches, and a middle of the line position has been taken by Thurlbeck,[440] who stated:

. . . to the pragmatist, the situation in ARDS is rather like a fire started by a match. The first priority is to put out the fire; to hell with worrying about finding the match that caused it. But being a pathologist, I am a match man and I think that where the cause of ARDS is known, the term should be applied. Where you don't know the cause, it is fine to use "adult RDS" but one should always be trying to determine the underlying and pathogenetic mechanism and disease state involved.

We agree with this point of view: for the experimental pathologist, splitting is a virtue, but for the vast majority of practicing physicians who deal with patients diagnosed as having ARDS, lumping is the only practical approach.

Following trauma, shock, sepsis, aspiration, or a variety of other direct or indirect pulmonary insults, a certain number of patients develop progressive respiratory distress characterized by tachypnea, dyspnea, cough, and the physical findings of airspace consolidation; the chest roentgenogram reveals diffuse airspace disease, blood gas analysis demonstrates severe arterial desaturation that is resistant to even high concentrations of inhaled oxygen, the lungs become stiff and difficult to ventilate, pulmonary vascular pressures and resistance increase, and it becomes necessary to institute prolonged ventilatory support. Pathologic changes are similar despite the varying inciting events and consist of a concatenation of abnormalities often called "diffuse alveolar damage." In the early stages, these consist of interstitial and alveolar edema, hyaline membrane formation, and destruction of Type I alveolar epithelial cells; after several days, there is proliferation of Type II alveolar cells and, in some patients, progressive interstitial fibrosis.[709] This constellation of clinical, roentgenographic, and pathologic findings constitutes a syndrome sufficiently homogeneous to refer to in general terms.[249]

The wide diversity of predisposing conditions has led to a multitude of synonyms for ARDS— shock lung, posttraumatic pulmonary insufficiency, hemorrhagic lung syndrome, Da Nang lung, stiff-lung syndrome,[441] respirator lung, pump lung, congestive atelectasis, oxygen toxicity, catastrophic pulmonary failure,[442] and acute respiratory distress in adults. Although the terminology to be applied to this complex condition is a matter of some contention,[438, 443] because of its familiarity and brevity, the designation ARDS will be employed throughout this text.

Pathogenesis

Although it may be convenient to regard ARDS as simply a form of pulmonary edema caused by increased microvascular permeability, it has become increasingly evident that it consists not only of an acute inflammatory condition that causes major alteration in structure and function of the lungs but also of a specific manifestation of a generalized permeability defect.[710] Although an increase in microvascular permeability and the development of interstitial and airspace edema are perhaps the major consequences of this acute inflammatory process, in most cases the injury goes far beyond a simple increase in capillary "pore" size and involves severe damage to endothelial and epithelial cells. The pathogenesis involves a complex series of inflammatory events, including participation of preformed plasma-derived inflammatory mediators and newly generated arachidonic acid mediators from both the cyclooxygenase and lipoxygenase pathways. Activation of the complement and blood clotting systems can also be involved in addition to recruitment of numerous inflammatory cell types. Despite the variety of precipitating events (see Table 10–5, page 1954) the pathologic characteristics common to all cases of ARDS suggest that either there is one common activating factor or the lung is capable of reacting to injury in only a limited manner.[444]

THE ROLE OF SHOCK

Episodes of hypotension, either brief or prolonged, are frequent in patients who subsequently develop ARDS and may be caused by either hypovolemia or a decrease in systemic vascular smooth muscle tone. Although shock frequently accompanies ARDS, it is difficult to cause lung damage by shock alone[445] and it is probable that other factors must be involved to produce the complete syndrome.

In an ultrastructural study of the lungs of dogs subjected to hemorrhagic shock by induction of either arterial hypotension or severe hypovolemia without hypotension, Connell and coworkers[446] found that the initial change was platelet adhesiveness and aggregation. These aggregates, to which leukocytes were soon added, caused extensive occlusion of the pulmonary microcirculation, followed shortly by swelling and fragmentation of vascular endothelium and disintegration and disappearance of the platelets; subsequently, the leukocytes also disintegrated, freeing their lysosomes into the microcirculation, particularly the capillaries and venules. Discontinuities appeared in Type I alveolar lining cells, and edema fluid and red blood cells began to accumulate in the interstitium and alveoli. Of major importance in these studies was the observation that the development of pathologic changes in the lungs was time-dependent: rapid bleeding of the dog followed by death within 20 minutes elicited platelet aggregation but no changes in the alveolar septa, whereas more prolonged hypotension or hypovolemia (up to one hour) permitted leukocytes to become incorporated into the aggregates, with subsequent disintegration and release of lysosomal granules. The investigators further observed that reinfusion of the withdrawn blood following the hypotensive episode increased the severity of the pulmonary lesions unless the blood was passed through a Dacron wool filter that removed platelet-leukocyte microemboli. By contrast, a study in sheep showed that hemorrhage and reinfusion of the shed blood produced no evidence of pulmonary microvascular injury.[447]

In another study of dogs made hypotensive by hemorrhagic shock, Todd and colleagues[278] measured the flow and protein concentration of lung lymph and the permeability of endothelium to the electron microscopic tracer, horseradish peroxidase. They found that although the calculated microvascular pressure decreased, lung lymph flow remained constant or increased and the protein concentration in lymph remained high, indicating an increase in microvascular permeability. Using horseradish peroxidase as a marker, they calculated the changes in pore size and number that would be required to produce the injury and found that the data could be explained best by a seven-fold increase in pore number and no change in average pore size. As the authors point out, this represents a very subtle injury and could easily not be recognized in an ultrastructural study.

THE ROLE OF POLYMORPHONUCLEAR LEUKOCYTES

There is considerable evidence derived from both experimental and clinical studies that the activated neutrophil is an important contributor to lung injury in many cases of ARDS. It is probable—if paradoxical—that many of the characteristics that make the neutrophil an effective agent in host defense also make it a potential mediator of host injury.

A large pool of marginated neutrophils reside within the normal human lung. These cells are normally inactive, and their presence in the pulmonary circulation may simply reflect the fact that they are larger and less deformable than red blood cells, mechanical constraints that slow their transit through the pulmonary microvasculature. The size of the marginated pool of leukocytes appears to be dependent on regional pulmonary blood flow, at least in some species; for example, in the dog[448, 449] and rabbit,[450] the regional retention of leukocytes in a single passage through the lung is dependent on regional blood flow. A vertical gradient exists in white blood cell retention so that more white cells are removed in a single pass through the nondependent lung (where blood flow per unit lung volume is low) than at the lung base (where blood flow per unit lung volume is high). Similarly, if pulmonary blood flow is transiently decreased, white cells accumulate within the lung but are released again without the development of lung damage when cardiac output is increased. This phenomenon appears to explain the leukocytosis that occurs in man following exercise and catecholamine infusion.[451] Thus, it is possible that blood flow can play an important role in the development of leukocyte-induced lung injury.

Circulating or marginated neutrophils can respond to numerous substances, called *chemotaxins,* that cause a directed migration to extravascular sites. These chemotaxins include factors such as the bacterial lipopolysaccharide endotoxins, the complement anaphylatoxin C5a, leukotrienes, prostaglandins, immunoglobulin fragments, fibrinogen fragments, macrophage products, and platelet activating factor. These substances and chemical compounds such as N-formylated peptides (f-MLP) and phorbol esters (such as PMA) cause not only migration of neutrophils but also their activation, presumably as a preparatory step to dealing with invading microorganisms. Activation results in an increased generation of *oxygen free radicals,* lysosomal enzymes, and arachidonate metabolites and in their eventual penetration through junctions between endothelial cells.[452] When activated, neutrophils undergo a respiratory burst that appears to be related to the stimulation of a membrane-bound nicotinamide-adenine dinucleotide phosphate (reduced form) (NADPH) oxidase and is characterized by increased oxygen consumption, increased hexose-monophosphate shunt activity, and the production of several species of oxygen radicals, including superoxide $(O_2\cdot^-)$, hydrogen peroxide (H_2O_2), and the hydroxyl radical $(OH\cdot)$. Oxygen radical generation by activated neutrophils is necessary for its bactericidal action on ingested microorganisms. The importance of the ability of neutrophils to produce oxygen radicals is amply demonstrated in the disorder chronic granulomatous disease (*see* page 803): the neutrophils of affected patients are normal except for their inability to undergo a respiratory burst; the polymorphonuclear leukocytes can phagocytose normally but are ineffective in killing ingested microorganisms, resulting in frequent, often severe, bacterial infections.

In addition to oxygen radicals, neutrophils can also release from their granules products of arachidonate metabolism and enzymes that are designed for bacterial digestion. Neutrophil granules contain a variety of enzymes, including elastase, collagenase, cathepsins, cationic proteins, lysozyme, lactoferrin, and myeloperoxidase, many of which can attack and degrade normal proteins and cells; regurgitation of these toxic enzymes during bacterial phagocytosis, either successful or attempted, may be an important mechanism of tissue injury. Leukocytes have all the metabolic machinery to produce prostaglandins, thromboxanes, and leukotrienes.

Evidence in support of a role for leukocytes in the development of ARDS includes the following:

1. Animal models of acute lung injury that are dependent on the presence of neutrophils.

2. The presence of numerous neutrophils in some lung biopsy specimens and postmortem lung specimens from patients with established ARDS.[453, 454]

3. The presence of increased numbers of neutrophils and of neutrophil-derived products such as neutrophil elastase in BAL fluid of similarly affected patients.

4. The recognition that many of the risk factors for ARDS are associated with complement activation and leukopenia secondary to sequestration of leukocytes within the lungs.

5. The demonstration that severe, acute leukopenia frequently predates the onset of clinical ARDS.[455–457]

6. Animal models in which chemotactic agents such as C5a have been shown to attract leukocytes to the pulmonary microvasculature with resulting pulmonary microvascular injury.

7. The production of leukopenia has been shown to protect against certain lung injuries.

Infusion of gram-negative bacteria[458] or microemboli[459] can cause an increase in microvascular permeability in sheep in which lung lymph flow and protein concentration are used to assess microvascular permeability. Neutrophils are necessary for the development of these permeability changes because prior administration of chemotherapeutic agents in doses sufficient to cause neutropenia protects against the development of lung injury.[459–461] Neutrophils are necessary for the development of pulmonary edema resulting from the injection of phorbol myristate acetate (PMA), a substance that causes increased neutrophil adhesiveness, aggregation, degranulation, and the production of oxygen radicals. In the presence of leukocytes, PMA causes pulmonary edema in rabbit lungs, an effect that can be attenuated when dimethylthiourea (an oxygen free radical scavenger) is administered in conjunction with the PMA.[462, 463]

In experimental animals, endotoxin causes preferential neutrophil sequestration in the pulmonary vascular bed. Low doses of endotoxin apparently exert a direct effect on the leukocytes rather than on the pulmonary microvascular endothelium itself. A combination of minute doses of bacterial lipopolysaccharide endotoxin and chemotactic factors, such as complement fragments, results in prolonged sequestration of neutrophils within the pulmonary microvascular compartment and increased microvascular permeability.[464] Endotoxin infusion in sheep causes leukopenia, pulmonary arterial hypertension, and increased pulmonary vascular permeability;[465] a blocker of the cyclooxygenase pathway of arachidonic acid metabolism blocks the pulmonary hypertensive effect but not the leukopenia or increased permeability.

In patients with established ARDS, BAL fluid

not only shows a considerable increase in the differential count of neutrophils but also contains chemotactic factors for human neutrophils.[466] Peripheral circulating leukocytes show signs of activation characterized by an increased chemotactic index, increased metabolic activity, and increased superoxide anion generation,[467, 468] although they may not show increased adherence in vitro.[469] In one study,[470] BAL fluid was obtained from nine intubated control subjects without ARDS, 12 patients who had risk factors for the development of ARDS (aspiration or sepsis), and 11 patients with established ARDS caused chiefly by aspiration or sepsis: there was a significant increase in the total number of cells recovered from BAL fluid in the latter two groups, the percentage of neutrophils increasing from approximately 1 per cent in the control group to 53 per cent in those at risk, to 70 per cent in patients with established ARDS. In addition, there was a ten-fold to 40-fold increase in the protein content of the lavage fluid, indicating a considerable increase in alveolar epithelial permeability to proteins. Finally, these investigators[470] found that there was an unidentified substance in the BAL fluid from patients at risk and those who had established ARDS that promoted an increase in neutrophil adherence to plastic surfaces. In another study,[471] BAL was performed on four mechanically ventilated control subjects, 12 normal volunteers, and 11 patients with ARDS: the percentage of neutrophils in the lavage fluid was 4, 0.8, and 68, respectively, and in the patients with ARDS the percentage correlated with the severity of their gas exchange impairment. Eosinophils may also participate in the lung injury of ARDS; eosinophil cationic protein, a toxic granule component of eosinophils, has been demonstrated in the BAL fluid of patients with ARDS, as has myeloperoxidase derived from polymorphonuclear leukocytes.[472, 473]

In 40 patients at high risk for the development of ARDS, Thommasen and colleagues[457] monitored the peripheral blood leukocyte count every 6 hours; ARDS developed in ten patients; in eight of these patients, the clinical diagnosis was *preceded* by the development of transient leukopenia (defined as a total leukocyte count less than 4,200 cells/ml). Only four of the 30 patients in whom ARDS did not develop showed a similar leukopenia. It has also been shown that patients with fully developed ARDS—or even those with factors such as sepsis that predispose to ARDS—sequester increased numbers of radiolabeled polymorphonuclear leukocytes in their lungs.[474]

Although these experimental and clinical studies provide strong support for the important contribution that neutrophils make to the pulmonary damage in ARDS, there is also convincing evidence that the syndrome can occur in the absence of circulating or tissue neutrophils.[475, 476] In one retrospective study,[477] 11 patients were identified in whom ARDS was accompanied by an absence of circulating neutrophils; in five of these, lung biopsy specimens showed changes typical of ARDS unassociated with a neutrophilic infiltrate. In another clinical study of six leukopenic patients, ARDS developed in the absence of circulating neutrophils but worsened appreciably when the bone marrow had recovered from chemotherapeutic suppression.[478]

THE ROLE OF SURFACTANT

Both qualitative and quantitative abnormalities of surfactant function have been demonstrated in alveolar fluid obtained from patients with ARDS,[479–481] abnormalities that could be caused by either dilution of the normal amount of surface active phospholipid by the exudate of serum that floods the alveoli or by a deficiency in phospholipid production resulting from epithelial injury and Type II cell death. Studies of animals subjected to acute lung injury by subcutaneous injection of N-nitroso-N-methylurethane have shown a progressive decrease in lung compliance coincident with a reduction in levels of desaturated phosphatidylcholine (DSPC) in alveolar lavage fluid during the early phase of the injury.[482] It has also been shown that in addition to a reduction in the amount of surface active phospholipid that can be recovered by lavage, a decrease in intracellular DSPC also occurs, suggesting that impaired synthesis rather than increased degradation is the major cause of the deficiency.[483]

In the respiratory distress syndrome of newborn infants, a deficiency of surfactant production with a loss of the ability of alveolar lining fluid to lower surface tension is believed to be the primary cause of lung injury. By contrast, it is probable that the abnormalities of surfactant function and synthesis that occur in adults with acute alveolar damage and ARDS are the result rather than the cause of the injury. This is not to say that the disruption of the surfactant layer and the resultant increase in surface tension are not important mechanisms contributing to the development of alveolar edema in ARDS; Albert and associates[312] have shown that disruption of surfactant by itself can increase lung water, presumably by increasing the surface tension at the alveolar fluid-air interface, resulting in the suction of water from the interstitial space.

THE ROLE OF COMPLEMENT

One of the components of complement activation by either the classical or alternate pathway is the "anaphylatoxin" C5a. Biologically, C5a is a highly active peptide that, in addition to having a direct effect on pulmonary capillary permeability, can release histamine from mast cells, cause contraction of smooth muscle, and act as a chemotactic agent for white blood cells.[484] Administration of this substance in experimental animals induces an intense, acute inflammatory lung injury.[485] Both trauma and infection can cause activation of the complement system, resulting in hyperemia, increased vascular permeability, adherence of neutrophils to the vascular endothelium, and emigration of neutrophils into the inflamed tissue. Although activation of complement is designed primarily to initiate inflammation as part of the protective response against invading microorganisms, it is clear that in some circumstances, complement activation can result in host damage. Complement may have a direct toxic effect on certain cells; neutrophil activation can then cause a release of enzymes and oxygen radicals that can secondarily damage host cells and tissues.[486] Both the blood and BAL fluid of patients with ARDS have been shown to contain increased levels of the complement component C5a.[487, 711, 712] Systemic complement activation accompanied by leukopenia can also be demonstrated following extracorporeal circulation during hemodialysis,[488] following cardiopulmonary bypass for coronary artery grafting,[489] and following plasmapheresis.[490] When patients with established ARDS are supported by extracorporeal membrane oxygenation, further activation of complement and a decrease in the circulating leukocyte count occur.[491]

The hypothesis that complement activation might be the initiating event in the pathogenesis of ARDS was first suggested by Hammerschmidt and associates in 1980.[492] However, the central role played by this mechanism has been questioned;[493] for example, it has been shown that a large percentage of patients with sepsis and other risk factors for the development of ARDS manifest complement activation *in vivo* unaccompanied by the subsequent development of pulmonary dysfunction.[494, 495]

THE ROLE OF THE CLOTTING SYSTEM

The role of the blood clotting system in causing increased pulmonary microvascular permeability has been reviewed by Malik[496] and by Saldeen.[497] In a study in which thrombin was infused intravenously in sheep and dogs, a transient increase in pulmonary arterial pressure and a sustained increase in pulmonary microvascular permeability occurred, indicated by increased lung lymph flow and lung lymph protein concentration.[498, 499] The increase in microvascular permeability was associated with a decrease in peripheral blood fibrinogen levels, an increase in blood fibrin split products, and a decrease in the number of circulating leukocytes and platelets. Morphologic examination of the lungs of these experimental animals showed polymerized fibrin within pulmonary vessels, and neutrophils and platelets trapped within the meshwork of fibrin; in addition, there was evidence of interstitial and alveolar edema.[498, 499] The microvascular injury associated with thrombin infusion is dependent on activation of the coagulation cascade, since defibrinogenation prior to fibrin infusion attenuates both

the vascular and permeability effects.[500] The permeability response can also be attenuated or abolished if polymorphonuclear leukocytes[501] or complement[502] is depleted before thrombin challenge or if there is interference with activation of the fibrinolytic pathway.[500] Some studies, however, have shown that lung damage is increased when fibrinolysis is blocked.[503]

The results of these experiments have suggested the following hypothesis for the pathogenesis of the vascular injury following thrombin infusion:

1. Fibrin is generated from fibrinogen.
2. Fibrin activates the fibrinolytic system, resulting in the formation of plasmin from plasminogen.
3. Plasmin breaks down fibrin and causes cleavage of complement proteins and the formation of the chemotactic peptides C3a and C5a.
4. The complement fragments cause sequestration of neutrophils within the lung.
5. Neutrophil activation eventually results in vascular injury and pulmonary edema.[498]

There is also ample evidence that ARDS is associated with disseminated intravascular coagulation (DIC), also known as consumption coagulopathy, diffuse intravascular thrombosis, and defibrination syndrome. This syndrome has been observed in a wide variety of clinical disorders and has been implicated as a major pathogenetic feature of ARDS.[445, 446, 504–508] For example, in a study of 30 consecutive patients with ARDS, Bone and colleagues detected definite evidence of DIC in seven (23 per cent).[509] The diagnosis of DIC can be made in the laboratory by detecting a deficiency of clotting factors (primarily fibrinogen), thrombocytopenia, and excessive fibrinolysis (indicated by increased blood levels of fibrin degradation products). It is unclear whether the association of DIC with ARDS is causative (i.e., the activation of the coagulation cascade results in pulmonary microvascular injury) or is secondary. Coagulation can be initiated by clotting on the surface of damaged vascular endothelium or by the entry into the circulation of a procoagulant substance such as tissue thromboplastin. The widespread coagulation process that follows would cause platelet aggregation, thrombocytopenia, and consumption of fibrinogen and other clotting factors, particularly factors II, V, VIII, X, and XIII.[504]

Patients with established ARDS frequently have elevated blood levels of fibrin degradation products.[510] Activation of the coagulation system is particularly evident when ARDS follows major trauma. In one study, 18 severely injured patients were evaluated prospectively for the development of ARDS and for biochemical evidence of coagulation and fibrinolysis;[511] the eight patients (44 per cent) who fulfilled the criteria for the diagnosis of ARDS were found to have levels of antithrombin III, fibrinogen, and plasminogen that were significantly lower than those in whom the pulmonary complications of trauma did not develop. In a study of 29 patients who had major trauma, five of whom fulfilled the clinical criteria for the diagnosis of ARDS (a PaO_2 ratio of less than or equal to 38), Alberts and associates[512] found that the five patients had a lower platelet count and decreased levels of antithrombin III, fibrinogen, and plasminogen; they suggested that following acute trauma, a decrease in platelet count may be a sensitive predictor of the development of ARDS.[512]

Examination of BAL fluid from patients with ARDS reveals increased levels of a procoagulant that is capable of activation of factor X;[513] this augmented activity of the extrinsic coagulation pathway within the alveolar compartment may partly explain the presence of extravascular fibrin deposition and hyaline membrane formation in ARDS. Additional evidence that the coagulation process may participate in the pathogenesis of ARDS comes from the morphologic observation of considerable intra-alveolar fibrin deposition and capillary obliteration by fibrin clots during the acute phase.[514] In the two cases of DIC following severe trauma described by Putman and his colleagues,[505] histologic studies of the lungs revealed occlusion of the lumen of small vessels by platelet and fibrin thrombi.

DIC appears to be strongly associated with the development of ARDS in patients who are affected by heat stroke. During the 1985 pilgrimage to Mecca, El-Kassimi and associates[515] studied 52 consecutive patients with heat stroke. Of these, 12 (23 per cent) developed ARDS and nine died; all of the 12 patients with ARDS demonstrated biochemical evidence of DIC, whereas only one of the 40 patients without ARDS showed evidence of activation of the coagulation system.[515]

Thrombocytopenia occurs in at least half the patients in whom ARDS develops, almost certainly caused by the consumption of platelets rather than by their decreased production. In a study in which radiolabeled platelets were injected into patients with ARDS, platelet life span was lower than normal and the platelets were found to be sequestered in the pulmonary vasculature.[516] Radiolabeled fibrinogen accumulates rapidly in the lungs of patients with established ARDS but not in the lungs of patients who are equally ill but do not have ARDS.[517]

Endothelial cells, including those in the lungs, are the source of factor VIII, and the fact that pulmonary endothelial cells are the putative site of major injury in ARDS creates another reason why there may be alterations in the normal hemostatic balance in patients with this condition. In a study of 100 patients with ARDS, Carvalho and associates[518] demonstrated increased levels of antigenically determined factor VIII, although its coagulant ability was within the normal range; they suggested that endothelial damage may result in the release of a defective factor VIII molecule.

Clotting can be initiated by either the intrinsic or the extrinsic system. Exposure of collagen following pulmonary microvascular injury could activate the intrinsic system, whereas tissue thromboplastin generated from damaged lung could activate the extrinsic system. Activation results in the production of thrombin and fibrin, both of which have been shown experimentally to result in endothelial cell damage and increased pulmonary vascular permeability. In addition, fibrin monomers can stimulate pulmonary vasoconstriction through the arachidonic acid metabolism pathway. Once fibrin is generated, the plasminogen system is activated and fibrin is degraded by plasmin into fibrin split products, which themselves can damage the pulmonary microvascular endothelium.[509]

THE ROLE OF OXYGEN RADICALS

Oxygen is the very stuff of life, but like most good things, it has its sinister side. Short-lived unstable species of oxygen molecules, termed *oxygen free radicals*, are generated by neutrophils, by certain specific enzymes normally present within the body, and by a variety of toxic substances. The cytotoxic oxygen species include the superoxide radical ($O_2{}^{-}$), hydrogen peroxide (H_2O_2), hydroxyl radical ($OH^{\cdot}$), singlet oxygen ($O_2{}^{*}$), and peroxide radicals generated by peroxidation of lipids. These highly toxic species are generated by enzymes, such as xanthine oxidase, and by the normal mitochondrial energy transfer reactions. However, under normal conditions, the body is equipped with a battery of antioxidant defense mechanisms that include specific enzymes, such as (1) *superoxide dismutase*, which catalyzes the conversion of $O_2{}^{-}$ to hydrogen peroxide; (2) *catalase*, which catalyzes the conversion of hydrogen peroxide to oxygen and water; and (3) *glutathione peroxidase*, which converts peroxide radicals to nontoxic lipids (see figure below).

In addition to these specific enzymes that can inactivate oxygen free radicals, nonspecific "free radical scavengers," such as ascorbic acid, betacarotene, and glutathione, can also neutralize these radicals. Oxygen free radicals damage the lung by denaturation of lipids associated with the plasma membrane, inactivation of sulfhydryl-containing protein enzymes, depolymerization of polysaccha-

$$O_2 \longrightarrow O_2^- \xrightarrow[\text{dismutase}]{\text{superoxide}} H_2O_2 \longrightarrow OH^{\circ} \longrightarrow H_2O$$

catalase

glutathione peroxidase

rides, and strand breakages in molecules of deoxy-ribonucleic acid (DNA) with resultant mutations. Oxygen free radicals can be generated within the lung as a result of exposure to very high levels of inspired oxygen and of the inhalation of photochemical smog, ozone, nitrogen dioxide, and phosgene. Oxygen free radical formation is probably also responsible for the lung damage induced by x-rays; the herbicide paraquat; chemotherapeutic agents, such as bleomycin and doxorubicin (Adriamycin); the antimicrobial nitrofurantoin; and drugs such as alloxan and streptozotocin.[519] Lung toxicity associated with agents that produce oxygen free radicals is enhanced by hyperoxic and lessened by hypoxic conditions. In many animal models, the specific enzymes that metabolize oxygen free radicals and the drugs that are known to scavenge them can protect against lung injury; the protection is afforded in models in which the injurious agent appears to damage the endothelium directly by generating radicals and in those in which neutrophil sequestration and activation within the lung appear to be a prerequisite for the development of injury. Experimental studies suggest that oxygen free radical damage may be the final common pathway in a variety of acute lung injuries, whether they are related to direct toxicity or to neutrophil-mediated toxicity.[520] However, it is difficult to gather direct evidence that incriminates oxygen free radical formation in the pathogenesis of ARDS in humans. Oxygen free radicals are extremely short-lived, and no direct methods are available either to identify them or to quantify them. Indirect evidence for their presence in the lung derives from studies that have shown an increased amount of oxidized substances, such as 1 proteinase inhibitor, in the BAL fluid of patients with ARDS.[521]

THE ROLE OF ENZYMES AND MEDIATORS

There is considerable evidence that both the mediators of inflammation and a variety of enzymes can play important roles in initiating or modifying lung injury in ARDS. The products of arachidonic acid metabolism can either cause or protect against lung injury. Arachidonic acid is a membrane-derived, free fatty acid that can be metabolized via the cyclooxygenase pathway to the prostaglandins and thromboxanes or via the lipoxygenase pathway to the leukotrienes. Thromboxane causes platelet aggregation and pulmonary vascular constriction, whereas prostacyclin is a potent pulmonary arterial dilator and is capable of causing disaggregation of platelets. The leukotrienes are a varied group of mediators that can cause edema either directly by increasing vascular permeability or indirectly by inducing vascular smooth muscle contraction and chemotaxis of leukocytes to the site of mediator release. Most cells have the enzymatic capacity to produce prostaglandins and leukotrienes, although different cell types preferentially generate particu-

lar products. There may be complex interactions between various arachidonic acid–derived mediators; for example, leukotriene D_4, a lipoxygenase-derived product, causes pulmonary arterial hypertension that can be blocked by the cyclooxygenase blocker indomethacin, suggesting that the leukotriene exerts its vascular effect by stimulating prostaglandin production.[522]

Although plasma levels of prostaglandins are not increased in patients with ARDS,[523] increased levels of leukotrienes (including leukotriene D_4) have been identified in the pulmonary edema fluid of such patients but not in those with hydrostatic edema of similar severity.[524] There is also evidence for decreased pulmonary removal of certain prostaglandins such as prostaglandin E_1 (PGE_1), probably secondary to the diffuse endothelial injury that constitutes the basic feature of ARDS.[525, 713]

Attempts have been made to alter the natural course of ARDS by modulating the synthesis of arachidonic acid products; for example, in a small controlled study of ten patients, a thromboxane A_2 synthesis blocker was effective in decreasing blood levels of thromboxane A_2 but had no influence on the clinical course or outcome of the treated patients.[526] Prostaglandin E_1 is a potent pulmonary vasodilator and theoretically could be of benefit in the treatment of ARDS: in one study, infusion of PGE_1 decreased pulmonary arterial pressure, increased cardiac output, and improved gas exchange;[527] in another controlled study, the survival rate of a PGE_1-treated group was significantly better than a placebo-treated group.[528]

Prekallikrein is the inactive precursor of plasma kallikrein, which is both a component of the coagulation and fibrinolytic systems and an activator of the kinin system. There is some evidence for prekallikrein activation in the blood and BAL fluid of patients with ARDS;[529, 530] in addition, in animal models of acute lung injury,[531] bradykinin generation has been demonstrated and has been accompanied by increased pulmonary vascular permeability. Greatly increased concentrations of elastase[530, 532–534] and other neutrophil-derived enzymes[535] can be detected in the blood and BAL fluid of patients with ARDS. It is likely that these increased enzyme levels represent a marker of leukocyte activation, although it is possible that the enzymes themselves cause tissue injury. Increased levels of the enzyme phospholipase A_2 have been demonstrated in the blood of patients with gram-negative sepsis, the levels being particularly high in those who develop ARDS.[536] If the phospholipase gained access to the alveolar compartment, it could cause degradation of surfactant and thus contribute to the decreased lung compliance characteristic of ARDS.

Pathologic Characteristics

The pathologic changes in the lungs of patients with ARDS are virtually the same regardless of

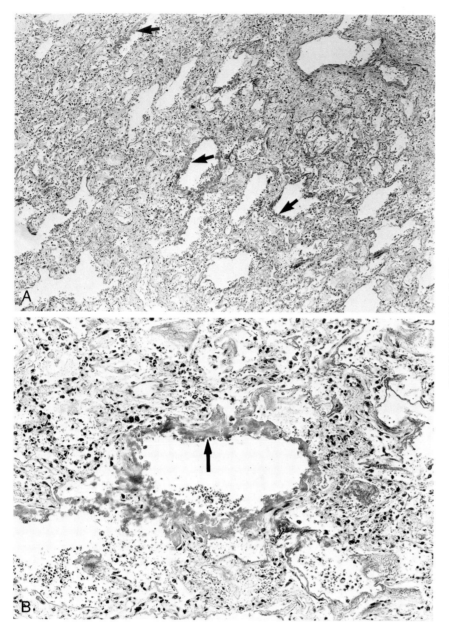

Figure 10–61. Diffuse Alveolar Damage: Exudative Phase. A histologic section of lung in the early exudative phase of diffuse alveolar damage (A) shows filling of almost all alveolar airspaces by a proteinaceous exudate containing scattered red blood cells. These changes are seen to better advantage in a section with higher magnification (B). Inflammatory cells are few in number and there is a mild to moderate degree of interstitial edema. Hyaline membranes (arrows) are present in several transitional airways. (A, × 40; B, × 120.)

etiology[445, 505, 537–541] and are frequently described by the term diffuse alveolar damage. Although a continuum of histologic abnormalities exists, for purposes of discussion the changes can conveniently be described in three phases: exudative, proliferative, and fibrotic.[538, 684, 685]

The Exudative Phase. In the early exudative phase, which in most cases occurs within hours after the initial pulmonary insult, the lungs are heavy and airless and often deep red-purple. Histologically, there is interstitial edema (affecting perivascular and interlobular interstitium as well as the alveolar wall), capillary congestion, and extensive airspace filling by a proteinaceous exudate and a variable number of red blood cells (Fig. 10–61); inflammatory cells are usually scarce. Fibrin thrombi may be present in capillaries and small arterioles

and venules.[437, 505, 538] There is considerable evidence that widespread destruction of Type I alveolar epithelial cells constitutes the major mechanism for the massive alveolar edema.[542]

Somewhat later in the course of the exudative phase (2 to 7 days), the intra-alveolar edema appears more compact and eosinophilic and may contain macrophages; similar material in alveolar ducts and distal respiratory bronchioles tends to become flattened against the airway wall, producing hyaline membranes (Fig. 10–61). Ultrastructurally, these membranes are composed of necrotic cellular debris and fibrin;[686, 687] immunohistochemically, they contain immunoglobulin (predominantly IgG), fibrinogen, surfactant apoprotein, and, in the later stages, fibronectin.[686] During this period, Type II alveolar epithelial cells undergo proliferation, resulting in a relining of alveolar surfaces. Such hyperplastic cells are often large and can show markedly reactive nuclear features.

The Proliferative Phase. Although it is not possible to put a precise time on the end of the exudative phase, changes of the proliferative phase usually become apparent anywhere from 7 to 28 days after the initial pulmonary insult. This process is characterized by fibroblast (myofibroblast) proliferation, predominantly within alveolar airspaces[686] but also in the parenchymal interstitium. Proximal transitional airways are often spared, creating a highly characteristic gross appearance of multiple, evenly distributed spaces (representing the lumens of proximal transitional airways) separated by more or less solid white-gray tissue (representing consolidated lung parenchyma) (Fig. 10–62). Mononuclear inflammatory cells, predominantly lymphocytes, may be apparent within the interstitium; in addition, focal areas of bronchopneumonia caused by bacterial superinfection are fairly common.

The Fibrotic Phase. In many cases the end result of the first two stages is the deposition of mature collagen and resulting chronic interstitial fibrosis. In some patients, however, presumably those with relatively mild disease, much of the fibroblastic proliferation resolves without functionally significant residual fibrosis.

Vascular Abnormalities

Pulmonary vascular abnormalities are also common and are sometimes extensive.[688, 689] They probably result from several causes, including microvascular thrombosis initiated by the initial pulmonary insult, thromboembolism, and necrotizing vasculitis secondary to superimposed infection.[688] Such processes result in vascular remodeling characterized by tortuous arteries and veins, a decreased number of pulmonary capillaries, intimal fibrosis, increased muscle in arterial media, and extension of muscle into arterioles (neomuscularization).

Gas-Exchange Studies

Lamy and associates[543] correlated the pathologic features with physiologic studies of gas exchange in 45 patients, most of whom were referred for extracorporeal membrane oxygenation because of severe ARDS of varying etiology. Pathologic material was obtained from either lung biopsy or necropsy. Three distinct groups were defined:

1. Patients with severe hypoxia, which responded poorly to positive end-expiratory pressure (PEEP), and with a fixed shunt at all fractions of inspired oxygen; pathologically, the lungs showed consolidation from severe edema and hemorrhage.

2. Patients with less severe hypoxia, which responded moderately well but slowly to PEEP; pathologically, there was evidence of extensive fibrosis.

3. Patients with the least hypoxia, which responded rapidly to PEEP. The pathologic findings in this group were similar to but less severe than those in group 1. Prognosis was best in group 3 patients (ten of 21 survived) and dismal in groups 1 and 2 (only two of 11 and three of 13 patients survived).

Roentgenographic Manifestations

Remarkably good correlation has been reported between the roentgenographic patterns observed during life and the pathologic changes observed at necropsy.[505, 537–539, 541]

Up to 12 Hours. All observers report a characteristic delay of up to 12 hours from the clinical onset of respiratory failure to the appearance of abnormalities on the chest roentgenogram. This lucid roentgenographic interval may be of some importance in differential diagnosis, since the major condition to be differentiated in the appropriate clinical setting is massive pulmonary embolism. However, since the chest roentgenogram can be normal in the latter condition as well, differentiation may not be possible short of a lung scan. According to Joffe,[537] roentgenographic evidence of interstitial pulmonary edema is remarkably infrequent and was observed in only five of his 75 patients. However, in two other series,[538, 539] interstitial edema was seen frequently (Fig. 10–63).

Twelve to 24 Hours. Patchy, ill-defined opacities appear throughout both lungs. The appearance is similar to airspace edema of cardiac origin, except that heart size is usually normal; in addition, the edema tends to show a more peripheral distribution (Fig. 10–64). Although upper zone vessels are usually more prominent than normal, this sign is of no value as evidence of pulmonary venous hypertension since the majority of patients will have been radiographed in the supine position.

Twenty-four Hours to 4 Days. The patchy zones of consolidation rapidly coalesce to a point of massive airspace consolidation of both lungs (Fig. 10–65). Characteristically, involvement is diffuse, affecting all lung zones from apex to base and to the extreme periphery of each lung; in our experience, this widespread distribution can be of considerable value in distinguishing ARDS from cardiogenic pulmonary edema, whose distribution is seldom as extensive. Similarly, in contrast to cardiogenic edema, an air bronchogram is frequently visible. Pleural effusion is characteristically absent; its presence should strongly suggest a complicating acute pneumonia or pulmonary infarction.

Four to 7 Days. Characteristically, improvement in the roentgenographic picture occurs, the homogeneous consolidation becoming inhomogeneous, suggesting diminution of the amount of alveolar edema (Fig. 10–65). It is during this period that superimposed bacterial pneumonia frequently

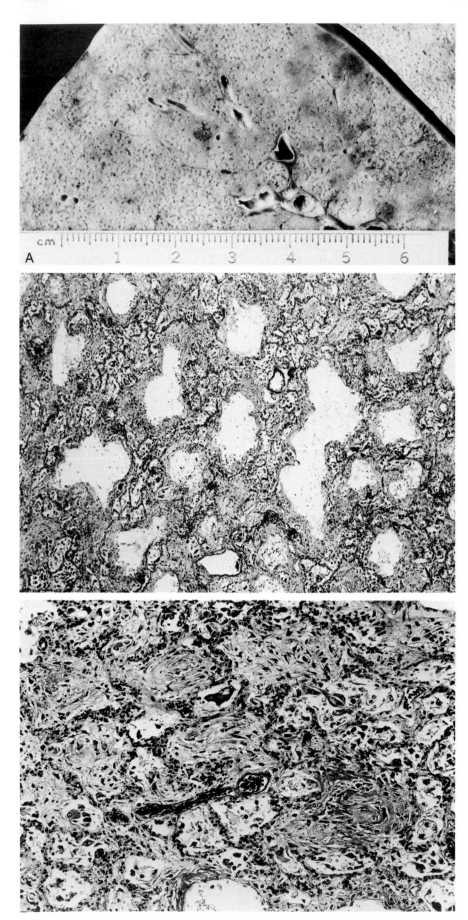

Figure 10–62. Diffuse Alveolar Damage: Organizing Phase. A magnified view of the superior segment of a lower lobe (*A*) shows diffuse, fairly uniform parenchymal consolidation associated with numerous minute interspersed "holes." A histologic section (*B*) reveals that the "holes" consist of residual patent alveolar ducts and respiratory bronchioles. At higher magnification (*C*), the intervening lung parenchyma is seen to be almost completely consolidated by loose connective tissue containing fibroblasts and macrophages. Alveolar walls are clearly recognizable and are only slightly thickened, indicating that the fibroblastic reaction is occurring within alveolar airspaces. (*B*, × 40; *C*, × 120.)

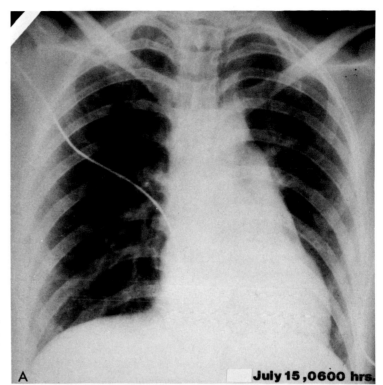

Figure 10–63. Acute Respiratory Insufficiency Associated with Gram-Negative Septicemia (ARDS). Several hours before the roentgenogram illustrated in *A*, a 31-year-old woman had noted the onset of respiratory distress, which had increased in severity in this interval; arterial blood gas analysis revealed a Po_2 of 58 and a Pco_2 of 49. This roentgenogram reveals diffuse interstitial edema but no evidence of air-space edema or of major pulmonary consolidation. Twenty-four hours later (*B*), the right upper lobe and the whole of the left lung were extensively consolidated by acute air-space edema.

Illustration continued on following page

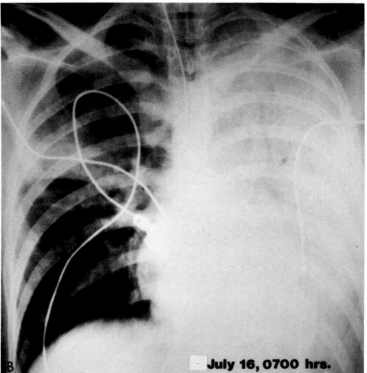

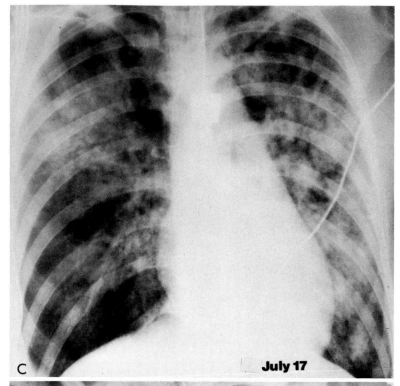

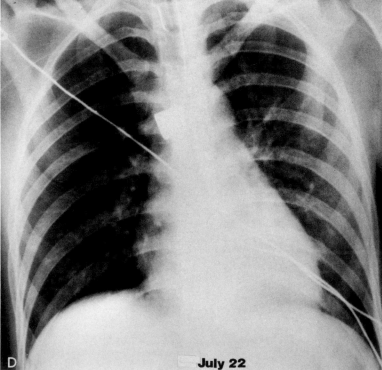

Figure 10–63 *Continued* Forty-eight hours later (*C*), the lungs were uniformly involved, although in more patchy distribution. With the institution of vigorous supportive therapy and positive end-expiratory pressure ventilation (PEEP), the patient's condition improved slowly to a point where 5 days later (*D*) the lungs were almost clear. Gram-negative septicemia following laparotomy.

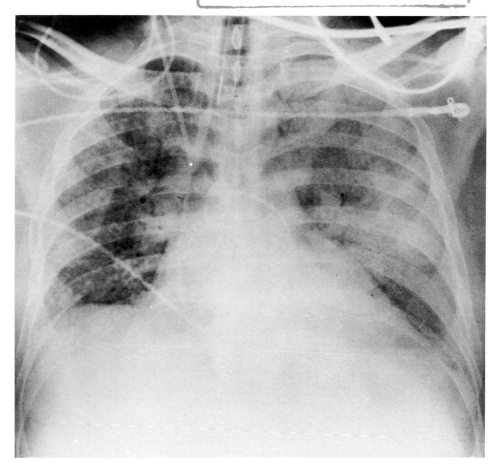

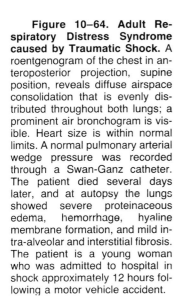

Figure 10–64. Adult Respiratory Distress Syndrome caused by Traumatic Shock. A roentgenogram of the chest in anteroposterior projection, supine position, reveals diffuse airspace consolidation that is evenly distributed throughout both lungs; a prominent air bronchogram is visible. Heart size is within normal limits. A normal pulmonary arterial wedge pressure was recorded through a Swan-Ganz catheter. The patient died several days later, and at autopsy the lungs showed severe proteinaceous edema, hemorrhage, hyaline membrane formation, and mild intra-alveolar and interstitial fibrosis. The patient is a young woman who was admitted to hospital in shock approximately 12 hours following a motor vehicle accident.

becomes evident in the form of local areas of consolidation. In cases of gram-negative pneumonia, the presence of microabscesses makes the consolidation appear mottled, like Swiss cheese.[537]

It is vital to be aware of the potential effects of mechanical ventilation and PEEP on roentgenographic appearances: as emphasized by Zimmerman and his colleagues,[544] the institution of PEEP can result in dramatic variations in the appearance of parenchymal opacities in technically identical roentgenograms exposed over a 10- to 15-minute period; in fact, patients who demonstrate roentgenographic evidence of diffuse pulmonary edema in the absence of mechanical ventilation can show an almost complete disappearance of roentgenographic abnormality within minutes of the institution of PEEP therapy (Fig. 10–65). It is obvious that knowledge of ventilator settings is essential to the correct interpretation of the severity of pulmonary abnormalities in patients with ARDS. Continuous positive pressure ventilation can also lead to diffuse interstitial emphysema that may be readily visible against the background of extensive parenchymal consolidation. It is important to recognize this development because of the frequency of impending pneumomediastinum or pneumothorax, or both.

Over 7 Days. The lungs remain diffusely abnormal, but the pattern tends to become reticular[538]

or "bubbly."[539] Of the 46 cases reported by Ostendorf and associates, eight who had a relatively long survival and continuous assisted ventilation developed a coarse reticular pattern. It is likely that this pattern represents diffuse interstitial and airspace fibrosis so characteristic of the end-stage picture observed pathologically (Fig. 10–66).

In roentgenologic differential diagnosis, the major conditions to be considered are severe cardiogenic pulmonary edema and widespread bacterial pneumonia. Cardiogenic pulmonary edema may present a similar picture roentgenographically, although involvement of the lungs is seldom as widespread and uniform as in ARDS. There are other features that aid in distinguishing cardiogenic edema from ARDS, and these are discussed in the next section. In the most severe cases, differentiation can be made only by measuring the pulmonary arterial wedge pressure with a Swan-Ganz catheter, bearing in mind that left ventricular failure and consequent elevation of the wedge pressure can also occur as a complication of ARDS itself.

Pulmonary edema caused by aspiration of liquid gastric contents (Mendelson's syndrome) can usually be differentiated by the fact that roentgenographic changes occur immediately after the acute insult rather than showing the usual 12-hour delay of ARDS. Massive pneumonia may be impossible to

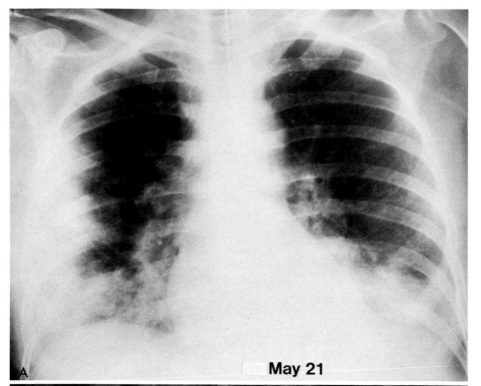

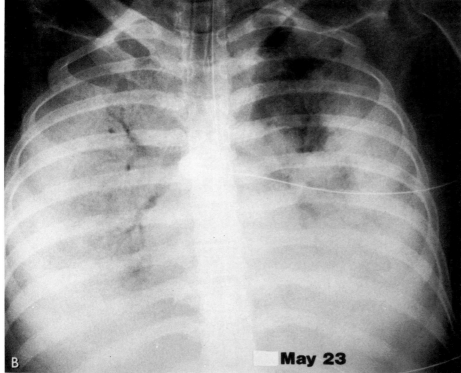

Figure 10–65. Acute Posttraumatic Respiratory Insufficiency ("Shock Lung," ARDS). This 18-year-old girl was admitted to the intensive care unit in severe shock following a motor vehicle accident. A roentgenogram the day after admission (*A*) revealed homogeneous consolidation of the left lower lobe and the axillary portion of the right lung. Two days later (*B*), both lungs were massively consolidated by pulmonary edema; note the prominent air bronchogram.

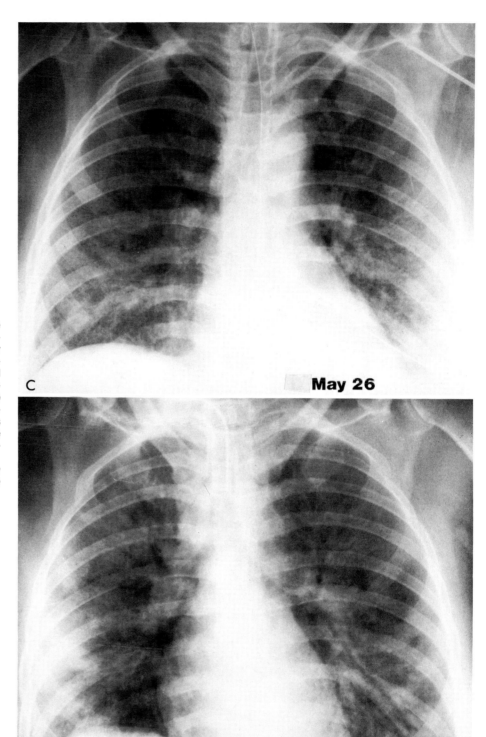

Figure 10–65 *Continued C,* Three days later, following vigorous supportive therapy and positive end-expiratory pressure (PEEP) ventilation, the patient's condition improved slightly and a roentgenogram revealed considerable clearing of the diffuse air-space edema. Three days later (*D*), the roentgenographic appearance of the lungs had once again deteriorated and there was evidence of patchy airspace consolidation.

*Illustration continued on
following page*

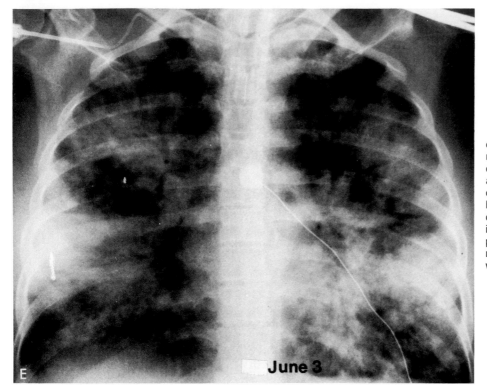

Figure 10–65 *Continued* Five days later (*E*), both lungs had become massively consolidated in a pattern compatible with combined edema and acute airspace pneumonia. The patient died shortly thereafter. At necropsy, both lungs were found to be massively consolidated and very heavy. Histologically, there was extensive fibroblastic proliferation and collagen deposition, not only within the interstitium but within alveoli.

differentiate from ARDS except on clinical grounds. Traumatic fat embolism is impossible to distinguish from other forms of ARDS on roentgenographic evidence. However, the typical clinical triad associated with lipuria usually permits early diagnosis.

Perhaps not unexpectedly, the pathologic, roentgenographic, and clinical manifestations of ARDS in children are little different from those in adults.[545]

ROENTGENOGRAPHIC DIFFERENTIATION OF CARDIOGENIC AND PERMEABILITY EDEMA

Although, as pointed out above, the differentiation of high-pressure (cardiogenic) and low-pressure (permeability) edema often requires the measurement of pulmonary arterial wedge pressure, the roentgenographic pattern of edema frequently permits the distinction to be made with a high degree of accuracy. Milne and his colleagues[546] carried out an independent two-observer study in which 216 chest roentgenograms obtained on 119 patients with pulmonary edema were reviewed with respect to the presence or absence of nine features; 61 of the patients had cardiac disease, 30 had renal failure or overhydration, and 28 had ARDS. Three principal and six ancillary roentgenographic features were identified, all of which permitted the cause of the edema to be determined correctly in a high percentage of patients. The highest accuracy was obtained in distinguishing ARDS from the other two varieties of edema (in 91 per cent of cases), and the lowest accuracy in distinguishing chronic cardiac failure from renal failure (in 81 per cent of pa-

tients). Of the nine features to be described below, the first three were principal and the remaining six ancillary.

Distribution of Pulmonary Blood Flow. Of the three patterns of blood flow distribution, normal, balanced and inverted, 50 per cent of patients with cardiogenic edema showed an inverted flow and 40 per cent a balanced distribution; 80 per cent of patients with renal failure had a balanced distribution and 20 were normal; and 40 per cent of those with capillary permeability had normal distribution and 50 per cent a balanced distribution. Of note is the fact that in none of the patients with renal failure and in only 10 per cent of those with ARDS was pulmonary blood flow inverted.

Distribution of Pulmonary Edema. Although there were many variations in the distribution of edema, all could be grouped into three principal categories—even, central, and peripheral. Ninety per cent of patients with cardiogenic edema showed an even distribution pattern (more or less homogeneous from chest wall to heart) and only 10 per cent were predominantly central; in these cases, the distribution of edema was clearly affected by gravity, being most marked at the lung bases. In the renal failure patients, central edema predominated (70 per cent of cases) and in none was a peripheral pattern observed. In contrast to these two patterns, in 45 per cent of patients with ARDS a peripheral distribution was shown and in 35 per cent it was widespread from chest wall to mediastinum; the pattern was often patchy with small intervening unaffected regions of lung parenchyma.

Width of the Vascular Pedicle. Three possible

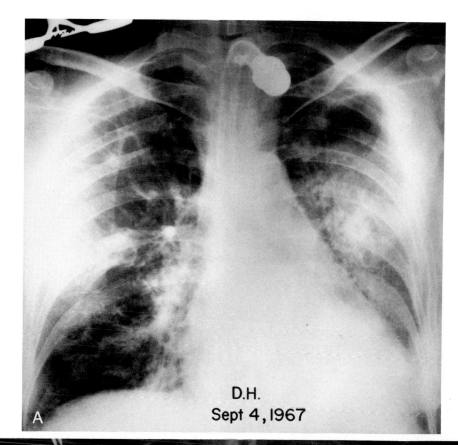

Figure 10–66. Adult Respiratory Distress Syndrome (ARDS) with a Prolonged Course and Partial Resolution. Twenty-four hours after admission of a young woman with multiple bone fractures sustained in a motor vehicle accident, a roentgenogram of the chest in anteroposterior projection, supine position (A) shows a mixture of reticular and airspace opacities asymmetrically distributed throughout the lungs. Endotracheal intubation is present. Four days later, a repeat roentgenogram (B) demonstrates worsening of the airspace consolidation, a progression that is common in ARDS.

Illustration continued on following page

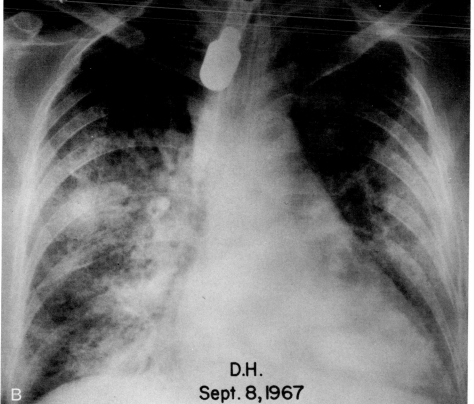

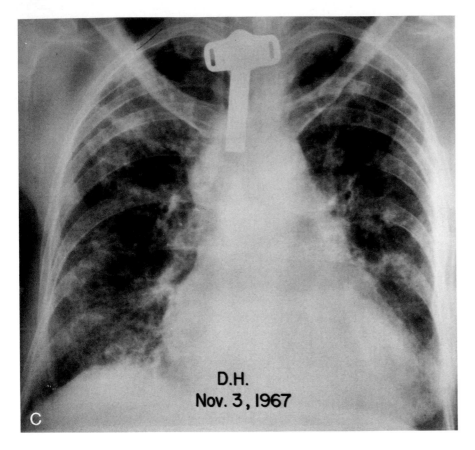

D.H.
Nov. 3, 1967

C

Figure 10–66 *Continued* Approximately 2 months later, a predischarge roentgenogram (*C*) shows that most of the airspace component has resolved; however, the lungs are the site of persistent coarse reticulation that almost certainly represents residual parenchymal fibrosis. Follow-up films over the ensuing months demonstrated only modest further improvement.

variations of vascular pedicle width are possible—decreased, normal, or increased. (For a description of the normal and abnormal vascular pedicle, *see* page 242). In the cardiac failure group, 60 per cent of patients showed an increased vascular pedicle width and 40 per cent were in the normal range. In the renal-overhydration group, 85 per cent of patients showed a widened vascular pedicle and only 15 per cent were normal. Of the patients with capillary permeability edema, 35 per cent had a normal pedicle and 35 per cent a narrowed pedicle. Of note with respect to the ARDS group is the fact that 60 per cent of patients were radiographed in the supine position, which increased the vascular pedicle width by an average of 20 per cent.[547]

Pulmonary Blood Volume. This parameter was assessed by estimating the size of visible lung markings, there being three possible variations—diminished, normal, or increased. A decrease in blood volume was seen in a small number of patients with ARDS on PEEP and in a few cardiac cases with very low cardiac output. In general, the pulmonary blood volume tended to be increased in patients with renal failure or overhydration (70 per cent) but in only 40 per cent of those with cardiogenic edema and 20 per cent of those with permeability edema; it was normal in 80 per cent of patients with ARDS.

Septal Lines and Peribronchial Cuffing. Septal lines were observed in approximately 30 per cent of patients with either cardiac or renal-overhydration edema but were identified in none of the ARDS patients. Peribronchial cuffing was observed in the majority of the renal and cardiac patients but in only a small number of patients with ARDS.

Air Bronchograms. This sign was identified frequently in patients with capillary permeability edema (70 per cent) but in only 20 per cent of the cardiac and renal-overhydration cases.

Pleural Effusion. Pleural effusion was identified in approximately 40 per cent of patients with cardiac edema and in 30 per cent of those with renal edema but in only about 10 per cent of those with permeability edema.

Lung Volume. Lung volume was usually normal or slightly increased in patients with renal-overhydration edema, reduced in patients with cardiac edema (reflecting diminished compliance), and normal in patients with ARDS (except in patients on PEEP).

Heart Size. Following application of a 12.5 per cent correction factor necessitated by the supine position of patients, the anteroposterior projection, and the shortened 40-inch distance, cardiac enlargement was identified in 85 per cent of patients with renal-overhydration edema, in 72 per cent of patients with cardiogenic edema, but in only 32 per cent of those with capillary permeability edema.

A summation of all these statistically significant factors in distinguishing the three types of edema is given in Table 10–4.

In a subsequent study by this same group headed by Miniati,[681] 119 roentgenograms of patients with pulmonary edema caused by left heart decompensation (Group 1, N = 56), renal failure (Group 2, N = 19), and microvascular injury (Group 3, N = 44) were retrospectively analyzed to assess the value of the chest roentgenogram in distinguishing these types of pulmonary edema. Two trained observers who were unaware of the clinical diagnosis assigned chest roentgenograms to the corresponding group with an accuracy of 86 and 90 per cent, respectively. In addition, roentgenographic findings were used as input variables for discriminant analysis: when the three groups are considered together, computer-generated numerical functions identified the etiology of pulmonary edema with an accuracy of 88 per cent; when groups were compared as pairs, percentages of correct classification were 91 (Group 1 versus Group 2), 93 (Group 1 versus Group 3), and 100 (Group 2 versus Group 3).

Two other studies designed to identify roentgenographic features that permit differentiation of different etiologies of pulmonary edema have been carried out in recent years, one of which more or less supports the conclusions reached in the Milne and Miniati studies and the other of which refutes them. Smith and his colleagues[548] compared the conventional chest roentgenograms of 94 critically ill patients with different types of pulmonary edema—49 cardiogenic, 33 permeability, and 12 renal-overhydration. On the basis of a standardized score sheet of findings, these authors found that patients with cardiogenic edema had enlarged hearts, vascular engorgement, septal lines, and absence of an air bronchogram significantly more often than patients with permeability pulmonary edema. Patients with renal failure–overhydration had enlarged hearts significantly more often than patients with permeability edema. Of particular interest in this study was the fact that heart size and the presence or absence of septal lines could have been used to distinguish cardiogenic from permeability edema in 83 per cent of patients. By contrast, a study by Aberle and her colleagues[682] concluded that chest roentgenograms are of limited value in the differentiation of types of pulmonary edema in severe cases. These authors studied 45 patients with severe pulmonary edema, roughly evenly divided between hydrostatic and permeability types. Chest roentgenograms were classified as showing hydrostatic, increased permeability, or mixed edema by three independent observers without knowledge of the clinical diagnosis. Overall, 87 per cent of patients with hydrostatic edema but only 60 per cent of those with increased permeability edema were correctly identified. A patchy, peripheral distribution of edema was the single most discriminating criterion, occurring in 50 per cent of patients with permeability edema but in only 13 per cent of those with the hydrostatic type. Considerable overlap was found with various signs, including the vascular pedicle, pleural effusion, peribronchial cuffs, and septal lines.

In summary, despite the rather dismal results obtained by Aberle and her colleagues,[682] on the basis of personal observation of many cases over several years and on the strength of the findings in the other three studies,[546, 548, 681] we believe that it is possible to distinguish cardiogenic from permeability edema with a reasonable degree of accuracy in the majority of patients. However, there is no question that the measurement of pulmonary arterial wedge pressure is almost always necessary to provide an objective criterion on which to estimate the presence or absence of increased pressure in the left atrium and pulmonary veins; this is perhaps particularly so in patients with severe ARDS in whom superimposed left ventricular failure can modify the therapeutic regimen.

Clinical and Physiologic Manifestations

The clinical manifestations of ARDS can develop either insidiously, hours or days after the initiating event (e.g., sepsis or fat emboli), or acutely, coincident with the event (e.g., aspiration of liquid gastric contents). Typical symptoms are dyspnea, tachypnea, dry cough, retrosternal discomfort, and agitation; cyanosis may be present. The expectora-

Table 10–4. Radiographic Features of Pulmonary Edema*

	CARDIAC	RENAL	INJURY
Heart size	Enlarged	Enlarged	Not enlarged
Vascular pedicle	Normal or enlarged	Enlarged	Normal or reduced
Pulmonary blood flow distribution	Inverted	Balanced	Normal or balanced
Pulmonary blood volume	Normal or increased	Increased	Normal
Septal lines	Not common	Not common	Absent
Peribronchial cuffs	Very common	Very common	Not common
Air bronchogram	Not common	Not common	Very common
Lung edema, regional distribution (horizontal axis)	Even	Central	Peripheral
Pleural effusions	Very common	Very common	Not common

*From Milne ENC, Pistolesi M, Miniati M, et al: The radiologic distinction of cardiogenic and noncardiogenic edema. AJR *144*:879, 1985.

Note: Each factor listed has been shown to have statistical significance in determining which type of edema is present.

tion of copious blood-tinged fluid signifies the presence of the full-blown syndrome. Examination of the chest reveals coarse crackles and bronchial breath sounds. Arterial blood analysis shows severe hypoxemia and a normal or decreased arterial P_{CO_2}. The hypoxemia is difficult or impossible to correct even with the use of very high concentrations of inspired oxygen. Clinical deterioration is usual, requiring endotracheal intubation to maintain adequate oxygenation (O_2 saturation greater than 90 per cent). The chest roentgenogram at this stage typically reveals widespread airspace consolidation, raising the question as to whether the edema is cardiogenic or permeability in type. Although the roentgenographic features described above can aid differentiation, the measurement of pulmonary vascular pressures is an essential discriminating test.

The measurement of pulmonary arterial wedge pressure, using a balloon-tipped, flow-directed catheter is frequently used in the investigation of patients with pulmonary edema.[549] When correctly measured, the wedge pressure provides an accurate estimate of the filling pressure of the left ventricle and is therefore a reflection of left ventricular preload; in addition, it provides information concerning the hydrostatic pressure in pulmonary fluid-exchanging microvessels. The principle behind the measurement is as follows: inflation of a balloon in a pulmonary artery to a size sufficient to occlude flow results in a static column of blood that extends from the tip of the catheter to the point where the pulmonary vein subserved by that artery joins the other pulmonary veins before their entrance into the left atrium. Because the pulmonary circulation is an end-arterial system with no collateral perfusion, the wedge pressure provides an accurate reflection of pulmonary venous pressure at the confluence of the pulmonary veins close to the left atrium. Since an elevated left ventricular filling pressure is the hallmark of cardiogenic pulmonary edema, the finding of a normal wedge pressure provides convincing evidence that the edema is the result of increased permeability (provided that therapy with diuretics and cardiac stimulating agents has not been instituted). Central venous pressure measurement does not provide similar information because the right and left ventricles often differ considerably in their performance characteristics and filling pressures.[550]

Correct measurement of the arterial wedge pressure as an estimate of pulmonary venous pressure requires that a column of blood extend from the peripheral end of the wedged catheter to the pulmonary venous system. When the lung is in Zone I or II conditions and alveolar pressure exceeds pulmonary arterial or pulmonary venous pressure (or both), the pulmonary wedge pressure may not be an accurate reflection of pulmonary venous pressure.[549] This artefact can occur when there is an increase in alveolar pressure (e.g., in the presence of PEEP) or when there is a decrease in intravascular pressure (e.g., in the presence of shock). The application of PEEP, a procedure frequently used in critically ill patients with pulmonary edema, can also influence the measurement of pulmonary capillary wedge pressure in another way: by increasing pleural pressure around the heart and pulmonary veins, PEEP can provide an erroneously elevated estimate of pulmonary venous pressure. Normally, about half of the externally applied PEEP is transmitted to the pleural space; as a result, the pulmonary wedge pressure increases by approximately half of the PEEP pressure that is added. The proportion of externally applied PEEP that is transmitted to the pleural space—and therefore to the wedge catheter measurement—is dependent on the relative compliances of the lung and chest wall. If the lung is very stiff, as in patients with ARDS, less of the externally applied PEEP is "seen" in the pleural space. Whether or not the pulmonary artery catheter is in Zone III can be determined by obtaining a lateral roentgenogram of the chest with a horizontal x-ray beam. If the mean pulmonary artery pressure (referenced to midthorax) and the alveolar pressure at end-expiration are known, the vertical level at which Zone I flow conditions will begin can be calculated. In addition, if the catheter is wedged in Zone I or II, the pressure will show very little cardiogenic fluctuation but will have considerable respiratory swings.

The pulmonary wedge pressure provides an accurate reflection of left atrial pressure, provided there is no major venous obstruction between the confluence of pulmonary veins and their point of entry into the left atrium; obstructive lesions in large veins occasionally result in an elevated pulmonary venous pressure and a normal left atrial pressure.[549] If there is no mitral valvular obstruction, pulmonary wedge pressure also provides an accurate reflection of left ventricular end-diastolic pressure. Following pneumonectomy, the pulmonary wedge pressure can provide a falsely low estimate of left atrial pressure.[551]

In addition to giving an accurate estimate of left ventricular filling pressure, the pulmonary wedge pressure provides information concerning the microvascular pressure in the exchanging vessels. As discussed above, pulmonary capillary pressure is dependent on the relative resistance of the arterial and venous systems. During occlusion of the pulmonary artery, any pressure drop between the pulmonary microvessels and the major pulmonary veins disappears so that pulmonary wedge pressure will underestimate pulmonary capillary pressure. The latter must be somewhat higher than pulmonary wedge pressure, and the magnitude of this difference is related directly to the pulmonary venous resistance. Since pulmonary venous resistance is relatively low and since few conditions selectively increase it, in most cases it is reasonable to use the pulmonary wedge pressure as an estimate of pulmonary microvascular pressure. The one condition in which this assumption is invalid and can lead to diagnostic errors is pulmonary veno-occlusive disease: when small pulmonary veins are obstructed, pulmonary capillary pressure can be substantially higher than pulmonary venous pressure during conditions of flow; however, when the wedge catheter is inserted, the large pressure drop between pulmonary capillary and pulmonary vein disappears, and as a consequence, the wedge pressure gives an erroneously low estimate of the functional pulmonary capillary pressure.

In addition to its use as a method of determining whether pulmonary edema is caused by increased microvascular pressure or increased permeability, the measurement of wedge pressure can be a very effective management tool in testing the effectiveness of agents and therapies designed to lower intravascular pressure. In the presence of increased microvascular permeability, edema formation is critically dependent on microvascular pressure; although an increase in microvascular pressure is not the *primary* cause of edema in such circumstances, transient or prolonged elevation of microvascular pressure can significantly exaggerate the formation of edema (Fig. 10–67); by contrast, a very low microvascular pressure, such as may be present in severe shock, could conceivably diminish the amount of edema formed.

In the presence of pulmonary edema, normal or low pulmonary arterial wedge pressure provides strong, indirect evidence that endothelial damage and increased permeability are the cause of the edema. A number of *direct* tests of endothelial integrity have been devised, and although none of these is practical for general clinical use, they are of considerable theoretical interest. Radioactive tracers can be nebulized or instilled into the lung and their appearance in the blood monitored over time as a measure of permeability.[552–555] In some of these studies, an increase in permeability has been demonstrated before the manifestations of ARDS became evident clinically, suggesting that tests of permeability may be useful in predicting the probability of the development of ARDS. Similar results are obtained when radiolabeled tracers are administered intravenously and their accumulation in the lung is monitored, either with external counters[555, 556] or by measuring them in BAL fluid.[557, 558] The pulmonary endothelium normally metabolizes both propranolol and serotonin during their passage through the pulmonary microvasculature; pulmonary extraction of radiolabeled propranolol and serotonin has been shown to be impaired in patients with ARDS, the degree of impairment correlating with the severity of the pulmonary damage.[559]

In patients with pulmonary edema who are intubated, sampling of the pulmonary edema fluid through the endotracheal tube permits measurement of the protein concentration in the edema fluid and comparison with simultaneously measured protein concentration in the serum. In a study in which patients with clinically diagnosed cardiogenic pulmonary edema were compared with those with permeability edema, the ratio of protein concentration in edema fluid to that in serum was significantly higher in patients with permeability edema, permitting clear separation of the two entities in patients in whom the diagnosis was not obvious.[560]

Once a diagnosis of ARDS has been established, it is necessary to follow the severity of the lung injury with a quantitative measurement of the pul-

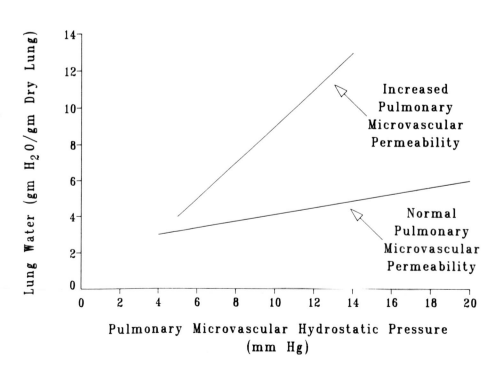

Figure 10–67. Lung Water versus Pulmonary Microvascular Pressure. Lung water, expressed as grams of water per gram of dry lung, is plotted against mean pulmonary microvascular pressure. When pulmonary microvascular permeability is normal, increased microvascular pressure causes a modest increase in lung water (hydrostatic edema); when microvascular permeability is increased, the same changes in pressure cause a marked accumulation of lung water.

monary edema. Roentgenographic methods to assess the severity of edema have already been discussed (*see* page 1899). A number of other methods have been developed to measure the amount of extravascular lung water, using the double indicator dilution technique[561–563] in which the volume of distribution of a tracer is based on the relationship between flow, volume of distribution, and transit time according to the formula

$$\text{volume of distribution} = \text{flow} \times \text{transit time}$$

If a tracer is injected into the pulmonary artery and its arrival in the aorta is determined, the volume of its distribution between those two points can be measured if the total flow through the system is known (i.e., cardiac output) and if the transit time between the injection and sensing site can be measured. If two tracers are injected simultaneously, one of which remains confined to the intravascular space and the other diffuses throughout the interstitial space of the lung, measurement of both in the left heart or aorta reveals the difference between the volumes of distribution of the diffusible and nondiffusible tracer and constitutes a measure of pulmonary extravascular water. The most practical method involves the intravenous injection of a cold green dye, with subsequent detection of the dye and measurement of blood temperature (using a thermocouple) in the arterial circulation. The green dye remains confined to the intravascular space and serves as a nondiffusible indicator while the temperature dissipates readily in the entire pulmonary extravascular space. By measuring the appearance times of the dye and the cold with a specially designed catheter inserted into a systemic artery,[564–566] the quantity of extravascular lung water can be estimated. Using a similar principle, lung water can also be quantified by inhaling gases of different solubility such as acetylene and dimethyl ether.[567]

The most important pathophysiologic effect of the edema in patients with ARDS is on gas exchange, the profound hypoxemia rather than the ventilatory failure being the major indication for intubation and mechanical ventilation. The hypoxemia is caused by intrapulmonary shunting of blood through edematous lung regions. By employing the multiple inert gas technique[568, 569] or the classic method of 100 per cent O_2 ventilation,[570] it has been shown that the predominant pathogenesis of hypoxemia is pure shunt rather than other forms of ventilation-perfusion mismatching. It is the distinct impression of many physicians who care for patients with ARDS that the gas-exchange impairment is worse than in patients with cardiogenic pulmonary edema of equal severity, an effect that is possibly the result of a failure of the mechanisms that normally tend to minimize ventilation-perfusion mismatching. As discussed above, these mechanisms could be either a failure of interstitial pressure to

increase and thus occlude vessels in the edematous lung regions or a failure of hypoxic pulmonary vasoconstriction. In 14 patients with ARDS, Brigham and associates[571] measured extravascular lung water, gas-exchange abnormalities, and the permeability-surface area product, and found that the more abnormal gas exchange and poorer prognosis related better to an increased permeability-surface area product than to increased lung water. They suggested that preservation of pulmonary vascular constriction improves gas exchange and survival in patients with ARDS. Other studies have also shown that pulmonary vascular tone improves gas exchange.[714] The intrapulmonary shunt in patients with ARDS increases when total pulmonary blood flow is increased,[572, 573] an effect that is probably related to an increase in mixed venous PO_2 and decreased hypoxic vasoconstriction.

In addition to the obvious defect in pulmonary gas exchange that occurs in patients with ARDS, there is evidence that peripheral oxygen uptake may also be impaired. In normal subjects, oxygen consumption by the body is not dependent on oxygen delivery (cardiac output $\times$ arterial O_2 content); if the oxygen content of arterial blood decreases, peripheral oxygen extraction increases, resulting in a larger difference in arterial-to-venous oxygen content and thus preserving total oxygen consumption. Not until oxygen delivery decreases to approximately 8 ml/minute/kg does oxygen consumption diminish in normal subjects.[574] By contrast, in patients with ARDS most[575–578] but not all[579] studies have shown that O_2 consumption decreases linearly with O_2 delivery, even when it exceeds 20 ml/minute/kg. Although the mechanism of this defect in tissue oxygen extraction is incompletely understood, it suggests that ARDS is a generalized abnormality, possibly of microvascular regulation.

ARDS is often accompanied by pulmonary arterial hypertension[580] and the resultant increase in right ventricular afterload usually causes right ventricular dysfunction. Abnormalities of right ventricular contractility have been demonstrated by radionuclide techniques[581, 582] and by two-dimensional echocardiography.[583] There is also evidence that right ventricular dysfunction can result in left ventricular dysfunction, most likely related to a shift in the shared interventricular septum.[582]

Risk Factors and Prognosis in ARDS

It has been estimated that there are 150,000 new cases of ARDS each year in the United States and that the mortality rate is invariably over 50 per cent.[584, 585] The major risk factors for the development of ARDS include sepsis (or "sepsis syndrome"), aspiration of liquid gastric contents, multiple trauma (including long bone and pelvic fractures and lung contusion), multiple blood transfusions, overwhelming pneumonia, and DIC (often associated with sepsis).[586] Fowler and associates[587] prospectively studied 993 patients who had at least one of eight risk factors known to predispose to the development of permeability pulmonary edema; 57 of the 993 patients (5.7 per cent) had more than one risk factor. ARDS was defined as acute respiratory failure requiring mechanical ventilation, accompanied by the acute onset of widespread airspace opacities on the chest roentgenogram; physiologic criteria included a pulmonary wedge pressure less than 12 mm Hg, a respiratory system compliance less than 50 ml cm H_2O, and an arterial-to-alveolar partial pressure ratio of 0.2 or less. Of the 993 patients, 67 (6.8 per cent) developed ARDS, the incidence increasing to 24 per cent in the 57 patients who had two or more risk factors. Over the period of study, the syndrome developed in 20 additional patients from causes other than those identified for prospective evaluation, including drug overdose, pancreatitis, thoracic trauma, and presumed sepsis. In this study, the factor with the highest incidence of ARDS was aspiration, 16 (35.6 per cent) of 45 patients being so affected. Sixty-five per cent of patients who developed the syndrome died, and in 90 per cent of these, death occurred within 14 days of the onset of symptoms.[587] Clinical features and laboratory data recorded at the time of diagnosis of the syndrome were analyzed in an attempt to identify predictors of survival and mortality: the only factors that were significantly related to increased mortality were a decreased number of band-form polymorphonuclear leukocytes, a low arterial blood pH, and a low concentration of arterial blood bicarbonate ion; direct measurements of the severity of the pulmonary injury such as arterial blood gas tensions, gas-exchange abnormalities, and pulmonary hemodynamic derangements were not predictive of survival. This study suggests that factors other than the severity of the pulmonary injury itself may be important in determining prognosis following the development of ARDS.

In a cooperative, prospective study of 713 patients with severe respiratory failure, multiple organ failure was an important contributing factor to the 61 per cent mortality rate:[588] only 40 per cent of those with pulmonary insufficiency alone died, whereas patients with two, three, four, and five organs involved showed mortality rates of 54, 72, 84, and 100 per cent, respectively. Coincident renal failure is a particularly important complication: in one study,[589] the mortality rate increased from 40 per cent in patients with pulmonary involvement alone to 89 per cent in those with combined renal and respiratory failure. Sepsis is also a frequent, fatal complication of ARDS in addition to being the most common initiator of the syndrome; infection is most often caused by gram-negative organisms and the most frequent sites of infection are the lung and abdominal cavity.[590]

The suggestion that mortality in ARDS is related to functional derangement of multiple organs more closely than to specific pulmonary dysfunction has been supported by another study of risk and mortality in 207 patients who were prospectively identified as being at risk for the development of ARDS.[591] The specific risk factors included the "sepsis syndrome" (see farther on), documented aspiration of gastric contents, near-drowning, pulmonary contusion, multiple long bone fractures, multiple transfusions (more than 10 units of blood over 6 hours), and hypotension (systolic blood pressure less than 90 mm Hg for more than 2 hours). ARDS was defined as a $PaO_2:FiO_2$ ratio less than 150, roentgenographic evidence of diffuse airspace consolidation, a pulmonary artery wedge pressure less than 18 mm Hg, and no other findings to explain these abnormalities. Forty-seven (23 per cent) of the 207 patients developed ARDS and 32 (68 per cent) of these died; by contrast, only 55 (34 per cent) of the 160 patients died who had similar risk factors but did not develop ARDS. Only five of the 32 ARDS patients died of irreversible respiratory failure, most of the deaths that occurred during the first 3 days after entry into the study being attributed to the underlying illness or injury, and most of those that occurred after 3 days being related to unremitting sepsis. In this and other studies, the "sepsis syndrome" was defined as the presence of systemic bacterial infection accompanied by evidence of a deleterious systemic effect of the infection; criteria for the diagnosis of infection included significant hyperthermia or hypothermia, appreciable leukopenia or leukocytosis, and a positive blood culture of an accepted pathogen (or the identification of a suspected source of systemic infection from which a known pathogen was cultured); evidence for deleterious systemic effects included hypotension or a decrease in systemic vascular resistance (or both) and unexplained metabolic acidosis.[591]

The results of these studies are in contrast to those of the multicenter randomized trial of extracorporeal membrane oxygenation sponsored by the National Heart, Lung, and Blood Institute of the United States.[592] In that trial, 82 of 90 patients died; 40 were thought to have had a respiratory-related death and only 22 per cent of these developed sepsis. The differences observed in the results of this study and the one previously cited[591] are probably related to their design: in the membrane oxygenation study, patients with severe gas-exchange abnormalities were preferentially selected, whereas those with significant disease involving other organs tended to be excluded.

The results of these studies[591, 592] permit three important conclusions:

1. Maintenance of normal arterial blood gases throughout the period of acute lung injury does not guarantee eventual survival because lung repair and reversal of the injury do not necessarily occur.

2. Multiple organ failure and death from causes unrelated to, or only secondarily related to, the primary pulmonary insult are the rule rather than the exception.

3. The prognosis is dismal despite intensive

medical management, and survival may depend in large measure on the institution of early prophylactic therapeutic interventions in order to prevent rather than treat this devastating condition.

In one prospective study of patients with ARDS, changes in body weight and balance of fluid intake and output were important predictors of survival;[593] patients who had a progressive weight gain were less likely to survive than those who lost weight, an effect that was present even after correction for serum albumin levels and renal status. There are two possible explanations for these observations:

1. Patients who did not survive had a continued generalized microvascular capillary leak that resulted in progressive fluid accumulation.

2. Their hemodynamic instability was sufficiently severe to require excessive fluid transfusion.

Patients who die of pulmonary insufficiency usually show a progressive decrease in lung compliance and worsening gas exchange; in the terminal stages, in addition to barotrauma hypercapnia may develop despite an enormous minute ventilation. Pathologic examination of the lungs in these patients reveals extensive interstitial and intra-alveolar fibrosis; biochemical analysis demonstrates the presence of increased lung collagen.[594] Fibrosis can occur over an extremely short time course;[595] we have observed the development of ossification of pulmonary tissue over a period of 2 weeks following the onset of the syndrome. The rapidity of development of exuberant fibrosis and the unfavorable prognosis associated with it have suggested that the early institution of corticosteroid therapy might be beneficial in arresting the fibrotic process; however, despite isolated reports of success,[596] most controlled trials have produced negative results.[597, 715]

Patients who survive ARDS manifest surprisingly little long-term impairment of lung function;[598–600] they may have mild restrictive impairment and gas-exchange deficit[598] and occasionally can exhibit partly reversible airway obstruction.[601] Long-term abnormalities of function are more likely to be present in patients who have had the most severe disturbances in lung mechanics and gas exchange during their acute illness and in those treated for prolonged periods with an FiO_2 greater than 0.5.[602, 603]

SPECIFIC FORMS OF PERMEABILITY EDEMA

High-Altitude Pulmonary Edema

Many individuals develop a variety of symptoms while becoming acclimatized to high altitudes. This symptom complex, known as mountain or altitude sickness,[604] includes headache, giddiness, dizziness, tiredness, weakness, body aches, anorexia, nausea, vomiting, abdominal pain, insomnia, rest-

lessness, cough, dyspnea on exertion, and occasionally fever. Physical examination of some patients reveals rales, which may persist and even increase as long as the individuals remain at high altitude. Diastolic blood pressure and pulse rate increase and maximal breathing capacity and peak expiratory flow rates decrease. All symptoms and signs characteristically disappear on descent to sea level. A small percentage of persons arriving at high altitude develop overt pulmonary edema, which occasionally proves fatal.[605] This is a relatively rare occurrence, however, as illustrated by one study in which edema developed in only one of 200 persons.[612]

The illness may become manifest on both acute[616] and prolonged[617] exposure at 3,500 to 4,000 meters (11,500 to 13,000 feet). Usually, the move from sea level to high altitude is abrupt—all but three of 101 patients reported by Menon[612] had arrived at an altitude of 3,500 meters (11,500 feet) by airplane. It is rare for edema to develop at altitudes of less than 3,350 meters (11,000 feet), but reports have originated in the United States of cases developing at 2,750 meters (9,000 feet).[618, 619]

Characteristically, the patients are young and healthy; some have arrived at high altitudes for the first time but the condition appears to show a predilection for former residents who are returning after being at sea level for a few days to several weeks.[607, 608, 612, 615] In one study,[615] 75 per cent of affected patients were returning to high altitude, having lived at heights for 6 to 9 months followed by a sojourn of 30 to 60 days on the plains. Edema usually develops within 2 to 3 days and almost always within the first month after arrival at high altitude. Physical exertion and cold weather are considered precipitating factors in some cases,[606, 609, 611] but the majority of Menon's patients were employed in sedentary occupations.[612]

The pathophysiology of high-altitude pulmonary edema is unknown. One study[620] has clearly demonstrated that increased capillary permeability is a contributing factor; however, the fact that the edema usually occurs in constitutionally predisposed individuals who develop an inordinate degree of pulmonary arterial hypertension following exposure to normally tolerable levels of hypoxia suggests that increased intravascular pressure is also important.[251, 716] Despite this, some patients who have experienced high-altitude edema demonstrate completely normal pulmonary vascular responsiveness to hypoxemia.[477] In one study, a group of men who were known to have developed high-altitude pulmonary edema months before were compared with a control group;[615] it was found that the susceptible persons had shorter chests, smaller lung volumes, and higher pulmonary arterial pressures and pulse rates than the controls. Hypoxic breathing lowered the oxygen saturation of the arterial blood and raised the pulmonary arterial pressures to a greater extent in the susceptible than in the normal subjects.

The pathophysiology of acute mountain sickness, high-altitude pulmonary edema, and high-altitude cerebral edema are probably interrelated.[621, 622, 717] Small but significant changes in vital capacity can be demonstrated in individuals who manifest symptoms of acute mountain sickness in the absence of overt pulmonary edema.[623] People who experience altitude sickness have lower minute ventilation and higher values of end-tidal P_{CO_2} at high altitude and also show a decreased ventilatory response to hypoxia when studied at sea level.[624] Hyers and colleagues[625] made careful measurements of gas exchange in seven individuals with a previous history of high-altitude pulmonary edema and nine subjects who tolerated altitude without pulmonary symptoms: at a simulated altitude of 4,150 meters, the former showed significantly lower P_{O_2} and higher P_{CO_2} values; the hypoxemia could not be attributed solely to decreased ventilation, since the $(A - a) D_{O_2}$ was also increased. In normal individuals, the mechanical properties of the lungs do not change significantly during acclimatization to altitude;[626] there occurs a slight loss of elastic recoil and a slight increase in maximal expiratory flow rates, presumably as a result of the decreased density of air at high altitude.

Hultgren and Flamm[608a] suggested that the cause of high-altitude pulmonary edema is intense vasoconstriction of a large fraction of the pulmonary arterial vessels, forcing blood flow at high pressures through the remaining patent vessels. This explanation requires the presence of regional inhomogenicities in pulmonary capillary pressures owing to nonuniform populations of precapillary resistances, so that the extraordinary pulmonary arterial hypertension affects some pulmonary capillary pressures more than others. Just how or why this occurs is not known, although Viswanathan and associates[627] proposed a combination of mechanisms including increased capillary permeability, luminal occlusions distal to spastic arterioles, and severe contraction of muscular arterioles resulting in wider opening of perpendicular muscular arterioles. These authors[627] also suggested that the hypertrophied muscle of the high-altitude native involutes only partially and nonuniformly during the stay at sea level, thus accounting for the nonuniform intensity of precapillary vasoconstriction upon return to high altitude. Viswanathan and coworkers[628] reproduced this form of edema in animals and found the characteristic spasm of the muscular arterioles as well as electron microscopic evidence of disruption of the alveolar-capillary membrane. Visscher[629] suggested that obstruction of 75 per cent of the pulmonary vascular bed in dogs resulted in pulmonary edema because of the high pressures necessary to produce adequate flow through the remaining microvascular bed.

The evidence that high-altitude pulmonary edema is primarily related to increased microvascular permeability derives from clinical studies of vascular pressures and the characteristics of the edema fluid. Right heart catheterization studies have revealed raised pulmonary arterial pressure but normal pulmonary wedge pressure.[609, 610, 718] The measurements of the constituents of pulmonary edema fluid derive from studies performed by Schoene and associates[620, 630, 631] at a high-altitude research facility situated at 4,400 meters on Mount McKinley in Alaska. In a tented camp equipped with bronchoscopes, ventilators, and oxygen, these investigators studied climbers with high-altitude pulmonary edema, using unaffected climbers as control subjects; they showed that pulmonary edema fluid obtained by BAL possessed a high protein content. When compared with the lavage fluid from nonaffected climbers, the fluid was also shown to contain increased numbers of macrophages and neutrophils, and increased amounts of arachidonic acid metabolites (including leukotriene B_4), complement fragments, and a variety of proteolytic enzymes.

Considerable interest has been shown in the limits to exercise at very high altitudes. The ambient and arterial P_{O_2} at the summit of Mount Everest are so low that maximal exercise capacity is severely diminished because of reduced oxygen delivery.[632] Climbers with a brisk hypoxic ventilatory response are particularly successful at extreme altitudes, presumably because the extra ventilation gives them a slightly higher arterial P_{O_2} and increases their V_{O_2} max.[633] Exercise at altitude is associated with a moderate retention of fluid and sodium, a factor that in addition to increased microvascular permeability may contribute to the development of pulmonary edema.[634] A significant relationship exists between the symptoms of acute mountain sickness and weight gain during ascent to high altitude.[635] High-altitude climbers develop striking episodes of periodic breathing and apnea during sleep, associated as expected with severe hypoxemia.[636] Acetazolamide stimulates breathing and decreases the nocturnal hypoventilation by producing a mild metabolic acidosis.

The roentgenographic appearances are typical of acute pulmonary edema, although the distribution tends to be rather irregular and patchy, possibly reflecting the pathogenesis of inhomogeneous distribution of precapillary resistances. Although the central pulmonary vessels may be prominent as a result of acute pulmonary hypertension, cardiac enlargement has not been noted. CT scans of the brain usually show cerebral edema.[718, 719]

Symptoms develop within 12 hours to 3 days after arrival at high altitude[608, 612] and consist of cough, dyspnea, weakness, and hemoptysis, often associated with substernal discomfort. Common findings include cyanosis and tachycardia, and rales may be heard throughout the lungs. Papilledema and retinal hemorrhages have been described.[718] Fever occurs in about one third of patients and leukocytosis is common, ranging from 13,000/mm³ to as high as 30,000/mm^3.[614, 618, 627] The ECG may show nonspecific changes such as right atrial enlargement or right axis shifts but is usually normal.[618]

Patients respond rapidly to the administration of oxygen or to a return to sea level, and the results in one series suggested that a similar response occurs after digitalis therapy without oxygen.[612] The chest roentgenogram clears within 24 to 48 hours.[607]

Diffuse pulmonary edema, with focal hemorrhages and many thrombi in the smaller branches of the pulmonary artery, was found at necropsy in two cases.[608]

Re-expansion of Lung at Thoracentesis

Numerous case reports have appeared in the literature[637–649] of unilateral pulmonary edema developing following rapid removal of air or liquid from the pleural space in the presence of pneumothorax or hydrothorax. In their review of 12 cases, Waqaruddin and Bernstein[642] regarded three features as being common to almost all cases: (1) the pneumothorax or hydrothorax is moderate or large in size (amounting to at least 50 per cent); (2) the pulmonary edema is strictly localized to the ipsilateral lung; and (3) the pneumothorax or hydrothorax has been present for a considerable period of time, usually several days, prior to rapid re-expansion. In the 12 recorded cases, the duration of pneumothorax, as judged from the onset of dyspnea, averaged 18 days, with a minimum of 3 days. It is clear, however, that the duration of pneumothorax is not a critical issue as illustrated by the case reported by Humphreys and Berne[637] in which edema developed 1 hour after accidental induction of pneumothorax from placement of a central venous catheter, and a similar case seen by us in which the pneumothorax was present for a brief half hour. Others[720] have also reported a relatively short time interval. The development of edema is often preceded by a feeling of tightness in the chest and by spasmodic coughing. When such symptoms develop, thoracentesis should be discontinued. Typically, the edema resolves spontaneously within a few days.

The pathogenesis of this form of edema has not been firmly established. Increased capillary permeability would appear to be at least one factor as judged by the protein content of the edema fluid that has been shown to be at a level usually associated with permeability rather than hydrostatic influences.[650, 651] In addition, a normal microvascular pressure is common to the four current theories of pathogenesis:

1. The sudden increase in negative intrapleural pressure[637] (in the case reported by Ziskind and associates,[640] the lungs were exposed inadvertently to a negative pressure of 120 mm Hg).

2. A delay in venous or lymphatic return caused by stasis in the pulmonary venules and lymphatics during prolonged collapse.[371]

3. The alteration in alveolar surface tension that may accompany prolonged relaxation atelectasis.[638, 643]

4. A reperfusion injury to the pulmonary endothelium caused by the local production of toxic oxygen free radicals.

At one time, a direct anoxic effect on the pulmonary capillaries was considered a possible mechanism, but although this theory may seem attractive, Staub[254] has stated that hypoxia has no direct effect, either alone or in conjunction with other forces, in producing pulmonary edema.

The most logical explanation for re-expansion pulmonary edema is the rapid onset of negative pressure to which the pleural space is subjected. Since the negative pressure is instantaneously transferred to the alveoli and the interstitium, it might be expected to alter the Starling forces in a manner favoring transudation of fluid from the microvasculature. However, the negative pressure will also be transmitted to the pulmonary microvessels and it is not at all clear that a net change in transvascular hydrostatic pressure would occur. In addition, the negative pressure hypothesis does not explain the finding of increased protein in the edema fluid characteristic of re-expansion edema.[651] It is certain, however, that the rapidity of re-expansion influences the development of edema. In experiments on Rhesus monkeys, Miller and associates[652] produced ipsilateral pulmonary edema within 2 hours in all animals in which 80 to 100 per cent pneumothorax had been maintained for 3 days and in which rapid re-expansion was obtained by applying suction of -10 cm Hg; by contrast, edema did not develop in those animals whose lungs were re-expanded after 1 hour with the application of negative pressure to the pleural space, or in those in which underwater drainage of the pneumothorax was applied after 3 days' collapse.

Pavlin and associates[653] have used a rabbit model to study the pathogenesis of re-expansion pulmonary edema. They found that rapid re-inflation with a very negative pleural pressure was required to produce edema; further, by using radiolabeled tracers to measure protein flux into the extravascular, extracellular space, they showed that the edema was associated with increased permeability. When a lung is collapsed as a result of pneumothorax or hydrothorax, perfusion to that lung decreases because of the mechanical collapse of extra-alveolar vessels and the hypoxic vasoconstriction that accompanies the reduction in ventilation.[654] When the lung is re-expanded, there occurs a rapid but incomplete return of blood flow, and it is this sudden reperfusion that may cause endothelial damage.[654] It has been shown that reperfusion of the heart and kidneys causes organ damage; similarly, rapid reperfusion of lung made ischemic by pulmonary artery occlusion has been shown to cause fever, leukopenia, and pulmonary edema.[655] Although the mechanism of perfusion injury of the lung is unknown, it is possibly related to the generation of oxygen free radicals by tissue enzymes that were depleted of substrate and O_2 during ischemia and are suddenly presented with an abundance of both. It is also possible that leukocytes play a role in the reperfusion injury, since rapid reexpansion of collapsed lung can be associated with the acute development of leukopenia.

It is almost certain that pulmonary edema from this cause occurs much more commonly than reports indicate. It is important to be aware of this potential complication of rapid thoracentesis in pneumothorax or hydrothorax, since fatalities have been reported[638, 657, 720] and since it may be prevented by slow withdrawal of gas or liquid by underwater drainage. Two cases have been reported[658] in which pulmonary edema developed in the lung contralateral to a pneumothorax caused by resuscitation following cardiac arrest. It was postulated that the cause was left ventricular failure, although no wedge pressure measurements were obtained. Another plausible explanation is that the severe hypoxemia associated with the arrest could have increased capillary permeability, so that with

restoration of the cardiac output (most of which would go through inflated lung), edema would occur only unilaterally.

Pulmonary Edema Associated with Severe Upper Airway Obstruction

The pathogenesis of the diffuse pulmonary edema that occurs sometimes in patients with *severe upper airway obstruction* is somewhat controversial but in any event is almost certainly a permeability phenomenon. It has been observed in both children and adults and occurs exclusively in lesions affecting the extrathoracic airway from the nasopharynx to the thoracic inlet (Fig. 10–68).[410, 659, 683] Since airway obstruction above the thoracic inlet is predominantly inspiratory, efforts to inspire are associated with an increase in negative intrathoracic pressure—in effect, a sustained Mueller maneuver—that can conceivably alter the Starling equation to effect transudation of liquid from capillaries into interstitium and airspaces. In 1942, Warren and associates[660] showed in experiments on dogs that a

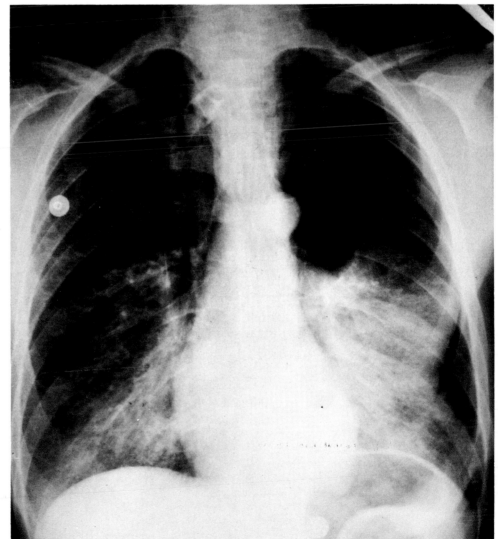

Figure 10–68. Acute Pulmonary Edema Presumed Due to Prolonged Excessive Negative Intra-alveolar Pressure. A 52-year-old woman was brought to the emergency room in severe respiratory distress and was found to have a huge mass (subsequently proved to be a primary carcinoma) almost completely obstructing the larynx. An emergency tracheostomy was performed. Shortly thereafter, a roentgenogram showed diffuse interstitial and airspace pulmonary edema and a moderate-sized left pneumothorax. Cardiac size and configuration were within normal limits. It is assumed that the edema resulted from prolonged, sustained negative intrathoracic pressure occasioned by the patient's futile attempts to inspire beyond the laryngeal obstruction—in essence a sustained Mueller maneuver. The edema disappeared in less than 24 hours following tracheostomy.

large increase in negative intrathoracic pressure drew fluid from pulmonary capillaries into parenchyma and that under extreme conditions not only plasma but red blood cells left the capillaries.

Although the theory of maximally sustained negative intrathoracic pressure resulting in edema *before* the obstruction is relieved seems attractive, it has been questioned by Young and coworkers[661] and by Sofer and associates:[662] these authors studied several children whose chest roentgenograms appeared normal just before bypass of severe upper airway obstruction but who developed edema *after* tracheal intubation. The theoretical explanation they provide for this phenomenon is that the high negative intrapulmonary pressures generated during inspiration before the obstruction is relieved are counteracted by an expiratory component akin to a modified Valsalva maneuver; when the obstruction is relieved, the counteracting force is no longer present, pulmonary blood flow rapidly increases, and pulmonary edema occurs because of the increased permeability of damaged capillaries (analogous to the proposed mechanism of re-expansion edema). Pulmonary edema developing following the relief of upper airway obstruction has also been reported in adults.[663, 664]

Regardless of the mechanism of this form of edema, its recognition is of obvious importance since vigorous treatment usually results in prompt resolution.[665, 666]

Miscellaneous Causes of Permeability Edema

The multiple direct and indirect pulmonary insults that have been associated with the development of ARDS are listed in Table 10–5. The clinical features, pathophysiology, and roentgenographic appearance of most of these conditions are described in the sections of this text dealing directly with these etiologic agents: pulmonary edema in association with aspiration of liquids is discussed in Chapter 13, that associated with the use of drugs and chemicals and the inhalation of toxic fumes is covered in Chapter 14, and the pulmonary infections that can cause ARDS are discussed in detail in Chapter 6. Some of the causes that are not dealt with elsewhere are discussed briefly in the following sections.

PANCREATITIS

In a small but significant proportion of patients with acute pancreatitis, ARDS develops, unassociated with other precipitating causes such as sepsis or aspiration (Fig. 10–69). In one large autopsy study, the pulmonary complications of acute pancreatitis were the most common cause of death in the first 7 days after admission.[667] The mechanisms by which this disorder causes pulmonary edema remain speculative. In experiments on both sheep[668] and dogs,[669] it has been shown that pancreatitis

Table 10–5. Causes of Adult Respiratory Distress Syndrome

DIRECT PULMONARY INSULTS
  Inhalation or aspiration
    Smoke
    Toxic chemicals (e.g., NO_2)
    Gastric acid
    Oxygen toxicity
    Water (near-drowning)
  Drugs and chemicals
    Paraquat
    Heroin
    Salicylates[690]
    Bleomycin[691]
    Amiodarone[692]
    Ethylene glycol[693]
    Lithium[694]
    Ethchlorvynol
    Methadone
    Propoxyphene
  Infection
    Viral
    Rickettsial[695]
    Bacterial
    Fungal
    Tuberculous[696]
    Protozoal (pneumocystis, malaria)[697]
  Fat emboli
  Amniotic fluid emboli
  Air emboli
  Decompression sickness[698]
  Pulmonary contusion
  Radiologic contrast media[680–682]
  Thoracic irradiation[699]
  Chronic eosinophilic pneumonia[700]

INDIRECT PULMONARY INSULTS
  Sepsis
  Anaphylaxis[701]
  Multisystem trauma
  Multiple transfusions
  Antilymphocyte globulin therapy[702]
  Disseminated intravascular coagulation
  Pancreatitis
  Pheochromocytoma[674–676]
  Diabetic ketoacidosis[677, 678]
  Cardiopulmonary bypass
  High altitude
  Rapid lung re-expansion
  Neurogenic
  Sickle-cell crisis[703]
  Hyperthermia[704]
  Extreme physical exertion[705]

results in increased transvascular fluid and protein flux related to an alteration in lung endothelial permeability. It has been proposed that the pancreatic enzymes in the blood could cause activation of the coagulation pathway, generation of kinins,[671] or activation of the complement system.[672]

It has also been suggested that patients with ARDS of diverse etiologies can develop secondary pancreatic injury.[673] In a study in which patients with ARDS were compared with patients with bronchopneumonia, cardiogenic pulmonary edema, or shock without ARDS, it was found that those with ARDS had increased blood levels of trypsin and lipase that followed rather than preceded the onset of their symptoms. These results suggest that mi-

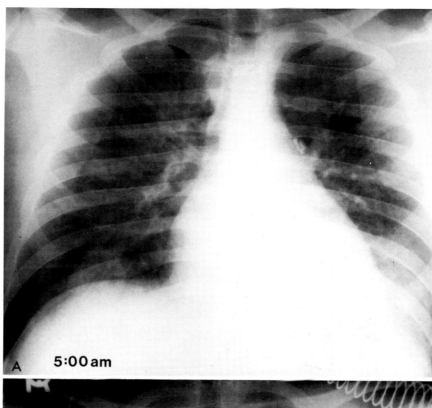
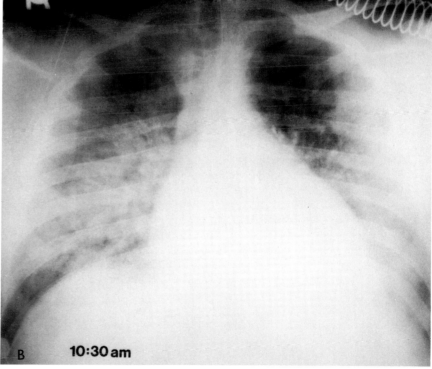

Figure 10–69. Acute Respiratory Insufficiency (ARDS) Associated with Acute Pancreatitis. This acutely ill 23-year-old man was admitted from the emergency room with a typical clinical presentation of acute pancreatitis. An anteroposterior roentgenogram at 5 A.M. (*A*) revealed homogeneous consolidation of the base of the left lung and a much smaller area of consolidation in the right lower lobe. Five hours later (*B*), both lungs had become extensively consolidated in a pattern consistent with severe airspace edema. He succumbed shortly thereafter from acute respiratory failure. At necropsy, the lungs revealed extensive hemorrhagic edema and necrosis of alveolar lining cells characteristic of the acute respiratory insufficiency syndrome. In addition, there was severe acute hemorrhagic pancreatitis.

crovascular injury may be diffuse in patients with ARDS and that such injury may result in secondary pancreatic damage.

FAT EMBOLISM

ARDS frequently occurs following major trauma, particularly in the presence of multiple pelvic and long bone fractures (Fig. 10–70). As discussed in the section on pulmonary fat embolism in Chapter 9 (*see* page 1782), the contribution of this condition to post-traumatic ARDS remains unresolved; patients with multiple trauma are frequently hypotensive, have massive transfusions, or develop sepsis, each of which by itself is a risk factor for the development of ARDS, and it is not certain

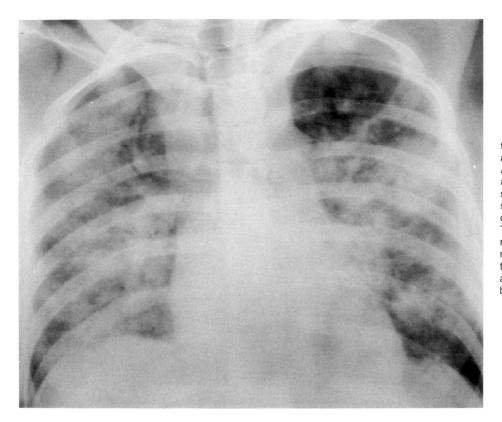

Figure 10–70. Adult Respiratory Distress Syndrome Associated with Traumatic Fat Embolism. A roentgenogram of the chest in anteroposterior projection, supine position, shows diffuse airspace consolidation with some peripheral predominance. Cardiac size is normal. The patient, a young woman with multiple leg fractures sustained in a motor vehicle accident, died shortly thereafter. At autopsy, the arterioles and capillaries were widely occluded by fat.

to what extent fat emboli themselves contribute to pulmonary damage.

PHEOCHROMOCYTOMA

Some patients with pheochromocytoma present with episodes of acute pulmonary edema; by the time they are examined, signs of left ventricular failure or elevated pulmonary microvascular pressure are usually absent, and the clinical syndrome has all of the features of permeability pulmonary edema. It is possible that the mechanism of pulmonary edema formation in these patients is similar to that which occurs from neurogenic causes—massive adrenergic stimulation that results in a considerable (transient) increase in pulmonary microvascular pressure and subsequent pulmonary vascular leak.[674–676]

DIABETIC KETOACIDOSIS

Rarely, patients with diabetic acidosis develop noncardiogenic pulmonary edema that does not appear to be related to other well-defined predisposing factors such as sepsis.[677–679] The mechanism of edema formation is unknown; in one case,[679] severe leukopenia developed prior to the onset of the clinical picture of pulmonary edema, suggesting to the authors that complement activation associated with severe acidosis could have caused pulmonary sequestration of leukocytes and resultant lung injury.

PARENTERAL CONTRAST MEDIA

Pulmonary edema has been described following the parenteral administration of two different forms of contrast media, the oil-based medium used for lymphangiography and the water-based media employed in urography and arteriography. The first of these consists of pulmonary edema that develops some days after the lymphatic injection of ethiodized oil.[680] It has been shown that the injection of an oil-based contrast medium in rabbits results in hemorrhagic pulmonary edema several days after embolization; the fatty acids used in ethiodized oil are esterified, and although a major proportion of the content of this material is oleic acid, esterification makes it less toxic than the free fatty acid. It is possible that the oil microemboli are acted upon by esterases in the lung, causing a breakdown of the esterified compounds to free fatty acids and resultant pulmonary capillary damage.[680] The second form of pulmonary edema associated with contrast media accompanies the anaphylactic shock that occasionally occurs after intravenous administration for urography or arteriography;[656, 670] the onset of pulmonary edema is characteristically acute, occurring minutes to hours after the injection, and is associated with evidence of systemic hypotension and complement activation.[670]

The pulmonary edema that develops occasionally following aspiration of hypertonic contrast media used for examination of the upper gastrointestinal tract is discussed in Chapter 13.

REFERENCES

1. Cumming G: The structure of the pulmonary circulation. *In* Scadding G, Cumming G, Thurlbeck WM (eds): Scientific Foundations of Respiratory Medicine. London, Heinemann, 1981, 71.
2. Horsfield K: Morphometry of the small pulmonary arteries in man. Circ Res 42:593, 1978.
3. Culver BH, Butler J: Mechanical influences on the pulmonary microcirculation. Annu Rev Physiol 42:187, 1980.
4. Chen JTT, Capp MP, Johnsrude IS, et al: Roentgen appearance of pulmonary vascularity in the diagnosis of heart disease. Am J Roentgenol 112:559, 1971.
5. Simon M: The pulmonary vessels: Their hemodynamic evaluation using routine radiographs. Radiol Clin North Am 1:363, 1963.
6. Jacobson G, Turner AF, Balchum OJ, et al: Vascular changes in pulmonary emphysema: The radiologic evaluation by selective and peripheral pulmonary wedge angiography. Am J Roentgenol 100:374, 1967.
7. Schwedel JB, Escher DW, Aaron RS, et al: The roentgenologic diagnosis of pulmonary hypertension in mitral stenosis. Am Heart J 53:163, 1957.
8. Fleming PR, Simon M: The haemodynamic significance of intrapulmonary septal lymphatic lines (lines B of Kerley). J Fac Radiol 9:33, 1958.
9. Harley HRS: The radiological changes in pulmonary venous hypertension, with special reference to the root shadows and lobular pattern. Br Heart J 23:75, 1961.
10. Melheim RE, Dunbar JD, Booth RW: The "B" lines of Kerley and left atrial size in mitral valve disease: Their correlation with the mean left atrial pressure as measured by left atrial puncture. Radiology 76:65, 1961.
11. Viamonte M Jr, Parks RE, Barrera F: Roentgenographic prediction of pulmonary hypertension in mitral stenosis. Am J Roentgenol 87:936, 1962.
12. Milne ENC: Physiological interpretation of the plain radiograph in mitral stenosis, including a review of criteria for the radiological estimation of pulmonary arterial and venous pressures. Br J Radiol 36:902, 1963.
13. Lieber A, Rosenbaum HD, Hanson DJ, et al: Accuracy of predicting pulmonary blood flow, pulmonary arteriolar resistance and pulmonary venous pressure from chest roentgenograms. Am J Roentgenol 103:577, 1968.
14. Turner AF, Lau FYK, Jacobson G: A method for the estimation of pulmonary venous and arterial pressures from the routine chest roentgenogram. Am J Roentgenol 116:97, 1972.
15. Abedin Z, Bidwai PS, Sodhi JS, et al: Relationship between radiologically measured trans-pulmonary artery distance and the mean pulmonary artery pressure in patients with mitral stenosis. Australas Radiol 18:297, 1974.
16. Baumstark A, Svensson RG, Hessel SJ, et al: Evaluating the radiographic assessment of pulmonary venous hypertension in chronic heart disease. AJR 141:877, 1984.
17. Fowler Noble O, Westcott RN, Scott RC: Normal pressure in the right heart and pulmonary artery. Am Heart J 46:264, 1953.
18. Sasamoto H, Hosono K, Katayama K, et al: Electrocardiographic findings in patients with chronic cor pulmonale. Respir Circ 9:55, 1961.
19. Heath D, DuShane JW, Wood EH, et al: The structure of the pulmonary trunk at different ages and in cases of pulmonary hypertension and pulmonary stenosis. J Pathol Bacteriol 77:443, 1959.
20. Moore GW, Smith RRL, Hutchins GM: Pulmonary artery atherosclerosis. Correlation with systemic atherosclerosis and hypertensive pulmonary vascular disease. Arch Pathol Lab Med 106:378, 1982.
21. Wagenvoort CA, Wagenvoort M: Smooth muscle content of pulmonary arterial media in pulmonary venous hypertension compared with other forms of pulmonary hypertension. Chest 81:581, 1982.
22. Meyrick B, Reid L: Ultrastructural findings in lung biopsy material from children with congenital heart defects. Am J Pathol 101:527, 1980.
23. Smith P, Heath D: Electron microscopy of the plexiform lesion. Thorax 34:177, 1979.
24. Wagenvoort CA: Open lung biopsies in congenital heart disease for evaluation of pulmonary vascular disease. Predictive value with regard to corrective operability. Histopathology 9:417, 1985.
25. Shepherd JT, Wood EH: The role of vessel tone in pulmonary hypertension. Circulation 19:641, 1959.
26. Lupi-Herrera E, Bialostozky D, Sobrino A: The role of isoproterenol in pulmonary artery hypertension of unknown etiology (primary). Short- and long-term evaluation. Chest 79:293, 1981.
27. Richards DW: The J Burns Amberson Lecture: The right heart and lung: With some observations on teleology. Am Rev Respir Dis 94:691, 1966.
28. Harvey RM, Enson Y, Ferrer MI: A reconsideration of the origins of pulmonary hypertension. Chest 59:82, 1971.
29. Youssef HH, Edeen HE, Elgammal MY: Hypercapnic pulmonary hypertension. (A preliminary report.) Dis Chest 53:328, 1968.
30. Vogel JHK, Blount SG Jr: The role of hydrogen ion concentration in the regulation of pulmonary artery pressure. Observations in a patient with hypoventilation and obesity. Circulation 32:788, 1965.
31. Fritts HW Jr, Harris P, Clauss HH, et al: The effect of acetylcholine on the human pulmonary circulation under normal and hypoxic conditions. J Clin Invest 37:99, 1958.
32. Penazola D, Sime F: Chronic cor pulmonale due to loss of altitude acclimatization (chronic mountain sickness). Am J Med 50:728, 1971.
33. Harrison DA, Sasahara AA, Bushueff B, et al: Angiographic demonstration of segmental vascular response to acetylcholine in the lung. Am J Roentgenol 120:805, 1974.
34. Rounds S, Hill NS: Pulmonary hypertensive diseases. Chest 85:397, 1984.
35. Harris P, Heath D: The Human Pulmonary Circulation: Its Form and Function in Health and Disease. Baltimore, Williams & Wilkins, 1962.
36. Friedman PJ: Direct magnification angiography and correlative pathophysiology in experimental pulmonary hypertension. Invest Radiol 7:474, 1972.
37. Milne ENC: Some new concepts of pulmonary blood flow and volume. Radiol Clin North Am 16:515, 1978.
38. Hinchcliffe WA, Greenspan RH: Study of the dynamics of pulmonary veins by a new method. Preliminary report. Invest Radiol 6:310, 1971.
39. Ormond RS, Poznanski AK, Templeton AW: Pulmonary veins in congenital heart disease in the adult. Radiology 76:885, 1961.
40. Mallamo JT, Baum RS, Simon AL: Diffuse pulmonary artery calcifications in a case of Eisenmenger's syndrome. Radiology 99:549, 1971.
41. Baltaxe HA, Amplatz K: The normal chest roentgenogram in the presence of large atrial septal defects. Am J Roentgenol 107:322, 1969.
42. Doyle AE, Goodwin JF, Harrison CV, et al: Pulmonary vascular patterns in pulmonary hypertension. Br Heart J 19:353, 1957.
43. Rees RSO, Jefferson KE: The Eisenmenger syndrome. Clin Radiol 18:366, 1967.
44. Rees S: The chest radiograph in pulmonary hypertension with central shunt. Br J Radiol 41:172, 1968.
45. Friedman VF, Braunwald E, Morrow AG: Alterations in regional pulmonary blood flow in patients with congenital heart disease studied by radioisotope scanning. Circulation 37:747, 1968.
46. Cuen JTT, Robinson AE, Goodrich JK, et al: Uneven distribution of pulmonary blood flow between left and right lungs in isolated valvular pulmonary stenosis. Am J Roentgenol 107:343, 1969.
47. Dollery CT, West JB, Wilcken DEL, et al: A comparison of the pulmonary blood flow between left and right lungs in normal subjects and patients with congenital heart disease. Circulation 24:617, 1961.
48. Kerley P: Lung changes in acquired heart disease. Am J Roentgenol 80:256, 1958.
49. Whitley JE, Rudhe U, Herzenberg H: Decreased left lung vascularity in congenital left to right shunts. Acta Radiol 1:1125, 1963.
50. Davies H, Dow J: Differential pulmonary vascularity and the orientation of the right ventricular outflow tract with special reference to corrected transposition. Br J Radiol 44:258, 1971.
51. Nordenström B, Grim S: A method for determination of blood flow with use of roentgen contrast medium. Radiology 84:644, 1965.
52. Wheatley D, Coleman EN, Reid JM: Coronary artery fistula: Report of three cases. Thorax 30:535, 1975.
53. Ferencz C: The pulmonary vascular bed in tetralogy of Fallot. I. Changes associated with pulmonic stenosis. II. Changes following a

systemic-pulmonary arterial anastomosis. Bull Johns Hopkins Hosp *106*:81, 1960.

54. Puyau FA, Meckstroth GR: Evaluation of pulmonary perfusion patterns in children with tetralogy of Fallot. Am J Roentgenol *122*:119, 1974.

55. von Bernuth G, Ritter DG, Schattenberg TT, et al: Severe pulmonary hypertension after Blalock-Taussig anastomosis in a patient with tetralogy of Fallot. Chest *58*:380, 1970.

56. Muster AJ, Paul MH, Nikaidoh H: Tetralogy of Fallot associated with total anomalous pulmonary venous drainage. Chest *64*:323, 1973.

57. Haroutunian LM, Neill CA, Dorst JP: Pulmonary pseudofibrosis in cyanotic heart disease. A clinical syndrome mimicking tuberculosis in patients with extreme pulmonic stenosis. Chest *62*:587, 1972.

58. von Bernuth G, Ritter DG, Schattenberg TT, et al: Severe pulmonary hypertension after Blalock-Taussig anastomosis in a patient with tetralogy of Fallot. Chest *58*:380, 1970.

59. Roisman ML, Beller BM, O'Keefe JD: Irreversible pulmonary hypertension after correction of tetralogy of Fallot. Chest *62*:34, 1972.

60. Dresdale DT, Schultz M, Michtom RJ: Primary pulmonary hypertension I. Clinical and haemodynamic study. Am J Med *11*:686, 1951.

61. Fishman AP, Pietra GG: Primary pulmonary hypertension. Annu Rev Med *31*:421, 1980.

62. Hughes JD, Rubin LJ: Primary pulmonary hypertension: an analysis of 28 cases and a review of the literature. Medicine *65*:56, 1986.

63. Yu N: Primary pulmonary hypertension: Report of six cases and review of literature. Ann Intern Med *49*:1138, 1958.

64. Heath D, Whitaker W, Brown JW: Idiopathic pulmonary hypertension. Br Heart J *19*:83, 1957.

65. Evans W: The less common forms of pulmonary hypertension. Br Heart J *21*:197, 1959.

66. Evans W, Short DS, Bedford DE: Solitary pulmonary hypertension. Br Heart J *19*:93, 1957.

67. Rich S, Dantzker DR, Ayres SM, et al: Primary pulmonary hypertension: a national prospective study. Ann Int Med *107*:216, 1987.

68. Shinnick JP, Cudkowicz L, Blanco G, et al: A problem in pulmonary hypertension. Part 1: The clinical course. Chest *65*:69, 1974.

69. Shinnick JP, Cudkowicz L, Saldana M, et al: A problem in pulmonary hypertension. Part 2: The final course and autopsy findings. Chest *65*:192, 1974.

70. Shane SJ, Aterman K, Roy DL, et al: Primary pulmonary hypertension: A review and report of five cases. Can Med Assoc *91*:145, 1964.

71. Elkayam U: Vasodilator therapy in primary pulmonary hypertension. Chest *79*:254, 1981.

72. Melmon KL, Braunwald E: Familial pulmonary hypertension. N Engl J Med *269*:770, 1963.

73. Tsagaris TJ, Tikoff G: Familial primary pulmonary hypertension. Am Rev Respir Dis *97*:127, 1968.

74. Porter CM, Creech BJ, Billings FT Jr: Primary pulmonary hypertension occurring in twins. Arch Intern Med *120*:224, 1967.

75. Kingdon HS, Cohen LS, Roberts WC, et al: Familial occurrence of primary pulmonary hypertension. Arch Intern Med *118*:422, 1966.

76. Loyd JE, Primm RK, Newman JH: Familial primary pulmonary hypertension—clinical patterns. Am Rev Respir Dis *129*:194, 1984.

77. Thompson P, McRae C: Familial pulmonary hypertension, evidence of autosomal dominant inheritance. Br Heart J *32*:758, 1970.

78. Inglesby TV, Singer JW, Gordon DS: Abnormal fibrinolysis in familial pulmonary hypertension. Am J Med *55*:5, 1973.

79. Gurtner HP, Gertsch M, Salzmann C, et al: Häufen sich die primär vaskulären formen des chronischen cor pulmonale? Schweiz Med Wochenschr *98*:1579, 1968.

80. Follath F, Burkart F, Schweizer W: Drug-induced pulmonary hypertension? Br Med J *1*:265, 1971.

81. Kay JM, Smith P, Heath D: Aminorex and the pulmonary circulation. Thorax *26*:262, 1971.

82. Garcia-Dorado D, Miller DD, Garcia EJ, et al: An epidemic of pulmonary hypertension after toxic rapeseed ingestion in Spain. J Am Coll Cardiol *1*:1216, 1983.

83. Blount SG Jr, Vogel JHK: Pulmonary hypertension. Mod Concepts Cardiovasc Dis *36*:61, 1987.

84. Gurtner HP: Pulmonary hypertension "plexigenic pulmonary arteriopathy," anti-appetite depressant drug Aminorex: post or propter. Bull Eur Physiopathol Respir *15*:897, 1979.

85. Kay JM, Heath D, Smith P, et al: Fulvine and the pulmonary circulation. Thorax *26*:249, 1971.

86. Kay JM, Smith P, Heath D: Electron microscopy of *Crotalaria* pulmonary hypertension. Thorax *24*:511, 1969.

87. Wagenvoort CA, Wagenvoort N, Dijk HJ: Effect of fulvine on pulmonary arteries and veins of the rat. Thorax *29*:522, 1974.

88. Heath D, Shaba J, Williams A, et al: A pulmonary hypertension-producing plant from Tanzania. Thorax *30*:399, 1975.

89. Lebrec D, Capron JP, Dhumeaux D, et al: Pulmonary hypertension complicating portal hypertension. Am Rev Respir Dis *120*:849, 1979.

90. Kibria G, Smith P, Heath D, et al: Observations on the rare association between portal and pulmonary hypertension. Thorax *35*:945, 1980.

91. McDonnell PJ, Toye PA, Hutchins GM: Primary pulmonary hypertension and cirrhosis: are they related? Am Rev Respir Dis *127*:437, 1983.

92. Berliner S, Schoenfeld Y, Dean H, et al: Primary pulmonary hypertension: A facet of a diffuse angiopathic process? Respiration *43*:76, 1982.

93. Bunch TW, Tancredi RG, Lie JT: Pulmonary hypertension in polymyositis. Chest *79*:1, 105, 1981.

94. Perez HD, Kramer N: Pulmonary hypertension in systemic lupus erythematosus: report of four cases and review of the literature. Semin Arthritis Rheum *11*:117, 1981.

95. Salerni R, Rodman GP, Leon DF, et al: Pulmonary hypertension in the CREST syndrome variant of progressive systemic sclerosis. Ann Intern Med *86*:394, 1977.

96. Trell E: Pulmonary hypertension in systemic sclerosis. Ann Rheum Dis *30*:30, 1971.

97. Walcott G, Burchell HB, Brown AL Jr: Primary pulmonary hypertension. Am J Med *49*:70, 1970.

98. Chang CH: The normal roentgenographic measurement of the right descending pulmonary artery in 1,085 cases. Am J Roentgenol *87*:929, 1962.

99. Kuriyama K, Gamsu G, Stern RG, et al: CT-determined pulmonary artery diameters in predicting pulmonary hypertension. Invest Radiol *19*:16, 1984.

100. Boxt LM, Rich S, Fried R, et al: Automated morphologic evaluation of pulmonary arteries in primary pulmonary hypertension. Invest Radiol *21*:906, 1986.

101. Sleeper JC, Orgain ES, McIntosh HD: Primary pulmonary hypertension. Review of clinical features and pathologic physiology with a report of pulmonary hemodynamics derived from repeated catheterization. Circulation *26*:1358, 1962.

102. Williams MH Jr, Adler JJ, Colp C: Pulmonary function studies as an aid in the differential diagnosis of pulmonary hypertension. Am J Med *47*:378, 1969.

103. Scharf SM, Feldman NT, Graboys TB, et al: Restrictive ventilatory defect in a patient with primary pulmonary hypertension. Am Rev Respir Dis *118*:409, 1978.

104. Horn M, Ries A, Neview C, et al: Restrictive ventilatory pattern in precapillary pulmonary hypertension. Am Rev Respir Dis *128*:163, 1983.

105. Dantzker DR, Bower JS: Mechanisms of gas exchange abnormality in patients with chronic obliterative pulmonary vascular disease. J Clin Invest *64*:1050, 1979.

106. Dantzker DR, D'Alonzo GE, Bower JS, et al: Pulmonary gas exchange during exercise in patients with chronic obliterative pulmonary hypertension. Am Rev Respir Dis *130*:412, 1984.

107. Williams JO: Death following injection of lung scanning agent in a case of pulmonary hypertension. Br J Radiol *47*:61, 1974.

108. Child JS, Wolfe JD, Tashkin D, et al: Fatal lung scan in a case of pulmonary hypertension due to obliterative pulmonary vascular disease. Chest *67*:308, 1975.

109. Caldini P, Gensini GG, Hoffman MS: Primary pulmonary hypertension with death during right heart catheterization: A case report and a survey of reported fatalities. Am J Cardiol *4*:519, 1959.

110. Nicod P, Peterson K, Levine M, et al: Pulmonary angiography in severe chronic pulmonary hypertension. Ann Intern Med *107*:565, 1987.

111. Rich S, Levy PS: Characteristics of surviving and non-surviving patients with primary pulmonary hypertension. Am J Med *76*:573, 1984.

112. de Soyza NDB, Murphy ML: Persistent post-embolic pulmonary hypertension. Chest *62*:665, 1972.

113. Rich S, Levitsky S, Brundage BH: Pulmonary hypertension from chronic pulmonary thromboembolism. Ann Intern Med *108*:425, 1988.

114. Sperling DR, Patrick JR, Anderson FM, et al: Cor pulmonale secondary to ventriculoauriculostomy. Am J Dis Child *107*:308, 1964.

115. Lai KS, McFadzean AJS, Yeung R: Microembolic pulmonary hypertension in pyogenic cholangitis. Br Med J *1*:22, 1968.

116. Clinicopathologic Conference: A fifty-six year old woman with jaundice and pulmonary hypertension. Am J Med *47*:287, 1969.

117. Bower JS, Dantzker DR, Naylor B: Idiopathic pulmonary hypertension associated with nodular pulmonary infiltrates and portal venous thrombosis. Chest *78*:111, 1980.

118. Moser KM, Spragg RG, Utley J, et al: Chronic thrombotic obstruction of major pulmonary arteries. Results of thromboendarterectomy in 15 patients. Ann Intern Med *99*:299, 1983.

119. Sofawora EO: Pulmonary heart disease in Ibadan. Thorax 26:339, 1971.

120. Rowley PT, Englander D: Hemoglobin S-C disease presenting as acute cor pulmonale. Am Rev Respir Dis 98:494, 1968.

121. Starkie CM, Harding LK, Fletcher DJ, et al: (The Birmingham eclampsia study group): Intravascular coagulation and abnormal lung-scans in pre-eclampsia and eclampsia. Lancet 2:889, 1971.

122. Littler WA, Redman CWG, Bonnar J, et al: Reduced pulmonary arterial compliance in hypertensive pregnancy. Lancet 1:1274, 1973.

123. Rich S, Pietra GG: Primary pulmonary hypertension: radiographic and scintigraphic patterns of histologic subtypes. Ann Intern Med 105:499, 1986.

124. Woodruff WW III, Hoeck BE, Chitwood WR Jr, et al: Radiographic findings in pulmonary hypertension from unresolved embolism. AJR 144:681, 1985.

125. Lisbona R, Kreisman H, Novales-Diaz J, et al: Perfusion lung scanning: differentiation of primary from thromboembolic pulmonary hypertension. AJR 144:27, 1985.

126. Powe JE, Palevsky HI, McCarthy KE, et al: Pulmonary arterial hypertension: value of perfusion scintigraphy. Radiology 164:727, 1987.

127. Nadel JA, Gold WM, Burgess JH: Early diagnosis of chronic pulmonary vascular obstruction. Value of pulmonary function tests. Am J Med 44:16, 1968.

128. Wagenvoort CA, Beetstra A, Spijker J: Capillary hemangiomatosis of the lung. Histopathology 2:401, 1978.

129. Tron V, Magee F, Wright JL, et al: Pulmonary capillary hemangiomatosis. Hum Pathol 17:1144, 1986.

130. Wagenvoort CA: Pathology of congestive pulmonary hypertension. Prog Respir Res (Karger, Basel), 9:195, 1975.

131. Magee F, Wright JL, Kay JM, et al: Pulmonary capillary hemangiomatosis. Am Rev Respir Dis 139:922, 1985.

132. Arvidsson H, Karnell J, Möller T: Multiple stenosis of the pulmonary arteries associated with pulmonary hypertension, diagnosed by selective angiocardiography. Acta Radiol 44:209, 1955.

133. Dighiero J, Fiandra O, Barcia A, et al: Multiple pulmonary stenoses with pulmonary hypertension: Report of a case. Acta Radiol 48:439, 1957.

134. Gyllenswärd A, Lodin H, Lundberg A, et al: Congenital, multiple peripheral stenoses of the pulmonary artery. Pediatrics 19:399, 1957.

135. Orell SR, Karnell J, Wahlgren F: Malformation and multiple stenoses of the pulmonary arteries with pulmonary hypertension. Acta Radiol 54:449, 1960.

136. Gay BB Jr, Franch RH, Shuford WH, et al: The roentgenologic features of single and multiple coarctations of the pulmonary artery and branches. Am J Roentgenol 90:599, 1963.

137. Winfield ME, McDonnel GM, Steckel RJ: Multiple coarctations of the pulmonary arteries with associated infundibular pulmonic stenosis. Case report with serial right-heart catheterization studies obtained at a three-year interval. Radiology 83:854, 1964.

138. del Castillo JJ, Gianfrancesco H, Mannix EP Jr: Pulmonic stenosis due to compression by sternal chondrosarcoma. J Thorac Cardiovasc Surg 52:255, 1966.

139. Tikoff G, Bloom S: Complete interruption of the aortic arch in an adult associated with a dissection aneurysm of the pulmonary artery. Am J Med 48:782, 1970.

140. Best J: Dissecting aneurysm of the pulmonary artery with multiple cardiovascular abnormalities and pulmonary hypertension. Med J Austral 2:1129, 1967.

141. Nasraliah A, Goussous Y, El-Said G, et al: Pulmonary artery compression due to acute dissecting aortic aneurysm: Clinical and angiographic diagnosis. Chest 67:228, 1975.

142. Buja LM, Ali N, Fletcher RD, et al: Stenosis of the right pulmonary artery: A complication of acute dissecting aneurysm of the ascending aorta. Am Heart J 83:89, 1972.

143. Cheris DN, Dadey JL: Fibrosing mediastinitis. An unusual cause for cor pulmonale. Am J Roentgenol 100:328, 1967.

144. Baum GL, Fisher FD: The relationship of fatal pulmonary insufficiency with cor pulmonale, rightsided mural thrombi and pulmonary emboli: A preliminary report. Am J Med Sci 240:609, 1960.

145. Emirgil C, Sobol BJ, Herbert WH, et al: Routine pulmonary function studies as a key to the status of the lesser circulation in chronic obstructive pulmonary disease. Am J Med 50:191, 1971.

146. Steckel RJ, Bein ME, Kelly PM: Pulmonary arterial hypertension in progressive systemic sclerosis. Am J Roentgenol 124:461, 1975.

147. Fry WA, Archer FA, Adams WE: Long-term clinical-pathologic study of the pneumonectomy patient. Dis Chest 52:720, 1967.

148. Massumi RA, Sarin RK, Pooya N, et al: Tonsillar hypertrophy, airway obstruction, alveolar hypoventilation, and cor pulmonale in twin brothers. Dis Chest 55:110, 1969.

149. Leading Article: Obstruction by tonsils and adenoids. Br Med J 4:5, 1968.

150. Levin DL, Muster AJ, Pachman LM, et al: Cor pulmonale secondary to upper airway obstruction. Cardiac catheterization, immunologic, and psychometric evaluation in nine patients. Chest 68(Suppl):166, 1975.

151. Gerald B, Dungan WT: Cor pulmonale and pulmonary edema in children secondary to chronic upper airway obstruction. Radiology 90:679, 1968.

152. Levy AM, Tabakin BS, Hanson JS, et al: Hypertrophied adenoids causing pulmonary hypertension and severe congestive heart failure. N Engl J Med 277:506, 1967.

153. Marks CE Jr, Goldring RM: Chronic hypercapnia during methadone maintenance. Am Rev Respir Dis 108:1088, 1973.

154. Bindelglass IL, Trubowitz S: Pulmonary vein obstruction: An uncommon sequel to chronic fibrous mediastinitis. Ann Intern Med 48:876, 1958.

155. Stovin PGI, Mitchinson MJ: Pulmonary hypertension due to obstruction of intrapulmonary veins. Thorax 20:106, 1965.

156. Singshinsuk SS, Hartmann AF Jr, Elliott LP: Stenosis of the individual pulmonary veins: a rare cause of pulmonary hypertension? Radiology 87:514, 1966.

157. Symmers WSC: Necrotizing pulmonary arteriopathy associated with pulmonary hypertension. J Clin Pathol 5:36, 1952.

158. Wagenvoort CA: Morphologic changes in intrapulmonary veins. Hum Pathol 1:205, 1970.

159. Heath D, Edwards JE: Histological changes in the lung in diseases associated with pulmonary venous hypertension. Br J Dis Chest 53:8, 1959.

160. Heard BE, Path FC, Steiner RE, et al: Oedema and fibrosis of the lungs in left ventricular failure. Br J Radiol 41:161, 1968.

161. Simon M: The pulmonary veins in mitral stenosis. J Fac Radiol 9:25, 1958.

162. Milne ENC: Pulmonary blood flow distribution. Invest Radiol 12:479, 1977.

163. West John B, Dollery CT, Heard BE: Increased pulmonary vascular resistance in the dependent zone of the isolated dog lung caused by perivascular edema. Circ Res 17:191, 1965.

164. Ritchie BC, Schauberger G, Staub NC. Inadequacy of perivascular edema hypothesis to account for distribution of pulmonary blood flow in lung edema. Circ Res 24:807, 1969.

165. Muir AL, Hall DL, Despas P, et al: Distribution of blood flow in the lungs in acute pulmonary edema in dogs. J Appl Physiol 33:763, 1972.

166. Hughes JMB, Glazier JB, Maloney JE, et al: Effect of interstitial pressure on pulmonary blood-flow. Lancet 1:192, 1967.

167. Surette GD, Muir AL, Hogg JC, et al: Roentgenographic study of blood flow redistribution in acute pulmonary edema in dogs. Invest Radiol 10:109, 1975.

168. Burko H, Carwell G, Newman E: Size, location, and gravitational changes of normal upper lobe pulmonary veins. Am J Roentgenol 111:687, 1971.

169. Simon G: The value of radiology in critical mitral stenosis—an amendment. Clin Radiol 23:145, 1972.

170. Lavender JP, Doppman J, Shawdon H, et al: Pulmonary veins in left ventricular failure and mitral stenosis. Br J Radiol 35:293, 1962.

171. Doppman JL, Lavender JP: The hilum and the large left ventricle. Radiology 80:931, 1963.

172. Tattersfield AE, McNicol MW, Shawdon H, et al: Chest x-ray film in acute myocardial infarction. Br Med J 3:332, 1969.

173. Simon M: The pulmonary vessels in incipient left ventricular decompensation: Radiologic observations. Circulation 24:185, 1961.

174. Chait A, Cohen HE, Meltzer LE, et al: The bedside chest radiograph in the evaluation of incipient heart failure. Radiology 105:563, 1972.

175. McHugh TJ, Forrester JS, Adler L, et al: Pulmonary vascular congestion in acute myocardial infarction: Hemodynamic and radiologic correlations. Ann Intern Med 76:29, 1972.

176. Bryk D: Dilated right pulmonary veins in mitral insufficiency. Chest 58:24, 1970.

177. Legge DA, Miller WE, Ludwig J: Pulmonary findings associated with mitral stenosis. Chest 58:403, 1970.

178. Heath D, Scott O, Lynch J: Pulmonary veno-occlusive disease. Thorax 26:663, 1971.

179. Galloway RW, Epstein EJ, Coulshed N: Pulmonary ossific nodules in mitral valve disease. Br Heart J 23:297, 1961.

180. Wilson WR, Sasaki R, Johnson CA: Disseminated nodular pulmonary ossification in patients with mitral stenosis. Circulation 19:323, 1959.

181. Whitehouse G: Tracheopathia osteoplastica: Case report. Br J Radiol 41:701, 1968.

182. Fleming HA, Robinson CLN: Pulmonary ossification with cardiac calcification in mitral valve disease. Br Heart J 19:532, 1957.

183. Seningen RP, Chen JTT, Peter RH, et al: Roentgen interpretation of postoperative changes (clinical and hemodynamic) in pure mitral stenosis. Am J Roentgenol 113:693, 1971.

184. Wagenvoort CA, Wagenvoort N: Pathology of Pulmonary Hypertension. New York, John Wiley and Sons, 1977.

10

185. Shilkin KB, Low LP, Chen BTM: Dissecting aneurysm of the pulmonary artery. J Pathol 98:25, 1969.
186. Gutierrez FR, Moran CJ, Ludbrook PA, et al: Pulmonary arterial calcification with reversible pulmonary hypertension. Am J Roentgenol 135:177, 1980.
187. Gupta BD, Moodie DS, Hodgman JR: Primary pulmonary hypertension in adults. Cleve Clin Q 47:275, 1980.
188. Matthay RA, Schwarz MI, Ellis JH Jr, et al: Pulmonary artery hypertension in chronic obstructive pulmonary disease: determination by chest radiography. Invest Radiol 16:95, 1981.
189. Austin JHM, Young BG Jr, Thomas HM, et al: Radiologic assessment of pulmonary arterial pressure and blood volume in chronic, diffuse, interstitial pulmonary diseases. Invest Radiol 14:9, 1979.
190. Ramirez A, Grimes ET, Abelmann WH: Regression of pulmonary vascular changes following mitral valvuloplasty. An anatomic and physiologic case study. Am J Med 45:975, 1968.
191. Gorlin R, Gorlin SG: Hydraulic formula for calculation of the area of the stenotic mitral valve, other cardiac valves, and central circulatory shunts. I. Am Heart J 41:1, 1951.
192. Symbas PN, Abbott OA, Logan WD, et al: Atrial myxomas: Special emphasis on unusual manifestations. Chest 59:504, 1971.
193. Rosenow EC III, Harrison CE Jr: Congestive heart failure masquerading as primary pulmonary disease. Chest 58:28, 1970.
194. Thadani U, Burrow C, Whittaker W, et al: Pulmonary veno-occlusive disease. Q J Med 44:133, 1975.
195. Palmer WH, Gee JBL, Mills FC, et al: Disturbances of pulmonary function in mitral valve disease. Can Med Assoc J 89:744, 1963.
196. Singh T, Dinda P, Chatterjee SS, et al: Pulmonary function studies before and after closed mitral valvotomy. Am Rev Respir Dis 101:62, 1970.
197. MacIntosh DJ, Sinnott JC, Milne IG, et al: Some aspects of disordered pulmonary function in mitral stenosis. Ann Intern Med 49:1294, 1958.
198. Donald KW, Bishop JM, Wade OL, et al: Cardiorespiratory functions two years after mitral valvotomy. Clin Sci 16:325, 1957.
199. Carrington CD, Liebow AA: Pulmonary veno-occlusive disease. Hum Pathol 1:322, 1970.
200. Wagenvoort CA: Pulmonary veno-occlusive disease: entity or syndrome? Chest 69:82, 1976.
201. Thadani U, Burrow C, Whitaker W, et al: Pulmonary veno-occlusive disease. Q J Med 44:133, 1975.
202. Heath D, Segal N, Bishop J: Pulmonary veno-occlusive disease. Circulation 34:242, 1966.
203. Wagenvoort CA, Wagenvoort N: Pulmonary veno-occlusive disease. In Wagenvoort CA, Wagenvoort N (eds): Pathology of Pulmonary Hypertension. New York, John Wiley and Sons, 1977, p 217.
204. Rambihar VS, Fallen EL, Cairns JA: Pulmonary veno-occlusive disease: Antemortem diagnosis from roentgenographic and hemodynamic findings. Canad Med Assoc J 120:1519, 1979.
205. Shackelford GD, Sacks EJ, Mullins JD, et al: Pulmonary veno-occlusive disease. Case report and review of the literature. Am J Roentgenol 128:643, 1977.
206. McDonnell PJ, Summer WR, Hutchins GM: Pulmonary veno-occlusive disease. Morphological changes suggesting a viral cause. JAMA 246:667, 1981.
207. Case records of the Massachusetts General Hospital. Case 14–1983. N Engl J Med 308:825, 1983.
208. Weisser K, Wyler F, Gloor F: Pulmonary veno-occlusive disease. Arch Dis Child 42:322, 1967.
209. Hasleton PS, Ironside JW, Whittaker JS, et al: Pulmonary veno-occlusive disease. A report of four cases. Histopathology 10:933, 1986.
210. Leinonen H, Pohjola-Sintonen S, Krogerus L: Pulmonary veno-occlusive disease. Acta Med Scand 221:307, 1987.
211. Kuipers JRG, Elema JD: Familial pulmonary veno-occlusive disease: a case report. Thorax 32:763, 1977.
212. Alpert LI: Veno-occlusive disease of the liver associated with oral contraceptives: case reports and review of literature. Hum Pathol 7:709, 1976.
213. Hensby CN, Dollery CT, Barnes PJ, et al: Production of 6-oxo-PGF$_1$ alpha by human lung in vivo. Lancet 2:1162, 1979.
214. Stuart KL, Bras G: Veno-occlusive disease of the liver. Q J Med 26:219, 1957.
215. Mehta MJ, Karmody AM, McKneally MF: Mediastinal veno-occlusive disease associated with herbal tea ingestion. NY State J Med 86:604, 1986.
216. Shrivastava S, Moller JH, Edwards JE: Congenital unilateral pulmonary venous atresia with pulmonary veno-occlusive disease in contralateral lung: an unusual association. Pediatr Cardiol 7:213, 1986.
217. Bates DV, Macklem PT, Christie RV: Respiratory Function in Disease: An Introduction to the Integrated Study of the Lung. 2nd ed. Philadelphia, WB Saunders Co, 1971.
218. Rambihar VS, Fallen EL, Cairns JA: Pulmonary veno-occlusive disease: antemortem diagnosis from roentgenographic and hemodynamic findings. Can Med Assoc J 120:1519, 1979.
219. Wiedmann HP: Wedge pressure in pulmonary veno-occlusive disease (letter). N Engl J Med 315:1233, 1986.
220. Swischuk LE, L'Heureux PL: Unilateral pulmonary vein atresia. Am J Roentgenol 135:667, 1980.
221. Report (reprinted from World Health Organization Technical Report Series No. 213): Chronic cor pulmonale. Report of an expert committee. Circulation 27:594, 1963.
222. Stevens PM, Terplan M, Knowles JH: Prognosis of cor pulmonale. N Engl J Med 269:1289, 1963.
223. Sherman WT, Ferrer MI, Harvey RM: Competence of the tricuspid valve in pulmonary heart disease (cor pulmonale). Circulation 31:517, 1965.
224. Sepúlveda G, Ríos E, León J, et al: Clinico-pathologic correlation in chronic cor pulmonale. Dis Chest 52:205, 1967.
225. World Health Organization, Report of an Expert Committee: Definition and diagnosis of pulmonary diseases with special reference to chronic bronchitis and emphysema. In Chronic Cor Pulmonale, WHO Technical Report Series No. 213, 1961, pp 14–19.
226. Deterling RA Jr, Clagett OT: Aneurysm of the pulmonary artery: review of the literature and report of a case. Am Heart J 34:471, 1947.
227. Charlton RW, Du Plessis LA: Multiple pulmonary artery aneurysms. Thorax 16:364, 1961.
228. Baum D, Khoury GH, Ongley PA, et al: Congenital stenosis of the pulmonary artery branches. Circulation 29:680, 1964.
229. Plokker HWM, Wagenaar S, Bruschke AVG, et al: Aneurysm of a pulmonary artery branch: An uncommon cause of a coin lesion. Chest 68:258, 1975.
230. Challis TW, Fay JE: Isolated dilatation of the main pulmonary artery: A report of three cases and a review of the literature. J Can Assoc Radiol 20:180, 1969.
231. Chiu B, Magil A: Idiopathic pulmonary arterial trunk aneurysm presenting as cor pulmonale: Report of a case. Hum Pathol 16:947, 1985.
232. Tung H, Liebow AA: Marfan's syndrome. Lab Invest 1:382, 1952.
233. Symbas PN, Scott HW Jr: Traumatic aneurysm of the pulmonary artery. J Thorac Cardiovasc Surg 45:645, 1963.
234. Sevitt S: Arterial wall lesions after pulmonary embolism, especially ruptures and aneurysms. J Clin Pathol 29:665, 1976.
235. Salyer WR, Salyer DC, Hutchins GM: Local arterial wall injury caused by thromboemboli. Am J Pathol 75:285, 1974.
236. Meyer JS: Thromboembolic pulmonary arterial necrosis and arteritis in man. Arch Pathol 70:63, 1960.
237. Auerbach O: Pathology and pathogenesis of pulmonary arterial aneurysm in tuberculous cavities. Am Rev Tuberc 39:99, 1939.
238. Ungaro R, Saab S, Almond CH, et al: Solitary peripheral pulmonary artery aneurysms. J Thorac Cardiovasc Surg 71:566, 1976.
239. Kauffman SL, Lynfield J, Hennigar GR: Mycotic aneurysms of the intrapulmonary arteries. Circulation 35:90, 1967.
240. Jaffe RB, Condon VR: Mycotic aneurysms of the pulmonary artery and aorta. Radiology 116:291, 1975.
241. Choyke PL, Edmonds PR, Markowitz RI, et al: Mycotic pulmonary artery aneurysm: Complication of aspergillus endocarditis. AJR 138:1172, 1982.
242. Navarro C, Dickinson PCT, Kondlapoodi P, et al: Mycotic aneurysms of the pulmonary arteries in intravenous drug addicts. Am J Med 76:1124, 1984.
243. Slavin RE, de Groot WJ: Pathology of the lung in Behçet's disease. Am J Surg Pathol 5:779, 1981.
244. Luchtrath H: Dissecting aneurysm of the pulmonary artery. Virchows Arch (Pathol Anat) 391:241, 1981.
245. Shilkin KB, Low LP, Chen BTM: Dissecting aneurysm of the pulmonary artery. J Pathol 98:25, 1968.
246. Hughes JP, Stovin PGI: Segmental pulmonary artery aneurysms with peripheral venous thrombosis. Br J Dis Chest 53:19, 1959.
247. Kopp WL, Green RA: Pulmonary artery aneurysms with recurrent thrombophlebitis. The "Hughes-Stovin syndrome." Ann Intern Med 56:105, 1962.
248. Teplick JG, Haskin ME, Nedwich A: The Hughes-Stovin syndrome: Case report. Radiology 113:607, 1974.
249. Ashbaugh DG, Bigelow DB, Petty TL, et al: Acute respiratory distress in adults. Lancet 2:319, 1967.
250. Petty TL, Ashbaugh DG: The adult respiratory distress syndrome. Clinical features, factors influencing prognosis and principles of management. Chest 60:233, 1971.
251. Fishman AP: Pulmonary edema: The water-exchanging function of the lung. Circulation 46:390, 1972.
252. Robin ED, Carroll EC, Zelis R: Pulmonary edema (first of two parts). N Engl J Med 288:239, 1973.
253. Robin ED, Carroll EC, Zelis R: Pulmonary edema (second of two parts). N Engl J Med 288:292, 1973.

254. Staub NC: 'State of the art' review. Pathogenesis of pulmonary edema. Am Rev Respir Dis 109:358, 1974.

255. Staub NC: Pulmonary edema. Physiol Rev 54:678, 1974.

256. Staub NC: Pulmonary edema due to increased microvascular permeability. Ann Rev Med 32:291, 1981.

257. Staub NC: Pathophysiology of pulmonary edema. In Staub NC, Taylor AE (eds): Edema. New York, Raven Press, 1984, p 719.

258. Staub NC: Pathways for fluid and solute fluxes in pulmonary edema. In Fishman AP, Renkin EM (eds): Pulmonary Edema. Baltimore, Williams and Wilkins, 1979, p 113.

259. Pritchard JS: Edema of the lung. Springfield, Ill, Charles C Thomas, Publisher, 1982.

260. Effros RM: Pulmonary microcirculation and exchange. In Renkin EM, Michel CG (eds): Handbook of Physiology—the Cardiovascular System. IV. Oxford, Oxford University Press, 1984, pp 865–915.

261. Snashall PD: Pulmonary oedema. Br J Dis Chest 74:2, 1980.

262. Staub NC (ed): Lung Water and Solute Exchange. In Lenfant C (executive ed): Lung Biology in Health and Disease. New York, Marcel Dekker Inc, 1978.

263. Weibel ER: Morphometry of the human lung. New York, Academic Press, 1963.

264. Weibel ER: Morphological basis of alveolar-capillary gas exchange. Physiol Rev 53:419, 1973.

265. Iliff LD: Extra-alveolar vessels and edema development in excised dog lungs. Circ Res 28:524, 1971.

266. Albert RK, Lakshminarayan S, Charan NB, et al: Extra-alveolar vessel contribution to hydrostatic pulmonary edema in in situ dog lungs. J Appl Physiol 54:1010, 1983.

267. Albert RK: Sites of leakage in pulmonary edema. In Said SI (ed): The Pulmonary Circulation and Acute Lung Injury. New York, Futura Publishing Company, Inc, 1985, p 189.

268. Bo G, Hauge A, Nicolaysen G: Alveolar pressure and lung volume as determinants of net transvascular fluid filtration. J Appl Physiol 42:476, 1977.

269. Cottrell TS, Levine OR, Senior RM, et al: Electron microscopic alterations at the alveolar level in pulmonary edema. Circ Res 21:783, 1967.

270. Schneeberger EE: Barrier function of intercellular junctions in adult and foetal lungs. In Fishman AP, Renkin EM (eds): Pulmonary Edema. Baltimore, Williams and Wilkins Company, 1979.

271. Claude P, Goodenough DA: Fracture faces of zonulae occludentes from "tight" and "leaky" epithelium. J Cell Biol 58:390, 1973.

272. Walker DC, MacKenzie A, Hulbert WC, et al: A reassessment of the tricellular region of epithelial cell tight junctions. Acta Anat 122:35, 1985.

273. Blake LH, Staub NC: Pulmonary vascular transport in sheep, a mathematical model. Microvasc Res 12:197, 1976.

274. Blake LH: Mathematical modelling of steady state fluid and protein exchange in lung. In Staub NC (ed): Lung Water and Solute Exchange. New York, Marcel Dekker, Inc, 1978, p 99.

275. McNamee JE, Staub NC: Pore models of sheep lung microvascular barrier using new data on protein tracers. Microvasc Res 10:229, 1979.

276. Harris TR, Roselli RJ: A theoretical model of protein, fluid, and small molecule transport in the lung. J Appl Physiol 50:1, 1981.

277. Brigham K: Lung edema due to increased vascular permeability. In Staub NC (ed): Lung Water and Solute Exchange. New York, Marcel Dekker, Inc, 1978, p 235.

278. Todd TRJ, Baile E, Hogg JC: Pulmonary capillary permeability during hemorrhagic shock. J Appl Physiol 45:298, 1978.

279. Renzoni A: Importanza del plesso venoso peribronchiale nel cane. Arch Ital Anat Embryol 60:111, 1955.

280. Pietra GG, Fishman AP: Bronchial edema. In Staub NC (ed): Lung Water and Solute Exchange. In Lenfant C (executive ed): Lung Biology in Health and Disease. New York, Marcel Dekker, Inc, 1978, p 407.

281. Pietra GG, Szidon JP, Leventhal MM, et al: Histamine and interstitial pulmonary edema in the dog. Circ Res 29:323, 1971

282. Nakahara K, Ohkuda K, Staub NC: Effect of infusing histamine into pulmonary or bronchial artery on sheep pulmonary fluid balance. Am Rev Respir Dis 120:875, 1979.

283. Staub NC, Nagano H, Pearce ML: Pulmonary edema in dogs, especially the sequence of fluid accumulation in lungs. J Appl Physiol 22:227, 1967.

284. Parker JC, Falgout HJ, Parker RE, et al: The effect of fluid volume loading on exclusion of interstitial albumin and lymph flow in the dog lung. Circ Res 45:440, 1979.

285. Bert JL, Pearce RH: The interstitium and microvascular exchange. In Renkin EM, Michel CG (eds): Handbook of Physiology—the Cardiovascular System. IV. Oxford, Oxford University Press, 1984, pp 521–547.

286. Gee MH, Williams DO: Effect of lung inflation on perivascular cuff fluid volume in isolated dog lung lobes. Microvasc Res 17:192, 1979.

287. Pare PD, Warriner B, Baile EM, et al: Redistribution of pulmonary

288. extravascular water with positive end-expiratory pressure in canine pulmonary edema. Am Rev Respir Dis 127:590, 1983.

288. Malo J, Ali J, Duke K, et al: Effects of PEEP on lung liquid distribution and pulmonary shunt in canine oleic acid pulmonary edema. Clin Res 28:703, 1980.

289. Schneeberger-Keeley EE, Karnovsky MJ: The ultrastructural basis of alveolar-capillary membrane permeability to peroxidase used as a tracer. J Cell Biol 37:781, 1968.

290. Egan EA: Effect of lung inflation on alveolar permeability to solutes. In Lung Liquids. Ciba Symposium. (New Series) 38, New York, Excerpta Medica, 1976.

291. Gil J, Weibel ER: Morphological study of pressure volume hysteresis in rat lungs fixed by vascular perfusion. Respir Physiol 15:190, 1972.

292. Lauweryns JM, Boussauw L: The ultrastructure of pulmonary lymphatic capillaries of newborn rabbits and of human infants. Lymphology 2:108, 1969.

293. Renkin EM: Lymph as a measure of the composition of interstitial fluid. In Fishman AP, Renkin EM (eds): Pulmonary Edema. Baltimore, Williams and Wilkins, 1979, p 145.

294. Pump KK: Lymphatics in the pulmonary alveoli: preliminary report. Chest 58:140, 1970.

295. Lauweryns JM, Baert JH: Alveolar clearance and the role of the pulmonary lymphatics. Am Rev Respir Dis 115:625, 1977.

296. Tobin CE: Lymphatics of the pulmonary alveoli. Anat Rec 120:625, 1954.

297. Lauweryns JM: The juxta-alveolar lymphatics in the human adult lung. Histologic studies in 15 cases of drowning. Am Rev Respir Dis 102:877, 1970.

298. Leak LV, Burke JF: Ultrastructural studies on the lymphatic anchoring filaments. J Cell Biol 36:129, 1968.

299. Paré PD, Brooks LA, Baile EM: Effect of systemic venous hypertension on pulmonary function and lung water. J Appl Physiol 51:592, 1981.

300. Starling EH: On the absorption of fluids from the connective tissue spaces. J Physiol (London) 19:312, 1896.

301. Dawson CA, Grimm DJ, Linehan JH: Effects of lung inflation on longitudinal distribution of pulmonary vascular resistance. J Appl Physiol 43:1089, 1977.

302. Hakim TS, Dawson CA, Linehan JH: Hemodynamic responses of dog lung lobe to lobar venous occlusion. J Appl Physiol 47:145, 1979.

303. Bhattacharya J, Staub MC: Direct measurement of microvascular pressures in the isolated perfused dog lung. Science 210:327, 1980.

304. Goshy M, Lai-Fook SJ, Hyatt RE: Perivascular pressure measurements by wick catheter technique in isolated dog lobes. Appl Physiol 46:950, 1979.

305. Inoue H, Inoue C, Hildebrandt J: Vascular and airway pressures and interstitial edema affect peribronchial fluid pressure. J Appl Physiol 48:177, 1980.

306. Lai-Fook SJ: Perivascular interstitial fluid pressure measured by micro-pipettes in isolated dog lung. J Appl Physiol 52:9, 1982.

307. Landis EN, Pappenheimer JR: Exchange of substances through the capillary wall. In Hamilton WS, Dow P (eds): Washington DC, American Physiological Society, 1963, p 261.

308. Nitta S, Ohnuki T, Okkuda K, et al: The corrected protein equation to estimate plasma colloid osmotic pressure and its development on a nomogram. Tohoku J Exp Med 135:43, 1981.

309. Prather JW, Gaar KA, Guyton AC: Direct continuous recording of plasma colloid osmotic pressure of whole blood. J Appl Physiol 24:602, 1968.

310. Olver RE, Strang LB: Ion fluxes across the pulmonary epithelium and the secretion of lung liquid in the foetal lamb. J Physiol 241:327, 1974.

311. Olver RE: Ion transport and water flow in the mammalian lung. In Lung Liquids. Ciba Symposium (New Series) 38, New York, Excerpta Medica, 1976.

312. Albert RK, Lakshminarayan S, Hildebrandt J, et al: Increased surface tension favours pulmonary edema formation in anesthetized dogs' lungs. J Clin Invest 63:115, 1979.

313. Brigham KL, Woolverton WC, Staub NV: Increased pulmonary vascular permeability after Pseudomonas aeruginosa bacteremia in unanesthetized sheep. Fed Proc 32:440, 1973.

314. Dumont AE, Clauss RH, Reed GE, et al: Lymph drainage in patients with congestive heart failure. N Engl J Med 269:949, 1963.

315. Sampson JJ, Leeds SE, Uhley HN, et al: Studies of lymph flow and changes in pulmonary structures as indexes of circulatory changes in experimental pulmonary edema. Isr J Med Sci 5:826, 1969.

316. Uhley HN, Leeds SE, Sampson JJ, et al: Some observations on the role of the lymphatics in experimental acute pulmonary edema. Circ Res 9:688, 1961.

317. Uhley HN, Leeds SE, Sampson JJ, et al: Role of pulmonary lymphatics in chronic pulmonary edema. Circ Res 11:966, 1962.

318. Leeds SE, Uhley HN, Sampson JJ, et al: Significance of changes in

10

the pulmonary lymph flow in acute and chronic experimental pulmonary edema. Am J Surg 114:254, 1967.

319. Rusznyák L, Földi M, Szabó G: Lymphatics and lymph circulation: Physiology and pathology. In Youlten L (ed). 2nd English ed., Oxford, Pergamon Press, 1967.

320. Magno M, Szidon JP: Haemodynamic pulmonary edema in dogs with acute and chronic lymphatic edema. Am J Physiol 231:1777, 1976.

321. Cross CE, Shaver JA, Wilson RJ, et al: Mitral stenosis and pulmonary fibrosis: Special reference to pulmonary edema and lung lymphatic function. Arch Intern Med 125:248, 1970.

322. Turino GM, Edelman NH, Senior RM, et al: Extravascular lung water in cor pulmonale. Bull Physiopathol Respir 4:47, 1968.

323. O'Reilly G, Jefferson K: Septal lines in pure right heart failure. Br J Radiol 49:123, 1976.

324. Erdmann AJ, Vaughan TR, Brigham KL, et al: Effect of increased vascular pressure on lung fluid balance in unanesthetized sheep. Circ Res 37:271, 1975.

325. Montaner JSG, Tsang J, Evans KG, et al: Alveolar epithelial damage: a critical difference between high pressure and oleic acid—induced low pressure pulmonary edema. J Clin Invest 77:1786, 1986.

326. West JB, Dollery CT, Heard BE: Increased vascular resistance in the lower zone of the lung caused by perivascular oedema. Lancet 2:181, 1964.

327. Muir AL, Hall DL, Despas P, et al: Distribution of blood flow in the lungs in acute pulmonary edema in dogs. J Appl Physiol 33:763, 1972.

328. Vreim CE, Staub NC: Protein composition of lung fluid in acute alloxan edema in dogs. Am J Physiol 230:376, 1976.

329. Vreim CE, Snashall PD, Staub NC: Protein composition of lung fluid in anesthetized dogs with acute cardiogenic edema. Am J Physiol 231:1466, 1976.

330. Staub NC: Alveolar flooding and clearance. Am Rev Respir Dis 127 (part 2) S:44, 1983.

331. Stender HS, Schermuly W: Das interstitielle lungenödem im röntgenbild. (Roentgen findings in interstitial pulmonary edema.) Fortschr Roentgensstr 95:461, 1961.

332. Slutsky RA, Higgins CB: Intravascular and extravascular pulmonary fluid volumes II. Response to rapid increases in left atrial pressure and the theoretical implications for pulmonary radiographic and radionuclide imaging. Invest Radiol 18:33, 1983.

333. Dodek A, Kassebaum DG, Bristow JD: Pulmonary edema in coronary-artery disease without cardiomegaly. Paradox of the stiff heart. N Engl J Med 286:1347, 1972.

334. Heitzman ER: The Lung: Radiologic-Pathologic Correlations. St. Louis, The CV Mosby Co, 1973, pp 127-134.

335. Don C, Johnson R: The nature and significance of peribronchial cuffing in pulmonary edema. Radiology 125:577, 1977.

336. Grainger RG: Interstitial pulmonary oedema and its radiological diagnosis. A sign of pulmonary venous and capillary hypertension. Br J Radiol 31:201, 1958.

337. Heitzman ER, Ziter FM: Acute interstitial pulmonary edema. Am J Roentgenol 98:291, 1966.

338. Meszaros WT: Cardiac roentgenology: Plain Films and Angiocardiographic Findings. Springfield, Ill, Charles C Thomas, 1969, p 103.

339. Heikkilä J, Hugenholtz PG, Tabakin BS: Prediction of left heart filling pressure and its sequential change in acute myocardial infarction from the terminal force of the P wave. Br Heart J 35:142, 1973.

340. Bennett ED, Rees S: The measurement of radiological changes in the lungs in acute myocardial infarction. Br J Radiol 47:879, 1974.

341. McCredie M: Measurement of pulmonary edema in valvular heart disease. Circulation 36:381, 1967.

342. Hedlund LW, Vock P, Effmann EL, et al: Hydrostatic pulmonary edema. An analysis of lung density changes by computed tomography. Invest Radiol 19:254, 1984.

343. Gamsu G, Kaufman L, Swann SJ, et al: Absolute lung density in experimental canine pulmonary edema. Invest Radiol 14:261, 1979.

344. Ahluwalia BD, Brownell GL, Hales CA: An index of pulmonary edema measured with emission computed tomography. J Comput Assist Tomogr 5:690, 1981.

345. Tamaki N, Itoh H, Ishii Y, et al: Hemodynamic significance of increased lung uptake of thallium-201. Am J Roentgenol 138:223, 1982.

346. Skalina S, Kundel HL, Wolf G, et al: The effect of pulmonary edema on proton nuclear magnetic resonance relaxation times. Invest Radiol 19:7, 1984.

347. Wexler HR, Nicholson RL, Prato FS, et al: Quantitation of lung water by nuclear magnetic resonance imaging. A preliminary study. Invest Radiol 20:583, 1985.

348. Schmidt HC, McNamara MT, Brasch RC, et al: Assessment of severity of experimental pulmonary edema with magnetic resonance imaging. Effect of relaxation enhancement by Gd-DTPA. Invest Radiol 20:687, 1987.

349. Carroll FE Jr, Loyd JE, Nolop KB, et al: MR imaging parameters in the study of lung water. A preliminary study. Invest Radiol 20:381, 1985.

350. Gleason DC, Steiner RE: The lateral roentgenogram in pulmonary edema. Am J Roentgenol 98:279, 1966.

351. Richman SM, Godar TJ: Unilateral pulmonary edema. N Engl J Med 264:1148, 1961.

352. Nessa CG, Rigler LG: The roentgenological manifestations of pulmonary edema. Radiology 37:35, 1941.

353. Azimi F, Wolson AH, Dalinka MK, et al: Unilateral pulmonary edema—differential diagnosis. Australas Radiol 19:20, 1975.

354. Calenoff L, Kruglik GD, Woodruff A: Unilateral pulmonary edema. Radiology 126:19, 1978.

355. Gyves-Ray KM, Spizarny DL, Gross BH: Case Report. Unilateral pulmonary edema due to postlobectomy pulmonary vein thrombosis. AJR 148:1079, 1987.

356. Leeming BWA: Gravitational edema of the lungs observed during assisted respiration. Chest 64:719, 1973.

357. Kieffer SA, Amplatz K, Anderson RC, et al: Proximal of a pulmonary artery: Roentgen features and surgical correction. Am J Roentgenol 95:592, 1965.

358. Saleh M, Miles AI, Lasser RP: Unilateral pulmonary edema in Swyer-James syndrome. Chest 66:594, 1974.

359. Amjad H, Bigman O, Tabor H: Unilateral pulmonary edema. JAMA 229:1094, 1974.

360. Albers WH, Nadas AS: Unilateral chronic pulmonary edema and pleural effusion after systemic-pulmonary artery shunts for cyanotic congenital heart disease. Am J Cardiol 19:861, 1967.

361. Salem MR, Masud KZ, Tatooles CJ, et al: Unilateral pulmonary oedema following aorta to right pulmonary artery anastomosis (Waterston's operation). Br J Anaesth 43:701, 1971.

362. Felman AH: Neurogenic pulmonary edema: Observations in 6 patients. Am J Roentgenol 112:393, 1971.

363. Royal HD, Shields JB, Donati RM: Misplacement of central venous pressure catheters and unilateral pulmonary edema. Arch Intern Med 135:1502, 1975.

364. Flick MR, Kantzler GB, Block AJ: Unilateral pulmonary edema with contralateral thoracic sympathectomy in the adult respiratory distress syndrome. Chest 68:736, 1975.

365. Robin ED, Thomas ED: Some relations between pulmonary edema and pulmonary inflammation (pneumonia). Arch Intern Med 93:713, 1954.

366. Zimmerman JE, Goodman LR, St. Andre AC, et al: Radiographic detection of mobilizable lung water: the gravitational shift test. Am J Roentgenol 138:59, 1982.

367. Hodson CJ: Pulmonary oedema and the 'batswing' shadow. J Fac Radiol 1:176, 1950.

368. Hughes RT: The pathology of butterfly densities in uraemia. Thorax 22:97, 1967.

369. Steckel RJ: The radiolucent kinetic border line in acute pulmonary oedema and pneumonia. Clin Radiol 25:391, 1974.

370. Herrnheiser G, Hinson KFW: An anatomical explanation of the formation of butterfly shadows. Thorax 9:198, 1954.

371. Rigler LG, Surprenant EL: Pulmonary edema. Semin Roentgenol 2:33, 1967.

372. Prichard MML, Daniel PM, Ardran GM: Peripheral ischaemia of the lung. Some experimental observations. Br J Radiol 27:93, 1954.

373. Reeves JT, Tweeddale D, Noonan J, et al: Correlations of microradiographic and histological findings in the pulmonary vascular bed. Technique and application in pulmonary hypertension. Circulation 34:971, 1966.

374. Borgström KE, Ising U, Linder E, et al: Experimental pulmonary edema. Acta Radiol 54:97, 1960.

375. Gibson DG: Hemodynamic factors in the development of acute pulmonary oedema in renal failure. Lancet 2:1217, 1966.

376. Crosbie WA, Snowden S, Parsons V: Changes in lung capillary permeability in renal failure. Br Med J 4:388, 1972.

377. Fleischner FG: The butterfly pattern of acute pulmonary edema. Am J Cardiol 20:39, 1967.

378. Wrinch J, Thurlbeck WM, Hogg J, et al: The pathogenesis of the "butterfly" shadow in pulmonary edema: A study of the effect of the lymphatic drainage. Unpublished data.

379. Frank NJ: Influence of acute pulmonary vascular congestion on the recoiling forces of excised cats' lungs. J Appl Physiol 14:905, 1959.

380. Cooke CD, Mead J, Schreiner GL, et al: Pulmonary mechanics during induced pulmonary edema in anesthetized dogs. J Appl Physiol 14:17, 1969.

381. Said SI, Longacre JW, David RK, et al: Pulmonary gas exchange during induction of pulmonary edema in anesthetized dogs. J Appl Physiol 19:403, 1964.

382. Levine OR, Mellins RB, Fishman AP: Quantitative assessment of pulmonary edema. Circ Res 17:414, 1965.

383. Sharp JG, Griffith GD, Bunnell IL, et al: Ventilatory mechanics in pulmonary edema in man. J Clin Invest 37:111, 1958.

384. Hogg JC, Agarawal JB, Gardiner AJF, et al: Distribution of airway

resistance with developing pulmonary edema in dogs. J Appl Physiol 32:20, 1972.

385. Collins JV, Cochrane SN, Davis J, et al: Some aspects of pulmonary function after rapid saline infusion in healthy subjects. Clin Sci Molec Med 45:407, 1973.

386. Hales CA, Kazemi H: Small airway function in myocardial infarction. N Engl J Med 290:761, 1974.

387. Zidulka A, Despas DJ, Milic-Emili J, et al: Pulmonary function with acute loss of lung water by hemodialysis in patients with chronic uremia. Am J Med 55:134, 1973.

388. West JB, Dollery CT, Heard BE: Increased pulmonary vascular resistance in the dependent zone of the isolated dog lung caused by perivascular edema. Circ Res 17:191, 1965.

389. West JB: Perivascular oedema: a factor in pulmonary vascular resistance. Am Heart J 70:570, 1965.

390. Dawson A, Kaneko K, McGregor M: Regional lung function in patients with mitral stenosis studied with 133 XE during air and oxygen breathing. J Clin Invest 44:999, 1965.

391. Paintal AF: Mechanism of stimulation of Type J pulmonary receptors. J Physiol 203:511, 1969.

392. Aberman A, Fulop M: The metabolic and respiratory acidosis of acute pulmonary edema. Ann Intern Med 76:173, 1972.

393. Fulop M, Horowitz M, Aberman A, et al: Lactic acidosis in pulmonary edema due to left ventricular failure. Ann Intern Med 79:180, 1973.

394. Anthonisen NR, Smith HJ: Respiratory acidosis as a consequence of pulmonary edema. Ann Intern Med 62:991, 1965.

395. Agostoni A: Acid-base disturbances in pulmonary edema. Arch Intern Med 120:307, 1967.

396. Avery WG, Samet P, Sackner MA: The acidosis of pulmonary edema. Am J Med 48:320, 1970.

397. Miller A, Chusid EL, Samortin TG: Acute, reversible respiratory acidosis in cardiogenic pulmonary edema. JAMA 216:1315, 1971.

398. Wilson JG: Pulmonary oedema in acute glomerulonephritis. Arch Dis Child 36:661, 1961.

399. Macpherson RI, Banerjee AK: Acute glomerulonephritis: A chest film diagnosis? J Can Assoc Radiol 25:58, 1974.

400. Lee HY, Stretton TB, Barnes AM: The lungs in renal failure. Thorax 30:46, 1975.

401. Zidulka A, Despas PJ, Milic-Emili J, et al: Pulmonary function with acute loss of excess lung water by hemodialysis in patients with chronic uremia. Am J Med 55:134, 1973.

402. Cooperman LH, Price HL: Pulmonary edema in the operative and postoperative period. Ann Surg 172:883, 1970.

403. daLuz PL, Weil MH, et al: Pulmonary edema related to changes in colloid osmotic and pulmonary artery wedge pressure in patients after acute myocardial infarction. Circulation 51:350, 1975.

404. Stein L, Beraud J, Cavonilles J, et al: Pulmonary edema during fluid infusion in the absence of heart failure. JAMA 229:65, 1974.

405. Westcott JL, Rudick MG: Cardiopulmonary effects of intravenous fluid overload: radiologic manifestations. Radiology 129:577, 1978.

406. Luft FC, Klatte EC, Weyman AE, et al: Cardiopulmonary effects of volume expansion in man: radiographic manifestations. AJR 144:289, 1985.

407. Philipps E, Fleischner FG: Pulmonary edema in the course of a blood transfusion without overloading the circulation. Dis Chest 50:619, 1966.

408. Ward HN: Pulmonary infiltration associated with leukoagglutinin transfusion reactions. Ann Intern Med 73:688, 1970.

409. Thompson JS, Severson CD, Parmerly MJ, et al: Pulmonary "hypersensitivity" reactions induced by transfusion of non-HL-A leukoagglutinins. N Engl J Med 284:1120, 1971.

410. Lewis RW, Rudd N, Pittman JA: Blood transfusion complications: leukoagglutinin reactions. Obstet Gynecol 65:785, 1985.

411. Levy GJ, Shabot MM, Hart ME, et al: Transfusion-associated non-cardiogenic pulmonary edema. Report of a case and a warning regarding treatment. Transfusion 26:278, 1986.

412. Popovsky MA, Moore SB: Diagnostic and pathogenetic considerations in transfusion-related acute lung injury. Transfusion 25:573, 1985.

413. Ruff F, Hughes JBM, Stanley M, et al: Regional lung function in patients with hepatic cirrhosis. J Clin Invest 50:2403, 1971.

414. Trewby PN, Warren R, Contini S, et al: Incidence and pathophysiology of pulmonary oedema in fulminant hepatic failure. Gastroenterology 74:859, 1978.

415. Harris GBC, Neuhauser EBD, Giedion A: Total anomalous pulmonary venous return below the diaphragm: The roentgen appearances in three patients diagnosed during life. Am J Roentgenol 84:436, 1960.

416. Lucas RV Jr, Adams P Jr, Anderson RC, et al: Total anomalous pulmonary venous connection to the portal venous system: A cause of pulmonary venous obstruction. Am J Roentgenol 86:561, 1961.

417. Hacking PM, Simpson W: Partially obstructed total anomalous pulmonary venous return. Clin Radiol 18:450, 1967.

418. Sande MA, Alonso DR, Smith JP, et al: Left atrial tumor presenting with hemoptysis and pulmonary infiltrates. Am Rev Respir Dis 102:258, 1970.

419. Montreal General Hospital Case Records: Dyspnea and lymphadenopathy in a patient with two PH-1 chromosomes. N Engl J Med 289:524, 1973.

420. Sarnoff SJ: Massive pulmonary edema of central nervous system origin: Hemodynamic observations and the role of sympathetic pathways. Fed Proc 10:118, 1951.

421. Sarnoff SJ, Kaufman HE: Elevation of left auricular pressure in relation to ammonium pulmonary edema in the cat. Proc Soc Exp Biol Med 78:829, 1951.

422. Cameron GR, De SN: Experimental pulmonary oedema of nervous origin. J Pathol Bacteriol 61:375, 1949.

423. Ducker TD, Simmons RL: Increased intracranial pressure and pulmonary edema. Part II. Hemodynamic response of dogs and monkeys to increased intracranial pressure. J Neurosurg 28:118, 1968.

424. Worthen M, Argano B, Siwadiowski W, et al: Mechanisms of intracisternal veratrine pulmonary edema. Dis Chest 55:45, 1969.

425. Harari A, Rapin M, Regnier B, et al: Normal pulmonary capillary pressures in the late phase of neurogenic pulmonary edema. Lancet 1:494, 1976.

426. Melon E, Bonnet F, Lepresle E, et al: Altered capillary permeability in neurogenic pulmonary oedema. Intensive Care Med 11:323, 1985.

427. Ducker TD: Increased intracranial pressure and pulmonary edema. Part I. Clinical study of 11 patients. J Neurosurg 28:112, 1968.

428. Theodore J, Robin E: Speculations on neurogenic pulmonary edema. Am Rev Respir Dis 113:404, 1976.

429. Wray NP, Nicotra MB: Pathogenesis of neurogenic pulmonary edema. Am Rev Respir Dis 118:783, 1978.

430. Van der Zee H, Malik AB, Lee BC, et al: Lung fluid and protein exchange during intracranial hypertension and role of sympathetic mechanisms. J Appl Physiol 48:273, 1980.

431. Bowers RE, McKeen CR, Park BE, et al: Increased pulmonary vascular permeability follows intracranial hypertension in sheep. Am Rev Respir Dis 119:637, 1979.

432. Bonbrest HC: Pulmonary edema following an epileptic seizure. Am Rev Respir Dis 91:97, 1965.

433. Huff RW, Fred HL: Postictal pulmonary edema. Arch Intern Med 117:824, 1966.

434. Chang CH, Smith CA: Postictal pulmonary edema. Radiology 89:1087, 1967.

435. Teplinsky K, Hall J: Post-ictal pulmonary edema. Report of a case. Arch Intern Med 146:801, 1986.

436. Schumacker PT, Rhodes GR, Newell JC, et al: Ventilation-perfusion imbalance after head trauma. Am Rev Respir Dis 119:33, 1979.

437. Petty TL, Ashbaugh DG: The adult respiratory distress syndrome. Clinical features, factors influencing prognosis and principles of management. Chest 60:233, 1971.

438. Murray JF: The adult respiratory distress syndrome (may it rest in peace). Am Rev Respir Dis 111:716, 1975.

439. Fishman AP: Shock lung. A distinctive nonentity. Circulation 47:921, 1973.

440. Thurlbeck WM: Conference summary. Chest 66(Suppl):40, 1974.

441. Addington WW, Cugell DW, Bayley ES, et al: The pulmonary edema of heroin toxicity—an example of the stiff lung syndrome. Chest 62:199, 1972.

442. Briscoe WA, Smith JP, Bergofsky E, et al: Catastrophic pulmonary failure. Am J Med 60:248, 1976.

443. Petty TL: The adult respiratory distress syndrome (confessions of a "lumper"). Am Rev Respir Dis 111:713, 1975.

444. Blennerhassett JB: Shock lung and diffuse alveolar damage: pathological and pathogenetic considerations. Pathology 17:239, 1985.

445. Blaisdell FW, Schlobohm RM: The respiratory distress syndrome: A review. Surgery 74:251, 1973.

446. Connell RS, Swank RL, Webb MC: The development of pulmonary ultrastructural lesions during hemorrhage shock. J Trauma 15:116, 1975.

447. Demling RH, Niehaus G, Will JA: Pulmonary microvascular response to hemorrhagic shock, resuscitation and recovery. J Appl Physiol 46:498, 1979.

448. Thommasen HB, Martin BA, Wiggs B, et al: The effect of pulmonary blood flows on white blood cell uptake and release by the dog lung. J Appl Physiol 56:966, 1984.

449. Hogg JC, Martin BA, Lee S, et al: Regional differences in red blood cell transit in normal lungs. J Appl Physiol 59:126, 1985.

450. Doerschuk CM, Allard MF, Martin BA, et al: Marginated pool of neutrophils in rabbit lungs. J Appl Physiol 63:1806, 1987.

451. Muir AL, Cruz M, Martin BA, et al: Leukocyte kinetics in the human lung: role of exercise and catecholamines. J Appl Physiol 57:711, 1984.

452. Cochrane CG: The enhancement of inflammatory injury. Am Rev Respir Dis 136:1, 1987.

10

453. Bachofen N, Weibel ER: Alterations of the gas exchange apparatus in adult respiratory insufficiency associated with septicemia. Am Rev Respir Dis 116:589, 1977.

454. Elliott CG, Zimmerman GA, Orme JF, et al: Granulocyte aggregation in adult respiratory distress syndrome (ARDS)—serial histologic and physiologic observations. Am J Med Sci 289:70, 1985.

455. Tate RM, Repine JE: Neutrophils and the adult respiratory distress syndrome. Am Rev Respir Dis 128:552, 1983.

456. Thommasen HB: The role of the polymorphonuclear leukocyte in the pathogenesis of the adult respiratory distress syndrome. Clin Invest Med 8:185, 1985.

457. Thommasen HB, Russell JA, Boyko WJ, et al: Transient leukopenia associated with adult respiratory distress syndrome. Lancet 1:809, 1984.

458. Brigham KL, Woolverton WC, Blake LH, et al: Increased sheep lung vascular permeability caused by pseudomonas bacteremia. J Clin Invest 54:792, 1974.

459. Flick MR, Perel G, Staub NC: Leukocytes are required for increased lung microvascular permeability after microembolism in sheep. Circ Res 48:344, 1981.

460. Heflin AJ, Brigham KL: Prevention by granulocyte type depletion of increased vascular permeability of sheep lung following endotoxemia. J Clin Invest 68:1253, 1981.

461. Johnson A, Malik AP: Effect of granulocytopenia on extravascular lung water content after micro-embolization. Am Rev Respir Dis 122:561, 1980.

462. Shasby DM, Fox RB, Harada RN, et al: Reduction of the edema of acute hypoxic lung injury by granulocyte depletion. J Appl Physiol 52:1237, 1982.

463. Shasby DM, Van Benthuysen KM, Tate RM, et al: Granulocytes mediate acute edematous lung injury in rabbits and isolated rabbit lungs perfused with phorbol miristate acetate: Role of oxygen radicals. Am Rev Respir Dis 125:443, 1982.

464. Worthen GS, Haslett C, Rees AJ, et al: Neutrophil-mediated pulmonary vascular injury: synergistic effect of trace amounts of lipopolysaccharide and neutrophil stimuli on vascular permeability and neutrophil sequestration in the lung. Am Rev Respir Dis 136:19, 1987.

465. Snapper JR, Bernard GR, Hinson JM, et al: Endotoxemia-induced leukopenia in sheep—correlation with lung vascular permeability and hypoxemia but not with pulmonary hypertension. Am Rev Respir Dis 127:306, 1983.

466. Parsons PE, Fowler AA, Hyers TM, et al: Chemotactic activity in bronchoalveolar lavage fluid from patients with adult respiratory distress syndrome. Am Rev Respir Dis 132:490, 1985.

467. Zimmerman GA, Renzetti AD, Hill HR: Functional and metabolic activity of granulocytes from patients with adult respiratory distress syndrome—evidence for activated neutrophils in the pulmonary circulation. Am Rev Respir Dis 127:290, 1983.

468. Miyata T, Torisu M: Plasma endotoxin levels and functions of peripheral granulocytes in surgical patients with respiratory distress syndrome. Jpn J Surg 16:412, 1986.

469. Zimmerman GA, Renzetti AD, Hill HR: Granulocyte adherence in pulmonary and systemic arterial blood samples from patients with adult respiratory distress syndrome. Am Rev Respir Dis 129:798, 1984.

470. Fowler AA, Hyers TM, Fisher BJ, et al: The adult respiratory distress syndrome: cell populations and soluble mediators in the air spaces of patients at high risk. Am Rev Respir Dis 136:1225, 1987.

471. Weiland JE, Davis WB, Holter JF, et al: Lung neutrophils in the adult respiratory distress syndrome. Clinical and pathophysiologic significance. Am Rev Respir Dis 133:218, 1986.

472. Hallgren R, Samuelsson T, Venge P, et al: Eosinophil activation in the lung is related to lung damage in adult respiratory distress syndrome. Am Rev Respir Dis 135:639, 1987.

473. Modig J, Hallgren R: Lethal adult respiratory distress syndrome after meningococcal septicemia biochemical markers in bronchoalveolar lavage. Resuscitation 13:159, 1986.

474. Warshawski FJ, Sibbald WJ, Driedger AA, et al: Abnormal neutrophil-pulmonary interaction in the adult respiratory distress syndrome. Qualitative and quantitative assessment of pulmonary neutrophil kinetics in humans with in vivo 111 Indium neutrophil scintigraphy. Am Rev Respir Dis 133:797, 1986.

475. Maunder RJ, Hackman RC, Riff E, et al: Occurrence of the adult respiratory distress syndrome in neutropenic patients. Am Rev Respir Dis 133:313, 1986.

476. Braude S, Apperley J, Krausz T, et al: Adult respiratory distress syndrome after allogeneic bone-marrow transplantation: evidence for a neutrophil-independent mechanism. Lancet 1:1239, 1985.

477. Ognibene RP, Martin SE, Parker MM, et al: Adult respiratory distress syndrome in patients with severe neutropenia. N Engl J Med 315:547, 1986.

478. Rinaldo JE, Borovetz H: Deterioration of oxygenation and abnormal lung microvascular permeability during resolution of leukopenia in patients with diffuse lung injury. Am Rev Respir Dis 131:579, 1985.

479. Hallman M, Spragg R, Harrell JH, et al: Evidence of lung surfactant abnormality in respiratory failure. J Clin Invest 70:673, 1982.

480. Petty TL, Reiss OK, Paul GW, et al: Characteristics of pulmonary surfactant in adult respiratory distress syndrome associated with trauma and shock. Am Rev Respir Dis 115:531, 1977.

481. Petty TL, Silvers DW, Paul GW: Abnormalities in lung elastic properties and surfactant function in adult respiratory distress syndrome. Chest 75:571, 1979.

482. Liau DF, Barrett CR, Bell ALL, et al: Functional abnormalities of lung surfactant in experimental acute alveolar injury in the dog. Am Rev Respir Dis 136:395, 1987.

483. Ryan SF, Liau DF, Bell ALL, et al: Correlation of lung compliance and quantities of surfactant phospholipids after acute alveolar injury from N-nitroso-N-methylurethane in the dog. Am Rev Respir Dis 123:200, 1981.

484. Muller-Eberhard HJ: Complement. Annu Rev Biochem 44:697, 1975.

485. Shaw JO, Henson PM, Henson J, et al: Lung inflammation induced by complement derived chemotactic fragments in the alveolus. Lab Invest 42:547, 1980.

486. Till GO, Ward PA: Complement-induced lung injury. In Said SI (ed): The Pulmonary Circulation and Acute Lung Injury. Mount Kisco, NY, Futura Publishing Company, Inc, 1985, p 387.

487. Robbins RA, Russ WD, Rasmussen JK, et al: Activation of the complement system in the adult respiratory distress syndrome. Am Rev Respir Dis 135:651, 1987.

488. Knudsen P, Nielsen AH, Pedersen JD, et al: Adult respiratory distress-like syndrome during hemodialysis: relationship between activation of complement, leukopenia, and release of granulocyte elastase. Int J Artif Organs 8:187, 1985.

489. Lew PD, Forster A, Perrin LH, et al: Complement activation in the adult respiratory distress syndrome following cardiopulmonary bypass. Bull Eur Physiopathol Respir 21:231, 1985.

490. Boogaerts MA, Roelant C, Goossens W, et al: Complement activation and adult respiratory distress syndrome during intermittent flow apheresis procedures. Transfusion 26:82, 1986.

491. Gardinali M, Cicardi M, Frangi D, et al: Studies of complement activation in ARDS patients treated by long term extracorporeal CO_2 removal. Int J Artif Organs 8:135, 1985.

492. Hammerschmidt DE, Weaver LJ, Hudson LD, et al: Association of complement activation and elevated plasma C5a with adult respiratory distress syndrome. Pathophysiologic relevance and possible prognostic value. Lancet 1:947, 1980.

493. Rinaldo JE, Rogers RM: Adult respiratory distress syndrome. N Engl J Med 315:578, 1986.

494. Weinberg PF, Matthay MA, Webster RO, et al: Biologically active products of complement and acute lung injury in patients with sepsis syndrome. Am Rev Respir Dis 130:791, 1984.

495. Duchateau J, Haas M, Schreyen H, et al: Complement activation in patients at risk of developing the adult respiratory distress syndrome. Am Rev Respir Dis 130:1058, 1984.

496. Malik AB: Mediators of pulmonary vascular injury and edema after thrombin. In Said SI (ed): The Pulmonary Circulation and Acute Lung Injury. Mount Kisco, NY, Futura Publishing Company, Inc, 1985, p 429.

497. Saldeen T: Clotting, microembolism, and inhibition of fibrinolysis in adult respiratory distress. Surg Clin North Am 63:285, 1983.

498. Malik AB: Pulmonary microembolism. Physiol Rev 63:1114, 1983.

499. Saldeen T: The microembolism syndrome. In Saldeen T (ed): The Microembolism Syndrome. Stockholm, Almquist and Wiksell International, 1979, p 7.

500. Johnson A, Tahamont MB, Malik AB: Thrombin-induced lung vascular injury: Role of fibrinogen and fibrinolysis. Am Rev Respir Dis 128:38, 1983.

501. Tahamont MB, Malik AB: Granulocytes mediate the increase in pulmonary vascular permeability after thrombin embolism. J Appl Physiol 54:1489, 1983.

502. Johnson A, Blumenstock FA, Malik AB: Effect of complement depletion on lung fluid balance after thrombin. J Appl Physiol 55:1480, 1983.

503. Lo SK, Perlman MB, Niehaus GD, et al: Thrombin-induced alterations in lung fluid balance in awake sheep. J Appl Physiol 58:1421, 1985.

504. Kwaan HC: Disseminated intravascular coagulation. Med Clin North Am 56:177, 1972.

505. Putman CE, Minagi H, Blaisdell FW: The roentgen appearance of disseminated intravascular coagulation (DIC). Radiology 109:13, 1973.

506. Unger KM, Shibel EM, Moser KM: Detection of left ventricular failure in patients with adult respiratory distress syndrome. Chest 67:8, 1975.

507. Horwitz CA, Ward PCJ: Disseminated intravascular coagulation, nonbacterial thrombotic endocarditis and adult pulmonary hyaline membranes—an interrelated triad? Report of a case following small bowel resection for a strangulated inguinal hernia. Am J Med 51:272, 1971.

508. Bone RC, Francis PB, Pierce AK: Intervascular coagulation associated with the adult respiratory distress syndrome. Am J Med 61:585, 1976.

509. Carlson RW, Schaeffer RC, Carpio M, et al: Edema fluid and coagulation changes during fulminant pulmonary edema. Chest 79:43, 1981.

510. Haynes AB, Hyers TM, Giclas PC, et al: Elevated fibrin(ogen) degradation products in the adult respiratory distress syndrome. Am Rev Respir Dis 122:841, 1980.

511. Modig J, Bagge L: Specific coagulation and fibrinolysis tests as biochemical markers in traumatic-induced adult respiratory distress syndrome. Resuscitation 13:87, 1986.

512. Alberts KA, Norén I, Rubin M, et al: Respiratory distress following major trauma. Predictive value of blood coagulation tests. Acta Orthop Scand 57:158, 1986.

513. Idell S, Gonzalez K, Bradford H, et al: Procoagulant activity in bronchoalveolar lavage in the adult respiratory distress syndrome. Contribution of tissue factor associated with factor 7. Am Rev Respir Dis 136:1466, 1987.

514. Bachofen M, Weibel ER: Structural alterations of lung parenchyma in the adult respiratory distress syndrome. Clin Chest Med 3:35, 1982.

515. El-Kassimi FA, Al-Mashhadani DCP, Abdullah AK, et al: Adult respiratory distress syndrome and disseminated intravascular coagulation complicating heat stroke. Chest 90:571, 1986.

516. Schneider RC, Zapol WM, Carvalho AC: Platelet consumption and sequestration in severe, acute respiratory failure. Am Rev Respir Dis 122:445, 1980.

517. Quinn DA, Carvalho AC, Geller E, et al: ^{99m}Tc-fibrinogen scanning in adult respiratory distress syndrome. Am Rev Respir Dis 135:100, 1987.

518. Carvalho ACA, Bellman SM, Saullo VJ, et al: Altered factor 8 in acute respiratory failure. N Engl J Med 307:1113, 1982.

519. Frank L: Oxidant injury to pulmonary endothelium. In Said SI (ed): The Pulmonary Circulation and Acute Lung Injury. Mount Kisco, NY, Futura Publishing Company, Inc, 1985, p 283.

520. Taylor AE, Martin DJ, Townsley MI: Oxygen radicals and pulmonary edema. In Said SI (ed): The Pulmonary Circulation and Acute Lung Injury. Mount Kisco, NY, Futura Publishing Company, Inc, 1985, p 307.

521. Cochrane CG, Spragg R, Revak SD: Pathogenesis of the adult respiratory distress syndrome—evidence of oxidant activity in bronchoalveolar lavage fluid. J Clin Invest 71:754, 1983.

522. Ahmed T, Marchett B, Wanner A, et al: Direct and indirect effects of leukotriene—D4 on the pulmonary and systemic circulations. Am Rev Respir Dis 131:554, 1985.

523. Slotman GJ, Burchard KW, Yellin SA, et al: Prostaglandin and complement interaction in clinical acute respiratory failure. Arch Surg 121:271, 1986.

524. Matthay MA, Eschenbacher WL, Goetzl EJ: Elevated concentrations of leukotriene D4 in pulmonary edema fluid of patients with the adult respiratory distress syndrome. J Clin Immunol 4:479, 1984.

525. Gillis CN, Pitt BR, Widemann HP, et al: Depressed prostaglandin E1 and 5-hydroxytryptamine removal in patients with adult respiratory distress syndrome. Am Rev Respir Dis 134:739, 1986.

526. Reines HD, Halushka PV, Olanoff LS, et al: Dazoxiben in human sepsis and adult respiratory distress syndrome. Clin Pharmacol Ther 37:391, 1985.

527. Shoemaker WC, Appel PL: Effects of prostaglandin E1 in adult respiratory distress syndrome. Surgery 99:275, 1986.

528. Holcroft JW, Vassar MJ, Weber CJ: Prostaglandin E1 and survival in patients with the adult respiratory distress syndrome. A prospective trial. Ann Surg 203:371, 1986.

529. Schapira M, Gardaz JP, Py P, et al: Prekallikrein activation in the adult respiratory distress syndrome. Bull Eur Physiopathol Respir 21:237, 1985.

530. Idell S, Kucich U, Fein A, et al: Neutrophil elastase-releasing factors in bronchoalveolar lavage from patients with adult respiratory distress syndrome. Am Rev Respir Dis 132:1098, 1985.

531. O'Brodovich HM, Stalcup SA, Pang LM, et al: Bradykinin production and increased pulmonary endothelial permeability during acute respiratory failure in unanesthetized sheep. J Clin Invest 67:514, 1981.

532. McGuire WW, Spragg RG, Cohen AB, et al: Studies on the pathogenesis of the adult respiratory distress syndrome. J Clin Invest 69:543, 1982.

533. Nuytinck JK, Goris JA, Redl H, et al: Posttraumatic complications and inflammatory mediators. Arch Surg 121:886, 1986.

534. Lee CT, Fein AM, Lippmann M, et al: Elastolytic activity in pulmonary lavage fluid from patients with adult respiratory-distress syndrome. N Engl J Med 304:192, 1981.

535. Johnson AR, Coalson JJ, Ashton J, et al: Neutral endopeptidase in serum samples from patients with adult respiratory distress syndrome. Comparison with angiotensin-converting enzyme. Am Rev Respir Dis 132:1262, 1985.

536. Vadas P: Elevated plasma phospholipase A2 levels: correlation with the hemodynamic and pulmonary changes in gram-negative septic shock. J Lab Clin Med 104:873, 1984.

537. Joffe N: The adult respiratory distress syndrome. Am J Roentgenol 122:719, 1974.

538. Ostendorf P, Birzle H, Vogel W, et al: Pulmonary radiographic abnormalities in shock. Roentgen-clinical pathological correlation. Radiology 115:257, 1975.

539. Dyck DR, Zylak CJ: Acute respiratory distress in adults. Radiology 106:497, 1973.

540. Webb WR: Pulmonary complications of nonthoracic trauma: Summary of the National Research Council Conference. J Trauma 9:700, 1969.

541. Greene R: Adult respiratory distress syndrome: Acute alveolar damage. Radiology 163:57, 1987.

542. Weibel ER: Looking into the lung: what can it tell us. Am J Roentgenol 133:1021, 1979.

543. Lamy M, Falatt RJ, Koeniger E, et al: Pathologic features and mechanisms of hypoxemia in adult respiratory distress syndrome. Am Rev Respir Dis 114:267, 1976.

544. Zimmerman JE, Goodman LR, Shahvari MBG: Effect of mechanical ventilation and positive end-expiratory pressure (PEEP) on chest radiograph. Am J Roentgenol 133:811, 1979.

545. Effmann EL, Merten DF, Kirks DR, et al: Adult respiratory distress syndrome in children. Radiology 157:69, 1985.

546. Milne ENC, Pistolesi M, Miniati M, et al: The radiologic distinction of cardiogenic and noncardiogenic edema. AJR 144:879, 1985.

547. Pistolesi M, Milne EWC, Miniati M, et al: The vascular pedicle of the heart and the vena azygos. Part II: Acquired heart disease. Radiology 152:9, 1984.

548. Smith RC, Mann H, Greenspan RH, et al: Radiographic differentiation between different etiologies of pulmonary edema. Invest Radiol 22:859, 1987.

549. O'Quin R, Marini JJ: Pulmonary artery occlusion pressure: Clinical physiology, measurement, and interpretation. Am Rev Respir Dis 128:319, 1983.

550. Touissant GP, Burgess JH, Hampson LG: Central venous pressure and pulmonary wedge pressure in critical surgical illness. A comparison. Arch Surg 109:265, 1974.

551. Wittnich C, Trudel J, Zidulka A, et al: Misleadiang "pulmonary wedge pressure" after pneumonectomy: its importance in postoperative fluid therapy. Ann Thorac Surg 42:192, 1986.

552. Jones J, Grossman RF, Berry M, et al: Alveolar-capillary membrane permeability. Correlation with functional, radiographic, and postmortem changes after fluid aspiration. Am Rev Respir Dis 120:399, 1979.

553. Jones JG, Minty BD, Royston D: Alveolar barrier permeability and ARDS. Eur J Respir Dis 64:9, 1983.

554. Tennenberg SD, Jacobs MP, Solomkin JS, et al: Increased pulmonary alveolar-capillary permeability in patients at risk for adult respiratory distress syndrome. Crit Care Med 15:289, 1987.

555. Braude S, Nolop KB, Hughes JMB, et al: Comparison of lung vascular and epithelial permeability indices in the adult respiratory distress syndrome. Am Rev Respir Dis 133:1002, 1986.

556. Spicer KM, Reines DH, Frey GD: Diagnosis of adult respiratory distress syndrome with Tc-99m human serum albumin and portable probe. Crit Care Med 14:669, 1986.

557. Anderson R, Holliday L, Driedger A, et al: Documentation of pulmonary capillary permeability in the adult respiratory distress syndrome accompanying human sepsis. Am Rev Respir Dis 119:869, 1979.

558. Glauser FL, Millen JE, Falls R: Effects of acid aspiration on pulmonary alveolar epithelial membrane permeability. Chest 76:201, 1979.

559. Morel DR, Dargent F, Bachmann M, et al: Pulmonary extraction of serotonin and propranolol in patients with adult respiratory distress syndrome. Am Rev Respir Dis 132:479, 1985.

560. Sprung CL, Long WM, Marcial EH, et al: Distribution of proteins in pulmonary edema: the value of fractional concentrations. Am Rev Respir Dis 136:957, 1987.

561. Rinaldo JE, Borovetz HS, Mancini MC, et al: Assessment of lung injury in the adult respiratory distress syndrome using multiple indicator dilution curves. Am Rev Respir Dis 133:1006, 1986.

562. Vuorela AL: Measurement of regional extravascular lung water using the double indicator-dilution isotope technique. Ann Clin Res 17:3, 1985.

10

563. Laggner A, Kleinberger G, Haller J, et al: Bedside estimation of extravascular lung water in critically ill patients. Comparison of the chest radiograph and the thermal dye technique. Intensive Care Med 10:309, 1984.

564. Eisenberg PR, Hansbrough JR, Anderson D, et al: A prospective study of lung water measurements during patient management in an intensive care unit. Am Rev Respir Dis 136:662, 1987.

565. Sibbald WJ, Short AK, Warshawski FJ, et al: Thermal dye measurements of extravascular lung water in critically ill patients. Intravascular Starling forces and extravascular lung water in the adult respiratory distress syndrome. Chest 87:585, 1985.

566. Feeley TW, Mihm FG, Halperin BD, et al: Failure of the colloid oncotic-pulmonary artery wedge pressure gradient to predict changes in extravascular lung water. Crit Care Med 13:1025, 1985.

567. Overland ES, Gupta RN, Huchon GJ, et al: Measurement of pulmonary tissue volume and blood flow in persons with normal and edematous lungs. J Appl Physiol 51:1375, 1981.

568. Dantzker DR, Brook CJ, Dehart P, et al: Ventilation-perfusion distributions in the adult respiratory distress syndrome. Am Rev Respir Dis 120:1039, 1979.

569. Ralph DD, Robertson HT, Weaver LJ, et al: Distribution of ventilation and perfusion during positive end-expiratory pressure in the adult respiratory distress syndrome. Am Rev Respir Dis 131:54, 1985.

570. Lemaire F, Matamis D, Lampron N, et al: Intrapulmonary shunt is not increased by 100% oxygen ventilation in acute respiratory failure. Bull Eur Physiopathol Respir 21:251, 1985.

571. Brigham KL, Kariman K, Harris TR, et al: Correlation of oxygenation with vascular permeability surface area but not with lung water in humans with acute respiratory failure and pulmonary edema. J Clin Invest 72:339, 1983.

572. Lynch JP, Mhyre, JG, Dantzker DR: Influence of cardiac output on intra-pulmonary shunt. J Appl Physiol 46:315, 1979.

573. Breen PH, Schumacker PT, Hedenstierna G, et al: How does increased cardiac output increase shunt in pulmonary edema? J Appl Physiol 53:1273, 1982.

574. Shiabutani K, Komatsu T, Kubal K, et al: Critical level of oxygen delivery in anesthetized man. Crit Care Med 11:640, 1983.

575. Danek SJ, Lynch JP, Weg JG, et al: The dependence of oxygen uptake on oxygen delivery in the adult respiratory distress syndrome. Am Rev Respir Dis 122:387, 1980.

576. Rashkin MC, Bosken C, Baughman RP: Oxygen delivery in critically ill patients. Relationship to blood lactate and survival. Chest 87:580, 1985.

577. Kariman K, Burns SR: Regulation of tissue oxygen extraction is disturbed in adult respiratory distress syndrome. Am Rev Respir Dis 132:109, 1985.

578. Mohsenifar Z, Goldbach P, Tashkin DP, et al: Relationship between O_2 delivery and O_2 consumption in the adult respiratory distress syndrome. Chest 84:267, 1983.

579. Annat G, Viale JP, Percival C, et al: Oxygen delivery and uptake in the adult respiratory distress syndrome. Lack of relationship when measured independently in patients with normal blood lactate concentrations. Am Rev Respir Dis 133:999, 1986.

580. Zapol WM, Snider MT: Pulmonary hypertension in severe acute respiratory failure. N Engl J Med 296:476, 1977.

581. Sibbald WJ, Short AI, Driedger AA, et al: The immediate effects of isosorbide dinitrate on right ventricular function in patients with acute hypoxemic respiratory failure. A combined invasive and radionuclide study. Am Rev Respir Dis 131:862, 1985.

582. Sibbald WJ, Driedger AA, Cunningham DG, et al: Right and left ventricular performance in acute hypoxemic respiratory failure. Crit Care Med 14:852, 1986.

583. Jardin F, Gueret P, Dubourg O, et al: Right ventricular volumes by thermodilution in the adult respiratory distress syndrome. A comparative study using two-dimensional echocardiography as a reference method. Chest 88:34, 1985.

584. Respiratory Diseases. Task Force Report on Problems, Research Approaches, Needs. National Heart and Lung Institute. DHEW Pub. No. NIH 73–432, 1972, pp 167–80.

585. Bernard GR, Brigham KL: The adult respiratory distress syndrome. Annu Rev Med 36:195, 1985.

586. Petty TL: Indicators of risk, course, and prognosis in adult respiratory distress syndrome (ARDS). Am Rev Respir Dis 132:471, 1985.

587. Fowler AA, Hamman RF, Good JT, et al: Adult respiratory distress syndrome: Risk with common predisposition. Ann Intern Med 98:593, 1983.

588. Bartlett RH, Morris AH, Fairley HB, et al: A prospective study of acute hypoxic respiratory failure. Chest 89:684, 1986.

589. Gillespie DJ, Marsh HM, Divertie MB, et al: Clinical outcome of respiratory failure in patients requiring prolonged (greater than 24 hours) mechanical ventilation. Chest 90:364, 1986.

590. Seidenfeld JJ, Pohl DF, Bell RC, et al: Incidence, site, and outcome of infections in patients with the adult respiratory distress syndrome. Am Rev Respir Dis 134:12, 1986.

591. Montgomery AB, Stager MA, Carrico CJ, et al: Causes of mortality in patients with the adult respiratory distress syndrome. Am Rev Respir Dis 132:485, 1985.

592. National Heart, Lung, and Blood Institute: Extracorporeal support for respiratory insufficiency: collaborative study. Washington, DC: National Heart, Lung, and Blood Institute, December, 1979.

593. Simmons RS, Berdine GG, Seidenfeld JJ, et al: Fluid balance and the adult respiratory distress syndrome. Am Rev Respir Dis 135:924, 1987.

594. Zapol WM, Trelstad RL, Coffey JW, et al: Pulmonary fibrosis in severe acute respiratory failure. Am Rev Respir Dis 119:547, 1979.

595. Auler JO, Calheiros DF, Brentani MM, et al: Adult respiratory distress syndrome: evidence of early fibrogenesis and absence of glucocorticoid receptors. Eur J Respir Dis 69:261, 1986.

596. Ashbaugh DG, Maier RV: Idiopathic pulmonary fibrosis in adult respiratory distress syndrome. Diagnosis and treatment. Arch Surg 120:530, 1985.

597. Weigelt JA, Norcross JP, Borman KR, et al: Early steroid therapy for respiratory failure. Arch Surg 120:536, 1985.

598. Elliott CG, Morris AH, Cengiz M: Pulmonary function and exercise gas exchange in survivors of adult respiratory distress syndrome. Am Rev Respir Dis 123:492, 1981.

599. Buchser E, Leuenberger P, Chiolero R, et al: Reduced pulmonary capillary blood volume as a long-term sequel of ARDS. Chest 87:608, 1985.

600. Towne BH, Lott IT, Hicks DA, et al: Long-term follow-up of infants and children treated with extracorporeal membrane oxygenation (ECMO): a preliminary report. J Pediatr Surg 20:410, 1985.

601. Simpson DL, Goodman M, Spector SL, et al: Long-term follow-up and bronchial reactivity testing in survivors of the adult respiratory distress syndrome. Am Rev Respir Dis 117:449, 1978.

602. Fanconi S, Kraemer R, Weber J, et al: Long-term sequelae in children surviving adult respiratory distress syndrome. J Pediatr 106:218, 1985.

603. Elliott CG, Rasmusson BY, Crapo RO, et al: Prediction of pulmonary function abnormalities after adult respiratory distress syndrome (ARDS). Am Rev Respir Dis 135:634, 1987.

604. Wilson R: Acute high-altitude illness in mountaineers and problems of rescue. Ann Intern Med 78:421, 1973.

605. Hurtado A: Some clinical aspects of life at high altitudes. Ann Intern Med 53:247, 1960.

606. Houston CS: Acute pulmonary edema of high altitude. N Engl J Med 263:478, 1960.

607. Hultgren HN, Spickard WB, Hellriegel K, et al: High altitude pulmonary edema. Medicine 40:289, 1961.

608. Hultgren H, Spickard W, Lopez C: Further studies of high altitude pulmonary oedema. Br Heart J 24:95, 1962.

608a. Hultgren HN, Flamm MD: Pulmonary edema. Mod Concepts Cardiovasc Dis 31:1, 1969.

609. Fred HL, Schmidt AM, Bates T, et al: Acute pulmonary edema of altitude. Clinical and physiologic observations. Circulation 25:929, 1962.

610. Hultgren HN, Lopez CE, Lundberg E, et al: Physiologic studies of pulmonary edema at high altitude. Circulation 29:393, 1964.

611. Singh I, Kapila CC, Khanna PK, et al: High-altitude pulmonary oedema. Lancet 1:229, 1965.

612. Menon ND: High-altitude pulmonary edema. A clinical study. N Engl J Med 273:66, 1965.

613. Editorial: High-altitude pulmonary edema. N Engl J Med 273:108, 1965.

614. Singh I, Khanna PK, Srivastava MC, et al: Acute mountain sickness. N Engl J Med 280:175, 1969.

615. Viswanathan R, Jain SK, Subramanian S, et al: Pulmonary edema of high altitude. II. Clinical, aerohemodynamic, and biochemical studies in a group with history of pulmonary edema of high altitude. Am Rev Respir Dis 100:334, 1969.

616. Kamat SR, Banerjil BC: Study of cardiopulmonary function on exposure to high altitude. I. Acute acclimatization to an altitude of 3500 to 4000 meters in relation to altitude sickness and cardiopulmonary function. Am Rev Respir Dis 106:404, 1972.

617. Kamat SR, Rao TL, Sama BS, et al: Study of cardiopulmonary function on exposure to high altitude. II. Effects of prolonged stay at 3500 to 4000 meters and reversal on return to sea level. Am Rev Respir Dis 106:414, 1972.

618. Kleiner JP, Nelson WP: High altitude pulmonary edema. A rare disease? JAMA 234:491, 1975.

619. Leading Article: Pulmonary oedema of mountains. Br Med J 3:65, 1972.

620. Schoene RB: Pulmonary edema at high altitude. Review, pathophysiology, and update. Clin Chest Med 6:491, 1985.

621. Sutton JR, Lassen N: Pathophysiology of acute mountain sickness

and high altitude pulmonary oedema: an hypothesis. Bull Eur Physiopathol Respir 15:1045, 1979.

622. Hackett PH, Rennie D, Grover RF, et al: Acute mountain sickness and the edemas of high altitude: a common pathogenesis? Respir Physiol 46:383, 1982.

623. Anholm JD, Houston CS, Hyers TM: The relationship between acute mountain sickness and pulmonary ventilation at 2,835 meters (9,300 ft.). Chest 75:33, 1979.

624. Moore LG, Harrison GL, McCullough RE, et al: Low acute hypoxic ventilatory response and hypoxic depression in acute altitude sickness. J Appl Physiol 60:1407, 1986.

625. Hyers TM, Scoggin CH, Will DH, et al: Accentuated hypoxemia at high altitude in subjects suceptible to high-altitude pulmonary edema. J Appl Physiol 46:41, 1979.

626. Gautier H, Peslin R, Grassino A, et al: Mechanical properties of the lungs during acclimatization to altitude. J Appl Physiol 52:1407, 1982.

627. Viswanathan R, Jain SK, Subramanian S: Pulmonary edema of high altitude: III. Pathogenesis. Am Rev Respir Dis 100:342, 1969.

628. Viswanathan R, Jain SK, Subramanian S, et al: Pulmonary edema of high altitude. I. Production of pulmonary edema in animals under conditions of simulated high altitude. Am Rev Respir Dis 100:327, 1969.

629. Visscher MB: The pathophysiology of lung edema: A physical and physicochemical problem. Lancet 82:43, 1962.

630. Schoene RB, Hackett PH, Henderson WR, et al: High-altitude pulmonary edema. Characteristics of lung lavage fluid. JAMA 256:63, 1986.

631. Schoene RB, Roach RC, Hackett PH, et al: High altitude pulmonary edema and exercise at 4,400 meters on Mount McKinley. Effect of expiratory positive airway pressure. Chest 87:330, 1985.

632. West JB, Hackett PH, Maret KH, et al: Pulmonary gas exchange on the summit of Mt. Everest. J Appl Physiol 55:678, 1983.

633. Schoene RB, Lahiri S, Hackett PH, et al: Relationship of hypoxic ventilatory response to exercise performance on Mount Everest. J Appl Physiol 56:1478, 1984.

634. Whithey WR, Milledge JS, Williams ES, et al: Fluid and electrolyte homeostasis during prolonged exercise at altitude. J Appl Physiol 55:409, 1983.

635. Hackett PH, Rennie D, Hofmeister SE, et al: Fluid retention and relative hypoventilation in acute mountain sickness. Respiration 43:321, 1982.

636. Sutton JR, Houston CS, Mansell AL, et al: Effect of aceta-zolamide on hypoxemia during sleep at high altitude. N Engl J Med 301:1329, 1979.

637. Humphreys RL, Berne AS: Rapid reexpansion of pneumothorax: A cause of unilateral pulmonary edema. Radiology 96:509, 1970.

638. Trapnell DH, Thurston JGB: Unilateral pulmonary oedema after pleural aspiration. Lancet 1:1367, 1970.

639. Carlson RI, Classen KL, Gollan F, et al: Pulmonary edema following the rapid reexpansion of a totally collapsed lung due to a pneumothorax: A clinical and experimental study. Surg Forum 9:367, 1959.

640. Ziskind MM, Weill H, George RA: Acute pulmonary edema following the treatment of spontaneous pneumothorax with excessive negative intrapleural pressure. Am Rev Respir Dis 92:632, 1965.

641. Childress ME, Moy G, Mottram M: Unilateral pulmonary edema resulting from treatment of spontaneous pneumothorax. Am Rev Respir Dis 104:119, 1971.

642. Waqaruddin M, Bernstein A: Re-expansion pulmonary oedema. Thorax 30:54, 1975.

643. Ratliff JL, Chavez CM, Jamchuk A, et al: Re-expansion pulmonary edema. Chest 64:654, 1973.

644. Saini GS: Unilateral pulmonary oedema after drainage of spontaneous pneumothorax. Br Med J 1:615, 1974.

645. Grant MJA: Acute unilateral oedema following re-expansion of a spontaneous pneumothorax: Case report. NZ Med J 74:250, 1971.

646. Murphy K, Tomlanovich MC: Unilateral pulmonary edema after drainage of a spontaneous pneumothorax: case report and review of the world literature. J Emerg Med 1:29, 1983

647. Kassis E, Philipsen E, Clausen KH: Unilateral pulmonary edema following spontaneous pneumothorax. Eur J Respir Dis 62:102, 1981.

648. Mahajan VK, Simon M, Huber GL: Reexpansion pulmonary edema. Chest 75:192, 1979.

649. Shaw TJ, Caterine JM: Recurrent re-expansion pulmonary edema. Chest 86:784, 1984.

650. Buczko GB, Grossman RF, Goldberg M: Re-expansion pulmonary edema: evidence for increased capillary permeability. Canad Med Assoc J 125:459, 1981.

651. Sprung CL, Loewenherz JW, Baier H, et al: Evidence for increased permeability in reexpansion pulmonary edema. Am J Med 71:497, 1981.

652. Miller WC, Toon R, Palat H, et al: Experimental pulmonary edema following re-expansion of pneumothorax. Am Rev Respir Dis 108:664, 1973.

653. Pavlin JD, Nessly ML, Cloney FW: Increased pulmonary vascular permeability as a cause of re-expansion edema in rabbits. Am Rev Respir Dis 124:422, 1981.

654. Yamazaki S, Ogawa J, Shohzu A, et al: Pulmonary blood flow to rapidly reexpanded lung in spontaneous pneumothorax. Chest 81:1, 1982.

655. Bishop MJ, Boatman ES, Ivey TD, et al: Reperfusion of ischaemic dog lung results in fever, leukopenia and lung edema. Am Rev Respir Dis 134:752, 1986.

656. Solomon DR: Anaphylactoid reaction and non-cardiac pulmonary edema following intravenous contrast injection. Am J Emerg Med 4:146, 1986.

657. Henderson AF, Banham SW, Moran F: Re-expansion pulmonary oedema: a potentially serious complication of delayed diagnosis of pneumothorax. Br Med J 291:593, 1985.

658. Steckel RJ: Unilateral pulmonary edema after pneumothorax. N Engl J Med 289:621, 1973.

659. Lagler U, Russi E: Upper airway obstruction as a cause of pulmonary edema during late pregnancy. Am J Obstet Gynecol 156:643, 1987.

660. Warren MF, Peterson DK, Drinker CK: The effects of heightened negative pressure in the chest, together with further experiments upon anoxia in increasing the flow of lung lymph. Am J Physiol 137:641, 1942.

661. Young LW, Bowen A, Oh KS, et al: Postintubation pulmonary edema (abstr). Invest Radiol 16:428, 1981.

662. Sofer S, Bar-Ziv J, Scharf SM: Pulmonary edema following relief of upper airway obstruction. Chest 86:401, 1984.

663. Randour P, Joucken K, Collard E, et al: Pulmonary edema following acute upper airway obstruction. Acta Anaesthesiol Belg 37:225, 1986.

664. Tami TA, Chu F, Wildes TO, et al: Pulmonary edema and acute upper airway obstruction. Laryngoscope 96:506, 1986.

665. Lorch DG, Sahn SA: Post-extubation pulmonary edema following anesthesia induced by upper airway obstruction. Are certain patients at increased risk? Chest 90:802, 1986.

666. McGonagle M, Kennedy TL: Laryngospasm induced pulmonary edema. Laryngoscope 94:1583, 1984.

667. Renner IG, Savage WT, Pantoja JL, et al: Death due to acute pancreatitis. A retrospective analysis of 405 autopsy cases. Dig Dis Sci 30:1005, 1985.

668. Tahamont MV, Barie PS, Blumenstock FA, et al: Increased lung vascular permeability after pancreatitis and trypsin infusion. Am J Pathol 109:15, 1982.

669. Falls R, Millen JE, Galuser FL, et al: Pulmonary alveolar epithelial permeability in surgically induced hemorrhagic pancreatitis in dogs. Respiration 40:213, 1980.

670. Boden WE: Anaphylactoid pulmonary edema ("shock lung") and hypotension after radiologic contrast media injection. Chest 81:759, 1982.

671. Satake K, Rozmanith JS, Appert H, et al: Hemodynamic change and bradykinin levels in plasma and lymph during experimental acute pancreatitis in dogs. Ann Surg 178:659, 1973.

672. Minta JO, Man D, Movat HZ: Kinetic studies on the fragmentation of the third component of complement (C_3) by trypsin. J Immunol 118:2192, 1977.

673. Nicod L, Leuenberger P, Seydoux C, et al: Evidence for pancreas injury in adult respiratory distress syndrome. Am Rev Respir Dis 131:696, 1985.

674. deLeeuw PW, Waltman FL, Birkenhager WH: Noncardiogenic pulmonary edema as the sole manifestation of pheochromocytoma. Hypertension 8:810, 1986.

675. Blom HJ, Karsdorp V, Birnie R, et al: Phaeochromocytoma as a cause of pulmonary oedema. Anesthesia 42:646, 1987.

676. Feldman JM: Adult respiratory distress syndrome in a pregnant patient with a pheochromocytoma. J Surg Oncol 29:5, 1985.

677. Brun-Buisson CJ, Bonnet F, Bergeret S, et al: Recurrent high-permeability pulmonary edema associated with diabetic ketoacidosis. Crit Care Med 13:55, 1985.

678. Botha J, van Niekerk DJ, Rossouw DJ, et al: The adult respiratory distress syndrome in association with diabetic keto-acidosis. A case report. S Afr Med J 71:535, 1987.

679. Russell J, Follansbee S, Matthay M: Adult respiratory distress syndrome complicating diabetic ketoacidosis. West J Med 135:148, 1981.

680. Silvestri RC, Huseby JS, Rughani I, et al: Respiratory distress syndrome from lymphangiography contrast medium. Am Rev Respir Dis 122:543, 1980.

681. Miniati M, Pistolesi M, Paoletti P, et al: Objective radiographic criteria to differentiate cardiac, renal, and injury lung edema. Invest Radiol 23:433, 1988.

10

682. Aberle DR, Wiener-Kronish JP, Webb WR, et al: Hydrostatic versus increased permeability pulmonary edema: diagnosis based on radiographic criteria in critically ill patients. Radiology 168:73, 1988.

683. Rivera M, Hadlock FP, O'Meara ME: Pulmonary edema secondary to acute epiglottitis. Am J Roentgenol 132:991, 1979.

684. Hasleton PS: Adult respiratory distress syndrome—a review. Histopathology 7:307, 1983.

685. Blennerhasset JB: Shock lung and diffuse alveolar damage. Pathological and pathogenetic considerations. Pathology 17:239, 1985.

686. Fukuda Y, Ishizaki M, Masuda Y, et al: The role of intraalveolar fibrosis in the process of pulmonary structural remodeling in patients with diffuse alveolar damage. Am J Pathol 126:171, 1987.

687. Nash G, Langlinais PC: Pulmonary interstitial edema and hyaline membranes in adult burn patients. Electron microscopic observations. Hum Pathol 5:149, 1974.

688. Tomashefski JF Jr, Davies P, Boggis C, et al: The pulmonary vascular lesions of the adult respiratory distress syndrome. Am J Pathol 112:112, 1983.

689. Snow RL, Davies P, Pontoppidan H, et al: Pulmonary vascular remodeling in adult respiratory distress syndrome. Am Rev Respir Dis 126:887, 1982.

690. Suarez M, Krieger BP: Bronchoalveolar lavage in recurrent aspirin-induced adult respiratory distress syndrome. Chest 90:452, 1986.

691. Gilson AJ, Sahn SA: Reactivation of bleomycin lung toxicity following oxygen administration. A second response to corticosteroids. Chest 88:304, 1985.

692. Wood DL, Osborn MJ, Rooke J, et al: Amiodarone pulmonary toxicity; report of two cases associated with rapidly progressive fatal adult respiratory distress syndrome after pulmonary angiography. Mayo Clin Proc 60:601, 1985.

693. Catchings TT, Beamer WC, Lundy L, et al: Adult respiratory distress syndrome secondary to ethylene glycol ingestion. Ann Emerg Med 14:594, 1985.

694. Lawler PG, Cove-Smith JR: Acute respiratory failure following lithium intoxication. A report of two cases. Anaesthesia 41:623, 1986.

695. Gotloib L, Barzilay E, Shustak A, et al: Hemofiltration in severe high microvascular permeability pulmonary edema secondary to rickettsial spotted fever. Resuscitation 13:25, 1985.

696. Dyer RA, Chappel WA, Potgieter PD: Adult respiratory distress syndrome associated with miliary tuberculosis. Crit Care Med 13:12, 1985.

697. Feldman RM, Singer C: Noncardiogenic pulmonary edema and pulmonary fibrosis in falciparum malaria. Rev Infect Dis 9:134, 1987.

698. Zwirewich CV, Muller NL, Abboud RT, et al: Noncardiogenic pulmonary edema caused by decompression sickness: rapid resolution following hyperbaric therapy. Radiology 163:81, 1987.

699. Fulkerson WJ, McLendon RE, Prosnitz LR: Adult respiratory distress syndrome after limited thoracic radiotherapy. Cancer 57:1941, 1986.

700. Ivanick MJ, Donohue JF: Chronic eosinophilic pneumonia: a cause of adult respiratory distress syndrome. S Med J 79:686, 1986.

701. Lazar A: Pulmonary oedema following scorpion sting. J Assoc Physicians India 33:489, 1985.

702. Dean NC, Amend WC, Matthay MA: Adult respiratory distress syndrome related to antilymphocyte globulin therapy. Chest 91:619, 1987.

703. Haynes J, Allison RC: Pulmonary edema. Complication in the management of sickle cell pain crisis. Am J Med 80:833, 1986.

704. Stark P, Guthrie AM, Bull J: Thoracic radiographic changes after systemic hyperthermia for advanced cancer. Radiology 154:55, 1985.

705. Young M, Sciurba F, Rinaldo J: Delirium and pulmonary edema after completing a marathon. Am Rev Respir Dis 136:737, 1987.

706. Shive ST, McNally DP: Pulmonary hypertension from prominent vascular involvement in diffuse amyloidosis. Arch Intern Med 148:687, 1988.

707. Pietra GG, Ruttner JR: Specificity of pulmonary vascular lesions in primary pulmonary hypertension. A reappraisal. Respiration 52:81, 1987.

708. Calandrino FS Jr, Anderson DJ, Mintun MA, et al: Pulmonary vascular permeability during the adult respiratory distress syndrome; a positron emission tomographic study. Am Rev Respir Dis 138:421, 1988.

709. Nerlich AG, Nerlich ML, Muller PK: Pattern of collagen in acute post-traumatic pulmonary fibrosis. Thorax 42:863, 1987.

710. Kreuzfelder E, Joka T, Keinecke HO, et al: Adult respiratory distress syndrome as a specific manifestation of a general permeability defect in trauma patients. Am Rev Respir Dis 137:95, 1988.

711. Weigelt JA, Chenoweth DE, Borman KA, et al: Complement and the severity of pulmonary failure. J Trauma 28:1013, 1988.

712. Langlois PF, Gawryl MS: Accentuated formation of the terminal C5b-9 complement complex in patient plasma precedes development of the adult respiratory distress syndrome. Am Rev Respir Dis 138:368, 1988.

713. Cox JW, Andreadis NA, Bone RC, et al: Pulmonary extraction and pharmacokinetics of prostaglandin E 1 during continuous intravenous infusion in patients with adult respiratory distress syndrome. Am Rev Respir Dis 137:5, 1988.

714. Melot C, Naeije R, Mols P, et al: Pulmonary vascular tone improves pulmonary gas exchange in the adult respiratory distress syndrome. Am Rev Respir Dis 136:1232, 1987.

715. Bone RC, Fisher CJ Jr, Clemmer TP, et al: Early methyl-prednisolone treatment for septic syndrome and the adult respiratory distress syndrome. Chest 92:1032, 1987.

716. Hackett PH, Roach RC, Schoene RB, et al: Abnormal control of ventilation in high-altitude pulmonary edema. J Appl Physiol 64:1268, 1988.

717. Schoene RB, Swenson ER, Pizzo CJ, et al: The lung at high altitude: bronchoalveolar lavage in acute mountain sickness and pulmonary edema. J Appl Physiol 64:2605, 1988.

718. Kobayashi T, Koyama S, Kubo K, et al: Clinical features of patients with high altitude pulmonary edema in Japan. Chest 92:814, 1987.

719. Koyama S, Kobayashi T, Kubo K, et al: The increased sympathoadrenal activity in patients with high altitude pulmonary edema is centrally mediated. Jpn J Med 27:10, 1988.

720. Mahfood S, Hix WR, Aaron BL, et al: Reexpansion pulmonary edema. Ann Thorac Surg 45:340, 1988

Diseases of the Airways

GENERAL CONSIDERATIONS

This chapter is concerned with several lung diseases that are grouped together because of their common characteristics of hypersecretion from and obstruction of the airways. Airway obstruction may be acute or chronic. Acute episodes may be isolated or recurrent. Obstruction can occur in either the upper or the lower airways, and in the latter site it may be local or diffuse. Although the clinical manifestations of obstruction of the upper airways (defined as that portion of the conducting system from the mouth or nose to the tracheal carina) are usually sufficiently distinctive to permit prompt recognition, an appreciable number of cases of chronic upper airway obstruction are misdiagnosed as asthma or chronic obstructive pulmonary disease (COPD). Since appropriate roentgenographic procedures and physiologic measurements readily distinguish upper from lower airway obstruction, these examinations should be performed in all cases of obstructive airway disease to prevent needless—and sometimes life-threatening—misdiagnosis. Lower airway obstruction results from a large number of entities of varying etiology and pathogenesis whose clinical manifestations may overlap. It is important to recognize that although the term obstructive airway disease usually connotes *general* obstruction of the conducting system of the lungs, *local* obstructing diseases (e.g., an endobronchial neoplasm obstructing a segmental bronchus) also may represent examples of obstructive airway disease. Although confusion seldom arises in distinguishing local from general obstructive disease, it is of some importance from a conceptual point of view to recognize both as types of obstructive airway disease.

As a result of correlative clinical, pathologic, roentgenologic, and physiologic studies, our knowledge of diseases characterized by chronic lower airway obstruction has been greatly extended, but with the better understanding has come the realization that precise differentiation of the individual diseases often is difficult. This has resulted in the use of such terms as "chronic nonspecific lung disease," "general obstructive lung disease," and "chronic obstructive pulmonary disease" to describe all those conditions that come within this category. Such broad categorization does have merit, since it is clear that the clinical, roentgenologic, and physiologic manifestations of these diseases frequently overlap so that precise placement in one or another disease category is impossible.

The majority of patients with "chronic obstructive pulmonary disease" have chronic bronchitis with airway narrowing, intractable asthma, emphysema, bronchiectasis, or a combination of these conditions. However, the term is not restricted to these four disorders. Other diseases can give rise to similar clinical and physiologic manifestations. Cystic fibrosis and familial dysautonomia (Riley-Day syndrome), diseases of the exocrine glands and their autonomic nerve supply that result in abnormal bronchial secretions, present both clinically and functionally as airway obstruction. Similarly, laryngeal or tracheal obstruction may be responsible for symptoms and signs that closely mimic chronic bronchitis and emphysema (although such patients have stridor). Even more rarely, multiple airways may be partially or completely blocked by endobronchial masses such as papillomas, sarcoid granulomas, or amyloid deposits.

In recent years, the term chronic obstructive pulmonary disease has been used in a more narrow sense to describe those patients with largely irreversible obstruction to expiratory flow in whom a specific diagnosis cannot be made. These patients are usually heavy cigarette smokers, and the airway obstruction is related to a combination of loss of lung elasticity and inflammatory narrowing of the membranous and respiratory bronchioles. For the most part, use of the term COPD in this text refers to this more restrictive definition.

The recognition of diseases within the broad category of "chronic obstructive pulmonary disease" implies identification of increased resistance to air flow in the conducting system. In the later stages of these diseases or in acute exacerbations, airway obstruction is judged clinically to be present on the basis of rhonchi or continuous wheezing, prolonged expiration, and decreased breath sounds. Dyspnea is a frequent complaint, although diffuse rhonchi may be present in patients who are asymptomatic. In this latter group, the chest roentgenogram almost invariably is normal, and in these patients as well as those who manifest neither physical signs nor roentgenologic evidence of airway obstruction the diagnosis must be based on tests of pulmonary function. Emphysema can be assessed fairly accurately roentgenologically when the disease is advanced, and roentgenologic studies may sometimes present convincing evidence of its presence even when there is little or no clinical evidence of obstructive pulmonary disease. In many of these latter cases, the roentgenographic examination is part of a screening procedure and subsequent direct questioning reveals evidence of deteriorating exercise tolerance or cough.

In no other area of pulmonary disease is a close correlation of the clinical, roentgenologic, and pulmonary function parameters so vital in the overall assessment of the patient as in chronic obstructive airway disease.

This chapter is divided into two major sections: diseases of the upper airways (pharynx, larynx, and trachea) and the much larger group of diseases that affect the lower airways.

OBSTRUCTIVE DISEASE OF THE UPPER AIRWAYS

The upper airway can be considered as the conduit for inspired and expired gas, extending from the external nares (during nose breathing) or the lips (during mouth breathing) to the carina. Thus, the upper airway consists of a varied and complex system of channels arranged in series. Functional or anatomic obstruction is possible at any level. Although the following pages deal largely with anatomic abnormalities that cause upper airway obstruction, there also exist a number of conditions characterized by abnormal contraction of the muscles designed to maintain upper airway patency.[1]

ACUTE UPPER AIRWAY OBSTRUCTION

This disorder occurs most commonly in infants and young children because of the small intraluminal caliber and greater compliance of their upper airways. Regardless of etiology, the cardinal symptom is a sudden onset of dyspnea or even suffocation, sometimes requiring emergency tracheostomy. The cause of respiratory distress usually is readily apparent from the history. For example, patients with acute upper respiratory infections generally have fever and cough, although in one series of 97 patients with acute epiglottitis cough was present in only one third.[2] Similarly, patients with angioneurotic edema may give a history of allergy, with or without familial occurrence, and have usually experienced previous episodes dating back to childhood. Stridor is common, but its presence does not necessarily constitute an indication for immediate tracheostomy. However, the presence of stridor warrants immediate direct or indirect visualization of the larynx, a procedure that is of major importance in distinguishing edema from tracheobronchitis in patients who have been exposed to smoke in fires.[3]

Roentgenographic manifestations vary somewhat according to the specific etiology (*see* farther on), although there exist a number of unusual and unexpected manifestations, particularly in infants and children, which should alert the radiologist to the possibility of upper airway obstruction. Whereas chronic obstruction of the intrathoracic trachea or of the lower airways characteristically results in pulmonary overinflation, acute obstruction of the upper airways may be associated with lungs of normal or even small volume; at the same time, the airway *proximal* to the site of obstruction will be unusually distended during inspiration. This combination of changes—distention of the proximal airway and lungs of normal or small volume—should be readily apparent on lateral views of the soft tissues of the neck and thorax and constitutes highly suggestive evidence of acute upper airway obstruction.[4] A paradoxical change in heart size between inspiration and expiration (cardiac diameter greater on inspiration than expiration) may also be observed, but is a more common manifestation of chronic upper airway obstruction (*see* farther on).

The causes of acute upper airway obstruction include infection, edema, hemorrhage, foreign body aspiration, and faulty placement of endotracheal tubes.

Infection

Infection may cause severe narrowing of the upper airways in infants and young children. Acute pharyngitis and tonsillitis, which may be complicated by retropharyngeal abscess, most commonly are caused by β-hemolytic streptococci[5] and less often by adenoviruses[6, 7] and coxsackieviruses.[8, 9] Acute laryngotracheitis (croup) is caused by parainfluenza or respiratory syncytial viruses and results in a characteristic narrowing of the subglottic trachea. A variant of this usual picture is seen in so-called membranous croup, in which the inflammatory narrowing of the upper trachea is associated with the presence of adherent or semiadherent mucopurulent membranes that cause marked irregularity of contour of the proximal tracheal mucosa;[10] the membranes can cause a severe degree of obstruction and sometimes require endoscopic removal.

Acute epiglottitis usually is caused by *Haemophilus influenzae* and occasionally by *Staphylococcus aureus* or *Streptococcus pneumoniae*.[2] Although it most commonly affects infants and young children, it also occurs in adults, in whom it is often unrecognized:[11, 12] of 47 cases of acute epiglottitis reported by Schabel and his colleagues,[11] ten (21 per cent) were in adults and of these an initial diagnosis of epiglottitis was made in only four. Roentgenographic findings include swelling of the epiglottis, aryepiglottic folds, arytenoids, uvula, and prevertebral soft tissues; the hypopharynx and oropharynx tend to be ballooned and the valleculae obliterated. Narrowing of the subglottic trachea, simulating croup, occurs in roughly a quarter of affected children.[13] The presenting symptoms are severe sore throat and difficulty in breathing. Stridor was noted in six of the ten adult patients described by Schabel and associates and hoarseness in four; emergency tracheostomy was required in five of the ten patients. All patients were much improved after 72 hours on appropriate therapy and none died.

In the syndrome known as whooping cough, *Bordetella pertussis* and adenovirus types I, II, III, and IV are the causative agents.[14, 15] Acute retropharyngeal abscess can result in severe upper airway obstruction in both infants and adults (Fig. 11–1), and can extend into the mediastinum and cause an acute mediastinal abscess. A congenital laryngocele can become infected, with resulting laryngopyocele formation and acute upper airway obstruction.[16]

Edema

As a cause of acute upper airway obstruction, edema of noninfective origin characteristically affects the larynx. Underlying causes include trauma, the inhalation of irritant noxious gases, and angioneurotic edema. The last named is perhaps the commonest cause of acute upper airway obstruction and includes a variety of subgroups, some with an allergic etiology (anaphylaxis), some inherited, and others of idiopathic origin.[17, 18] The laryngeal edema is often associated with multiple pruritic and usually nonpainful swellings in the subcutaneous tissues of the face, hands, feet, and genitalia; some patients develop urticaria. Although many patients are atopic, with or without a familial history, the precise

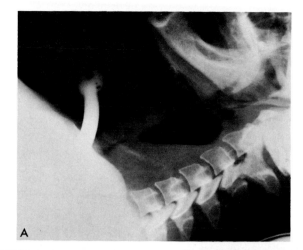

Figure 11–1. Acute Retropharyngeal and Mediastinal Abscess. A 29-year-old woman was admitted to the hospital with an 8-day history of increasing dyspnea, difficulty in swallowing, and loss of voice. An emergency tracheostomy was performed. Lateral roentgenography of the soft tissues of the neck with a horizontal x-ray beam *(A)* revealed a large accumulation of gas and fluid in the retropharyngeal space associated with complete obliteration of the airspace of the hypopharynx and anterior displacement of the cervical trachea.

Illustration continued on following page

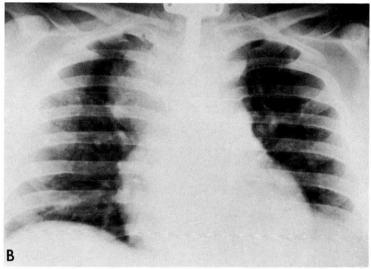

mechanism for the development of angioedema is identified in less than one fifth of cases. In a minority, acute episodes are provoked by certain foods, inhalants, bee stings, or drugs; in this type, antigen combines with IgE resulting in the release from mast cells of histamine, leukotrienes, and eosinophil-chemotactic factor of anaphylaxis (ECF-A), with consequent local vasodilatation and escape of edema fluid (Type I reaction). Type III reactions of a less acute nature may be caused by antiserum, certain drugs such as penicillin, and some radiographic contrast media. Antigen-antibody complexes are formed with immunoglobulin G (IgG), complement is activated, and chemical mediators are released from damaged endothelial cells. Certain drugs such as aspirin may cause nonimmunologic histamine release, particularly in adults with nasal polyps.

The hereditary form of angioneurotic edema usually begins in childhood and is characterized by recurrent attacks, often in association with abdominal cramps.[19] These attacks are not precipitated by allergens, but may follow local trauma such as tonsillectomy or tooth extraction[19] or may be associated with emotional upsets.

The form of inheritance of angioneurotic edema is autosomal dominant. The underlying defect is absence of a serum $alpha_2$ globulin esterase inhibitor of the first component of complement, the increase in C1 being reflected in a decrease in C2 and C4. It is believed that the byproducts of the complement cascade are responsible for the release of vasoactive substances, which in turn produce angioedema. In approximately 10 to 15 per cent of patients, the $alpha_2$ globulin inhibitor is present in normal quantity but is nonfunctional. The prognosis in the hereditary form of angioneurotic edema is very grave, with approximately one third of affected family members dying from suffocation.[17, 18] Careful management and long-term prophylactic measures can save a considerable number of lives.[19]

Thermal injury and edema of the upper airway are frequent complications of smoke inhalation. Hot air and smoke inhalation account for 50 per cent of the fire-related deaths reported annually in the United States.[20] The burning or singeing of nasal hairs in a smoke-exposed patient indicates that mucosal damage is likely at the level of the larynx and that life-threatening airway obstruction due to

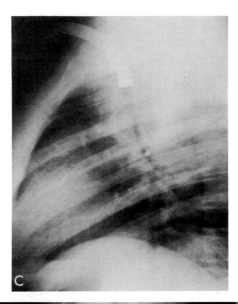

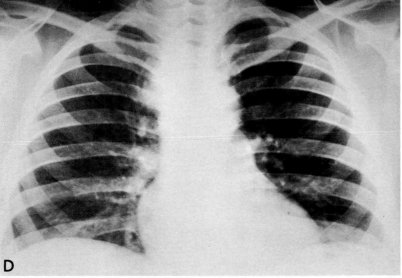

Figure 11–1. *Continued.* Anteroposterior *(B)* and lateral *(C)* roentgenograms of the chest showed a large mediastinal mass projecting predominantly to the right of the midline, situated mainly behind the trachea and causing anterior displacement and narrowing of this structure. The retropharyngeal and mediastinal abscesses were evacuated and drained surgically; 3 weeks later the mediastinal silhouette was almost normal *(D).*

edema, hyperemia, and ulceration may develop hours after the smoke inhalation. Hoarseness is a clue that the larynx may be damaged and that fiberoptic laryngoscopy is indicated.[20] Inspiratory and expiratory flow-volume loops can be of help in assessing the presence of upper airway involvement and the need for intubation.[21] Although upper airway obstruction caused by smoke inhalation usually occurs within 24 hours, late tracheal stenosis has been reported.[22] An unusual mechanism for the development of late upper airway obstruction consists of cutaneous burns that result in severe scar contractures of the neck; affected patients may manifest upper airway obstruction when endotracheal intubation is attempted.[23] A case has been reported in which acute upper airway obstruction developed in an infant as a result of retropharyngeal edema secondary to idiopathic thrombosis of the superior vena cava and brachiocephalic veins.[24] Another rare cause is inflammatory edema of the uvula.[25]

Retropharyngeal Hemorrhage

Acute upper airway obstruction can result from hemorrhage into the retropharyngeal space from a variety of causes, including neck surgery, external trauma, carotid angiography, transbrachial retrograde catheterization,[26] and erosion of an artery secondary to infection. Hemorrhage can occur spontaneously in hemophiliacs or in patients with acute leukemia or receiving anticoagulant therapy.[27–30] Acute upper airway obstruction has also been reported in a patient with polycythemia rubra vera in whom retropharyngeal hemorrhage developed.[31]

Foreign Bodies

Obstruction of the air and food passages by foreign bodies occurs most frequently in infants and young children and tends to affect the esophagus and major bronchi much more commonly than the upper airway.[32] The objects most frequently aspirated by children are peanuts, coins, plastic bullets, and screws, whereas in adults meat and bones are the commonest offending agents (Fig. 11–2).[32] The aspiration of partly masticated meat and its lodgment in the larynx is the most common cause of the "café-coronary syndrome." As might be anticipated, obstruction from foreign bodies occurs more often in patients with pre-existing dysfunction of pharyngeal muscles. Candies inhaled by young children can cause severe edema of the airway mucosa as a result of the hyperosmolar viscid fluid produced as they dissolve.[33] In children, dilatation of the esophagus secondary to achalasia has been reported to compress and obstruct the intrathoracic trachea.[34] Large esophageal foreign bodies can occasionally cause upper airway obstruction in adults.[35]

Faulty Placement of Endotracheal Tubes

Complications of endotracheal intubation are infrequent and occur more often in association with emergency resuscitation than with more routine respiratory therapy.[36] The incidence in one large series of patients on inhalation therapy was 10 per cent.[37] The chief complication is large airway obstruction resulting from malpositioning of the tube too low in the trachea and major bronchi. In the vast majority of instances, the endotracheal tube enters the right main bronchus (in 27 of 28 cases in one series[36]) and the orifice of the left main bronchus is occluded by the balloon cuff of the endotracheal tube, resulting in complete obstruction and atelectasis of the left lung (Fig. 11–3). If the tube is advanced sufficiently far down the right main bronchus, the right upper lobe bronchus may be occluded, with resultant atelectasis of this lobe as well as the left lung (Fig. 11–4) or of the right middle lobe alone. The latter complication occurred in one patient in the Twigg and Buckley series of 28 patients.[36] Occasionally the tube enters the left rather than the right mainstem bronchus, leading to obstruction of the latter. The rate at which atelectasis occurs depends on the gas content of the lung at the moment of occlusion. Total collapse requires 18 to 24 hours if the parenchyma is air-containing, but may occur in a matter of minutes if the lung contains 100 per cent oxygen (often the case in acute respiratory emergencies). Withdrawal of the tube typically results in rapid re-expansion of the collapsed lung or lobe. According to Twigg and Buckley,[36] the ideal location of the tip of an endotracheal tube is 3 cm distal to the vocal cords. However, since in our experience the vocal cords are infrequently visualized on bedside roentgenograms, the carina seems a much more logical point from which to establish reference. Conrardy and associates[38] recommended that with the head and neck in a neutral position, the ideal distance between the tip of the endotracheal tube and the carina is 5 ± 2 cm. These authors also showed that flexion and extension of the neck cause a 2-cm descent and ascent, respectively, of the tip of the endotracheal tube; if the position of the neck can be established from the roentgenogram (through visualization of the mandible), the ideal distance between the tip of the endotracheal tube and the carina should be 3 ± 2 cm with the neck flexed and 7 ± 2 cm with the neck extended. As pointed out by Goodman and his colleagues,[39] if the carina is not visualized, it is sufficient to establish the relationship of the tip of the endotracheal tube to the fifth, sixth, or seventh thoracic vertebral body, this relationship pertaining in 92 of 100 patients whose bedside chest roentgenograms were studied. In infants, Todres and his associates[40] have emphasized the importance of correlating the position of the tip of the endotracheal tube with the position of the patient's head. In a study of 16 intubated newborn infants in whom chest roentgenograms were obtained with the head fully flexed and fully extended, movement of the tip of the endotracheal tube ranged from 7 to 28 mm, being closest to the carina in full flexion.

The roentgenographic findings are typical and should present no difficulty in interpretation. Clinically, the examining physician should not be misled by hearing breath sounds transmitted from the normal or overinflated contralateral lung through the collapsed lung.

CHRONIC UPPER AIRWAY OBSTRUCTION

In contrast to acute upper airway obstruction, the cause of which is generally apparent, chronic obstructive disease of the pharynx, larynx, and trachea frequently is misdiagnosed as asthma or bronchitis. Dyspnea is the usual presenting complaint, often first noted on exertion and sometimes exacerbated when the patient assumes a recumbent position. In a minority of patients, obstruction results in serious impairment of alveolar ventilation, cor pulmonale, and sleep disturbance. Although the symptoms may mislead the physician into a false interpretation of acute or chronic lower airway obstruction, the application of standard and specialized roentgenographic procedures and the discovery of characteristic physiologic disturbances on pulmonary function testing will readily permit identification of the offending lesion in the majority of cases. The intermittent nocturnal obstruction of the hypopharynx that occurs in obstructive sleep apnea is the most common form of chronic upper airway obstruction, but represents a sufficiently distinct syndrome to be considered separately (*see* page 2006).

Etiology

A wide variety of conditions affecting all levels of the upper airway, from the nasopharynx to the

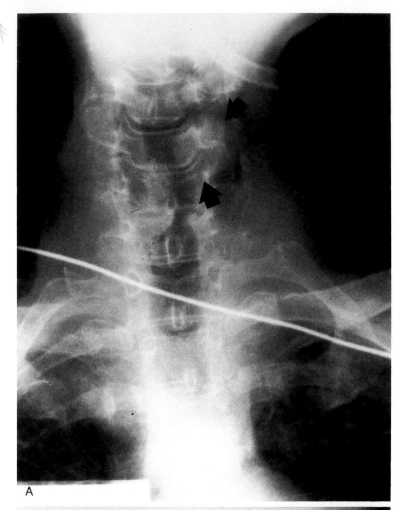

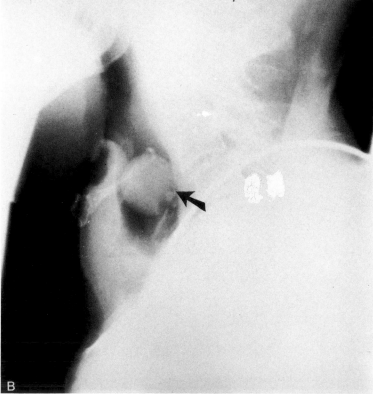

Figure 11–2. Acute Upper Airway Obstruction Caused by a Foreign Body. A roentgenogram of the neck in anteroposterior projection *(A)* reveals a grape-sized opacity *(arrows)* situated in the region of the left pyriform sinus immediately above the false vocal cords. The object can be seen with greater clarity *(arrow)* on a detail lateral view of the soft tissues of the neck *(B)*. This 71-year-old woman presented in acute respiratory distress; she was cyanotic and stuporous. Direct laryngoscopy revealed a grape, the removal of which resulted in prompt improvement. (Courtesy of Dr. John Fleetham, University of British Columbia, Vancouver.)

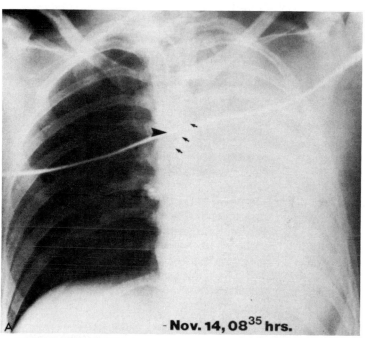

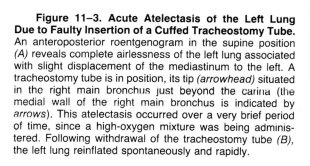

Figure 11–3. Acute Atelectasis of the Left Lung Due to Faulty Insertion of a Cuffed Tracheostomy Tube. An anteroposterior roentgenogram in the supine position *(A)* reveals complete airlessness of the left lung associated with slight displacement of the mediastinum to the left. A tracheostomy tube is in position, its tip *(arrowhead)* situated in the right main bronchus just beyond the carina (the medial wall of the right main bronchus is indicated by *arrows*). This atelectasis occurred over a very brief period of time, since a high-oxygen mixture was being administered. Following withdrawal of the tracheostomy tube *(B),* the left lung reinflated spontaneously and rapidly.

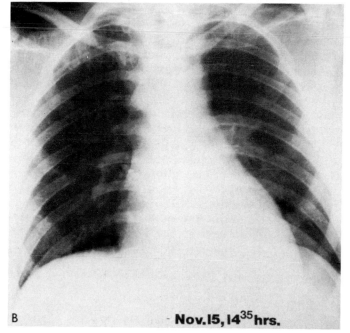

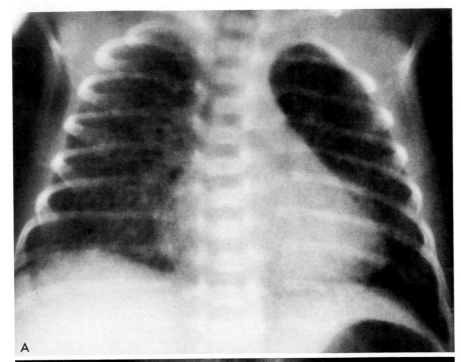

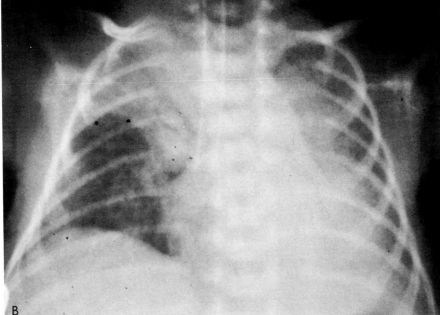

Figure 11–4. Atelectasis Caused by Malpositioning of an Endotracheal Tube in a Newborn Infant. The initial roentgenogram of this newborn premature infant *(A)* reveals a coarse reticular pattern throughout both lungs that was considered to be caused by aspiration. The patient was in severe respiratory distress and tracheal intubation was carried out. A follow-up roentgenogram *(B)* shows the tip of the endotracheal tube in the right bronchial tree. The right upper lobe is airless and there is marked reduction in air content of the left lung, indicating progressive atelectasis. Affected lung parenchyma expanded rapidly following withdrawal of the endotracheal tube. In infants of this size, the endotracheal tube itself is capable of occluding the tiny airways.

tracheal carina, can cause chronic upper airway obstruction. The following list is by no means comprehensive but contains the most common causes: hypertrophy of the tonsils and adenoids, vocal cord paralysis, tracheal stenosis following tracheostomy or prolonged tracheal intubation, primary neoplasms, extrinsic compression of the airway, sclerosing mediastinitis, and a number of rare primary diseases of the trachea such as relapsing polychondritis, "saber-sheath" trachea, tracheobronchomegaly, and tracheobronchopathia. Disturbance in the dynamic activity of the trachea as a result of increased compliance of its walls—tracheomalacia—may occur as a part of some of these conditions.

Each of these possesses fairly characteristic roentgenographic manifestations that permit their differentiation, and each is discussed in some detail further on. However, certain roentgenologic, clinical, and physiologic manifestations are common to all, regardless of their precise nature, and these will be described first.

Physiologic Manifestations

Of major importance in a consideration of upper airway obstruction is the degree to which a lesion is *fixed* or *variable* in its dynamic effects. "Fixed" obstructions are those in which the cross-sectional area of the airway is unable to change in response to transmural pressure differences; thus, they may be situated in either extrathoracic or intrathoracic airways without observed differences in their physiologic effects. By contrast, in "variable" obstructions the airway is capable of responding to transmural stress, and since such stresses are different in the extrathoracic and intrathoracic airways, the physiologic (and to lesser extent roentgenographic) effects depend to a considerable extent on the anatomic location of the lesion.

In contrast to inspiratory flow, which is effort-dependent at all lung volumes from residual volume (RV) to total lung capacity (TLC), forced expiratory flow from TLC is effort-dependent only over the upper 20 to 30 per cent of vital capacity, being independent of effort over the remaining 70 to 80 per cent down to residual volume. The effort-dependent portion of maximal expiratory flow is influenced by alveolar pressure (elastic recoil pressure plus pleural pressure) and the resistance of the airways. At lower lung volumes flow depends on the elastic recoil of the lungs, the resistance of the smaller intrathoracic airways, and the collapsibility of the airway at the site of flow limitation. Flow is limited in such a way that an increase in effort with increased pleural pressure will also compress airways. The increased resistance caused by upper airway obstruction will be reflected in a reduction in flow at high lung volumes where flow is effort-dependent and may not be identified in measurements that measure flow at low lung volumes where flow is effort-independent.[43–45]

An excellent method of portraying how physiologic determinants of flow can be affected by various obstructing lesions of the conducting system is the flow-volume loop, which combines maximal expiratory and inspiratory curves from TLC and RV, respectively (Fig. 11–5). It can be seen that in normal subjects the maximal or peak expiratory flow rate (PEFR) occurs early in the effort-dependent portion of the curve and that a flow ratio between expiratory and inspiratory limbs at mid-vital capacity (50 per cent) is approximately 1.[45, 46] The flow-volume loop is altered by having normal subjects breathe through fixed external resistances.[45, 47–49] Miller and Hyatt[45] found that the most sensitive test to detect the obstruction under these circumstances was peak expiratory flow, which did not increase significantly until the orifice was 10 mm in size; this finding correlates well with the clinical observation that dyspnea on exertion occurs only when the caliber of the tracheal air column is reduced to half normal.[50] Breathing through an external orifice of 6 mm reduces peak flows and produces plateaus on both inspiration and expiration (Fig. 11–5), a loop pattern closely resembling that of fixed airway obstruction. Asthma and COPD are predominantly diseases of the small airways; reduction in flow is apparent mainly in the effort-independent portion of the expiratory loop, the mid-VC expiratory-inspiratory ratio usually being less than 0.5 (Fig. 11–5). By contrast, in upper airway obstruction, the reduction in flow is proportionately greater in the effort-dependent portion of the loop (both inspiratory and expiratory), one or both limbs tending to plateau.

The dynamic effects of lesions of the upper airway depend in part on the extent to which the obstruction is "fixed" (the airway is unable to change cross-sectional area in response to transmural pressure differences—usually produced by circumferential benign strictures) or "variable" (the airway responds to transmural pressure—most often re-

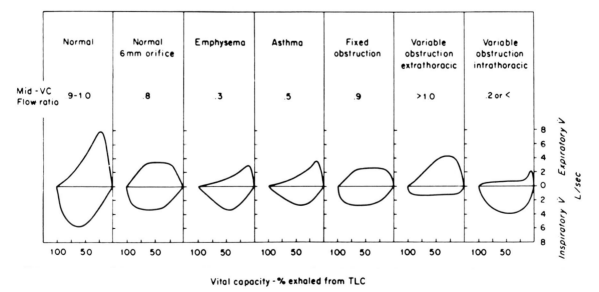

Figure 11–5. Flow-Volume Loops of Various Obstructive Conditions Compared with Normal. Volume is given as a percentage of vital capacity exhaled from total lung capacity. Representative mid-vital capacity flow ratios are given. (Reproduced from Miller RD, Hyatt RE, Mayo Clin Proc 44:145, 1969, with permission of the authors and editor.)

sulting from neoplasms that arise from the wall of the airway and create a crescentic lumen, thus permitting a variable cross-sectional diameter throughout the forced ventilatory cycle). Characteristic flow-volume loop patterns are produced by fixed and variable lesions (Fig. 11–5). Since fixed upper airway obstructions, either intrathoracic or extrathoracic, are not influenced by transmural pressure gradients, both inspiratory and expiratory flow are proportionately lowered. When a lesion is variable, however, its location (intrathoracic or extrathoracic) becomes important because the airway responds to transmural pressure. During inspiration the extrathoracic airway has a transmural pressure favoring narrowing because intraluminal pressure is subatmospheric while extraluminal pressure is approximately atmospheric.

Experimental studies in normal adults[48] have indicated that the reduction in air flow occasioned by extrathoracic obstructions results from transmural pressure at the site of the lesion rather than distal to it, the trachea below being too well stabilized to undergo dynamic compression. However, such is not the case in infants, who may develop considerable narrowing in the extrathoracic trachea just distal to an obstruction.[51] The pressure surrounding the extrathoracic trachea may not be as close to atmospheric pressure as was once believed. Several studies have shown that pleural pressure may be transmitted to the tissue spaces in the neck; to the extent that *negative* pleural pressure is transmitted to the neck, the dynamic compression of the trachea associated with upper airway obstruction will be decreased.[52, 53]

In contrast to the dynamic events that occur during inspiration in variable extrathoracic lesions, during expiration intraluminal pressure is positive relative to extraluminal pressure, thus tending to dilate the airway and obscure the presence of the lesion. Thus, *a variable extrathoracic lesion tends to cause predominant decrease in maximal inspiratory flow and relatively little effect on maximal expiratory flow.*[45]

This situation is reversed when a variable lesion is intrathoracic in location. During inspiration, extraluminal pressure (equivalent to pleural pressure) is negative relative to intraluminal pressure so that transmural pressure favors airway dilatation. By contrast, during expiration extraluminal pressure is positive relative to intraluminal pressure so that airway narrowing occurs. Thus, *a variable intrathoracic lesion results in a predominant reduction in maximal expiratory flow with relative preservation of maximal inspiratory flow* (Fig. 11–5).[45] The usefulness of comparing maximal flows on inspiratory and expiratory flow-volume curves has been confirmed in a study in which lesions were localized with tantalum bronchograms.[54] It was shown that expiratory-inspiratory flow ratios near 1.0 may be seen when the tracheal stenosis is near the thoracic inlet and that increased ratios may be observed with extrathoracic tracheomalacia. Periodic flow oscillations that can

be identified on either volume-time or flow-volume recordings and that correspond to a fluttering of upper airway structures, either passively or as a result of periodic muscle contraction, may be an important indicator of an abnormality of control of upper airway caliber.[55, 56] The identification of such flow oscillations should lead to the investigation of the upper airway and its surrounding musculature, since these changes may be an early indicator of disorders that can eventually lead to symptomatic upper airway obstruction.

Since the clinical and roentgenologic diagnosis of upper airway obstruction may be exceedingly difficult, it is of vital importance to recognize the basic physiologic changes caused by lesions in this area and to know how they are reflected in pulmonary function tests. In their study of normal subjects breathing through fixed resistances (the equivalent of fixed upper airway obstruction), Miller and Hyatt[45] found that forced vital capacity (FVC) was not reduced by an orifice as small as 4 mm and that forced expiratory volume in 1 second (FEV_1) did not decrease until orifice size was reduced to 6 mm in diameter; these two measurements have also been found to be normal in symptomatic patients with tracheal stenosis.[45, 57] Lesions of the larynx and trachea that produce a predominantly inspiratory obstruction may be recognized by comparing forced inspiratory (FIF) with forced expiratory (FEF) flow rates;[49, 58] these are usually measured at mid-VC and produce an FEF-FIF ratio greater than 1. However, since in many laboratories neither flow-volume loops nor FIF measurements are routine procedures, it is pertinent to compare the results of tests that measure effort-dependent expiratory flow with those that reflect the effort-independent flow contribution. The diagnosis may be suggested by finding a PEFR that is reduced proportionately greater than FEV_1.[43, 44, 47] Some investigators advocate measurement of other ratios of flow at small to large lung volumes, such as FEV_1-$FEV_{0.5}$.[47] A comparison of FEV_1 and FEF_{25-75} may be of particular benefit in detecting upper airway obstruction when flow-volume loops are not available. In the absence of airflow obstruction, the numerical values of FEV_1 and FEF_{25-75} are roughly comparable but as lower airway obstruction (asthma, COPD) develops, the FEF_{25-75} becomes disproportionately lowered. In upper airway obstruction, the FEV_1 (reflecting both effort-dependent and effort-independent flow) is decreased to the same extent as FEF_{25-75}, which reflects effort-independent flow only.[59] The maximal voluntary ventilation (MVV) or maximal breathing capacity (MBC), formerly a routine procedure in many laboratories, can be very useful in the detection of upper airway obstruction since it measures both inspiratory and expiratory flow; reduced values are particularly significant if the FEV_1 is within the normal range.[43, 47] Tests measuring the distribution (mixing) of inspired gases and the response to bronchodilators have been said to be useful in distinguishing upper from lower airway obstruction, patients with the former showing normal distribution and being unresponsive to bronchodilators. However, these observations were not borne out in the patients studied by Miller and Hyatt,[60] although it is possible that their patients had associated bronchitis. It would be anticipated that patients with upper airway obstruction, in contrast to those with emphysema, would have normal diffusing capacity, and a limited number of reports suggest that this is so.[57, 61]

The breathing of helium-oxygen mixtures can also differentiate between upper and lower airway obstruction.[43, 62] The resistance caused by turbulent flow in the larger bronchi is reduced by the breathing of this less dense gas mixture, whereas laminar flow in peripheral airways remains unchanged (Fig. 11–6). In patients with chronic upper airway obstruction, the presence of hypoxemia and hypercarbia at rest is usually indicative of an extreme degree of airway narrowing; however, exercise may decrease P_{O_2} in those patients who complain of dyspnea on exertion.[47]

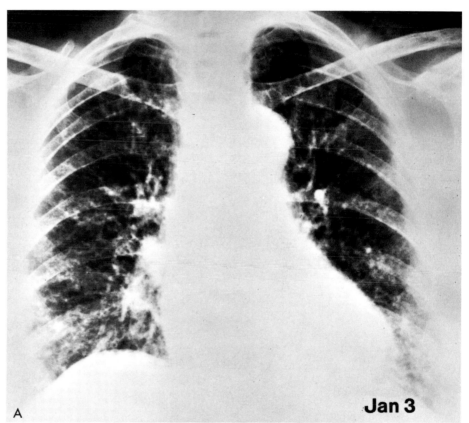

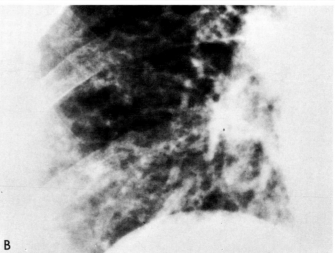

Figure 11–6. Severe Airway Obstruction Caused by Widespread Submucosal Lymphoma: Value of Helium Breathing in Distinguishing Large from Small Airway Obstruction. This 71-year-old woman presented for the first time with a 4-month history of increasing dyspnea on mild exertion. There was an audible expiratory wheeze and prolonged expiration. The initial roentgenogram (A) revealed a rather coarse reticular pattern throughout both lungs, seen to better advantage in a magnified view of the lower portion of the right lung (B). Pulmonary function studies revealed a marked reduction in FEV_1 and an FEV_1/FVC value of 50 per cent. A single-breath N_2 test revealed a normal closing volume and a normal slope of phase 3. The flow-volume curve with the patient breathing helium was much better than when she was breathing air, indicating obstruction in large airways.

Illustration continued on following page

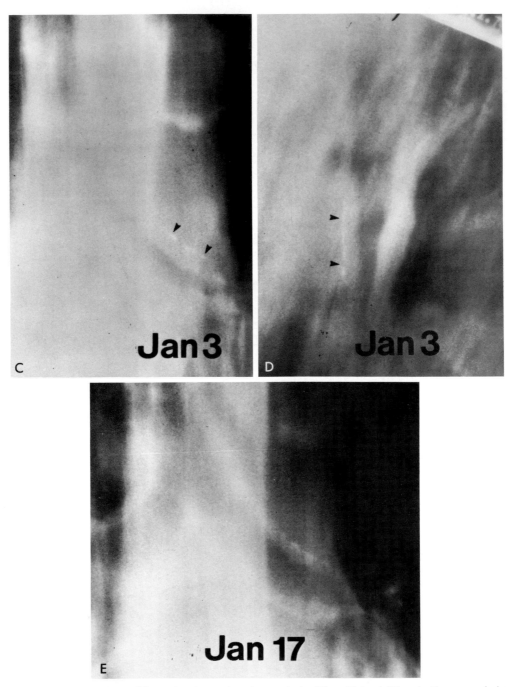

Figure 11–6. *Continued.* Tomograms of the major airways in anteroposterior *(C)* and lateral *(D)* projections revealed marked narrowing of the airways of the main bronchi. The small *arrowheads* point to calcified cartilaginous rings of the bronchi, indicating marked increase in soft tissue thickness between these rings and the airways due to thickening of the submucosa. A transbronchial biopsy revealed lymphocytic lymphoma. Antineoplastic therapy was begun immediately, and 2 weeks later the submucosal thickening had diminished considerably *(E)*.

Roentgenographic Manifestations

As in acute upper airway obstruction, these vary somewhat, according to the specific etiology (*see* farther on), although there are certain unusual manifestations, particularly in infants and children, which should alert the radiologist to the possibility of upper airway obstruction.

Although theoretically the effects on lung volume of variable intrathoracic and extrathoracic obstructing lesions should be different (the former being associated with expiratory air trapping and overinflation while the latter is not), the assessment of pulmonary overinflation on standard posteroanterior and lateral roentgenograms is subject to so much individual variation as to be of questionable

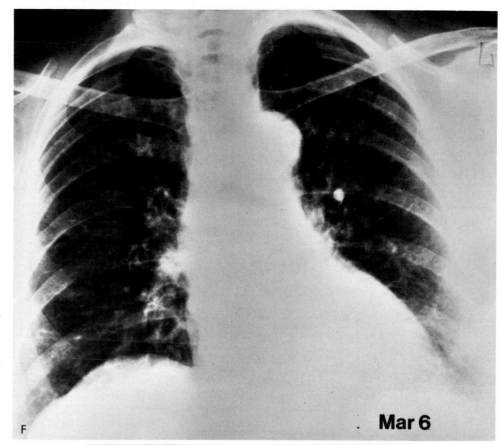

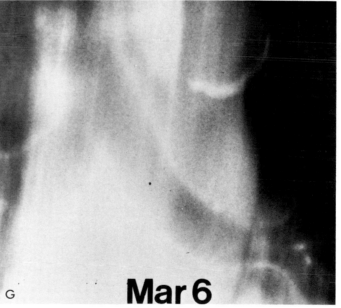

Figure 11–6. *Continued.* Two months after the institution of therapy, the chest roentgenogram *(F)* and tomogram *(G)* had returned to normal. Similarly, values for FEV₁ and FVC had returned to normal predicted levels and the FEV₁/FVC value was 80 per cent. (Courtesy of The Royal Adelaide Hospital, Adelaide, Australia, and Dr. Peter Macklem, The Royal Victoria Hospital, Montreal.)

value. However, unequivocal evidence of pulmonary overinflation, particularly in a young patient, should immediately raise the suspicion of upper airway obstruction, especially since overinflation is such a surprisingly infrequent manifestation of spasmodic asthma.

Obviously of much greater importance than this indirect sign of obstructive airway disease is the narrowing of the airway, and it is in this area that the roentgenologist can play a very useful—and sometimes vital—role. Unfortunately, frequently such lesions go unrecognized. The reasons are twofold:

1. The trachea is all too often a "blind spot" for the radiologist, a deficiency that can be corrected only by paying constant attention to those areas on a roentgenogram that are known to "hide" significant disease.

2. In our experience, the frequency with which posteroanterior roentgenograms of the chest are underexposed is so high that the lack of appreciation of tracheal narrowing is readily understandable.

As pointed out elsewhere, roentgenographic underexposure places an intolerable restriction on roentgenologic interpretation, since there is no method by which lack of identification of important structures can be compensated for (as one can compensate for overexposure by viewing with a bright light). As discussed in Chapter 2, the only technique that permits both adequate penetration of the mediastinum and proper exposure of the lungs employs high kilovoltages. In institutions in which the high kilovoltage technique is not employed, the trachea can be adequately seen on all posteroanterior roentgenograms only by the use of a third overpenetrated film, an addition that most would regard as economically unacceptable. However, even in the absence of adequate penetration of the mediastinum in posteroanterior projection, the lateral view often permits identification of the tracheal air column to good advantage, and it is perhaps on this view that the majority of lesions in the lower two thirds of the trachea are recognized. The inadequacy of standard posteroanterior roentgenograms in revealing tracheal disease was well illustrated in a Mayo Clinic report of 53 patients with primary cancer of the trachea,[63] of whom only 13 had a demonstrable tracheal abnormality on routine posteroanterior roentgenograms.

Once a lesion has been identified, its more precise anatomic nature can be established by tomography, either conventional or computed (CT). In the Mayo Clinic series of 53 primary cancers of the trachea,[63] conventional tomography was performed in 18 patients and was of diagnostic assistance in 16; of some interest is the fact that in 13 of these 16 patients, tomograms revealed lesions that were not evident on standard roentgenograms of the chest. In their CT study of 39 patients with various diseases of the trachea, Gamsu and Webb[64] found that in patients with tracheal stenosis, CT did not provide additional information over that obtained in more conventional studies; however, in patients with primary or secondary neoplasms involving the trachea, CT was more accurate in defining the intraluminal presence of tumor, the degree of airway compression, and, most importantly, the presence or absence of extratracheal extension of neoplasm. The superiority of CT over conventional tomography in these circumstances has also been emphasized by Kittredge.[65]

Other roentgenographic techniques that may be of value in selected cases include lateral roentgenograms of the soft tissues of the neck (particularly in infants and young children, in whom such abnormalities as hypertrophied tonsils and adenoids may be responsible for upper airway obstruction) and studies of the dynamic activity of the trachea with either cineradiographic or videotape recording to assess the fixed or variable nature of an obstruction (e.g., tracheomalacia). Positive contrast laryngography or tracheography may be diagnostically useful in some cases; powdered tantalum has been strongly recommended as the contrast medium of choice for these studies,[66] perhaps particularly in evaluating the precise length of trachea involved in post-intubation stenosis; however, at the time of writing, this substance has not been approved by the Food and Drug Administration (FDA) for clinical use in the United States. Another technique that might prove useful in some circumstances is cine CT. Ell and his colleagues[67] employed this technique with its very rapid imaging capabilities in the evaluation of eight adult patients with suspected nonfixed upper airway obstruction: seven showed intermittent obstruction, and only one was judged to be normal. The authors concluded that cine CT has the potential of providing information rapidly and noninvasively regarding upper airway dynamics.

Three unusual roentgenographic manifestations of chronic upper airway obstruction relate to the heart and pulmonary circulation. The first is *pulmonary edema*, a complication that can have ominous consequences; it is thought to be caused by the sustained maximal negative intrathoracic pressure created by attempted inspiration against an obstruction (the Mueller maneuver), although, as pointed out in Chapter 10 (*see* page 1953), there is evidence that in some patients the edema develops only after the obstruction has been relieved. The second unusual manifestation is *cardiac enlargement* (cor pulmonale) that results from pulmonary arterial hypertension secondary to chronic hypoxemia and acidosis;[68] in fact, some children with certain forms of chronic upper airway obstruction, such as hypertrophied tonsils, can present for the first time to their physician in frank right ventricular failure. The third unusual manifestation consists of a paradoxical change in heart size between inspiration and expiration. Normally, cardiac diameter is greater on expiration than inspiration; in the presence of chronic (and sometimes acute) upper airway obstruction, the heart is smaller on expiration than inspiration, a paradox that also occasionally occurs in association with chronic *lower* airway obstruction such as in emphysema. This can be explained on the basis of the Valsalva and Mueller maneuvers. In the presence of upper airway obstruction, expiration constitutes an effective Valsalva maneuver, raising intrathoracic pressure and reducing venous return to the thorax; the heart becomes smaller. By contrast, inspiration against the obstruction creates a Mueller maneuver, with greater negativity of intrathoracic pressure and increased venous return to the thorax; in addition to increasing venous return, the very negative intrathoracic pressure functions as an afterload on the left ventricle which must pump blood out of the thorax into the systemic circulation, which is unaffected by the negative pressure.

Clinical Manifestations

Obviously, the symptoms and signs of chronic upper airway obstruction will vary with the nature of the underlying lesion and, to some extent, with the age of the patient. As might be expected, the major complaint is dyspnea, either during exercise or at rest, depending on the severity of obstruction. Stridor also may be noted either at rest or during exercise, and its timing may be inspiratory, expiratory, or both. Nonproductive cough is common.

Hypertrophy of Tonsils and Adenoids

Hypertrophy of the palatine tonsils results in a characteristic roentgenographic appearance of a smooth, well-defined, elliptical mass of unit density extending downward from the soft palate into the hypopharynx (Fig. 11–7); hypertrophy of the nasopharyngeal adenoids is a commonly associated condition. Both should be readily apparent on lateral roentgenograms of the soft tissues of the neck. The major effect of the chronic upper airway ob-

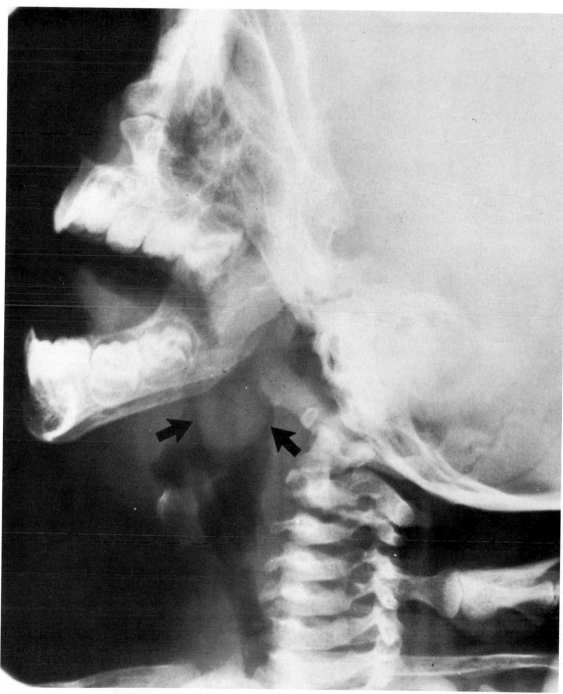

Figure 11–7. Hypertrophied Tonsils Resulting in Upper Airway Obstruction. A view of the soft tissues of the neck in lateral projection reveals a large soft tissue mass *(arrows)* protruding downward into the hypopharynx from the oropharynx. This represents huge hypertrophied tonsils. There is in addition evidence of moderate enlargement of the nasopharyngeal adenoids. This 3-month-old girl was experiencing severe respiratory distress. (Courtesy of Dr. Bernard Epstein, University of Texas, San Antonio.)

struction is alveolar hypoventilation, with resultant hypoxia, hypercapnia, and pulmonary arterial hypertension and cor pulmonale.[69-75] In the patient reported by Levy and associates,[76] pulmonary arterial pressure was near systemic levels; this pressure was halved shortly after intubation.

A similar picture is seen in obese subjects as a result of obstruction of the pharynx by the tongue when the patient is recumbent.[43, 77-80]

Laryngeal Dysfunction

The upper airway site with the greatest potential for deranged function is the larynx. There are 24 sets of skeletal muscles that surround the upper airway and are involved in stabilization and closure of the airway, and most of these are laryngeal muscles under both voluntary and involuntary control; they are involved in speech, song, cough, defecation, and so on.[1] The major laryngeal dilator muscle (abductor) is the posterior cricoarytenoid, and the major constrictors (adductors) are the thyroarytenoid and lateral cricoarytenoid. These muscles are respiratory, in that they receive phasic neural output from brainstem respiratory neurons. During inspiration, the posterior cricoarytenoid dilates the larynx and in some instances expiratory adductor activation narrows it. The alae nasi are also inspiratory muscles, and during periods of increased ventilation, their phasic inspiratory contraction prevents collapse of the external nares.[81] Paralysis of the laryngeal abductors causes fixed obstruction of the upper airway,[60, 82, 83] whereas unopposed action of laryngeal adductors results in "laryngospasm." Bulbar involvement in generalized neuromuscular disease causes weakness of the upper airway muscles that may be associated with inspiratory upper airway obstruction and characteristic flow oscillations on flow-volume curves.[84]

One of the principal causes of respiratory obstruction during the neonatal period is collapse of the hypotonic larynx, caused chiefly by infolding of the arytenoid cartilages during inspiration;[85] the result is congenital laryngeal stridor. Congenital hypoplasia of laryngeal structures and redundancy of the mucous membranes of the larynx and subglottic segment of the trachea result in dyspnea and inspiratory-expiratory stridor. Congenital cleft larynx is another rare cause of upper airway obstruction.[86] In a report of 34 cases of vocal cord paralysis or paresis in infants and children, Williams and his associates[87] suggested that this entity is not as rare as has been previously reported. Although the presence of upper airway obstruction may be apparent roentgenographically from the general signs previously described, none of the roentgenologic findings observed by Williams and colleagues were felt to be specific for the diagnosis of vocal cord paralysis. The presence of chronic upper airway obstruction as a result of vocal cord paralysis has also been reported by others.[60, 82, 88, 89]

Interruption of the superior laryngeal nerves at the time of thyroidectomy is the most common cause of bilateral vocal cord paralysis in the adult. It can also occur in rheumatoid disease or poliomyelitis, following viral infections, in association with Guillain-Barré syndrome, or for no apparent reason (idiopathic). Vocal cord paralysis predominantly affects inspiratory flow rates; in ten patients, the mean expiratory to inspiratory flow ratio at 50 per cent vital capacity was 1.65.[83] Some degree of obstruction can also be caused by unilateral vocal cord paralysis; in one study, polytef (Teflon) injection of the paralyzed cord improved inspiratory flows.[90]

A syndrome that mimics asthma termed "emotional laryngeal wheezing" occurs in emotionally disturbed patients and is caused by expiratory glottic narrowing.[91] Such narrowing, uninfluenced by general anesthesia, has also been reported in a single asthmatic patient.[92] Episodic, paradoxical inspiratory laryngeal narrowing and stridor results in a syndrome in adults that resembles croup;[93] in this condition, the abnormal laryngeal muscle activity has been documented by videorecording of bronchoscopic images; it was precipitated by respiratory tract infection and histamine inhalation and abolished by continuous positive airway pressure.

Laryngeal narrowing can also occur in association with lower airway obstructive diseases such as asthma and COPD.[94] In many asthmatic subjects, inspiratory resistance is paradoxically greater than expiratory resistance, and inspiratory pressure-flow curves are more curvilinear and density-dependent, suggesting that the upper airway is the site of the excessive inspiratory narrowing.[95] The reasons for this are unclear. In normal and asthmatic subjects, histamine-induced airway obstruction is associated with expiratory glottic and oropharyngeal narrowing.[96, 97] The glottic narrowing is not caused by a direct effect on the laryngeal musculature, since the larynx contains no smooth muscle, and skeletal muscles do not contract in response to histamine; it may be caused by stimulation of afferent receptors and a reflex effect. It is puzzling as to why the glottis should narrow in response to lower airway obstruction; one explanation that has been suggested is that the glottic narrowing slows expiratory flow, producing dynamic increase in FRC, thus sparing the inspiratory muscles the task of maintaining hyperinflation.[97]

Glottic inspiratory and expiratory dimensions are decreased and upper airway resistance is increased in patients with COPD, the decreased laryngeal dimensions correlating with the severity of expiratory flow limitation.[98, 99] The expiratory glottic narrowing in COPD may function in a manner similar to pursed-lip breathing, preventing airway closure and contributing to hyperinflation. Functional upper airway obstruction can also occur in patients with a variety of extrapyramidal neurologic disorders. Vincken and associates[2748] reported abnormal flow-volume curves in 24 of 27 patients with extrapyramidal disorders, including essential tremor and Parkinson's disease. It appears that the obstruction in these individuals was caused by rhythmic or irregular involuntary contractions of the laryngeal adductors. Endoscopy during performance of flow-volume loop studies showed either rhythmic or irregular changes in the glottic area as a result of alternating abduction and adduction of the vocal cords and supraglottic structures.

Tracheal Stenosis

Even when predicted on the basis of age, height, and sex, there is considerable variation in maximal expiratory flow among normal subjects. Since central airways (trachea to segmental bronchi) are the site of flow limitation over most of the vital capacity in normal subjects,[100, 101] part of this variation is caused by differences in the size of the central airways.[102, 103]

Tracheal cross-sectional areas can be evaluated from posteroanterior and lateral chest roentgenograms or from CT scans.[104, 105] As reviewed in Chapter 1 (see page 36), the caliber of the tracheal air column in normal men and women is as follows: assuming a normative range that encompasses three standard deviations about the mean (i.e., pertaining to 99.7 per cent of the normal population), the upper limits of normal for coronal and sagittal diameters in men ranging in age from 20 to 79 years are 25 mm and 27 mm; in women they are 21 mm and 23 mm, respectively.[106] The lower limits of normal for both dimensions are 13 mm in men and 10 mm in women. These measurements were obtained from conventional posteroanterior and lateral chest roentgenograms of 808 patients with no clinical or roentgenographic evidence of respiratory disease; there were 430 men and 378 women. All roentgenograms were exposed at total lung capacity, and measurements were made at a point 2 cm above the projected top of the aortic arch. Deviation from these figures indicates the presence of pathologic widening or narrowing, respectively, of the caliber of the tracheal air column. Of some interest was the observation that no statistically significant correlation was found between tracheal caliber, body weight, or body height.

One of the most common causes of chronic upper airway obstruction is tracheal stenosis occurring as a complication of intubation or tracheostomy, a reflection of the ever increasing tendency to support ventilation in seriously ill patients. In one study of 342 patients who required prolonged endotracheal intubation,[107] 5 per cent manifested stridor following extubation and 1.8 per cent required reintubation or tracheostomy. Although reversible laryngeal edema and inflammation were the major causes of the stridor, stricture developed as a result of fibrosis in four patients.

Tracheal stenosis following the prolonged use of cuffed tracheostomy or endotracheal tubes may occur at the level of the stoma, at the level of the inflatable cuff, or, rarely, where the tip of the tube impinges on the tracheal mucosa. The frequency with which stenosis occurs at these sites seems to vary from series to series; in one group of 25 clinically significant tracheal strictures, 18 occurred at the stoma and seven at the inflatable cuff;[108] by contrast, in another group of 55 patients,[109] the incidence of stoma (24 cases) and inflatable cuff (23 cases) stenosis was almost equal (the remaining eight cases were at various other locations, mostly in the cervical trachea).

Plastic tubes with inflatable high-compliance balloons are now the most commonly used endotracheal and tracheostomy devices. Once the tube is in position, the cuff is inflated with sufficient air to occlude the tracheal lumen in order to provide an air-tight system at the maximum ventilatory pressure required by the patient. The cuff is usually situated 1.5 cm or more distal to the stoma.[110, 111] Since the trachea is not circular in cross section, the circumferential cuff can attain an air-tight seal only by expanding the tracheal lumen and deforming its wall (Fig. 11–8). The tracheal mucosa is easily compressed between the cuffed balloon and the nonyielding tracheal cartilage, and since the pressure may easily exceed capillary pressure, blood supply to the mucosa is compromised, resulting in ischemic necrosis. The most susceptible portion of the trachea is where the mucosa overlies rigid cartilaginous rings, and it is here that necrosis occurs most often.[110] The lesion begins as a superficial tracheitis and progresses to shallow mucosal ulcerations, usually 2 or more days following the inflation of the cuff. As the tracheal mucosa becomes eroded, the cartilaginous rings are exposed and become softened, split, fragmented, and eventually completely destroyed.[110] Following deflation of the cuff and removal of the tracheostomy tube, fibrosis occurs in the damaged tracheal wall, resulting in cicatricial stenosis (Fig. 11–9; see also Fig. 8–88, page 1504).

Experimental studies on dogs have demonstrated both the immediate effects of intubation[112] and the effects of prolonged use of cuffed tracheostomy tubes.[113] In the former study, dog tracheas examined by scanning electron microscopy 2 hours after intubation showed nearly complete ciliary denudation along the tract of tubal insertion. When cuffs were inflated, more widespread changes were observed, especially over tracheal rings. Seven days later, regeneration was nearly complete, although isolated areas of denudation could still be identified. In the experimental study carried out by Goldberg and Pearson,[113] both cuffed and uncuffed tracheostomy tubes were maintained in position for 2 weeks at low and high pressures. Changes were assessed by bronchoscopy and tracheography and by histologic examination following sacrifice 8 weeks after extubation. It was found that the greater the

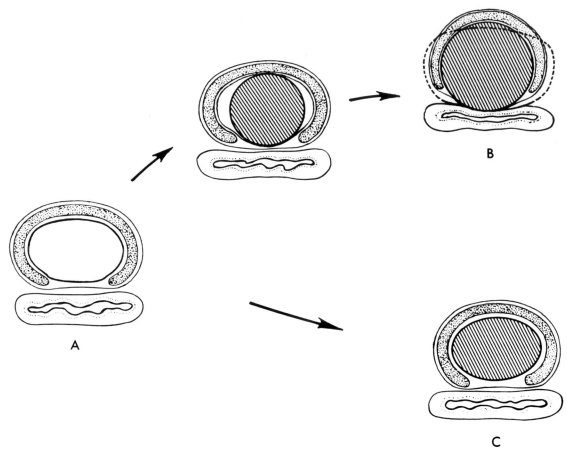

Figure 11–8. Diagrammatic Views of the Trachea in Cross Section with Varied Inflation of a Balloon Cuff. *A,* Without the balloon cuff; *B,* overinflation of the balloon with increased pressure on the tracheal wall; *C,* normal inflation of the balloon. (Reproduced from James AE Jr, MacMillan AS Jr, Eaton SB, Grillo HC: Am J Roentgenol *109*:455, 1970, with permission of the authors and editor.)

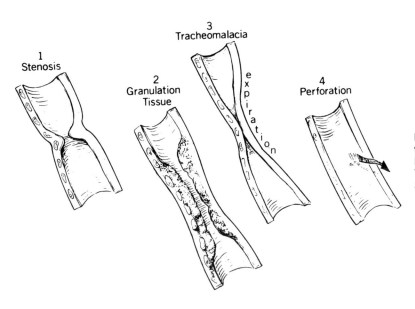

Figure 11–9. Diagrammatic Representation of Distal Posttracheostomy Lesions That Occur in the Area of the Balloon Cuff. (Reproduced from MacMillan AS Jr, James AE Jr, Stitik FP, Grillo HC: Thorax *26*:696, 1971, with permission of the authors and editor.)

size of the tracheostomy tube relative to tracheal diameter and the greater the inflating pressure, the more severe the resultant stenosis. In another experimental study on dogs, Leverment and associates[114] assessed the merits of two low-pressure cuffs and found that both produced little visible damage to the tracheal wall of dogs intubated continuously over a 2-week period. Tracheal stenosis at the cuff level following extubation occurred far less frequently than when the stiff, unyielding, low-residual-volume cuffs were used.

Roentgenologically, the narrowing of the tracheal lumen typically begins 1 to 1.5 cm distal to the inferior margin of the tracheostomy stoma and involves 1.5 to 2.5 cm of tracheal wall (including two to four cartilaginous rings).[110] James and his colleagues described three different roentgenographic appearances: (1) the tracheal lumen is circumferentially narrowed over a distance of approximately 2 cm; (2) a thin membrane or diaphragm (caused by granulation tissue rather than mature fibrous tissue) may project almost at right angles from the tracheal wall; and (3) a long, thickened, eccentric opacity of soft tissue density compromises the tracheal lumen. The last named results most often from impingement of the tip of the tracheostomy tube on the tracheal wall (or from an eccentric cuff), so that mucosal necrosis and resultant cicatrization are local rather than circumferential. Adequate roentgenographic assessment can usually be made by standard films of the chest (the posteroanterior roentgenograms preferably being at full inspiration and maximal expiration), along with tomography in anteroposterior and lateral projections. Occasionally, precise delineation of the length of stenosis may require opacification (Fig. 11–10). In such cases insufflation with powdered tantalum is preferable to instillation of liquid contrast media because of the greater tendency of the latter to occlude the tracheal lumen.

Occasionally, thinning of the trachea results in tracheomalacia rather than cicatricial stenosis, usually as a result of excessive removal of cartilage at the time of tracheostomy or destruction of cartilage by pressure necrosis and infection.[115, 116] In such circumstances, the increased compliance of the affected tracheal segment can be appreciated by fluoroscopic examination or cinefluorography.

Clinically, most patients are symptom-free for a variable period following removal of the tracheostomy tube, although edema of the tracheal wall may be present. Eventually, they experience increasing difficulty in raising secretions and note shortness of breath on exertion; these symptoms may progress to stridor and marked dyspnea on minimal exertion.[110] Stridor may not be present at rest but may be noticed with exercise or be brought on by hyperventilation. Symptoms and signs of upper airway obstruction may not become apparent for several weeks, during which time the edema subsides and progressive fibrosis occurs.

Resection of the stenotic segment with primary end-to-end anastomosis appears to be the definitive treatment of choice. As pointed out by Grillo,[117, 118] more than half of the trachea may be resected and primary anastomosis performed.

Tracheal Neoplasms

Neoplasms of the upper airway were discussed in some detail in Chapter 8. Compared with the larynx and bronchi, the trachea is a rare site of primary cancer. At the Mayo Clinic,[63] only 53 primary cancers of the trachea were diagnosed over a period of 30 years, the relative incidence compared with laryngeal cancer being one to 75 and with lung cancer one to 180. It has been speculated that protection is provided by a vigorous cough reflex, effective ciliary action, and the large diameter of the trachea, factors that prevent trapping of mucus containing carcinogens.[119] The commonest primary cancer of the trachea is squamous cell carcinoma (Fig. 11–11), constituting 50 per cent or more of cases in various series and being approximately four times as common in men as in women.[63, 120, 121] Adenoid cystic carcinoma is slightly less common and shows no sex predilection. Other tumors such as lymphoma, leukemia, plasmacytoma, benign and malignant soft tissue neoplasms, and other types of primary and secondary carcinoma are much less common.[57, 82, 122–126]

Patients with tracheal neoplasms often are treated for asthma for considerable periods of time before the correct diagnosis is made.[50, 57, 63, 122–124, 127, 128] Although initially dyspnea may be noted only on exertion, eventually its paroxysmal occurrence at night may suggest the diagnosis of asthma. Hoarseness, cough, and wheeze are common, and when associated with hemoptysis virtually eliminate the possibility of spasmodic asthma. A characteristic wheeze (stridor) may be heard with or without a stethoscope placed over the trachea. The timing of the wheeze is characteristically inspiratory with extrathoracic lesions and expiratory with intrathoracic lesions. Rarely, granulomas and neoplasms of the trachea may occasion hypoventilation, hypoxemia, hypercarbia, pulmonary hypertension, and cor pulmonale.[75, 127]

"Saber-Sheath" Trachea

In cross section the resting trachea is roughly horseshoe-shaped, the open end of the cartilage rings being closed by the compliant posterior sheath. Considerable variation exists in the shape of the tracheal cartilage rings, the commonest being a C shape; however, U and V shapes also occur.[129, 130] On posteroanterior and lateral roentgenograms, the coronal and sagittal diameters of the tracheal air column are roughly equal; as pointed out in Chapter 1 (see page 36), however, the sagittal diameter is normally slightly greater than the co-

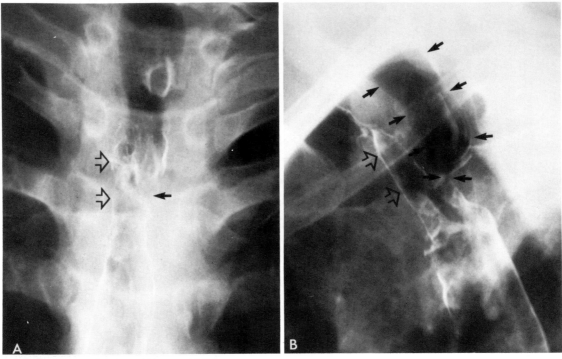

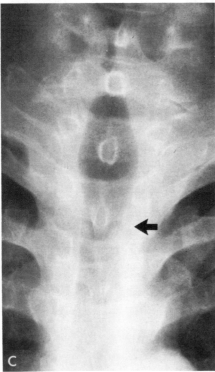

Figure 11–10. Severe Tracheal Stenosis at the Site of Insertion of a Tracheostomy Tube. Following instillation of contrast medium through a permanent tracheostomy opening, views of the upper portion of the trachea in anteroposterior *(A)* and oblique *(B)* projections reveal opacification of the tract of the tracheostomy tube *(open arrows* in both projections). In *B,* the *solid arrows* point to the air column of the trachea proximal to a severe degree of stenosis situated at the point of the lowest *arrows* (and also indicated by the single *arrow* in *A*). Note that the stenosis is at the point of entry of the tracheostomy tube rather than at the site of the tracheostomy cuff. The stenosis was resected and end-to-end anastomosis performed; the tracheostomy tract was closed. Several weeks later, an anteroposterior view of the tracheal air column *(C)* reveals little more than a slight narrowing at the site of anastomosis *(arrow).*

Figure 11–11. Primary Carcinoma of the Trachea. At the time of the normal roentgenogram illustrated in *A,* the patient, a 55-year-old man, had no chest symptoms. Approximately 1 year later, during which time he had noted increasing dyspnea on effort, a roentgenogram *(B)* revealed an increased thoracic volume, the diaphragm being approximately 2 cm lower than on the previous film. In addition, the air column of the cervical trachea approximately 2 cm distal to the larynx had become markedly narrowed. A large mass can be identified arising from the right wall of the trachea and extending over a distance of at least 3 cm of its length.

Illustration continued on following page

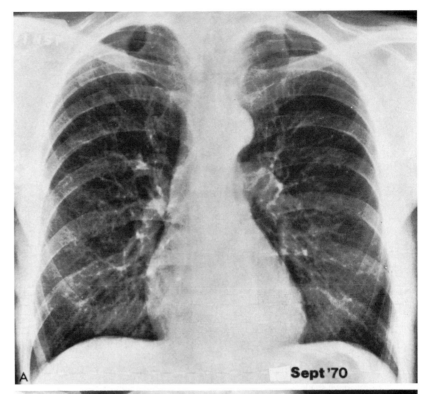

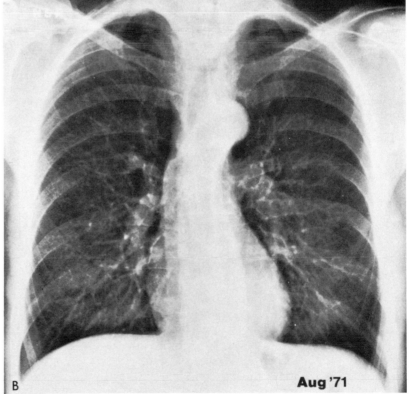

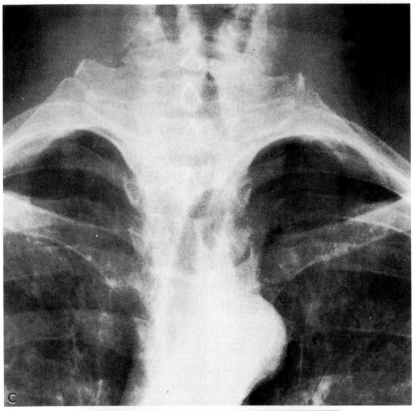

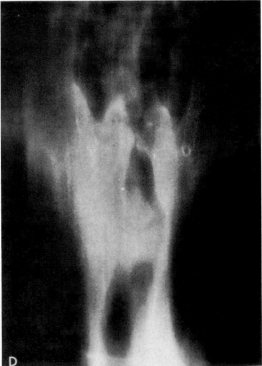

Figure 11–11. *Continued.* A detail view *(C)* and an anteroposterior tomogram *(D)* reveal the lesion to better advantage and show the severe compromise of the tracheal air column. A sleeve resection was carried out with end-to-end anastomosis. Proven squamous cell carcinoma.

ronal. Very occasionally, the coronal diameter is markedly reduced and the sagittal diameter correspondingly increased, a condition called "saber-sheath" trachea by Greene and Lechner.[131] These authors reported 13 patients with this condition, the only criterion for selection being an internal coronal diameter of the intrathoracic trachea one-half or less the corresponding sagittal diameter; measurements were made 1 cm above the level of the top of the aortic arch. All patients were men ranging in age from 52 to 75 years. Coronal tracheal diameter ranged from 7 to 13 mm (mean 10.5 mm), the "tracheal index" (the ratio of coronal to sagittal diameter) ranging from 0.5 to 0.25 (mean 0.4). Generally, the narrow coronal diameter extended the entire length of the intrathoracic trachea from carina to thoracic outlet, at which point the coronal diameter abruptly widened and the sagittal diameter narrowed, the air column thus assuming a normal configuration. This abrupt change in tracheal configuration from intrathoracic to extrathoracic trachea was a consistent finding and almost certainly reflected the influence of intrathoracic transmural pressures (Fig. 11–12).

Obvious tracheal ring calcification was identified in ten of the 13 patients and the lateral tracheal walls seemed relatively thick in comparison with normal dimensions. Necropsy examination of one patient who died from unrelated causes revealed extensive ossification of the cartilaginous rings associated with a rather rigid "saber-sheath" deformity. These findings would suggest that the deformity is fixed rather than variable.

All of Greene and Lechner's 13 patients[131] were heavy smokers; seven had a primary diagnosis of COPD and ten an "associated diagnosis of chronic bronchitis." Despite this apparent association between chronic airflow limitation and the saber-sheath tracheal configuration, the authors felt insecure in establishing a definite relationship between the two conditions because of the small number of patients involved. Since this original report, however, Greene[132] carried out a study of 60 male patients with the saber-sheath tracheal configuration and 60 control subjects 50 years of age or older: of the 60 patients, 57 (95 per cent) had clinical evidence of obstructive airway disease compared with only 18 per cent of the control subjects. Of considerable diagnostic importance was the finding that 26 (45 per cent) of the 57 patients with COPD lacked conventional roentgenographic evidence of obstructive airway disease; thus, the saber-sheath deformity provided a clue to the presence of COPD when other signs were absent. Although it was not stated whether flow-volume loops were obtained on these patients, it is probable that they would not have been particularly informative in any event: the almost universal presence of obstructive disease of the lower airways would likely have skewed the results such that a fixed upper airway obstruction would not have been recognized.

Chronic sclerosing mediastinitis could conceivably produce local or general circumferential narrowing of the tracheal lumen similar to the saber-sheath configuration, although the more usual sites of airway involvement are the main bronchi.

Relapsing Polychondritis

This unusual and interesting systemic disease affects cartilage in many anatomic sites throughout the body, including the ribs, tracheobronchial tree, ear lobes, nose, and central or peripheral joints.[133–136] A poor prognostic feature is said to be involvement of the cartilages of the upper airways; respiratory complications have accounted for 50 per cent of the reported deaths, although they are infrequently the presenting problem.[137, 138] The condition has been reported in association with cryptogenic cirrhosis,[139] systemic lupus erythematosus (SLE),[140] and Wegener's granulomatosis,[141] and as a complication of hydralazine therapy.[142] It is now firmly recognized as one of the autoimmune connective tissue diseases, and its characteristics were described in detail in Chapter 7 (see page 1238); it is discussed here only briefly.

One of the most important roentgenographic manifestations of relapsing polychondritis is narrowing of the tracheal and major bronchial airway columns.[135] In one patient we observed, the major involvement was of the left mainstem bronchus, bronchography revealing marked irregular narrowing of its air column. This narrowing was fixed and did not vary with forced inspiration or expiration, as observed cinefluorographically. The left lung showed severe air trapping on expiration and was diffusely oligemic, reflecting hypoxic vasoconstriction as a result of hypoventilation. It appears that the effects on the major airways may be fixed (as in our patient) or variable (as in the patient reported by Gibson and Davis).[138] Variable obstruction is the result of increased compliance and flaccidity, so that the airway readily collapses on expiration; this effect may be of sufficient severity to cause fatal expiratory airway obstruction.

In the patient reported by Gibson and Davis,[138] the degree of airflow obstruction as judged by the FEV_1 and conductance was severe and did not improve with a bronchodilator. Inspiratory flow rates were reduced less than the expiratory measurements, the typical pattern of intrathoracic large airway obstruction.[45] In another study of pulmonary function in five patients with relapsing polychondritis, flow-volume loops showed a flattening of the expiratory limb compatible with intrathoracic upper airway obstruction, but in most subjects there was also a decrease in inspiratory flow.[137, 143]

The diagnosis is made on the basis of recurrent inflammation of two or more cartilaginous sites, most commonly the ears and nose. In addition to chondritis, other manifestations include episcleritis, iritis, hearing impairment, cataracts, anemia, abnor-

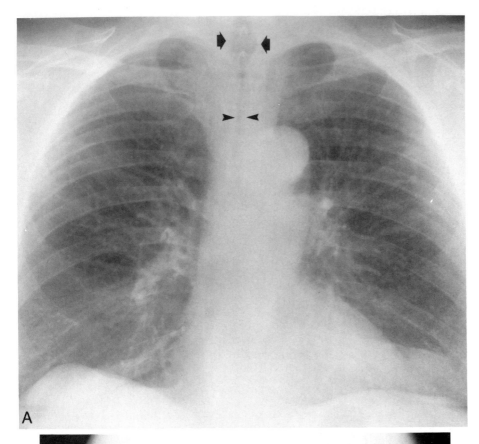

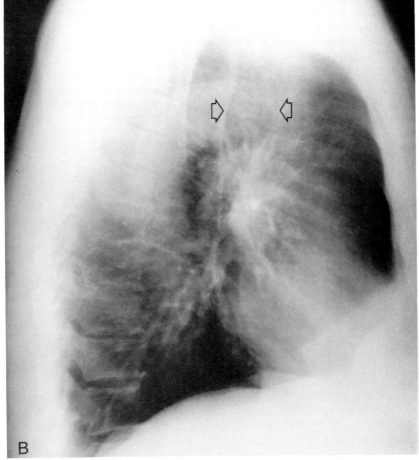

Figure 11–12. Saber-Sheath Trachea. Posteroanterior *(A)* and lateral *(B)* chest roentgenograms reveal severe narrowing of the intrathoracic trachea in the coronal plane *(arrowheads)* and widening in the sagittal plan *(open arrows),* resulting in an abnormal "tracheal index" of 0.20 or less *(see* text). Note that the extrathoracic trachea *(arrows)* is normal, the narrowing beginning at the thoracic inlet.

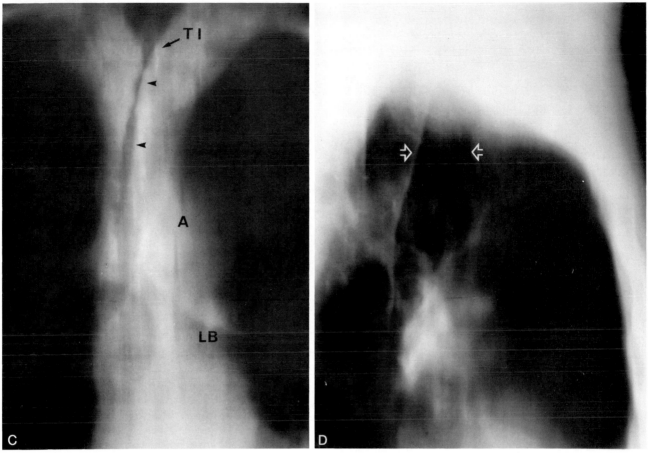

Figure 11–12. *Continued.* Linear tomograms in anteroposterior *(C)* and lateral *(D)* projections confirm the narrowing and lobulation *(arrowheads)* and show that the most severe reduction in caliber extends from the thoracic inlet (TI) to a point slightly above the aortic arch (A). Note that the diameter of the left main bronchus (LB) exceeds that of the trachea. In *D*, the sagittal diameter *(open arrows)* is greater than normal. The patient is a 65-year-old man.

malities of liver function, myocarditis, and aortic valvular insufficiency.[134, 135] Chondrolysis of the joints may lead to severe arthritis. The airway involvement can be rapidly progressive and severe, and since a beneficial effect of corticosteroid therapy has been reported, prompt recognition and institution of therapy is vitally important.[144] The active airway lesions have been reported to take up gallium 67, which may be helpful in localizing the site and assessing the activity of the disease.[145] Rarely, an airway lesion resembling relapsing polychondritis can develop without evidence of other cartilaginous involvement or a connective tissue disease.[146]

Tracheobronchomegaly

Tracheobronchomegaly is a condition consisting of a "cystic" dilatation of the tracheobronchial tree that may extend all the way from the larynx to the periphery of the lung.[147, 148] Originally described by Mounier-Kuhn,[149] it is reported to have a familial incidence.[147] Campbell and Young[150] found this condition to be a relatively common although seldom recognized form of obstructive lung disease, and

we agree that the incidence is undoubtedly much higher than is indicated by the 1973 review of the subject by Bateson and Woo-Ming,[151] who found only 55 cases reported in the literature and added two of their own. According to these authors, the disease occurs predominantly in males, the majority of whom are in their third and fourth decades of life. Few patients present over the age of 50 or in childhood, although a case has been reported in an 18-month-old child.[152]

In tracheobronchomegaly, the increased compliance of the trachea results in abnormal flaccidity and easy collapsibility during forced expiration and cough. In normal subjects, all central airways narrow during coughing and the resultant increase in the linear velocity of expired air aids in the transport and expectoration of mucus and sputum; however, in tracheobronchomegaly the trachea is the only portion of the tracheobronchial tree that narrows when pleural pressure increases during coughing.

Pathologically, both the cartilaginous and membranous portions of the trachea and bronchi are affected, having thin atrophied muscular and elastic tissue.[153, 154] Campbell and Young[150] described 25 patients in whom tracheobronchial collapse was observed bronchoscopically during forced expiration or cough. In one case, marked widening and flaccidity of the posterior membranous sheath of the right main bronchus and, to a lesser extent, the left main bronchus were found at necropsy.

The etiology and pathogenesis of this condition are unclear. The association of the abnormality with Ehlers-Danlos syndrome has been reported in adults[155, 156] and with congenital cutis laxa in children,[157] suggesting the presence of an underlying defect in elastic tissue. An acquired form of the condition has recently been reported as a complication of diffuse pulmonary fibrosis.[2772] A localized form has been reported in association with end-stage relapsing polychondritis.[136]

Roentgenologically, the diagnosis of tracheobronchomegaly is usually apparent at a glance (Fig. 11–13). The caliber of the trachea and major bronchi generally is increased, and the air columns have an irregular corrugated appearance caused by the protrusion of redundant mucosal and submucosal tissue between the cartilaginous rings (sometimes called tracheal diverticulosis). This appearance is often best visualized in lateral projection.[147, 148] Both CT and magnetic resonance imaging (MRI) can be used to demonstrate the abnormal tracheal and bronchial dilatation (Fig. 11–13).[158] The inefficient cough mechanism leads to retention of mucus with resultant recurrent pneumonia, emphysema, bronchiectasis, and parenchymal scarring. Increased large airway compliance is not limited to patients with enlarged central airways: at bronchoscopy, many patients with COPD who do not have an abnormally dilated trachea appear to have an increase in tracheal compliance manifested by large changes in the tracheal cross-sectional area during the respiratory cycle. It is unclear whether this is a manifestation of a more collapsible airway or simply reflects the larger pleural pressure swings in these obstructed patients.

Symptoms of tracheobronchomegaly are usually indistinguishable from those caused by chronic bronchitis or bronchiectasis. The presence of prolonged cough and a loud, harsh, rasping sound on auscultation in a patient who complains of inability to expectorate secretions should arouse suspicion of the diagnosis.[154] Pulmonary function tests typically show decrease in bronchial flow rates,[147] an enlarged dead space, and increased tidal volume.[151]

Tracheobronchopathia Osteochondroplastica

Tracheobronchopathia osteochondroplastica (*synonyms*: tracheo-osteoma, tracheitis chonica ossificans, tracheopathia osteoplastica)[159] is a rare condition characterized by the development of nodules or spicules of cartilage and bone in the submucosa of the trachea and bronchi.[160–164] It occurs almost exclusively in men over the age of 50. In the majority of reported cases, the condition is diagnosed only at necropsy, having been unsuspected during life;[161] for example, in a prospective bronchoscopic study of 2180 patients over an 8-year period, the abnormality was recognized in only nine.

The etiology and pathogenesis are unknown. At least three reports have associated the disease with tracheobronchial amyloidosis,[165–167] and in view of the common occurrence of calcification and ossification in this condition,[168] it has been speculated that tracheobronchopathia osteochondroplastica may represent an end stage of this condition.[165, 167] However, since the majority of cases of the classic disease[169] as well as occasional examples of apparently early disease[170] show no evidence of amyloid deposition, it seems unlikely that this is a valid explanation. A more likely hypothesis is that the nodules develop as enchondroses from the tracheobronchial cartilage rings.[169]

Pathologically, the nodules are usually confined to those portions of the tracheal and bronchial walls that normally contain cartilage, showing little or no tendency to develop in the posterior membranous sheath. The cartilaginous and bony masses are submucosal and produce numerous sessile and polypoid elevations that give the trachea and bronchi a beaded appearance at both autopsy and bronchoscopy. Histologically, the nodules are composed of cartilage alone or of bone with a variable amount of marrow. Serial sections invariably demonstrate continuity with the perichondrium of the underlying cartilage rings. The rings themselves are often normal but may show focal metaplastic bone formation. The mucous membrane usually is intact, although it may show squamous metaplasia; rarely, ulceration results in hemoptysis.[161, 171–173]

Roentgenologically, the findings are variable and are chiefly those resulting from bronchial obstruction.[161] Tomography should clearly reveal the irregular nodular appearance of the tracheal and bronchial air columns (Fig. 11–14) and permit identification of bone formation. CT has been said to reveal the tracheal deformity to excellent advantage (Fig. 11–15);[174] coronal and sagittal MRI should demonstrate the deformity even more clearly, as should dual energy digital radiography.

The majority of patients are asymptomatic, the degree of osteochondromatous proliferation being insufficient to cause clinically significant airway narrowing. Occasionally, there is dyspnea, hoarseness, cough, expectoration, wheezing, and hemoptysis.[175] Pulmonary function studies in one case revealed an increase in TLC and RV and a decrease in FEV_1 and MBC.[176] The diagnosis is made most easily at bronchoscopy, the spicule-like formations of bone and cartilage producing a grating sensation as the instrument is passed. When the disease affects the more distal cartilaginous bronchi, the submucosal masses may be large enough to obstruct lumens with resultant atelectasis or obstructive pneumonitis. In fact, death from such bronchial obstruction has been reported.[176]

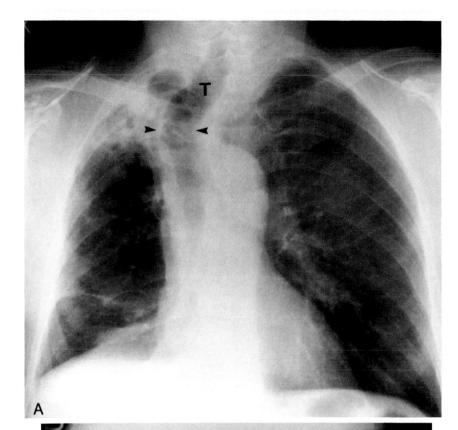

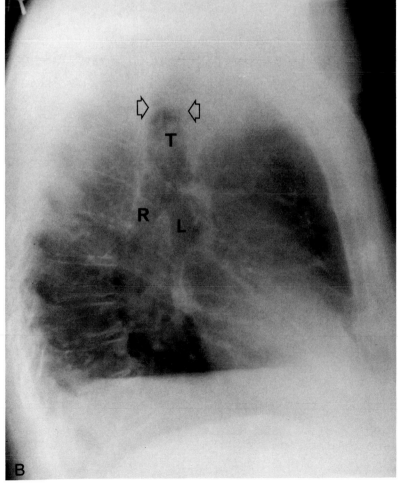

Figure 11–13. Tracheobronchomegaly. Posteroanterior *(A)* and lateral *(B)* chest roentgenograms show an increased diameter of the trachea (T) and the right (R) and left (L) main bronchi in both coronal *(arrowheads)* and sagittal *(open arrows)* planes (the tracheal air column measured approximately 27 mm in both planes). There is moderate deviation of the trachea to the right as a result of right upper lobe fibrosis from presumed prior granulomatous infection. The hila are asymmetric, the right being diminutive.

Illustration continued on following page

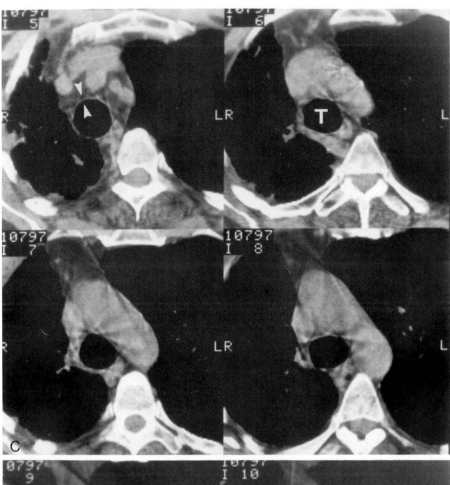

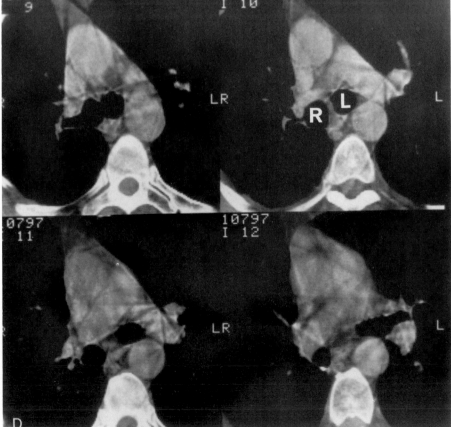

Figure 11–13. *Continued.* A series of CT scans, 10 mm thick, from the upper trachea *(C)* to the intermediate/left main bronchial level *(D)* show that the tracheal dilatation (T) extends distally into the right (R) and left (L) main bronchi. The tracheal wall *(between arrowheads)* is thin. The patient is a middle-aged man.

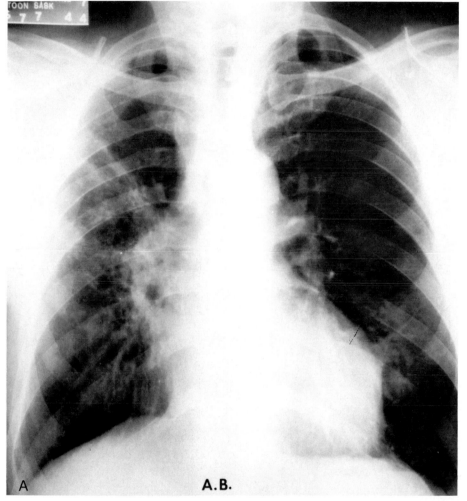

Figure 11–14. Tracheobroncho-pathia Osteochondroplastica. A posteroanterior chest roentgenogram *(A)* reveals general overinflation and oligemia indicating diffuse emphysema.

Illustration continued on following page

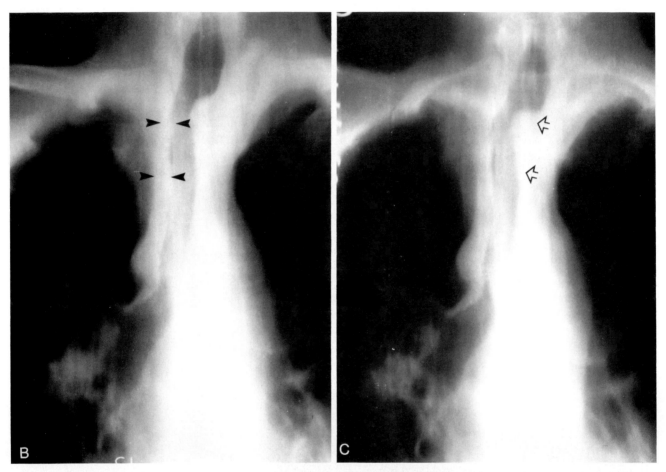

Figure 11–14. *Continued.* Linear tomograms through the trachea (*B* and *C*) reveal an eccentric mass *(open arrowheads)* distorting the tracheal air column; there is more diffuse mural thickening of the trachea caudally *(arrowheads)*. At autopsy, squamous metaplasia of the luminal epithelium, atrophy of submucosal glands, and submucosal nodular deposits of bone containing bone marrow were seen as a haphazard but diffuse change within the trachea and major bronchi. The patient is an elderly man with a long history of a chronic nonproductive cough.

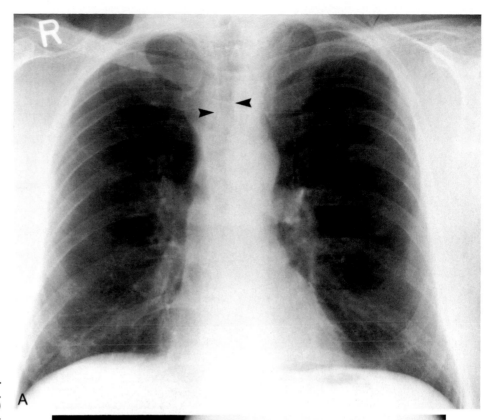

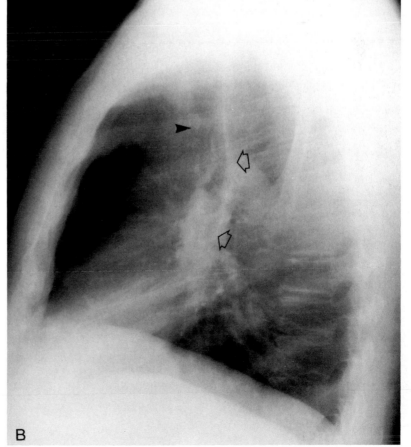

Figure 11–15. Tracheobronchopathia Osteochondroplastica. Posteroanterior *(A)* and lateral *(B)* chest roentgenograms show a narrowed and irregular contour of the tracheal air column *(arrowheads)*; the intermediate stem line is thickened *(open arrowheads)*.

Illustration continued on following page

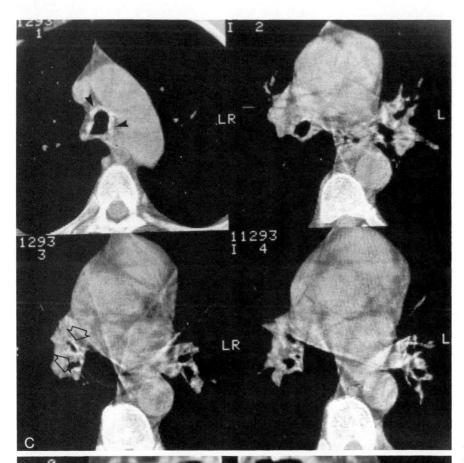

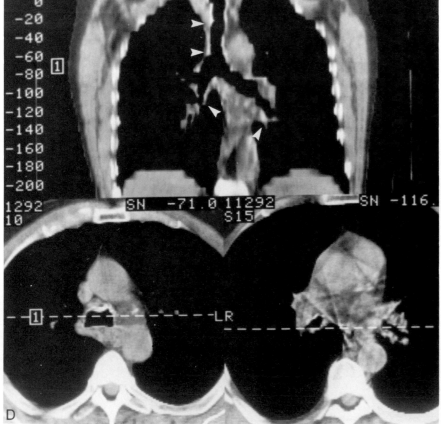

Figure 11–15. *Continued.* A series of CT scans through the tracheobronchial tree *(C)* demonstrate a diffusely thickened and irregularly calcified wall of the trachea and lobar and segmental bronchi. The calcification involves the anterior and lateral wall of the trachea *(arrowheads)* but spares the posterior wall; however, in the lobar and more distal bronchial walls, it is circumferential *(open arrows).*

Illustration continued on opposite page

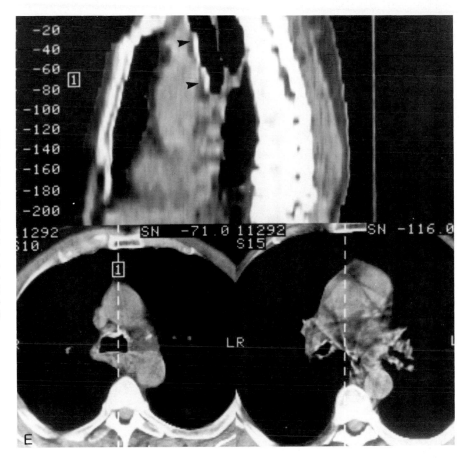

Figure 11–15. *Continued.* Coronal *(D)* and sagittal *(E)* CT reformations (and their appropriate transverse images) through the carina confirm the extensive tracheal and bronchial wall calcification *(arrowheads)*. The tracheal lumen is irregular and slightly narrowed anteriorly and on its right lateral wall. At bronchoscopy, the epithelium was thickened and thrown into undulating folds. A mucosal biopsy disclosed squamous metaplasia; submucosal tissue was not included in the specimen. With these roentgenographic findings, the differential diagnosis should include diffuse tracheobronchial amyloidosis. The patient is a 62-year-old man with a chronic nonproductive cough.

Tracheomalacia

Tracheomalacia (tracheobronchomalacia) is a descriptive term that refers to weakness of the tracheal walls and supporting cartilages with resultant easy collapsibility. It is most often acquired, secondary usually to intubation or COPD but occasionally to trauma, chronic or recurrent infection, or relapsing polychondritis.[177] It can also be seen as a primary condition, most often in children and usually associated with a deficiency of cartilage in the tracheobronchial tree.[178, 179] In such circumstances, it may be associated with other anomalies such as laryngomalacia and cleft palate.[180, 181] As with tracheobronchomegaly, abnormal flaccidity causes inefficiency of the cough mechanism, resulting in the retention of mucus, recurrent pneumonitis, and bronchiectasis. Symptoms include stridor and shortness of breath. In both tracheomalacia and tracheobronchomegaly, bronchography reveals dilatation of the conducting airways during inspiration and their premature collapse during expiration.[150, 179, 180] During fiberoptic bronchoscopy of conscious normal subjects, a voluntary cough produces less than 40 per cent narrowing of the anteroposterior tracheal diameter. In acquired tracheomalacia, the narrowing is greater than 50 per cent and in the presence of severe disease the anterior and posterior walls can actually come in contact.[182] These changes in tracheobronchial dynamics may be particularly well illustrated cinefluorographically. With the exception of those patients in whom tracheomalacia follows tracheostomy or endotracheal intubation, we suspect that this condition is related to the increased compliance and premature collapse of major airways usually associated with severe COPD *(see* page 2144).

Miscellaneous Causes of Upper Airway Obstruction

Vascular malformations of the great vessels can cause obstruction of the trachea and main bronchi, the commonest being double and right-sided aortic arch; aberrant subclavian, innominate, or common carotid arteries have also been reported to cause airway compression,[183] as have aneurysms of the ascending aorta.[184] Ankylosis of the cricoarytenoid joint in patients with long-standing rheumatoid arthritis can result in severe airway obstruction.[185] Sarcoidosis,[186] amyloidosis (Fig. 11–16),[187] and substernal goiter[188] should also be borne in mind when evaluating a patient with chronic upper airway obstruction. Additional rare causes of upper airway narrowing include acromegaly,[189] cervical osteophytes, diffuse ankylosing spondylitis of the cervical spine,[190, 191] intratracheal thymus,[41] and epidermolysis bullosa dystrophica.[42] In Africa, South America,

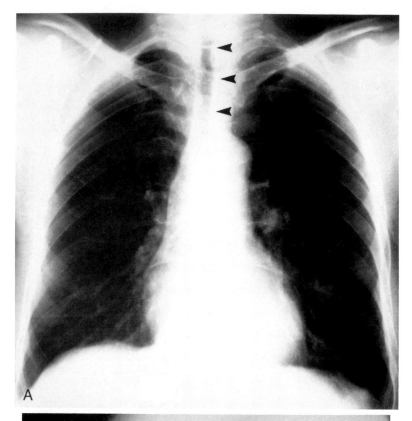

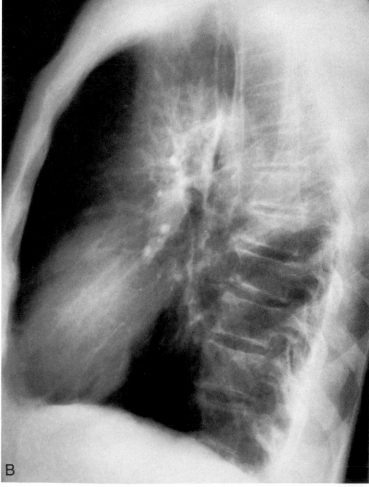

Figure 11–16. Laryngotracheobronchial Amyloidosis. Posteroanterior *(A)* and lateral *(B)* chest roentgenograms reveal diffuse narrowing and internal lobulation of the tracheal air column *(arrowheads)*. The lungs are slightly overinflated, but the pulmonary vasculature is normal.

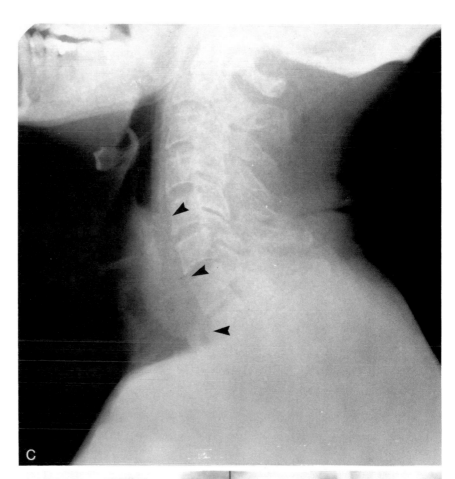

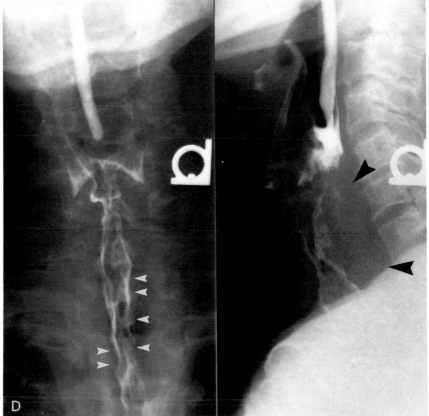

Figure 11–16. *Continued.* A lateral view of the neck *(C)* shows a posteriorly located laryngotracheal soft tissue mass *(arrowheads).* Faint stippled calcification is suggested within the lesion. Detail views of the larynx and trachea from a laryngotracheogram in anteroposterior and lateral projections *(D)* confirm the presence of an intraluminal soft tissue mass *(large black arrowheads),* encroaching upon the sagittal diameter of the tracheal air column; note the more diffuse nodular coronal narrowing of the proximal and middle parts of the trachea *(small white arrowheads).* A biopsy of the proximal mass disclosed amyloidosis. The patient is a middle-aged man with a forced expiratory wheeze.

and Asia, chronic granulomatous infection with *Klebsiella rhinoscleromatis* can cause obstruction of the larynx and trachea.[136] Benisch and his colleagues[192] have described an apparently unique case of focal muscular hypoplasia of the posterior tracheal wall associated with dysphagia and shortness of breath.

OBSTRUCTIVE SLEEP APNEA

Our knowledge of this relatively common disorder has increased exponentially over the past 15 years, and the diagnosis and management of affected patients has achieved virtual subspecialty status among respiratory physicians. To understand its pathophysiology, it· is necessary to have some knowledge of the physiologic interactions of sleep and breathing. Sleep has profound effects on respiratory system mechanics, the control of breathing, metabolism, and hemodynamics.

Sleep is categorized as either non–rapid eye movement (NREM) or rapid eye movement (REM) based on the electroencephalographic (EEG) pattern and on the presence or absence of rapid phasic eye movements on an electro-oculogram. NREM sleep is subdivided into four stages in which progressively slower EEG activity is associated with specific events called *sleep spindles* and *K complexes*:[193] stages 1 and 2 make up *light sleep*, during which breathing is unsteady and irregular; stages 3 and 4 make up *slow-wave sleep*, during which breathing is at its most regular.

During the initial 10 to 60 minutes of sleep, frequent changes occur between wakefulness and stages 1 and 2; this unsteady phase of NREM sleep is associated with periodic breathing. Major cyclic variations occur in tidal volume and the breathing pattern may resemble Cheyne-Stokes or Biot breathing. The periods of relative hyperpnea may be followed by brief central apneas, i.e., without respiratory effort. The oscillations in breathing patterns correlate with oscillations in sleep stage and are probably related to differences in the setpoint for regulation of ventilation in the awake and asleep states.[193] During unsteady NREM sleep, the average minute ventilation (VE) decreases and alveolar and arterial P_{CO_2} increase slightly.

With the onset of steady NREM sleep (stages 3 and 4), breathing becomes remarkably regular, although VT and overall VE decrease further as a result of a decrease in VT/TI (mean inspiratory flow) with little or no change in the ratio of inspiratory time to total respiratory cycle time (duty cycle). The decrease in ventilation ranges from 5 to 30 per cent of awake VE, and although part of this is related to a decreased metabolic rate, there is net alveolar hypoventilation because end-tidal and arterial P_{CO_2} increase from 2 to 7 mm Hg.[194–196] The decrease in tidal volume during NREM sleep is not caused by a decrease in respiratory muscle electromyographic (EMG) activity; in fact, EMG activity of

the intercostal muscles may actually increase during this stage of sleep.[197] Despite preserved muscle activation, a decrease in VE suggests increased impedance; during sleep, upper airway resistance increases by over 50 per cent whereas lower airway resistance does not change.[198] The increased upper airway resistance is caused by decreased activation of the upper airway dilating and stabilizing muscles—the superior and inferior hyoid, the genioglossus, and the tensor palati.

Coincident with the onset of REM sleep, breathing becomes irregular again. Tidal volume decreases concomitantly with the development of episodes of rapid eye movements, and an irregular pattern of rapid shallow breathing is observed. In contrast to NREM sleep, there is a substantial decrease in intercostal EMG activation and in the contribution of the rib cage to tidal volume. Although diaphragmatic EMG activity may increase, there is an overall decrease in VE despite considerable fluctuation in breath-by-breath alveolar ventilation. The decreased intercostal activation is secondary to the generalized supraspinal inhibition of alpha–motor neuron drive and the depression of fusimotor function that occurs during REM sleep. The resultant muscular atonia affects most skeletal muscles, including those in the upper airways, resulting in a further increase in upper airway resistance.[193]

Ventilatory chemosensitivity decreases during all stages of sleep, both hypoxic and hypercapnic ventilatory responses being depressed. The slope describing the relationship between change in arterial O_2 saturation and ventilation is a useful index of ventilatory chemosensitivity to hypoxia; the slope can decrease by a third to a half of its value during wakefulness, a drop that is particularly prominent in men.[199] Depression in the slope of the relationship between changes in P_{CO_2} and changes in ventilation that characterizes the hypercapnic response is similar in both men and women. In general, the depression in chemosensitivity is more pronounced during REM than during NREM sleep.

During wakefulness, the addition of an external resistive load results in rapid adjustment in ventilatory drive so that VT and VE are restored to their preload values; this load detection is dependent on lung and chest wall afferent input. During sleep, the compensatory response to added external resistive loads is diminished. Load compensation during loaded breathing is tested for by occluding the airway and measuring the pressures generated in the first 0.1 second (P0.1) of the occluded breath; during resistive loading, P0.1 does not increase as much during sleep as it does during the awake state.[199]

Thus, sleep is a time of particular vulnerability for the respiratory system—the resistance of the system is increased and at the same time both chemical and mechanical sensors of trouble are depressed. The ultimate safeguard is arousal, which results in a rapid decrease in upper airway resistance and an increased sensitivity of the chemical and mechanical responses.[200] Surprisingly, alteration in arterial blood gases is relatively ineffective in causing arousal during sleep;[199, 201, 202] for example, in some individuals, arterial Po_2 values of 40 mm Hg do not induce arousal. Arousal is defined as the simultaneous presence of EMG activation, eye movements, and alpha EEG activity—i.e., a short neurologic awakening. When these persist for longer than 15 seconds, they constitute a true awakening. To induce wakefulness in normal individuals, an increase in Pco_2 of 15 mm Hg or more may be required. Considerable individual variation exists in the threshold for arousal in response to changes in blood gases or in response to added loads, a variation in responsiveness that may be an important risk factor for obstructive sleep apnea.

Diagnostic Techniques

The diagnosis of obstructive sleep apnea requires the study of breathing during sleep. The techniques of polysomnography have been reviewed;[203, 204] for physicians interested specifically in respiration, these include sleep staging and the measurement of respiratory effort, air flow, and changes in arterial blood gas tensions. Sleep staging is accomplished by recording the EEG (usually two electrode positions), the electro-oculogram, and the EMG of a skeletal muscle (usually submental muscle). The frequency and amplitude of the brain waves are the most important signals used in sleep staging.

During wakefulness, the EEG is dominated by rapid, relatively low-amplitude waves called *alpha waves* (7 to 16 cycles/second). At the onset of stage 1 sleep, periods of lower-frequency activity are interspersed with alpha waves. During stage 2 sleep, the low-amplitude, mixed-frequency EEG activity continues but is mixed with brief episodes of high-frequency, low-amplitude rhythmic bursts (sleep spindles) and with well-defined, higher-amplitude negative deflections that are followed by sharp positive waves (K complexes). Tonic EMG activity is slightly decreased during stages 1 and 2 sleep, and there are no eye movements. Approximately 50 per cent of sleep is spent in stage 2. Stages 3 and 4 are called *slow-wave sleep* and are characterized by high-amplitude, low-frequency periods of EEG activity (0.1 to 3 cycles/second). Stage 4 is distinguished from stage 3 by a greater amount of time occupied by the low-frequency pattern, slow waves constituting over 50 per cent. During stages 3 and 4, EMG activity decreases further and there are no eye movements. Between 8 and 20 per cent of sleep is characterized by slow waves. The onset of REM sleep is signaled by a return to low-amplitude, rapid-frequency EEG waves and by episodic bursts of rapid eye movements detected by electro-oculography. The EMG shows virtual absence of activity with the exception of bursts of activity during rapid eye movement. Approximately 20 to 25 per cent of sleep is spent in REM sleep. Stages vary throughout sleep, and on average about 40 changes occur between stages during a sleep of 7.5 hours' duration.

Sleep is staged by visually scoring the polysomnographic record and categorizing short time periods (called *epochs*) into the appropriate stage based on the EMG, electro-oculogram, and EEG. In addition to the stages, it is possible to determine the total time asleep, sleep latency, sleep efficiency, and the number of arousals. Sleep latency is the time taken to fall asleep, and sleep efficiency is the time spent asleep divided by the time in bed. With normal aging, sleep efficiency decreases and sleep latency and the number of awakenings increase.

During sleep, respiration is assessed by measuring airflow and respiratory movement. Respiratory effort can be determined with devices that measure rib cage and/or abdominal movement or changes in intrathoracic pressure. Chest and abdominal movements can be measured with a circumferential strain gauge, by transthoracic impedance pneumography, or, more commonly, by respiratory inductance plethysmography (Respitrace). It is important to measure rib cage and abdominal motion separately because the paradoxical chest wall motion that occurs during obstructive sleep apnea can result in little change in net volume; i.e., as the rib cage expands, there is an equal and opposite inward motion of the abdominal wall. Respiratory effort can be sensitively detected by measuring changes in esophageal pressure, but this is invasive and not used routinely.

Respiratory air flow can be measured with a thermistor, a microphone, a pneumotachograph, or an expired CO_2 sensing device. The thermistor is a thermally sensitive electrical resistor that, when properly positioned, changes its electrical resistance in response to inspiratory cooling and expiratory warming, causing a signal that is in phase with flow. A thermistor must be positioned over the nose and mouth to detect breathing through these orifices. A microphone placed over the trachea provides a simple but effective signal of respiratory airflow.[212] A CO_2 sensor positioned over the nose or mouth detects expired CO_2 and is a useful noninvasive means of sensing respiratory air flow. A pneumotachograph requires the use of a face mask that can interfere with sleep and with the breathing pattern during sleep; however, only this device provides an estimate of tidal volume.

Changes in arterial blood gas concentration and arterial oxygen saturation can be monitored noninvasively, the most commonly used device being a pulse-type or transmittance-type ear oximeter. A probe applied to the ear or finger provides a continuous reading of arterial oxygen saturation. There are also devices which can measure mean capillary Po_2 and Pco_2 transcutaneously. The final measurements that complete a polysomnographic record are an electrocardiogram (ECG) to record cardiac dysrhythmias and an audio signal to detect snoring.

A complete overnight sleep study with full polysomnography is expensive and time-consuming. The results of one study suggest that an accurate estimate of apnea index, total apnea time, mean apnea time, mean oxygen saturation, sleep efficiency, and sleep staging can be achieved by examining as little as 20 per cent of an overnight sleep record.[213] The increasing recognition of patients with sleep-disordered breathing has put a heavy burden on sleep laboratories, and there is much incentive to develop easier and cheaper screening techniques.[214] Ambulatory monitoring systems are commercially available[204] although at present none of these provides sufficiently accurate data to replace overnight monitoring.[215, 216] Observation of a patient during sleep either directly or on a video recording can provide valuable qualitative information about breathing during sleep and can be used to diagnose obstructive sleep apnea but not to assess its severity.

Pathogenesis

Obstructive sleep apnea is the clinical syndrome of asphyxia and sleep fragmentation caused by repeated episodes of upper airway obstruction. The episodes of obstruction and apnea occur during all stages of sleep but especially during stage 2 of NREM sleep and during REM sleep, when the apneas tend to be the longest and the resultant arterial desaturation most severe.[217] The precise mechanism(s) that cause the obstruction are not completely understood, although its usual anatomic location at the level of the oropharynx has been well established. The factors that have been implicated in pathogenesis include an anatomically narrowed airway, an abnormally collapsible airway (increased compliance), decreased neural drive to upper airway dilating muscles, decreased chemoreceptor stimulation and load compensation of upper airway dilating muscles,[218] and uncoordinated activation of the upper airway muscles.[219]

STRUCTURAL NARROWING

Structural narrowing of the upper airway is a definite predisposing factor in obstructive sleep apnea and may be caused by congenital or acquired abnormalities. In some patients, the narrowing is caused by pathologic abnormalities such as enlarged adenoids and tonsils (particularly in children), macroglossia in myxedema, or acromegaly and micrognathia in facial dysmorphia (e.g., in the Pierre Robin syndrome) (Table 11–1).[220] Although the obstruction of sleep apnea usually occurs at the level of the oropharynx, it can be precipitated by airway narrowing upstream (such as in the nasal passages) by virtue of the more negative downstream inspiratory pressures that must be generated.[221] Nasal

Table 11–1. Unusual Causes of Obstructive Sleep Apnea

ENDOCRINE DISORDERS
  Macroglossia in myxedema
  Macroglossia in acromegaly
FACIAL DYSMORPHIA
  Micrognathia
  Retrognathia
  Pierre Robin syndrome
  Crouzon's disease
  Treacher-Collins syndrome[205]
  Frontal metaphyseal dysplasia
  Hallermann-Streiff syndrome[205]
NEUROMUSCULAR DISORDERS
  Chiari malformations
  Syringobulbia
  Cerebral palsy
  Myotonic dystrophy
  Shy-Drager syndrome[206]
  Chronic alcoholism[207]
  Phrenic and/or recurrent laryngeal nerve paralysis[208]
OTHER
  Hypertrophy of adenoids and tonsils
  Tonsillar lymphoma[209]
  Oropharyngeal malignancy
  Oral cysts[210]
  Retrosternal goiter[211]

obstruction necessitates mouth breathing, which itself can precipitate obstructive apnea. In normal men, mechanical nasal obstruction during sleep causes apneas and episodic arterial oxygen desaturation.[222, 223] The effect of nasal obstruction may be related in part to the bypassing of nasal flow and temperature receptors because stimulation of these receptors may cause reflex activation of upper airway dilating muscles; this hypothesis has been strengthened by the observation that nasal and oropharyngeal anesthesia unassociated with obstruction can induce nocturnal apnea in normal subjects.[224, 225]

Besides these well-defined causes for anatomic narrowing of the upper airway, CT studies of the oropharyngeal airway sometimes show a narrowing of the airway not attributable to any specific cause. Tongue size also has a wide normal range, and individuals with large tongues may be at risk of developing obstructive sleep apnea. The tongue forms the anterior wall of the oropharynx; both the supine posture and opening of the mouth tend to displace the tongue posteriorly and encourage airway closure.

Felman and his colleagues[226] performed cinefluorography of the upper airways of nine children during sleep and found that during inspiration the tongue and hypopharyngeal soft tissues approximated, obliterating the hypopharyngeal airspace and causing intermittent and almost complete obstruction to air flow. In two other reported cases, cinefluorography of the upper airways during sleep revealed recurrent rhythmic posterior retraction of the tongue with each inspiratory effort, the tongue coming into apposition with the posterior pharyngeal wall.[77]

Lowe and associates[227] studied the upper airway anatomy of 25 adult men with obstructive sleep apnea using three-dimensional CT reconstructions (Fig. 11–17). In the majority of subjects, measurement of the cross-sectional area of the upper airway at different levels revealed the narrowest point to be in the orophyarnx (0.52 ± 0.18 cm^2); in some subjects, however, a second narrowing was seen at the level of the hypopharynx. The investigators also measured the volume of the tongue and found that subjects with larger tongues experienced more severe obstructive sleep apnea and had a smaller airway lumen.

Similar images can be obtained with MRI without radiation exposure. Because MRI is sensitive in detecting water content, it may prove useful in determining whether significant soft tissue swelling contributes to the upper airway narrowing (Fig. 11–18).[228]

In patients with obstructive sleep apnea, ceph-

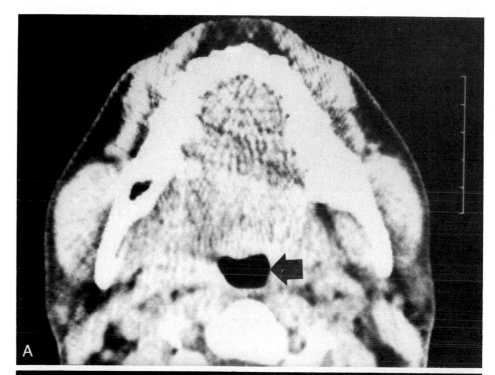

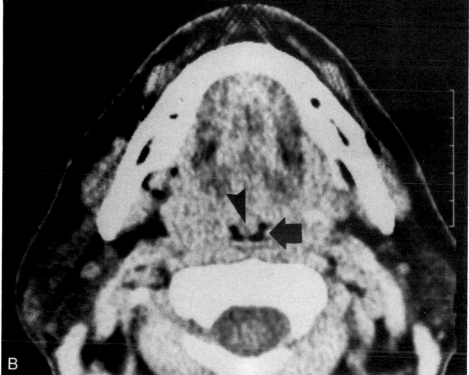

Figure 11–17. Computed Tomography (CT) of the Upper Airway in a Normal Subject and a Patient with Obstructive Sleep Apnea. A CT slice at the level of the oropharynx in a normal subject *(A)* reveals a widely patent oropharynx *(arrow).* In a patient with obstructive sleep apnea, a CT slice at approximately the same level *(B)* shows a markedly reduced cross-sectional area of the airway *(arrowhead)* and a prominent uvula *(arrow).*

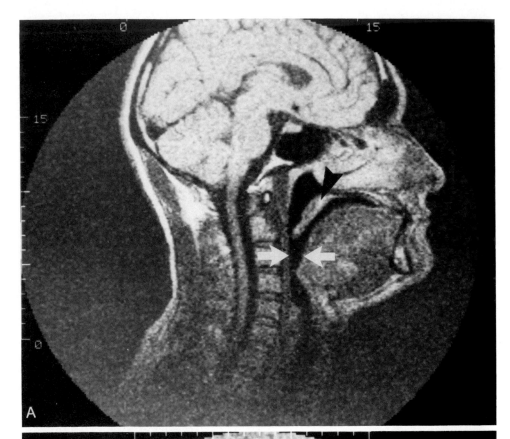

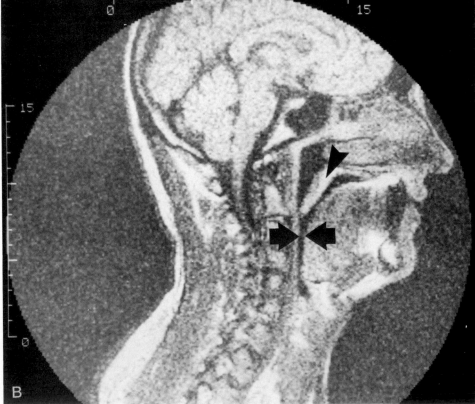

Figure 11–18. Magnetic Resonance Imaging (MRI) of the Upper Airway in a Normal Subject and a Patient with Obstructive Sleep Apnea. A sagittal reconstructed magnetic resonance image of the head and neck of a normal subject *(A)* demonstrates the uvula *(arrowhead)* and hypopharyngeal airway *(arrows)*. A similar image of a patient with obstructive sleep apnea *(B)* reveals a slightly enlarged uvula *(arrowhead)* and a markedly narrowed hypopharyngeal airway *(arrows)*. These images were obtained at 8:00 A.M. following an overnight sleep study.

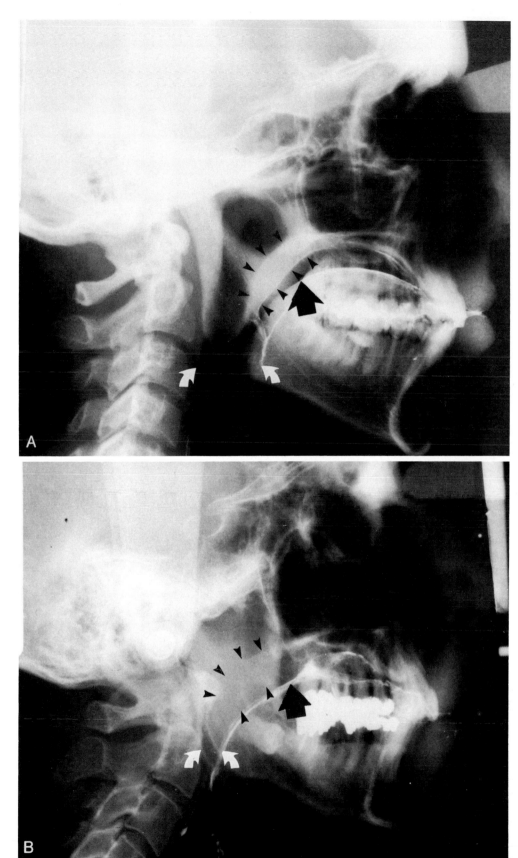

Figure 11–19. Lateral Roentgenography of the Upper Airway in a Normal Subject and a Patient with Obstructive Sleep Apnea.
A lateral roentgenogram of the face and neck *(A)* of a normal subject after ingestion of barium paste to outline the top of the tongue *(large arrows)* reveals a widely patent airway. A similar view in a patient with obstructive sleep apnea *(B)* shows a markedly narrowed oropharynx *(large arrow)* and hypopharynx *(curved arrows)* and a very large uvula *(arrowheads)*.

alometric roentgenograms of the face demonstrate a high incidence of skeletal abnormalities in addition to the soft tissue abnormalities described above (Fig. 11–19). When compared with a reference population, 150 of 155 patients with obstructive sleep apnea exhibited at least two significant abnormalities of cephalometric landmarks;[229] the most common abnormalities were retroposition of the mandible and inferior displacement of the hyoid bone.

It is possible that some of the pharyngeal narrowing seen in patients with obstructive sleep apnea occurs as a result of the obstruction rather than the cause; many patients have swollen pharyngeal walls and soft palate as well as a pendulous uvula,[219] and it is possible that chronic obstruction and snoring could cause edema of these structures because of the very negative intrapharyngeal pressures that are engendered. If swelling does occur because of these mechanisms, it could exacerbate obstructive apnea.

These anatomic causes of narrowing of the upper airway may be suggested by abnormalities of inspiratory and expiratory flow-volume curves.[230] In one study of 60 patients referred for investigation of possible obstructive sleep apnea, 14 of 35 with confirmed obstructive sleep apnea had a ratio of maximal mid-expiratory to mid-inspiratory flow greater than 1:

$$Vmax_{50}E/Vmax_{50}I > 1.0$$

In only two of the 25 patients without demonstrable obstruction was the ratio greater than 1.[231] The measurement of inspiratory and expiratory flow-volume curves in the supine position increases the sensitivity of distinguishing patients with and without obstructive sleep apnea. The presence of a "saw-toothed" curve was 92 per cent specific in differentiating 17 patients with obstruction and 13 non-affected individuals (Fig. 11–20).[232] "Saw-toothing"

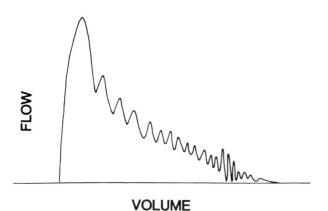

VOLUME

Figure 11–20. A "Saw-Toothed" Flow-Volume Curve. This flow-volume curve was obtained in a patient with Parkinson's disease. It shows reduced maximal expiratory flow and a rhythmic fluctuation in flow throughout expiration caused by the "tremor" in the upper airways and expiratory muscles.

and mid–vital capacity flow ratios greater than 1 correlate with pharyngeal airway narrowing detected during fiberoptic nasopharyngoscopy.[233] Snorers may exhibit flow-limited inspiration during sleep as a result of a flow-limiting segment in the oropharynx similar to the flow-limiting airway collapse that occurs in the intrathoracic airways during maximal expiratory flow maneuvers.[234]

INCREASED COMPLIANCE

Increased compliance of the upper airway is the second major factor that has been implicated in the pathogenesis of obstructive sleep apnea. The compliance of the upper airway can be measured during sleep by applying negative pressure at the airway opening and determining the negative pressure that will result in airway closure.[235–237] In normal subjects, negative pressures less than -25 cm H_2O can be applied before closure occurs; in patients with obstructive sleep apnea, however, closure occurs with pressures as small as -0.5 cm H_2O. The airway is most compliant during REM sleep, during which the average closing pressure is -2.4 cm H_2O; it is most stable during slow-wave sleep, when the average closing pressure is -4.2 cm H_2O. It has been shown that closing pressure is less negative in the supine than in the lateral decubitus position.[237] In snoring subjects with and without obstructive sleep apnea, Brown and associates[238] measured pressure-area curves of the pharynx using the acoustic reflection technique. They found that the specific compliance of the oropharynx was 2.5-fold greater in individuals with nocturnal obstruction.

Bradley and associates[239] measured pharyngeal cross-sectional area and compliance in normal subjects and in snorers with and without obstructive sleep apnea; they found that although airway size was decreased in all the snorers, those with obstructive sleep apnea also had unstable hypercollapsible pharyngeal airways at low lung volumes. Once the airway closes, the pressure necessary to re-establish patency increases as a result of surface adhesive forces.[240] In human infant cadavers, the oropharynx closes when -0.04 cm H_2O pressure is applied, whereas much more negative pressure is required to close the nasopharynx and hypopharynx; pressures as low as -60 cm H_2O are necessary to close the larynx.[241] Although the principal site of airway narrowing in obstructive sleep apnea is the oropharynx, there is evidence that the nasopharyngeal airway is also narrower and more compliant.[242] The site of the major increase in resistance can differ from patient to patient, which may explain why a single surgical procedure is not universally successful therapy.[243]

NEUROMUSCULAR DYSFUNCTION

Neuromuscular dysfunction of the upper airway muscles is the third factor that contributes to the development of obstructive sleep apnea. Twenty-three pairs of muscles encircle the pharyngeal airway, the majority of which dilate and stabilize the pharynx when they contract. These dilating muscles include the paired genioglossi, the geniohyoid, the hypoglossus, the tensor palati, and the thyrohyoid. Contraction of these muscles stiffens the walls of the oropharynx, counteracting the tendency of the airway to narrow in response to the negative intraluminal pressure that develops during inspiration. They display tonic and phasic respiratory EMG activity. Their inspiratory activation (via the 12th cranial nerve) typically precedes phrenic activity by 50 to 100 milliseconds so that the upper airway is dilated and stiffened before the onset of the negative intraluminal pressure that develops with inspiratory air flow.[244, 245]

Periodic and parallel fluctuations in diaphragmatic and genioglossal muscle EMG activity occur during sleep, the nadirs of these cycles occurring simultaneously with hypopneic episodes and central or obstructive apneas.[246, 247] The onset of REM sleep is associated with maximally decreased activation (hypotonia) of upper airway muscles, and since the decrease in diaphragmatic activation is less, REM sleep represents the period of maximal vulnerability for airway closure.[248] Periodic breathing can be induced with hypoxic inspiratory gas mixtures and in otherwise normal subjects can cause both episodic increase in upper airway resistance and apneas.[249] Patients with Cheyne-Stokes breathing also show an increased incidence of obstructive sleep apnea, supporting the contention that periodic breathing is important in the genesis of this condition.[250]

The activity of the upper airway dilating muscles is influenced by a number of inputs including changes in lung volume, changes in chemical drive, and input from upper airway receptors.[221] The increasing lung volume that occurs during inspiration suppresses the neural drive of the upper airway muscles. The afferent information about changes in lung volume comes from lung mechanoreceptors that run in the vagal nerve. The airway obstruction that occurs as a result of sleep apnea would be expected to increase the neural input because the inhibitory effect of lung inflation would be absent.[221] The neural drive to upper airway muscles also increases in response to hypercapnia and hypoxia.[251-253] Receptors in the upper airway mucosa can also reflexly influence pharyngeal muscle activation. There are receptors that respond to pressure, temperature, and muscle contraction, stimulation of which results in increased neural drive.[221]

Pharyngeal patency is promoted by input from all the factors discussed above. If the airway narrows, the more negative intraluminal pressure induced by inspiration stimulates mechanoreceptors; should the obstruction persist, a decrease in tidal volume and changes in arterial blood gas content augment muscle activity, thus tending to restore upper airway patency. These protective mechanisms

are depressed during sleep and by alcohol and sedative drugs.[254-258] It is still unclear whether a primary abnormality of these protective mechanisms is responsible for some cases of obstructive sleep apnea. An abnormality in neuromuscular control of upper airway caliber could be the factor that explains the familial tendency for the development of obstructive sleep apnea; in fact, a definite decrease in genioglossal activation during sleep has been reported in one family with the affliction.[259]

The sleep deprivation and hypoxia that result from obstructive sleep apnea can cause depression of phasic respiratory activity in the upper airway muscles and can lead to a vicious circle of worsening obstruction and more fragmented sleep.[221, 260, 261, 264] Evidence for this observation derives from direct recordings of genioglossal EMG activity[261] and from clinical studies in which the prolonged use of nasal positive pressure causes improvement in sleep apnea, even when patients are studied without nasal positive pressure.[221] This improvement may be the result of the beneficial effect of adequate sleep on the respiratory control centers. However, other explanations, such as a relief of pharyngeal edema, can also explain these observations. It is conceivable that fatigue could develop in the upper airway muscles if they were exposed to very negative intraluminal pressures, but there is no evidence that this occurs. However, there is some evidence to suggest that patients with obstructive sleep apnea have decreased central ventilatory drive and impaired load compensation in addition to decreased activation of upper airway muscles,[262] but it is unclear whether this impairment is a result of the disorder or a predisposing factor for its development.

The importance of coordinating the muscular dilatation and stabilization of the oropharynx with the muscular contraction of the respiratory pump is illustrated by case reports of patients in whom obstructive sleep apnea develops during diaphragmatic pacing.[263] During pacing the diaphragmatic contraction is not associated with synchronous activation of upper airway muscles, and if the patient does not have a tracheostomy, upper airway closure can develop. A similar sequence results in the airway closure that accompanies a hiccup.

The pathophysiologic sequence that results in obstructive sleep apnea has been described by Kuna and Remmers.[221] Oropharyngeal narrowing is caused by either structural changes or a diminution of the force generated by the muscles that maintain airway patency. The narrowing results in an increase in pharyngeal resistance that causes more negative intrapharyngeal inspiratory pressures and airway closure. Although airway closure increases the neural input to the pharyngeal dilator muscles, it also increases drive to the diaphragm and intercostal inspiratory muscles, thus generating more negative intra-airway pressures that keep the oropharynx closed. The only escape from such a vicious circle is arousal accompanied by higher center activation of the upper airway dilator muscles and consequent relief of the obstruction. For any given upper airway geometry, upper airway patency is dependent on the balance of activity of upper airway dilator muscles and the thoracic inspiratory muscles:[265] when the upper airway is narrowed to begin with, it becomes essential for activation of the upper airway muscles to be greater than that of the thoracic muscles in order to maintain airway patency. It is possible that in some individuals the primary problem is a narrow upper airway; in others, it may be decreased neural activation of upper airway muscles. Brief periods of central hypoventilation or apnea frequently precede and initiate the obstructive episodes in patients with obstructive sleep apnea; the mechanism of these central depressions may be the periods of hyperventilation that terminate the previous obstructive apneic episodes. The hypocapnia that results can depress the respiratory center and initiate the next apneic episode, thus setting up a vicious circle.[266] Activation of upper airway dilating muscles is depressed by alcohol[267] and by hypnotic sleeping pills,[268] both of which are known to exacerbate snoring and obstructive sleep apnea. Interestingly, narcotics that decrease ventilatory drive do not appear to increase the incidence of sleep apnea.[269]

It is not known which stimulus causes arousal during apneic episodes. Although hypoxemia seems to be the most obvious candidate, administration of oxygen does not invariably prolong the apneic episodes. Arousal frequently occurs when the amount of tension generated by the inspiratory muscles against the occluded upper airway approaches the amount of tension that causes muscle fatigue, suggesting that a message from inspiratory muscles may be an important arousal stimulus.[270]

Prevalence

The prevalence of obstructive sleep apnea in the general population is unknown. This uncertainty relates to the lack of a precise definition of the condition and to the time and expense involved in surveying a large population with formal polysomnography. One definition of obstructive sleep apnea—more than five apneas per hour of sleep, apnea being defined as the cessation of breathing for greater than 10 seconds—was derived from studies by Guilleminault and associates,[271, 272] which showed that normal individuals ranging in age from 18 to 60 years experienced fewer than 25 apneas a night, whereas every patient with symptomatic obstructive sleep apnea experienced more than 45 apneas per night. Using more than five apneas per hour as the diagnostic criterion, Lavie[273] found an incidence of obstructive sleep apnea of 1.26 per cent among 1,262 male industrial workers. More recent surveys suggest that this arbitrary definition may overestimate the true prevalence of the condition, especially in the older population;[274, 275] for example, in one study, 80 per cent of elderly subjects suffered more than five apneas an hour but only a small number of these had symptoms suggesting the presence of significant clinical consequences.[275] In one small "population" study of 46 healthy snoring males, 13 per cent had an apnea index (number of apneic episodes per hour of sleep) of more than 5; however, even in this "asymptomatic" group, apneic severity correlated with elevated blood pressures and with subjective evidence of sleepiness and napping frequency, suggesting that even "subclinical" levels of sleep apnea may not be completely benign.[276]

The factors that predispose to the development of obstructive sleep apnea are shown in Figure 11–21. Predominant risk factors are obesity and masculinity.[277] The condition develops six to ten times more frequently in men than women,[204] and in women it usually occurs in the postmenopausal period. Women with obstructive sleep apnea have elevated androgen levels, and administration of androgens can induce the abnormal state in previously unaffected men and women.[278–280] Androgen therapy in women can cause an increase in upper airway resistance, suggesting that these drugs can exert an effect on the structural configuration of the oropharynx.[281] These observations, together with the known ventilatory stimulant effect of medroxyprogesterone, have lead scientists to suggest that the male predominance is related to a detrimental effect of the hormone testosterone and the lack of a protective effect of the hormone progesterone.[278]

Pharyngeal cross-sectional area measured with the acoustic-reflection technique reveals no significant difference between men and women,[282] although one report suggests that pharyngeal resistance in men (4.6 cm H_2O/liter/second) is higher than in women (2.3 cm H_2O/liter/second) and that it tends to increase with increasing weight and height.[283] It is not clear how the sex hormones influence the caliber of the upper airway. Men and women normally breathe through the nose during sleep, although in older men a significantly greater proportion of nocturnal breathing is through the mouth.[284]

The relationship between obesity and obstructive sleep apnea is complex. The association of obesity with ventilatory abnormalities antedates the knowledge that nocturnal airway obstruction was the basic pathophysiologic problem. The association became fixed in medical teaching with the rediscovery of Dickens' classic clinical description of the fat boy who snored and had right ventricular failure.[285] The fat boy, Joe, in Dickens' *The Posthumous Papers of the Pickwick Club*, published in 1836, had all the features of what we now recognize as florid obstructive sleep apnea—he was an obese, plethoric, hypersomnolent snorer who had dropsy. In 1956, Burwell and his colleagues[285] described patients who had a similar syndrome and they called the clinical

Predisposing Factors	Underlying Mechanisms	Primary Events	Secondary Events	Clinical Complications
• Alcohol • Sedatives • Sleep loss	• ↓ Upper airway muscle activity	• Sleep onset	• Vibration of soft palate	• Snoring
• Obesity • Male gender • Testosterone • Familial history • Hypothyroidism • Acromegaly • Facial dysmorphia	• ↓ Oropharyngeal size	• Upper airway narrowing	• Pulmonary arterial vasoconstriction	• Pulmonary hypertension • Right heart failure
• Obesity	• ↑ Oropharyngeal compliance	• Obstructive apnea	• Systemic arterial vasoconstriction	• Systemic hypertension
• Nasal obstruction • Chronic rhinitis • U.R.T.I.	• ↑ Upstream airflow resistance	• ↓ PO_2, ↑ PCO_2 • ↓ pH	• Vagal bradycardia • Cardiac ischemia and irritability	• Cardiac arrhythmias • Sudden unexplained death
• Respiratory stimulants • Diaphragmatic pacemaker	• ↑ Negative inspiratory pressure	• Arousal from sleep	• Cerebral vascular dilation	• Morning headache
		• Resumption of airflow	• Hypothalmic - pituitary-testicular dysfunction	• Reduced libido • Impotence
• Obesity • Respiratory disease • Air travel • Altitude	• ↓ Baseline PO_2	• Return to sleep	• Stimulation of erythropoiesis	• Polycythemia
• Sedatives	• ↓ Peripheral chemoreceptor activity • ↓ CNS arousability		• Cerebral impairment and/or damage	• Excessive daytime sleepiness • Intellectual deterioration • Personality changes • Behavioral disorders
			• Sleep fragmentation • Loss of deep sleep	
			• Excessive motor activity	• Nocturnal "epilepsy"

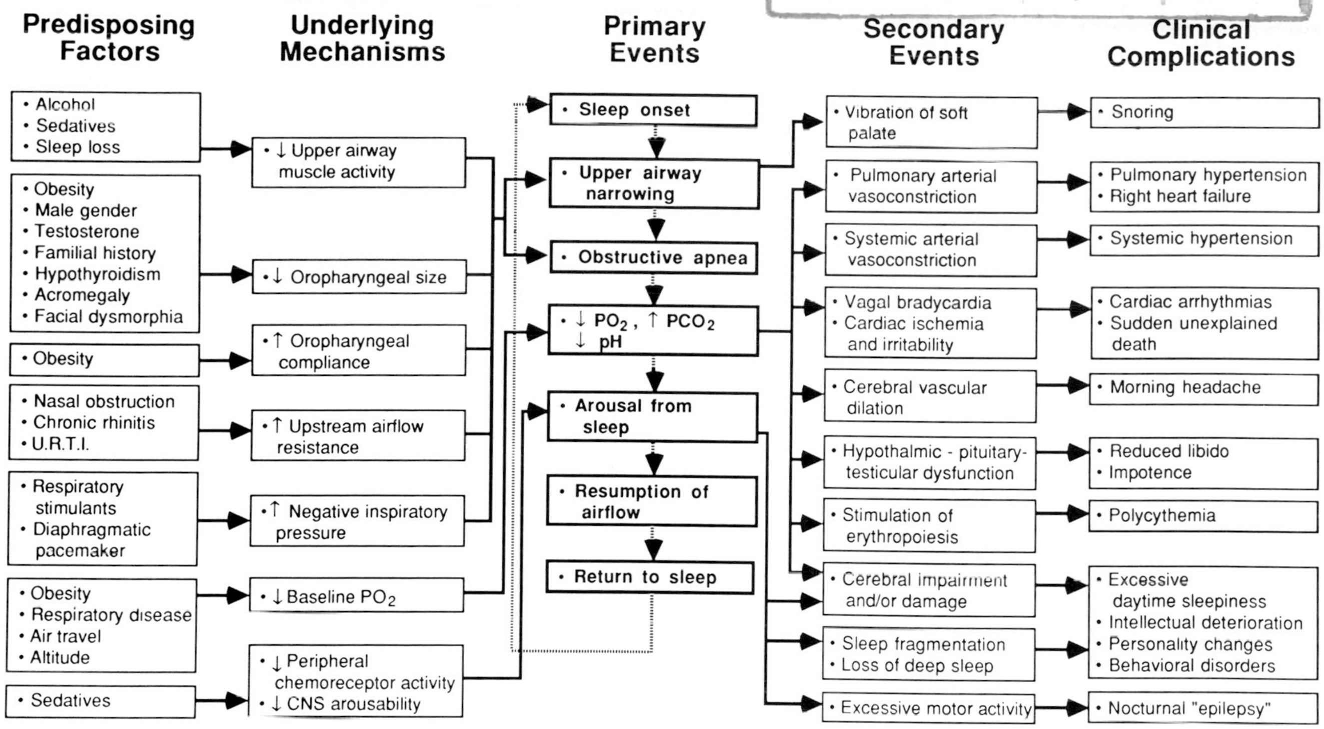

Figure 11–21. The Pathogenesis of Obstructive Sleep Apnea. (Modified from a table constructed by Dr. John Fleetham, Health Sciences Centre Hospital, University of British Columbia, Vancouver.)

constellation of obesity, hypoventilation, hypersomnolence, and right ventricular failure the "pickwickian syndrome." Even at that time, the pivotal role of nocturnal apnea was not appreciated; it was believed that obesity caused ventilatory depression and hypercapnia by increasing the mechanical load on the respiratory system and that it was the hypercapnia which caused the excessive daytime somnolence. It was also suggested that some primary hypothalamic defect might contribute to both the obesity and the decreased central respiratory drive.[285] Now that the pathophysiology of obstructive sleep apnea is understood, the retrospectoscope has allowed identification of individuals whose personalities and behavior were shaped by obstructive sleep apnea; for example, Phillipson has suggested that the giant in *Jack and the Beanstalk* suffered from the disorder because he was fat and irritable and snored during sleep and fell asleep during the day.[286]

Although early reports suggested that obstructive sleep apnea occurs typically in very obese individuals, the diagnosis is now made more frequently in patients who are of normal weight or are only slightly overweight.[219] However, obesity is associated with a higher incidence and more severe form of the disorder. In individual patients the severity of obstructive sleep apnea is logarithmically related to body weight; i.e., a small decrease in body weight can result in a large decrease in the apnea index.[219, 287, 288] Similarly, from a prospective study of eight patients with obstructive sleep apnea before and after dietary-induced weight loss, Suratt and his

colleagues[289] concluded that moderate weight loss improves oxygenation during both sleep and wakefulness, decreases the number of disordered breathing events, and decreases the collapsibility of the nasopharyngeal airway.

The relationship between obesity and obstructive sleep apnea is complex and incompletely understood. It is possible that it increases the risk of the condition developing by affecting upper airway geometry. Deposition of adipose tissue in the submucosal connective tissue surrounding the oropharynx and in the soft palate can narrow the upper airway and increase its compliance. Using an acoustic reflection technique, Hoffstein and associates[290] showed that the pharyngeal cross-sectional area of obese patients with obstructive sleep apnea is less than that of equally obese patients without the disorder. Obesity also decreases FRC, especially in the supine posture; should FRC fall to below closing capacity, nocturnal hypoxemia would result, thus contributing to more severe arterial oxygen desaturation during apneic episodes. There is also a possibility that the converse of the obesity–obstructive sleep apnea relationship might occur; i.e., the sleep apnea might itself contribute to the development of obesity. Sullivan has shown that the successful treatment of obstructive sleep apnea by continuous positive nasal pressure facilitates subsequent weight reduction. He hypothesized that prolonged hypoxemia, hypercapnia, and sleep fragmentation could cause changes in hypothalamic-pituitary function, which favor the development of obesity.[219]

The interaction between obesity and gender

was demonstrated in one study in which seven male and seven female patients who were referred for surgery for morbid obesity participated in overnight sleep studies. Six of the seven men had apneic periods and significant arterial oxygen desaturation, whereas none of the women did; the one man in whom obstruction and desaturation did not develop had hypogonadism![291]

Clinical Manifestations

An almost invariable sign in patients who suffer from obstructive sleep apnea is snoring. However, the presence of snoring is by no means a sensitive indicator of the presence of the disorder. In a survey of 4,713 people, Lugaresi and associates[292] found that 41 per cent of men and 28 per cent of women were occasional or habitual snorers; the incidence in men and women over 60 years of age was higher—60 and 40 per cent, respectively. Despite these figures, only 1 to 2 per cent of the population suffers from symptomatic sleep apnea. The snoring of patients with the disorder tends to be loud, irregular, and very disturbing to bed partners, roommates, or others in the household. In the absence of obstructive sleep apnea, snoring appears to be a separate predictor of systemic arterial hypertension[293] and to increase the risk of cerebrovascular accidents.[294] In patients with obstructive sleep apnea, snoring is typically interrupted by frequent periods of silent apnea, during which progressively greater inspiratory efforts are expended against a completely closed airway. The apneic periods are terminated by loud snorting and motor activity associated with arousal. With resumption of sleep, rhythmic snoring returns, punctuated by frequent apneas, explosive snorts, and arousals.

Obtaining a history of snoring and a description of the snoring pattern is an important diagnostic step in the investigation of patients with suspected obstructive sleep apnea. Because patients cannot describe their own snoring, it is necessary to interview a spouse or bed partner. A history of loud snoring, interspersed with quiet periods, and ending with a loud snort and motor activity is strong evidence for the presence of the condition; a more rhythmic crescendo and decrescendo pattern indicates simple heavy snoring without apnea.[219] The loud and disturbing snoring and frequent arousals associated with obstructive sleep apnea can cause considerable disruption in the personal life of affected individuals; spouses cannot sleep in the same bed or in the same room (or occasionally in the same house!) and may actually be injured during the erratic motor activity that accompanies arousal. It is not surprising that marital problems are a frequent occurrence among patients with this disturbing disorder.

A characteristic symptom of obstructive sleep apnea, second in incidence only to snoring, is excessive daytime sleepiness. Its severity correlates with the intensity of nocturnal apnea and sleep deprivation and can be estimated by careful history taking.[219] There are three clinical levels of increasing severity.

In *Category 1*, or mild sleepiness, the individual falls asleep only when reading, watching television, or listening to lectures; although the sleepiness is more severe when the subject is overtired, it does not completely disappear despite a "good" night's sleep. The patient and his family do not view the sleepiness as a problem, nor does it interfere with the patient's work.

Category 2 is characterized by unequivocal hypersomnolence; the patient falls asleep not only while relaxing but also while engaged in activities such as driving. The patient and his family are aware that excessive sleepiness is a problem and is interfering with the individual's work.

Category 3 involves extreme sleepiness; the patient falls asleep while talking, eating, or relating his medical history. He is unable to work or drive a car.

The frequency and duration of nocturnal apneas and the severity of nocturnal arterial oxygen desaturation correlate well with the severity of hypersomnolence. Subjects in Category 1 typically experience 30 to 60 apneas per night, and arterial saturation rarely falls below 80 per cent. Individuals in Category 3 have more than 400 apneic episodes a night, and arterial oxygen saturation falls below 80 per cent during each episode; these patients spend most of the night either obstructed or awake. Pathologic hypersomnolence is easy to recognize in patients in Categories 2 and 3, but it can be difficult to make a diagnosis in those patients who have mildly excessive sleepiness (Category 1) in whom the symptoms may be difficult to distinguish from the normal sleepiness caused by "overtiredness"[219] or postprandial lethargy.

In addition to the clinical characterization of excessive sleepiness, hypersomnolence can be estimated quantitatively by the "multiple sleep latency test," which measures the rapidity with which a patient can fall asleep. The patient is given the opportunity to fall asleep during several daytime nap periods of 20 minutes each and is evaluated by EEG, EMG, and electro-oculography. The "latency" to sleep is defined as the time until the beginning of any sleep stage. The tendency to fall asleep quickly is indicative of pathologic hypersomnolence.[215]

The precise cause of the hypersomnolence of obstructive sleep apnea is not known. Although sleep fragmentation during the night is likely to contribute to hypersomnolence, it may not be the sole explanation. In one study, four patients with severe sleep apnea and hypersomnolence were compared with patients whose sleep apnea was equally severe but was unassociated with hypersomnolence: the former patients were more obese and demonstrated significantly more severe arterial oxygen desaturation while asleep and awake.[295] It is thus possible that the hypoxemia contributes to sleepiness;[296, 297] however, although hypersomnolence is rapidly corrected by tracheostomy or the use of continuous nasal positive pressure,[223] it is not improved by administration of long-term nocturnal oxygen therapy.[298]

Episodic hypoxemia and profound sleep fragmentation are also the most likely causes of the changes in personality and behavior that can accompany severe obstructive sleep apnea. Confusion with a psychiatric disorder is likely if the excessive sleepiness is attributed to depression. There is a striking incidence of severe psychosocial disruption in the lives of patients with sleep apnea that affects their family, social interactions, and work situations.[299]

The arterial oxygen desaturation associated with apneic episodes causes pulmonary arterial hypertension and an increase in right ventricular afterload.[300] Since prolonged pulmonary hypertension can result in irreversible vascular narrowing, the pulmonary hypertension may eventually persist during the waking hours, despite correction of hypoxemia; the almost inevitable result is cor pulmonale and ultimately right ventricular failure.[301] Patients in whom right ventricular failure develops experience not only severe arterial oxygen desaturation at night but also arterial oxygen desaturation and hypercapnia during the day.[302] In some patients, daytime hypoventilation is attributable partly to concomitant obstructive pulmonary disease[303] and partly to the central ventilatory depression that may be occasioned by prolonged sleep deprivation and hypoxemia.[304, 305]

The severity of nocturnal desaturation depends not only on the length of apneic periods but also on lung function while the patient is awake and on the pre-obstruction arterial Po_2. Because of the shape of the oxygen dissociation curve, considerable hypoxemia can occur without much desaturation if arterial Po_2 is normal to begin with. If significant hypoxemia precedes the apneic episodes, as it may in individuals with intrinsic pulmonary disease, a similar duration of apnea will cause more profound desaturation.[306] This may be another of the interactions of obesity with obstructive sleep apnea: because obesity causes a decrease in FRC in the supine position, it tends to diminish baseline, pre-apneic Po_2 and thus to exaggerate the asphyxic effects of an apnea.

Patients with obstructive sleep apnea may also present with systemic arterial hypertension[307–309] because nocturnal hypoxemia and respiratory acidosis cause smooth muscle contraction in the systemic as well as the pulmonary circulation. Sleep apnea must be considered a diagnostic possibility in hypertensive patients, especially when they are male, are obese, and have symptoms of hypersomnolence and snoring.[301] The abnormalities of arterial blood gas tensions not only affect vascular smooth muscle

function but can also affect cardiac muscle action. Although hypoxemia and hypercapnea cause tachycardia during wakefulness,[310] in sleep apnea they are more often associated with bradycardia and on rare occasions with serious conduction defects (e.g., heart block, sinus arrest) or dysrhythmias (e.g., ventricular tachycardia).[301, 311] Serious cardiac dysrhythmias are an important indication for prompt and definitive treatment because these patients are at risk for sudden unexplained nocturnal death.[312]

Prolonged hypoxemia and hypercapnia can cause decreased libido and impotence. Although, as discussed previously, testosterone is a risk factor for the development of sleep apnea, the presence of severe obstructive sleep apnea itself causes reduced serum testosterone levels, and successful treatment results in a return toward normal levels.[313] Nocturnal hypoxemia can also stimulate erythropoietin secretion and may cause secondary polycythemia, particularly in individuals with baseline arterial hypoxemia; in fact, nocturnal accentuation of arterial desaturation makes an important contribution to the polycythemia of obstructive pulmonary disease.[310]

The therapy of obstructive sleep apnea includes weight reduction, administration of respiratory stimulants, the use of continuous positive nasal pressure during sleep, oropharyngeal surgery, and tracheostomy. The choice of proper therapy depends on the careful assessment of severity.[2773] Moderate weight loss and a change in sleeping posture from supine to erect or lateral decubitus can be beneficial in alleviating the symptoms but are seldom sufficient to reverse moderate symptoms completely.[314, 315] In mild cases, medroxyprogesterone or tricyclic antidepressants may be tried but are incompletely effective in the vast majority of patients.[278] Nasal positive pressure is very effective therapy for obstructive as well as central sleep apnea (Fig. 11–22),[316, 317] but the major problem with this therapy is the compliance of the patients in continuing to use the device after the symptoms have been somewhat alleviated. In some patients, surgical removal of part of the uvula, soft palate, and pharyngeal wall (uvulopalatopharyngoplasty) causes long-term relief of symptoms; however, in others this procedure is ineffective and the challenge remains to select those patients who will benefit from it. The variation in response is probably related to the variable site of upper airway narrowing. The prospective use of cephalometric roentgenograms, somnofluoroscopy,[318] and CT reconstruction of the upper airway[2774] may prove to be beneficial in identifying those patients who will benefit from surgery and may aid in the planning of individual surgical procedures.[227, 319–321] Observation of the upper airway during fiberoptic nasopharyngoscopy during a Mueller maneuver can also aid in predicting a beneficial effect of uvulopalatopharyngoplasty.[322] Additional therapeutic benefits can be obtained

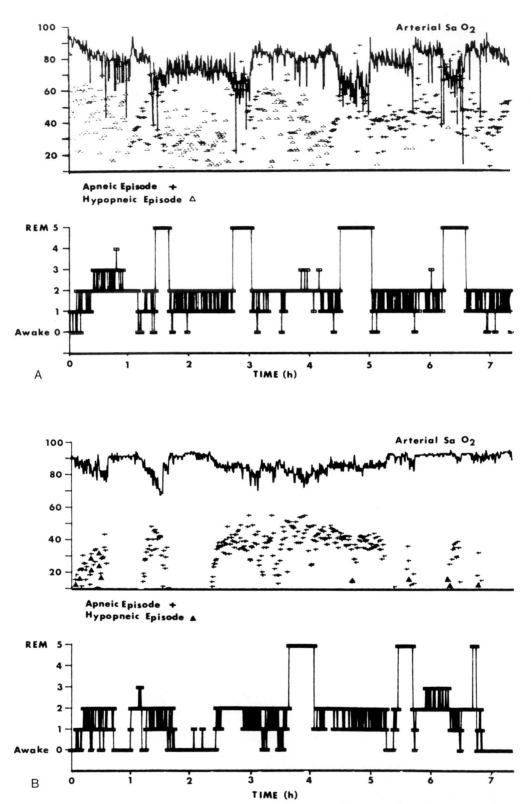

Figure 11–22. Overnight Sleep Studies in Patients with Obstructive Sleep Apnea. The upper panel in *A* depicts the variation in arterial oxygen saturation measured with an ear oximeter during a 7-hour overnight sleep study in a patient with severe obstructive sleep apnea. The vertical axis indicates the arterial saturation and the duration in seconds of apneic episodes (indicated by a plus sign) and hypopneic episodes (indicated by an open triangle). Note that frequent periods of severe desaturation occurred in association with the numerous hypopneic and apneic episodes. In the lower panel is depicted sleep staging, stage 0 being the awake state and state 5 rapid eye movement (REM) sleep. It is apparent that this subject spends much of his time awake or in stages 1 and 2 sleep. There are only brief episodes of REM sleep and these correspond with periods of more severe arterial desaturation.

A similar overnight sleep study *(B)* in an individual with less severe but still substantial obstructive sleep apnea shows the variation in arterial oxygen saturation and the duration of apneic and hypopneic episodes.

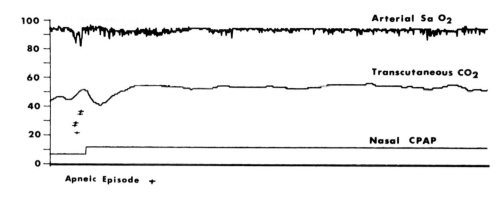

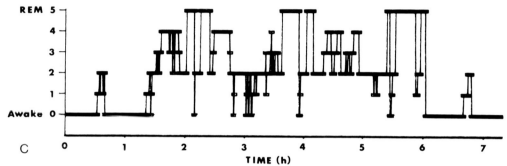

Figure 11-22. *Continued.* Compare the results with those obtained in the same individual in a repeat overnight sleep study *(C)* during application of nasal continuous positive airway pressure (CPAP). The upper panel shows transcutaneous carbon dioxide in addition to oxygen saturation and also depicts the application of nasal CPAP in cm H_2O. With the application of 7.5 cm H_2O CPAP, there was still slight desaturation and apnea; however, when CPAP was increased to 10 cm H_2O, there was a complete absence of apneic episodes, no periods of severe arterial saturation, and significantly increased REM sleep duration during the remainder of the night.
(Courtesy of Dr. John Fleetham, Health Sciences Centre Hospital, University of British Columbia, Vancouver.)

from maxillofacial surgery and the application of mandibular appliances that prevent the tongue from occluding the airway.[323]

ASTHMA

DEFINITIONS

Asthma is a disease characterized by wide variations over short periods of time in resistance to air flow in intrapulmonary airways.[324] The changes in severity of airway narrowing can occur spontaneously or as a result of therapy. In addition, asthmatic subjects show an increased responsiveness of the tracheobronchial tree to a variety of stimuli.[325]

The airway narrowing that occurs in asthma is intermittent and variable; complete remission can occur between attacks, although some abnormality of function is often detectable with sensitive tests.[326, 327] During attacks, widespread narrowing of the bronchi results in diffuse wheezing, often associated with dyspnea, even at rest. Although the reversibility of airway obstruction may be suspected from the clinical history, it should always be evaluated objectively by measurement of airway function after administration of a bronchodilator.[328]

Like COPD, the definition of asthma is functional and clinical and does not imply structural change or etiology.[324] The term is frequently mis-

used, being applied to "bronchospasm" or "wheezing" despite the recognition of other clinical entities that can produce intermittent airway obstruction. Asthma should be a diagnosis of exclusion. Several well-recognized diseases can present a clinical picture simulating asthma—acute bronchitis and bronchiolitis, chronic bronchitis, emphysema, bronchiectasis, lymphangitic carcinomatosis, cardiac disease associated with intermittent attacks of left-sided heart failure, and anatomic or functional upper airway obstruction. To apply the term "asthma" to the bronchial narrowing manifested by patients with these disorders is incorrect and inevitably results in confusion.

Although there may be some overlap, asthma can generally be characterized as falling into two major categories, extrinsic and intrinsic.

EXTRINSIC ASTHMA

Extrinsic asthma occurs in patients who are *atopic*, a term used to refer to the genetic predisposition to respond to antigenic challenge with excessive IgE production. The inheritance is complex but usually incomplete, increasing greatly if both parents are atopic. For example, of 13 children born of two allergic parents, 11 developed atopy over a 4-year follow-up period; viral upper respiratory infection frequently predated the onset of allergic manifestations, suggesting that interaction of viral infections with genetic predisposition may be important.[329] At least two separate gene loci, one of which is HLA-associated, appear to be involved.[330, 331] The reason for the high incidence of atopy (which appears to be harmful to the individual affected) is not clear. It has been hypothesized that the ability to respond with IgE antibody may have survival benefit in offering protection against parasitic infestations.[330] The genetic predisposition to IgE production may come about because of abnormalities in suppressor cell activity; a specific suppressor cell population keeps IgE production under control, and in animals an experimental reduction in suppressor cell function results in increased IgE levels. The suppressor cells of asthmatic patients may have a decreased responsiveness to some stimuli.[332] Allergen-specific IgE sensitivity can be transferred by bone marrow transplantation.[2775]

The prevalence of atopy increases until approximately age 20, when it gradually declines. Peak IgE levels occur at age 14; in infants and young children, atopy and asthma are twice as common in males.[330, 333, 334] Besides demonstrating increased blood levels of IgE, atopic individuals are characterized by immediate skin test responses to a variety of antigens and a high incidence of eczema, rhinitis, and asthma. However, atopy is not synonymous with asthma: the former occurs in over 30 per cent of the population, whereas the incidence of asthma (although variable) is generally less than 5 per cent. Although affected identical twins invariably develop atopy, their allergic manifestations and development of asthmatic symptoms and nonspecific bronchial responsiveness are discordant.[335, 336]

Patients with extrinsic, or atopic, asthma are distinguished by (1) a family history of atopy, (2) onset in the first three decades of life, (3) seasonal symptoms, (4) elevated blood levels of IgE, (5) positive skin and bronchial challenge tests to specific allergens, and (6) a tendency for the disease to remit in later life.[324, 336] A second category, called *extrinsic nonatopic* asthma,[324] includes patients in whom exposure to a specific external agent can be clearly shown to be the cause of reversible bronchoconstriction but in whom specific IgE does not mediate the response or in whom there is no tendency for excessive IgE production. Patients in this category are usually those with occupational asthma that occurs in response to powerful sensitizers such as plicatic acid or toluene diisocyanate.[337] Certain antigens are powerful inducers of IgE production and can result in IgE-mediated airway responses in the absence of a genetic atopic predisposition.[337]

INTRINSIC ASTHMA

Intrinsic, or cryptogenic, asthma refers to patients in whom atopy or specific external triggers of bronchoconstriction cannot be identified. The term "intrinsic" was initially coined because it was believed that these patients were responding to antigens from microbial agents released in their tracheobronchial tree. Patients with intrinsic asthma are characterized by (1) being in an older age group, (2) having no family history of asthma or allergic disease, (3) an absence of elevated blood levels of IgE or positive skin or bronchial response to allergen challenge, (4) increased blood and sputum eosinophil counts, (5) an increased incidence of autoantibodies to smooth muscle, (6) an increased incidence of autoimmune disease, (7) decreased responsiveness to therapy, and (8) a tendency to persistent and progressive disease resulting in fixed airflow obstruction.[324, 338, 339]

ADDITIONAL TERMS

Exercise-induced asthma is not a separate category because the majority of patients in the above categories will develop exaggerated bronchoconstriction during exercise.

The excessive bronchial lability seen in some patients with chronic bronchitis, COPD, bronchiectasis, and cystic fibrosis should not be called asthma; although these conditions fulfill some of the features of asthma, each has a clearly defined etiologic basis.

INCIDENCE

Asthma is a common disease, estimates of prevalence in children ranging from less than 1 per cent up to 20 per cent in different countries.[340–343] The first attack can occur at any age, although the onset of extrinsic asthma is invariably before the age of 30 years and that of the intrinsic variety is more commonly in middle life. When the two major varieties of asthma are taken together, onset is as frequent after as before the age of 15 years.[344, 345] Characteristics of severe asthma in children include onset in the first 3 years of life, a high frequency of attacks during the initial year, clinical and physiologic evidence of persisting airway obstruction, pulmonary hyperinflation, chest deformity, and impairment of growth.[346] Although the majority of 586 asthmatic children in one study were found to have IgE-mediated extrinsic asthma, 12 per cent were considered to have intrinsic disease, which appeared to be more severe and more rapidly progressive. In very young children, it may be difficult to distinguish infective bronchiolitis from asthma; indeed, early infection may predispose to later symptoms of wheeze and nonspecific airway hyper-responsiveness.[347, 348]

There are considerable racial and geographic variations in the prevalence of the disease, although it is unknown whether this is purely genetic or is related to climate or to prevalence of antigen exposure.[349–351] The lower incidence of asthma in some tropical countries is believed by some[343, 351, 352] but not all[353] to be related to a protective effect of high serum IgE levels induced by parasitic infestation. In a study of the prevalence of asthma in different Latin American countries, marked variability was found; the lowest rate was 0.4 per cent of the population of Peru, and the highest was 4.3 per cent of the population of Brazil. That the prevalence of asthma within a population can change is illustrated by the dramatic increase in the number of Papua–New Guinea Melanesians who have acquired the disease during the past decade.[355–358] The increase in the prevalence of asthma from 0.1 to 7.3 per cent of this population during this period may be related to the intensity of house dust mite infestation.[2776]

The severity of asthma can vary widely; for the majority it is a mildly troublesome disorder that interferes only slightly with physical activities and only rarely requires treatment. At the other end of the spectrum are the few patients who have repeated episodes of life-threatening airway obstruction and who never achieve normal predicted lung function despite the constant heavy use of therapeutic agents. In any research or clinical study involving asthmatic subjects, it is important to characterize the virulence of the disease in the population being studied.

PATHOLOGIC CHARACTERISTICS

The basic pathophysiologic abnormality that determines the functional and symptomatic status of an asthmatic patient is airway narrowing. This can occur by three main mechanisms: (1) airway smooth muscle contraction and shortening, (2) edema and congestion of the airway wall, and (3) mucous hypersecretion and plugging of the airway lumen. For the most part, it is difficult if not impossible to determine in a given patient at a given time what proportion of airway obstruction is caused by each of these mechanisms. As a generalization, however, it can be reasonably concluded that when obstruction is rapidly reversible following inhalation of cholinergic antagonists or beta-adrenergic agonists, the pathogenesis is smooth muscle shortening, whereas when it responds over a period of days to steroids and other therapeutic interventions, it is caused by edema and mucous plugging.[359, 360]

Although it might be expected that the pathogenesis of airway obstruction in asthma could be appreciated from descriptions of airway morphology, since much of our knowledge of the morphologic characteristics of asthma derives from studies at necropsy, the changes that have been described likely represent the effects of prolonged severe disease; thus, generalization to milder forms of disease could be questioned. Despite this, evidence provided by analysis of bronchial biopsy specimens and sputum samples suggests that although morphologic changes can diminish between attacks,[361] considerable epithelial, muscular, and microvascular abnormalities can persist.[362–364] Although it is impossible to follow the sequence of pathologic changes that occur in the airways of asthmatic subjects, animal models allow more precise chronology of morphologic features, at least following antigen challenge. In allergic rabbits, the immediate reaction (30 minutes later) is characterized by edema alone; at 6 and 48 hours, there develops a combination of edema, congestion, and cellular infiltration.[382]

At autopsy, the lungs of patients who die of asthma are distended and typically project above the cut ends of the ribs and across the midline of the thorax when the chest is opened. Focal depressions bounded by interlobular septa are evident on the pleural surface,[365] representing areas of subsegmental atelectasis caused by bronchiolar obstruction. Cut sections show the bronchi and bronchioles to be plugged with large amounts of viscid, tenacious mucus, which in some cases extends into the trachea. Focal cystic bronchiectasis, often in the upper and middle lobes, has been reported in some patients.[365]

Histologically, although mucous plugs are most frequent in bronchi and larger membranous bronchioles, they usually extend to the level of respiratory bronchioles.[365] The plugs themselves are composed of both mucoid and proteinaceous material and typically completely fill the airway lumen (Fig. 11–23). Scattered within them is a variable number of cells, most of which are eosinophils or ciliated cells derived from the airway epithelium. The ciliated cells can occur singly or in clusters of up to 100 cells, termed *Creola bodies*.[367] Also present in both airway plugs and sputum[363] are *Charcot-Leyden crystals* and *Curschmann spirals*. The former are variably sized, colorless crystals ranging in length from 20 to 40 μm and in width from 2 to 4 μm (Fig. 11–24) and are believed to be composed predominantly of lysophospholipase (phospholipase B) derived from eosinophilic granules.[369] Curschmann spirals are convoluted strands of mucus composed of a relatively compact central core surrounded by numerous delicate fibrils (Fig. 11–24); they range in size from microscopic to 2 cm and are believed to be formed within small airways. Although characteristic of asthma, neither Charcot-Leyden crystals nor Curschmann spirals are pathognomonic of the condition.[369, 370]

Histologic changes in the bronchial and bronchiolar walls are characteristic of asthma.[364, 365] Although the epithelium may be focally normal, goblet cell hyperplasia is frequent[364] and is sometimes so marked that large segments of the airway surface are composed solely of these cells (Fig. 11–25). In addition, in many areas the surface epithelial cells are detached, leaving only a layer of cuboidal basal cells (Fig. 11–26); this feature can be present in both autopsy[364, 365] and biopsy[373] specimens. The pathogenesis of this epithelial damage and shedding

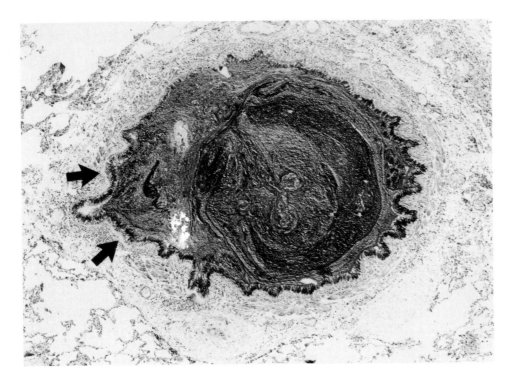

Figure 11–23. Asthma: Mucous Plugging. A histologic section of a small bronchus shows it to be completely occluded by a dense plug of strongly periodic acid–Schiff (PAS)-positive mucus; variation in cellularity of the mucus causes a somewhat laminated appearance. The bronchial wall contains a moderate number of inflammatory cells; even at this magnification, thickening of the basement membrane is evident as a lightly stained subepithelial stripe *(arrows)*. Note the strong PAS positivity of the epithelium, indicating extensive goblet cell hyperplasia. The patient was a 43-year-old male who died of severe asthma (PAS, × 40).

is unclear. Dunnill[365] has suggested that it may be caused by transudation of fluid from the lamina propria to the airway lumen. The possibility that epithelial damage may be the result of eosinophil or mast cell degranulation has also been suggested;[373] ultrastructural abnormalities of ciliated epithelial cells have been described both in patients whose disease was in remission and in those with severe persistent asthma,[364, 373] lending some support to the degranulation hypothesis. Thompson[367] reported a remarkable case of a patient with an ovarian teratoma who died of asthma; the tumor contained bronchial mucosa that showed all the pathologic changes typically found in pulmonary airways in asthma, including shedding of surface epithelial cells. This suggests that the pathogenesis of the epithelial abnormalities is not necessarily a local phenomenon. Whatever the mechanism of epithelial damage and shedding, it is likely that the resulting loss of ciliary function is at least partly responsible for the presence of the extensive intraluminal mucus found at autopsy.

Other bronchial wall abnormalities characteristic of asthma include basement membrane thickening,[364, 365, 374] edema and vascular congestion of the lamina propria and submucosa, and a more or less intense mural infiltrate of eosinophilic leukocytes (Fig. 11–26); the basement membrane thickening is possibly caused by repeated bouts of epithelial damage[375] and in one study[364] was considered to result from collagen deposition beneath the basement membrane. Rarely, local exaggeration of the submucosal inflammatory reaction results in the formation of endobronchial polyps similar to those found in the nares of patients with allergic rhini-

tis.[376] Some authorities believe that the bronchial mucous glands are increased in size,[364, 377] although others have not found evidence for this.[365] Similar results have been reported with respect to smooth muscle, although most authors consider this tissue to be clearly increased in amount.[364, 365, 377, 2777] In one necropsy study,[378] the muscle from two bronchi of the left lower lobe of five male asthmatic subjects and three control subjects was quantified. The absolute area and volume of bronchial muscle in the asthmatic subjects were approximately three times that of the control subjects; a count of the nuclei of muscle cells in the sections showed that there were almost three times as many muscle cells in the airways of the asthmatic subjects, indicating that the increased muscle volume was chiefly the result of hyperplasia and only slightly of hypertrophy. In contrast to these rather impressive results, another postmortem study of six elderly nonsmoking asthmatic subjects who died of other causes revealed no significant increase in smooth muscle mass.[379]

Of particular interest is the location and number of mast cells in the lungs of asthmatic patients: they can be situated in the submucosa, airway epithelium, and airway lumen; in the last two locations, they can be particularly important because of their potential for interacting with inhaled allergens prior to epithelial penetration.[362, 380] The bronchi of patients who have died of asthma have been reported to contain a sparsity of mast cells in comparison with bronchi of nonasthmatic control subjects or asthmatic patients who have died from other causes,[381] an observation that may reflect a failure to recognize such cells after degranulation.

Figure 11–24. Asthmatic Sputum: Charcot-Leyden Crystals and Curschmann Spiral. A sputum specimen from a 20-year-old man with an exacerbation of asthma (A) shows multiple variably sized but uniformly shaped Charcot-Leyden crystals. Bilobed nuclei, some showing degenerative changes, indicate the presence of eosinophils (arrows). Elsewhere in the same specimen (B), a convoluted Curschmann spiral is evident. The dense central core and lightly stained filamentous periphery are characteristic. (Papanicolaou stain; A, B, × 325.)

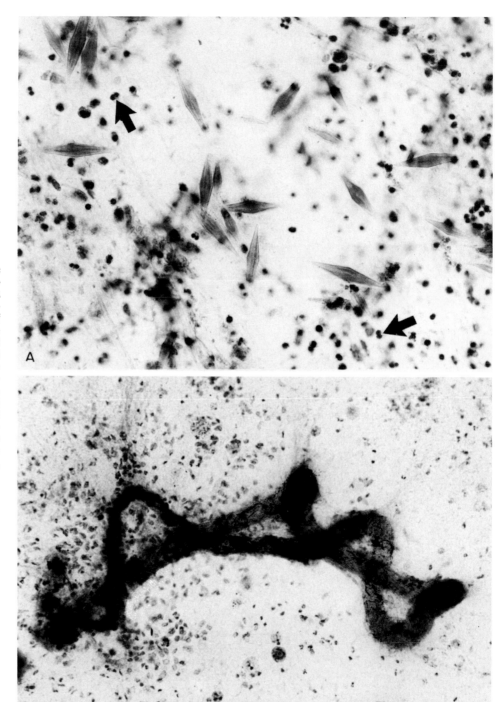

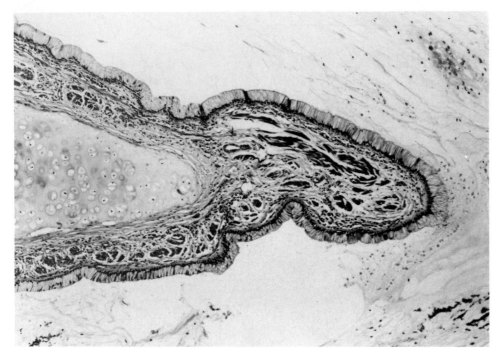

Figure 11–25. Asthma: Goblet Cell Hyperplasia. A histologic section of bronchial wall at the bifurcation of two airways shows an epithelium that is composed almost entirely of goblet cells. Specimen obtained at autopsy of the same patient as illustrated in Figure 11–23 (× 60).

MUCUS AND MUCOCILIARY CLEARANCE IN ASTHMA

Excessive mucus production and mucous plugging are characteristic features of asthma, and attempts have been made to identify a specific biochemical or rheologic abnormality in the sputum and mucus from patients with this condition.[383] Generally, studies have shown that the glycoprotein content and viscoelastic properties of mucus in patients with asthma and other airway diseases relate more to the type of sputum (i.e., mucoid, mucopurulent, or purulent) than to the specific disease entity. Patients with asthma tend to have "mucoid" sputum. Sputum samples from patients with so-called intrinsic asthma demonstrate a variable glycoprotein content and possess viscoelastic properties closely related to the sputum of patients with chronic bronchitis; by contrast, patients with extrinsic asthma are a more homogeneous group with sputum possessing less variability in biochemical and viscoelastic properties.[383] A long list of putative mediators of asthma are known to increase the quantity of mucous secretion, including histamine, the prostaglandins (E, F_2, D_2, and I), alpha-adrenergic agonists, and lipoxygenase products of arachidonic acid metabolism.[384]

Radioaerosol techniques reveal impaired mucociliary clearance rates in patients with stable asthma. This is true despite the fact that asthmatics tend to show more central deposition of inhaled radiolabel, a fact that should favor faster clearance rates.[385, 386] When the Teflon disk method is used to measure mucociliary clearance, asthmatics in remission show tracheal mucous velocities as low as 55 per cent of normal.[387]

In allergic asthmatics and in sheep with specific allergy to *Ascaris suum*, antigen challenge further decreases mucous transport, an effect that is prevented by pretreatment with either cromolyn sodium or the SRS-A (leukotriene)-blocking agent FPL55712.[388–392] The observation that histamine inhalation alone stimulates mucociliary clearance and that leukotriene-blocking drugs and cromolyn sodium block the antigen-induced decrease in mucociliary clearance suggests that the impaired clearance is a result of leukotrienes. In support of this hypothesis is experimental evidence that antigen challenge increases clearance after pretreatment with FPL55712, suggesting that the inhibitory effect is attributable to the leukotrienes whereas other released mediators may be stimulatory.[392] Despite these observations, *in vitro* antigen challenge of ciliated epithelial cells of allergic sheep has resulted in a stimulation of ciliary activity and an increase in ciliary beat frequency;[391] also, the addition of leukotrienes to airway explants *in vitro* results in a dose-dependent stimulation of ciliary beat frequency. This occurs despite the fact that nebulized leukotrienes result in depressed mucociliary clearance.[388]

These studies suggest that the chemical mediators of allergic asthma exert their deleterious effect on mucociliary function by altering the quantity and perhaps the rheologic properties of airway secretions. The role of antigen and the resulting mediators in modulating the secretion of the liquid in the sol phase is incompletely understood, but it is possible that these mediators interfere with epithelial water transport.[388] *Ascaris suum* challenge of sheep trachea *in vitro* stimulates the production of glycoprotein secretion and transiently increases Na^+ and Cl^- flux across the respiratory epithelium.[393]

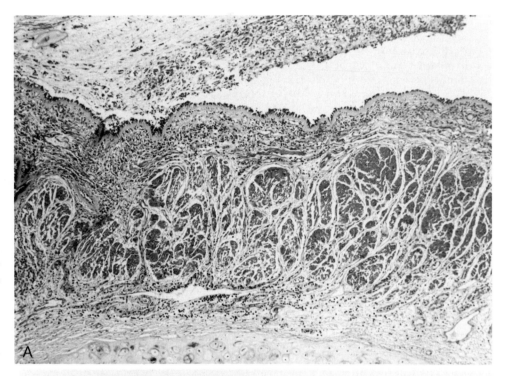

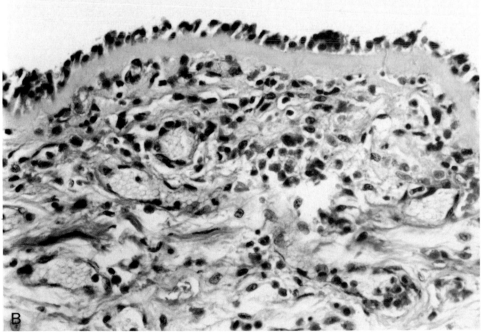

Figure 11–26. Asthma: Bronchial Wall Abnormalities. A histologic section of bronchial wall *(A)* shows marked thickening of the muscularis mucosa, numerous inflammatory cells, and a uniformly thickened basement membrane (compare with Figure 1–13, page 14). The bronchial epithelium is composed only of a row of cuboidal basal cells, the ciliated and goblet cells having been shed into the overlying mucus. A section with greater magnification reveals to better advantage the residual epithelium, thickened basement membrane, and inflammatory cell infiltrate. Section is from the same patient as in Figure 11–23. *(A,* × 40; *B,* × 300.)

The effect on mucociliary clearance of a single antigen challenge may be very prolonged.[394] In allergic sheep, antigen challenge has been shown to result in an increase in pulmonary resistance, a decrease in arterial Po_2, and impairment of tracheal mucous velocity (measured by the radiopaque Teflon disk method).[394] The abnormalities of pulmonary mechanics and gas exchange return to normal by 2 to 3 hours, but mucociliary clearance continues to worsen, reaching the lowest value between 5 and 7 hours and remaining depressed for up to 7 days.

Some asthmatics have been found to have a ciliary inhibitory compound in their sputum that possesses a low molecular weight (6,000 to 8,000 daltons). The inhibitory effect has been demonstrated in human bronchial explants and is more common in the sputum of asthmatics during clinical exacerbation; it is readily reversible on removal of the specific sol phase.[395] Prolonged therapy of asthmatics with corticosteroids for 4 weeks has been shown to result in improved mucociliary clearance, despite more peripheral deposition of the inhaled radiolabel.[396]

NONSPECIFIC BRONCHIAL RESPONSIVENESS

In the previous edition of this text, the concept of nonspecific bronchial responsiveness (NSBR) and the association of increased NSBR and asthma were mentioned only briefly. Since that time, there has been an increasing interest in the phenomenon, to the extent that many authorities now believe that the presence of nonspecific bronchial hyper-responsiveness (NSBH) is a *sine qua non* of asthma.[397] NSBH (*synonyms:* bronchial hyper-reactivity, bronchial hyperexcitability) represents the exaggerated airway narrowing that occurs in response to inhalation of a variety of nonallergenic, usually pharmacologic stimuli. We shall use "nonspecific bronchial responsiveness" as the generic term for this phenomenon and "nonspecific bronchial hyper-responsiveness" for the exaggerated responsiveness of asthmatic patients.[398] Although all the stimuli used to demonstrate NSBH result in some degree of airway narrowing in normal subjects, it is the excessive narrowing at very much lower doses or concentrations that characterizes NSBH.

Exaggerated bronchial narrowing in response to pharmacologic agents was described many years ago, but only during the last 10 years has the importance of NSBH been recognized and techniques to demonstrate and quantify it been developed. In 1921, Alexander and Paddock reported that pilocarpine resulted in "asthmatic breathing" in asthmatic patients but not in normal subjects;[2749] they also observed exaggerated vagal effects, such as salivation and sweating, and suggested that asthma might be secondary to increased vagal tone ("vagatonics"). In 1929 and 1932, Weiss and his associates demonstrated a decrease in vital capacity in response to intravenous histamine in emphysematous and asthmatic subjects at concentrations that had no effect on the lungs of normal subjects.[399, 400] In 1949, Curry administered histamine and acetyl-beta-methylcholine by both inhaled and intravenous routes to normal subjects and patients with rhinitis and asthma: in addition to showing an exaggerated response in asthmatics, he demonstrated concordance of the response to both agents and was therefore the first to note the nonspecific nature of the hyper-responsiveness.[401] Despite these important advances, it was Tiffeneau in the 1950s who first recognized the potential importance of NSBH and who systematically and quantitatively began to study NSBH in patients with asthma and allergic rhinitis, employing acetylcholine and histamine as provocative agents.[402, 403] Since the mid-1970s, interest in NSBH has increased dramatically and the condition has been discussed extensively in the literature.[404–407]

The nonspecific nature of the exaggerated response has become increasingly apparent, and the list of substances to which asthmatic patients respond excessively is continually enlarging; among the pharmacologic agents, it includes histamine, pilocarpine, methacholine, carbachol, acetylcholine, serotonin, bradykinin, prostaglandin $F_{2\alpha}$, leukotrienes C_4 and D_4, and adenosine.[404, 408, 409] Asthmatics also show excessive airway narrowing in response to inhalation of atmospheric pollutants, dust, and cold and dry air, and to certain respiratory maneuvers such as a deep inspiration or forced expiration to RV.[404] Although edema of airway walls and mucous plugging of lumens almost certainly contribute to the airway obstruction in spontaneous asthmatic episodes, the responses that result from tests of NSBR are caused predominantly by airway smooth muscle shortening because they are rapid in onset and readily reversible with bronchodilators.[404] However, in allergic airway disease, hyper-responsiveness may extend beyond the smooth muscle; for example, patients with allergic rhinitis show increased mucous secretion and protein exudation in response to administration of intranasal methacholine.[410, 411]

The fact that NSBH is such a characteristic feature of asthma raises a question: does it represent a basic defect in the control of bronchial caliber that precedes and predisposes to the development of the asthmatic state, or is it a consequence of it? The demonstration that bronchomotor response to pharmacologic agents by various nonasthmatic animal species as well as by man is highly variable raises the possibility that the exaggerated airway narrowing in asthma simply represents one end of a wide biologic susceptibility.[412–414] Certain canine species such as the basenji-greyhound exhibit markedly increased NSBR,[415] whereas some strains of rats can be bred to manifest exaggerated bronchoconstriction;[416] in addition, a percentage of clinically healthy, first-degree relatives of children with asthma demonstrate NSBH.[417] These observations support the concept that a genetically determined airway responsiveness might predispose to asthma. However, studies of monozygotic and dizygotic twins have shown similar inter-twin variability of response to methacholine, supporting the role of environmental factors as determinants of nonspecific responsiveness.[418] It is now clear that NSBH is not a static phenomenon; an individual's responsiveness can change considerably with the duration of exposure to infectious agents,[419] environmental pollutants,[420] and specific antigens or sensitizing agents.[421] For example, in a group of patients with occupational asthma secondary to western red cedar exposure, nonspecific airway responsiveness decreased gradually over a period of months following cessation of exposure and increased again following re-exposure.[422] These related studies make it likely that airway hyper-responsiveness is a *result* of asthma rather than a genetic risk factor for it.

Patients with allergic rhinitis but without pulmonary symptoms do not invariably demonstrate NSBH.[423, 424] The increased NSBR manifested by some patients with atopy and isolated nasal symptoms has been interpreted as indicating the presence of subclinical asthma.[423]

NSBH is so characteristic of asthma that it is questionable whether a diagnosis can be made in its absence.[397] Rarely, patients with occupational asthma or nonoccupational allergic asthma do not show increased NSBR at the time of diagnosis but develop increased responsiveness with prolonged exposure.[425–428] Although NSBH is virtually 100 per cent sensitive in the *diagnosis* of asthma, it is far from being specific: for example, it has been demonstrated in patients with sarcoidosis,[429, 430] extrinsic allergic alveolitis,[431–433] and COPD,[434–436] although in these conditions it appears to be related to a baseline decrease in airway caliber.[429, 431, 435] In a comparison study of patients with asthma and COPD, NSBH was found to be unrelated to baseline FEV_1 in the former but to be significantly related to prechallenge FEV_1 in the latter.[435] Similarly, in occupational surveys of airway responsiveness, the incidence of NSBH is higher than that of clinically diagnosed asthma, suggesting an appreciable false-positive rate.[437, 438]

Of 876 adults in western Australia, the incidence of bronchial hyper-responsiveness (defined as PC_{20} FEV_1 of less than 3.9 μM) was approximately 11 per cent[439] whereas the incidence of asthma (defined as symptoms consistent with asthma in addition to bronchial hyper-responsiveness) was only 5.9 per cent. Bronchial hyper-responsiveness was significantly related to respiratory symptoms, atopy, smoking, and abnormal lung function. The prevalence of NSBH was even higher (19 per cent) in 1,400 Australian school children between 8 and 10 years of age;[440] not all children who had symptoms compatible with asthma (or asthma diagnosed by a physician) were hyper-responsive and, conversely, only about 60 per cent of the individuals with NSBH had symptoms of asthma.

Measurement

The various methods that have been used to quantify nonspecific airway responsiveness are described in detail in Chapter 3 (*see* page 443). Briefly, airway narrowing is measured by one of a variety of tests, those most often employed being the measurement of FEV_1, PEFR, airway resistance (RAW), or specific airway conductance (SGAW), although pulmonary resistance, oscillatory respiratory system resistance, and instantaneous expiratory flow rates from partial or incomplete flow-volume curves have also been used.[441–446] Asthmatics show exaggerated airway narrowing in whatever test is employed, but better separation between asthmatic and normal subjects can be achieved by using a test that involves a maximal inspiratory maneuver (FEV_1, PEFR, and maximal expiratory flows); this is so because in addition to exhibiting exaggerated narrowing, asthmatics appear to bronchodilate less after a big breath.[447]

Airway response can be quantified by measuring the degree of narrowing produced by a single dose of the agonist but can be ascertained more accurately by obtaining a partial or complete dose-response curve. Increasing doses or concentrations of inhaled agonists are administered until a predetermined decrease in flow or increase in resistance is observed or until an arbitrary maximal dose or concentration has been used.[448] Considerable controversy exists as to how best to analyze and quantify the results of *in vivo* airway dose-response curves.[449, 450] Techniques of dose-response curve analysis used by pharmacologists for *in vitro* smooth muscle have been applied to *in vivo* data, although the relationship is clearly much more complicated than the dose-dependent development of isometric tension in an organ bath.[451] *Sensitivity* (or potency) is generally measured by determining the lowest dose associated with a measurable change and has been distinguished from *reactivity*, which is represented by the degree of change for a given arithmetic or logarithmic increase in concentration or dose of agonist.[452] It has been observed that plateaus in the dose-response relationship can be elicited *in vivo*, at least in some subjects, and this has provided another numerical value—the maximal effect (efficacy) (Fig. 11–27).[453–455]

The most frequently used numerical estimate of NSBR is the dose or concentration of inhaled histamine or methacholine that causes a 20 per cent decrease in FEV_1 (PC_{20}) or a 35 per cent decrease in specific airway conductance. These measurements do not separate sensitivity and reactivity; in fact, altered sensitivity or reactivity could produce a similar change in these estimates of responsiveness. Although in theory the separation of sensitivity

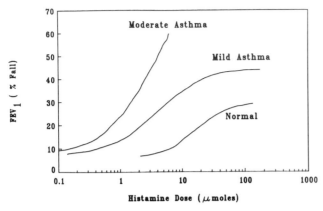

Figure 11–27. Histamine Dose-Response Curves. The percentage fall in the forced expiratory volume in 1 second (FEV₁) is plotted against the dose of inhaled histamine for a normal subject and patients with mild and moderate asthma. In the normal subject and the patient with mild asthma, a plateau is reached on the dose-response curve. In the patient with moderate asthma, there is no plateau despite a 60 per cent decrease in FEV₁. Asthma is characterized by a shift of the dose-response curve to the left and an increase in the maximal response. (Modified from Woolcock AJ, Salome CM, Yan K: Am Rev Respir Dis *130*:71, 1984.)

and reactivity could provide additional insight into the mechanism that results in exaggerated broncho-constriction,[452, 456] separation of the two has actually added little to our understanding of asthma and NSBH.[457–459] Whether separation of "sensitivity" and maximal response clarifies anything remains to be seen; theoretically, a low threshold for response is not necessarily accompanied by an increased maximal response and *vice versa*.[451]

Histamine and methacholine are the most frequently used pharmacologic agonists for investigative or clinical testing of NSBH, and with few exceptions[460] the concordance between the provocative doses of the two agents on a molar basis is excellent.[461–463] Correlation with other pharmacologic agents (e.g., methacholine versus PGF₂) may not be as good.[464] Histamine has the disadvantage of causing flushing when concentrations greater than 8 mg/ml are inhaled;[465] however, the bronchoconstrictive effect of methacholine is two to three times more prolonged.[461, 466] Both agents are thought to act directly on specific receptors on airway smooth muscle—methacholine at the post-ganglionic muscarinic receptor and histamine at a different site. Although histamine can potentially stimulate reflexes as well as smooth muscle directly, it is primarily the direct effect that functions in clinical testing. The effects of histamine are not altered by the mast cell stabilizing agent, disodium cromoglycate.[467] Methacholine has been reported to cause a late or prolonged response after inhalation of very high doses, suggesting that a mechanism other than smooth muscle shortening such as mucus or edema might be responsible.[468] Tests with both agents show very good short- and long-term reproducibility, provided patients remain clinically stable between tests.[446, 462, 469–473]

Other triggers that have been used to demonstrate airway hyper-responsiveness include exercise, isocapnic hyperventilation of cold and/or dry air, and the inhalation of ultrasonically generated hypotonic or hypertonic solutions.[474–477]

A different approach to the measurement of nonspecific bronchial responsiveness has been the study of diurnal variation in airway function and the "responsiveness" to a bronchodilating rather than a bronchoconstricting stimulus. Spontaneous diurnal variation in peak expiratory flow rates, as well as exercise-induced lability and bronchodilator response to a beta-adrenergic agonist, has shown excellent correlation with responsiveness to inhaled histamine, although the histamine response was more sensitive and specific for asthma.[478, 479] The concordance between the responsiveness to such a wide variety of stimuli in asthmatic patients emphasizes the nonspecific nature of the hyper-responsiveness. Any theory to explain the pathogenesis of airway hyper-responsiveness must take this nonspecificity into account.

Pathogenesis of Nonspecific Bronchial Hyper-responsiveness

The various links in the chain between airway smooth muscle stimulation, airway narrowing, and an increase in airway resistance are shown in Figure 11–28. Abnormalities at any level of this cascade could theoretically produce an exaggeration of airway narrowing in response to a given stimulus; an increase in smooth muscle shortening or a deficiency in one of the inhibitory relaxant systems could result in NSBH. The factors that have been proposed to explain NSBH will be considered individually.

STARTING AIRWAY CALIBER

Because airway resistance is alinearly related to airway radius, the effect of a given degree of narrowing is greater in previously narrowed airways; in fact, resistance is related to the fourth power of the radius with both laminar and turbulent flow regimes. In addition, turbulent flow is more likely to occur with prior airway narrowing and could produce a further alinear relationship between pressure and flow. These observations have led to the theory that decreased starting airway caliber could be a major contributor to NSBH. In normal subjects, narrower airways have been suggested as the cause of the increased methacholine response observed in the very young[483] and in women.[484]

The prechallenge dimensions of the tracheobronchial tree could be decreased in asthmatic subjects for a variety of reasons:

1. The airway wall could be edematous as a result of the mucosal and submucosal inflammation characteristic of asthma.

2. The resting airway smooth muscle length

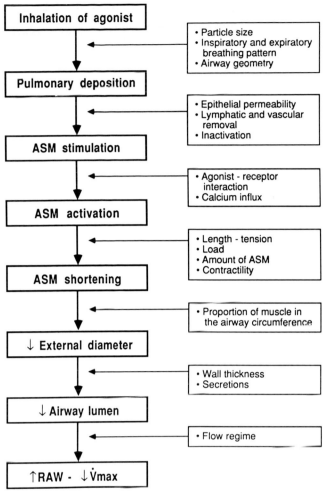

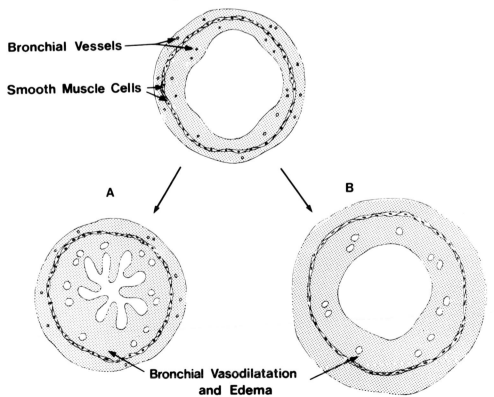

Figure 11–28. Airway Responsiveness Cascade. See text for description.

Figure 11–29. Airway Wall Edema: Diagrammatic Representation. A normal bronchial wall is depicted at top. With an increase in airway thickness as a result of the accumulation of edema fluid, there may be encroachment upon the lumen (A) or an enlargement of the airway wall with a relative sparing of luminal area (B). (See text for discussion.)

could be shorter than normal as a result of increased vagal tone, increased muscle response to normal vagal tone, or smooth muscle response to inflammatory mediators.

3. Mucus could narrow or occlude the lumen of airways.[451]

If starting airway caliber were an important contributor to NSBH, a relationship would be expected between the baseline resistance or expiratory flow rates and the responsiveness with challenge. Although such a relationship has been clearly shown in patients with COPD and other nonasthmatic diseases associated with NSBH,[429, 431] studies in asthmatic subjects have generally failed to show such a relationship.[478, 485] However, these negative studies do not exclude an important role for starting airway narrowing as a contributor to NSBH, since theoretical calculations suggest that minor and possibly unmeasurable differences in initial airway size may have a profound influence on the subsequent response.[451, 472] Although it has not been quantified, edema of the airway wall is clearly a prominent pathologic feature of asthma and could theoretically enhance the effect of a given degree of airway smooth muscle shortening; this could occur with or without altering starting airway size, depending on whether the fluid accumulates at the expense of airway lumen narrowing or airway smooth muscle lengthening.[451, 472] Both possibilities are shown in Figure 11–29. A similar mechanical explanation has been advanced to explain the exaggerated vascular responsiveness of essential hypertension.[486]

Some degree of airway smooth muscle shortening is undoubtedly present in the majority of patients with moderate-to-severe asthma because they show a greater than normal response to inhaled bronchodilators. However, baseline smooth muscle shortening would not necessarily result in the greater maximal shortening characteristic of asthma; in fact, the results of studies designed to test this possibility suggest that increased baseline "tone" does not lead to exaggerated responsiveness.[487] The importance of starting airway caliber in general and airway wall thickening caused by edema and/or smooth muscle hypertrophy in particular awaits quantitative studies of airway morphometry in normal and diseased airways.[451, 482]

ALTERED AEROSOL DEPOSITION

In vivo airway responses are quantified by measuring the effect of a given nebulized dose or concentration of inhaled agonist. A more accurate relationship between dose and response could be obtained if the amount of the agonist deposited in the lung or (ideally) reaching smooth muscle could be calculated. In fact, the fraction of nebulized drug that reaches the tracheobronchial tree may be small, and the amount and distribution of the inhaled agonist can vary considerably with the breathing pattern.[488, 489] Although it is convenient to think of the tracheobronchial tree as a single resistor and the airway narrowing in response to inhaled agonist as the response of a single tissue, in reality the airway is made up of a multitude of resistors joined in series and in parallel. The response to inhaled agonists is dependent on the fractional distribution of aerosol to a given airway generation, the surface area of wall at that level of the airway, and the relative importance of that generation of airways to overall airway resistance or flow limitation. Deposition of aerosol particles of the size used for testing airway responsiveness is dependent predominantly on impaction;[490] since impaction increases when linear velocity and turbulence are increased, altering baseline airway caliber and the airflow rates during aerosol inhalation will change the site of deposition of an inhaled drug. For example, rapid inspiratory[488] or expiratory[489] flow rates result in more central deposition of aerosol; this concentration of drug at a site that contributes importantly to total airway resistance and to flow limitation can shift the inhaled concentration-response curve leftward, creating an apparent hyper-responsiveness. Even asymptomatic asthmatic subjects can show more central deposition of inhaled aerosol, but the importance of the resulting localized concentration of agonist as a determinant of NSBH is unknown. The exaggerated responsiveness to cold and dry air in asthmatics cannot be explained by altered deposition because the penetration of such air into the tracheobronchial tree would be unaffected by starting airway caliber.

INCREASED BRONCHIAL MUCOSAL PERMEABILITY

To have any effect, inhaled agonists must cross a layer of respiratory tract secretions, bronchial epithelium, and submucosa to reach receptor sites on smooth muscle. Similarly, agents that cause reflex bronchoconstriction through the network of irritant nerve endings must penetrate the bronchial epithelium through tight junctions between epithelial cells.[491] The amount or concentration of drug that reaches the smooth muscle will be dependent on the balance between penetration of these barriers and the removal of agonist by the bronchial vasculature, lymphatics, and enzymatic degradation. Since the respiratory epithelium is characteristically damaged and sloughed in patients with asthma, it seems reasonable to assume that a greater proportion of inhaled agonist might reach receptors on vagal afferents and smooth muscle.[491] One study of a small group of asthmatics showed a relationship between NSBR and quantitative estimates of epithelial damage;[492] similarly, patients with sarcoidosis and extrinsic allergic alveolitis with NSBH have epithelial damage and hyperpermeability.[493, 494]

Although animal studies have shown that NSBR increases with epithelial damage induced by cigarette smoke[495] and antigen exposure,[496] studies in humans have shown no relationship between airway mucosal hyperpermeability and NSBH.[497, 498] In one study in which disappearance from the lung of inhaled ^{99m}Tc diethylenetriaminepenta-acetate (DTPA) was employed as a marker of epithelial permeability, no differences were observed between two groups of normal and asthmatic subjects despite marked differences in airway responses to inhaled histamine.[497, 498] The lack of relationship between lung epithelial permeability and NSBR was further illustrated by the demonstration in current cigarette smokers of hyperpermeability without hyper-responsiveness.[498] The inhalation of hypotonic distilled water fog produces transiently increased permeability in both normal and asthmatic subjects, but airway narrowing in response to this challenge occurs only in asthmatics.[499, 500] In baboons that have been heavy cigarette smokers (two packs a day for 3 years), airway responsiveness to inhaled methacholine was *decreased* in comparison to nonsmoking control animals,[501] an effect that could be related to a protective action of a thickened layer of tracheobronchial mucus.[502]

Difference in the rate of removal of inhaled or locally released mediator is an additional factor that could be altered in patients with asthma and that has the potential to contribute to apparent NSBH. Very little is known about the mechanisms contributing to mediator removal, but in peripheral airways at least, both the pulmonary and bronchial circulations appear to contribute to this removal.[503]

ABNORMALITIES OF NEUROHUMORAL CONTROL

Airway smooth muscle is innervated by the autonomic nervous system and is equipped with membrane receptors for a wide variety of circulating excitatory and inhibitory substances.[404] Exaggerated excitatory or deficient inhibitory control could result in NSBH. Before the possible abnormalities that have been regarded as important in asthma are detailed, a review of the neurohumoral control of airway smooth muscle seems appropriate.

The major excitatory innervation is from cholinergic *postganglionic fibers* that arise from neurons in the ganglia of the airway wall. *Preganglionic fibers* from the brainstem descend in the vagus nerve to synapse with the postganglionic fibers; stimulation of this *efferent system* results in acetylcholine release and smooth muscle contraction. Efferent excitatory cholinergic activity is stimulated by a wide variety of afferent inputs to the brainstem.

Stimulation of *afferent receptors* in the nose, larynx, and lung all cause reflex bronchoconstriction by this pathway; in addition, connections between chemoreceptors and baroreceptors and the efferent vagal system have been demonstrated.[404] The lung irritant receptors are potentially the most important with respect to NSBH. The afferents begin as a network of free nerve endings located immediately below the tight junctions of the respiratory epithelium; they are probably mainly mechanoreceptors that respond to local irritation but are also stimulated by inhalation of dust, by pollutants, by altered local osmolarity, by drugs such as histamine, and by bronchoconstriction itself. In addition to producing reflex bronchoconstriction, stimulation of these nerve endings results in a subjective sensation of irritation, cough, and—at least in animals—an altered pattern of breathing termed *rapid shallow breathing*.[404, 504, 505] The reflex bronchoconstriction can be blocked by vagal section or atropine, but atropine does not abolish the cough or altered breathing pattern.[404] In addition to their role as the afferent limb of reflex bronchoconstriction, afferent receptors in the airway may have a more direct pathophysiologic role because they contain inflammatory neuropeptides, including substance P and calcitonin gene-related peptide, that are potent inflammatory mediators that cause increased vascular permeability and edema as well as direct smooth muscle stimulation.[506–508] Excessive afferent nerve stimulation could theoretically cause airway narrowing in the absence of a central nervous system connection via the so-called axon reflex.

The presence of a synapse between preganglionic and postganglionic cholinergic fibers within the ganglia of the airway wall allows for the possibility of presynaptic modulation of efferent cholinergic activity. In various animal species, norepinephrine-induced inhibition[509] and substance P–induced enhancement[510] of cholinergic excitation have been demonstrated. The distribution of vagal efferent fibers within the tracheobronchial tree varies between animal species and in individuals within a species.[404] The autoradiographic demonstration of cholinergic receptors has allowed determination of receptor density and suggests denser innervation of central airways and sparse or absent innervation of bronchioles,[511] consistent with functional studies. There is some efferent cholinergic tone in normal people that is demonstrated by anticholinergic-induced bronchodilatation.[512] Airway hyper-responsiveness may be the result of exaggerated vagal tone caused by increased afferent stimulation from lung receptors or of increased efferent activity in response to a normal afferent input. Earlier studies suggesting that much of the histamine-induced and even antigen-induced airway narrowing was vagally mediated supported the concept that exaggerated reflex bronchoconstriction could explain the entire phenomenon of NSBH.[404, 513] However, more recently it has become clear that the major effect of histamine is directly on smooth muscle.[514, 515] In addition, asthmatic patients manifest increased bronchoconstriction in response to methacholine, a substance that has little effect on vagal afferents.[504, 505] NSBH cannot be attributed to reflex bronchoconstriction because it fails to explain the nonspecificity of the exaggerated response; asthmatic subjects show exaggerated responsiveness to agents that do not act via efferent cholinergic pathways. Despite this, it appears that there may be abnormalities of the parasympathetic system in asthmatic patients; for example, they show exaggerated reflex bradycardia in response to a deep breath or simulated dive, and this increased cholinergic reactivity correlates with nonspecific airway responsiveness.[516, 517] Atropine does not block the accentuated NSBR that occurs after antigen exposure in allergic asthmatics.[518]

The major inhibitory or bronchodilating influence on airway smooth muscle is stimulation of *beta-adrenergic receptors*. The beta-adrenergic receptors on human airway smooth muscle are not related to adrenergic innervation: adrenergic postganglionic fibers originating in the stellate ganglion enter the lung at the hila but in man appear to supply only vascular smooth muscle, both pulmonary and bronchial. As noted above, adrenergic fibers can also innervate airway ganglia and modulate cholinergic activity, but direct airway smooth muscle innervation has not been demonstrated.[519] Human lung beta-receptors have been identified autoradiographically;[520] these can be demonstrated and subtyped on alveolar and bronchial epithelium and glands as well as on airway and vascular smooth muscle. Consistent with their function, the receptors on airway smooth muscle are largely of the β_2 subtype, receptor density being greater on peripheral than on central airways.[521]

The most persistent hypothesis to explain airway hyper-responsiveness is the theory of *partial beta-adrenergic blockade* proposed by Szentivanyi in 1968.[522] This hypothesis was originally based on observations made in rodents that developed exaggerated susceptibility to histamine and impaired beta-adrenergic responses when immunized with heat-killed pertussis vaccine. The hypothesis received support from numerous studies that demonstrated defective beta-adrenergic responsiveness in patients with asthma[523] and decreased beta-receptor number and function in isolated blood leukocytes from asthmatic subjects.[524–527] In some studies in which investigators have studied the ability of beta-adrenergic agonists to relax contracted normal and asthmatic airway smooth muscle *in vitro*, the results have shown deficient beta-adrenergic relaxation in the asthmatic subjects, although theophylline was equally potent in the two groups.[528] Some recent studies suggest that the decreased beta responsiveness is the result of exogenous beta-adrenergic administration, with resulting down-regulation of beta-receptor number and function in blood cells[529–531] and airway smooth muscle.[532–535] It appears that beta-receptor number and, therefore, responsiveness are not static but vary over time in response to various stimuli; stable asthmatics receiving no beta-adrenergic therapy show normal numbers of beta-receptors on leukocytes (and presumably on airway smooth muscle), but prolonged beta-agonist therapy[530] or acute antigen exposure[536, 537] decreases the receptor number. Thirty days after discontinuing beta-adrenergic drug therapy, 30 young atopic asthmatic patients demonstrated normal leukocyte beta-receptor number and function, although their cardiovascular sensitivity to infused isoproterenol was decreased.[538] In addition to beta-adrenoceptor tachyphylaxis related to down-regulation of receptor numbers, circulating antibodies or antibody-like substances directed at beta-receptors have been demonstrated in the blood of some asthmatic patients.[539–541]

Although these data provide convincing evidence that the partial beta blockade of asthma is an acquired phenomenon, they do not negate its possible contribution to NSBH. If a normal response to bronchoconstricting stimuli was endogenous release of bronchodilating beta-agonist, impaired beta responses could result in an apparent increase in airway sensitivity and maximal narrowing. If this were true, one would expect pharmacologic beta blockade to produce NSBH in normal subjects—which is not the case. Exaggerated bronchoconstriction does not develop in normal subjects in response to nonspecific stimuli, even when profound beta-adrenergic blockade is produced by systemic or inhaled beta-blocking agents.[414, 542–545] Despite partial beta blockade to start with, asthmatic patients paradoxically can show profound bronchoconstriction following administration of beta-blocking drugs.[546–548] Clearly, then, despite decreased beta-receptor numbers, airway patency in asthmatics is partly dependent on tonic beta-receptor stimulation, which counteracts a tendency to ongoing bronchoconstriction. The fact that cholinergic blockade alleviates the beta-blocker effect suggests that vagal tone is at least part of the ongoing constrictor activity.[546, 547] An additional potential mechanism for bronchial narrowing resulting from beta blockade is inhibition of endogenous beta-agonist–induced depression of mast cell mediator release. However, plasma histamine levels do not increase following propranolol infusion in asthmatic patients;[549] because airway patency is partly dependent on tonic beta-adrenergic input, one would expect their airways to respond to factors that alter circulating catecholamine levels.

In addition to abnormalities of beta-receptors, there is some evidence to suggest that endogenous release of catecholamines may be abnormal in asthmatic patients. Although stable asthmatics show normal levels of circulating catecholamines at rest, data from some studies suggest that exercise-induced increase in blood levels is impaired and that the response to the acute stress of an asthmatic attack is blunted.[549–551] There is no detectable increase in levels of circulating plasma epinephrine or norepinephrine in response to inhaled methacholine in normal or asthmatic subjects, making it unlikely that differences in catecholamine release are important in NSBH.[552]

The role of *alpha-adrenergic receptors* in the control of normal and asthmatic airway caliber is confusing and controversial.[404, 553] The agonist norepinephrine does not contract normal human airway smooth muscle *in vitro* unless the tissue is pretreated with histamine or potassium chloride; by contrast, postmortem specimens of airway smooth muscle from patients with a variety of lung diseases respond with contraction to alpha stimulation without pretreatment.[554] These data suggest that human airway smooth muscle is equipped with alpha-receptors, but that to be effective the receptors must be modified or unmasked in some way.

The results *in vivo* have been conflicting; in one study, phenylephrine did not produce bronchial obstruction in asthmatic patients even after beta blockade was induced to negate any possible beta-agonist effect of this largely alpha-agonist agent,[555] but inhalation of methoxamine consistently produced airway narrowing in some subjects.[556–558] It is possible that airway narrowing induced by alpha-agonist is secondary to stimulation of alpha-receptors at sites other than smooth muscle. Alpha-adrenergic stimulation of mast cells may increase mediator release, whereas activation of bronchial vascular smooth muscle may produce vasoconstriction, thus decreasing the removal of mediators.

Finally, alpha-agonists may exert their effect at the level of the airway ganglia.[558] Data from studies showing exaggerated alpha-adrenergic cutaneous vascular constriction and pupillary dilatation in asthmatic and atopic patients suggest that a systemic derangement in alpha-receptor function may be important.[559, 560] Alpha-adrenergic blocking agents do not appear to have a bronchodilating effect when given alone[561] although they tend to attenuate the airway response to histamine,[562] exercise,[563] and isocapnic hyperventilation of dry air.[564] Clearly, the ultimate importance of the alpha-adrenergic component of the sympathetic nervous system in the control of airway patency requires further study, but it is safe to say that unopposed alpha-receptor stimulation is not a major mechanism of NSBH.

A third component of the autonomic nervous system in the airway is the so-called *nonadrenergic inhibitory system* (NAIS). The NAIS was originally described in the gut, where it is the major inhibitory system and where a deficiency is believed to be responsible for Hirschsprung's disease.[565, 566] Subsequent *in vitro* studies have demonstrated the presence of this bronchodilating system in the airways of most mammals, including man,[404, 567–569] and the intriguing possibility has been suggested that a defective NAIS may be responsible for NSBH.[404] In the cat, nonadrenergic bronchodilatation has been demonstrated *in vitro*; stimulation of the vagus nerve in beta-adrenergic blocked animals has been shown to reverse serotonin-induced bronchoconstriction.[570, 571] Since the neural mediator released from nerve endings of the NAIS is unknown and since no effective specific antagonist has been developed, there have been few *in vivo* studies to discern the importance of this system in normal and asthmatic subjects. *In vitro*, the potent neurotoxin tetrodotoxin can be used to block the system and to quantify its importance. In airway tissue from a small number of patients with COPD and varying NSBR *in vivo*, the magnitude of nonadrenergic smooth muscle relaxation was small in comparison to beta-adrenergic relaxation and showed no correlation with *in vivo* responsiveness to methacholine.[571, 572] Maximal NAIS stimulation produced only 10 to 20 per cent of maximal theophylline-induced relaxation in human tissue, whereas it accounted for 70 per cent of maximal relaxation in the guinea pig airway.[573]

Michoud and her colleagues have been able to demonstrate the presence of the nonadrenergic inhibitory system in human subjects *in vivo*.[573] They have also quantified its importance in bronchodilatation and compared its effectiveness in normal and asthmatic subjects.[574, 2750] They mechanically stimulated the larynx during histamine-induced bronchoconstriction and showed an abrupt but transient fall in pulmonary resistance that was not mediated through the beta-adrenergic system. Although these results clearly demonstrate the presence of nonadrenergic bronchodilatation, there was incomplete relaxation of the airway smooth muscle and no significant differences in the effectiveness of the bronchodilatation between normal and asthmatic subjects.[2750]

A clear picture of the possible role of deficient nonadrenergic inhibitory innervation in the pathogenesis of NSBH awaits the definitive characterization of the neurotransmitter and the development of a specific antagonist. Current evidence strongly supports vasoactive intestinal polypeptide as the neurotransmitter,[575–577] although this conclusion is not unanimous.[569]

Histamine produces bronchoconstriction in human airways by stimulating H_1 receptors. The demonstration in animals that H_1-contracting and H_2-relaxing histamine receptors could be present in the same airway tissue has raised the possibility that an imbalance in receptor number or affinity could result in the increased histamine response of asthma.[578] Despite extensive study, however, the presence and importance of H_2 receptors in human airways has not been clearly determined.[578] Although data from *in vitro* studies suggest the presence of smooth muscle–relaxing H_2 receptors, at least in large airways,[579] the expected increase in histamine-induced bronchoconstriction *in vivo* in the presence of specific H_2 blockers has not been consistent.[580–584] Whatever the role of H_1 and H_2 receptors, receptor imbalance cannot be an important contributor to NSBH because it can account for exaggerated responses only to this specific agonist.[578]

Another, and theoretically more important, role for H_2 receptors is histamine-induced feedback inhibition of mediator release from mast cells.[585, 586] If this were an important mechanism that modulated mediator release, H_2 blocker administration would be expected to worsen asthmatic symptoms and signs and increase the response to inhaled antigen, neither of which adverse effects of therapeutic doses of H_2 blockers has been reported.[583, 587] These results are of practical as well as theoretical importance, considering the widespread therapeutic use of H_2 blocking agents for peptic disease.

ABNORMALITIES OF SMOOTH MUSCLE

In pharmacologic parlance, hyper-reactivity or supersensitivity can be prejunctional or postjunctional, the junction referring to the neural (receptor) muscle cell interface. Prejunctional supersensitivity occurs when receptor number is increased or when a greater proportion of an administered or released drug is available to interact with receptors (increased input). Postjunctional supersensitivity occurs with augmentation of excitation-contraction coupling, i.e., a greater response or output for a given prejunctional input. Postjunctional supersensitivity is characteristically nonspecific;[588, 589] the nonspecificity of asthmatic airway hyper-responsiveness suggests that augmentation of excitation-contraction coupling may be important. Alternatively, a given degree of contraction could result in greater smooth muscle shortening and airway narrowing if there were an alteration in the smooth muscle length-tension relationship.[451]

To understand how changes in excitation-contraction coupling or smooth muscle length-tension relationships could result in NSBH, a brief review of the biochemistry and mechanics of airway smooth muscle contraction is desirable. The generation of tension and shortening by smooth muscle is believed to be related to actin and myosin filament interaction, similar to that which produces skeletal and cardiac muscle contraction. The initiating event is influx of free intracellular calcium from a sequestered source; calcium interacts with calmodulin, activating specific enzymes that mediate the actin and myosin cross-bridge formation, which is responsible for tension development and shortening. Calcium is normally sequestered extracellularly in a concentration 1,000 times greater than intracellular levels; this active exclusion of calcium is accomplished by an energy-requiring ion pump. In addition, calcium is stored in an inactive form within intracellular membrane–bound organelles, such as mitochondria and the sarcoplasmic reticulum. Calcium can be released into the intracellular space to initiate contraction through transmembrane channels that respond to cell depolarization (voltage-dependent channels) or through separate channels that open in response to specific receptor activation (receptor-activated channels).[590] Calcium channel blockers inhibit smooth muscle contraction by blocking the voltage-dependent channels but have little effect on receptor-operated channels or intracellular organelle sources of Ca^{++}. Once calcium is released into the cytoplasm and contraction is initiated, the free calcium is resequestered to terminate the contractile process. Cyclic adenosine monophosphate (cAMP) within the cell accelerates the removal of Ca^{++}, and bronchodilating drugs may exert their effect by increasing levels of this substance.[590] Airway hyper-responsiveness may occur as a result of either increased calcium availability from one of its sources or decreased removal of intracellular calcium. Increased contraction of the actin-myosin chain in response to Ca^{++} release is another possible cause of postjunctional supersensitivity.[588] An alteration in calcium handling could play a pivotal role in the pathogenesis of asthmatic airway obstruction at sites other than smooth muscle. The same process of calcium sequestration and release initiates both mucous secretion and mast cell mediator release, each of which is known to be abnormal in asthma. Although an abnormality of calcium handling by asthmatic airways is an intriguing possible pathogenetic mechanism of asthma, it is purely speculative at the present.

Smooth muscle can be activated in two ways:

1. So-called single-unit smooth muscle shows spontaneous oscillations in membrane potential and the development of action potentials that spread from cell to cell via electrical interconnectors between cells called gap junctions; single-unit smooth muscle is sparsely innervated but exhibits myogenic control, responding to external forces such as stretch or distention.

2. Smooth muscle can also be of a multi-unit type in which cells are densely innervated and possess little cell-to-cell communication; this type of muscle is believed to be entirely under nervous control, its mechanical activation being dependent on the magnitude and distribution of nerve firing.[591]

Although normal human tracheobronchial smooth muscle possesses some gap junctions, it behaves as the multi-unit type, being dependent on excitatory innervation to induce contraction. However, the type of smooth muscle is not static and it is possible that inflammatory mediators alter smooth muscle function and structure toward those of single-unit muscle; since activation of a single unit can enhance the response by spreading the effect of activation over many muscle units, hyper-responsiveness would be expected.[591] Single-unit behavior is a possible explanation for the bronchoconstriction that characteristically occurs in asthmatics following a deep inspiration.[592] An inspiratory capacity maneuver dilates airways and stretches the smooth muscle; if the stretch results in contraction as it does in single-unit muscle, airway narrowing would ensue. Such a myogenic response to stretch has been demonstrated in isolated smooth muscle from dogs sensitized to ovalbumin; the trachealis muscle of the sensitized dogs also demonstrates increased isometric tension with maximal stimulation and a degree and velocity of isotonic shortening that is greater than in matched controls.[593]

DECREASED SMOOTH MUSCLE LOAD

Once activated, smooth muscle narrows the airway by shortening. The degree to which the smooth muscle shortens in response to a given stimulus depends on a number of factors, including prejunctional ones such as receptor number and occupancy, the effectiveness of excitation-contraction coupling, and the load against which the muscle must shorten.

Isometric contraction occurs when smooth muscle contracts against an immovable load and the energy of contraction results in tension without shortening; by contrast, a purely *isotonic* contraction occurs when smooth muscle is completely unloaded so that the total energy is transferred into shortening. As smooth muscle is progressively loaded, both the speed and magnitude of shortening progressively decrease, the ultimate load resulting in a purely isometric contraction. The magnitude of shortening of stimulated smooth muscle is also dependent on its initial length in relation to the length-tension curve of the muscle. All muscle—smooth, striated, and cardiac—displays a characteristic length-tension relationship, there being a unique length at which stimulation will result in the greatest shortening or tension generation. This optimal length (Lmax) is determined by the optimal relationship for interaction between actin and myosin filaments within the muscle; at lengths longer or shorter than Lmax, the same stimulus will result in less shortening or tension.[594, 595]

The loads and operating lengths of smooth muscle *in vivo* are largely unexplored areas. Airway smooth muscle at optimal length *in vitro* will shorten 70 per cent when allowed to contract isotonically.[596] If airway smooth muscle completely surrounds the tracheobronchial airway, is at optimal length, and contracts isotonically, it can be calculated that muscle shortening of approximately 45 per cent could close the airways. Because maximal pharmacologic stimulation in normal subjects results in only a tenfold to 15-fold increase in resistance (approximately 30 per cent smooth muscle shortening), it is unlikely that isotonic contraction from Lmax can occur *in vivo*.[451] The vast potential for airway narrowing that these mechanical considerations imply has led Macklem to speculate that the key to understanding the hyper-responsiveness of asthma is an understanding of the apparent hyporesponsiveness of normal subjects.[597] What limits airway smooth muscle shortening in normal people? The most likely explanation is that contraction is not isotonic because the muscle is contracting against loads that impede shortening and therefore airway narrowing. In large cartilaginous airways, the muscle is clearly loaded by the outward recoil of airway cartilage,[598] whereas in smaller intraparenchymal airways it is the elastic recoil of the lung that imparts the elastic load. As the airway narrows, local lung parenchyma becomes distorted, increasing transmural pressure and converting more of the smooth muscle activation to tension generation rather than to shortening.[451]

The load dependency of smooth muscle shortening is most graphically illustrated by the effect of lung volume on maximal airway narrowing: although airway resistance varies only slightly with lung volume in the absence of smooth muscle stimulation, marked changes in resistance occur with lung volume (and therefore lung recoil changes) when smooth muscle is contracted.[599] These mechanical details of airway smooth muscle contraction suggest additional potential explanations for NSBH; if airway smooth muscle length was moved toward Lmax *in vivo* or if the loads impeding shortening were decreased, a similar activation would produce greater narrowing.

It is possible that changes in smooth muscle afterload could be important in the airway hyper-responsiveness of patients with COPD in whom the loss of lung elastic recoil and decrease in cartilage would be expected to increase the potential for shortening;[600] however, it is more difficult to envisage how the resting length or afterload could be deranged in the airways of patients with asthma.

The degree of shortening of smooth muscle in response to a stimulus depends on both muscle strength and its starting length and load. If in fact muscle shortening is limited by elastic loads, hyperplasia produced by adding fibers in series would increase the shortening for a given stimulus while not necessarily altering the maximally obtainable shortening of unloaded muscle. The effect of the increased smooth muscle strength that accompanies hyperplasia and hypertrophy is separate from the effect of increasing wall thickness discussed above but is possibly additive.[451, 486] There is morphologic evidence that the volume of smooth muscle in asthmatic airways is increased;[601, 602] if the increased muscle mass functions normally, an exaggerated shortening and airway narrowing would be expected for a given stimulus and afterload.

IN VIVO/IN VITRO COMPARISONS

The conjecture that the basic defect underlying NSBH might reside postjunctionally at the level of the smooth muscle contractile apparatus has prompted a number of investigators to compare *in vivo* airway responses to *in vitro* smooth muscle function. These studies have generally been conducted on smokers with COPD of variable severity who were undergoing operative resection of lung tissue for pulmonary carcinoma; although these subjects showed a wide range of responsiveness to inhaled bronchoconstrictors preoperatively, resected large airway tissue showed much less variability in response and no *in vivo/in vitro* correlation.[572, 603–607] All these studies have been associated with similar deficiencies:

1. All patients had COPD rather than asthma, and, as discussed above, the mechanisms of NSBH may be quite different.

2. The amount, orientation, and operating length of the smooth muscle were unknown and uncontrolled.

3. Isometric tension rather than shortening was measured.

Of some interest was a similar study of naturally hyper-responsive basenji-greyhound dogs in which no *in vivo/in vitro* relationship was apparent, although tissue amount was controlled and isotonic shortening was measured with a fixed pre-load.[608]

In the few studies in which human asthmatic airway tissue has been available for pharmacologic study, the results have also been disappointing.[2778] Although a small number of asthmatic patients appeared to have supernormal contractile responses to histamine,[609] in most the potency and efficacy of contractile agonists were the same as in tissue from nonasthmatic subjects. A decrease in relaxant responses to beta-adrenergic agonists has been reported, but it is unknown whether this is acquired as a result of chronic endogenous or exogenous beta stimulation *in vivo*.[528, 607, 610]

INFLAMMATION

Although it was initially believed that NSBH was a genetically determined phenomenon that predisposed to the development of asthma, it is becoming increasingly clear that NSBH is acquired *as a consequence of* rather than a *risk factor for* asthma.[404, 611] Normal airway responses have been observed in asymptomatic monozygotic twins of asthmatic patients with airway hyper-responsiveness.[335, 418] Bronchial hyper-responsiveness develops in normal subjects following viral respiratory tract infections[612] or exposure to ozone or other atmospheric pollutants.[420] NSBH also increases with infection and pollutant exposure in asthmatic subjects and is enhanced following specific antigen challenge[613–615] and inhalation of ultrasonically nebulized distilled water.[616, 617] The increased responsiveness associated with antigen exposure occurs following challenge in a laboratory as well as to natural antigen. The enhanced NSBH appears to be dependent on the development of a late response to antigen; patients with an isolated immediate response do not show a change although NSBH may be increased in the interval between the immediate and delayed response.[613, 618–620, 2779] NSBH increases during the pollen season in asthmatic subjects who are sensitive to ragweed and grass.[621]

Perhaps the clearest demonstration of acquired airway hyper-responsiveness occurs in occupational asthma.[622] The NSBH that occurs with the development of sensitivity to plicatic acid in western red cedar sawdust can be profound. Similarly, toluene diiosocyanate in the plastic and paint industries induces increased airway responsiveness in sensitive individuals; the delayed response to this substance and the subsequent increase in NSBR can be blocked by prednisone but not by indomethacin.[623] In the majority of affected individuals, the hyper-responsiveness decreases slowly after cessation of exposure to these substances.[404, 422] The ability to enhance or produce hyper-responsiveness on exposure to a variety of substances has led to the suggestion of a new terminology for bronchoactive agents.[624] *Inciters* are considered to be the agents of primary response, the most commonly employed being histamine, methacholine, exercise, and isocapnic dry air hyperventilation; an inciter produces bronchoconstriction without altering subsequent responses to bronchoactive agents. *Inducers* are substances or processes that augment the nonspecific response to inciters, usually after producing their own bronchoconstrictive effect; included among the inducers are the late asthmatic response, occupational exposure, endotoxin, and viral infection.

Airway hyper-responsiveness can be induced in animals by exposure to cigarette smoke, ozone, toluene diiosocyanate, or antigen.[420, 625, 626] Animal models have allowed investigation of the mechanisms by which these various exposures cause NSBH. A feature common to all agents that induce hyper-responsiveness is the development of airway inflammation,[627] characterized by an initial exudative phase during which mucosal and vascular permeability is increased; this is followed by a cellular phase during which acute inflammatory cells migrate from the circulation into the airway wall, particularly the epithelium. This is accompanied by sloughing of epithelial cells and by mucous hypersecretion.[420]

The mechanisms by which inflammation results in hyper-responsiveness remains conjectural, but a number have been postulated. As discussed above, the increased permeability of endothelium and epithelium may result in greater exposure of airway smooth muscle and irritant receptors to inhaled or injected agonist. However, failure to demonstrate hyperpermeability in stable but hyper-responsive asthmatic patients makes this unlikely as the sole explanation for the phenomenon of NSBH.[497] Alternatively, the increased vascular permeability caused by the inflammatory process could result in airway wall edema;[628] by the geometric factors discussed above, the resulting thickening may enhance the airway narrowing effect of a given degree of smooth muscle shortening. Finally, the release of secondary mediators from inflammatory cells could directly alter smooth muscle responsiveness.[420, 629]

The relationship between inflammation and increased smooth muscle response has been described in animals exposed to ozone and antigen. The evidence suggests that ozone causes acute airway epithelial damage and that the damaged epithelium responds by producing leukotriene-derived chemotactic substances such as leukotriene B_4. The chemotaxin causes neutrophil accumulation in the airway wall, and prostaglandin products released from these cells act on smooth muscle to enhance its responsiveness to challenges subsequently administered. This schema has been suggested following a careful series of studies designed to identify the pertinent events in ozone-induced hyper-responsiveness:

1. Increased airway responsiveness is coincident with an inflammatory cell influx into the airway wall, observed in both biopsy specimens and bronchial lavage fluid.

2. Although neutrophil depletion does not change the initial epithelial injury produced by ozone, it blocks the cellular phase of the inflammatory response and the subsequent hyper-responsiveness;

3. Indomethacin, an inhibitor of prostaglandin production, diminishes the hyper-responsiveness but not the influx of neutrophils.

Except for the neutrophil depletion study, many of these same experiments have been repeated and confirmed in man following ozone exposure.[420] For example, in a study of ten normal subjects,[630] an increase in NSBR was observed following exposure to 0.4 or 0.6 parts per million (ppm) ozone; bronchoalveolar lavage demonstrated an increase in the number of neutrophils and of concentrations of PGE_2, $PGF_{2\alpha}$, and thromboxane B_2. A similar chain of events is possible following antigen challenge in sensitive subjects. Neutrophil depletion decreases airway responses to aerosolized histamine in sheep and in passively sensitized rabbits.[631] Chemotactic substances may be released from mast cells as well as from epithelial cells.

The role of prostaglandin products in the modification of airway response to other agonists has been confirmed in human studies. When administered by inhalation prior to histamine or methacholine, $PGF_{2\alpha}$ and PGD_2 have been shown to increase the response to these agonists, an effect that could not be explained by decreased baseline airway caliber since the dose of prostaglandin was sufficiently low that it did not produce detectable bronchoconstriction on its own.[336, 632, 633] In normal subjects, indomethacin treatment has been shown to decrease airway responsiveness in stable asthmatic subjects and to block the increased responsiveness attendant on viral infection.[612, 634] Although prostaglandin produced by inflammatory cells may enhance airway responsiveness, prostaglandin secreted by normal respiratory epithelium may actually decrease the smooth muscle response. Canine bronchial preparations have shown exaggerated contraction in response to acetylcholine and histamine when stripped of epithelium prior to challenge.[635] The aerosol administration of platelet-activating factor (PAF) has been shown to enhance subsequent airway responsiveness to nonspecific agents in both animals and humans.[636, 637] PAF causes intense and prolonged inflammation of the airways, increased microvascular permeability, and edema.[637]

Experiments such as those discussed above illustrate the importance of considering the environment of the airway smooth muscle. The bronchoconstrictive response of muscle *in vivo* is much more complex than the response that occurs in an organ bath. Mediators to which smooth muscle is exposed *in vivo* or which are released from inflammatory, epithelial, or other cells in response to bronchoconstricting influences can modify the subsequent response in a way that is not possible *in vitro*.

Although inflammation-induced modification of smooth muscle response is an attractive theory, a word of caution seems appropriate. In normal subjects, the increase in NSBR caused by manipulations that produce airway inflammation is small compared with the large increases in sensitivity and maximal response apparent in asthmatic patients. In addition, the small changes in sensitivity and response that can be produced in normal subjects are transient whereas the NSBH of asthmatic subjects is prolonged.

The suggestion that chronic airway inflammation might be the underlying pathophysiologic inducer of NSBH has resulted in a number of studies designed to decrease hyper-responsiveness with chronic anti-inflammatory therapy. In these studies, prolonged (weeks to months) treatment with inhaled sodium cromoglycate[638–640] or inhaled[641, 642] or oral[643] corticosteroids has generally shown some decrease in NSBH; however, the degree of improvement has been disappointing and has been difficult to separate from simple improvement in baseline airway caliber.[644]

Consequences of Nonspecific Bronchial Hyper-responsiveness

Although the pathogenesis of NSBH is not completely understood, its physiologic and clinical

manifestations have been clearly established. NSBH renders asthmatic subjects susceptible to excessive airway narrowing in response to a wide variety of otherwise trivial exposures. The importance of NSBH as a determinant of symptomatic asthma is most clearly defined for allergic reactions. It was the studies of Killian[645] and Cockcroft[646] and their colleagues who first showed that the magnitude of the airway response to inhaled specific allergen in allergic asthmatic patients was related to the severity of allergy, assessed by the size of the skin response to a given dose of allergen and the degree of NSBH measured by a histamine dose-response curve. The severity of antigen-induced bronchoconstriction can be appreciated better by a combination of NSBH and skin test response than by either alone (Fig. 11–30), an observation that has been confirmed by a number of investigators.[647–649] These studies point out the vicious circle of specific and nonspecific airway responses that tend to perpetuate and potentiate the asthmatic state: on the one hand, allergen exposure induces increased nonspecific airway response; on the other, the degree of response is related to the NSBH. It is probable that the majority of everyday symptoms experienced by asthmatic patients are secondary to excessive airway narrowing in response to otherwise trivial inhalational exposures. These nonspecific episodes occur on a

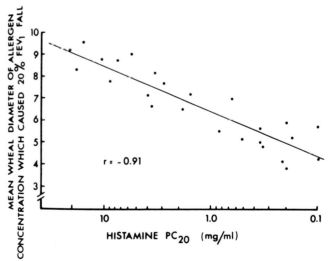

Figure 11–30. Relationship of Allergic and Nonallergic Airway Responsiveness. The magnitude of the airway allergic response is determined by an individual's degree of sensitization to the inhaled antigen and by nonspecific bronchial hyperresponsiveness. This plot shows the mean wheal diameter raised by a skin test using the concentration of allergen that caused a 20 per cent fall in FEV_1 during inhalation challenge in individual asthmatic subjects versus the nonspecific bronchial hyperresponsiveness as determined by the histamine concentration that provoked a 20 per cent decrease in FEV_1. Individuals with increased nonspecific bronchial responsiveness (low valves for PC_{20}) require only low concentrations of inhaled antigen, whereas those without increased nonspecific bronchial responsiveness (higher values for PC_{20}) require a larger concentration of antigen. (From Cockcroft DW, Ruffin RE, Frith PA, et al: Am Rev Respir Dis *120*:1053, 1979.)

background of episodic exposure to inducing inflammatory agents, such as allergens, viruses, and atmospheric pollution.[627, 650, 651]

Clinical Usefulness of Nonspecific Bronchial Hyper-responsiveness

NSBH correlates with the severity of asthma. Patients with greater nonspecific responsiveness tend to experience greater diurnal variation in lung function, greater increases in flow rates with inhaled bronchodilators, and symptoms that are more difficult to control.[652] The measurement of nonspecific airway response can be used in epidemiologic studies and as a test in the investigation of the basic mechanisms of asthma. Clinically, it is employed to make the diagnosis of asthma and to follow its severity in relation to treatment or exposure to occupational sensitizing substances.

Although the diagnosis of asthma is usually made from history, spirometry, and the response to bronchodilating drugs, there are patients in whom the history may not be clear and who demonstrate normal spirometric values at the time of examination, thus precluding assessment of bronchodilator response; in these subjects, NSBH (defined, for example, by a PC_{20} of less than 8 mg/ml) is a very useful adjunct to diagnosis.[653] Tests of nonspecific airway responsiveness are particularly useful in patients with the isolated symptom of chronic cough; this can be the sole presenting symptom in some patients with asthma, and the demonstration of increased nonspecific airway responsiveness is useful in predicting whether the patient will respond symptomatically to the inhalation of beta-adrenergic agents.[653, 654] However, as discussed earlier, the lack of nonspecific airway hyper-responsiveness does not completely exclude the diagnosis of asthma; rarely, some patients, especially those with seasonal symptoms or occupational asthma, may develop detectable hyper-responsiveness only following exposure to sufficient inducing agents.[653] Similarly, NSBH alone does not confirm the diagnosis of asthma, particularly if baseline airway function is abnormal.[429, 431] Although tests of NSBR may be useful in diagnosing asthma in patients with normal or near-normal baseline lung function, they are of less help and potentially dangerous in those who are already severely obstructed; in such patients, the history and response to bronchodilators are usually diagnostic.[655] Because NSBH can be altered by treatment, it is theoretically possible to use it as an indicator of the effectiveness of therapy and the need for more or less intensive therapy (e.g., decreasing systemic corticosteroid dosage as NSBH decreases); in fact, Woolcock[656] has suggested that the measurement of NSBR should be a routine part of the clinical assessment of patients with asthma as an indicator of severity and as a guide to therapeutic response. In an occupational setting, serial measurement of NSBH may be of particular value; i.e., the development or worsening of NSBH with occupational exposure and its gradual improvement following withdrawal of exposure is strong evidence that the symptoms are work-related.[657] A rapid method has been developed to test for NSBH and has been used in epidemiologic investigation of the prevalence of asthma.[655]

Purpose of Airway Smooth Muscle

The harmful effects of excessive airway smooth muscle contraction lead naturally to speculation as to what useful function the muscle serves normally. Unlike in the gut or urinary bladder, in which smooth muscle is vital for normal organ function, the presence of smooth muscle in the human lung might be considered a mere vestigial nuisance; in fact, however, smooth muscle in the airways may serve a number of useful, if not vital, homeostatic functions. The most important may be to protect against impurities in the inspired air: by narrowing the airway and increasing the linear velocity of inspired air, bronchoconstriction encourages impaction of inspired particles on central airways where effective mucociliary clearance and cough can readily expel the offending substance. In mammals that live in the ocean, airway smooth muscle is highly developed and may actually be able to close large airways completely to prevent the accidental aspiration of salt water. Like pulmonary vascular smooth muscle, airway smooth muscle may also play a part in the matching of ventilation and perfusion; regional alveolar hypocapnia as a consequence of a high $\dot{V}_A/\dot{Q}$ ratio tends to cause bronchoconstriction, thus decreasing the regional overventilation. In addition, the action of vagal tone on parenchymal smooth muscle contributes to the static recoil of the normal human lung; unevenness of vagal tone or regional variation in the response to it serves to improve the uniform distribution of inspired air.[658, 659] Airway smooth muscle contraction in the trachea and mainstem bronchi may decrease the collapsibility of these structures by preventing invagination of their posterior membranous portion and allowing the tips of the cartilaginous rings to abut.[660]

Summary

Nonspecific bronchial hyper-responsiveness is the exaggerated airway narrowing demonstrated by asthmatic individuals in response to inhalation of pharmacologic bronchoconstricting agents and a variety of irritant substances. It can be quantified by measuring the dose or concentration of inhaled histamine or methacholine that causes a 20 per cent decrease in FEV_1. Bronchial hyper-responsiveness is almost invariable in patients with asthma and is a useful diagnostic test.

Rather than being a congenital defect that increases the risk of developing asthma, NSBH is probably an acquired abnormality; however, its pathogenesis remains unknown despite considerable research. Although numerous hypotheses have been proposed to account for NSBH, the most plausible theory is that it is a consequence of the chronic inflammatory reaction in the airway mucosa of asthmatic patients. Inflammation may cause hyper-responsiveness by producing epithelial damage and increased airway permeability, by causing airway wall edema and thickening, and by altering the amount and contractility of airway smooth muscle. Although characteristic of asthma and virtually diagnostic when the baseline FEV_1 is normal, increased bronchial responsiveness also occurs in other airway diseases associated with baseline airway narrowing such as COPD, cystic fibrosis, and bronchiectasis.

In patients with asthma, NSBH is important not only because it is a diagnostic and investigative test but also because it is probably responsible for the majority of symptoms.

PROVOKING FACTORS

Susceptible individuals are prone to episodic airway obstruction that can be precipitated in a variety of ways. The most thoroughly studied of these provoking factors is the inhalation of antigenic material by a sensitized individual, resulting in an extrinsic allergen-induced asthmatic attack. Bronchospasm can also occur in association with anaphylaxis, which consists of a generalized allergic reaction precipitated by ingestion, inhalation, or parenteral administration of a specific allergen. Infection or exercise can initiate attacks in patients with either intrinsic or extrinsic asthma. In some asthmatics—usually middle-aged and nonatopic—certain analgesics, notably acetylsalicylic acid (ASA), can cause severe, even fatal, bronchoconstriction. Exposure to nonspecific irritants in the atmosphere, food additives, ingested antigens, and altered climatic conditions can all induce attacks. Occupational exposure to sensitizing agents, some of which act by classic IgE-mediated allergic pathways, is becoming increasingly important. Psychophysiologic factors are probably responsible for some attacks, and there is evidence that the severity of airway obstruction in response to a variety of agents can be worsened or alleviated by suggestion.

Allergens

Specific antigens provoke asthmatic attacks in sensitized persons who frequently suffer from other allergic manifestations, such as hay fever and eczema, and who usually manifest positive prick or intradermal skin tests to a variety of allergens. Despite these indications for a state of hypersensitivity, however, the antigen responsible for a specific attack of bronchoconstriction is often not identified.

In a minority of patients with extrinsic asthma, the timing of attacks coincident with exposure to certain antigens leaves little doubt as to the cause of the attacks, particularly antigens such as pollens, animal dander, and some foods. More frequently, incrimination of a suspected allergen requires confirmation by more reliable means such as radioallergosorbent test (RAST)[661, 662] or inhalation challenge.[662] RAST is an *in vitro* radioimmunoassay in which anti-IgE prepared in animals is used to detect IgE antibodies to specific allergens in human serum.[662] The RAST has the advantage of preventing risk or discomfort for the patient.

Tests for the detection of specific antigens responsible for asthma measure tissue-bound or serum IgE reagin. This immunoglobulin, first described in 1966,[663] is believed to bind to tissue mast cells and circulating basophils from which chemical mediators are released after interaction with specific antigens. Although many asthmatics have raised levels of total IgE,[664, 665] there is considerable overlap with values obtained in normal subjects.[665] Serum levels of IgE do not distinguish asthmatics from control populations nearly as well as do skin tests and radioallergosorbent tests,[666] nor are levels significantly different in allergic and nonallergic asthmatics.[667] The serum concentration of IgE gives little indication of the severity of the disease; in fact, very high levels of IgE (such as are found in patients with parasitic infestation) are thought to block the binding sites on the mast cells from specific IgE molecules and thus to protect against asthma.[352] In population studies, peak IgE levels occur between 6 and 14 years of age and decline progressively thereafter. Males have higher levels than females, and subjects with positive skin responses to antigens have levels four to five times higher than non–skin test–sensitive subjects.[668] Although there is general agreement that antigen activation of an IgE-sensitized target releases mediators by a noncytotoxic secretory process with the initiation of immediate anaphylaxis, some workers[669, 670] have also demonstrated immediate reactions to skin prick and inhalation challenge with the house mite *Dermatophagoides pteronyssimus*, mediated by a short-term sensitizing IgG.

Potential antigens in our environment are innumerable. Exposure to a variety of organic and inorganic materials often is governed by geographic and seasonal variation. Allergenic and industrial sensitization is an increasing and poorly understood problem urgently requiring investigation and control. Surveys of the population at large with immediate skin test reactivity to a variety of antigens indicate that approximately 30 per cent demonstrate a positive prick test response to at least one allergen.[671-673] Many of these sensitive individuals are asymptomatic, and those with allergies usually suffer from only seasonal or perennial rhinitis. Positive skin test reactions show a definite age relationship, the peak incidence being in the third decade and decreasing rapidly after the age of 50.[671] A number of surveys of atmospheric pollens and fungal spores (and skin test reactions to them) reveal geographic variation. Grass and tree pollens are universal and are the most common causes of hay fever.[671, 674–676] These antigens cause positive skin reactions and inhalation challenge in many atopic asthmatics[677, 678] but are not thought to be common causes of asthmatic attacks. In fact, seasonal asthma caused by pollens usually is not severe. Ragweed pollen grains are approximately 20 μm in diameter and are in the nonrespirable range; thus, only fragmented pollen grains can gain access to the lower respiratory tract.[679] In addition to pollens, fungal spores are a major source of airborne allergens, usually outnumbering pollen spores by up to 1,000:1. The most commonly recognized forms are the imperfect fungi, which include *Alternaria, Aspergillus, Cladosporium, Mucor,* and *Penicillium*; however, additional entire families have been relatively ignored and may be important.[680]

A variety of foods, especially eggs, fish, shellfish, nuts, spices, and chocolate, tend to cause immediate wheal and erythematous skin reactions to intracutaneous skin testing, particularly in children. Evidence of hypersensitivity to the specific food may be corroborated by the occurrence of an asthmatic attack following ingestion of the food in question and sometimes by the absence of attacks when the specific allergens are avoided. By contrast, some young people who manifest positive skin test reactions to specific food allergens can consume these foods repeatedly with apparent impunity.

A substantial proportion (approximately 11 per cent) of chronic hemodialysis patients develop IgE antibody in response to human serum albumin—ethylene oxide conjugates. Ethylene oxide is used in sterilization of the dialysis equipment. Some of these patients develop chronic asthma, and others experience anaphylactoid reactions during dialysis.[681]

Animal dander from a variety of household pets, including gerbils and guinea pigs in addition to the more ubiquitous cat and dog, can cause ocular and nasal symptoms as well as asthma.[680]

Certain insects such as the caddis fly (mayfly) and the mushroom fly have been held responsible for epidemic asthma in certain areas during the spring and autumn.[682, 683] Support for the theory that insects can act as allergens has been provided in recent years by evidence incriminating house mites as a responsible allergen in house dust. Many asthmatics show positive skin test reactions to house dusts, and although such dusts contain many substances, including potentially allergenic molds and disintegrating fibers, a number of studies have shown that various house mites, notably *D. pteronyssimus*, are present in large numbers, particularly in dust from mattresses.[684–687] The house mite measures approximately 300 μm in length and thrives in homes that are usually damp. Several reports[684, 688, 689] have shown that individuals sensitive to house dust also manifest increased sensitivity to extracts of house mites, although desensitization with house mite extracts is not always therapeutically efficacious.[686] Thirty per cent of patients whose skin tests are positive to house dust do not react to *D. pteronyssimus*, but most of these respond to animal danders present in the dust.[690]

A particularly serious and sometimes fatal manifestation of anaphylaxis in humans can occur following administration of drugs.[691, 692] The reaction usually occurs when the drug is administered intravenously or intramuscularly, although oral, percutaneous, or even respiratory exposure may produce a response in highly sensitive individuals. The drug most commonly implicated in this reaction is penicillin. In a study of 809 cases of anaphylactic shock resulting from parenteral administration of antibiotics, Welch and his associates[693] judged all but 16 to be due to penicillin; 74 (9.1 per cent) of these patients died. Sensitive individuals may develop asthmatic attacks from inhaled medications, including acetylcysteine,[694] pancreatic dornase,[695] lidocaine,[696] and even disodium cromoglycate[697, 698] and beclomethasone dipropionate[699] administered for the relief of bronchospasm itself.

Another cause of potentially fatal anaphylaxis is a sting from one of the insects of the *Hymenoptera* order, including bees, wasps, hornets, and yellow jackets.[692] In the United States, stings from these insects are said to cause as many deaths as do snake bites.[692] Usually, the victim has an atopic background;[700] in one study of 249 affected patients, 53 per cent had a history of rhinitis, asthma, or cutaneous allergy.[692]

Other substances that occasionally cause systemic anaphylactic reactions in humans include heterologous proteins in the form of antiserum, hormones, enzymes, extracts, foods, and diagnostic agents such as iodinated contrast media and sulfobromophthalein (Bromsulphalein, BSP).[700] A rare cause is passive sensitization by blood transfusion from an atopic donor.[701, 702] Typically, an anaphylactic reaction develops rapidly, reaching a maximum within 5 to 30 minutes. Early symptoms include nausea and vomiting, pruritus, and substernal tightness; these are followed quickly by generalized urticaria, angioedema, shortness of breath, weakness, hypotension, choking, and loss of consciousness. The commonest cause of death is asphyxia due to laryngeal edema or acute bronchoconstriction, although sometimes the clinical presentation may be one of circulatory collapse and hypovolemia.[703, 704] Anaphylactic sensitivity in humans is mediated largely by IgE antibodies and perhaps occasionally by some IgG subclass antibodies.

Although IgE-mediated extrinsic asthma is generally recognized as the allergic form of this disease, this does not necessarily imply that allergic factors can be excluded in nonatopic asthma. In one study of 656 asthmatic patients,[705] 554 of whom had positive and 102 negative skin prick tests, more than half (52 per cent) of the former group were under

10 years of age at the time of onset of asthma, whereas an almost equal percentage (56 per cent) of the negative response group were over 30 years of age at the time of onset. Of the larger group with positive skin test results, 70 per cent reported a history of rhinitis and 29 per cent of infantile eczema, compared with 48 per cent and 9 per cent, respectively, in the skin test–negative group. Symptoms attributed to house dust, pollens, and animal dander were noted two to three times more frequently in the atopics. Also, a larger percentage of the patients with negative skin test results had been treated with corticosteroid drugs.[705]

In contrast to patients with extrinsic asthma in whom sensitization is due to specific antigens, those with a typical clinical picture of intrinsic asthma (i.e., negative skin tests, negative allergic histories, some eosinophilia, and long-term severe bronchospasm requiring steroid therapy) have lymphocytes that are sensitive *in vitro* to a large variety of nonspecific antigens, as judged by the production of macrophage inhibitory factor.[706]

The interaction of allergen and specific IgE on mast cells and basophils brings about the release of preformed granule-associated mediators and the production of a variety of membrane-derived products. The immediate asthmatic response as well as the late phase or delayed response is believed to be a consequence of this initial event. Inhaled antigen first comes in contact with mast cells in the respiratory epithelium. Mediator released from these superficial mast cells can alter epithelial permeability, allowing penetration of antigen through the mucosal barrier, where it can interact with IgE on tissue mast cells and circulating basophils. In the nose, migration of mast cells into the epithelium appears to be induced by exposure to specific antigen.[707, 708] In 12 patients who were allergic to birch pollen,[709] the total number of mast cells in nasal biopsy specimens did not change during the pollen season although the percentage in the nasal epithelium was increased.

When a sensitized individual inhales antigen, there occurs an immediate or early response characterized by bronchoconstriction, which reaches a maximum in 15 to 30 minutes and is followed by a return toward normal lung function even without treatment.[710] In some patients, the early response is followed by a late or delayed response that comes on between 3 and 10 hours after the initial challenge and may persist for 48 hours (Fig. 11–31). In some patients, a single-antigen inhalation challenge is followed by recurrent nocturnal episodes of asthma.[709] Occasional individuals develop only a delayed response to inhaled antigen. Although it was initially believed that the late response might be mediated by IgG antibody, it is now accepted that it is a delayed result of the immediate IgE–

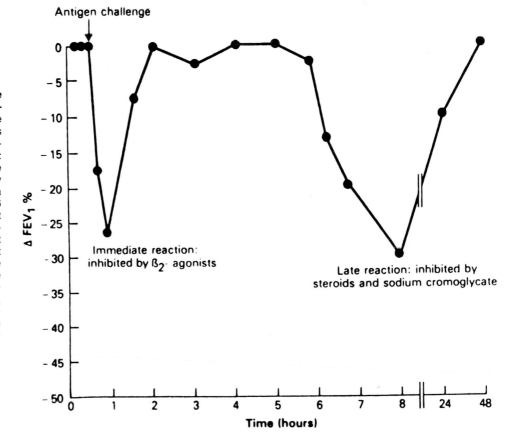

Figure 11–31. Immediate and Late Allergic Airway Response. This graph reveals the response when asthmatic patients are challenged with a specific antigen to which they are allergic: they can develop an immediate bronchoconstriction that generally wanes by 1 hour, followed by a late reaction that begins 4 to 6 hours after challenge and can last as long as 24 hours. Beta-adrenergic agonists effectively inhibit the immediate allergic reaction but have less effect on alleviating the late response. Both the immediate and late responses can be inhibited by sodium cromoglycate, whereas steroid therapy attenuates the late response but has no influence on the immediate response.

mast cell interaction. A delayed response to antigen also occurs with nasal and dermal antigen skin challenge.

Besides being more prolonged, the late asthmatic response differs from the immediate response with respect to modulation by pharmacologic interventions. Beta-adrenergic agonists in sufficient concentration effectively block the immediate response but are much less effective against the delayed response; corticosteroids do not influence the immediate response but attenuate the late response; and sodium cromoglycate blocks both the immediate and the late responses.[711] Increased blood levels of histamine and of neutrophil chemotactic factor of anaphylaxis can be found during the immediate response and a second peak occurs coincident with the delayed response in those individuals in whom it develops.[712] The physiologic changes associated with the immediate and late responses are similar; however, there is evidence of more peripheral airway participation during the delayed response, in which the pulmonary function changes closely resemble those found in spontaneous exacerbations of asthma.[713] The delayed response in human skin and in the airways of animals is characterized by edema and a mixed cell inflammatory infiltrate that creates perivascular cuffing.[382, 714] Some indication of the mechanisms involved in the induction of the late asthmatic response can be obtained by bronchoalveolar lavage during this phase of the allergic response. Lam and associates[715] demonstrated an increase in the amount of albumin and in the number of eosinophils and neutrophils in the lavage fluid during the late response; in addition, they showed the presence of epithelial damage as evidenced by an increased number of desquamated epithelial cells.

The similarity of the pathology of the late phase response to that of chronic asthma suggests that the former may be the link between immediate hypersensitivity reactions and the subacute or chronic airway disease that characterizes the majority of patients with asthma. Repeated late responses to antigen can result in chronic structural and functional changes in the airway; a similar common final pathway of airway inflammation may explain the similarity of airway function and pathology in asthmatic patients in whom asthma is triggered by nonallergic mechanisms.[359, 716]

Mediators and Cells

HISTAMINE

In humans, histamine originates from mast cells and basophils. It produces airway smooth muscle contraction by a direct action on the muscle and by stimulation of afferent receptors that cause reflex bronchoconstriction.[717]

Allergic subjects challenged with allergens develop increased levels of histamine in mixed venous

and atrial blood, although arterial levels are higher, indicating that histamine is metabolized in its passage through the systemic circulation.[718] Sensitized dogs challenged with an aerosol of A. suum antigen develop measurable concentrations of histamine in arterial plasma, levels correlating with the degree of airflow obstruction; however, when very dilute antigen is inhaled, bronchoconstriction still occurs despite undetectable levels of histamine in arterial plasma, thus indicating the importance of the local effects of chemical mediators.[719] The importance of local tissue concentrations has also been observed in studies in which the effects of aerosol and intravenous histamine have been compared:[720] histamine administered intravenously to asthmatic patients results in less bronchial response than when it is administered as an aerosol, even though the intravenous route produces systemic symptoms such as flushing and a throbbing headache. In both animals and humans, large doses of histamine administered intravenously can produce contraction of smooth muscle in alveolar ducts and bronchioles, causing decrease in static compliance.[721] It is unknown whether histamine-induced parenchymal smooth muscle contraction occurs in humans with asthma. By stimulating afferent lung receptors, locally released histamine can also induce cough and changes in the breathing pattern.[722, 723]

The recent demonstration of the existence of two types of histamine receptors (H_1 and H_2) has resulted in renewed interest in this substance. Although stimulation of H_2 receptors on the smooth muscle of various animal species results in bronchodilatation or attenuation of the H_1 constrictor response, the presence of significant H_2 receptor–induced relaxation of smooth muscle in humans remains doubtful.[578] On the other hand, H_2 receptors located on cells other than smooth muscle may be important modulators of the allergic response; for example, H_2 receptors on suppressor cell lymphocytes may allow histamine-induced modulation of IgE production.[332] Both H_1 and H_2 receptors may be present on mast cells so that histamine release can feedback to modulate subsequent mediator release through cyclic nucleotide induction.[724, 725] In sheep, the effects of histamine H_1 and H_2 receptor stimulation on bronchial vascular smooth muscle have been shown to be different: stimulation of H_1 receptors results in bronchoconstriction without bronchial vascular dilatation, whereas H_2 stimulation increases bronchial blood flow without inducing airway smooth muscle contraction.[726] Increased bronchial blood flow may modulate airway responses by removing locally produced mediators.

Parenteral H_1 receptor blockade does not significantly decrease the airway response to inhaled antigen because the blocker is ineffective in antagonizing mediators that are released locally and because other released mediators are not inhibited.[727, 728]

CHEMOTACTIC FACTORS

Neutrophil chemotactic factor of anaphylaxis (NCFA) is a slightly acidic macromolecule of large molecular weight (greater than 750,000 daltons) that is specifically chemotactic for polymorphonuclear leukocytes and eosinophils. NCFA is released from antigen-challenged human lung fragments[729] and can be detected in the peripheral circulation shortly after induction of the immediate allergic airway response.[730, 731] Blood levels can remain elevated for 24 hours or more and can undergo a secondary increase during delayed bronchoconstrictive responses.[732, 733] NCFA is believed to be released from mast cells as a preformed mediator because pretreatment with sodium cromoglycate blocks the increase in blood levels. NCFA can also be detected in peripheral blood during exercise-induced asthmatic attacks.[734] In addition to attracting leukocytes to the site of release, NCFA can also activate leukocytes.[735]

Eosinophil chemotactic factor of anaphylaxis (ECFA) is a small-molecular-weight (300 to 3000 daltons) substance released from mast cells preformed and is obviously chemotactic for eosinophils.[736] Both NCFA and ECFA as well as small-molecular-weight chemotaxins derived from lipoxygenase metabolism of arachidonic acid may be important in the induction of the late asthmatic response; the latter is characterized by the presence of inflammatory cells at the site of the initial mediator release.[737]

PLATELET-ACTIVATING FACTOR

Platelet-activating factor (PAF) is a phospholipid that is released from mast cells and basophils during antigen challenge. It can also be produced by macrophages and its release stimulated by endotoxin.[738] In addition to causing platelet aggregation and degranulation, PAF is associated with a wide variety of biologic activities that may be important in the pathogenesis of asthma. In the presence of platelets, PAF causes airway smooth muscle contraction; by itself it increases vascular permeability and in aerosol form causes prolonged inflammation and eosinophilia in animals. PAF may also release or generate mitogenic factors that could lead to airway smooth muscle hypertrophy or hyperplasia and the development of nonspecific bronchial hyper-responsiveness.[739, 738]

In contrast to its effect on animals, antigen challenge of sensitive asthmatic patients does not result in pulmonary sequestration of platelets, although deleterious effects of PAF may occur in the absence of platelets.[740] Platelet kinetics are abnormal in asymptomatic asthmatics, there being an almost 50 per cent decrease in the circulating half-life, but the lung does not appear to be the preferred sequestration site.[741, 742] The recent demonstration that inhalation of an aerosol containing PAF results in a prolonged increase in nonspecific airway responsiveness in normal subjects is an exciting development.[637]

ADDITIONAL PREFORMED MEDIATORS

Basophils contain and may release a kallikrein-like enzyme on antigen challenge. The enzyme can react with human plasma kininogen and generate kinins that can provide an additional link between immediate anaphylaxis and the delayed response and chronic inflammation of asthma.[743, 744] In asthmatic patients, nebulized bradykinin causes prolonged cough, retrosternal discomfort, and bronchoconstriction.[745] Mast cell granules also contain heparin, neutral proteases, and acid hydrolases (such as N-acetyl-beta-glucosaminidase, beta-glucoronidase, and aryl sulfatase). The role that these enzymes play in the allergic response is unknown, but it is possible that they contribute to tissue damage.[736]

The other major source of inflammatory mediators that may play a role in asthma is the cell membrane–derived products of arachidonic acid metabolism. Antigen-antibody interaction in addition to other stimuli can result in activation of intramembranous methyltransferases that convert phosphatidylethanolamine to phosphatidylcholine. This process results in calcium influx, activating intramembranous phospholipase A_2 that in turn catalyses the generation of arachidonic acid from phosphatidylcholine; arachidonic acid is then acted upon by enzymes of the cyclooxygenase or lipoxygenase pathway to produce prostaglandins or leukotrienes, respectively.[736]

PROSTAGLANDINS

Although virtually all cells have the ability to generate prostaglandins, the amount and type produced are dependent on the enzyme content of the individual cell type. Prostaglandins can both contract and relax airway smooth muscle. In normal subjects, PGE_1 and PGE_2 usually cause bronchodilatation, although low concentrations result in bronchoconstriction.[746, 747] In asthmatic patients, administration of PGE_2 by aerosol produces either bronchoconstriction or dilatation.[747] Prostaglandin F_2 is the best known of the bronchoconstricting prostaglandins; asthmatic patients are up to 8,000 times more sensitive to PGF_2 than are healthy normal subjects,[748–750] although some asthmatic individuals show a paradoxical bronchodilatation or tachyphylaxis with high concentrations of the inhaled drug.[751, 752] When infused intravenously, PGF_2 has little effect on airway function in normal or asthmatic subjects, although it causes some smooth muscle contraction in alveolar ducts, especially in asthmatics.[744, 753] Despite these results, the therapeutic administration of PGF_2 to women with normal lung function for purposes of abortion has been shown to result in greatly reduced midexpiratory flow rates, air trapping, and hypoxemia.[754] Prostaglandin D_2 is released in substantial amounts after IgE challenge of human lung and is a potent bronchoconstrictor in normal and asthmatic subjects.[755]

Because antigen challenge of lung fragments from sensitized individuals[756] and inhalation of specific allergens by asthmatic patients[757] result in the release of prostaglandins and their metabolites, there is much potential for prostaglandin contribution to allergic airway responses. However, since sodium cromoglycate is unable to inhibit bronchospasm induced by PGF_2[757, 758] whereas it blocks antigen responses, it is unlikely that bronchoconstricting prostaglandins play a major role in IgE-mediated asthma. In fact, in allergic nonasthmatic subjects (such as those with allergic rhinitis), pretreatment with indomethacin has been shown to increase bronchoconstriction in response to inhaled antigen, suggesting that in some individuals production of bronchodilator prostaglandins may be an important negative feedback mechanism.[759]

ASA, indomethacin, and other analgesics provoke asthma and anaphylaxis in some individuals, and it is thought that this is related to the ability of these agents to block cyclooxygenase, the first enzyme in the pathway of prostaglandin synthesis.[760] The effectiveness of these agents in inhibiting prostaglandin synthesis *in vitro* has been shown to correlate with the degree of bronchoconstriction produced *in vivo*,[761] and it has been postulated that asthmatic subjects who are sensitive to analgesics produce large amounts of the bronchodilating PGE_2 to compensate for their airway narrowing; a sudden drop in PGE_2 synthesis in response to these medications precipitates an acute asthmatic attack.[760] The recent demonstration that the bronchoconstricting leukotrienes are also derived from arachidonic acid metabolism suggests an alternative hypothesis—that cyclooxygenase blockade results in increased substrate for the lipoxygenase pathway and increased leukotriene synthesis.

LEUKOTRIENES

The remarkable increase in our understanding of the leukotrienes over the past several years illustrates the rapidity with which scientific knowledge is progressing in the modern era. Since the last edition of this text, the chemical structures of the elusive slow-reacting substances of anaphylaxis (SRS-A) have been discovered and these substances have been synthesized. In addition, pharmacologic blockers have been made and sensitive techniques of assay have been developed.

Like the prostaglandins, the leukotrienes are derived from the metabolism of arachidonic acid; the initial enzymatic step in the biosynthetic sequence is a lipoxygenase, and a large number of substances are generated by subsequent enzymatic action. The substances that fulfill the functional characteristics of SRS-A are the leukotrienes C_4, D_4, and E_4 (LTC_4, LTD_4, and LTE_4); these produce bronchial smooth muscle contraction, increased vascular permeability, and increased mucus production.[762, 763] Although the leukotrienes (C_4 and D_4) cause more severe bronchoconstriction in asthmatic than in normal individuals, they are relatively more potent in normal subjects than is methacholine or histamine.[409] In addition, LTB_4 is a powerful chemotaxin and can attract both eosinophils and neutrophils to the site of its release.[764]

Leukotrienes can be synthesized by mast cells, airway epithelium, macrophages, and blood-derived inflammatory cells, but the proportion of the various leukotrienes produced varies in accordance with the enzyme complement of the cell. Since leukotrienes are released with antigen challenge of the respiratory tract[765] and with anti-IgE challenge of purified human lung mast cells,[766] they have the potential to be important mediators in the pathogenesis of asthma. An assessment of their importance has been hindered by the lack of specific and effective blocking agents of their synthesis or action. In sheep allergic to *A. suum*, the putative receptor antagonist FPL 55712 has been shown to decrease the delayed response to antigen inhalation, suggesting that the leukotrienes may be important in producing the delayed response.[767]

When administered by aerosol to human subjects, the bronchoconstricting leukotrienes cause dose-dependent airway narrowing that is maximal at 3 minutes and resolves over 1 to 3 hours, a duration of action that is longer than that produced by histamine.[768] Asthmatic patients are some 25 to 100 times more sensitive to the effects of LTD_4 than are normal subjects, whereas patients with allergic rhinitis are only slightly more sensitive (three to four times). In normal and asthmatic subjects, the response of the airways to LTD_4 correlates with the response to methacholine, although on a molar basis LTD_4 is 250 to 800 times more potent than methacholine.[768–770]

OTHER MEDIATORS

Serotonin (5-hydroxytryptamine) is not present in human lung mast cells or blood-derived inflammatory cells. It is produced by the neuroendocrine cells of the gastrointestinal and respiratory tracts but is not considered to play a significant role in causing anaphylaxis or asthma in humans, although it appears to be an important mediator in some mammals. However, in the carcinoid syndrome, serotonin can be liberated in large quantities and can cause severe bronchospasm by its direct action on bronchial smooth muscle.

There is no evidence that complement activation[771] or circulatory immune complexes are important in human asthma, although elevated blood levels of IgE and IgG have been reported in atopic and nonatopic asthmatic patients.[772] Oxygen radicals, specifically hydrogen peroxide (H_2O_2), can cause smooth muscle contraction.[773]

Afferent nerve endings in the airway wall contain the polypeptide substance P. Substance P can produce smooth muscle contraction and increased vascular permeability of the airway and can be released locally with afferent nerve stimulation. The release of substance P from afferent nerve fibers is thought to be responsible for the flare portion of cutaneous "wheal and flare" responses, and a similar axonal reflex that results in airway mucosal swelling is also possible in asthma. However, it has been shown that inhalation of capsicin, the active ingredient of hot peppers that acts by stimulating substance P release from afferent nerves, causes only slight and transient bronchial narrowing in normal subjects.[774]

MAST CELLS AND BASOPHILS

Mast cells and basophils are thought to be the most important mediator-releasing cells in allergic airway disease. There is evidence that basophils from asthmatic patients can release mediators more readily in response to nonantigenic stimuli than those of normal subjects.[775, 776]

Although mast cells and basophils have received the most attention in the study of the pathogenesis of allergic asthma, it has become increasingly evident that other cells can also play an important role. Alveolar macrophages have membrane receptors that bind IgE; allergen binding by IgE may stimulate mediator release from these macrophages.[777–779] Alveolar macrophages can also produce a factor that releases histamine from basophils and lung mast cells,[780] and can produce LTB_4, the potent leukotriene chemotaxin that could in turn amplify the allergic reaction by attracting blood-derived inflammatory cells.[781]

EOSINOPHIL AND POLYMORPHONUCLEAR LEUKOCYTES

Blood and tissue levels of eosinophils are increased in both intrinsic and extrinsic asthma, so that their presence is not necessarily related to an IgE-mediated immune response.[782] In sensitized individuals, antigen challenge produces an initial fall in the blood eosinophil count followed by a rise.[783]

Although there is controversy concerning the beneficial or harmful role that eosinophils play in asthma, the bulk of evidence suggests that they play a harmful role by damaging airway epithelium. However, they can also exert a salutary effect through their production of enzymes and proteins that are potentially beneficial. These enzymes include aryl sulfatase B, phospholipase D, and histaminase, agents that can deactivate leukotrienes, PAF, and histamine, respectively, in a dose-dependent fashion in vitro, thereby damping the allergic response. The epithelial cell damage is caused by three toxic proteins contained in eosinophils that are of major importance in the protection against

parasitic infestation: (1) major basic protein (MBP), MW 9,300; (2) eosinophil catonic protein (ECP), MW 21,000; and (3) eosinophil protein X (EPX), MW 19,000; however, they can also cause damage to and detachment of epithelial cells in vitro.[782, 784] When stimulated with the calcium ionophore A23187, eosinophils from patients with either intrinsic or extrinsic asthma generate three times more leukotriene C_4 than the cells of normal subjects.[785] Products derived from eosinophils may also damage alveolar macrophages.[786] Elevated levels of eosinophils and ECP can be detected in the sputum and bronchoalveolar lavage of patients with active asthma, levels decreasing with successful treatment.[787, 788] Although the blood eosinophil count decreases with antigen challenge, the serum level of ECP rises, a sequence that suggests that eosinophils sequester in the lung and then release ECP. There may be a secondary increase in serum levels of ECP coincident with a delayed asthmatic response.[782, 783] Patients with asthma and hypereosinophilic syndromes have greater numbers of circulating hypodense eosinophils, suggesting an increase in their turnover rate or activation.[789]

There is also evidence that circulating polymorphonuclear leukocytes of asthmatic subjects are altered. These cells show an increased number of IgG and complement receptors and release more histamine and superoxide anion in response to activation with calcium ionophore than do the leukocytes of normal individuals.[790–792] The use of bronchoalveolar lavage has extended our knowledge of the contribution of the cellular phase of the acute inflammatory reaction in asthma;[793–795] when a small volume of lavage fluid is used to wash proximal airways before and after antigen inhalation, an increase in the number of epithelial cells, eosinophils, and polymorphonuclear leukocytes can be demonstrated at 24 and 48 hours following the challenge.[795, 796]

Determinants of the Allergic Response

The severity of the bronchoconstriction resulting from inhaled antigen in a sensitized person is related to the degree of allergy and the nonspecific bronchial responsiveness.[645, 646, 797] The degree of allergy can be determined by quantitative skin testing[646] or RAST testing[797] and relates to the amounts of specific IgE and mediator released for a given antigen dose. The severity of NSBH determines the degree of bronchial narrowing that will occur when a given amount of mediator is released (see Fig. 11–28, page 2029).

The amount of mediator released during antigen challenge of the nasal and intrapulmonary airways can be modulated pharmacologically. In the lung, beta-adrenergic agonists not only decrease the amount of smooth muscle contraction produced by mediators (via a direct smooth muscle effect) but also appear to decrease the amount of mediator released, presumably by stabilizing mast cells.[798, 799] A similar protective effect has been demonstrated for disodium cromoglycate.[800] Topical beta-agonists also decrease antigen-induced mediator release from the nose[801] but not from the skin, suggesting differences in mast cell function according to their location.[802, 803] The combination of antigen challenge and a hypertonic environment is synergistic in its effect on basophil mediator release.[804]

Exercise

Exercise-induced asthma (EIA) is the excessive airway narrowing and reduction in maximal expiratory flow rates that accompany moderate or vigorous exercise. Although it occurs in the majority of patients with asthma, the term EIA is unfortunate because it implies that exercise induces the asthmatic state; in fact, exercise is one of many provoking stimuli in patients *with* asthma. However, the label is so well established in the literature that any attempt to introduce a more reasonable nomenclature such as "exercise asthmatic response" would be futile.[398, 805–807] A decrease of 10 per cent or more of PEFR or FEV_1 or a greater than 35 per cent decrease in $SGAW$, FEF_{25-75}, or $Vmax_{50}$ following exercise is considered diagnostic of EIA. The maximal impairment in lung function characteristically occurs 5 to 12 minutes after rather than during exercise, and the lowest value is used to calculate the *Percentage Fall Index*:

$$\frac{\text{pre-exercise value} - \text{lowest post-exercise value}}{\text{pre-exercise value}}$$

Defined in this way, EIA occurs in 70 to 80 per cent of patients with asthma who exercise at 80 to 90 per cent of their maximal work load for 6 to 8 minutes.[805] An increase in nasal resistance has been reported to occur 15 to 20 minutes after exercise in 30 per cent of asthmatic children.[808] Exercise-induced asthma is equally common in highly trained athletes and unfit subjects.[809, 810]

In both normal and asthmatic subjects, bronchodilation occurs during the first few minutes of exercise, and the magnitude of bronchodilation is calculated as the *Percentage Rise Index*:[805, 811, 812]

$$\frac{\text{highest intra-exercise value} - \text{pre-exercise value}}{\text{pre-exercise value}}$$

Patients with asthma can show an excessive bronchodilation during exercise in addition to the exaggerated post-exercise bronchoconstriction. An increase in PEFR or FEV_1 greater than 22 per cent is considered abnormal. In general, the lower the asthmatic patient's starting flow rates, the greater will be the exercise-induced bronchodilation; however, the degree of bronchoconstriction cannot be predicted from baseline studies. The mechanism of exercise-induced bronchodilation is not completely understood but is in part related to decreased vagal tone and increased circulating catecholamines.[805, 812, 813]

An index of overall bronchial lability in response to exercise can be calculated by combining the Percentage Fall Index and the Percentage Rise Index, called the *Exercise Lability Index* (ELI):

$$\frac{\text{highest flow rate during exercise} - \text{lowest post-exercise value}}{\text{initial value}}$$

The ELI tends to be higher than normal both in patients with allergic rhinitis and in asymptomatic relatives of asthmatic subjects. In the latter group, the ELI is abnormal chiefly as a result of excessive exercise-induced bronchodilation; in patients with asthma, the main contributor is exaggerated bronchoconstriction.[814]

The bronchoconstriction of EIA peaks 5 to 12 minutes after the cessation of exercise and spontaneously remits within 30 to 60 minutes, although rarely the attack can be prolonged. The majority of patients are refractory to the induction of a second episode of EIA for approximately 2 hours. Late bronchoconstriction in response to exercise has been reported, particularly in children, although it is less frequent and severe than the late response following antigen challenge.[805, 806, 815]

The physiologic abnormalities of lung function and gas exchange that accompany EIA do not differ from those that occur with other inciters of asthmatic episodes.[805] A number of investigators have attempted to localize the site of the airway narrowing using density dependence of maximal expiratory flow[816, 817] and have found that both large and small airways participate; the degree of peripheral airway narrowing appears to be greater in patients with severe disease.[818] The uncertainty regarding the usefulness of density-dependence measurements in determining the site of obstruction and the poor reproducibility of the response in some patients with asthma at different times makes these conclusions questionable.[819]

MECHANISMS OF EXERCISED-INDUCED ASTHMA

Significant progress towards an understanding of the mechanism responsible for EIA has been made since the last edition of this text. The major advance came with the observation that airway narrowing could be completely abolished if the inspired air during exercise was warmed to body temperature and saturated with water vapor (37° C and a water content of about 46 mg/liter).[820–823] McFadden and his colleagues found that the degree of airway obstruction following identical exercise challenges could be modified by altering the inspired air conditions: the colder and drier the air breathed during exercise, the greater the subsequent response.[823, 824] Shortly after these important studies were published, it was recognized that exercise is not even necessary to produce EIA, the airway response being reproducible by the isocapnic hyperventilation of unconditioned air.[825-827] Hypocapnia must be prevented by adding CO_2 to the inspired gas because hypocapnia itself can produce bronchoconstriction.[608]

With identical inspired air conditions, there is a dose-response relationship between ventilation and the severity of bronchoconstriction in patients with asthma whether the ventilation is associated with exercise or with isocapnic hyperventilation. Although normal subjects show a similar dose response, much greater ventilation is required to produce much smaller changes in expiratory flow rates.[828-830] When the water content and temperature of inspired air are the same, the mode of exercise is not important as a determinant of obstruction in asthmatic patients; at matched levels of minute ventilation, the bronchoconstriction that occurs with treadmill walking, bicycling, or swimming is similar.[584, 587]

The fact that EIA is related in some way to the breathing of cold and/or dry air has rekindled interest in inspired air conditioning. Since inspired air temperature is almost always below body temperature and less than 100 per cent saturated with water vapor, and since alveolar gas is 100 per cent saturated at body temperature, the airways must give up heat and water to the inspired air. During resting ventilation and nasal breathing, the conditioning process is almost completed by the time inspired gas reaches the lower airways;[831] however, with the increased ventilation and mouth breathing that occur during exercise, incompletely conditioned air can penetrate deeply into the lung, especially if cold dry air is breathed.[832] The consequences are cooling and drying of the airway wall. The degree of cooling is determined by the amount of heat lost from the airway wall that is required to warm the inspired air (convective heat loss) and by the evaporative heat loss that results from the humidification of inspired air. The total heat lost from the respiratory tract can be calculated as

$$RHL = V_E \, HC \, (T_I - T_E) + V_E \, HV \, (WC_E - WC_I)$$

where RHL = total respiratory heat loss in kilocalories (kcal)/minute; V_E = minute ventilation in liters/minute; HC = the heat capacity of air (0.304×10^{-3} kcal/1° C), T_I and T_E = inspired and expired air temperature, HV = the latent heat of vaporization of water (0.58×10^{-3} kcal/mg), and WC_I and WC_E = the inspired and expired water content of the air (mg/liter).[824]

Obviously, total heat loss will be greater when inspired air is cooler or drier and expired air warmer or wetter. The temperature and water content of expired gas differ from that of alveolar gas because a countercurrent exchange mechanism serves to recover a portion of the heat and water added to inspired air. The upper airway mucosa cools during inspiration as a result of convective and evaporative heat loss, and the cooled mucosa recovers heat and water during expiration by cooling expired gas and condensing expired water vapor. The effectiveness of the countercurrent exchange is dependent on the surface area of the upper airway mucosa and its blood flow: an increase in mucosal blood flow by warming would decrease the extent of penetration of cool air into the lung but would result in a larger expired heat and water loss; and a decrease in mucosal blood flow would serve to cool the upper airway surface further, facilitating the recovery of heat and water from expired air but also resulting in deeper penetration of unconditioned air into the lung.[833]

It is not known how the upper airway vasculature responds to the inhalation of cool or dry air in man. An increase in tracheobronchial blood flow has been reported in the dog on inspiration of cold and/or dry air during isocapnic hyperventilation (ISH). Based on observations of blanching of the tracheobronchial mucosa during cold air breathing in man, it has been postulated that the bronchial vasculature constricts, although no direct measurements of airway blood flow have been made.[834] It is clear, however, that cooling of the airway occurs for a variable distance into the lung; although evidence for this was initially obtained indirectly by measuring retrotracheal esophageal temperature,[835] subsequent mapping of airway thermal profiles in man has shown that during cold air hyperventilation, temperature does not equilibrate with body temperature until the air reaches airways 2 mm in diameter.[836] Of some interest was the observation that airway cooling was identical for a given ventilation whether it was achieved during exercise or ISH, suggesting that variations in overall cardiac output do not affect inspired air conditioning.[824]

In individual patients with asthma, the degree of bronchoconstriction produced by exercise or ISH correlates with the calculated respiratory heat loss and with changes in retrotracheal esophageal temperature, although the slope of the relationship differs among subjects.[835, 837, 838] The bronchoconstriction that occurs in asthmatics in response to the ventilation of unconditioned air appears to result not from a defect in inspired air conditioning but rather from an abnormal response to a normal stimulus. Normal subjects do not seem to have more efficient air conditioning because they develop equivalent airway cooling at matched levels of ventilation and inspired air conditions.[835] With identical levels of ventilation and inspired air conditions, nasal breathing results in much less airway cooling and bronchoconstriction than that noted with oral breathing.[839, 840]

The observations that airways cool during exercise and ISH and that there is a dose-response relationship between cooling and bronchoconstriction suggest that in some way cooling of the airway is responsible for the bronchoconstriction.[831, 837] However, an alternative hypothesis is that airway drying is the inciting stimulus;[841–843] it has been difficult to separate the effects of cooling and drying because it is virtually impossible for one to be present without the other.

Cool air is by nature dry air, and evaporative heat loss is a major contributor to airway cooling. Even when dry air at body temperature is breathed during exercise or ISH, there is a substantial respiratory heat loss, and cooling of the airway can be demonstrated by measuring either retrotracheal esophageal temperature or tracheal tissue temperature.[843, 2751] Thus, drying cannot be achieved without cooling. Because the amount of water that air can contain as water vapor is directly related to the air temperature, it is also impossible to produce cooling of the airway without drying. Cool or cold air will not hold enough water to prevent evaporation and drying of the respiratory mucosa. Despite these difficulties, there is evidence that drying of the airway may be the important stimulus to bronchoconstriction in EIA- and ISH-induced bronchoconstriction. Dry air hyperventilation results in approximately equivalent bronchoconstriction regardless of its temperature.[824] When the temperature and water content of inspired air are varied so as to produce a range of total respiratory heat and water loss, the magnitude of bronchoconstriction correlates more closely with calculated water loss than with heat loss.[841, 842, 844] Of some interest was the observation that in the dog, the increase in airway blood flow that occurs during hyperventilation of cold-dry and warm-dry air also correlates more closely with calculated respiratory water loss than with total heat loss or mucosal cooling.

To the extent that water loss from the airway mucosa exceeds water replacement, the fluid lining the airway will develop hyperosmolarity. Anderson and her colleagues have postulated that it is the hyperosmolarity of the periciliary fluid that in some way mediates the bronchoconstriction of EIA and ISH.[828] This hypothesis has been strengthened by studies that have shown that inhalation of hypoosmolar or hyperosmolar aerosols elicit bronchoconstriction in patients with EIA.[2752, 2753] There is a significant relationship between the severity of EIA and the responsiveness to inhaled hypotonic aerosols.[845] Air saturated with water vapor in which the temperature is higher than the body can cause an airway response, possibly by condensation of the excess water on respiratory epithelium.[846]

How airway cooling or drying results in airway narrowing remains to be completely explained. Three possible mechanisms have been studied the most: (1) release of mediators from mast cells or other sources; (2) stimulation of afferent receptors with resultant reflex bronchoconstriction; and (3) a direct effect on smooth muscle.

Release of Mediators. Although there is some variation among studies, most investigators have been able to detect inflammatory mediators in the peripheral blood of patients with asthma following exercise or ISH and coincident with the induced bronchoconstriction.[847–849] The mediators that have been detected are histamine and the large-molecular-weight chemotactic substance, NCFA, both of which are thought to be derived from pulmonary mast cells.[805, 848] Their release appears to be causally related to the exercise-induced bronchoconstriction because a similar magnitude of methacholine-induced bronchial obstruction does not result in detectable levels of these mediators and since the breathing of warm humid air during exercise blocks both the bronchoconstriction and the mediator release.[850, 851] Patients with exercise-induced asthma also show an increase in neutrophil and monocyte complement rosettes and in neutrophil cytotoxicity following exercise.[851] Platelet release products, such as platelet factor IV, have been detected in the plasma of asthmatic subjects following exercise.[852] Exercise and ISH result in similar plasma histamine levels at matched ventilation, but the rise in NCFA is less or absent with ISH—one of the few differences between the two challenges.[853] Although normal subjects develop equivalent degrees of airway cooling (and presumably drying), they do not show increased plasma levels of histamine or NCFA with exercise; this suggests that the mast cells of asthmatic patients may release mediators more readily.[854] EIA cannot be explained simply by exaggerated airway narrowing for a given mediator release. Nasal challenge with cold dry air causes the release of histamine, PGD_2, kinins, and *t*oluene-*s*ulfo-*t*rypsin *a*rginine *m*ethyl *e*ster (TAME)—esterases, mediators that can be recovered by nasal lavage.[855]

Mediator release from mast cells in the airway may be triggered by the change in osmolarity accompanying evaporative water loss. Basophils and mast cells release preformed mediators *in vitro* in response to both hyperosmolar and hypo-osmolar challenges.[856–858] The release of mediators in response to osmolar stimuli is not associated with cell disruption or death; in fact, very high levels of osmolarity inhibit mediator release. Since cells from normal and asthmatic subjects appear to respond equally to alterations in osmolarity *in vitro*, the link with the abnormal increase in plasma mediators *in vivo* remains tenuous. Of some interest is the fact that the osmolar mediator release is dependent on temperature, the maximal effect occurring at 32° C—a temperature that can easily develop in the airway wall with exercise or ISH.[856] Breathing cold dry air through the nose has been shown to induce release of both preformed mediators and arachidonic acid metabolites.[859]

In some individuals, exercise appears to produce generalized release of mast cell mediators that results in anaphylaxis; this rare entity is associated with "generalized body warmth, pruritus, erythema and urticaria, laryngeal edema, hoarseness, gastrointestinal colic, and vascular collapse."[860] In these people, increased blood levels of histamine and degranulation of skin mast cells have been demonstrated.[860, 861] Surprisingly, the eating of celery before exercising can precipitate the syndrome in some subjects.[862] Bronchoconstriction can also accompany a less severe form of systemic mast cell mediator release known as cholinergic urticaria, characterized by generalized punctate wheals and itchiness that follow hot showers or accompany pyrexia.[863]

The release of vasoactive and chemotactic substances from the lung during exercise suggests the development of an inflammatory response. Mucosal inflammation with disruption and sloughing of bronchial epithelium develops in animals breathing dry air through a tracheostomy.[864] Additional evidence that the release of inflammatory mediators may be important in the genesis of exercise- and ISH-induced airway obstruction derives from studies in which anti-inflammatory drugs have proved effective in preventing bronchoconstriction. Mediator release from mast cells can be attenuated by administration of disodium cromoglycate, beta-agonists, or calcium channel blockers, each of which has proved to be an effective prophylactic for exercise- and ISH-induced asthma, especially the first two.[865, 866] Although beta-agonists and calcium channel blockers may produce an additional direct relaxant effect on smooth muscle, it has not been established whether this effect or inhibition of mediator release is the more important action. Finally, these agents could have a dilating effect on the bronchial vasculature, resulting in a decreased airway cooling for a given ventilation; however, this does not appear to be the case for disodium cromoglycate at least.[867]

Stimulation of Afferent Receptors. The second possible mechanism by which airway cooling or drying might produce bronchoconstriction is by cold or hyperosmolar stimulation of afferent nerve endings in the airway and resultant reflex bronchoconstriction. The evidence for such a mechanism comes largely from *in vivo* studies of pharmacologic blockade of the afferent or efferent vagal pathways, but the data relating to both limbs of the reflex are conflicting and controversial. For example, interruption of the afferent limb by inhalation of local anesthetic agents appears to decrease the subsequent airway response to exercise, at least in some studies.[868, 869] However, despite objective evidence of afferent interruption (decreased gag reflex and decreased citric acid–induced cough), other studies have shown no decrease in response at matched levels of ventilation.[870, 871] It is possible that airway anesthesia decreases ventilation at any level of exercise, thus decreasing the stimulus for EIA rather than the response to it.[869]

Interruption of the efferent limb of the reflex pathway has been produced by aerosol and parenteral administration of atropine. Although in most studies, inhaled atropine has attenuated the response to exercise or ISH, the effect is small and it is difficult to separate an "apparent" protection

(secondary to increased baseline airway size) from a direct effect.[872–874] Since parenteral administration of atropine is more effective in attenuating the airway response despite equivalent baseline bronchodilation, it has been suggested that complete cholinergic blockade is not achieved with the inhaled drug.[875, 876]

It is possible that in some subjects a cholinergic reflex is the major cause of obstruction whereas in others mediator release is more important. In one study, patients with asthma who were refractory to repeated ISH challenges derived no protective effect with inhaled ipratropium bromide whereas those who did not show a refractory period were helped by the inhaled anticholinergic agent.[877] Since the refractory period is thought to be caused by mediator release and depletion, mediators may be the major mechanism only in patients who show a refractory period and lack of anticholinergic protection.

Direct Effect on Smooth Muscle. Cooling and/or drying of the airway may have a direct contractile effect on airway smooth muscle. Cooling of animal and human airway smooth muscle has been studied *in vitro*, and although it was found to decrease the baseline tone, it potentiated the contractile response to some agonists.[879, 880] In one *in vitro* study of human airway tissue, hyper-osmolar and hypo-osmolar conditions did not produce smooth muscle contraction or alter the responsiveness to added agonists.[2754]

Although it is generally believed that airway smooth muscle contraction is the major cause of airway narrowing in EIA, the possibility has been suggested that at least some of the effect could be secondary to bronchial vascular reactivity and edema.[881] This concept deserves attention. In the nose, rapid changes in caliber can occur, and since no luminal encircling layer of smooth muscle exists, these changes are entirely attributable to vasomotion in the vascular bed of the nasal mucosa. Like the nose, the lower airway mucosa possesses a complex and extensive submucosal plexus of blood vessels,[882] and it is quite possible that vascular constriction induced by cold followed by vasodilation and mucosal edema could play a role in the airway obstruction of EIA.[881]

There is some evidence that the alpha-adrenergic receptors are important in the induction of EIA: alpha-adrenergic blocking drugs, such as phentolamine and prazosin, attenuate the response to exercise.[563, 564, 833] Norepinephrine, which has alpha-agonist activity, may be released during exercise[883] and acts as a bronchoconstricting agent in asthmatic patients but not in normal subjects.[556] As with the bronchial narrowing that is induced directly by alpha-agonists, it is not known whether the pertinent alpha-receptors are located in airway smooth muscle, airway ganglia, or vascular smooth muscle.

In addition to exhibiting disordered adrenergic airway responses, patients with asthma can show abnormal release of catecholamines during exercise, although the results of studies that have addressed this question have not all been in agreement. Although a number of investigators have found that asthmatic patients have an impairment in the normal exercise-induced increase in blood levels of cAMP, epinephrine, and norepinephrine,[550, 551, 884] others have shown normal responses when subjects were carefully matched for age and the intensity and duration of exercise.[883, 885] Whether or not catecholamine release is decreased, beta-adrenergic blocking drugs can severely exacerbate EIA.[886]

REFRACTORY PERIOD

From 50 to 80 per cent of asthmatic subjects who develop EIA show a refractory period following challenge; during this period, similar levels of exercise produce no response or an attenuated response.[815, 887] The degree of attenuation of the second response is dependent on the intensity of the initial exercise and on time; 30 minutes after an initial episode, EIA is considerably less; by 4 hours, however, the protective effect has completely disappeared.[887] A more prolonged protective effect can be achieved by using short bursts of cold air hyperventilation over a 12-week training period; however, in some subjects, this protocol caused a reduction of prechallenge expiratory flows and a worsening of symptoms.[888]

The possible explanations for the refractory period include:

1. Mediator depletion of the cells that respond to airway cooling and/or drying.

2. Decreased responsiveness of airway smooth muscle to released mediator.

3. Decreased respiratory heat and water loss despite similar exercise.

4. Decreased response resulting from exercise-induced sympathoadrenal activation.

5. Release of bronchodilating, secondary mediators such as prostaglandins.[805]

Some of these possibilities have been tested experimentally. Exercise produces refractoriness to subsequent antigen challenge in some patients with asthma[889] but does not affect methacholine and histamine responses;[890, 891] this suggests that mediator depletion may be important and virtually excludes a direct effect on smooth muscle responsiveness. Although mediator depletion is an attractive hypothesis, decreased blood levels have not been demonstrated by direct measurement of NCFA during an initial and subsequent challenge.[892]

The calculated heat and water loss is the same during the initial and second exercise period, making an adaptation of air-conditioning mechanisms unlikely.[893] Since ISH results in a refractory period without causing the increase in circulating catecholamines associated with exercise, a protective effect of beta-adrenergic stimulation is also unlikely to be the only explanation.[894] The fact that indomethacin

abolishes the refractory period supports the hypothesis that exercise-induced release of bronchodilating prostaglandins, such as PGE_2, is the cause of the refractory period;[895, 896] however, one would also expect attenuation of nonspecific airway responses.

There is controversy as to whether the refractory period depends on the development of bronchoconstriction during the initial exercise period. Some investigators have found that a refractory period persists even if bronchoconstriction is prevented during the initial exercise by breathing warm humid air,[897, 898] whereas others have shown the absence of a refractory period with a similar sequence of challenges.[899]

Although it has been suggested that hypoxia accentuates and hyperoxia attenuates EIA, in one study eucapnic hypoxia did not enhance the bronchoconstriction that occurs with dry air hyperventilation.[900] The hyperoxic attenuation of EIA may be caused by a decreased VE and therefore heat and water loss at similar exercise levels.[901, 902]

Body cooling without alteration in inspired air conditions may produce bronchoconstriction;[903, 904] even ingestion of cold drinks, while not producing direct effects on the airway, has been shown to enhance nonspecific responsiveness to histamine.[905] It is not known whether the airway narrowing that occurs with somatic cooling is related to EIA.

The refractory period is not only of theoretical interest—its study may help determine the basic mechanisms of EIA—but is also of some clinical interest in designing exercise programs for asthmatic patients; e.g., a warm-up period prior to exercise may be of benefit.[906, 2780]

DELAYED EXERCISE RESPONSES

Although a late or delayed bronchoconstrictive response has been reported following EIA (but not ISH), it does not appear as frequently (30 to 50 per cent) or result in as severe airway narrowing as the late response to antigen inhalation.[907–909] In children, the late response, which occurs from 4 to 12 hours after the initial reaction, is more marked following a severe initial response,[910] although this sequence does not occur in adults.[911] Another difference between the late exercise-induced and antigen-induced responses is the lack of change in subsequent nonspecific airway responsiveness following the former.[911, 912] In a recent, carefully controlled study, Rubinstein and associates[913] showed that a delayed exercise response is extremely uncommon.

EXERCISE-INDUCED ASTHMA AND NONSPECIFIC BRONCHIAL RESPONSIVENESS

In individual patients with asthma, the degree of bronchoconstriction in response to either exercise or ISH depends on the level of nonspecific bronchial responsiveness.[914–918] In fact, the responses correlate with NSBH so closely that exercise has been suggested as a test of NSBH, although it does not appear as sensitive as histamine and methacholine in separating normal from asthmatic subjects.[919]

EXERCISE-INDUCED COUGH

Exercise and isocapnic hyperventilation of cold and/or dry air causes cough as well as bronchoconstriction. The time course of the cough is very similar to that of bronchoconstriction, peaking 5 minutes after exercise or ISH and lasting for approximately 30 minutes. It correlates better with respiratory water loss than with heat loss and occurs in both normal and asthmatic subjects. Cough also occurs in response to inhaled hypertonic aerosols, suggesting that the stimulus is the change in airway fluid osmolarity attendant on evaporative water loss. Pretreatment with beta-agonist blocks bronchoconstriction but not cough, suggesting that the latter is not secondary to the bronchoconstriction induced by stimulation of irritant receptors.[920, 921]

SUMMARY

Exercise-induced asthma is the bronchial narrowing that occurs in association with vigorous exercise in asthmatic patients. It is common to all asthmatics and thus is not a specific form of the disease. Exercise-induced asthma can be mimicked in susceptible subjects by the hyperventilation of air that is not completely humidified or warmed to body temperature. It is believed that the stimulus for exercise-induced asthma is not exercise itself but the cooling or drying of the airway mucosa that occurs on inhalation of incompletely conditioned air; however, considerable controversy exists as to whether the pertinent stimulus is the cooling of the airway or the drying and subsequent development of hyperosmolarity in the surface lining liquid. In addition, the mechanism by which cooling or drying causes bronchoconstriction is unclear. It may be related to stimulation of irritant receptors within the airway wall, but there is evidence to suggest that release of bronchoconstricting mediators is also important. Following one episode of exercise-induced asthma, the majority of patients remain refractory in a second challenge for a period of up to 4 hours. Exercise-induced bronchospasm or cough may be the only clinical manifestations of the disease in some patients with asthma.

Infection

Viral respiratory tract infection can cause abnormal airway function in normal subjects, increased nonspecific bronchial responsiveness in normal and asthmatic subjects, and exacerbation of symptoms in patients with asthma. Although most normal subjects develop only cough without wheezing or dyspnea, abnormalities of airway function can be detected in the majority.[922] Children appear to be particularly susceptible to the development of airway narrowing, attributable to their relatively smaller peripheral airways.[922] The immaturity of the infant lung leaves it particularly vulnerable to long-term harmful effects of infection. Adenovirus subtypes 1, 3, 4, 7, and 21 are particularly devastating: in a 10-year follow-up study of 27 children who had had type 7 adenoviral pneumonia, six developed bronchiectasis and 16 had persistently abnormal lung function.[923] In otherwise normal adults, small but measurable transient changes in airway function and pharmacologic responsiveness can result from respiratory syncytial viral infection, influenza A viral infection, or vaccination with live attenuated virus;[924–927] killed virus vaccination is not associated with any change in lung function.[928] In asthmatic patients, heat-killed and live attenuated influenza vaccination as well as naturally occurring infection with respiratory syncytial virus, rhinovirus, and influenza A virus has been reported to cause increased NSBR.[419, 929–931]

Viral and mycoplasmal but not bacterial respiratory tract infection can also precipitate episodes of symptomatic exacerbation in patients with asthma,[932, 933] although its importance as a trigger of asthma varies in different series. In one study of 16 children aged 3 to 11 years who had a history of wheezing associated with apparent symptomatic respiratory infection, 42 (70 per cent) of 61 episodes of asthma were coincident with viral infections, mostly caused by rhinoviruses and the Hong Kong influenza A virus.[934] By contrast, in an adult population, careful sputum culture for bacterial and viral agents coupled with viral antibody titers showed that infection was a triggering stimulus in only 10.8 per cent of 111 exacerbations of asthma.[935] In one experimental study in which rhinovirus infection was induced in 19 patients with asthma, typical upper respiratory coryzal symptoms developed in 17 but a greater than 10 per cent decrease in FEV_1 developed in only four.[419] Increased levels of specific antibodies to *Mycoplasma pneumoniae* were detected in 21 per cent of 95 adult patients with acute exacerbations.[936] The duration of symptoms following exacerbations of asthma associated with respiratory infection is longer than that related to noninfectious exacerbations.[937]

Not only does bacterial infection fail to precipitate exacerbations of asthma but it does not appear to have an increased incidence in asthmatics. A comparative study of normal subjects and patients with bronchitis or asthma revealed bacterial precipitins in 50 per cent of those with bronchitis but in only 6 per cent of the atopic and nonatopic asthmatics, an incidence identical to that found in the normal control subjects.[938] The mechanism by which viral or mycoplasmal respiratory tract infection precipitates attacks of asthma is not clear. There is little evidence to support an immunologic mechanism. It is possible that airway wall edema and increased secretions within bronchial lumens further diminish the caliber of already narrowed airways. It is also possible that the mucosal inflammation associated with viral infection could result in airway smooth muscle contraction secondary to mediator release from inflammatory cells in the same way that is postulated for the airway response to ozone.[420]

Analgesics

Acetylsalicylic acid (ASA) and several other unrelated analgesics and anti-inflammatory agents are capable of provoking attacks in an appreciable proportion of patients with asthma. The incidence of ASA sensitivity in the nonasthmatic population is less than 1 per cent, whereas in the general asthmatic population it ranges from 3.8 to 28 per cent.[939–942] The typical ASA-sensitive asthmatic patient is a nonatopic woman over the age of 20 with a long history of perennial rhinitis and nasal polyps.[943] The incidence of migraine headaches is high (48 per cent).[953] Long-standing asthma and rhinitis usually precede the development of ASA sensitivity, and the intolerance increases with age, being six times more common after age 50 than before age 20.[941] Peripheral eosinophilia is observed in over 50 per cent of patients, although serum IgE levels are usually normal[940, 942] and specific IgE directed towards ASA is not detectable.[944]

Symptoms and signs develop anywhere from 20 minutes to 3 hours after ingestion. Two forms of response have been distinguished: a primarily respiratory pattern and an urticarial-angioedema form; rarely do both occur in the same individual.[942] The respiratory response is dominated by bronchoconstriction and can be severe and life-threatening; it is usually associated with rhinitis and conjunctivitis. In a study of patients with a history of ASA intolerance who were challenged orally, 72 per cent developed attacks of bronchial narrowing and 92 per cent of these showed concomitant nasal symptoms; 12 per cent showed rhinitis alone and 16 per cent had no response, indicating that tolerance can develop spontaneously.[945]

Tolerance or tachyphylaxis to the effects of ASA can be produced with a rapid oral densitization protocol: progressively increasing concentrations of oral ASA are administered over a 6-hour period or until a 25 per cent decrease in FEV_1 is observed.[946, 947] Tolerance can also be achieved without adverse reaction by progressively increasing a daily dose of ASA.[948] The refractoriness to ASA wanes over 2 to 4 days but will persist if a daily maintenance dose of 600 mg is administered.[946, 947]

Although ASA can occasionally act as an antigen and stimulate antibody production, there is abundant evidence that ASA-induced airway narrowing is nonallergic in nature.[760, 940, 944] Indirect evidence has been obtained that mast cell mediator release may play a role; neutrophil chemotactic factor (NCF) derived from mast cells can be detected in the blood 60 to 120 minutes after the ingestion of ASA, coincident with or following maximal bronchoconstriction.[949, 950] The fact that its appearance does not precede the airway narrowing raises the possibility that it is released secondary to the bronchoconstriction.[950] Disodium chromoglycate, which is believed to exert a beneficial effect by decreasing mast cell mediator release following antigen challenge, is also partly effective in decreasing ASA-induced and indomethacin-induced airway responses when administered prior to challenge.[951, 952]

The most likely mechanism by which ASA and other nonsteroidal anti-inflammatory agents cause bronchoconstriction is through their ability to block metabolism of arachidonic acid via the cyclooxygenase pathway. The drugs that show cross-reacting responses in ASA-sensitive subjects include indomethacin, aminopyrine, acetaminophen, mefenamic acid, dextropropoxyphene, and tartrazine, all of which inhibit prostaglandin synthesis. The degree of bronchoconstriction they induce *in vivo* has been shown to be proportional to their ability to retard prostaglandin synthesis *in vitro*.[761] It has been postulated that patients with ASA-sensitive asthma produce large amounts of the bronchodilator PGE_2 in compensation for continued bronchoconstriction; when ASA or other anti-inflammatory agents are administered, an acute drop in PGE_2 synthesis precipitates an acute asthmatic attack.[760] Alternatively, it has been suggested that blockade of the cyclooxygenase series of enzymes diverts more arachidonic acid toward the lipoxygenase metabolic pathway, resulting in excessive production of bronchoconstricting leukotrienes. In an *in vitro* study,[954] the platelets from ASA-sensitive asthmatic patients were activated when incubated in a medium containing nonsteroidal anti-inflammatory drugs (NSAIDs), an effect that was blocked by lipoxygenase inhibitors; the results of this study suggest that enhanced leukotriene production caused by cyclooxygenase blockers can activate platelets and that platelet products can cause bronchoconstriction.

From 10 to 30 per cent of patients with ASA-induced bronchoconstriction also show a paradoxical bronchial narrowing following intravenous administration of the corticosteroid hydrocortisone.[955, 956] Although it was initially believed that the effect might be caused by preservative additives, it clearly occurs with pure drug and may be secondary to an effect of the corticosteroid on prostaglandin metabolism. The effect is rarely marked and should not interfere with the therapeutic administration of systemic corticosteroids if they are otherwise indicated.[956, 957]

Gastroesophageal Reflux

Gastroesophageal reflux could trigger airway narrowing in susceptible individuals through reflex bronchoconstriction secondary to stimulation of esophageal vagal afferent nerves or by direct aspiration of a small amount of esophageal contents.[958–960] In an animal model of gastroesophageal reflux, minute quantities of acid instilled into the tracheobronchial tree caused considerably greater bronchoconstriction than acid in the esophagus,[959] suggesting that aspiration would be a powerful stimulus; however, there is no direct evidence that such aspiration occurs in patients with asthma.[961]

Simple reflux without aspiration is common in normal and asthmatic populations[958, 962] and may or may not[2781] precipitate airway narrowing. When acid is instilled into the esophagus of asthmatic patients, only those who develop symptoms of esophagitis exhibit bronchoconstriction.[961, 963–965] Gastroesophageal reflux can transiently increase NSBR as well as causing bronchoconstriction in its own right.[966] Antacids and the H_1 blocker cimetidine reduce the esophageal and respiratory symptoms caused by gastroesophageal reflux.[961, 967] In 11 of 13 asthmatics, surgical therapy for chronic gastroesophageal reflux resulted in an improvement in asthmatic symptoms and medication usage.[968] It has been suggested that since reflux is exacerbated during sleep as a result of recumbency and decreased tone in the lower esophageal sphincter, it tends to cause nocturnal asthma and morning dipping.[958, 969]

Emotion

It is difficult to evaluate the influence of psychological factors as provocative triggers of asthmatic attacks. Asthmatic patients may be emotionally unstable and dependent, but this is almost certainly a result of their disease rather than a factor predisposing to its development. Mild bronchoconstriction and bronchodilation can be produced by suggestion, presumably as a result of changes in cholinergic vagal activity.[970–972] In some of the studies designed to test the effect of suggestion,[973] it is possible that airway cooling or drying may have caused a true physiologic stimulus for bronchoconstriction. Children with asthma appear to manifest different psychological patterns: those whose symptoms remit rapidly on admission to the hospital tend to be rather neurotic, whereas those whose asthma is steroid-dependent tend to manifest less psychopathogenic behavior.[974] Hyperventilation provoked by anxiety is common in asthmatics; in fact, a vicious cycle can be established because the hyperventilation itself can cause bronchoconstriction as a result of hypocapnia and airway drying, thus tending to increase the anxiety.[975]

Although emotional distress can trigger an attack in a patient with asthma, it plays no role in the basic pathophysiologic process that causes the asthmatic state. The lifestyle of most asthmatics is hampered enough without their suffering the misapprehension that their emotional state might in some way be the cause of their illness.

Environment

The importance of air pollution and fluctuations in atmospheric temperature and humidity as triggers of asthmatic attacks is not known precisely, but it is clear that low levels of atmospheric chemical pollutants can cause functional abnormalities in patients with hyper-reactive airways. In southern Ontario, Canada, an area of heavy industrial air pollution, a comparison of hospital admission rates and levels of pollutants showed that admissions for acute respiratory disease are related to atmospheric levels of sulfate aerosol and ozone (O_3).[1513] In nonasthmatic subjects, cough and phlegm are more common in communities with high ambient sulfur dioxide (SO_2) levels;[976] in the ambient Los Angeles air that contains, among other things, 0.14 parts per million (ppm) O_3, exercise was found to cause a significant decrease in maximal expiratory flow when compared with similar exercise in purified air.[977, 978]

In another investigation of the relationship between air pollution and asthmatic attacks in the Los Angeles area, Schoettlin and Landau[1019] found the peak period of attacks to be during the early morning, despite the fact that maximal oxidant levels were recorded between 10 A.M. and 4 P.M. However, a significantly greater number of persons had attacks on days when oxidant levels were high enough to cause eye irritation and damage to plants. Studies in the New Orleans area showed a sharp increase in the incidence of asthmatic attacks during June and July and October and November, periods during which atmospheric pollution increased.[1013–1015]

The major respirable atmospheric chemicals that affect lung function are ozone and the oxides of sulfur and nitrogen. Like viral infections, these agents can cause mild airway obstruction and increased NSBR in normal subjects and can precipitate episodes of symptomatic exacerbation in patients with asthma. In normal subjects, SO_2 in concentrations of 0.5 to 1.0 ppm causes mild, transient, asymptomatic bronchoconstriction but only when the subjects exercise during the exposure, thereby increasing the dose of SO_2 reaching the airways.[979–981] The effect is partly blocked by atropine and disodium cromoglycate, so that both a reflex and a mediator-related mechanism may be operative.[982]

As might be expected, patients with asthma are more sensitive than normal subjects to the bronchoconstricting effects of SO_2; a concentration as low as 0.25 ppm can cause detectable obstruction during mild exercise,[983–986] and 5 minutes of heavy exercise in 0.4 or 0.5 ppm SO_2 can cause transient symptomatic exacerbation (followed by recovery within 24 hours).[987] There may be some tachyphylaxis with repeated bouts of exercise with the same concentration of SO_2;[986, 988] for the same level of ventilation and SO_2 exposure, nasal breathing is protective, presumably because the very soluble SO_2 dissolves in the fluid lining the nasal mucosa and fails to reach the lower respiratory tract.[989, 990] The bronchoconstriction caused by SO_2 and cold, dry air are synergistic: when cold, dry air is breathed, a concentration of SO_2 as low as 0.1 ppm will produce detectable airway obstruction.[991–993]

In summary, SO_2 can cause airway narrowing and symptoms in patients with asthma at concentrations well below accepted "standards." Such concentrations are frequently reached in urban industrial areas, and the effects are accentuated by exercise, mouth breathing, and cold, dry air.

In both normal and asthmatic subjects and at a concentration as low as 0.12 ppm (0.000012 per cent), ozone causes a dose-dependent decrease in expiratory flow rates and volumes as well as in TLC, making it the most potent irritant gas.[994–1004] As with SO_2, the effects of ozone are enhanced with exercise[994, 1002–1004] and tolerance can develop with repeated exposure.[998] Of more interest than direct O_3-induced airway narrowing is the ability of brief O_3 exposure to increase subsequent nonspecific airway responsiveness in normal subjects: 2 hours of exposure to 0.6 ppm O_3 increases the subsequent response to inhaled histamine and methacholine for at least 24 hours without significantly increasing baseline values of airway resistance.[1005, 1006] Atropine treatment blocks the effect of ozone on NSBR, suggesting that the effect could be related to increased reactivity of cholinergic postganglionic pathways; however, atropine also substantially reduces the baseline airway resistance (pre-histamine or pre-methacholine), creating difficulty in comparing these results with the non-atropine experiments.[1005] A more likely explanation for the ozone-induced increase in airway responsiveness is the airway inflammatory response that follows exposure. As discussed in the section on bronchial hyper-responsiveness, animal models and human studies of the ozone effect suggest that the enhanced NSBR is mediated by airway inflammation.[1007–1010] The degree of shift in histamine and methacholine response is small, and these exposures certainly do not alter the airway responsiveness of normal subjects to the same extent as in patients with spontaneous asthma; however, it is possible that the mechanism of the altered response is similar to that which occurs in asthma.

The oxides of nitrogen are another component of smog and industrial pollution that in low concentrations can precipitate symptomatic episodes in hyper-responsive individuals. A transient increase in nitrogen oxide levels to greater than 500 parts per billion (ppb) was blamed for an acute outbreak of asthma in Barcelona, Spain, in which 44 patients were admitted to hospital over a 2- to 3-hour period.[976] Inhalation of nitrogen dioxide (NO_2) (0.3 ppm) increases the severity of exercise-induced bronchoconstriction in asthmatic patients.[1011] In most studies, low-level NO_2 exposure (0.1 ppm for

1 hour or 910 $\mu g/M^3$ for 20 minutes) enhances nonspecific airway responsiveness in asthmatic but not in normal subjects.[977, 978, 1012]

A notable example of the relationship between air pollution and a syndrome characterized by acute respiratory distress resembling asthma has been reported in the Tokyo and Yokohama regions of Japan.[1016, 1017] This syndrome, which has been termed "Tokyo-Yokohama asthma," was observed in U.S. Service personnel in the area for the first time. The patients gave no history of previous respiratory disease, but almost all were heavy smokers.[1017] The bronchial obstruction responded poorly to bronchodilators but ceased when the patients were removed from the area.[1016] Comparison of the incidence of respiratory symptoms in permanent residents in the Tokyo and Yokohama regions with that in inhabitants of other areas of Japan with less air pollution showed a higher rate of chronic bronchitis in the former. However, Oshima and associates[1018] failed to discover in the permanent residents cases of the acute reversible airway obstruction previously described in the U.S. personnel. Since so many of the subjects who moved into the Tokyo-Yokohama area for the first time were heavy smokers, it is reasonable to assume that the "asthma" probably was an abrupt exacerbation of airway obstruction in patients with some degree of chronic bronchitis.

Deep Inspiration

The effect of a deep inspiration on airway caliber in normal and asthmatic subjects varies between subjects and is dependent on whether there is spontaneous or pharmacologically induced airway narrowing before the deep breath. Without previous administration of bronchoconstrictors, normal subjects show a transient decrease in airway resistance and an increase in anatomic dead space after a deep inspiration, suggesting that large central airways dilate.[1020] Maximal expiratory flows are not increased by a deep breath because partial and complete flow-volume curves can usually be superimposed (Fig. 11–32). When airway resistance is used as the test of airway caliber, many patients with asthma show a paradoxical airway narrowing and a decrease in dead space after a deep inspiration.[592, 1021] Maximal expiratory flows are not increased (complete versus partial flow-volume curves), even when the flows are abnormally low; in fact, in some subjects, the maximal flows can be less on a complete than on a partial flow-volume curve.[1022, 1023]

In normal subjects during pharmacologically induced airway narrowing, a deep breath has a profound bronchodilating effect, regardless of whether RAW or flows on a maximal flow-volume curve are used to estimate airway caliber (Fig. 11–32). With induced bronchoconstriction in patients with asthma, the bronchodilating effect of a deep

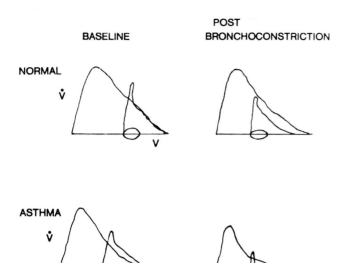

Figure 11–32. Effect of a Deep Inspiration on Maximal Expiratory Flow. Partial and complete flow-volume (V̇-V) curves before and after pharmacologically induced bronchoconstriction are shown for a normal subject and an asthmatic patient. At baseline, a deep inspiration does not increase maximal flow in the normal subject but causes a decrease in maximal flow in the asthmatic. Following bronchoconstriction, the normal subject shows marked reversibility following a deep inspiration, a feature shown by the asthmatic patient as well but to a lesser extent.

inspiration is generally less than in normal subjects and may not occur at all;[447, 1024, 1025] any bronchodilating effect is enhanced by a rapid deep inspiration and is attenuated by an end-inspiratory breath-hold.[1026, 1027]

To understand the possible mechanisms responsible for changes in airway size associated with deep inspiration, it is necessary to discuss the physiologic effects of a deep breath. A deep breath can stimulate airway irritant and stretch receptors, the former mediating reflex bronchoconstriction and the latter dilatation. It has been suggested that excessive stimulation of irritant receptors in patients with asthma is responsible for the paradoxical response to a deep breath in the nonchallenged condition; a study in which inhaled local anesthetic was shown to decrease the bronchoconstriction supports this hypothesis.[1027] In another study, cholinergic blockade in normal subjects did not decrease the bronchodilating effect of a deep inspiration, suggesting that withdrawal of vagal efferent activity is not responsible for the dilatation.[1028]

During a deep breath, lung recoil is increased, thereby stretching airway smooth muscle. This effect would be expected to dilate the airways and reverse pharmacologically induced muscle shortening; however, because of lung pressure-volume hysteresis, the lung recoil at functional residual capacity (FRC) is transiently decreased following a deep inspiration, thus tending to unload airway smooth muscle and allow increased shortening for a given neural input. It has been proposed that the variable response to a deep breath in asthmatic patients is

related to a variation in the ratio between smooth muscle stretch and parenchymal hysteresis.[1029] In subjects in whom a deep breath has little effect on smooth muscle tone but produces a decrease in lung recoil (and therefore smooth muscle load), narrowing of the airways would be expected. Bronchodilation would occur in those subjects in whom a deep inspiration stretches smooth muscle considerably but reduces recoil only slightly.

A third possibility to explain the differences in the effect of a deep breath in normal and asthmatic subjects is a change in the intrinsic smooth muscle response to stretch. Certain kinds of smooth muscle (such as the urinary bladder) show a "myogenic" response, consisting of a contraction following stretch. Although trachealis muscle in normal dogs relaxes when stretched, that from allergic dogs shows myogenic behavior. These data suggest that smooth muscle response to stretch could be altered in asthmatics.

It has been proposed that the absent or deficient bronchodilating effect of a deep breath may be a major contributor to the NSBH of asthma.[447, 1021] When histamine dose-response curves from atopic-asthmatic and nonasthmatic subjects were compared, much more overlap was found between the groups in decreases in expiratory flow and specific airway conductance measured before a deep inspiration than for isovolume flow and FEV₁ measured after a deep inspiration. These results led Fish to suggest that "airway hyperreactivity in asthma is perhaps less a reflection of enhanced end-organ responsiveness than of the impaired capacity to bronchodilate with increased lung volume."[447] Although the different effect of a deep inspiration in normal and asthmatic subjects can partly explain NSBH, it cannot be the only explanation because measurements such as pulmonary resistance obtained prior to a deep inspiration can be altered to a much greater extent in asthmatic subjects at much lower concentrations of an inhaled drug.

The effects of a deep inspiration can be summarized as follows:

1. Patients with asthma can show paradoxical bronchoconstriction following a deep inspiration when they are not pharmacologically bronchoconstricted.

2. Asthmatic patients demonstrate deficient bronchodilatation during a deep inspiration after induced bronchoconstriction.

3. These differences between asthmatic and normal subjects may be caused by a vagal reflex, an effect of a big breath on smooth muscle and lung parenchymal hysteresis, or a difference in the smooth muscle response to stretch.

Miscellaneous Provoking Factors

Alcohol-containing beverages have been reported to precipitate attacks of bronchoconstriction in some patients with asthma: in a questionnaire study of 168 patients, 32 per cent reported that alcohol, usually in the form of beer, wine, or whiskey, worsened their symptoms whereas 23 per cent suggested that they received some benefit, usually from whiskey or brandy.[1030] Although in some cases the bronchoconstriction is caused by the preservative metabisulfite, there are documented reports of adverse responses to pure ethanol administered orally. Patients develop rapid onset of flushing, nasal congestion, and wheeze; the response is attenuated by histamine H_1 and cyclooxygenase blockers but not by atropine.[1031, 1032] Asians who have a very high incidence of acetylaldehyde dehydrogenase deficiency, and who manifest vasomotor responsiveness to ethanol, may be particularly sensitive to its bronchoconstricting effects.[1031]

Certain food additives can precipitate acute bronchoconstriction in asthmatic subjects,[1033] the one most commonly implicated being metabisulfite salts; approximately 4 per cent of asthmatics demonstrate sensitivity to these salts.[1034] As a result of their antioxidant activity, these salts prevent discoloration and thus are used as preservatives in a wide variety of foods and beverages, including wine, beer, fruit juices, fresh fruits, vegetables, and seafood.[1035] They cause bronchoconstriction by producing SO_2, which is inhaled during swallowing. The response to wine depends on its SO_2 content; the higher the level, the greater the response.[1036] Sensitivity can be documented by careful oral challenges with capsules containing increasing amounts of metabisulfite.[1035] Paradoxical dose-dependent bronchoconstriction has been reported in response to a beta-adrenergic agonist containing sodium bisulfite.[1037] Monosodium glutamate and the food coloring additive tartrazine can also cause attacks.[1033, 2782] ASA-sensitive asthmatics frequently are also sensitive to tartrazine, suggesting that the mechanism of action of the two substances may be similar. A large number of asthmatics report a worsening of symptoms in the presence of certain odors, of which perfume and cologne are the most frequently mentioned offenders; in fact, exposure to these aromas has been associated with objective evidence of worsening airflow obstruction.[1038]

Patients with asthma frequently complain of an exacerbation of symptoms following exposure to passive cigarette smoke; in one study of ten subjects, "side-stream" smoke sufficient to increase carboxyhemoglobin by only 0.4 per cent resulted in an average 21 per cent decline in FEV_1.[1039] Despite this, 50 per cent of 106 asthmatics in one study were current or former smokers and among the former little change in flow rates was recorded after one cigarette.[1040] In fact, of 125 patients with asthma, 18 reported a worsening of their asthma following smoking cessation![1041] Despite these observations, it has been shown that asthmatic children of smoking mothers have more symptoms and lower expiratory flow rates than do children of mothers who do not smoke.[1042]

Up to 30 per cent of women with asthma complain of increased symptoms in the premenstrual period; symptoms are associated with a decrease in maximal expiratory flow and are not attributable to the use of ASA.[1043–1045] Severe asthma has been reported following ingestion of ergometrine maleate for the control of postpartum hemorrhage;[1046] since ergometrine in low concentration causes contraction of canine tracheal smooth muscle, its effect on human airway smooth muscle could be direct.[1046]

Outbreaks of asthma have been reported following thunderstorms and sudden changes in barometric pressure, temperature, and humidity. Heavy rain can cause a massive release of fungal spores, and this is more likely to be the triggering mechanism than the climatic changes themselves.[1047]

OCCUPATIONAL ASTHMA

Although it has long been appreciated that asthma can be caused or exacerbated by exposure to inhaled substances in the workplace, there has been a dramatic increase in the number of documented agents that can precipitate occupational asthma (Table 11–2).[337, 1048, 1049] The discovery of new occupations or compounds associated with asthma requires a high index of suspicion and careful history taking; it should not be forgotten that the offending exposure is not necessarily associated with the patient's primary occupation but may occur with hobbies. Unlike the usual atopic or nonatopic asthma, that related solely to occupational exposure is potentially completely reversible, making its early recognition especially important.

Various mechanisms contribute singly or in combination to the production of asthma during occupational exposure. In a comprehensive review, Chan-Yeung and Lam[337] defined categories based on four mechanisms: reflex, acute inflammatory, pharmacologic, and immunologic. The last-named was subdivided into (1) those exposures with proven allergic pathophysiology in which large-molecular-weight substances can be implicated and (2) those in which an immunologic mechanism is likely but unproven and in which small-molecular-weight substances are the offending agents.[337]

Reflex (Nonspecific) Bronchoconstriction

Patients with asthma that is unrelated to a specific occupational exposure can suffer episodic exacerbation of their symptoms when exposed to a variety of irritants in the workplace. As a result of NSBH, asthmatic workers exposed to nonspecific stimuli such as cold, dry air and gaseous or particulate industrial pollutants will develop work-related airway narrowing. Although the term "reflex" implies involvement of a vagal reflex arc, this may not be important in these nonspecific responses; in fact, "nonspecific occupational bronchoconstriction" might be better terminology. Because the reactions are no more than aggravations of pre-existing asthma, their inclusion within the definition of occupational asthma has been questioned.[337]

Inflammatory Bronchoconstriction

Acute exposure to a high concentration of certain gases, vapors, and smoke can produce severe bronchial and bronchiolar injury that causes narrowing and hyper-responsiveness of airways in the exposed worker.[337, 1101, 1102] This syndrome has been called "reactive airway dysfunction" and develops following a single exposure to a high concentration of gases, such as hydrogen sulfide, ammonia, diethylene diamine, and chlorine; fumes from plastics; or smoke from a variety of materials.[1102] Within 24 hours of exposure, airway obstruction develops and some degree of obstruction and exaggerated nonspecific airway responsiveness persist for months, usually followed by slow resolution. Although most such exposures occur in the workplace, a similar syndrome has been reported in a group of children exposed to a high concentration of chlorine in a swimming pool;[1103] we have seen one patient in whom it developed as a result of combustion of a plastic endotracheal tube during laser surgery. The mechanism by which a single exposure causes prolonged sequelae is unknown, but epithelial damage and airway wall inflammation were detected in a small number of patients with the syndrome in the absence of the basement membrane or smooth muscle changes of asthma.[1102]

Pharmacologic Bronchoconstriction

Some occupations involve exposure to substances that are thought to cause a direct, nonidiosyncratic airway effect in a dose-dependent fashion in all exposed workers.[337] The most common substances implicated in this category are cotton dust (byssinosis) and grain dust. Whether the syndrome that results should be called "asthma" is controversial; although workers clearly develop reversible airway obstruction, they fail to manifest the eosinophilia and diurnal lability of expiratory flow that are characteristic of asthma due to other causes.[1104] In addition, since fixed airflow obstruction can develop in both cotton and grain workers, it is possible that these exposures are more closely related to industrial COPD.[1105, 1106]

BYSSINOSIS

Byssinosis is a chronic airway disease that occurs in textile workers exposed to the dust of cotton, flax, hemp, and jute. In its early stages, it is characterized by acute dyspnea, cough, and wheeze on Monday mornings following a weekend away from the workplace; the symptoms decrease during the work week depite continued exposure. The inci-

dence and severity of symptoms and functional impairment are proportional to the exposure, both in duration and intensity.[337, 1107] Some bronchoconstriction can develop in normal subjects in response to an aerosol of cotton bract extract, the degree of bronchoconstriction possibly being related to their nonspecific airway responsiveness.[1108, 1109]

There is no evidence to support the presence of specific IgE- or IgG-mediated immunologic responses in the development of byssinosis. The two theories that best explain the pathogenesis are the presence of a histamine-releasing substance in cotton or the presence of a contaminating endotoxin.[337, 1110, 1111] Although histamine release by cotton has been demonstrated in vitro and blood levels of histamine increase in affected individuals during Monday morning attacks, the bulk of evidence supports endotoxin as the offending substance. Cotton dust is contaminated by endotoxin-containing bacteria and the magnitude of a worker's airway response to exposure correlates more closely with levels of endotoxin in the dust than with the concentration of dust.[1111, 1112] Endotoxin can activate complement in vitro and in guinea pigs can produce an acute airway response that subsequently exhibits tachyphylaxis similar to the Monday morning phenomenon in humans.[1113, 1114] This subject is discussed in greater detail in Chapter 7 (page 1272).

GRAIN FEVER

Because of the complex composition of grain dust, it is not surprising that a number of different syndromes and mechanisms are associated with exposure. Although specific IgE-mediated allergic responses to some components of grain dust have been documented (see later), many subjects show no specific airway or systemic responses. Stored grain can be contaminated with microorganisms, and extracts can release histamine and activate complement;[337] thus, some subjects may demonstrate a direct or pharmacologic airway effect similar to the cotton response.

Workers and nonworkers exposed experimentally to grain dust can develop a syndrome called *grain fever*, consisting of elevated temperature, flushing, headache, chest tightness, cough, dyspnea, an elevated white blood cell count, and a reduction in maximal expiratory flow.[1115, 1116] Workers can also develop leukocytosis and a significant decrease in maximal expiratory flow over a working shift.[1117] There is no evidence for an immunologic mechanism for these acute responses, and the possibility of contaminating endotoxin has again been suggested. Plicatic acid, the agent responsible for western red cedar asthma, has also been shown to activate complement in vitro.[1118]

OTHER OCCUPATIONAL HAZARDS

Occupational "asthma" has been described in factory workers exposed to the output from a con-

Table 11–2. Causes and Mechanisms of Occupational Asthma

PHARMACOLOGIC

Agent	*Occupation*
Cotton dust (byssinosis)	Textile workers
Grain dust	Grain elevator and storage workers, dock workers[1050]
Humidifier pollution or contamination	Factory workers[1051]
Organophosphate insecticides	Farm workers[1052, 1053]
"Red tide" (*Ptychodiscus brevis*)	Fishermen
Isocyanates (also see below)	Polyurethane industry
	Plastics manufacture
	Paint and varnish use and manufacture

PROVEN ALLERGIC

Animals and Animal Products	
Laboratory animals (rats, mice, rabbits, guinea pigs, and monkeys), hair, and urine	Laboratory workers, veterinarians, animal handlers[1054]
Birds (pigeons, chickens, budgerigars)	Bird breeders and poultry workers
Insects	
Poultry mites	Poultry workers[1055, 1056]
Grain mites, flour weevils	Grain and mill workers[1049]
Storage mites	Farmers[1057]
Locusts	Research laboratory
River fly	Power plants along rivers
Screw worm fly	Flight crews and entomologists
Cockroaches	Laboratory workers[1058]
Crickets	Field contact
Bee moth	Fish bait breeder
Moths, butterflies, and blow flies	Entomologists[1059, 1060]
Sewer flies	Sewer workers[1061]
Silkworm larvae	Sericulture[1059]
Honeybees and honeybee pollen	Apiary workers[1062, 1063]
Marine Animals	
Snow crabs and prawns	Crab and prawn processing[1064, 2804]
Hoya (sea squirt)	Oyster farming
Plants and Plant Products	
Grain dust	Grain elevator and storage workers, dock workers
Wheat, rye, and buckwheat flour	Bakers and millers[1065]
Green coffee beans	Coffee bean handlers[1066, 1067]
Castor bean, soybean	Oil industry, felt industry,[1068] and seamen[1069]
Tea	Tea workers
Tulips and narcissi	Gardeners[1049]
Tobacco leaf	Tobacco handling and cigarette manufacture
Baby's breath (*Gypsophila panniculata*)	Florists[1070]
Hops	Beer brewers
Garlic	Spice manufacture[1071, 1072]
Curry, coriander, and mace	Spice industry[1073]
Biologic Enzymes	
Bacillus subtilis	Detergent industry
Trypsin, pancreatin, papain, pepsin, flaviastase, bromelin, fungal amylase	Plastics, pharmaceutical, and laboratory personnel[1074, 1075]
Vegetables	
Gum acacia	Printers
Gum tragacanth	Gum manufacturing[1076]
Cellulase	

Table continued on opposite page

taminated humidifier;[1051, 1052] the syndrome was similar to grain fever and the Monday morning response in cotton workers, suggesting that a common agent (endotoxin?) may have been responsible. The predominant airway response was clinically distinguishable from extrinsic allergic alveolitis, which has been reported in association with *Micropolyspora faeni* contamination of air conditioners.[1119]

A pharmacologic mechanism is likely responsible for the acute "asthma" described in workers spraying organophosphate insecticides; these agents

act as anticholinesterases, permitting unopposed action of vagal tone.[337] The single-celled flagellated sea algae that contribute to "red tide" (*Pthcyodiscus brevis*) can become airborne in ocean spray, and the algal toxin can cause bronchoconstriction by direct acetylcholine release from cholinergic nerve endings.[1120]

Although the weight of evidence supports an allergic (or at least idiosyncratic) mechanism in the production of isocyanate-induced asthma,[1121, 1122] it is possible that pharmacologic dose-dependent in-

Table 11–2. Causes and Mechanisms of Occupational Asthma *Continued*

NOT PROVEN ALLERGIC

Agent	*Occupation*
Diisocyanates	
Toluene, 1,5-naphthylene, diphenylmethane, and hexamethylene diisocyanate	Polyurethane industry, plastics manufacture, foundry, paint, rubber, and varnish workers[1077-1082]
Anhydrides	
Phthalic, trimellitic, pyromellitic tetrachlorophalic and hexahydrophalic anhydride	Epoxy resin and plastics manufacture and use[1083-1085]
Wood Dusts	
Western red cedar, eastern white cedar, California redwood, cedar of Lebanon, Cocabolla, Iroko oak, Mahogany, abiruana, African maple, Tanganyika aningie, Central American walnut, kejaat, and African zebra wood	Carpenters, cabinet makers, construction and sawmill workers[1086, 1087]
Metals	
Platinum	Platinum refinery
Nickel	Metal plating; dental workers[1088]
Chromium	Tanning
Aluminum salts	Aluminum manufacture[1089-1091]
Cobalt, vanadium, and tungsten carbide	Hard metal workers, diamond polishers[1092]
Fluxes	
Aminoethyl ethanolamine	Aluminum soldering
Colophony	Electronics industry
Drugs	
Penicillin, cephalosporins, phenylglycine acid chloride, piperazine hydrochloride, psyllium, methyldopa, spiramycin, amprolium hydrochloride, tetracycline, sulfone chloramides	Pharmaceutical industry, chemists, nurses, brewers, poultry feed mixture
Other Chemicals	
Dimethyl ethanolamine	Spray painters
Persulfate salts and henna	Hairdressers[1093]
Ethylene diamine	Photographers
Azobisformanide	Plastics industry[1094]
Azodicarbonamide	Plastic and rubber industry[1094]
Dioazonium salt	Photocopying and dyeing[1095]
Glutaraldehyde, hexachlorophene and formalin	Hospital staff[1096]
Urea formaldehyde	Insulation and resin workers
Freon	Refrigeration
Paraphenylene diamine	Fur dyeing
Furfuryl alcohol	Foundry mold making[1097]
Methyl methacrylate and cyanoacrylate (crazy glue or super glue)	Dental workers[1098]
Polyvinylchloride	Plastics manufacture and meat wrappers[1099, 1100]
Oil mists	Machinists[2805]
Hydroquinones and methionine	Chemical workers[2806]
Acid vapors	Mineral analysis laboratory workers[2807]

hibition of various biologic enzymes and receptors (including beta-agonist receptors) might contribute to the airway response.[337, 1121, 1123]

Proven Allergic Bronchoconstriction

Table 11–2 contains a list of agents and occupations in which a specific IgE-induced allergic mechanism has been proven. For the most part, the antigens are large-molecular-weight proteins, polysaccharides, or glycoproteins derived from plants or animals. Sensitivity develops predominantly in workers with an atopic predisposition, and positive immediate skin test or specific IgE responses (RAST) can be demonstrated.

Up to 30 per cent of exposed laboratory workers develop specific IgE responses to proteins from the fur or urine of rats, mice, guinea pigs, or rabbits.

Symptoms begin within 4 years of initial exposure; conjunctivitis and rhinitis commonly precede the onset of bronchoconstriction.[337, 1124]

Grain dust is a complex mixture of insects, fungi, silicates, bacteria, herbicides, pesticides, and mammalian debris, and,[1125] not surprisingly, its inhalation can cause a variety of clinical syndromes. A small percentage of atopic workers develop IgE-mediated acute and delayed airway responses to specific antigens, such as grain mites and weevils, and to the specific grains themselves.[337, 1049] Interestingly, the incidence of atopy in grain elevator workers is less than in the general population, presumably because subjects with atopy, asthma, and increased nonspecific airway responsiveness avoid or drop out of the work force.[1126, 1127] Pre-employment respiratory symptoms, positive allergy skin test results, and increased NSBR are significantly associated with the development of work-related respiratory complaints in seasonal grain handlers.[1128]

Chronic exposure to grain dust may result in persistent functional derangement: of 587 grain elevator workers in one study,[1129] 288 had respiratory symptoms and 102 showed significant impairment of lung function. When 22 of the 102 patients were exposed to grain dust, six developed an immediate and/or late response typical of an IgE-mediated allergic airway reaction; the remaining 16 exhibited more fixed airway obstruction, presumably representing a form of industrial bronchitis or COPD.[1129]

The incidence of cough, sputum, wheeze, and airflow obstruction is higher in grain than in nonexposed workers, as is a more rapid rate of decline in FEV_1.[1125, 1130–1133] Grain workers with symptoms and lung function deficits are also more likely to show increased nonspecific airway responsiveness, but this probably represents a consequence of their impairment rather than a predisposing factor.[1127, 1133, 1134]

Between 7 and 20 per cent of bakers eventually develop symptoms of allergy (rhinitis and asthma).[337, 1135] Unlike the reactions in grain workers, specific cereal grain allergy revealed by positive skin tests and RAST to *cereal grains* (wheat, rye, barley, oats, and triticale) can be detected in the vast majority.

In one study of 14 subjects with long-term exposure to *pancreatic extracts* in the pharmaceutical industry, three patterns of response were distinguished:[1074] all showed positive immediate skin tests to pancreatic extracts and some had positive inhalation challenges; two of the 14 had documented extrinsic allergic alveolitis, and seven had clinical signs suggestive of emphysema. The possibility exists that enzymatic elastolytic destruction resulted in emphysema, but there was no documentation of loss of lung recoil or pathologic confirmation of emphysema.

In occupations in which allergic airway disease develops and in which the number of exposed workers is sufficient to calculate the prevalence of asthma, the incidence approaches 20 per cent, similar to the incidence of atopy in the general population.[1064, 1135] This suggests that with intense and prolonged exposure to reaginic antigens, most atopic subjects will develop manifestations of allergic airway disease. However, some antigens appear to be particularly capable of eliciting an IgE response, even in nonatopic individuals; for example, as many as 66 per cent of workers exposed to *Bacillus subtilis* enzymes in the detergent industry develop asthma.[1136, 1137]

Possible Allergic Bronchoconstriction

There is an ever increasing list of low-molecular-weight substances (1,000 daltons) that can induce asthma in exposed workers (*see* Table 11–2).

Many features are present in this form of industrial asthma that suggest an allergic mechanism:

1. Only about 5 per cent of exposed individuals develop asthma, and the occurrence of sensitivity is not dose-dependent. Both of these factors militate against a direct toxic or pharmacologic effect.

2. After a latent period, sensitization increases with the duration of exposure as in proven allergic airway syndromes.

3. Exposure to a minute concentration of the offending agent results in classic immediate and/or late bronchoconstrictive responses, the latter being followed by a prolonged increase in NSBH.

4. Hapten-specific IgE is present in some cases, with tissue and blood eosinophilia present in many.[337, 1121]

Although these four observations favor an allergic mechanism, there are at least three features that augur against classic Type I or III allergy as the cause of these syndromes: (1) the absence of positive skin responses and specific IgE or IgG in many cases; (2) the presence of specific IgE and IgG in asymptomatic workers; and (3) no difference in the prevalence of sensitization between atopic and nonatopic individuals.

The best studied single entity in this category is occupational exposure to plicatic acid, a component of *western red cedar (Thuja plicata)*. Although this condition was first recognized in Australian cabinet makers exposed to cedar sawdust,[1138] the clinical, epidemiologic, and pathophysiologic features of the syndrome have been most clearly documented by Chan-Yeung and associates in cedar saw-mill workers.[1139–1143] Approximately 4 per cent of exposed workers develop sensitivity to plicatic acid over an exposure period ranging from months to years. Nonatopics are equally as prone as atopics to develop sensitization, and there are no clinical or historical characteristics that permit prediction of which workers will be affected. Specific IgE antibody to plicatic acid–human serum albumin conjugate is found in approximately 40 per cent of patients tested. In one study of 185 patients,[1140] inhalation provocation testing showed isolated immediate airway reactions in only 7 per cent, isolated late reactions in 44 per cent, and dual reactions in 49 per cent. Patients with a dual response to inhalation of plicatic acid have significantly more severe occupational asthma characterized by a lower baseline FEF_{25-75} and a greater degree of nonspecific bronchial hyper-responsiveness.[1144] Nonspecific airway responsiveness can predict the response to plicatic acid and is increased in severity following development of a late response to western red cedar.[1139, 1145] Symptoms of cough and dyspnea can be insidious in onset and predominantly nocturnal, presumably as a result of the delayed response, making diagnosis difficult. Symptoms and pulmonary function abnormalities increase with the duration and intensity of exposure.[1146] A case has been reported of a saw-mill worker who was sensitive to eastern white cedar *(Thuja occidentalis)* and who showed cross-reactivity to western red cedar; eastern white cedar contains approximately half the plicatic acid present in the western red variety.[1087]

The prognosis for recovery following the development of western red cedar sensitivity is similar to that for other low-molecular-weight agents.[1147, 1148] Approximately 60 per cent of sensitive individuals have persistent symptoms for 4 years following cessation of exposure; those whose symptoms are of longer duration prior to diagnosis and whose pulmonary function is worse at diagnosis are less likely to recover completely.[1140, 1141, 1147, 1149, 1150] The PC_{20} methacholine at the time of diagnosis is also predictive of outcome, individuals who show no improvement having persisting NSBH.[1147, 1150]

The *anhydrides* are used in the production of epoxy resins, plastics, and adhesives. Exposure to the anhydrides can cause one of four clinical syndromes: (1) a simple irritant response, (2) asthma and rhinitis, (3) delayed airway obstruction accompanied by systemic symptoms, and (4), rarely, a pulmonary syndrome characterized by alveolar hemorrhage and anemia.[1151] Immunoglobulins directed against anhydride–protein conjugates have been implicated in the pathogenesis of the asthma-rhinitis syndrome (IgE) and the late systemic response (IgG).[1152–1154] A reduction in exposure levels in the workplace results in a decreased incidence of the late IgG-mediated syndrome but not of the IgE response.[1155]

Isocyanates are used as hardeners in paint, varnish, molds, and plastics, and exposure to them, particularly to toluene diisocyanate (TDI), is the most common cause of occupational asthma; up to 10 per cent of exposed workers develop airway sensitivity.[337] TDI hypersensitivity can cause prolonged asthma despite removal from occupational exposure.[1156, 1157] The clinical, epidemiologic, and pathophysiologic features are similar to those of plicatic acid sensitivity, although nonspecific irritant and allergic alveolitis-type syndromes have also been reported.[1158, 1159] An isolated negative methacholine challenge for NSBH does not exclude the presence of TDI hypersensitivity.[1160] As with plicatic acid, a delayed response to TDI results in a prolonged increase in nonspecific bronchial responsiveness.[421, 1161] When 114 subjects with TDI-induced asthma were challenged, an isolated immediate response developed in 24, a dual response in 40, and an isolated late response in 50;[1162] the patients with the dual response had a longer history of symptoms and more severe airway obstruction prior to challenge. Both the delayed response and the increased NSBR can be blocked with high doses of oral prednisone.[1163] Animal models have been used to study the mechanism of the enhanced nonspecific response: in guinea pigs, TDI causes severe airway inflammation and epithelial damage and can increase the sensitivity and maximal response of the trachealis muscle.[625, 1164]

Although *formaldehyde* was first reported as a cause of occupational asthma in 1939, its importance as a sensitizer is still unclear;[1165] of 28 patients who complained of respiratory symptoms related to exposure, only three had definite immediate responses, late responses, or both.[1165, 1166] Urea formaldehyde used as an insulator or binder in particle board has been reported to cause asthma.[1167, 1168]

The existence of "meat wrappers' asthma," thought to be caused by the cutting of *polyvinylchloride film* on a hot wire, is questionable because a number of careful studies of meat packers have failed to show objective evidence of airway narrowing despite ocular and bronchial symptoms.[1099, 1169]

The soldering agent *colophone*, a product of pine resin, has been used for over 100 years, although asthma secondary to exposure was not recognized until 1977.[1170–1172] In a retrospective study, many workers who left an electronics factory for respiratory health reasons had been exposed to solder flux, an illustration of how workers can self-select prior to diagnosis or medical intervention.[1173]

Of the metals and metal salts that induce asthma, *platinum* is the best documented; there is strong evidence that it is IgE-mediated.[1174] The mechanism and prevalence of asthma caused by *nickel, chromium, cobalt,* and *aluminum* have been less well established.[1089, 1090, 1175–1178]

Diagnosis

The diagnosis of occupational asthma requires the demonstration that the patient's symptoms are caused by asthma and are related to the work environment. As with nonoccupational asthma, diagnosis is established by a combination of clinical history, pulmonary function tests, bronchodilator response, and tests of nonspecific bronchial responsiveness. Documentation that the asthma is caused by work or hobby-related exposure requires a high index of suspicion. A carefully taken occupational history should be obtained from all patients with adult-onset asthma, remembering that in some cases occupational exposure can also exacerbate pre-existing asthma. It is especially helpful if symptoms develop during or immediately after exposure to a specific agent or if there is a high incidence of respiratory complaints in similarly exposed workers. However, symptoms can begin after working hours or can be solely nocturnal. Patients should be questioned concerning remission of their symptoms during weekends and holidays and exacerbation on return to work.

The documentation of positive skin tests to a battery of allergens proves atopy and makes it more likely that a patient will experience symptoms to large-molecular-weight agents that stimulate IgE production. A positive skin test or RAST result to a known occupational sensitizer is very suggestive of occupational asthma; however, skin tests can be positive in workers who are asymptomatic, especially those exposed to small-molecular-weight substances.

Patients with occupational asthma frequently manifest normal lung function at the time of presentation, and it may be necessary to document functional impairment related to work exposure. Recognized patterns of derangement include a greater than 20 per cent decline in PEFR or FEV_1 over a work shift and a progressive decline in flow rates over the work week with improvement shown on weekends.[1179-1181] Because of the potential for delayed responses, 24-hour records of PEFR with mini–peak flow meters may be particularly helpful in establishing the diagnosis.[337, 1180]

When first seen by the physician, the majority of patients manifest NSBR, although its absence does not exclude the diagnosis of occupational asthma.[426, 427] Besides helping to confirm the diagnosis, serial tests of NSBR can help document that the asthma is work-related.[337] An increase in NSBR during a period of exposure and a decrease during absence from work provide strong evidence for occupational sensitivity. Tests of NSBR can also help to predict the severity of the response to a challenge with a specific sensitizing agent.[1182]

Bronchial provocation testing with suspected specific occupational agents should not be undertaken lightly and need not be carried out in all patients to prove the diagnosis. Challenges should "be performed by experienced personnel in a hospital setting where resuscitation facilities are available and where frequent observations can be made."[337] Besides the danger of causing an immediate severe response, the possibility of delayed and prolonged effects from a single exposure exists; a delayed response is especially common following exposure to the small-molecular-weight agents, which can precipitate recurrent nocturnal asthma following a single exposure.[1183] Chan-Yeung and Lam[337] have suggested that challenge should be undertaken only to prove a new occupational sensitizer, to determine the specific agent in a complex exposure, or for medicolegal purposes. A significant airway response to a specific challenge remains the most definitive means of establishing a causative relationship, provided a nonspecific irritant response can be ruled out.

Summary

There is a rapidly increasing list of substances that can cause occupational asthma. Since this form of asthma is potentially reversible, a high index of suspicion and careful questioning concerning work exposure are vital to diagnosis.

Occupational asthma can be caused by one of four different mechanisms of bronchoconstriction—reflex or irritant, inflammatory, pharmacologic, or immunologic. The immunologic category comprises by far the largest of these and can be subdivided into (1) those agents that cause broncho-constriction by a proven allergic pathophysiology (large-molecular-weight substances) and (2) those in which the mechanism is probably immunologic (usually small-molecular-weight substances). A common cause of the proven allergic type of occupational asthma is that associated with exposure to laboratory animals; the prototype of occupation-induced asthma in which small-molecular-weight compounds produce hypersensitivity of presumed immunologic pathogenesis is exposure to western red cedar. An example of pharmacologically induced bronchoconstriction is that caused by the inhalation of cotton dust (byssinosis) or grain dust.

ROENTGENOGRAPHIC MANIFESTATIONS

The roentgenographic manifestations of bronchial asthma are more complex than customarily believed and in certain combinations may be highly suggestive, if not diagnostic.[2760] Notwithstanding, in many patients the chest roentgenogram is normal. As will be discussed later, the incidence of abnormality is influenced to a considerable degree by the age at onset of the asthma, its severity, and its constancy. In the presence of acute severe asthma or during prolonged, intractable asthmatic attacks, the most characteristic, although by no means invariable, roentgenographic signs are pulmonary overinflation and expiratory air trapping. In one series, hyperinflation, as manifested by anterior bowing of the sternum, increase in the depth of the retrosternal space, thoracic kyphosis, and diaphragmatic flattening or inversion, was identified in up to 72 per cent of 40 patients of varied age with bronchial asthma.[2760] The incidence varied somewhat, depending on the criterion of overinflation: in the adult the most frequent sign is an abnormal configuration of the diaphragm consisting of either flattening or inversion, an abnormality that can revert to normal following successful treatment (Fig. 11–33). (In adults a concave upper surface is more frequently the result of emphysema.) In children, additional signs of pulmonary overinflation include increased bowing of the sternum (perhaps related to the relative pliability of the bony thorax in the young patient) and widening of the retrosternal airspace (Fig. 11–34).

Cardiac size is almost invariably normal, although the long, narrow cardiac silhouette commonly seen in patients with emphysema is occasionally observed in asthmatics. Prominence of the main pulmonary artery and its hilar branches with rapid midlung attenuation is probably indicative of transient precapillary pulmonary arterial hypertension secondary to hypoxia and occurs in approximately 10 per cent of patients (Fig. 11–35).[2760] Vessels in the middle and peripheral lung zones are normal in up to 50 per cent of patients; abnormal patterns include diffuse narrowing and blood flow redistribution into the upper lobes, the latter in the absence

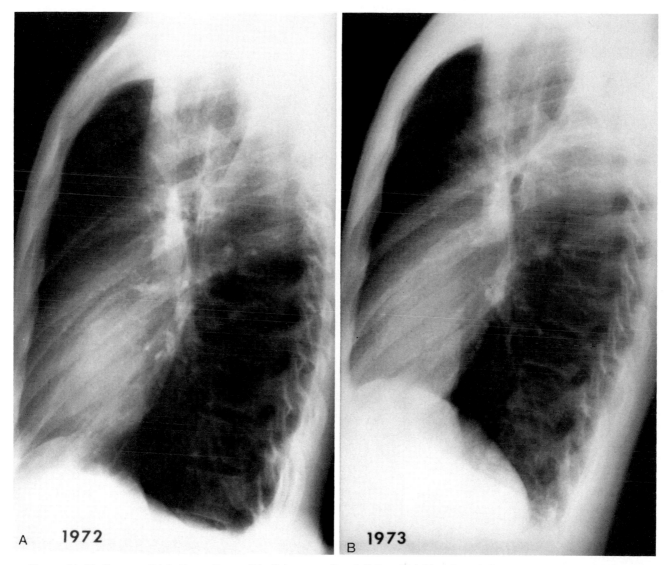

Figure 11–33. Spasmodic Asthma: Reversible Pulmonary Overinflation (Adult). A lateral chest roentgenogram *(A)* of an adult asthmatic during an attack of severe bronchospasm reveals a low position and flat configuration of the diaphragm, indicating severe pulmonary overinflation. Approximately 1 year later during a remission *(B)*, lung volume had returned to normal. Note that the curvature of the sternum and thoracic spine did not change, since these structures do not participate in acute hyperinflation in the adult.

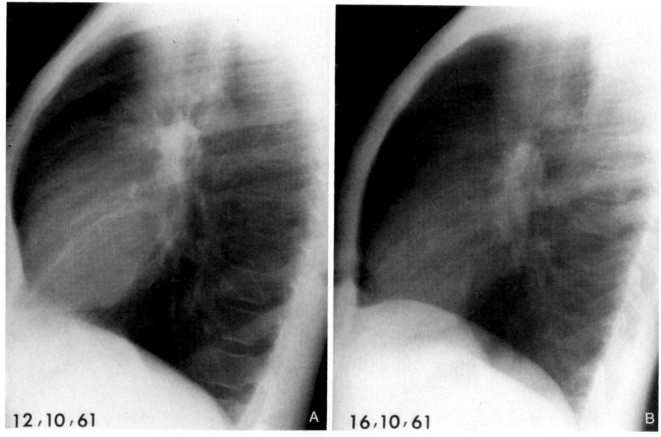

Figure 11–34. Spasmodic Asthma: Reversible Pulmonary Overinflation (Adolescent). A lateral chest roentgenogram *(A)* of a young asthmatic patient during an episode of severe, acute bronchospasm reveals an increase in the volume of the retrosternal and retrocardiac spaces, flattening of the diaphragm, anterior bowing of the sternum, and a slight kyphosis. Four days later following therapy *(B)*, the abnormal parameters have cleared except for persistence of an increased retrocardiac space. Note that hyperinflation tends to affect the bony skeleton to a greater extent in the young patient than in the adult, possibly as a result of more pliable cartilaginous and bony structures.

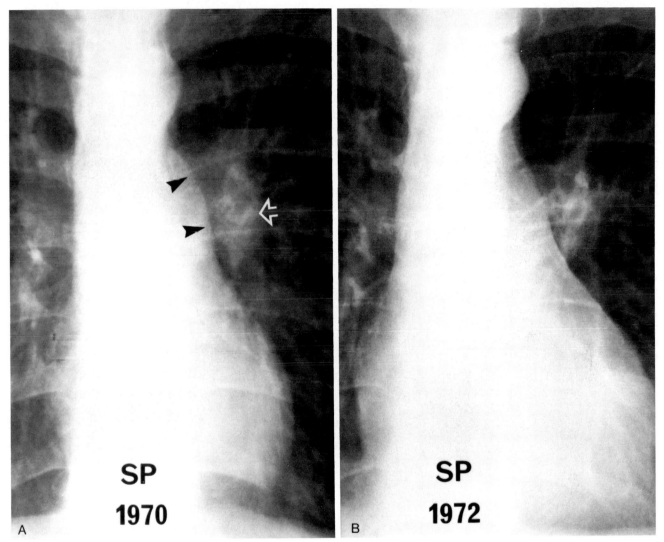

Figure 11–35. Spasmodic Asthma: Reversible Precapillary Pulmonary Hypertension. A detail view of the heart and left hilum from a posteroanterior roentgenogram *(A)* reveals enlargement of the main pulmonary artery *(arrowheads)* and left interlobar artery *(open arrows)*, consistent with the presence of pulmonary arterial hypertension. At the time of this study, this young man was experiencing a severe attack of acute bronchospasm. Approximately 2 years later during a period of remission, a repeat roentgenogram *(B)* demonstrates a return to normal of the configuration of the main and interlobar arteries. Note that the heart has increased in size during this interval, presumably reflecting the high transpulmonary pressure that existed during the acute attack and the consequent reduction in venous return.

of other signs of postcapillary hypertension. Focal or segmental arterial vasospasm can simulate acute thromboembolism clinically and can occur in the absence of roentgenographic abnormality, necessitating pulmonary angiography for certain distinction (Fig. 11–36).

A previously undescribed feature, seen on the posteroanterior chest roentgenogram in 13 (32.5 per cent) of the 40 patients in the previously cited study,[2760] consisted of a striking paucity of vessels in the outer 2 to 4 cm of the lungs (Fig. 11–37). This "subpleural oligemia" is especially evident when accompanied by an increased prominence of the hilar and midlung vessels and is reversible with treatment. Its pathogenesis probably relates to diffuse bronchiolar mucous plugging and spasm resulting in peripheral hypoventilation and hypoxic vasoconstriction, a hypothesis that is supported by both radionuclide and CT correlative studies (Fig. 11–38). However, the sign is not specific for bronchial asthma because we have also seen it in patients with cystic fibrosis, in Swyer-James syndrome, and following acute viral pneumonia.

Defects in perfusion associated with ventilation inequality may cause other abnormal scintigraphic patterns.[2761] One such pattern is the "stripe sign" described by Sostman and Gottschalk[2762] as indicative of nonembolic hypoperfusion (Fig. 11–39): it is manifested by a rim of normal perfusion in the cortex alternating with contiguous zones of hypoperfusion, central to which resides a zone of medullary hypoperfusion.[2762] It is the contention of these authors that this pattern effectively excludes thromboembolic disease as the cause of the oligemia, since thromboembolic deficits almost invariably extend to a pleural surface and hence must involve both the cortex and medulla simultaneously.

The influence of age at onset of asthma on the presence or absence of roentgenographic changes was illustrated graphically in a study by Hodson and associates[1184] of 117 asthmatic patients over 15 years of age. In this adult group, roentgenographic abnormalities were identified in 31 per cent of the patients whose asthma had its onset before the age of 15 years but in none of those in whom it occurred after 30 years of age. In this series, overinflation (with or without hilar enlargement) was identified in only 22 patients overall (19 per cent). The incidence of roentgenographic abnormalities is also affected by severity. In a study of 58 patients ranging in age from 10 to 69 years (mean age 32.7) in whom the asthma was categorized as "severe," evidence of pulmonary overinflation was detected in 42 (73 per cent).[1185] In this report, Rebuck[1185] drew attention to the rapidity with which signs of overinflation can disappear following appropriate ther-

Text continued on page 2075

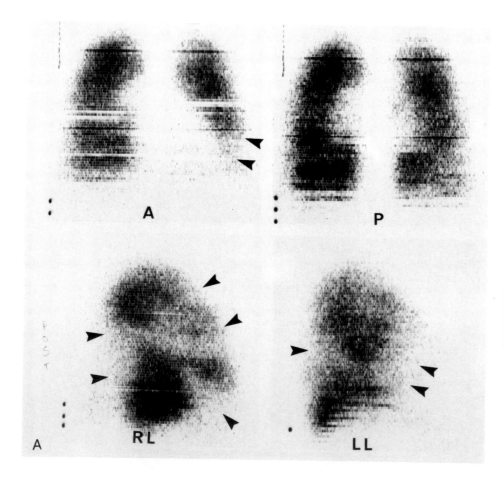

Figure 11–36. Spasmodic Asthma: Perfusion Abnormalities. A young obese woman with a history of atopic asthma was admitted to hospital complaining of severe dyspnea and wheezing; chest roentgenograms were normal. A perfusion lung scan was requested to evaluate the possibility of thromboembolism. Rectilinear perfusion scans *(A)* in anterior (A), posterior (P), right lateral (RL), and left lateral (LL) positions reveal multiple segmental flow deficits in both lungs *(arrowheads)* considered to be consistent with pulmonary embolism (a ventilation scan was not performed).

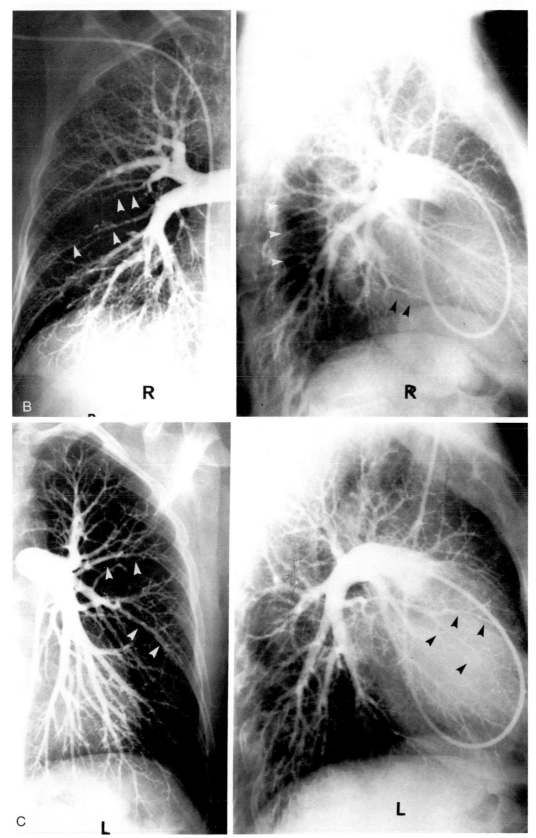

Figure 11–36. *Continued.* Detail views of the right *(B)* and left *(C)* lungs from selective right and left pulmonary angiograms reveal a patent arterial tree throughout both lungs, excluding the presence of thromboemboli. However, many of the segmental arteries are diffusely narrowed with a reduced number of side branches *(arrowheads)*, suggesting vasospasm as the cause of the perfusion scan findings.

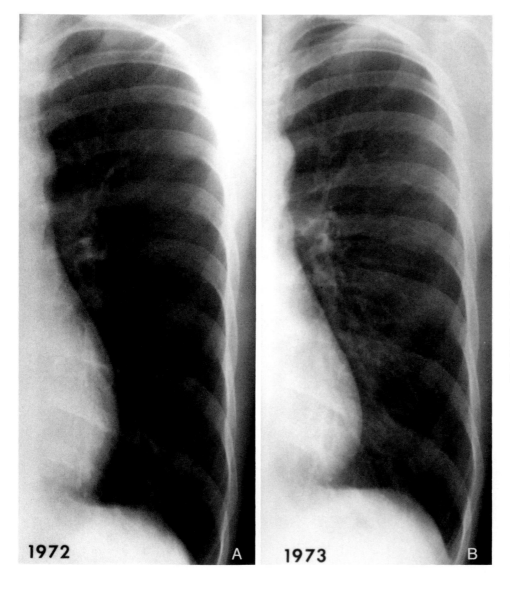

Figure 11–37. Spasmodic Asthma: Peripheral Oligemia. A detail view of the left lung from a posteroanterior chest roentgenogram *(A)* of a young man during an episode of acute bronchospasm reveals moderate hyperinflation. The vasculature in the outer 2 to 3 cm of lung is inconspicuous and barely visible, creating a subpleural shell of oligemic lung. A repeat study 1 year later during remission *(B)* shows less hyperinflation; the pulmonary vessels now taper normally, and most are visible well into the lung periphery.

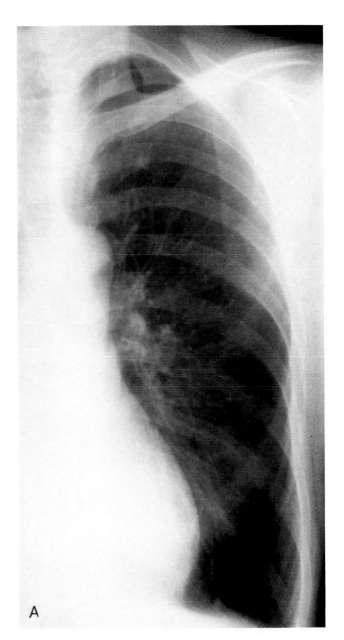

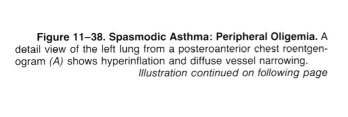

Figure 11–38. Spasmodic Asthma: Peripheral Oligemia. A detail view of the left lung from a posteroanterior chest roentgenogram *(A)* shows hyperinflation and diffuse vessel narrowing.

Illustration continued on following page

A

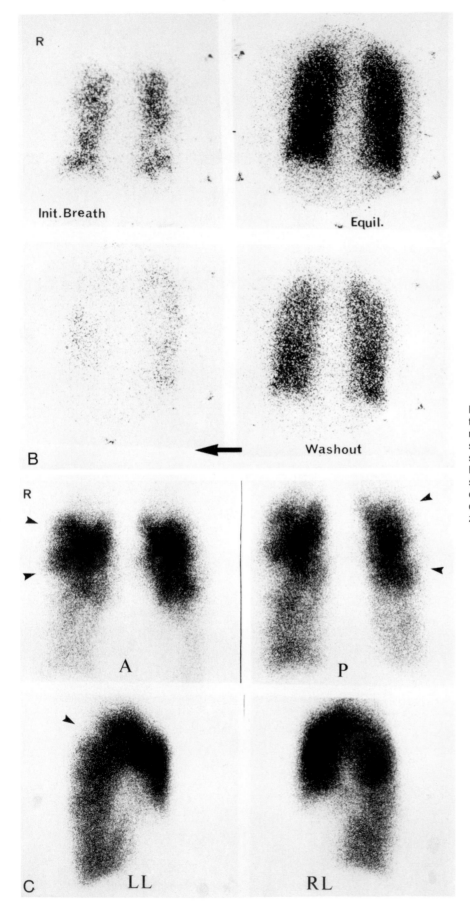

Figure 11–38. *Continued.* A ventilation lung scintigram *(B)* reveals poor filling on the initial breath, largely confined to the medulla; the end-stage of washout shows some peripheral air trapping. A perfusion scintigram *(C)* reveals poor perfusion of the lower lobes. Note the irregular subpleural shell of diminished perfusion *(arrowheads)*, corresponding with the subpleural oligemia on the conventional roentgenogram and the zone of air trapping on the ventilation scan.

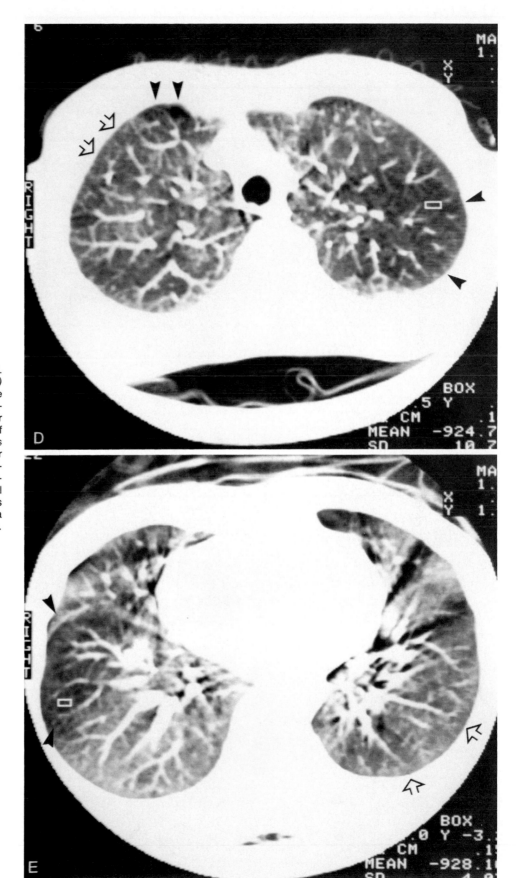

Figure 11–38. *Continued.* CT scans through the upper *(D)* and lower *(E)* lobes demonstrate low-density areas in the subpleural lung *(arrowheads)* (cursor boxes record measurements of −924 and −928 Hounsfield units in the left upper and right lower lobes, respectively). This CT finding is indicative of decreased perfusion; however, note that cortical perfusion is normal in some areas *(open arrows)*. The patient is a young woman with atopic asthma.

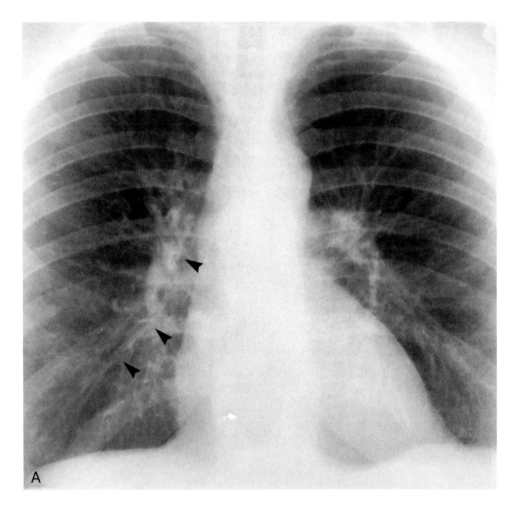

Figure 11–39. Spasmodic Asthma: The "Stripe Sign." A posteroanterior chest roentgenogram *(A)* is normal except for mild overinflation and bronchial wall thickening *(arrowheads)*.

Figure 11–39. *Continued.* A ventilation lung scintigram *(B)* reveals unequal deposition of the radioisotope in the central (medullary) parenchyma on the initial breath (IB), with relative sparing peripherally; equilibration (EQ) was eventually achieved centrally and peripherally, although air trapping occurred in both areas during the washout (WO) phase. A perfusion scan *(C)* in anterior (A), posterior (P), right lateral (RL), and left lateral (LL) positions demonstrates gross deficits in the perfusion pattern in the lower lobes and posterior parts of the upper lobes. Note the rim of maintained perfusion in the cortex *(1)* that alternates with adjacent regions of cortical hypoperfusion *(2)*; in both instances, the proximal medulla *(3)* is focally underperfused. The presence of maintained perfusion adjacent to contiguous medullary hypoperfusion on a scintigram is designated the "stripe sign," effectively excluding thromboembolic disease as the cause of the oligemia. The premise for this conclusion is that thromboembolism deficits almost invariably extend to the pleural surface, and hence they must affect the cortex and medulla simultaneously.

Illustration continued on following page

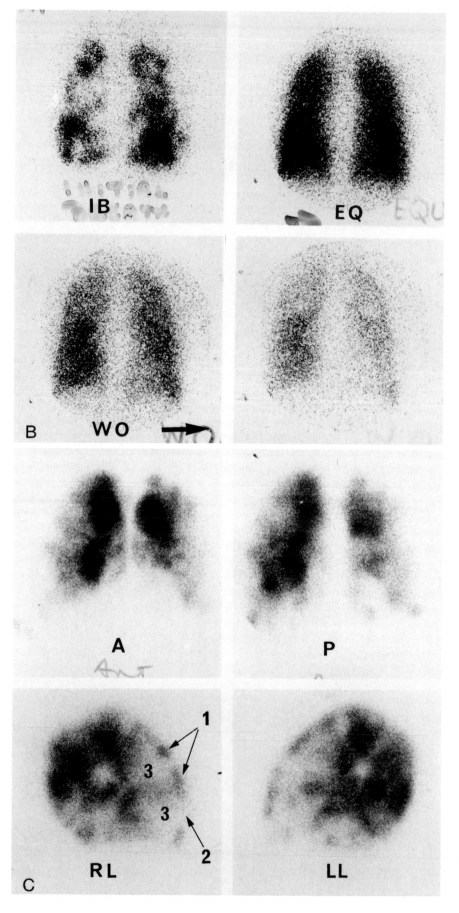

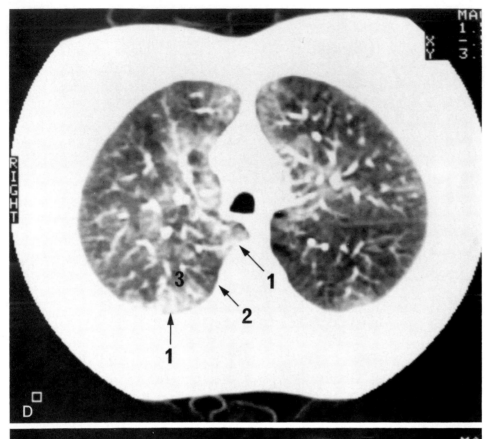

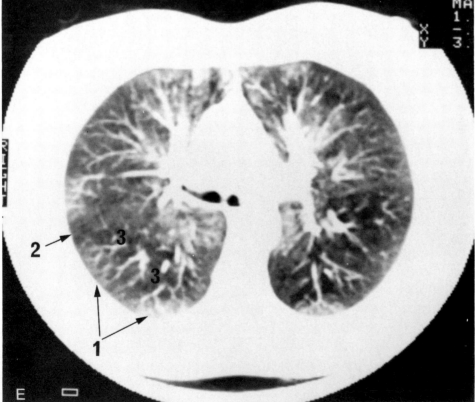

Figure 11–39. *Continued.* CT scans through the distal trachea *(D)* and carina *(E)* show features similar to those on the perfusion images: note the regions of maintained cortical perfusion *(1)*, deficient cortical perfusion *(2)*, and medullary hypoperfusion *(3)*, the CT equivalent of the stripe sign. The patient is a young woman with atopic asthma.

apy, sometimes in as short a time as 24 hours. The incidence of roentgenographic abnormalities also bears a relationship to the constancy or intermittent nature of symptoms. In a study of 218 children with asthma and a control group of 162 normal children, Simon and his colleagues[1186] found that the asthmatics with the most marked roentgenographic abnormalities were, without exception, suffering from severe or moderately severe *constant* asthma; those with *intermittent* symptoms usually had roentgenograms that appeared normal, even during asthmatic episodes. Overall, 73 per cent of the asthmatics were roentgenographically normal. Abnormalities consisted of overinflation and enlargement of hilar vessels, the latter sign being observed in almost half (44 per cent) the patients with overinflation.

In some patients with chronic asthma—usually those with a history of repeated episodes of infection—the bronchial walls are thickened, an abnormality sometimes detectable roentgenographically. In 1960, Hodson and Trickey[1187] drew attention to the frequency of tubular shadows in chest roentgenograms of children with asthma—a finding in 121 (64 per cent) of their 190 patients. They divided their patients into Group I, chronic infectious asthma *(sic)* (26); Group II, purely allergic asthma (58); and Group III, asthma of mixed etiology (106). Tubular shadows were identified in 88 per cent of those in Groups I and III and in only 9 per cent of those in Group II, and these authors therefore related bronchial wall thickening to the presence of chronic infection.

Bronchial wall thickening occurs in both segmental and subsegmental bronchi and can be seen either as ring shadows when viewed end-on or as tramline opacities when viewed *en face*. In contradistinction to the thickened and obviously dilated bronchial walls in cystic fibrosis and bronchiectasis, bronchial dilatation in asthma is absent or minimal (unless the asthma is associated with hypersensitivity bronchopulmonary aspergillosis). Smaller bronchi measuring 3 to 5 mm in diameter, normally invisible on conventional chest roentgenograms, may be identified (Fig. 11–40). These findings probably represent intramural and peribronchial thickening secondary to inflammation or fibrosis or both. Although the thickening is usually permanent, it may decrease or disappear entirely following treatment, suggesting that an inflammatory reaction and excessive surface epithelial mucus are responsible (Fig. 11–41). In our opinion, the combination of thickening of the walls of bronchi, diffuse vessel narrowing, and subpleural oligemia is highly suggestive, if not diagnostic, of bronchial asthma.

Mucous plugging of larger bronchi, with or without atelectasis, is rare;[2760] when present, it occurs most often in the upper lobes.[2763] Large inspissated mucous plugs may distend segmental bronchi, causing the syndrome of "mucoid impaction," which is indistinguishable from allergic bronchopulmonary aspergillosis. Of the 40 hospitalized patients with asthma studied by Genereux,[2760] 11 (27 per cent) developed focal areas of pneumonia; however, none showed the acute, diffuse bilateral bronchopneumonic pattern described by Felson and Felson.[2764]

The chief indication for chest roentgenography in patients with bronchial asthma is to exclude other conditions that cause diffuse wheezing throughout the chest—chronic bronchitis and emphysema, bronchiectasis, and obstructions of the trachea or major bronchi. Several studies have been carried out to evaluate the efficacy of roentgenographic examination in patients with asthma, and the conclusions are not by any means unanimous. Gillies and his associates[1188] reviewed the findings in 178 admissions of 142 children with acute asthma and found the frequency of complications sufficient to justify the routine use of chest roentgenography in this patient population: parenchymal consolidation (presumably acute pneumonia) was present in 21 per cent, atelectasis in 3 per cent, and pneumomediastinum in 2 per cent. In a similar study of 117 adults admitted to hospital with severe acute asthma, Petheram and associates[1189] found roentgenographic abnormalities that affected management in ten patients (9 per cent); in nine of these, the presence of consolidation or atelectasis was not detected on clinical examination. In this series, overinflation was common and correlated significantly with tachycardia, pulsus paradoxus, and a decrease in FEV_1; bronchial wall thickening was also common.

In contrast to the conclusion reached by these two groups—that routine chest roentgenography is useful in patients with acute asthma—Zieverink and her colleagues[1190] found to the contrary unless the patient is unresponsive to bronchodilators and is being admitted to hospital. These authors reviewed 528 chest roentgenograms of 122 adults (16 years of age or older), each film representing a separate acute asthmatic attack. Only 2.2 per cent of the roentgenograms revealed infiltrates *(sic)*, atelectasis, pneumothorax, or pneumomediastinum (pulmonary overinflation was not included as an abnormal finding). They also reviewed 464 chest roentgenograms of 188 children (15 years of age of younger) and found abnormalities in 13 per cent. Of considerable interest was the observation that the children with abnormal roentgenograms exhibited a high incidence of rales in addition to wheezing, suggesting to the authors that in the presence of such findings chest roentgenography may be useful in providing additional information.

Cinebronchography of bronchial tree dynamics reveals normal behavior (Fig. 11–42).[1191] Although the maximal inspiratory caliber may be slightly less than normal (particularly in the segmental and subsegmental bronchi), the reduction in caliber during forced expiration or cough is roughly proportional throughout the length of the visible bronchial

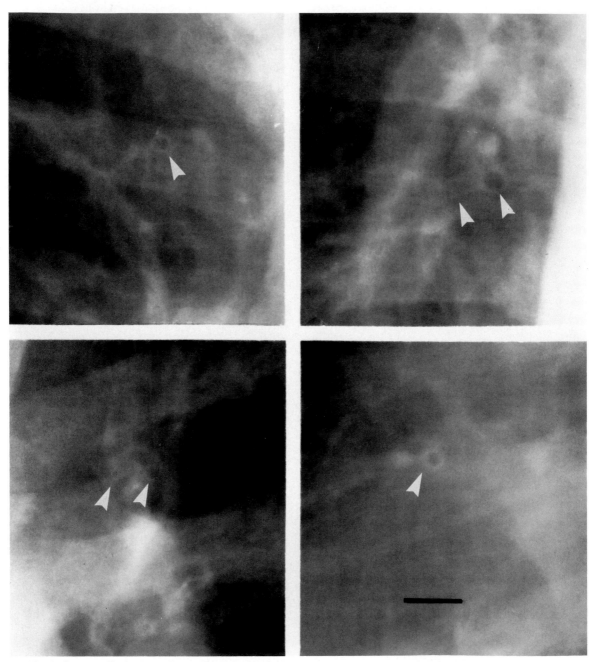

Figure 11–40. Spasmodic Asthma: Bronchial Wall Thickening. Detail views from four areas of the lungs from posteroanterior and lateral chest roentgenograms reveal thick-walled airways measuring 3 to 5 mm in diameter that are not normally visible *(arrowheads)*. The bar represents 1 cm. The patient is a young boy with atopic asthma.

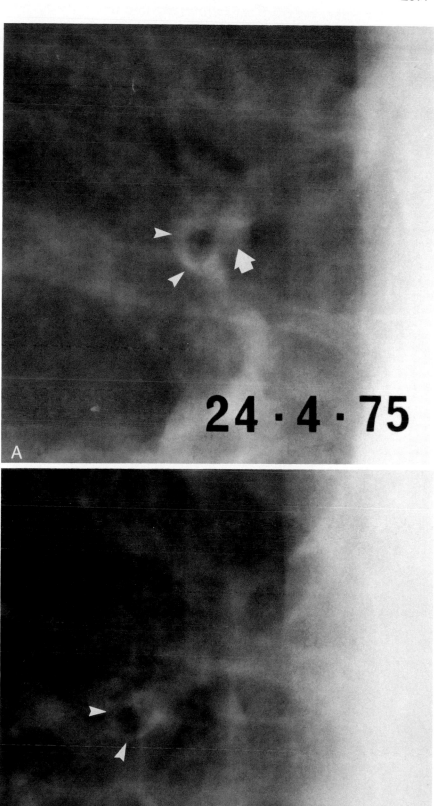

Figure 11–41. Spasmodic Asthma: Reversibility of Bronchial Wall Thickening. A detail view of the right hilar region from a posteroanterior chest roentgenogram (A) shows a moderately thickened wall of the anterior segmental bronchus of the upper lobe (arrowheads), adjacent to its companion artery (closed arrow). Approximately 1 year later (B), the bronchial wall was almost normal in thickness (arrowheads). The patient is a young woman who was hospitalized during a particularly severe episode of bronchospasm at the time of the roentgenogram (A) whereas in B she was in remission.

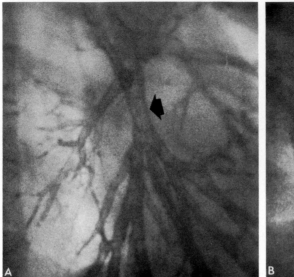
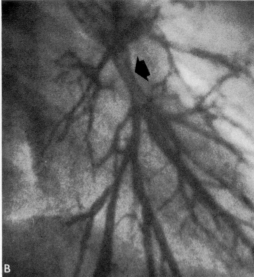

Figure 11–42. Airway Dynamics in Spasmodic Asthma. Single frames from a cinebronchographic study of a 35-year-old man with severe spasmodic asthma reveal a normal caliber of the major and segmental bronchi at full inspiration *(A)*. At forced expiration *(B)*, the minimum diameter also is normal, reduction in caliber of all segments being approximately 40 per cent. The main lower lobe bronchus *(arrow)* shows no evidence of the disproportionate collapse characteristic of chronic bronchitis or emphysema (compare with Figures 11–76 and 11–77).

tree, amounting to about 40 per cent of inspiratory caliber. This contrasts with the frequent finding of disproportionate collapse of the central bronchi during these two maneuvers in patients with chronic bronchitis and emphysema.

CLINICAL MANIFESTATIONS

The diagnosis of asthma is based largely on a history of periodic paroxysms of dyspnea, usually at rest as well as on exertion, with intervals of complete or nearly complete remission. Some patients have a more chronic form of the disease, but periodic exacerbation and remission occur in all cases. Cough can be a prominent symptom, and nonsmoking patients with asthma can fulfill the diagnostic criteria for chronic bronchitis.[1192] The diagnosis is strengthened by a history of eczema or hay fever or by a family history of allergic phenomena. Meticulous inquiry into circumstances initiating attacks, although time-consuming, undoubtedly constitutes the most important diagnostic procedure leading to rational therapy. If the patient is a child, questioning should be directed toward the possible association of food with the onset of attacks. Seasonal occurrence is of importance in suggesting either pollen sensitivity or allergic asthma precipitated by insects. Careful inquiry should be made into possible antigens in the home, especially domestic pets and feather pillows. The patient may have recognized an association between the onset of symptoms and exposure to a dusty environment at his or her place of work.

A history of drug intake should be looked for; drug allergy most often occurs in association with intravenous or intramuscular administration and often is associated with acute and sometimes fatal anaphylaxis. In highly sensitive persons, however, drugs taken by mouth or administered by aerosol inhalation can produce a maximum response within 5 to 30 minutes, manifested by nausea, vomiting, pruritus, substernal tightness, or dyspnea.[691] Rarely, exercise is the *only* provoking factor; in such circumstances the presence of the disease may go unrecognized if clinical examination and pulmonary function tests are not performed at appropriate times.[1193]

The patient should be questioned as to whether there is an association between the onset of asthmatic attacks and infections of the upper or lower respiratory tract, with particular emphasis on the occurrence of postnasal drip and facial pain. An attempt should be made to correlate the onset of attacks with emotional disturbance; if the patient is a child, this should include interview of the parents. Finally, the patient should be questioned as to the relationship between onset of attacks and exposure to cold air, irritating dusts, fumes, or odors, and the effects of changing temperature and humidity.

In both atopic and nonatopic patients, the original asthmatic episode commonly is termed acute bronchitis, with or without fever or upper respiratory symptoms. In such circumstances the diagnosis of asthma may not be suspected, particularly in elderly patients who are more prone to chronic bronchitis;[1194] in such patients wheezing and paroxysmal nocturnal dyspnea often are attributed to irreversible obstructive airway disease or left ventricular failure.[1195]

In the majority of patients, the onset of an attack of asthma is heralded by an unproductive cough and wheeze and only subsequently do the sensations of suffocation and tightness in the chest develop. The onset of dyspnea seldom is abrupt. The severity of airway narrowing that is required to cause dyspnea varies widely among asthmatic patients.[1196] Paroxysms occur most commonly at night; when paroxysms are severe, the patient may feel obliged to sit on the edge of the bed or to stagger to the window in the vain hope of obtaining more oxygen. Cough (with normal pulmonary function) may be the sole presenting symptom in some patients, and measurement of NSBR is helpful in identifying those patients in whom it is the initial symptom. Nocturnal breathlessness is a common symptom, and careful history taking may be necessary to distinguish asthma from paroxysmal nocturnal dyspnea.

Physical findings in asthma include hyperventilation, hyper-resonance on percussion, and auscultatory evidence of inspiratory and expiratory sonorous and sibilant rhonchi (low-pitched and high-pitched wheezes), decreased breath sounds, and prolonged expiration. In very severe attacks, wheezing may not be apparent, the clinical picture being one of air hunger; in such circumstances, there is evidence of the use of accessory muscles of respiration, diminished breath sounds without rhonchi, and often cyanosis.[1197, 1198] The correlation between physical findings suggestive of asthma, nonspecific airway responsiveness, and objective evidence of airway obstruction is not close, although FEV_1 can be roughly estimated with a combination of auscultation and palpation of the accessory muscles.[1199, 1200]

An abnormal degree of pulsus paradoxus has been correlated with severity of asthma.[1201-1203] On inspiration, the systolic arterial pressure of normal subjects decreases by up to 5 mm Hg, whereas in patients with asthma the pressure may drop by 10 mm Hg or more. This is probably the result of increased negative intrathoracic pressure consequent upon airway obstruction.[1204] The negative swings in intrathoracic pressure can decrease systolic pressure by two mechanisms:

1. The increased right ventricular volume caused by the negative pressure may result in a leftward shift of the interventricular septum and interfere with left ventricular diastolic filling.

2. The negative intrathoracic pressure acts as an afterload on the left ventricle because there is communication between the ventricle and the great vessels outside the thorax, which are not exposed to the negative pressure.[2755]

Correlation of clinical findings with physiologic dysfunction has indicated that the degree of pulsus paradoxus may be a valuable reflection of the severity of asthma.[1201-1204]

Although some patients present with attacks of asthma that develop over a period of hours, most have had progressive symptoms over days to weeks, often with a more rapid deterioration during the previous 24 hours.[1205] Younger, atopic subjects are more likely to present with exacerbations of rapid onset.[1206] Occasionally, the onset of asthma is so insidious that the diagnosis is not considered, particularly in elderly smokers; these patients are usually labeled as having COPD. Intensive therapy in such patients may result in a dramatic reversal of obstruction.[1207] When an attack persists beyond 12 hours and there is no therapeutic response to inhaled bronchodilators or subcutaneous injections of adrenalin, immediate hospitalization is required.[1208-1210] This phenomenon of beta-adrenergic blockade has been correlated with reduced responsiveness of adenylate cyclase activity and may reflect overactivity of the alpha-receptors, since the response to beta-adrenergic drugs may be restored to normal by concomitant treatment with the alpha-receptor–blocking drugs phentolamine and thymoxamine.[1211]

There is no doubt that an important contributing factor in the pathogenesis of intense and prolonged asthma ("status asthmaticus") is plugging of airways with mucus. Although little is known about the factors that govern the type and quantity of tracheobronchial mucus in asthma, a feature of prolonged asthmatic attacks is the presence of secretions that are more viscid than normal because of an increase in their protein content, particularly albumin.[1212, 1213] This proteinaceous mucus may revert to normal within 2 days of the institution of therapy with disodium cromoglycate. Since beta-adrenergic agonists can improve mucous clearance by increasing the frequency of ciliary beating,[1214-1216] the beta-adrenergic blockade phenomenon may play a role in the formation of mucous plugs by inhibiting mucociliary clearance.

Patients with acute severe asthma may be too dyspneic or exhausted to speak and may be stuporous or even comatose as a result of hypoxemia, hypercarbia, and perhaps water intoxication (see farther on under laboratory findings); they commonly manifest tachycardia (the heart rate is usually over 130 beats) and exaggerated pulsus paradoxus. As a result of airway obstruction and exhaustion, they usually exhibit such severe restriction of air flow that wheezing is absent and breath sounds are barely discernible.[1209, 1210] Arterial blood gas analysis is of particular value in the recognition of this state of emergency (see farther on).

Diurnal Variation and Morning Dipping

Both normal and asthmatic subjects show a circadian rhythm in airway caliber, but in asthmatics the diurnal variation is much more pronounced; the lowest values for expiratory flow are recorded in the early hours of the morning (2 to 4 AM).[1217, 1218] The magnitude of within-day variation in FEV_1 or PEFR correlates with nonspecific airway responsiveness, and although it is less sensitive than NSBR, it has been suggested as an alternative or additional diagnostic test of asthma.[1219]

The most prominent clinical manifestation of diurnal variation are the symptoms associated with the phenomenon of "morning dipping" in expiratory flow.[1220] Although an early morning exacerbation in asthmatic symptoms was described in 1698 by Sir John Floyer,[1221] interest in the phenomenon has been rekindled because of the demonstration of the severe obstruction associated with the symptoms.

Despite many investigations, the precise mechanism by which morning dipping occurs remains unclear. Rarely, the nocturnal asthma can be attributed to the development of hypersensitivity to antigens in bedding material, such as silkworm contamination of silk-filled bed quilts.[1222] The initial suggestion that nocturnal exposure to the house-dust mite was the inciting mechanism[685] can be ruled out because some nonatopic subjects also demonstrate the phenomenon. Other mechanisms that have been suggested include (1) a circadian rhythm in autonomic parasympathetic tone, (2) gastro-esophageal reflux, (3) decreased FRC during recumbency, (4) decreased nocturnal mucociliary clearance, (5) nocturnal airway cooling, (6) sleep itself, (7) a variation in circulating corticosteroid or catecholamine secretion, and (8) fluctuating endorphin levels.[1223–1225] The supine posture itself causes small decreases in expiratory flow, perhaps related to changes in lung volume.[1223]

Sleep itself is not a necessary factor because the obstruction develops, albeit somewhat less severely, when nocturnal sleep is prevented.[1226, 1227] The phenomenon is not related to either apneic episodes during sleep or any sleep state[1228] although the bronchoconstriction can be more severe during rapid eye movement (REM) sleep.[1229] Infusion of corticosteroids to block the normal nocturnal dip in circulating levels and administration of naloxone to prevent endorphin variations are ineffective in prevention.[1225, 1230]

The most likely mechanism for morning dipping is a nocturnal decrease in circulating catecholamines. Inhaled beta-agonists attenuate diurnal variation in expiratory flow,[1231] and there is a decrease in circulating epinephrine secretion that is related in time to the nocturnal decrease in PEFR.[1224, 1232] Decreased catecholamine levels would allow increased smooth muscle shortening and possibly an increase in mast cell mediator release.[1224] The severity of morning dipping varies within and between individual asthmatic subjects and may reflect disease activity.[1233]

Control of Breathing in Asthma

Most asthmatic patients appear to have normal or enhanced respiratory drive. Unlike that in patients with COPD, the ventilatory response to hypoxia and hypercapnea is normal despite alterations in baseline lung function. In fact, when more precise measurements of neural drive are employed, e.g., mouth occlusion pressure (P0.1) or mean inspiratory flow (V_T/T_I), asthmatic patients have increased respiratory drive at any given P_{O_2} or P_{CO_2}.[1234–1237] The preserved or increased drive to breathe observed in asthma has been variously attributed to either rapid fluctuations in respiratory impedance which prevent adaptive changes or increased stimulation of irritant receptors secondary to the chronic mucosal inflammation.[1234] Irritant receptor stimulation can increase respiratory drive even if reflex bronchoconstriction is blocked.[1236] It is likely that stimulation of afferent nerves from inspiratory muscles (muscle spindles and stretch receptors) is also an important input that maintains respiratory drive under load.[1238]

The preservation of drive to breathe in asthmatic patients has both beneficial and adverse effects. The normal drive is associated with an ability to detect and respond to increased loads on the respiratory system;[1239, 1240] at comparable loads (severity of obstruction), hypercapneic respiratory failure is much less likely to develop in asthmatic patients than in those with COPD. Unfortunately, the ability to perceive an increased respiratory impedance appears to be coupled to the sensation of dyspnea, and most asthmatic subjects experience more respiratory distress for a given degree of obstruction than do patients with COPD. During REM sleep, asthmatic patients may experience a decrease in intercostal muscle activity that results in paradoxical chest wall movement.[1241, 1242] Some asthmatic children show a tendency to develop ventilatory respiratory failure during acute attacks, and it has been shown that both they and their parents have reduced hypoxic ventilatory responses.[1243]

Cough in Asthma

The presence of the isolated symptom of persistent cough is a frequent reason for referring a patient to a respiratory specialist. Coughing, with or without sputum production, may be the sole or initial presenting symptom in patients with asthma.[1195, 1244, 1245] Of 182 patients who presented with unexplained cough and who were followed for a mean of 4.4 years, 29 (16 per cent) developed asthma over the follow-up period.[1247] Patients in whom asthma is the underlying cause of cough usually have an increase in nonspecific airway responsiveness, and the cough responds to treatment of the asthma. Measurement of the total eosinophil count may be useful screening technique to select patients in whom asthma is the underlying cause of coughing.[1246, 1247]

Coughing is thought to be initiated by stimulation of airway epithelial irritant receptors; these are the same receptors that mediate reflex bronchoconstriction. Despite this, the ability of some stimuli to initiate coughing and bronchoconstriction is clearly unrelated. The inhalation of hypo-osmolar and hyperosmolar aerosols causes both coughing and bronchoconstriction in asthmatic patients.[1248, 1249] The bronchoconstriction appears to be an effect of the abnormal osmolarity alone, but coughing is related to the ion content of the aerosol; lack of a permeant ion such as chloride or bromide causes coughing irrespective of the osmolarity of the solution.[1248] Nebulized hypo-osmolar and hyperosmolar solutions of citric acid cause coughing even if the bronchoconstriction is blocked, although both inhaled beta-agonist and anticholinergic agents decrease the severity of the coughing.[1248, 1250] Inhaled local anesthetic attenuates the coughing but not the bronchoconstriction associated with hypo-osmolar aerosols.[1251]

A coughing threshold can be measured by administering progressively increasing concentrations of citric acid aerosol and noting the lowest concentration that reproducibly causes coughing.[1252] A wide variability exists in the cough threshold among normal subjects;[1253] asthmatic patients do not have a lower threshold for provoked coughing in the same way that they have an increased tendency to bronchoconstrict. It has been suggested that postnasal drip can cause persistent coughing in some asthmatic patients and that pharyngeal inflammation can contribute to upper airway obstruction in these patients.[1254]

LABORATORY INVESTIGATION

The sputum expectorated by patients with uncomplicated bronchial asthma is characteristic, containing Curschmann's spirals up to several centimeters long, eosinophils, and, in some cases, Charcot-Leyden crystals. It should be emphasized, however, that sputum eosinophilia is not diagnostic of asthma; in one study of 115 patients with clinical evidence of either asthma or chronic bronchitis, no significant difference in sputum eosinophil count was found in the two groups.[1255] When infection is superimposed, as is often the case, the sputum becomes mucopurulent and, rarely, blood-streaked.

The white blood cell count usually is normal or slightly elevated, with slight eosinophilia in the majority of cases. Eosinophils usually do not exceed 10 per cent but may constitute up to 35 per cent of total white cell count. Peripheral eosinophilia may be a useful sign in differentiating primary bronchitis from infective asthma starting in middle age. In a comparative study of 40 children with bronchiectasis and 43 with asthma, significant peripheral eosinophilia was found in none of the former but in 37 (86 per cent) of the latter. Its degree was unrelated to the severity of the asthma, and it was often present between attacks.[1256] In adult asthmatics, peripheral blood eosinophilia is almost invariably present and absolute counts are recommended to monitor therapeutic effect.[1257, 1258] A decrease in eosinophilia correlates well with improvement of pulmonary function; it has been recommended that

a count of 85 cells or less per cubic millimeter be achieved in subjects treated with steroids.[1258]

An increase in the activity of several enzymes in the serum has been reported: high levels of serum glutamic-oxaloacetic transaminase (SGOT), lactate dehydrogenase (LDH), and creatine phosphokinase (CPK) usually are attributed to the effect of hypoxemia on tissues, although Karetzky[1259] has produced evidence that excessive muscular activity is responsible. Employing a more specific enzyme assay, Usher and associates[1260] found that isoenzyme patterns of LDH were largely LDH_3 and LDH_5, the former being derived from the lung and the latter from the liver. Serum alpha$_1$-antitrypsin levels have been found to be significantly higher in patients with intrinsic than in those with extrinsic asthma or in healthy subjects.[1261] In one study of seven patients in status asthmaticus, elevated levels of antidiuretic hormone (ADH) were found. The production of this substance is controlled by volume receptors believed to be located in the left atrium, by pressor receptors in the carotid body, and by osmoreceptors in the hypothalamus. The decreased pulmonary blood flow in asthma may stimulate atrial volume receptors, a possibility that should not be overlooked if water intoxication is to be avoided when planning fluid therapy.[1262] Such intoxication may be responsible for altered states of consciousness in patients in status asthmaticus.[1263, 1264]

Skin tests for various foods and inhalants are discussed in detail in Chapter 3 (see page 418). Application of the recommended dilutions of individual allergens may precipitate an attack. The patient must be watched carefully for reactions, and countermeasures should be at hand.[1265] Skin tests are particularly useful in confirming the responsibility of a specific allergen suspected by the patient. A positive reaction does not necessarily indicate that the specific allergen will cause bronchoconstriction, nor does a negative result exclude the specific substance as a causal agent in any individual case. Generally, however, a positive history shows a highly significant correlation with a positive prick test.[705] When the clinical situation indicates an obvious allergen of immediate type IgE-mediated hypersensitivity, confirmation may be obtained by the radioallergosorbent test for a specific IgE antibody in the serum[661, 662] or by passive sensitization by reaginic serum of human skin sections challenged with the suspected antigen.[1266]

An even more reliable method of identifying suspected antigens is bronchial (inhalational) provocation testing.[669, 1267] When skin test results are positive, the inhaled allergen should be well diluted and initially administered in small amounts. This method of testing may elicit immediate or delayed reactions that should be documented objectively by spirographic recordings made before and at intervals after the administration of the extract. Allergens that may be employed for this inhalation test include not only organic particles but also gases, vapors, and fumes.[669, 1267] The majority of immediate reactions are due to IgE, but some result from short-term sensitizing IgG. The delayed reactions are associated with IgE and may occur alone or in combination with an antecedent immediate reaction (dual reaction).[669] Inhalation challenge with specific antigens was discussed in Chapter 3 (see page 445) and with suspected occupational sensitizers in the section on occupational asthma (see page 2056). Nonspecific inhalation challenge with histamine or methacholine is an important diagnostic technique in some patients and may have value in following the response to long-term therapy.

Electrocardiographic changes may occur during severe episodes of bronchial asthma.[1268–1270] Sinus tachycardia is almost invariable; in addition, there may be right axis deviation, clockwise rotation of the heart, right ventricular hypertrophy, right atrial P waves, and S-T segment or T-wave abnormalities. These changes are closely associated with hypoxemia but not necessarily with pulmonary hypertension.[1202, 1268] Although pulmonary artery pressure may not be greatly elevated relative to atmospheric pressure, the transmural pulmonary artery pressure (pulmonary artery–pleural pressure) may be markedly increased as a result of the more negative swings in pleural pressure. It is the difference between the intravascular or intracardiac pressure and the surrounding pleural pressure that determines the load on the right ventricle.[1270]

ABNORMALITIES OF LUNG FUNCTION

As might be expected, aberrations in pulmonary function in asthma vary, depending largely upon whether the condition is in remission or exacerbation and, if the latter, upon the severity of the attack. Many patients whose asthma is in remission have normal pulmonary function,[1271–1273] with values being normal even when auscultation reveals wheezing.[1273] Even when maximal expiratory flows and volumes are within the normal predicted range, inhalation of a bronchodilator can result in a greater than 15 per cent increase in FEV_1 or FVC. However, pulmonary function test findings of symptom-free patients are not always normal;[326] for example, increased airway resistance and impaired distribution of inspired gas have been well documented during symptom-free periods.[327] The relationship between symptoms and function depends on the patient's ability to detect airway obstruction, and in fact some patients are unable to sense the presence of severe airway obstruction (FEV_1 less than 50 per cent predicted) after methacholine inhalation.[1274] Symptom-free adults who had asthma in childhood can manifest residual abnormalities of pulmonary function.[1275]

When direct and indirect measurement of airway size is completely normal, frequency dependence of dynamic compliance[1271, 1276] or increased closing volume[1277] may reveal small airway narrowing; with these techniques, reversible abnormalities of small airways have been identified during the hay fever season in patients with allergic rhinitis who have no pulmonary symptoms.[1278] In addition to the fact that patients with allergic rhinitis can have increased nonspecific airway responsiveness, these data suggest that subclinical airway disease may be present in these subjects.

Gas exchange may be impaired in symptom-free patients with asthma.[1279, 1280] Their hypoxemia is the result of $\dot{V}/\dot{Q}$ mismatching,[1279, 1281–1283] which in some cases is caused by a closing volume above FRC.[1277] In one study of 113 asthmatic children in remission, the PaO_2 was less than 90 per cent of the normal predicted value in 71 per cent.[1281] In asymptomatic asthmatic subjects who were studied by the multiple inert gas technique, the $\dot{V}/\dot{Q}$ distribution showed no shunt;[1282] however, there was a bimodal distribution of $\dot{V}/\dot{Q}$ ratios, one compartment having very low values, possibly as a result of collateral ventilation of lung regions in which the airways were completely occluded. Inhalation of a beta-adrenergic bronchodilator increased the perfusion to the low $\dot{V}/\dot{Q}$ region and lowered the arterial PO_2, suggesting pharmacologic reversal of hypoxic vasoconstriction in these regions.[1282] Similarly, 100 per cent O_2 increases $\dot{V}/\dot{Q}$ maldistribution, presumably by the same mechanism.[1284]

Airway narrowing is the basic functional abnormality of symptomatic asthma. Whether it is caused by smooth muscle shortening, mucus, or edema, the resulting increase in resistance leads to decreased flow, to hyperinflation, to gas trapping, and, ultimately, to an increase in the work of breathing. There has been much interest in determining which airways are the primary site of the increased resistance in asthma. The density dependence of maximal expiratory flow is frequently used to try to separate large central from small peripheral airway narrowing, and to the extent that this test is reliable, it appears that both central and peripheral airways may be narrowed.[1285–1289] Decreased density dependence of maximal expiratory flow, suggesting predominant small airway obstruction, occurs in older patients who have a long history of asthma,[1290] in asthmatics who smoke,[1291] and in those with a late allergic response to antigen challenge.[1292] Despite these studies, the recent demonstration that density dependence may be an unreliable method of detecting the site of obstruction leaves the question open as to which airways are involved in asthma.

Wherever the site of airway narrowing, it is most easily detected by measurements of maximal expiratory flow, derived from either volume-time or flow-volume plots.[1293, 1294] Maximal expiratory flow can be decreased as a result of one or more of the following changes—decreased lung elastic recoil, increased airflow resistance, and increased compressibility of airways; in asthmatic patients, the first of these is usually preserved while the last two have been shown to be important mechanisms.[1295]

In addition to decreasing flow during an asthmatic attack, the airway narrowing results in gas trapping manifested by an increase in RV and the RV/TLC ratio and by a decrease in VC.[1296-1299] The increase in RV is most probably related to airway closure resulting from altered pressure area behavior of the inflamed and narrowed peripheral airways.[1295, 1300] The increase in airway resistance is also associated with an increase in FRC.[1293, 1301] In normal subjects during tidal breathing, FRC is determined by the balance between the outward elastic recoil of the chest wall and the inward recoil of the lung; an increase in FRC could result from loss of lung recoil or from persistent inspiratory muscle activity during expiration, and the latter has been shown to contribute to the increase in FRC that occurs during pharmacologically induced bronchoconstriction.[1302, 1303] An additional mechanism for hyperinflation during an asthmatic attack is a dynamic resetting of FRC secondary to the prolonged expiratory phase of the respiratory cycle.[1304] Active laryngeal narrowing, by further slowing expiration, could contribute to hyperinflation and protect the inspiratory muscles.[97] The hyperinflation associated with induced asthma is caused predominantly by an increased volume of the rib cage rather than the abdominal compartment.[1305, 1306]

The hyperinflation associated with asthma and other obstructive pulmonary diseases possesses advantages and disadvantages:[1304] by increasing lung recoil, hyperinflation dilates the intraparenchymal airways and provides a load that impedes airway smooth muscle shortening;[451, 1307] in addition, it can improve the distribution of ventilation and prevent the phenomenon of tidal expiratory flow occurring on the maximal expiratory flow-volume curve.[1304] On the negative side, hyperinflation increases the elastic work of breathing and places inspiratory muscles on an inefficient part of their length-tension curve. Increased resistive work is normally considered the major load applied to inspiratory muscles in asthma, but in experimental studies elastic work has been shown to be more important.[1308] Although hyperinflation decreases resistive work by dilating the airways, it increases elastic work by moving the lung and chest wall to a less compliant portion of their pressure-volume curves.

Hyperinflation leads to inspiratory muscle shortening; since inspiratory muscles show a classic length-tension relationship, they are less able to develop tension at short lengths. Hyperinflation can also uncouple the parallel arrangement between the crural and costal portions of the diaphragm, forcing the two parts to contract in series; such an arrangement is less able to handle increased loads.[1304]

Although there is no question that RV and FRC increase with exacerbations of asthma, changes in TLC are more controversial. In some patients, Woolcock and Read[1301, 1309] demonstrated an in-

crease in TLC during an asthmatic attack and a return toward normal during recovery. Part of the apparent increase could have been an artefact secondary to an overestimation of TLC when measured plethysmographically in the presence of obstruction; however, increases were also observed when TLC was measured with the helium dilution technique. The acute changes in TLC that have been reported following induced bronchoconstriction in asthmatic patients can almost certainly be explained by errors in the plethysmographic method.[1310-1314]

Total lung capacity is determined by a balance between the elastic recoil of the lung and chest wall and the strength and shortening ability of the inspiratory muscles. An increase in TLC in subacute asthma could be caused by a reversible decrease in lung elastic recoil.[1315] It is also possible that breathing at high lung volumes for prolonged periods could alter surface or tissue forces as has been shown in a few normal subjects.[1316, 1317] Alternatively, there could be adaptive changes in the inspiratory muscles that allow greater than normal shortening. Serial plethysmographic measurements of TLC in asthmatic patients have not been reported since publication of the methods to overcome the potential errors. In a study of the long-term effect of asthma on TLC, Greeves and Colebatch[1318] compared ten patients in whom the disease had its onset before the age of 8 years with 8 patients in whom it began after the age of 18 years. It was found that TLC was significantly higher in the patients with childhood-onset asthma and that the pressure-volume curves of their lungs indicated loss of elastic recoil; the individuals with late-onset disease had normal values of TLC.

As an asthmatic episode resolves, there is improvement in expiratory flow and vital capacity and a decrease in FRC and RV. A decrease in symptoms may accompany the return of lung volumes to normal before changes in FEV_1 are observed, presumably as a result of the reversal of hyperinflation and gas trapping.[1307] Flow rates measured at low lung volumes (FEF_{25-75}, $\dot{V}_{50}$, $\dot{V}_{25}$) may take longer to improve or may never return to normal predicted values.[1296]

The steady-state diffusing capacity of the lungs ($DL_{CO}SS$) is normal in the majority of patients with asthma,[1293] although it may undergo progressive decline in the presence of severe obstruction.[1296, 1298, 1319] By contrast, the single-breath diffusing capacity ($DL_{CO}SB$) is often elevated during asthmatic attacks:[1319-1321] in one study of 163 asthmatic children in whom the mean FEF_{25-75} was 55 per cent of predicted, $DL_{CO}SB$ averaged 120 ± 18 per cent predicted.[1322] The most plausible explanation for this apparent paradox is a transient increase in pulmonary capillary blood volume that occurs as a result of the more negative inspiratory intrathoracic pressure secondary to obstruction of the airways. $DL_{CO}SB$ increased by an average of 18 per cent in ten normal subjects breathing through an inspiratory resistance and decreased appreciably after bronchodilatation in 31 asthmatic patients.[1322] An alternative explanation for the apparent increase in $DL_{CO}SB$ in asthma has been suggested by Graham and colleagues:[1323] in performing the single-breath DL_{CO}, it is sometimes assumed that CO uptake occurs only during breath-holding whereas in fact some CO is taken up during inspiration and expiration; in the presence of airflow obstruction, the inspiratory and expiratory times are prolonged, thus increasing CO uptake and resulting in a falsely elevated value for $DL_{CO}SB$.

Most patients with asthma have some degree of hypoxemia, whereas hypocapnia is observed during all but the most severe attacks. As airway obstruction increases in severity and the lungs become hyperinflated, $\dot{V}/\dot{Q}$ maldistribution worsens and hypoxemia increases.[1298, 1324] In one study of 101 patients with exacerbations of extrinsic asthma, 91 had some degree of hypoxemia, 73 had hypocapnia and respiratory alkalosis, and only ten with very severe airway obstruction had hypercapnea.[1325] Although hypoxemia is almost always observed in acute asthmatic attacks, the incidence of hypercapnia varies in different studies, being as high as 50 per cent of patients in some studies.[1326, 1327]

The mechanism of hypoxemia in asthma is related to ventilation-perfusion mismatch.[1328, 2783] Multiple inert gas studies frequently show a bimodal distribution of $\dot{V}/\dot{Q}$ ratios, with an increase in low $\dot{V}/\dot{Q}$ areas. There is variation in the degree of abnormality in $\dot{V}/\dot{Q}$ distribution with time, and this correlates with changes in arterial P_{O_2}. In patients with severe acute asthma who require mechanical ventilation, the pattern of $\dot{V}/\dot{Q}$ distribution is similar although a larger fraction of perfusion is to lower $\dot{V}/\dot{Q}$ areas.[2784]

Respiratory alkalosis is the only acid-base disturbance seen during mild asthmatic attacks, but metabolic and mixed acidosis can occur during severe exacerbations: in one study of 103 patients with "status asthmaticus," 23 were hypocapnic, 26 were eucapnic, 25 had a metabolic acidosis, and 14 had a mixed acidosis.[1329] The 38 per cent incidence of some degree of metabolic acidosis in this series is surprising; blood lactic acid levels were raised, and it is possible that anaerobic glycolysis in the failing respiratory muscles was the source of the lactate. In another study of 109 adults, 16.5 per cent of 164 episodes of acute asthma were associated with metabolic acidosis.[1330] In some patients the acidosis is not caused by excessive lactate levels but is of the non–anion-gap type.[2785]

The relationship between changes in PaO_2 and FEV_1 is not clear, some investigators finding that the two vary directly[1293, 1331, 1332] and others finding a poor correlation.[1208] Treatment can improve PaO_2 without producing a simultaneous increase in expiratory flow.[1333] In one study in which $\dot{V}/\dot{Q}$ distribution (as measured by the technique of multiple inert gases) and airway function were measured before and after exercise-induced bronchoconstriction, no correlation was found between the decrease in FEV_1 and the $\dot{V}/\dot{Q}$ maldistribution.[1334] When comparable degrees of obstruction (decreased S_{GAW}) were induced by inhaled methacholine and antigen, the antigen challenge was associated with more severe hypoxemia, suggesting more peripheral airway obstruction.[1335] Antigen-induced bronchoconstriction in dogs[1336] and exercise-induced asthma in children[1337] are associated with an initial widening in $\dot{V}/\dot{Q}$ distribution; with more severe obstruction, a bimodal distribution develops as has been reported in stable adult asthmatics.[1282]

In acute prolonged attacks, the PaO_2 has generally dropped to below 60 mm Hg,[1202, 1209] FEV_1 is less than 1, and peak flow is less than 60 liters/minute.[1208, 1209] As the severity and duration of obstruction increase, patients become exhausted, their respiratory muscles fatigue, and values of arterial P_{CO_2} rise into the hypercapnic range.[1298, 1338, 1324] In asthma, unlike COPD, hypercapnia is *never* a steady-state situation; the P_{CO_2} will generally decrease in response to therapy or will rise steeply within minutes or hours, and such patients should be under constant surveillance.[2786] At this stage, artificial ventilation should be considered if improvement is not prompt. The decision to ventilate will be influenced by the clinical state of the patient, especially level of consciousness, and by the elapsed time on therapy. Occasionally, patients without severe bronchoconstriction have CO_2 retention,[1339–1341] probably as a result of hyposensitivity of the respiratory center. As patients recover from severe acute attacks, the ventilatory response to CO_2 returns to normal in the majority, although some of those who present with hypercapnia fail to show improvement.[1339]

COMPLICATIONS

Complications of asthma are much more common in children than in adults and consist of pneumonia, atelectasis, mucoid impaction and mucous plugging, pneumomediastinum, and, rarely, arterial air embolism. In 479 roentgenographic examinations of 325 children with acute asthma,[1342] abnormalities (excluding hyperinflation) were apparent on 112, an overall incidence of complications of 23.3 per cent. In another study of 371 children who presented with asthma for the first time,[1343] only 5 to 6 per cent had roentgenographic evidence of complications; a similar study in adults revealed complications in only 1 per cent.[1344]

Lower respiratory tract infection occurs more frequently among patients with asthma than in the population at large, an observation that applies generally to all forms of obstructive airway disease. In a comparative study of the clinical course of Asian influenza among 161 nonallergic and 124 allergic patients, Bendkowski[1345] found the course of the disease to be generally more severe in the latter group. Bronchitis developed in the majority with or without exacerbation of asthma, and the incidence of pneumonia was twice that in the non-allergic group.

Atelectasis occurs predominantly in children and is the result of mucous plugging or mucoid impaction. It was noted by Luhr[1346] in 5.5 per cent of 217 children, by Lecks and associates[2787] in 7.4 per cent of 530 hospitalized asthmatic children, and in 15.7 per cent (51) of the 325 children studied by Eggleston and his colleagues.[1342] In the last-named series, the right middle lobe was most frequently involved. Although roentgenographically demonstrable atelectasis occurs very uncommonly in adult asthmatics (and then usually in association with mucoid impaction), it is probable that mucous plugging of smaller bronchi and bronchioles occurs much more frequently than is recognized. In such circumstances, it is assumed that pulmonary collapse distal to the obstructed airway is prevented by collateral air drift. In contrast to the central location of airway plugging in mucoid impaction, the obstruction in this variety of mucous retention is in the peripheral airways. This peripheral location was illustrated in a report by Dees and Spock[1347] of 30 children with right middle lobe atelectasis, 23 of whom had an associated allergic state. More than half of the children who underwent bronchoscopy showed no evidence of endobronchial obstruction, and it was assumed that plugging occurred in airways beyond bronchoscopic visibility.

Pneumomediastinum is an uncommon complication of asthma, being observed in only 16 (5 per cent) of the 325 asthmatic children studied by Eggleston and associates.[1342] It occurs predominantly in children[1348, 1349] and occasionally in young adults[1350] and is more common in males. The sudden onset of chest pain should arouse suspicion of the diagnosis.[1351] The presumed mechanism is alveolar rupture consequent upon the trapping of air beyond mucous plugs in the bronchioles, with subsequent dissection of air through the perivascular sheath to the hilum and mediastinum.[1352] In infants and young children there appears to be some form of anatomic resistance to the passage of air into the neck, so that gas may accumulate within the mediastinum and create "mediastinal air block."[1353] In infants, particularly, there is a tendency for the additional development of *pneumothorax*, the release of air into the pleural space relieving the pressure within the mediastinum.[1348, 1352] Should the pneumothorax fail to respond to chest-tube drainage and the ipsilateral lung is undergoing progressive loss of volume, obstruction of central airways by impacted mucus should be suspected.[1354] In older children[1349] and in adults,[1350] subcutaneous "emphysema" should be easily recognizable clinically. A precordial "click" or "crunch" synchronous with the heartbeat suggests the presence of pneumomediastinum but is not conclusive evidence of this. Contrary to the earlier belief that a precordial crunch (Hamman's sign) was diagnostic of pneumomediastinum, it is now recognized that this is heard in other conditions also, including pneumothorax and elevation of the left hemidiaphragm in association with gas in the gastric fundus. Occasionally, air will dissect along pulmonary vessels through the pericardial reflection, resulting in pneumopericardium.[1355] A single case has been reported of sudden death in "status asthmaticus" from arterial air embolism.[1356] Although air hunger is often implicated in such an event, the authors suggest that arterial air embolism may be the cause of sudden death in unexplained cases.

It is appropriate to consider here certain complications that occur as a result of therapy, although not strictly as a consequence of the disease itself. The influence on blood gases of the administration of bronchodilators, either parenterally or by aerosol, shows considerable variation.[1293, 1331, 1357-1364] Following relief of bronchospasm, some patients show a definite improvement in arterial PO_2, some show little change, and others have a worsening of hypoxemia, an observation originally made in 1959 by Halmagyi and Cotes.[1365] In a study of arterial PO_2 levels following the intravenous administration of 0.5 g of aminophylline, Rees and associates[1361] found values to range from an increase of 15 mm Hg to a decrease of 8 mm Hg, the response being unrelated to initial PaO_2 levels. In another series of 17 asthmatics who responded to aerosolized isoproterenol by a reduction in airway resistance, nine showed an increase in $(A-a)DO_2$, chiefly as a result of a fall in PaO_2.[1366] This effect was observed only in patients with modest hypoxemia and was of short duration. It has been postulated that pulmonary vascular resistance in smaller vessels is related to the degree of inflation of the lung unit being perfused. When airways dilate, local ventilation improves, thus decreasing hyperinflation and reducing vascular resistance. As a result, however, there is a reduction in $\dot{V}/\dot{Q}$ ratio caused by a disproportionate increase in perfusion.[1367, 1368] Alternatively, beta-adrenergic agonists may inhibit regional hypoxic vasoconstriction, thus increasing perfusion of poorly ventilated regions. It has been suggested that an increase in hypoxemia, combined with the cardiotoxic effect of beta-adrenergic sympathomimetic drugs such as isoproterenol, may have been responsible for the increase in mortality seen in asthmatic children in England during the 1960s.[1369] Fluorinated hydrocarbons (freons) inhaled from pressurized aerosol mixtures similarly have been implicated in producing cardiac arrhythmias. However, in one study[1370] peak serum concentrations of fluorocarbon-11 in chronic overusers of pressurized aerosols were not considered high enough to sensitize the heart to adrenergic compounds. In addition, the replacement of isoproterenol by selective β_2-adrenergic agonists has diminished the possibility of this potential complication.

Another iatrogenic method of worsening hypoxemia in asthmatics is the administration of sodium bicarbonate, and this drug should be avoided in critically ill patients who are not receiving artificial ventilation.[1371] Oral corticosteroid therapy is essential to the management of some cases of severe intractable asthma, and the benefits to be derived from these drugs far outweigh their potential hazards.[1372–1374] The common complications of such therapy include peptic ulcer, diabetes, mental disturbances, osteoporosis, and vertebral compression fractures. Although opportunistic infection is an uncommon complication, we have seen one asthmatic who developed active tuberculosis while receiving prednisone therapy. Another case has been reported of death resulting from disseminated strongyloidiasis, which developed as a complication of steroid therapy for asthma.[1375] The incidence of hyperlipidemia increases in asthmatic patients who are receiving long-term steroid therapy, and this may add to the risk of myocardial infarction.[1376] It is advisable to keep maintenance dosages of oral steroids to a minimum and whenever possible to substitute disodium cromoglycate or aerosolized steroid preparations for such therapy.

PROGNOSIS

Three issues need to be considered in determining prognosis: the determinants of recovery from an individual acute episode, the likelihood of achieving complete remission, and the chances of dying from asthma.

Recovery from Acute Asthmatic Episodes

Predicting the need for hospitalization and the rapidity of recovery from acute episodes of asthma has received considerable attention.[1377–1380] The requirement for hospitalization and slow (days to weeks) symptomatic and functional recovery in asthmatic patients are associated with (1) age greater than 40 years, (2) nonatopic asthma, (3) a longer duration of symptoms prior to admission, (4) poor long-term control of symptoms, and (5) use of maintenance steroids.[1378] The rapidity with which flow rates improve during the first 6 hours can also appreciably improve the prediction of a patient's recovery time.[1381] In one retrospective study, a scoring system based on pulse rate, respiratory rate, pulsus paradoxus, PEFR, the use of accessory muscles, and the severity of dyspnea and wheeze was 90 per cent effective in predicting the need for hospitalization and the relapse rate following discharge from the emergency room;[1380] however, application of the same scoring system prospectively to 114 acutely ill asthmatic patients failed to predict the need for admission or the likelihood of relapse.[1379]

Remissions

Determination of the ultimate long-term prognosis in asthma requires a long period of follow-up.

Studies in children[346, 666] have shown that a number of factors are associated with a poor prognosis—early onset of symptoms, multiple attacks in the initial year, clinical and physiologic evidence of persisting airway obstruction, pulmonary hyperinflation, chest deformity, and impairment of growth. The prognosis in patients whose asthmatic attacks are intermittent[1382] and who show evidence of lability[1383] is considerably better than in those whose symptoms are continuous and whose obstruction is relatively fixed. In this context, it is noteworthy that intermittent asthma usually has its onset before the age of 16 years whereas continuous bronchial obstruction usually begins later in life. Associated bronchitis worsens the prognosis significantly and is more common in patients with continuous asthma. Of 1,000 asthmatics followed over an average of 11 years, 60 per cent of those who acquired the disease before the age of 16 years were in good health whereas only 29 per cent of the late-onset group had recovered.[1384] Studies of asthmatic children support the high incidence of remission; 90 per cent of 449 patients whose asthma had its onset before the age of 14 years were assessed 20 years later, and only 30 per cent still suffered from the disease.[1385, 1386] In another study, 70 per cent of children with asthma were in apparent remission by the age of 10 years while 30 per cent continued to have asthmatic episodes.[341] The remissions experienced by adolescent and young adult asthmatics may not be permanent, however. In a 14-year follow-up of 441 children, the cumulative prevalence of asthma increased until the age of 7 years, then progressively decreased until the age of 17 to 18 years, at which time 70 per cent were "cured" (no symptoms or treatment for 1 year); however, subsequent "relapses" occurred, so that at an average age of 26 years only 57 per cent were still "cured."[1387] Additional relapses tend to occur with increasing age. Although a characteristic feature of asthma is some degree of reversibility of the airflow obstruction, it is clear that long-standing asthma can lead to a relatively fixed narrowing; in one study of 89 patients with long-standing asthma (mean duration 22 years), persistent functional impairment was present despite prolonged aggressive therapy with bronchodilators and corticosteroids.[1388] An 18-year follow-up case-control study of 92 asthmatic patients showed an accelerated age-related decline in FEV_1.[1389]

Mortality

Death from asthma occurs predominantly in adults ranging in age from 40 to 60 years[1390] and in children under the age of 2 years. During the years 1959 to 1966, an unexpected increase in mortality attributed to asthma was observed in the United Kingdom, New Zealand, and Australia, affecting patients aged 5 to 34 years and particularly those between 10 and 19 years of age.[1369, 1391–1394] The transient increase in mortality was initially attributed to the potent nonselective beta-adrenergic aerosol bronchodilators used during that period,[1391-1394] but retrospective analysis has not completely supported this explanation.[1395, 1396] Investigations into the circumstances surrounding the deaths from acute asthmatic attacks identified a number of risk factors, including a long history of asthma, previous hospital admissions for severe asthma, widely varying flow rates, delayed perception of the severity of the final attack, and underuse of corticosteroids.[1397] After 1966, death rates in the affected countries returned to "pre-epidemic" levels, but by 1977 they had increased again in New Zealand, confirmed in two studies.[1398, 1399] Death rates for Maoris (19 in 1,000 deaths) and Polynesians (nine in 1,000) were significantly higher than for patients of European origin (five in 1,000), but the death rate for the latter group was three times higher than that in the United Kingdom. The age at the time of death was bimodally distributed with a peak near 20 and another near 65 years. Seventy per cent of deaths occurred between 8:00 P.M. and 8:00 A.M., and more than half the people died at home. No single cause for the increase has been identified, although risk factors were similar to those observed in the previous studies, including under-use of corticosteroids.[1398-1400]

In 1980, death rates from asthma in patients aged 5 to 34 years ranged from 0.2 per 100,000 in the United States to three per 100,000 in New Zealand.[343] It is most unlikely that this large variation can be attributed to the unreliability of death certificates since in this age group, asthma is unlikely to be confused with COPD. There have been a number of studies that demonstrate an increase in death rates from asthma in Australia[2788] and the United States during the last decade,[1401, 1402, 2789] and another that supported a similar increase in England and Wales between 1974 and 1984.[1403] Patients who have life-threatening asthma have usually had symptoms of increasing severity over a period of days, although in one study eight of 26 patients deteriorated rapidly; in three of these, the attack was triggered by ASA.[1404] In a 2-year study of asthma deaths in New Zealand, Sears and associates[1405] found 11 asthma deaths in children aged 0 to 14 years. Seven of the children died in less than 3 hours from the onset of their final attack, and all died outside the hospital; the death rate in Maori children was five times that of European children. The factors that appeared to increase the risk of death in these children were similar to those described for adults. In a case-controlled study of asthma deaths in the 8- to 18-year-old age group, increased asthma symptoms in the week preceding death, a decrease in prednisone dosage, conflict between physician and parent, and a disregard of asthmatic symptoms were factors that contributed to the effectiveness of discrimination between cases and controls.[1406] In another case-controlled study, hospitalized patients who died from asthma were shown to have had inadequate management, including the use of sedatives, inadequate steroid and beta-adrenergic dosages, excessive theophylline dosage, and a failure to institute artificial ventilation.[1407] In a recent study of 75 deaths from asthma in New Zealand, it was shown that overreliance on the home use of nebulized bronchodilators may have been a contributing cause.[2790]

Both patients and physicians should be made more aware of the seriousness of this disease; patient education is the key to the prevention of deaths, and patients who are considered to be at risk of dying should be admitted to the hospital promptly when their clinical and physiologic findings indicate a severe attack.[1408] Patients at high risk for death from asthma can usually be identified, and if streamlined procedures are instituted for hospital admission of these individuals, death can often be prevented.[1409]

The sudden infant death syndrome (SIDS) that occurs most commonly at 2 to 3 months of age is probably attributable to a number of causes; in some cases it may be caused by allergy in the infants of atopic people. Levels of specific IgE antibodies to *D. pteronyssimus* (the house dust mite), *Aspergillus fumigatus*, and bovine beta-lactoglobulin were found to be significantly higher in a group of infants who died suddenly than in a control group of infants of the same age.[1410]

CHRONIC OBSTRUCTIVE PULMONARY DISEASE

Chronic respiratory disease related to cigarette smoking has made an enormous impact on society in this century. Death rates for respiratory disease doubled every 5 years between 1950 and 1970[1411] and have continued to rise. In the United States, age-adjusted death rates for the combined diagnoses of COPD, emphysema, and bronchitis showed a 22 per cent increase between 1968 and 1977. The increase in deaths caused by chronic respiratory disease is striking, considering the overall decline in death rates and the 22 per cent decline in deaths from heart disease over the same time period. In an 11-year follow-up study of 4,000 people aged 35 to 54 years, there was a two-fold to five-fold increase in death rates in smokers.[1412] In the United States, COPD represents the fifth most important cause of death, killing more Americans than does diabetes mellitus.

The high incidence of chronic respiratory disease has also had an important economic impact. There is good evidence that respiratory conditions constitute the most important cause of work incapacity and restricted activity in both the United States and the United Kingdom.[1413]

DEFINITIONS

In the previous edition of this book, chronic bronchitis and emphysema were discussed separately, since each was felt to contribute to the development of COPD. Although chronic bronchitis is a clinical diagnosis based on excessive mucous secretion, it was believed that in some patients mucous hypersecretion was associated with airway narrowing, whereas emphysema, defined by pathologic criteria, produced airway obstruction because of loss of lung elastic recoil. The classic follow-up study of Peto and associates refutes any connection between coughing and sputum production and the eventual development of airflow obstruction.[1414] On the basis of a questionnaire and spirometry, 2,718 men were studied and followed for 20 years. Over the follow-up period, there were 104 deaths from COPD and 103 from lung cancer. When adjusted for the initial FEV_1, the clinical diagnosis of chronic bronchitis had *no* predictive value for death from COPD and only a weak predictive value for lung cancer. Stated simply, patients were just as likely to die from COPD whether or not they coughed or expectorated. On the other hand, initial FEV_1 values had a powerful predictive value: an initial FEV_1 below two standard deviations of predicted normal was associated with a 52 times increased risk of death from COPD and a value between one and two standard deviations below normal was accompanied by a 20-fold increased risk (Fig. 11–43). In another long-term follow-up study of men and women who smoked, initial values of FEV_1/FVC and FEF_{25-75} were found to be related to longitudinal decline in lung function in the former but not in the latter.[1415]

Despite the disassociation between airflow obstruction and chronic coughing, it is clear that chronic airflow obstruction can develop in the absence of emphysema or loss of elastic recoil. In 1835 Laennec wrote: "In emphysema the air makes its escape from the air cell much slower than in a healthy state of the organ. This seems to indicate either more difficult communication between air contained in the air cells and that of the bronchi or else diminished elasticity of the air cells themselves."[1416]

What, then, are we to call the disease of patients with irreversible airflow obstruction, without proven emphysema or loss of elastic recoil? The nomenclature is in a state of transition and controversy.[1417; 1418] One suggestion is that the term "chronic bronchitis" should be reserved for patients with mucous hypersecretion and airflow obstruction.[1419] This leaves patients with airflow obstruction but no cough or phlegm without an appropriate category. Chronic obstructive "bronchitis" is also an inappropriate term because it is the bronchioles that are the main site of obstruction. "Small airway disease" was first suggested as the name for a specific clinical syndrome[1420] and does not communicate the basic functional derangement of obstruction. "Chronic obstructive bronchiolitis" is perhaps the best descriptive label but could be confused with other specific and nonspecific forms of bronchiolitis

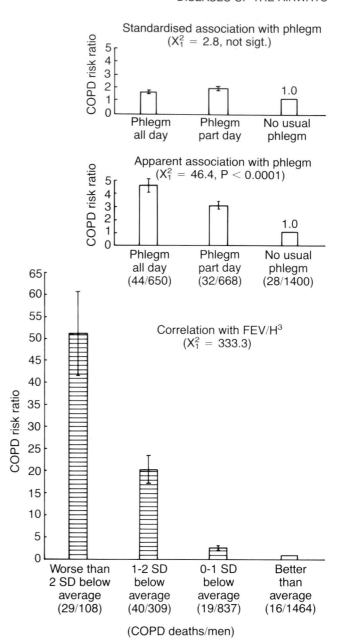

Figure 11–43. Risk Factors for the Development of Chronic Obstructive Pulmonary Disease (COPD). In a study of almost 3,000 men followed for 20 or more years to determine which factors predisposed to death from chronic obstructive pulmonary disease, the results as depicted in this graph showed that chronic cough and sputum production (standardized association with phlegm) did not increase risk but that the initial value for forced expiratory flow was strongly associated with subsequent death from COPD. Individuals in whom the initial FEV_1 was two standard deviations or more below the average value had a risk for death from COPD 52 times greater than those in whom the FEV_1 was equal to the average. (From Peto R, Speizer FE, Cochrane AL, et al: Am Rev Respir Dis 128:491, 1983.)

(*see* farther on). The problems with precise definition have led Fletcher and Pride[1418] to suggest the retention of a term such as "chronic obstructive lung disease" or "chronic airflow obstruction" to describe the disease in this group of patients. *For the purposes of this text, the following definitions will apply.*

CHRONIC BRONCHITIS

Chronic bronchitis is a clinical diagnosis based on a history of excessive mucus expectoration. Since standardization of the quantity of mucous production is necessary in order to compare populations, quantitative (and somewhat arbitrary) terms have been introduced; for example, "expectoration must occur on most days during at least 3 consecutive months for not less than 2 consecutive years."[1421] These criteria exclude persons with a chronic dry cough, although direct questioning of many of these patients will elicit the fact that they bring up small amounts of sputum on arising in the morning or that they swallow their bronchial secretions. Questionnaires administered by interviewers have been devised by the National Heart and Lung Institute (NHLI) and the British Medical Research Council (BMRC) for epidemiologic studies. Responses to these two questionnaires reveal very similar results and are reproducible. Slight modifications have been suggested for completion of the questionnaire without the use of an interviewer.[1422]

All other causes of chronic coughing and expectoration must be eliminated before a diagnosis of chronic bronchitis is recorded. In some cases it may be difficult to differentiate chronic bronchitis from asthma; however, the definition of asthma as a disease characterized by widespread reversible narrowing of the bronchial tree, changing relatively rapidly in severity either spontaneously or with treatment, is of differential value in the majority of patients. The term "asthmatic bronchitis" has been used to describe patients who fulfill the diagnostic criteria for both conditions.

Since the original definition of the term "chronic bronchitis" does not include airflow obstruction[1423] and since chronic coughing and sputum production are not necessarily associated with the development of airflow obstruction, the future of the term remains uncertain.

EMPHYSEMA

Emphysema is defined as a condition of the lungs characterized by abnormal permanent enlargement of airspaces distal to the terminal bronchioles, accompanied by destruction of their walls, and without obvious fibrosis.[1424] Strictly speaking, emphysema can be diagnosed only pathologically but certain clinical, pulmonary function, and roentgenographic features allow an *in vivo* estimation of its presence and severity. In general, emphysema is accompanied by a loss of lung elastic recoil, which is thought to cause airflow obstruction, hyperinflation, and gas trapping. However, as discussed below, loss of recoil can occur without the development of emphysema.

CHRONIC OBSTRUCTIVE PULMONARY DISEASE

Although the diagnosis of chronic bronchitis is made on the basis of clinical history and emphysema on the basis of morphology, COPD is characterized in functional terms. COPD consists of persistent, largely irreversible airway obstruction in which the underlying pathophysiology is not precisely known.[1418] To retain any usefulness, the term should exclude conditions characterized by persistent obstruction in which the mechanism of obstruction is known, such as asthma, bronchiectasis, bronchiolitis, cystic fibrosis, and alpha$_1$ protease inhibitor deficiency.

Since, in the vast majority of patients, irreversible airway obstruction cannot be easily attributed solely to loss of elastic recoil or airway narrowing, use of the term COPD or its synonyms has increased. In fact, a combination of intrinsic airway narrowing and loss of lung elasticity coexists in most patients with COPD. Synonyms for COPD include chronic obstructive lung disease (COLD), chronic airflow obstruction (CAO), and chronic airflow limitation (CAL). COLD and CAO are acceptable, but CAL is misleading because it suggests that airflow limitation is unique to this entity; in fact, everyone has maximal expiratory airflow limitation—it is the *severity* of the limitation that is abnormal in COPD.

In the following pages, the incidence, etiology, pathogenesis, pathology, and clinical manifestations of COPD, rather than the separate entities of chronic bronchitis and emphysema, are discussed. When possible, the mechanisms and consequences of airway obstruction caused by intrinsic airway narrowing and those resulting from loss of elastic recoil are separated, recognizing that in many patients separation is not possible. Since COPD, as defined, is characterized in functional terms and since the chest roentgenogram reveals gross morphology, the approach taken in the roentgenology section (*see* page 2116) is of necessity different; here, the characteristics of chronic bronchitis and emphysema are considered separately.

EPIDEMIOLOGY

The confusion in terminology has led to difficulty in defining the incidence of COPD. In Britain, the combination of chronic cough and expectoration, dyspnea, and airflow obstruction has traditionally been labeled chronic bronchitis,[1425] whereas in North America, there has been a tendency to refer to this as emphysema. Three decades ago, the use of these different terminologies gave the false impression that the death rate from "chronic bronchitis" in England and Wales was approximately 40 times that in the United States.[1426] With general acceptance of standard definitions and of the classification of COPD proposed in the CIBA symposium in 1952,[1423] subsequent epidemiologic studies have shown that the incidence of the disease is very similar in the two countries.[1427] Misclassification of patients still occurs not infrequently. In a community study of 351 patients who received a new diagnosis of asthma, chronic bronchitis, or emphysema over an 8-year period, 45 per cent had a prior or concomitant diagnosis of another obstructive pulmonary disease;[1428] older men were more likely to be labeled with a diagnosis of emphysema, and younger women were more often called asthmatic.

Many of the early studies of prevalence and incidence concerned patients with a clinical diagnosis of chronic bronchitis based on cough and expectoration. However, since chronic bronchitis is not invariably associated with obstruction and since COPD can develop without cough and expectoration, many of these studies are of questionable significance.

A review of the sex incidence of COPD has shown a male predominance of approximately 10 to 1,[1429] a difference for which cigarette consumption is a major responsible factor.[1430] However, retrospective and prospective studies designed to analyze risk factors for the development of COPD show that men are at increased risk even when adjustment is made for the amount smoked.[1415, 1431–1435] Additional factors, such as genetic differences, occupational pollution, and methods of cigarette smoking, may also be responsible. A propensity for the development of COPD is seen in cigarette smokers who have the habit of retaining the cigarette in their mouth between puffs[1436] and who extinguish and relight cigarettes,[1437] behavioral characteristics that are more common in men. Studies that have compared the disease in men and women generally agree that it is more rapidly progressive and more severe in the former.[1415, 1438–1440]

COPD is generally more severe in white than in non-white cigarette smokers, a difference that cannot be explained by the amount or duration of cigarette smoking or by whether or not smoke is inhaled.[1441] Individuals of African origin also have been reported to be less susceptible than other ethnic groups to the emphysema-producing effect of cigarette smoking.[1442] Alcoholics[1443] and patients with coronary artery disease[1444] are particularly prone to the development of COPD, a propensity that is attributable to excessive cigarette smoking in the latter group but not in the former. Patients with COPD are more likely than control groups to have a family history of chest disease, a hereditary tendency that is stronger in women than in men.[1438, 1445]

ETIOLOGY

There is abundant evidence to incriminate several etiologic factors acting singly or in concert in the production of COPD. Clinical and epidemiologic studies have addressed the etiologic contributions of cigarette smoking, air pollution (occupational or urban), infection (especially in childhood illnesses), climate, heredity, social class, atopy, nonspecific airway hyper-responsiveness, and homozygous or heterozygous deficiency of alpha$_1$ protease inhibitor. In most patients, cigarette smoking is the most important of these factors; in fact, many of the others simply represent modifiers of the host response to cigarette smoke.

One way to test for factors that increase the risk of the development of symptomatic COPD is to measure longitudinal declines in FEV_1 over a period of years in large population groups, and to determine which features characterize those patients with an accelerated decline in lung function. Healthy people who are nonsmokers show a yearly decline in FEV_1 that is largely secondary to the age-related decrease in lung elastic recoil. Smokers show an exaggerated yearly decline in FEV_1, the rate of decline increasing with the intensity of cigarette smoking.[1446, 1415] In a 15-year follow-up study of 2,406 Belgian Air Force personnel, the rate of yearly decline in FEV_1 allowed the prediction that 4 per cent of heavy smokers and 0.5 per cent of nonsmokers would develop an FEV_1 of less than 1.2 liters by the age of 65.[1446]

The other major predictor of the rapid deterioration in lung function observed in these longitudinal studies is the state of lung function at the beginning of the study:[1446, 1447] patients with lower FEV_1 values to begin with show deterioration more rapidly, even when adjusted for the amount smoked and other potential risk factors. Just as the "rich get richer," the obstructed become more obstructed! This important phenomenon, called the "horse race effect," simply states that individuals whose lung function is impaired for any reason are at increased risk for the development of COPD (Fig. 11–44).

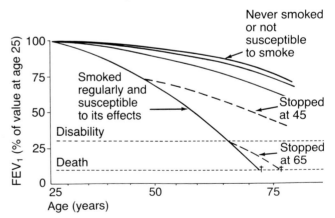

Figure 11–44. Changes in FEV$_1$ with Aging. This figure shows the percentage change of FEV$_1$ versus age for smokers and nonsmokers. Nonsmokers show a gradual decline in FEV$_1$ with age, and smokers who are not susceptible to the effects of cigarette smoke show a similar, although somewhat accelerated decline. Individuals who are susceptible to cigarette smoke and who smoke regularly demonstrate an accelerated decline in FEV$_1$, which increases in rapidity with increasing age ("horse race effect"). Smoking cessation returns the rate of decline to that observed in the nonsmoking or nonsusceptible population. (From Peto R, Speizer FE, Cochrane AL, et al: Am Rev Respir Dis 128:491, 1983.)

Cigarette Smoking

Cigarette smoking is overwhelmingly the most important contributor to the development of COPD, although other factors must play a role because many heavy smokers do not develop the disease.[1448] Clinical studies that have examined the incidence of respiratory disease in nonsmokers have shown that COPD is very rare.[1442–1444, 1449–1451] Comparative studies of the prevalence of coughing and expectoration in adult smokers and nonsmokers have shown a remarkable predominance among the former,[1452] the incidence in pipe and cigar smokers lying somewhere in between.[1453–1456] The symptoms of chronic cough and phlegm production can develop soon after commencement of the smoking habit, although symptomatic airflow obstruction usually does not become apparent until after the age of 50 years[1457] or until after 20 or 30 years of smoking.

Comparison of expiratory flow rates of smokers and nonsmokers has revealed an increase in airway obstruction in the former,[1458–1462] with the dose-response relationship between the degree of impairment of air flow and the amount smoked being statistically significant.[1433, 1463–1466] The duration and intensity of smoking are of equal importance in calculating a dose-response, factors that can be combined into a single index by calculating the pack-years (packages of 20 cigarettes/day × years smoked).[1466] In large cross-sectional population studies, an influence of smoking on lung function can be detected as early as 20 years of age;[1466] in one longitudinal study of children and adolescents, smoking diminished the rate of increase in expiratory air flow that normally occurs with growth.[1467] As outlined in the section on pulmonary function (see page 2155), smoking cessation is usually associated with some improvement in function and the symptoms of coughing and sputum expectoration often disappear completely; although the improvement in function may be small, the rate of annual decline in lung function diminishes or returns to normal.

Besides the total number of cigarettes smoked, the pattern of smoke inhalation can influence the total dose and the distribution within the lungs of the toxic gases and particles. Pulmonary symptoms and, to some extent, lung function correlate with the individual patient's subjective assessment of the depth of smoke inhalation.[1468] The breathing pattern and "inhaled puff volume" can be measured during smoking using the respiratory inductive plethysmograph,[1469] and it has been shown that there is wide variability in the depth and speed of inhalation and in the breath-hold time following inhalation.[1470, 1471] Slow, deep inhalation of smoke followed by breath-holding increases alveolar deposition of smoke and could favor the development of emphysema, whereas rapid shallow inspiratory puffs without breath-holding encourages airway deposition and could result in inflammation and narrowing of airways. The pattern of cigarette smoke exhalation can also influence the deposition of particles; coughing or flow-limited expiration tends to cause the accumulation of inhaled particles at the flow-limiting sites in central airways, presumably as a result of the increase in regional turbulence that develops.[1472]

A central location of particulate accumulation could explain the large airway changes of COPD and the tendency for bronchial carcinoma to occur in these airways. A vicious circle can be envisaged in which airflow obstruction results in more flow-limited breathing and thus in more localized particle deposition. Pipe smokers avoid pulmonary inhalation of smoke by closing off the oropharyngeal isthmus; smoke is puffed into the mouth then exhaled through the mouth and nose.[1473] It remains to be seen whether the pattern of smoke inhalation is an important variable in the individual response to cigarette smoke.

Tobacco smoke is a complex mixture of more than 100 volatile and particulate chemical substances, and it is not known which of the components are responsible for the changes of COPD. When other factors are controlled, the tar content of cigarette smoke does not appear to affect the progression of disease;[1474] in a cross-sectional study, the use of cigarette filters was also found to be unimportant.[1466] Some individuals develop immediate-type hypersensitivity to raw tobacco antigens; however, the manifestations show no correlation with their symptoms, and it is unlikely that allergy to cigarette smoke is an important mechanism in the pathogenesis of COPD.[1475, 1476]

In addition to the irreversible airway obstruction caused by prolonged cigarette smoking, a slight transitory bronchoconstriction has also been described,[1477–1484] as has nonuniform distribution of ventilation.[1481, 1482] In one study, heavy smokers tended to show more pronounced acute bronchoconstriction than did light smokers or nonsmokers.[1477] Despite these observations, there is no known relationship between this acute effect of cigarette smoking and the long-term deleterious effects.

As will be discussed, considerable interest has been shown in establishing whether the level of pre-existing, nonspecific airway responsiveness is a determinant of the long-term response to cigarette smoking; the antithesis, the effect of smoking on nonspecific responsiveness (NSBR), has also been addressed. Acute smoking (four cigarettes) has no effect on NSBR,[1485] although some young and middle-aged chronic asymptomatic smokers manifest significantly increased airway responsiveness when partial flow-volume curves are used as the test of airway narrowing.[1486–1488] The combination of smoking and atopy, manifested by allergic rhinitis, is sometimes additive in inducing hyper-responsiveness.[1489]

Although personal cigarette smoking is certainly the most important risk factor in the development of COPD, the possible harmful effects of passive or side-stream smoking have received considerable attention.[1490, 1491] Although the exposure is small compared with that experienced by "mainstream" smokers, nonsmoking individuals who are in the same room or house as smokers can show pulmonary deposition of smoke particles as well as increased blood levels of nicotine and carboxyhemoglobin.[1492, 1493] Infants and children living in the same household as parents or siblings who smoke are especially vulnerable to the effects of passive smoking. Epidemiologic studies have shown an increased incidence of respiratory illness and functional impairment in such individuals, the effect being greater with maternal than paternal smoking.[1490, 1494–1497] In one study, it was shown that exposure to cigarette smoke during the first years of life doubled the infant's risk of pneumonia or "bronchitis";[1501] however, it is possible that this association could have resulted from an increased incidence of infection in the parents and cross-infection between members of the family.

In infants exposed to passive cigarette smoke, normal lung growth and development can be affected; for example, in one longitudinal study of lung function in growing children, maternal smoking was associated with a 7 per cent less-than-expected increase in FEV_1 over a 7-year period.[1498] The effect on adults is less clear, although in some studies individuals passively exposed to cigarette smoke have shown a slight but significant decrease in maximal expiratory flow.[1499, 1500] Although in cross-sectional studies the magnitude of the impairment associated with passive cigarette smoking is small, extended longitudinal follow-up studies will be necessary to quantify the ultimate risk because slight changes in lung structure and function in children may predispose to later disease.[1490, 1491] Because the "horse race effect" predicts that a decrease in expiratory flow at an early age will contribute to a more rapid subsequent decline in function, any small changes in "starting lung function" may be critical.

Chronic airflow obstruction can also result from heavy and prolonged marijuana[1502, 1503] and opium[1504] smoking, the latter accompanied by widespread emphysema and pleuropulmonary fibrosis.

Air Pollution

The relationship between COPD and the breathing of polluted air has been investigated with reference to both urban atmospheric pollution from all sources and specific occupational exposure. There is no doubt that certain chemicals and dusts, if present in sufficient concentration, can cause acute and chronic airway damage and obstruction. However, except in heavily polluted regions and with certain industrial exposures, the effects are minor compared with the influence of cigarette smoking.[1505]

ATMOSPHERIC AIR POLLUTION

Urban air pollution can be divided into two major categories according to the chemicals involved: (1) reducing agents, consisting mainly of carbonaceous particulate matter and SO_2; and (2) oxidizing substances, including the hydrocarbons, oxides of nitrogen, pollutants of photochemical reactions (such as ozone, aldehydes, peroxyacetylnitrate), and other organic nitrates.

Although a sudden increase in the amount of air pollution, such as occurs with smog, can result in increased morbidity and mortality in patients with established COPD[1510–1512] or asthma,[1513] there is little evidence that urban air pollution per se causes obstructive pulmonary disease in nonsmokers.[1514, 1515] However, urban air pollution appears to play an additive role to that of cigarette smoke in the pathogenesis of COPD[1516, 1517] and may be partly responsible for progression of disability in patients already affected. The effects of a low concentration of SO_2, NO_2, and O_3 on lung function in normal subjects is discussed in the section on environmental provocation of asthma; acute exposure to these substances, especially when accompanied by exercise, results in transient pulmonary function abnormalities and, in some cases, prolonged enhancement of nonspecific airway responsiveness. In patients with COPD, exposure causes a similar transient impairment of lung function,[1518–1520] and it is probable that multiple repeated exposures, especially if combined with cigarette smoking, can cause permanent derangement. In one study in Milan, Italy, four different urban regions with varying SO_2 levels were compared. A correlation was found between SO_2 levels in the atmosphere, carboxyhemoglobin blood levels, and nonspecific airway responsiveness in both smokers and nonsmokers.[1521] Epidemiologic studies have revealed a higher incidence of chronic bronchitis among urban dwellers, implying that air pollution over cities is responsible for the increased incidence.[1018, 1522, 1523] A 1967 follow-up study of an adult population in Berlin, New Hampshire, originally surveyed in 1961, revealed a decrease in the prevalence of chronic bronchitis and COPD coincident with a decrease in air pollution;[1413, 1524, 1525] the improvement was noted even after the effects of aging and a change in cigarette smoking habits were taken into account.[1524] In a comparative study of rural and urban truck drivers, smoking habits played a much more significant role than that of atmospheric pollution in the development of chronic bronchitis.[1523] By contrast, another study showed significant impairment of pulmonary function in a large group of residents in the highly polluted Tokyo and Yokohama regions of Japan compared with residents of an area with less atmospheric pollution.[1526] The same study failed to find evidence in the Japanese population of the so-called "Tokyo-Yokohama asthma" described in American

Armed Forces personnel; however, this was a much more acute syndrome and was relieved by a change of environment (see page 2054).

Children with growing lungs may be particularly vulnerable to the effects of air pollution. The incidence of acute, lower respiratory tract infections is higher in children who live in environments with high levels of air pollution,[1527, 1528] and childhood infection is especially prone to impair subsequent lung function (see later). In addition to general atmospheric pollution, residential pollution can have an important deleterious effect on children's lungs. The use of natural gas in home cooking is associated with an increase in the incidence of childhood respiratory illness and pulmonary dysfunction, which is independent of the effects of parental smoking.[1529, 1530] Fires that are used indoors for domestic cooking are another source of residential air pollution: for example, in rural Nepal where indoor wood and dung fires are common, a very high incidence of obstructive lung disease, emphysema, and cor pulmonale has been observed in both men and women.[1531, 1532] Similarly, an increased incidence of "simple" chronic bronchitis has been reported in women who live in igloos and tents where there is heavy smoke pollution.[1533, 1534] Additional potential sources of air pollution in the home include house dust, hair sprays, insecticides, and soap powders. In a survey carried out in rural Western Australia,[1535] exposure to these substances was thought to play a role in the development of COPD.

OCCUPATIONAL AIR POLLUTION

There have been many attempts to relate occupational exposure to the development of COPD. These studies are fraught with many potential pitfalls because of other accepted or suspected etiologic factors that may coexist (e.g., cigarette smoking). In cross-sectional studies, errors can arise from the tendency of workers to move to different jobs within the occupational environment, particularly when those who take another job are physically fit and those who remain are disabled[1536, 1537] or when affected individuals drop out of the work force, leaving the healthy workers.[1538]

Becklake has reviewed results from cross-sectional and longitudinal studies that have addressed the importance of occupational dust exposure in the development of COPD.[1419] Although some controversy still exists as to the relative importance of smoking and exposure to dust in the workplace,[1505] she concluded that in some occupations there is unequivocal evidence for a significant effect of dust on lung function. Korn and associates[1539] studied a random sample of 8,515 adults from midwestern and eastern United States; after adjusting for smoking habits, age, sex, and city of residence, they found that subjects who had been exposed to dust, gases, and fumes showed a significantly increased incidence of respiratory symptoms and airflow obstruction (FEV_1/FVC ratio less than 0.6). An increased annual rate of decline in FEV_1 has been seen in workers exposed to inorganic dusts, coal and hard rock miners, foundry workers, and metal and chemical workers.[1419, 1510-1542] Chemicals such as TDI, which can cause occupational asthma in some individuals, can also produce a nonidiosyncratic acceleration of functional deterioration in occupationally exposed workers, both smokers and nonsmokers.[1541] Exposure to dusts that are known to produce fibrotic pneumoconioses can contribute to airflow obstruction in which the severity is not necessarily related to the amount of fibrosis. An explanation for the variation of pathologic response to single agents may be related to particle size and deposition pattern:[1543] for example, larger particles tend to impact on airways and cause airflow obstruction, whereas smaller particles reach alveolar airspaces where they induce fibrosis and a restrictive ventilatory defect.

In a 9-year longitudinal study of United States coal miners, the deleterious effect of dust exposure was found to be about a third to a half as important as that of smoking.[1541] Although exposure to asbestos dust is associated with abnormalities of small airway function,[1544] smoking is substantially more important to the development of significant symptomatic obstruction.[1545, 1546] A 5-year follow up study of 168 firefighters and 1474 control subjects revealed a significant acceleration in the rate of decline in FEV_1 in the firefighters when age, smoking history, and initial lung function were taken into account.[1547] However, not all studies have revealed a deleterious effect on function in firefighters (see Chapter 14). When rates were adjusted for the amount of smoking, miners showed more severe emphysema at autopsy than did nonexposed workers, and to the extent that emphysema is associated with airflow obstruction, this supports an independent effect of inorganic dust inhalation on airway function.[1419, 1548, 1549]

In a number of occupations, exposure to organic dust shows a dose-dependent effect on airway function that is separate from the effect of cigarette smoke. Although exposure to cotton and grain dust can produce a specific or nonspecific acute bronchoconstrictive response, chronic irreversible obstruction can also develop;[1105, 1106] the long-term effects of exposure to cotton and grain dust have been discussed in the section on occupational asthma (see page 2056). Inhalation of wood dust by pulp and paper mill workers can also contribute to the development of COPD.[1550]

Infection

There are a variety of possible relationships between lower respiratory tract infection and COPD:

1. Infection during childhood may increase the subsequent risk of COPD by affecting lung function, lung growth, or pulmonary defense mechanisms.

2. Respiratory infection in patients with established COPD may accelerate subsequent functional deterioration.

3. Established COPD may increase the incidence and severity of respiratory infection.

These possible relationships will be examined separately.

Retrospective studies have provided fairly conclusive evidence that lower respiratory tract infection in children is a significant risk factor for the subsequent development of COPD during adulthood.[1551–1554] Childhood "bronchitis," especially before the age of 2 years, is associated with persistently abnormal lung function and thus represents an important risk factor.[1555–1557] The question remains as to whether infection in childhood or "bronchitis" is the result of a genetic predisposition to respiratory illness (e.g., asthma) or is the initiating insult that causes the subsequent development of symptomatic airway obstruction.[1558] The interrelationship between infection, inhalation of pollutants, and host defense mechanisms is complex. Exposure to atmospheric or residential air pollution not only is associated with an increased incidence of childhood viral respiratory infections[1527, 1528, 1559] but also appears to have an independent detrimental effect on lung function.[1490, 1494] In addition, pollutants may interfere with macrophage efficiency, thus increasing susceptibility to infection.[1431, 1560]

One of the major risk factors for the development of symptomatic COPD is the initial lung function. Because of the "horse race effect," subjects with initially impaired lung function will show a more rapid decline in function. Thus, childhood respiratory infection may exert its long-term effect by producing slight functional impairment, which later predisposes to accelerated deterioration. In a study of 96 children 9 years after recovery from croup, a significant decrease in vital capacity and maximal expiratory flow rates and an increase in the RV/TLC ratio and nonspecific airway responsiveness were observed in comparison to age-matched control subjects.[1561] The regional death rate from COPD in England and Wales between 1959 and 1978 was strongly related to the infant mortality from bronchitis and pneumonia in the same regions between 1921 and 1925. Statistical analysis suggested that lower respiratory tract infection during early childhood was as important an influence as cigarette smoking in the geographical distribution of the COPD.[1562]

An initial proposal that a lack of secretory IgA is common in patients with chronic bronchitis and that it might predispose to infection and obstruction[1563] has not been confirmed. More recent studies have shown that levels of both secretory IgA (measured in saliva or in nasal or bronchial secretions) and serum IgA are within normal limits in the great majority of patients with COPD.[1564–1568] There is also no evidence for impaired cellular immunity as a risk factor in patients with COPD. Qualitative and quantitative cytologic and bacteriologic studies of the sputum of 60 patients with an acute exacerbation of COPD[1569] showed a normal pattern of neutrophil increase during the infection and the appearance of macrophages after the infection. Another study of 100 patients with COPD[1570] revealed normal cutaneous delayed hypersensitivity and phagocytic intracellular killing activity, but also showed a significant impairment in the ability of peripheral leukocytes to reduce nitroblue tetrazolium (NBT). High levels of mucous antibodies have been demonstrated in patients with chronic bronchitis, a finding that may simply reflect the presence of chronic infection and impaired mucociliary clearance that would permit abnormal reabsorption of mucous antigens.[1571]

Although airway function worsens acutely in patients with COPD as a result of intercurrent viral and bacterial respiratory infection, whether these infections produce permanent functional impairment and accelerate the natural course of the disease has not been established. Physiologic studies of airway function in normal subjects with naturally occurring[924–926, 1572, 1573] and experimentally induced[1574] viral infection have shown changes indicative of reversible airway obstruction and impaired gas exchange;[1575] however, it is possible that similar insults can cause a progression of irreversible airway obstruction in some patients with COPD.[1576] Smokers have been shown to be more susceptible than nonsmokers to the long-term sequelae of *Mycoplasma pneumoniae* infection.[1575] In a long-term study designed to assess the influence of *H. influenzae* infection on airway obstruction, the development of obstruction correlated with smoking habits but not with the infection itself.[1577] Despite a severe decline in pulmonary function during respiratory infections, most patients with COPD improve to their pre-exacerbation status after resolution of the infection, although irreversible deficits develop in some.[1578]

It is almost certain that the lower respiratory tract in healthy persons is sterile.[1579–1581] However, acute viral infections may extend into the lungs to involve a previously healthy lower respiratory tract, and it has been suggested that secondary infection from the upper respiratory tract by bacterial commensals may be superimposed upon this acute bronchitis-bronchiolitis.[1582] In addition, in chronic respiratory disease, such as COPD, and in the presence of obstructing endobronchial lesions, such as bronchogenic carcinoma, various microorganisms may be cultured from the lower respiratory tract.[1579, 1580] Growth of these organisms within the lung may be enhanced not only by destruction of the mucous membrane but also by other constitutional factors such as alcohol intake, hypoxia, starvation, and the administration of corticosteroid drugs.[1579] Infection results in acute episodes in which there is symptomatic and physiologic deterioration. The sputum often becomes purulent,[1583] cultures usually growing *H. influenzae* and sometimes *Streptococcus pneumoniae*;[1429, 1584–1587] antibodies to these organisms are found in the serum of many of these patients.[1577, 1588, 1589] In patients with acute exacerbations, detailed studies designed to distinguish nonencapsulated strains of *H. influenzae* from *H. parainfluenzae* have revealed positive cultures of the former organism (associated with a four-fold rise in antibody titer), whereas the latter appeared to act as a simple saprophyte.[1589] In a study of the changes in the bacterial flora in bronchitis, Cooper and her associates[1590] found that the frequency of acute exacerbations was not altered in patients receiving long-term antibiotic therapy but that they spent significantly less time in bed or away from work, indicating that morbidity from the superimposed bacterial infection was reduced.

Although several of the aforementioned studies suggest that bacteria may play a role in acute exacerbations of the disease, it is more likely that they act as a secondary invader following an acute viral infection of the lower respiratory tract. Viral infection is almost certainly responsible for the majority of clinical exacerbations in patients with COPD. Earlier studies that failed to demonstrate convincing evidence for a viral etiology of these acute flareups[1591, 1592] have been refuted by more recent investigations.[1593–1602] In one-third to two-thirds of acute exacerbations, viruses and, less commonly, *Mycoplasma pneumoniae* and the rickettsial organism responsible for Q fever, either have been isolated or their presence has been demonstrated by a four-fold increase in serum antibody titer.[1601–1603] Evidence for such infection is found far less frequently during periods of remission.[1601, 1602] The rhinoviruses and myxoviruses—the latter particularly during epidemics—appear to be the commonest etiologic agents.[1593, 1599, 1601, 1602] Identification of these organisms in conjunction with acute clinical exacerbations has clearly established their role as primary pathogens. Series differences in the percentage of acute episodes in which a specific virus is identified may depend upon the variety of tissue culture media employed, the extent of serologic testing, or a variation in the accepted definition of what constitutes an exacerbation. Another significant factor appears to be exposure of the adult with chronic bronchitis to schoolchildren in the family.[1600] In a study of six families, Stern[1600] identified a specific virus associated with acute exacerbations of COPD in 60 per cent of affected adults who were exposed to schoolchildren, but in only 29 per cent of those in households without schoolchildren.

In addition to the acute reversible exacerbations and perhaps the permanent bronchiolar obstruction that results from infection, it is likely that chronic granulomatous infection also may produce airway obstruction. In one study of 1,043 patients with tuberculosis,[1604] the data suggested that smoking and tuberculosis had an additive effect in producing airway obstruction.

Climate

Patients with COPD often relate exacerbations of their disease to climatic factors, particularly to extreme variations in humidity and temperature. It is possible that the effect of high humidity relates not only to the water vapor but also to the high level of air pollution that in many areas accompanies humid weather. In temperate climates, excessive air dryness during cold weather, particularly in apartments, seems to aggravate symptoms, and the use of a humidifier usually results in a decrease in cough and greater ease of expectoration. Fluid deprivation for 16 hours in the humid heat of Kerala, India, resulted in dehydration and a significant decrease in FEV_1, not only in patients with obstructive airway disease but in normal subjects.[1605] By contrast, short-term experimental studies in young healthy subjects exposed to a relative humidity ranging from 10 to 70 per cent at a constant temperature did not reveal any differences in nasal mucus flow.[1606] The increase in the number of emergency clinic visits by patients with COPD coincident with the onset of cold weather[1607] may be attributable to factors other than breathing cold air; for example, the excessive dryness created by hot-air heating or the inhalation of dust from convection currents around radiators may be contributory. In a study extending over the years 1952 to 1956 of the records of illness (absence from work for 4 or more days) attributed to bronchitis of nearly 60,000 London Transport employees, Cornwall and Raffle[1608] found a close relationship between the incidence of bronchitis and the number and density of fogs in any one year. In another survey of a large group of patients in which data were obtained by diaries,[1512] it was concluded that while exacerbations of COPD tended to occur with changing weather, it was air pollution rather than the adverse weather itself that was responsible for these episodes. Climate similarly may alter the clinical presentation; for example, it has been reported that in the warm, dry air of Tucson, Arizona, chronic cough is frequently nonproductive.[1609]

Some patients with chronic obstructive pulmonary disease appear to be abnormally sensitive to the inhalation of cold air.[1610, 1611] The degree of bronchoconstriction following cold air inhalation correlates with the magnitude of bronchodilation that occurs following inhalation of aerosol beta-adrenergic agonist[1612] and with nonspecific responsiveness to methacholine.[1613] Asthmatic patients with comparable starting values of FEV_1 develop more severe obstruction following cold or dry air breathing, suggesting that the mechanism of hyper-responsiveness is different in the two conditions.[1613]

Heredity

An inherited susceptibility to the effects of cigarette smoke may be as important a factor as smoking itself in the pathogenesis of COPD. The numerous studies of family members of patients with COPD support the presence of familial aggregation of airway obstruction and the results have been reviewed and summarized.[1614] The data show that first-degree relatives of patients with COPD have a likelihood of developing COPD 1.2 to 3 times that of the general population. However, a pattern to the familial association has not been demonstrated, and although heredity is the most likely explanation, the effects of a shared environment cannot be excluded from consideration. For example, the effect of parental smoking on their offspring's lung function can be a contributing factor and can confound attempts to establish a genetic basis for the familial aggregation of COPD. However, the fact that there is a greater concordance for indices of airway obstruction between the first-degree relatives than between spouses and between monozygotic twins than between dizygotic twins supports the influence of a genetic predisposition to COPD.[1614]

In the vast majority of cases, the underlying defect that constitutes the genetic predisposition for the development of COPD is unknown. Following the description in 1964 of the association between emphysema and alpha$_1$ protease inhibitor (PI) deficiency, it was believed that other inherited markers[1615] or deficiencies would be discovered to explain the genetic tendency for the development of COPD. Even though homozygous alpha$_1$ protease inhibitor deficiency (PiZZ) is associated with a 30-fold increased risk of symptomatic COPD developing, it accounts for less than 1 per cent of cases since the frequency of this genetic defect is only one in 2,000 to one in 4,000.[1616] Heterozygous deficiency (PiMS) is associated with serum alpha$_1$ PI levels that are approximately 60 per cent of normal but because this genetic makeup occurs more frequently (one in 100 to four in 100), an increased risk in such individuals could explain a greater familial tendency for the development of COPD.

As discussed farther on (see page 2163), it is accepted that the mechanism responsible for the development of COPD and emphysema in patients with severe protease inhibitor deficiency is an inability to counteract elastolysis caused by proteolytic enzymes, and it would seem logical to assume that patients with intermediate deficiency would be at increased risk for the development of COPD. Two types of cross-sectional studies have been used to address this hypothesis: (1) the prevalence of intermediate deficiency in a population of patients with COPD has been compared with that in a matched population without COPD; and (2) the prevalence of COPD in a population with intermediate deficiency has been compared with that in a population with normal protease inhibitor levels and phenotypes.[1617] The second type of study is more accurate but more difficult to perform. Numerous studies of both types have been carried out, and the bulk of evidence *does not* support the thesis that intermediate deficiency is a risk factor. Generally, studies that have found an association between heterozygous phenotype and pulmonary disease have been the less satisfactory type 1 variety[1618–1627] whereas those that have not supported an association have been predominantly the more definitive second type.[1488, 1626, 1628–1635]

Since decreased anti-elastase activity would predispose to airflow obstruction as a result of loss of lung elastic recoil, it is reasonable to hypothesize that loss of lung elasticity would be an early or sensitive sign; in fact, the results of a number of studies have suggested that intermediate alpha$_1$ PI deficiency does cause decreased lung elastic recoil when age and smoking factors are controlled.[1619, 1636] Despite the latter studies, it is safe to conclude that intermediate PI deficiency is not an important contributor to the familial aggregation of COPD; however, a definitive conclusion regarding the role of intermediate deficiency awaits longitudinal studies of large groups of subjects.[1637] The recent development of specific gene probes has allowed the examination of the alpha$_1$ PI gene in peripheral circulating white blood cells. A study has shown an incidence of genetic polymorphism in cells of patients with bronchiectasis and emphysema who do not have alpha$_1$ PI deficiency that is increased when compared with a group of healthy blood donors. Although this polymorphism may be a marker for genetic predisposition to chronic lung disease, it could also be a result of the pulmonary disease.[1638]

A genetic factor that could potentially influence the development of airway and lung damage is the enzymatic handling of chemical components in cigarette smoke. Aryl hydrocarbon hydroxylase (AHH) can generate toxic metabolites from hydrocarbons in cigarette smoke; if this enzyme were more readily induced in some individuals and families, more damage for a given dose of smoke would result. However, in one study, lymphocyte AHH was not more inducible in a group of patients with COPD than in a group of nonobstructed smokers.[1639]

There is some evidence that blood group antigens and salivary secretion of blood group antibody may be genetic markers, indicating an increased risk for the development of COPD. In a cross-sectional genetic-epidemiologic study of risk factors for COPD in 1787 adults, blood group A and family history were significantly related to airway obstruction.[1640] In a smaller population sample, the association with blood group A was present only in the women,[1447] and in a large longitudinal study, blood group A in men was associated with a slower decline in FEV_1.[1641] Subjects with blood group O, who do not secrete blood group antigens into the saliva, can be particularly susceptible to the detrimental effects of cigarette smoke.[1642]

A specific hereditary disease in which emphysema is an almost invariable component of a primary abnormality of connective tissue is cutis laxa (generalized elastolysis);[1643, 1644] other manifestations include diaphragmatic eventration and diverticula of the gastrointestinal and genitourinary tracts.

Socioeconomic Status

Epidemiologic studies have suggested an increased risk for the development of COPD in people of lower socioeconomic "class." The socioeconomic factor is small and is difficult to separate from related factors such as smoking habits, industrial exposure, passive smoking, and childhood infection.[1529] In Great Britain, people who live in homes without central heating have significantly worse lung function, and since central heating is more common in the homes of the well-off, this could represent one of the socioeconomic variables;[1645, 1646] however, it cannot represent the sole factor because in North America central heating is either universal or unnecessary and a socioeconomic risk factor still exists.[1647] In one large cross-sectional study, alcohol consumption was associated with lower values of FEV_1, but when corrected for smoking, age, sex, and socioeconomic status, the alcohol effect was not significant.[1647] In fact, in one autopsy study the incidence of centrilobular emphysema was lower in subjects with excessive consumption of alcohol, even after correcting for age and smoking history.[1648]

Mucus and Mucociliary Clearance in Chronic Bronchitis and COPD

Patients with chronic bronchitis have excess sputum production; biochemical analysis of the sputum shows an increased concentration of serum proteins and glycoproteins, indicating the presence in tracheobronchial secretions of serum transudate.[383] In the presence of infective exacerbations, the concentration of serum proteins is increased further and is accompanied by a decreased concentration of secretory IgA, indicating increased epithelial permeability and impaired epithelial secretion.[1649] Alteration in the viscoelastic properties of mucus occurs in patients with chronic bronchitis,[1650] but measurements of viscosity and elasticity *in vitro* do not invariably correlate well with measurements of mucous transport rate *in vitro*. However, in one study of 27 patients with chronic bronchitis,[1651] *in vivo* clearance and *in vitro* transport of sputum on a frog palate were significantly correlated.

The effect of cigarette smoking on mucociliary clearance has been examined in subjects without symptoms of chronic bronchitis. In a study in which mucociliary clearance and aerosol deposition were compared in 30 asymptomatic smokers (selected on the basis of an abnormal closing volume and volume of isoflow) and 20 nonsmokers without evidence of

small airway dysfunction, an increased scatter was observed in the deposition of radioaerosol in the smokers, suggesting nonuniform distribution of ventilation.[1652] In addition, asymptomatic smokers have delayed peripheral lung clearance.[1652, 1653] In another study,[1654] the tracheal mucous velocity technique was used to compare central airway clearance in young nonsmokers, elderly nonsmokers, young smokers without small airway disease, patients with chronic bronchitis, and patients with chronic bronchitis plus airflow obstruction: it was found that mucous velocity was decreased in older nonsmokers compared with young nonsmokers, and that central mucous velocity was significantly impaired in young smokers who manifested no evidence of small airway disease; ex-smokers showed some improvement in mucociliary clearance but not to normal levels. Patients with chronic bronchitis, with or without airway obstruction, showed marked reduction in tracheal mucous velocity.[1654]

In patients with COPD, the relationship between the amount smoked and decreased expiratory flow rate is closer than between the smoking history and impairment of mucociliary clearance, suggesting considerable interindividual variation in the effect of smoke on mucociliary clearance.[1655] In patients with similar smoking histories and similar degrees of airflow obstruction, those with pulmonary carcinoma show more severe impairment of mucociliary clearance rates.[1656]

Although it is generally agreed that smokers and patients with COPD have impaired mucociliary clearance, the magnitude of the impairment appears to relate to the measurement technique employed. For example, studies of central airway clearance show quite a marked decrease in clearance rates whereas much smaller differences are noted when whole lung studies are performed with radioaerosols. This probably results from the confounding variable of more central deposition in the obstructed patients, a fact that biases their results towards enhanced mucociliary clearance. Cough appears to be a more important and effective mechanism of mucociliary clearance in patients with chronic bronchitis than in normal subjects,[1657] and careful control of cough frequency is important in the study of mucociliary clearance in patients with obstructive airway disease.[1658, 1659]

Why cigarette smoking and chronic bronchitis impair mucociliary clearance is unknown. The number of ultrastructurally abnormal cilia in patients with chronic bronchitis is increased.[1660] In advanced disease, replacement of the normal ciliated epithelium by goblet cells and nonciliated squamous cells may be an important factor; in addition, the simple increase in the quantity of secreted mucus could disrupt the clearance mechanism. An *in vitro* study[1661] has shown that the particulate fraction of cigarette smoke can acutely decrease the electrical potential difference across dog tracheal epithelium and impair ion transport; such impairment could cause a reduction in the volume of sol-phase secretions, resulting in an imbalance between mucus and sol-phase constituents and impaired clearance.[1661]

The importance of increased mucous production and impaired mucociliary clearance in the pathogenesis of the airways obstruction associated with smoking is an interesting and difficult problem to address. The dyskinetic cilia syndrome (*see* page 2203) allows a comparison of airway function in patients with isolated defects of clearance. Mossberg and Camner[1662] measured mucociliary clearance and airway function in patients with ciliary dyskinesia, chronic bronchitis, cystic fibrosis, and emphysema secondary to homozygous alpha$_1$-antitrypsin deficiency: patients with ciliary dyskinesia showed marked impairment of mucociliary clearance, there being 92 per cent retention of a radioaerosol 2 hours after inhalation (the normal value is less than 35 per cent retention). In patients with COPD caused by smoking, impairment of clearance was less severe than in those with ciliary dyskinesia, retention amounting to 65 per cent at 2 hours. In patients with cystic fibrosis or asthma, clearance rates were also less abnormal than those in the ciliary dyskinesia group, although pulmonary function was significantly more impaired. Patients with alpha$_1$-antitrypsin deficiency showed no abnormality of mucociliary clearance, although they manifested marked airflow obstruction. The authors concluded that impaired mucociliary clearance may be a contributing mechanism in the production of obstruction in patients with COPD but that it is not the primary underlying cause.[1662] In most patients with ciliary dyskinesia mild chronic airway obstruction develops by the age of 25 to 40 years, indicating that severe dysfunction of mucociliary clearance can cause obstructive pulmonary disease.

In patients with COPD, tracheobronchial clearance of technetium-labeled particles is enhanced by the inhalation of hypertonic saline aerosol[1663] and by parenteral administration of beta-adrenergic agonists.[1664]

Nonspecific Bronchial Hyper-responsiveness (the Dutch Hypothesis)

In the 1960s, a group of Dutch investigators proposed a hypothesis for the selective development of COPD observed in some smokers. Termed the "Dutch hypothesis,"[1448, 1665] it states that patients with an atopic tendency and increased NSBR have a higher risk of developing irreversible airflow obstruction. It is not clear exactly how atopy and NSBH could cause COPD, but in individuals with hyper-responsive airways it is possible that repeated episodes of acute bronchoconstriction related to smoke inhalation might by themselves cause fixed narrowing. Alternatively, an exaggerated inflammatory response to smoke in atopic individuals may represent the basis of this association. A number of studies have supported the association of nonspe-

cific hyper-responsiveness and a more rapid annual decline in FEV$_1$.[1666–1669]

Interpretation of these studies is confounded by the established relationship between NSBR and the initial FEV$_1$ in COPD. Unlike that in asthmatic patients, in whom NSBH can occur in the presence of normal baseline measurements of lung function, NSBH in patients with COPD is associated with, and perhaps caused by, abnormal "prechallenge" lung function.[434–436] Since the initial FEV$_1$ is a known risk factor for the development of COPD, the relationship between NSBH and a decline in FEV$_1$ could be spurious:[1665, 1670] in a 3-year follow-up study of 985 patients with COPD, the rate of decline in FEV$_1$ was negatively related to the initial bronchodilator response,[1671] and to the extent that bronchodilator response reflects NSBH, this study argues against a relationship. On the other hand, a large cross-sectional analysis of a random population of 1,905 subjects by Rijcken and associates[1672] supports a relationship between airway hyper-responsiveness and pulmonary symptoms: even when cigarette smoking was controlled for, subjects with increased bronchial responsiveness to histamine were significantly more likely to have symptoms of respiratory disease.[1672] It is hoped that prospective follow-up longitudinal studies will prove or disprove an association.

Additional support for the Dutch hypothesis derives from population studies that have shown a positive relationship between decreased FEV$_1$ levels and skin test responses to allergens, blood eosinophilia, and elevated serum IgE levels.[1673–1676] Relatives of patients with COPD also have increased blood levels of IgE.[1677] Serum levels of IgE normally decline after 15 years of age but tend to remain elevated in smokers, even in the absence of skin test responsiveness; smoking cessation is accompanied by a decline in IgE levels to their normal range. It is unlikely that the increased IgE levels represent antibody production in response to components of tobacco, but they could be a consequence of increased respiratory mucosal permeability or smoke-induced inhibition of suppressor lymphocytes.[1676, 1678] In one study, 11 of 30 smokers but only two of 30 nonsmokers had detectable specific IgE directed against *S. pneumoniae*, an organism commonly recovered from the respiratory tract of smokers with chronic bronchitis.[1679] These data suggest that the elevated IgE levels in smokers are at least partly attributable to specific antibody directed against microorganisms that infect the airways.

Although there is abundant evidence that cigarette smoking, environmental and occupational air pollution, heredity, and socioeconomic status are predictive of the development of COPD, it is clear that our knowledge of these variables allows only an imprecise prediction. The majority of subjects, even with these risk factors, do not develop disabling obstructive pulmonary disease; even a retrospective study in which a small number of subjects with rapidly accelerating airflow obstruction were selected did not allow identification of the unknown variables that predict the development of significant disease.[1680]

PATHOGENESIS OF EMPHYSEMA

Emphysema results from the unchecked enzymatic destruction of the elastic and collagen framework of the lung.[1681–1683] Although in theory this can be caused by the action of proteolytic enzymes present in polymorphonuclear leukocytes, alveolar macrophages, and other inflammatory cells, the neutrophil is probably the most important source of elastase in emphysema. Human neutrophil elastase is a glycoprotein of 22,000 to 35,000 dalton molecular weight that is stored in neutrophil granules and is released following stimulation with chemotactic agents and during phagocytosis. Besides elastin and collagen, it degrades a broad spectrum of proteins, including fibronectin, immunoglobulins, complement components, clotting factors, and the glycoproteins that make up the interstitial ground substance of lung. Other elastases are probably less common but may be important in individual cases; a metalloprotease is synthesized and released by activated macrophages, and there are occasional examples of other incompletely defined elastolytic proteases; for example, a 20-year-old woman with cutis laxa and severe pulmonary emphysema was found to have very high levels of an unidentified protease that was capable of degrading elastin.[1684]

Lung elastin is normally protected from excessive elastolytic damage by alpha$_1$ PI. This is a glycoprotein of 54,000 dalton molecular weight that is synthesized in the liver and circulates in the blood. On serum protein electrophoresis it migrates with the alpha globulin band—hence its name; in fact, alpha$_1$ PI makes up the majority of the protein content of the alpha$_1$ band (normal = 180 to 200 mg/dl).

The level and electrophoretic mobility of alpha$_1$ PI are determined by an individual's genetic phenotype, and as discussed later (see page 2163), more than 30 of these exist. Most of the phenotypes are associated with normal blood levels of alpha$_1$ PI, but patients with the homozygous phenotypes ZZ or SS can have very low levels (<20 mg/dl) and those with the heterozygous phenotypes, MZ and MS, can have a mild-to-moderate decrease in blood levels (60 per cent of normal). Alpha$_1$ PI completely blocks the action of neutrophil elastase at equivalent molar concentrations by acting like a substrate for the enzyme and forming a stable complex with it; it is less effective against the macrophage-derived metalloprotease, which it only partly inhibits. Neutrophil and macrophage elastases can also be inhibited by a large-molecular-weight (800,000 daltons) circulating alpha$_2$ macroglobulin; however, the large molecular weight prevents escape of this substance from the vasculature, and since the site of elastolytic damage is the interstitial space of the lung, alpha$_2$ macroglobulin is not of major importance.[1685] Small-molecular-weight endogenous lung antiproteases that can be detected in airway mucus also exist.[1686, 1687]

The discovery by Laurell and Erikson[1615] that alpha$_1$ PI was virtually absent in some people and that this inherited deficiency was associated with a high incidence of severe emphysema raised hopes that other less severe defects in the antiproteolytic armamentarium would be discovered to explain individual susceptibility to emphysema and COPD. Although no other important specific deficiency has been discovered, there has been a growing interest in the balance between elastolytic and anti-elastolytic factors within the lung, and it is now accepted that an imbalance between these forces is the most important mechanism in the genesis of emphysema and loss of lung elasticity. The many factors that influence this dynamic balance are shown in Figure 11–45.

The lung possesses the enzymatic capacity to replace and repair damaged structural proteins, and there is normally a slow turnover of elastin and collagen in the lung. Normal synthesis and repair necessitate the presence of the enzyme lysyl oxidase, which catalyzes the cross-linking of collagen and elastin. In animals, beta-amino proprionitrite blocks lysyl oxidase and exaggerates the effects of elastase (see farther on). Cigarette smoke not only blunts the increase in lysyl oxidase that normally follows elastolytic injury[1682] but also increases the number of circulating and pulmonary neutrophils.[1688–1691] Not only is the peripheral blood count elevated in smokers but there is also a significant relationship between white blood cell count and lung function irrespective of smoking habit. Among smokers, former smokers, and nonsmokers, an inverse relationship exists between white blood cell count and the FEV$_1$,[1689] subjects with higher white blood cell counts showing a more rapid decline in FEV$_1$ over a 10-year follow-up period.[1688] In addition to increased leukocytes, the blood of smokers contains higher than normal amounts of acute "phase reactive" proteins, including the ninth component of complement, ceruloplasmin, and alpha$_1$ PI. These data support the concept that smoke induces a chronic low-grade inflammatory reaction.[1692] The increased number of pulmonary neutrophils in smokers has been demonstrated both in bronchoalveolar lavage fluid[1691, 1693] and histologically,[1690] although in one study there was no correlation between lavage and tissue neutrophils.[1694]

The dynamics of neutrophil transit through the lung are of considerable interest and potential importance in the pathogenesis of emphysema.[1695] A large number of so-called marginated leukocytes are present in the human lung, this marginating pool containing two to three times the number of

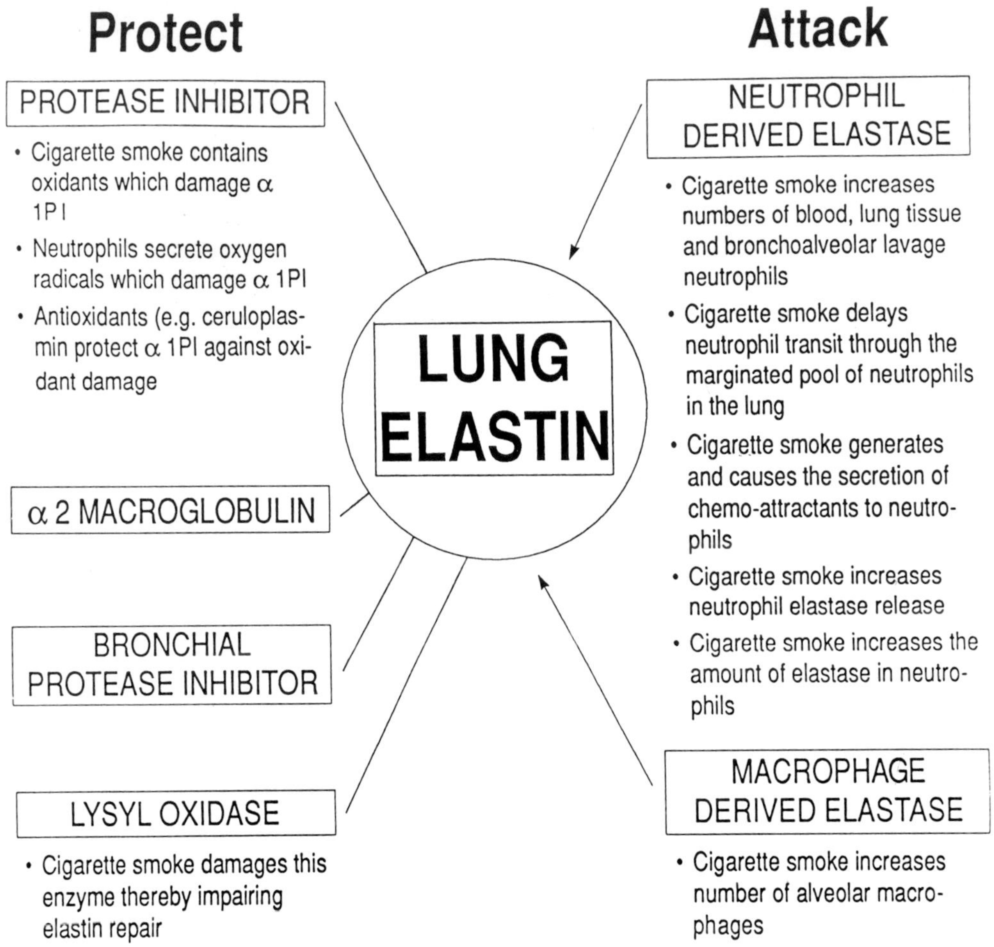

Protect

Attack

PROTEASE INHIBITOR

- Cigarette smoke contains oxidants which damage α 1PI
- Neutrophils secrete oxygen radicals which damage α 1PI
- Antioxidants (e.g. ceruloplasmin protect α 1PI against oxidant damage

α 2 MACROGLOBULIN

BRONCHIAL PROTEASE INHIBITOR

LYSYL OXIDASE

- Cigarette smoke damages this enzyme thereby impairing elastin repair

LUNG ELASTIN

NEUTROPHIL DERIVED ELASTASE

- Cigarette smoke increases numbers of blood, lung tissue and bronchoalveolar lavage neutrophils
- Cigarette smoke delays neutrophil transit through the marginated pool of neutrophils in the lung
- Cigarette smoke generates and causes the secretion of chemo-attractants to neutrophils
- Cigarette smoke increases neutrophil elastase release
- Cigarette smoke increases the amount of elastase in neutrophils

MACROPHAGE DERIVED ELASTASE

- Cigarette smoke increases number of alveolar macrophages

Figure 11–45. Pathogenesis of Emphysema. Cigarette smoke interacts with the proteolysis–anti-proteolysis balance at a number of sites. The overall effect is to promote increased breakdown of elastin and to interfere with repair.

cells in the circulating blood. The vast majority of the cells are within the pulmonary capillaries, and these turn over slowly with the circulating pool. Elegant *in vivo* studies in man have shown that approximately 20 per cent of labeled leukocytes are retained within the lung's marginating pool in a single pass through the pulmonary circulation.[1696] It is likely that the delay of leukocytes in their passage through the lung is partly a mechanical effect related to discrepancies in capillary segment diameter and the size and deformability of leukocytes,[1695] and partly an effect of regional blood flow and transit time. In regions where transit time is fast such as at the lung base, neutrophil delay is less than at the apex, where flow and transit time are slower.[1697] This delayed transit of white blood cells through the upper lung regions could contribute to the known upper lobe predominance of centrilobular emphysema. The longer a neutrophil remains in the pulmonary microvasculature, the more likely it is to interact with chemotactic or activating stimuli that could result in migration to the interstitium and release of elastase. Cigarette smoke may increase the pulmonary sequestration of leukocytes by delaying their transit through the lung.[1698]

Cigarette smoke and other inhaled substances may also increase the migration of leukocytes from

the vascular space to the interstitium by activating chemotaxins from a variety of sources and, in addition, can induce alveolar macrophages to secrete substances that are chemoattractants for neutrophils. Smoke has been shown in *in vitro* studies to activate complement and generate C5a, an extremely potent chemotactic substance.[1693, 1699] Collagen and elastin breakdown products may attract inflammatory cells to the site of injury, initiating a vicious circle.[1682] Patients with COPD have decreased levels of chemotactic factor inactivator, which could also increase the extravasation of activated leukocytes.[1700] In addition to attracting neutrophils, cigarette smoke can cause the release of elastase from neutrophils; it may stimulate neutrophils to actively secrete elastase or may simply damage the cell membrane, thereby releasing the enzyme.[1701] A number of studies have shown that in smokers with airway obstruction amounts of neutrophil elastase per cell are increased, but it is unclear whether it is the smoking that increases the levels.[1702–1704] The peripheral neutrophils of smokers also show a higher than normal content of myeloperoxidase, an enzyme that can oxidatively inactivate alpha$_1$ PI.[1705] Cigarette smokers also exhibit greatly increased numbers of alveolar macrophages[1706–1708] in which metabolic[1687] and elastolytic[1707, 1709] activity is increased. When stimulated, peripheral blood leukocytes of smokers with airflow obstruction accumulate greater amounts of intracellular and extracellular oxidants than the cells of smokers who are not obstructed.[2791]

Besides increasing the number and elastolytic capacity of inflammatory cells, smoke can tip the balance toward elastolysis by interfering with the ability of alpha$_1$ PI to inhibit any elastase that is released. The active site on alpha$_1$ PI is a methionine-serine bond that is susceptible to oxidation, and oxidant damage completely blocks the ability of alpha$_1$ PI to inhibit elastase.[1710] The gas phase of cigarette smoke is a rich source of oxidizing agents, and these substances have a direct effect on alpha$_1$ PI;[1711, 1712] in addition, activated neutrophils and macrophages release oxygen radicals that may have a similar effect. A relative inability to scavenge oxygen radicals may be a risk factor for elastolytic lung injury. In one study, the antioxidant activity of plasma was found to be deficient in subjects with a family history of lung disease and there was a significant relationship between antioxidant activity and the FEV_1/FVC ratio.[1713]

It has been difficult to prove that alpha$_1$ PI activity is decreased in the serum of smokers. Alpha$_1$ PI content and activity must be separately measured to show that there is a decrease in the active form. In some studies, circulating alpha$_1$ PI activity has been shown to be reduced whereas in others it is normal.[1714–1717] Acute heavy cigarette smoking causes a transient decrease in the anti-elastase capacity of circulating alpha$_1$ PI[1718] and an increase in the blood levels of elastase.[1719]

The concentration of oxidizing substances in the lung is likely to be much higher in the interstitium, where levels of smoke constituents and number of activated leukocytes are greatest. Since this is the site of elastase-induced injury,[1720] it is here that inactivation of alpha$_1$ PI would have the most harmful effect; studies of sputum and bronchoalveolar lavage fluid suggest that there is inactivation of alpha$_1$ PI in the lungs of smokers.[1721, 1722] Ceruloplasmin is an important circulating antioxidant and can theoretically protect alpha$_1$ PI from oxidative damage. Ceruloplasmin was detected in the bronchoalveolar lavage fluid of both smokers and nonsmokers, and although smokers had higher levels, it was less active as an antioxidant.[1723] Oxidative damage induced by smoke may also impair the anti-elastase activity of the low-molecular-weight bronchial mucus inhibitor.[1724]

There are no *in vivo* markers of accelerated elastolysis. Desmosine is an elastin-specific cross-linking molecule that is excreted in the urine; theoretically, the excretion should be increased if there is increased elastin digestion.[1725] Unfortunately, pathologic lung elastolysis may constitute too small a fraction of total body elastin turnover because elevated levels have not been detected in alpha$_1$ PI–deficient patients with emphysema.[1725]

EXPERIMENTAL EMPHYSEMA

Emphysema can be produced in animals by increasing proteolysis in the lung or by interfering with the synthesis and turnover of protein.

PROTEASE-INDUCED EMPHYSEMA

A variety of proteolytic enzymes have been used to produce emphysema in different animal species. In the initial studies, Gross and associates[1726] produced emphysema in rats by repeated intratracheal instillation of papain, a protease derived from the fruit of the papaw tree (*Carica papaya*). Administered intratracheally or by aerosol, papain has since been used experimentally in dogs, hamsters, and rabbits.[1620, 1727–1738] The resulting emphysema is usually mild unless excessive exposure causes pulmonary hemorrhage.

More recently, pancreatic elastase,[1739, 1740] homogenates of polymorphonuclear leukocytes and macrophages, and purified human neutrophil elastase have been shown to cause morphologic and physiologic changes comparable to those of human emphysema.[1736, 1741–1746] When administered via the airway, elastase is far more effective than when injected intravenously, presumably because antiproteases inactivate the enzyme when it is given parenterally. Physical exercise or mechanical ventilation following administration of elastase does not increase its effect.[1747, 1748] The emphysema that results from exogenous elastase is more severe if blood levels of antiprotease are decreased,[1749] but its development is completely inhibited if alpha$_1$ PI or synthetic elastase inhibitors are administered before elastase.[1732, 1738, 1750–1753] One dose of intratracheal elastase can cause progressive elastolytic damage; in dogs, elastin-derived peptide fragments can be detected in the blood for 40 days after the administration of a single dose.[1754] It is possible that elastase is taken up by macrophages and then slowly released to account for its prolonged action.[1682]

Guenter and associates[1755] have shown in dogs that repeated intravenous injection of bacterial endotoxin over 17 weeks causes sequestration of neutrophils in the pulmonary vasculature and mild emphysema (increased mean linear intercept and loss of lung recoil). Wittels and associates[1756] injected endotoxin intravenously into monkeys and observed sequestration of leukocytes in the pulmonary capillaries of lower lobes, accompanied by alveolar disruption; the daily injections of endotoxin were associated with a transient profound reduction in the number of circulating leukocytes, presumably as a result of pulmonary sequestration. These are important studies in the proteolysis-antiproteolysis theory of the pathogenesis of emphysema because they show that when neutrophils are activated and sequestered within the lung, an imbalance in favor of elastolysis may occur. A similar mechanism could explain the predominant lower zonal emphysema that develops in drug abusers who repeatedly inject talc-containing medications intravenously.[2792]

LATHYROGEN-INDUCED EMPHYSEMA

Cross-linking between collagen is necessary for normal connective tissue synthesis and repair. Defective bonding between collagen and elastin occurs in animals fed on the seed of *Lathyrus odoratus*,[1757] and a substance that interferes with the bonding process is therefore called a lathyrogen. Lysyl oxidase is the enzyme that catalyzes the cross-linking and the lathyrogen beta-aminoproprionitrile inhibits lysyl oxidase. Administration of beta-aminoproprionitrile to neonatal rats results in the development of large alveoli and increased compliance;[1758] when it is administered at the same time as elastase, it causes more severe emphysema than when elastase is given alone.[1682] Lysyl oxidase is dependent on minute concentrations of copper as a cofactor for its action, and it has been shown that copper-deficient rats[1759] and pigs[1760] develop larger airspaces and greater loss of lung elasticity than animals with normal copper levels. In one cross-sectional population study of 397 men, there was a significant relationship among nonsmokers between FEV_1 and the copper content of drinking water.[1761] Defective bonding between collagen and elastin is believed to be the underlying mechanism for the inherited emphysema-like changes found in the lungs of the "blotchy mouse."[1682, 1762]

CADMIUM-INDUCED EMPHYSEMA

Cadmium chloride in aerosol form has been reported to produce centrilobular emphysema in rats[1763] and hamsters,[1682] whereas it causes extensive fibrosis, irregular emphysema, and pulmonary overinflation in guinea pigs;[1764] beta-aminoproprionitrile enhances the emphysema formation in hamsters.[1682] In humans, cadmium can enter the body either in food, particularly seafood, or through environmental pollution and cigarette smoking. It has been shown that about 70 per cent of the cadmium content of cigarette tobacco passes into the smoke. Cadmium is stored in the liver; in one study,[1765] patients with a history of COPD were found to have a mean liver cadmium content more than three times that found in a control group, a level that may simply reflect the influence of cigarette smoking and air pollution. The association of lung disease and cadmium exposure in industry is dealt with at greater length in Chapter 14.

OTHER MODELS OF EMPHYSEMA

A morphologic and physiologic state simulating emphysema can be produced in animals by continuous exposure to moderately increased levels of NO_2.[1744, 1766–1768] Although with intermittent exposure to 15 ppm of NO_2 rats can live a normal life span, at autopsy they have voluminous lungs with a large FRC, obliteration of terminal bronchioles, and distention and loss of alveoli.[1768] Emphysema-like changes can also be produced in the lungs of certain animal species with chronic exposure to phosgene and cigarette smoke.[1744]

PATHOLOGIC CHARACTERISTICS

Because the vast majority of patients with chronic airflow obstruction have abnormalities in both the conducting airways and lung parenchyma, it is artificial to discuss the pathology of chronic bronchitis and emphysema separately. Consequently, in this section we describe the pathologic characteristics of the large airways, small airways, lung parenchyma, and pulmonary vasculature, recognizing that the changes in individual patients may be located predominantly in one of these sites.

Our understanding of the significance of the various pathologic abnormalities in patients with COPD has been greatly advanced by studies in which pulmonary function and structure have been compared. The main investigations have been three in type:

1. When patients have undergone pulmonary function tests during their lifetime and postmortem examination of their lungs after death, a comparison of pathology with function becomes possible: a potential disadvantage of such studies is that terminal events and a prolonged time interval between assessment of function and death can make the pathology unrepresentative of the lung morphology at the time the function studies were performed.

2. Certain lung function tests can be performed on lungs excised at autopsy and before pathologic examination, permitting close association in time between lung structure and function: the weakness of such studies consists of potential errors in extrapolating the function of excised lungs to the *in vivo* state.

3. Perhaps the most accurate method is a comparison of the pathology of excised lobes or lungs obtained at thoracotomy with lung function measured immediately preoperatively. Although this eliminates the problems associated with the first two forms of investigation, potential methodological limitations remain. These include (a) inadequate sampling due to the fact that only one lung or lobe can be examined and to the possibility of a nonuniform distribution of pathologic changes, and (b) potential inaccuracy due to the influence on airway pathology of the underlying lesion responsible for the resection.

The importance of comparing lung structure with function is increased by the trend to quantify pathologic abnormalities rather than just describe them; morphometric measurements of the extent of pathologic change and the relative volume or area of various tissues and airspaces have allowed quantitative comparison of structural abnormality and functional changes.

Large Airways

Abnormalities of the trachea and major bronchi are common in COPD and at some time in the course of this disease include involvement of virtually all tissue components—the epithelium, tracheobronchial glands, muscularis mucosa, interstitial tissue, and cartilage. Changes in the tracheobronchial glands have probably been the subject of greatest attention. Although it was known that hypertrophy and hyperplasia of these structures occurred in chronic bronchitis, it was Reid[1769] who first quantified the changes and correlated them with the clinical syndrome of excessive cough and mucus expectoration. The "yardstick" devised by Reid for the assessment of the presence and severity of gland hypertrophy consists of the ratio of the width of a mucous gland to the width of the adjacent bronchial wall measured from the airway epithelial basement membrane to the inner edge of the perichondrium (Fig. 11-46). This ratio, which is known as the *Reid Index*, is usually determined by averaging measurements of three to five trans verse sections from the main, lobar, or segmental bronchi. Although many studies have demonstrated reasonable correlation between the Reid Index and the presence and severity of mucous hypersecretion,[1769–1772] other investigations have shown that the correlation is better with morphometric estimate of the absolute area or volume of mucous glands.[1773–1775]

There are two major problems in relating measurement of the size of tracheobronchial glands to the pathogenesis of COPD. First, although very high and very low values for the Reid Index predict the presence or absence of chronic bronchitis with reasonable accuracy, intermediate values (which are found in the majority of both normal subjects and chronic bronchitics) possess virtually no predictive value.[1776–1779] Second, and perhaps more importantly, measurements of bronchial gland hypertrophy generally do not correlate with the severity of airway obstruction,[1773, 1780] a lack of association that is in keeping with the failure of the clinical syndrome of chronic bronchitis to predict the accelerated decline in expiratory flow rates that characterizes COPD.[1414] The absence of functional correlation with gland hypertrophy makes it very unlikely that mucus derived from tracheobronchial glands plays an important role in the pathogenesis of COPD.

The increase in size of tracheobronchial glands is sometimes apparent by simple observation of histologic sections of airways from patients with COPD (Fig. 11–46). The increase is probably related more to hyperplasia than to hypertrophy.[2765] The ratio of mucous cells to serous cells within the gland is also increased in some cases. The openings of the bronchial gland ducts into the airway lumen may be plugged with mucus and are often dilated,[1781] presumably reflecting the increase in volume of secretion. This can be appreciated on bronchograms as small depressions or diverticula on the airway luminal surface and can also be seen on scanning electron microscopy (Fig. 11–47). It has also been suggested that some diverticula are related to loss of subepithelial connective tissue and herniation of airway mucosa between smooth muscle bundles.[1781]

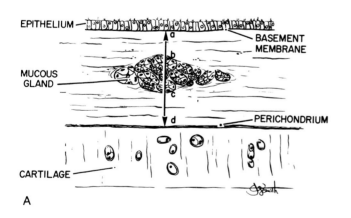

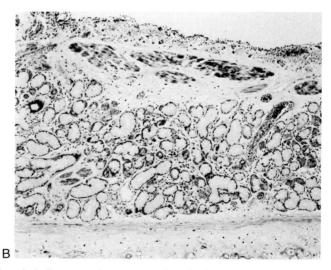

Figure 11–46. Bronchial Gland Hypertrophy and the Reid Index. *A*, A diagrammatic representation of a bronchial wall shows the measurements by which the Reid index is calculated: the maximum thickness of a bronchial gland internal to the cartilage (b to c) is divided by the distance from the basement membrane to the inner perichondrium. *B*, A section of segmental bronchus from a patient with chronic productive cough shows diffuse glandular hypertrophy, the Reid index being approximately 0.6. (*A* is from Thurbeck WM: Chronic Airflow Obstruction in Lung Disease. Philadelphia, WB Saunders Co, 1976, p 33.)

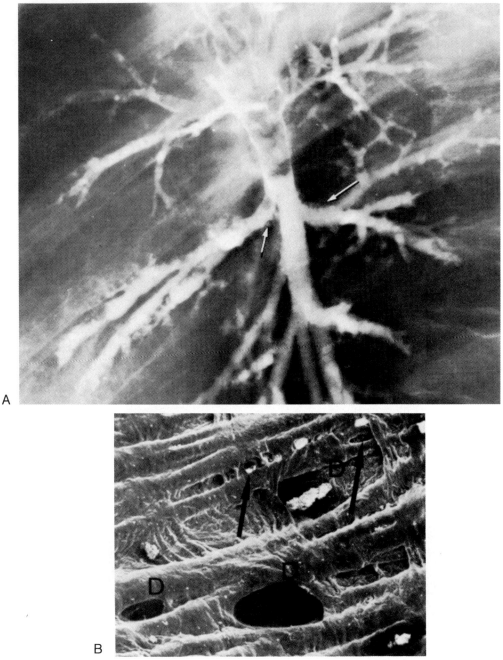

Figure 11–47. Bronchial Wall Diverticula in Chronic Obstructive Pulmonary Disease: Bronchographic and Scanning Micrographic Appearance. A lateral projection of the major and segmental bronchi from a right bronchogram *(A)* shows filling of several outpouchings or diverticula on the inferior aspect of the middle lobe bronchus and the upper surface of the superior segmental bronchus of the lower lobe *(arrows)*. Many of the segmental bronchi have lost their normal tapering, evidence of cylindrical bronchiectasis. A scanning electron micrograph *(B)* from a 64-year-old smoker shows several small *(arrows)* and large (D) diverticula. The longitudinal ridges consist of aggregates of subepithelial muscle cells. (*B,* × 34.) (*B* is from Wang N-S, Ling W-L: Hum Pathol *8*:304, 1977.)

The quantity of bronchial cartilage has been found to be decreased in patients with COPD in some[1782-1786] but not all[1779, 1789, 1790] investigations. The most severe deficiency has been seen in the segmental and subsegmental bronchi, and generally the changes have been more apparent in the lower than in the upper lobes. In both normal subjects and patients with COPD, maximal forced expiratory maneuvers result in flow-limiting collapse of segments of central cartilaginous airways (see page 2144).[1787, 1788] Since cartilage provides an important contribution to the relative incompressibility of these airways, its deficiency might be expected to result in more prominent collapse. In fact, studies of the relationship between pressure and cross-sectional area of the trachea in a small number of patients with COPD[1791] have shown increased "compliance," suggesting that the loss of cartilage observed histologically possesses a functional counterpart.

The pathogenesis of the cartilage deficiency is unclear. In experimental animals, damage to cartilage by proteolytic enzymes results in airflow obstruction unaccompanied by changes in lung elastic recoil or dimensions of small airways.[1558, 1792] It is possible that the chronic airway inflammation characteristic of COPD causes proteolytic damage to structural proteins in the large airways; to the extent that such damage increases the collapsibility of the large airways, maximal expiratory flow will be decreased. It has also been suggested that deficiency of airway elastic tissue may be caused by the same mechanism and can have the same functional consequences.[1793]

The amount of smooth muscle in the bronchial wall of patients with chronic bronchitis has been found to be increased in some studies[1794, 1795] but normal in others.[377] The relationship between such an increase and the presence of "asthmatic bronchitis" is not clear. Chronic inflammatory cells, especially lymphocytes, may be increased in number in the tracheobronchial wall;[1790] in one study,[1796] cough and sputum expectoration were shown to correlate more closely with the number of inflammatory cells in the airway wall than with gland volume, suggesting that inflammation of large airway mucosa and glands may be important in the pathogenesis of mucus production.

Epithelial changes in the trachea and major bronchi are fairly common in patients with COPD, and include hyperplasia of goblet and basal cells and squamous metaplasia, sometimes associated with dysplasia.[1797, 1798] Although such changes are not likely to contribute directly to airway obstruction, they may interfere with mucociliary clearance.

Small Airways

The demonstration by Hogg and his associates[1799] that airways smaller than 2 to 3 mm in internal diameter were the major site of increase in resistance to air flow in lungs removed at autopsy from patients with obstructive lung disease has focused attention on these airways. Although the exact mechanism for the increase in resistance is still incompletely understood, it appears to be related to a chronic inflammatory process that thickens, narrows, and obliterates the membranous and respiratory bronchioles.

Cosio and associates[1800] were the first to propose a semiquantitative grading system to assess the severity of different aspects of the inflammatory reaction in membranous bronchioles and to correlate the pathologic and physiologic abnormalities. With this system, bronchioles are examined microscopically and the following pathologic features of chronic inflammation are scored on a scale from 0 to 3: inflammatory cell infiltration, hyperplasia of goblet cells, squamous metaplasia of epithelial cells, fibrosis of the airway wall, hyperplasia of the airway smooth muscle, and pigment deposition in the airway wall. For the respiratory bronchioles, the system has been modified by deleting squamous cell metaplasia and goblet cell hyperplasia but including the accumulation of intraluminal macrophages.[2096] The grading is performed by comparing under the light microscope stained sections of individual membranous and respiratory bronchioles with a set of "standard" micrographs and assigning a grade of 0 to 3 on the basis of increasing severity of the abnormality.[1801] The total score for an individual patient is the observed score expressed as a percentage of the highest possible score (3, multiplied by the number of airways examined). Scores for each component of the inflammatory response are assigned, and a total pathology score is calculated as the sum of the component scores. Separate scores for membranous and respiratory bronchioles are determined. There are no "normal" values, but the system provides a method of ranking individual lungs for the severity of the different pathologic changes and of comparing this with altered pulmonary function when it is known.

More quantitative morphometric estimates of airway changes can also be used, such as measurements of the number of inflammatory cells/mm^2 of airway wall,[1802] the thickness of the airway wall,[1803] the ratio of airway size to the size of the accompanying pulmonary artery,[1804] and the number of airways per unit lung volume.[1805] These measurements are more difficult to make and more time-consuming than the grading system, and for the most part the correlations between them and the more subjective assessment of structural damage have been close.[1802, 1806, 1807]

Chronic inflammation can increase small airway resistance by one or more of four mechanisms:

1. Thickening of the wall at the expense of the lumen, caused by the actual bulk of inflammatory cells or by an increase in smooth muscle or fibrous tissue; an excessive amount of fibrous tissue can occasionally obliterate the lumen completely.

2. Mucous plugging, related at least partly to goblet cell hyperplasia. It is difficult to quantify the contribution that mucous plugging of small airways makes to obstruction in COPD, since the plugs may be lost when the lung is inflated with fixative. However, there is evidence that it is important; in a postmortem bronchographic study utilizing powdered tantalum, it was shown that the total number of patent small airways in patients with severe airflow obstruction was significantly reduced;[1808] subsequent histologic studies showed that the occluded airways were affected by a combination of obliteration and obstruction of their lumens by mucus and pus.

3. Interference with surface-active lipids, resulting in an alteration of the relationship between pressure and cross-sectional area in much the same way as the change in the pressure-volume curve of the lung occurs in the presence of pulmonary edema.

4. Disruption of the surrounding alveolar attachments, resulting in decreased radial traction.[1809] A significant relationship exists between the number of alveolar attachments to membranous bronchioles and the results of tests of airflow obstruction in human lungs at autopsy.[1809] The alveolar attachments also show enlarged fenestrae in subjects with decreased expiratory flow, suggesting that elastolytic disruption of the supportive framework of the small airways results from spill-over of the inflammatory process to adjacent alveolar walls.[1810]

When the lungs of smokers are compared with those of nonsmokers at autopsy, the former show narrowing and inflammatory changes in membranous and respiratory bronchioles;[1811] the airway narrowing is correlated with decreased maximal expiratory flow and increased total airway resistance.[1812, 1813] There have been a number of attempts to show a correlation between the "so-called" tests of small airway function (closing capacity, ΔN_2/liter, FEF_{25-75}, $\dot{V}max$ on helium/oxygen [He/O_2]), and the volume of isoflow on He/O_2 and air) and specific pathologic changes. The rationale behind these studies was the hope that these tests could detect small airway pathology at a potentially reversible stage (inflammatory cells and epithelial metaplasia) before fibrosis and obliteration occurred.

The majority of these studies have shown that closing volume, closing capacity, ΔN_2/liter, and maximal flows at low lung volumes do in fact correlate with the quantitative measurements and semiquantitative estimates of peripheral airway pathology.[1806, 1814–1819] It has been shown that in patients with an FEV_1 within the normal range but with significant abnormalities of small airway tests, inflammatory cell infiltration and goblet cell metaplasia are particularly evident but there is also increased fibrous tissue in the walls of the respiratory bronchioles.[1818, 1820] Decreased expiratory flows are associated with a decrease in the amount of muscle in peripheral airways, suggesting that smooth muscle

atrophy rather than hypertrophy may occur.[1818, 1822] Theoretically, the density dependence of maximal expiratory flow and the volume of isoflow on air and He/O_2 flow-volume curves should be tests of peripheral airway function, but the correlation between abnormalities in these tests and peripheral airway pathology has been disappointing.[1815, 1823] Many subjects show well-preserved density dependence despite a substantial decrease in maximal expiratory flow and severely inflamed small airways,[1823] perhaps because flow-limiting segments remain in central airways despite the increase in peripheral airway resistance.

In many studies, an association has been found between the severity of small airway changes and the presence and degree of emphysema,[1807, 1824, 1825] and it is possible that the inflammation that results in thickening and narrowing of the small airways also causes destruction of alveolar walls.[1807] The two processes are not invariably associated, however; many patients with airway obstruction and small airway pathologic abnormalities have no morphologic emphysema. In addition, membranous and respiratory bronchiolar inflammation is significantly worse in the lower lobes while centrilobular emphysema is invariably more severe in the upper lobes.[1826, 1827] The term "small airway disease" has been used not only to describe the pathologic abnormalities of small airways in patients with COPD but also to describe a distinct variant of the clinical presentation of a small number of patients with COPD.[1828, 1420] We feel that the use of the term in the latter context should be abandoned because it only leads to confusion; disease of the small airways is one of the abnormalities that leads to airway obstruction in COPD, not a disease in its own right.

Parenchyma

The basic pathologic abnormality of the lung parenchyma in COPD is destruction of alveolar walls and the formation of enlarged airspaces. As described in Chapter 1, the acinus consists of all tissue distal to the terminal bronchiole, comprising three or more generations of respiratory bronchioles, followed by alveolar ducts, alveolar sacs, and alveoli (Fig. 11–48). Selective involvement of the acinus at the level of the first and second generations of respiratory bronchioles (proximal acinar or centrilobular emphysema) causes a proportionately greater degree of loss of function than when destruction takes place predominantly in the alveolar sacs and alveoli (distal acinar or paraseptal emphysema). In addition, there is substantial evidence that there are several pathogenetic mechanisms of emphysema and that the pathologic and physiologic patterns vary with them. It is because of these relationships between structure and both function and pathogenesis that different morphologic types of emphysema have been defined. Such definitions have traditionally been related to the

Figure 11–48. Component Parts of the Acinus. This diagrammatic representation of the acinus shows a terminal bronchiole, respiratory bronchioles of the first (RB₁), second (RB₂), and third (RB₃) orders, an alveolar duct (AD), and an alveolar sac (AS). The acinus is that part of the lung distal to a terminal bronchiole, and emphysema is defined in terms of the acinus. (From Thurlbeck WM: Chronic Airflow Obstruction in Lung Disease. Philadelphia, WB Saunders Co, 1976, p 15.)

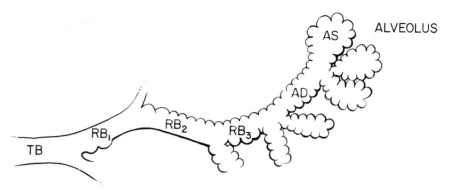

acinus and have resulted in four categories: (1) proximal acinar (centrilobular [CLE]), (2) panacinar (panlobular [PLE]), (3) distal acinar (paraseptal), and (4) irregular (scar) emphysema.

PROXIMAL ACINAR (CENTRILOBULAR) EMPHYSEMA

This form of emphysema results from destruction of parenchymal tissue in the region of the proximal respiratory bronchioles (Fig. 11–49). Although the term centrilobular is frequently used to refer to this, the fact that each lobule contains multiple acini means that instead of disease being located precisely in the center of the lobule, it is characteristically distributed in a multifocal fashion within it (Fig. 11–50). The term centriacinar has also been used to describe this form of emphysema; however, as Thurlbeck has pointed out,[1829] the central portion of the acinus (comprising predominantly the alveolar ducts) is not affected until disease is relatively advanced. For these reasons, both of these terms are inaccurate. Thurlbeck has proposed that the more descriptive term proximal acinar emphysema be used.[170] However, because of its widespread use, the term centrilobular emphysema will be used throughout this text.

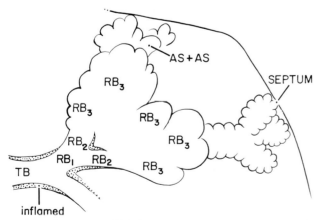

Figure 11–49. Centrilobular Emphysema. In centrilobular (proximal acinar) emphysema, respiratory bronchioles are selectively and dominantly involved. (From Thurlbeck WM: Chronic Airflow Obstruction in Lung Disease. Philadelphia, WB Saunders Co, 1976, p 15.)

Of those forms of emphysema that possess clinical and functional significance, this is the most common; it is found predominantly in cigarette smokers. A morphologically similar disease occurs in association with the inhalation of particulate foreign material (particularly coal dust) and is commonly known as focal dust emphysema; this variety is discussed in greater detail in Chapter 12.

The pathology of the early stages of centrilobular emphysema has not been well established. Pump[1830] made corrosion models of human lungs post mortem from patients with emphysema and described the early features of the disease as consisting of enlargement of alveoli in the acinus and loss of alveoli arising from respiratory bronchioles. The reason for the localization of early disease to parenchyma around respiratory bronchioles may be the "spillover" into this site of inflammatory cells centered on these airways.[1809, 1831] The earliest microscopic lesion in the progression to visible emphysematous spaces may be fenestrae or holes that can be seen in the alveolar walls adjacent to small airways (Fig. 11–51);[1810, 1832] theoretically, as these fenestrae increase in size and number they coalesce, so that eventually the alveolar wall disappears. Morphometric studies have shown that the number of alveolar walls attached to the small airways decreases in emphysema, supporting this concept. These early morphologic abnormalities are associated with a loss of lung elasticity and decreased maximal expiratory flow, and they can occur in the absence of the gross pathologic changes traditionally labeled as emphysema.[423, 429]

With progression of the disease, pathologic abnormalities become more clearly evident. The earliest change is dilatation of respiratory bronchioles, usually the two distal orders, accompanied by loss of adjacent parenchymal tissue; the peripheral elements of the acinus—alveolar ducts, alveolar sacs, and alveoli—are spared (Fig. 11–52). As destruction progresses, a number of respiratory bronchioles become confluent, both in series and in parallel, creating a common pool supplied by a terminal bronchiole proximally and leading to relatively normal alveolar tissue distally.[1833–1835] At this point, the disease is clearly visible grossly as multiple, regularly spaced foci of tissue destruction. Because of the association of centrilobular emphysema

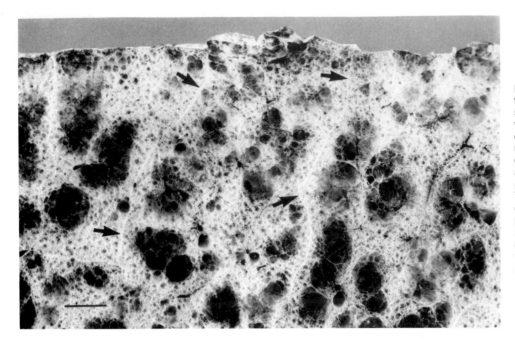

Figure 11–50. Centrilobular Emphysema: Anatomic Location within the Acinus. A cut section of lung parenchyma reveals multiple foci of emphysema distributed in a patchy fashion; most are associated with anthracotic pigment. The parenchyma adjacent to the interlobular septa *(arrows)* is essentially normal. The emphysematous spaces are clearly not limited to the central portion of the lobule but rather are scattered within it in a distribution corresponding approximately to the location of the proximal respiratory bronchioles. Bar = 8 mm.

with cigarette smoking, there is usually a prominent anthracotic pigment deposition; because this also occurs predominantly in relation to the proximal respiratory bronchioles, the emphysematous foci are typically black, resulting in a distinctive "checkerboard" appearance (*see* Fig. 11–50).

With further progression, the relatively discrete foci of earlier disease become confluent so that an entire lobule or even whole segments of lung parenchyma are eventually affected (Fig. 11–53). Although empty spaces several centimeters in diameter can be formed in this way, blood vessels or fine strands of residual lung parenchyma typically traverse the emphysematous spaces. At this point, it may be difficult to distinguish centrilobular from panacinar emphysema; however, except in the most advanced cases, centrilobular emphysema typically affects the parenchyma unevenly so that areas showing early changes diagnostic of the condition can usually be found (Fig. 11–54).

This variable severity is most obvious during examination of whole lung slices in which the disease can be seen to show considerable upper zonal predominance, particularly affecting the apical and posterior segments of the upper lobes and the superior segment of the lower lobes (*see* Fig. 11–

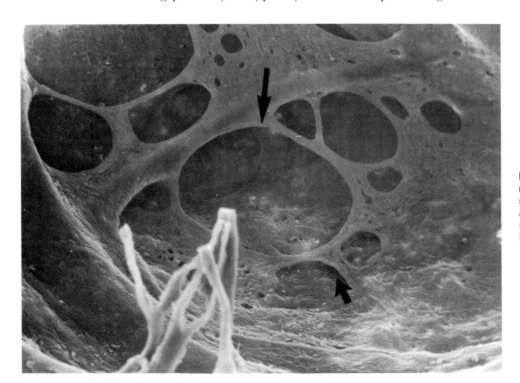

Figure 11–51. Alveolar Wall Fenestrae. A scanning electron micrograph of an alveolar wall shows multiple small *(short arrow)* and large *(long arrow)* fenestrae. (Courtesy of Dr. N.-S. Wang, McGill University, Montreal.)

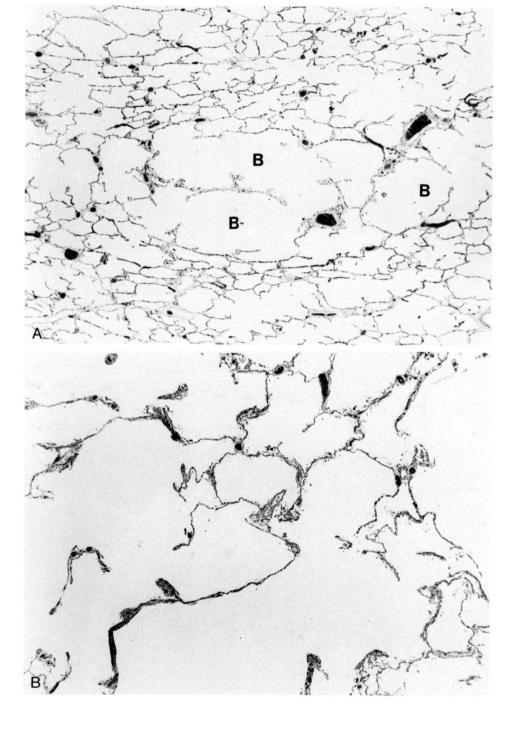

Figure 11–52. Centrilobular Emphysema: Comparisons of Mild and Severe. A histologic section of lung parenchyma *(A)* reveals early centrilobular emphysema; note the slight dilatation of respiratory bronchioles *(B)* associated with blunting and loss of alveolar septa. The adjacent parenchyma is normal. *B,* A section of lung parenchyma photographed at the same magnification as *A* showing advanced emphysema, almost no residual alveolar airspaces being identifiable. *(A, B,* × 25.)

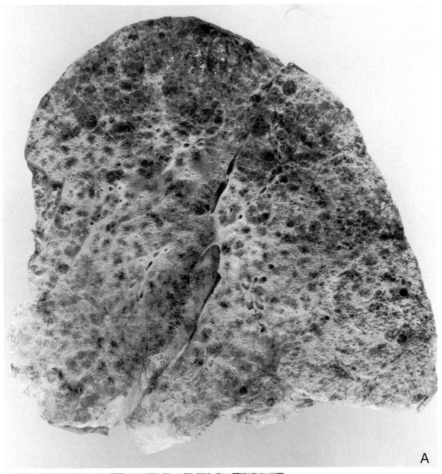

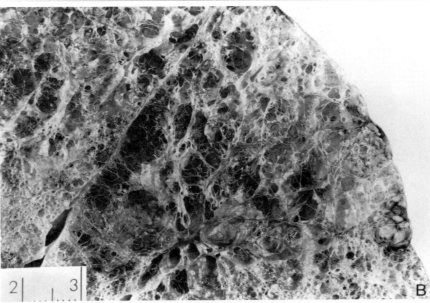

Figure 11–53. Centrilobular Emphysema: Moderately Advanced. A slice of right lung *(A)* shows moderately advanced centrilobular emphysema. The tendency to greater involvement of the apex of the upper lobe and superior segment of the lower lobe is clearly evident. A magnified view of the superior segment of the lower lobe *(B)* shows the majority of lung parenchyma to be totally destroyed and represented only by thin strands traversing emphysematous spaces.

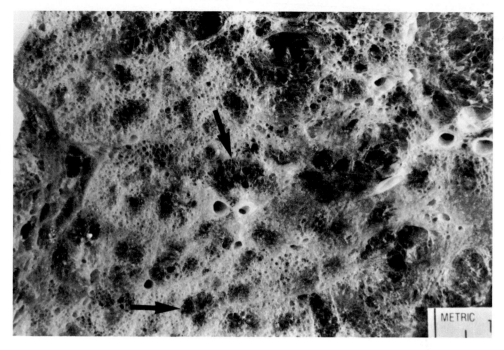

Figure 11–54. Centrilobular Emphysema: Mild. A magnified view of an upper lobe shows multiple foci of very mild centrilobular emphysema *(arrows)*. More advanced disease is present in the upper right.

53).[1834, 1836 1838] Although it is uncertain precisely why this is so, there are a number of factors that may contribute to this distribution:[1839]

1. The upper lobes are underperfused relative to their ventilation. If the development of emphysema is dependent on a balance between inflammation caused by the deposition of inhaled gases and the delivery of alpha$_1$ PI (*see* farther on), the upper lobes will be relatively undersupplied with anti-elastase.

2. Transit time of leukocytes through the upper lobes is slower than through the lower lobes, allowing a longer time for the leukocyte elastase to be released.

3. Particulate material appears to be deposited preferentially in upper lobes despite the gradient in ventilation distribution, perhaps because the caliber of airways is greater and the linear velocity of airflow is less than in the lower lobes; these differences can result in deeper penetration of inhaled particles in the upper lobes.

4. The deposition of pigment in nondependent lung regions observed at autopsy could be caused by less effective clearance of deposited material from the upper lobes.

5. Finally, the more negative pleural pressure and resultant relative hyperinflation of nondependent lung regions exert a mechanical stress on the alveolar walls in these regions, making disruption of elastic fibers more likely; the upper lobes are more compliant than the lower lobes, even in normal subjects without emphysema.[1840, 1841]

PANACINAR EMPHYSEMA

Panacinar (panlobular or diffuse) emphysema has also been called "unselective" because the acinus and secondary lobules are involved diffusely rather than selectively as is the case in proximal and distal acinar disease (Fig. 11–55). As with centrilobular emphysema, the initial morphologic changes have been poorly documented. Examination of thick sections of lung reveals abnormal fenestrations approximately 20 μm in diameter in the walls of the dilated alveoli.[1842] These are similar to those seen in proximal acinar emphysema, and as with this form, it is possible that they represent the initial abnormality. It has been suggested by some authors that the earliest abnormality is dilatation of alveolar ducts.[1843, 1844]

Macroscopically, early panacinar disease is manifested by a change in the normal architecture of the lobule, consisting of a loss of contrast between the larger, rounded alveolar ducts and the smaller, multifaceted alveoli. This is difficult, if not impos-

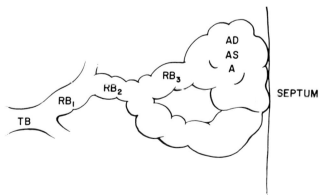

Figure 11–55. Panacinar Emphysema. In panacinar emphysema, the enlargement and destruction of airspaces involve the acinus more or less uniformly. (From Thurlbeck WM: Chronic Airflow Obstruction in Lung Disease. Philadelphia, WB Saunders Co, 1976, p 15.)

sible, to appreciate with the naked eye and is best seen by examination of barium-impregnated slices through the dissecting microscope. As disease progresses, the loss of parenchymal tissue may be evidenced by curling of the pleura into the lung and by the projection of bronchovascular bundles above the cut surface. In severe disease, affected parenchyma consists of no more than large airspaces through which strands of tissue and blood vessels pass like struts—the so-called cotton-candy lung. The appearance in this advanced stage is indistinguishable from that in advanced proximal acinar emphysema.

Panacinar emphysema characteristically shows a predilection for the lower lobes and anterior lung zones, although it can occur in more or less random distribution throughout the lungs.[1834, 1836, 1845] It may be associated with typical centrilobular emphysema, in which circumstance the lower lobe predominance may be less obvious.

Panacinar emphysema is the form characteristically seen in the presence of alpha$_1$ antiprotease deficiency. Although often associated with cigarette smoking, such exposure may be absent or minimal, resulting in relatively little anthracotic pigment deposition. In fact, this is the emphysema of nonsmokers; in one study,[1846] macrosections of lungs from 80 nonsmokers ranging in age from 37 to 94 years showed some degree of parenchymal dilatation and disruption in 24, mostly of mild degree but occasionally moderate in severity. In another study of whole lung sections from 200 autopsies, some emphysema was found in 70 per cent of men and 42 per cent of women. Emphysema was more frequent in smokers (70 per cent) than in nonsmokers (38 per cent); in smokers it was much more severe and was predominantly centrilobular.[1847]

DISTAL ACINAR EMPHYSEMA

Distal acinar (paraseptal or linear) emphysema selectively involves the alveolar ducts and sacs in the peripheral portion of the acinus (Fig. 11–56). Grossly, it is usually focal and consists of small

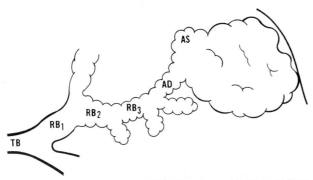

Figure 11–56. Paraseptal Emphysema. In paraseptal (distal acinar) emphysema, the peripheral part of the acinus (alveolar ducts and sacs) is dominantly or selectively involved. (From Thurlbeck WM: Chronic Airflow Obstruction in Lung Disease. Philadelphia, WB Saunders Co, 1976, p 16.)

emphysematous spaces in a more or less continuous zone of variable length located in the periphery of the lung adjacent to the pleura or along interlobular septa (Fig. 11–57). In some cases, there is an increase in collagen in the vicinity of the emphysema, suggesting that it is caused by a localized inflammatory process (possibly infectious pneumonia in which there have been both tissue destruction and healing fibrosis). Bullae may develop from coalescence of distended, destroyed alveoli and usually are multiple; in fact, paraseptal emphysema is thought to represent the basic lesion of bullous lung disease. Distal acinar emphysema is fairly common if diligently searched for in autopsy specimens, but in the vast majority of cases it is limited in extent and, with the exception of the occasional occurrence of spontaneous pneumothorax, gives rise to no symptoms.

IRREGULAR EMPHYSEMA

As the name suggests, irregular (paracicatricial or scar) emphysema shows no consistent relationship to any portion of the acinus (Fig. 11–58). It is always associated with fibrosis; thus, according to the recent modification of the definition of emphysema suggested by a workshop of the National Heart, Blood and Lung Institute, it should not even be classified as emphysema.[1848] As with some cases of distal acinar emphysema, the association of irregular emphysema with fibrosis suggests a relationship with inflammation. In some instances such as remote foci of granulomatous inflammation, this association is clearly evident (Fig. 11–59A); in others, it can only be assumed (Fig. 11–59B). Because of its association with scars, irregular emphysema is probably the most common form seen pathologically; typically, however, it is limited in extent and results in no functional or clinical abnormalities.

Structure-Function Correlation in Emphysema

The association of emphysema and airflow obstruction is thought to be caused by a loss of lung elasticity. Because maximal expiratory flow is dependent on lung elastic recoil as well as on airway size and collapsibility and since emphysema is often associated with a loss of normal elasticity, it has come to be accepted that emphysema causes loss of lung elasticity and that this is the cause of the decreased expiratory flow. However, it is clear that loss of lung elasticity can occur in the absence of obvious emphysema.[1849, 1850] These observations have led to the idea that loss of lung elasticity and emphysema may be essentially unrelated.[1851, 1852] Our recent understanding of the inconsistent relationship between emphysema and loss of elasticity comes from studies of structure and function: lung elasticity is assessed by measuring the elastic-recoil pressures at fixed percentages of total lung volume

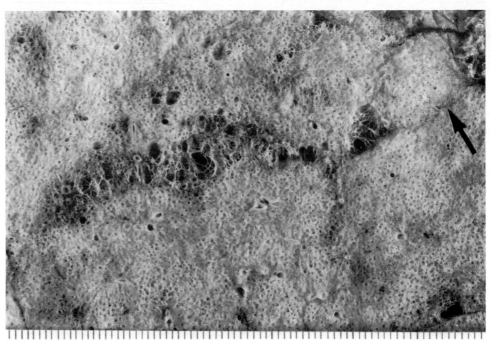

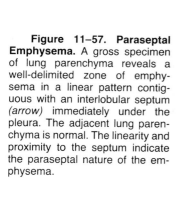

Figure 11–57. Paraseptal Emphysema. A gross specimen of lung parenchyma reveals a well-delimited zone of emphysema in a linear pattern contiguous with an interlobular septum *(arrow)* immediately under the pleura. The adjacent lung parenchyma is normal. The linearity and proximity to the septum indicate the paraseptal nature of the emphysema.

or by characterizing the shape of the entire pressure-volume curve with an exponential constant (K) (*see* Fig. 3–5, page 434). Although the lungs of patients with morphologic emphysema tend to have increased values for K and low lung recoil pressures,[1849, 1853–1855] this is by no means universal.

Studies of lung pressure-volume (P-V) behavior and its relationship to lung structure in a variety of animal species have shown that the shape of the P-V curve is strongly influenced by the average size of the airspaces contributing to the expired volume.[1856] Airspace size is measured by the mean linear intercept (Lm). Species with small alveoli (small Lm) have relatively stiff lungs (low K), whereas species with large alveoli have relatively compliant lungs (high K).

There is also an association between K and Lm in human lungs examined at autopsy.[1857] The P-V curve reflects the mean alveolar size of the airspaces that contribute to the expirate but does not reflect the P-V curve of emphysematous spaces. In lungs

removed at autopsy, Hogg characterized the P-V curve of centrilobular emphysematous spaces radiographically using lead dust to outline the spaces:[1858] the P-V curve of the centrilobular emphysematous spaces was compared with that of the whole lung in which the emphysema existed and to that of normal whole lungs (Fig. 11–60). He showed that the centrilobular emphysematous spaces did not contribute much to the total expired volume and that the P-V behavior of the spaces was less compliant than that of the lungs in which the spaces were found; in fact, it was even less compliant than normal lungs. The loss of elasticity and increased compliance found in the lungs of patients with emphysema must therefore represent the P-V behavior of airspaces other than the centrilobular emphysematous spaces. In one study in which preoperative lung P-V curves were compared with postoperative morphology, it was shown that the shape of the P-V curve correlated with the average size of airspaces (Lm) away from centriacinar emphysematous areas in the excised lobes and lungs. K correlated with Lm irrespective of the presence of emphysematous spaces.[1849]

The sequence of events in the development of COPD and emphysema probably begins with the simultaneous development of inflammatory changes in the small airways and adjacent alveolar septa. The inflammation results in narrowing of the lumen of the small airways, accentuated by the loss of alveolar attachments. As individual alveolar walls are disrupted, alveoli coalesce and the average size of airspaces increases, resulting in a loss of elasticity (increased K) and an increase in TLC.[1821] If the destruction of alveolar walls progresses, the enlarged airspaces coalesce to form visible centrilobular emphysematous areas; however, as this stage

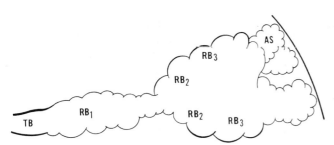

Figure 11–58. Irregular Emphysema. In irregular emphysema, the acinus is irregularly involved. This form is often accompanied by scarring in the lung. (From Thurlbeck WM: Chronic Airflow Obstruction in Lung Disease. Philadelphia, WB Saunders Company, 1976, p. 17.)

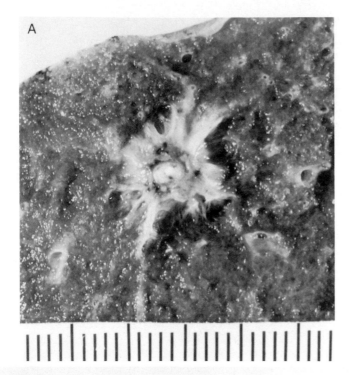

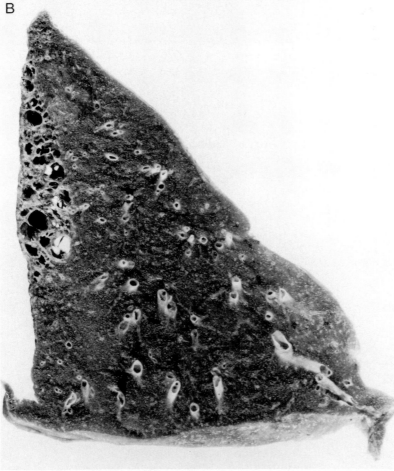

Figure 11–59. Irregular Emphysema. A slice of lung parenchyma *(A)* reveals a small, round focus of necrotic material (long-standing histoplasmosis) surrounded by irregular projections of fibrous tissue and small emphysematous spaces. The latter are caused by destruction of lung tissue during the initial inflammatory reaction to *Histoplasma capsulatum*. In another section of the lower lobe *(B)*, a well-defined zone of emphysema is present in the posterior subpleural region. The remaining lung parenchyma is normal. Note that the tissue between the emphysematous spaces is thickened as a result of fibrosis (compare with the fine strands seen in Figure 11–53). Both the fibrous tissue and the location suggest that the emphysema is related to remote pneumonia.

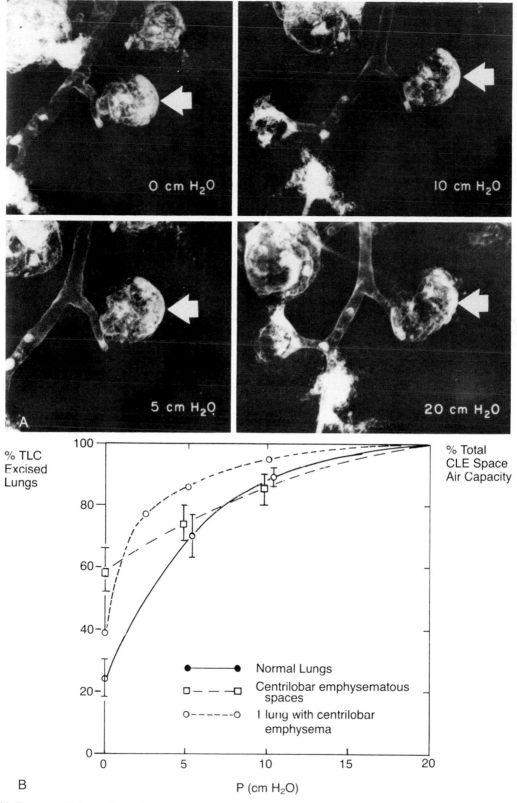

Figure 11–60. Pressure-Volume Behavior of the Centrilobular Emphysematous (CLE) Space. *A,* Four roentgenograms of a CLE space whose wall has been coated with insufflated lead *(arrow).* At increasing transpulmonary pressures of 0, 5, 10, and 20 cm H_2O, the volume of the centrilobular space changes little despite large changes in transpulmonary pressure. *B,* Pressure-volume curves of normal lung, a lung with centrilobular emphysema, and a CLE space. Volume is expressed as per cent of volume at total lung capacity (TLC). Although the whole lung with emphysema shows a decrease in lung elastic recoil at most lung volumes, the shape of the pressure-volume curve of the CLE space shows a flat curve with apparent decrease in compliance. (From Hogg JC, Nepszy SJ, Macklem PT, et al: J Clin Invest *48*:1306, 1969.)

progresses, these spaces contribute less to the expired air volume and to the P-V characteristics of the lungs and more to the "trapped gas" in the lung. Both the intrinsic narrowing of airways and the loss of elasticity contribute to the obstruction to air flow, and in the absence of detectable emphysema both mechanisms may be important.[1849]

Associated Vascular and Cardiac Manifestations

An increase in pulmonary vascular resistance occurs in patients with COPD and causes pulmonary hypertension, especially during exercise; the hypertension provides an increased afterload to right heart ejection and leads to the development of right ventricular hypertrophy and failure.[1859] The severity of pulmonary hypertension relates to the severity of abnormalities of gas exchange, including both the decrease in PaO_2 and increase in $PaCO_2$. The increased vascular resistance is related to a combination of loss of vascular bed, hypoxia-induced vascular smooth muscle contraction, and narrowing of small intrapulmonary vessels caused by thickening of their walls and loss of parenchymal support.[2793] Smokers and patients with mild airflow obstruction have an increased number of small muscular arteries and an increased thickness of the intima and media of pulmonary vessels,[1825, 1860, 1861] changes that correlate with the severity of small airway inflammation and the extent of emphysema.[1825, 1862, 2794]

Almost all patients with COPD who show evidence of pulmonary hypertension and cor pulmonale during life have morphologic changes in their pulmonary arteries at necropsy. These changes are not in any way specific and occur in pulmonary arterial hypertension of other etiology. A study in which the vasculature of normal and emphysematous lungs was injected with India ink showed a severe reduction in the alveolar-capillary bed in the lungs with emphysema.[1863] In advanced COPD and emphysema, there is a marked increase in anastomoses between the systemic and pulmonary circulations that may contribute to the development of pulmonary hypertension.[1864, 1865]

ROENTGENOGRAPHIC MANIFESTATIONS

As discussed in the section on Definitions (see page 2087), chronic bronchitis is defined clinically, emphysema pathologically, and COPD functionally. As a diagnostic tool that predominantly reveals morphologic abnormalities, the chest roentgenogram can demonstrate changes attributable to chronic bronchitis or emphysema but can disclose variations caused by COPD only by inference. In the following pages, therefore, only the first two of these will be addressed.

Chronic Bronchitis

The roentgenographic appearances in uncomplicated chronic bronchitis are inadequately documented, mainly because no large series has been reported of an assessment of premortem roentgenograms of known bronchitics who have been shown to have no emphysema at necropsy. As in spasmodic asthma, the main roentgenologic requirement is to exclude other conditions, such as bronchiectasis, that may mimic the disease clinically. We wish to emphasize at the outset that *chronic bronchitis cannot be diagnosed roentgenologically*. Changes may be observed in the lungs that *suggest* that bronchitis may be present, but on the basis of plain roentgenograms it is never appropriate to do more than indicate that the findings are compatible with or suggestive of that diagnosis.

In the three largest reported studies of the roentgenographic features of chronic bronchitis, of particular interest is the classification of "completely normal" for less than 50 per cent in each group: 41 per cent of 857 patients,[1866] 21 per cent of 184 patients,[1867] and "nearly half" of over 1,000 patients.[1868] The lower figure (21 per cent) recorded by Bates and colleagues[1867] reflects their inclusion of "tramlines" as an abnormality. These tubular shadows are discussed farther on. It is highly probable that the figure of 50 per cent is much too low. If one were to obtain chest roentgenograms of a number of cigarette smokers picked at random from passers-by on the street, each of whom satisfied the clinical criteria for the diagnosis of chronic bronchitis, it is very likely that the great majority would show no changes suggesting that diagnosis.

In our experience, there are only two roentgenographic abnormalities that suggest the presence of chronic bronchitis: (1) thickened bronchial walls (viewed either *en face* or end-on) and (2) prominent lung markings.

Tubular shadows, consisting of parallel or slightly tapering line shadows outside the boundary of the pulmonary hila, are probably always abnormal, although they are identified in some supposedly normal asymptomatic persons. These "tramlines" were identified in 80 (42 per cent) of the 184 cases studied by Bates and his associates[1867] but were not reported in either of the two series from the United Kingdom.[1866, 1869] In fact, Simon[1869] does not regard them as a roentgenographic feature of "chronic bronchitis" as defined in that country. Two possible explanations for this discrepancy are apparent:

1. In many of the cases reported by Bates and his colleagues,[1867] lung tomograms were available, doubtless giving improved visibility of tubular shadows.

2. The element of observer variability, by which one observer might have interpreted pulmonary line shadows as typical tubular shadows and another as normal vascular markings.

To reconcile this disturbing discrepancy and to reassess the overall accuracy of the roentgenologic diagnosis of chronic bronchitis, we undertook a study of the chest roentgenograms of approximately 300 men, made up of roughly equal numbers of normal subjects and patients with chronic obstructive pulmonary disease.[1870] Emphasis was placed on the thickness of bronchial walls visualized end-on in the parahilar zones, identified in roughly 80 per cent of both groups. Since a "tramline" represents a bronchus viewed longitudinally, roentgenographic visibility of this air-containing tube depends upon the absorptive power of its tissue in tangent (*see* Fig. 4–122, page 632). Therefore, because the image of the tangential wall thickness fades off at the margins, causing loss of definition, the *total* wall thickness cannot be accurately appreciated. However, when the bronchus is viewed end-on, in cross section, a substantially greater amount of tissue is traversed by the x-ray beam, particularly at the periphery, thus producing a sharp air-tissue interface and a well-defined margin. These end-on bronchi represent branches of the anterior or posterior segmental bronchi of the upper lobes or the superior segmental bronchi of the lower lobes (Fig. 11–61). They range in diameter from approximately 3 to 7 mm and thus represent different stages in bronchial subdivision. Their accompanying arteries are nearly always identifiable but, because of slight angulation, may not be sharply defined. Thickening of these bronchial shadows viewed end-on can usually be easily identified (*see* Fig. 4–121, page 631). In the study by Fraser and his coworkers,[1870] stepwise discriminant analysis of six variables showed that the median estimate of bronchial wall thickness was of some value in discriminating normal subjects from chronic bronchitics; however, the presence of thickening could not be used as an absolute criterion for the presence of chronic bronchitis, nor could its absence be construed as evidence against that diagnosis.

Prominent lung markings, or the "dirty chest," consist of a general accentuation of linear markings throughout the lungs. In a radiologic-pathologic correlative study of lungs obtained from consecutive autopsies, Feigin and Abraham[1871] found good correlation between the roentgenographic appearance of increased pulmonary markings and histologic evidence of edema, chronic inflammatory cell infiltration, and mild fibrosis in the perivenous interstitium. Although this roentgenographic sign is admittedly a very subjective finding, we consider it useful evidence in support of a diagnosis of chronic bronchitis. The appearance is similar to the "increased marking" pattern of emphysema (*see* page 2135), the major difference being the absence of pulmonary arterial hypertension and cor pulmonale in the uncomplicated chronic bronchitic.

In summary, it is emphasized that *chronic bronchitis is not a roentgenologic diagnosis*. Changes may be observed on the plain chest roentgenogram suggesting that bronchitis may be present, but it is inappropriate for the radiologist to do other than

indicate that the findings are compatible with or suggestive of that diagnosis. Estimation of wall thickness of bronchi visualized end-on in the parahilar zones can strengthen the conviction that chronic bronchitis is present.

Much has been written about the *bronchographic appearances* in chronic bronchitis. Although certain signs are virtually diagnostic, bronchography is indicated in patients with clinically suspected chronic bronchitis only to exclude potentially curable bronchiectasis. Not only does the instillation of contrast material significantly impair already disturbed pulmonary function (however temporarily),[1872, 1873] but the diagnostic yield is small or nil.

Emphysema

Traditionally, there have been three roentgenologic signs of emphysema:[1874] (1) excess air in the lungs; (2) alterations in the pulmonary vasculature (oligemia) and in some cases the cardiac contour; and (3) bullae. In 1970, however, Thurlbeck and his colleagues[1875] published a report that cast doubt on restricting the diagnosis to these three signs alone. They described 61 patients, the large majority of whom had morphologically proved emphysema, in whom clinical, pulmonary function, and roentgenologic data were correlated with morphologic findings and showed that application of only the three traditional roentgenologic criteria would have excluded almost half the patients with severe emphysema.

To be included in the survey, the cases had to meet the following criteria:

1. At least one lung had been adequately examined morphologically in the inflated state (one was a pneumonectomy specimen and all others were obtained at necropsy).

2. The patient had undergone complete pulmonary function testing.

3. There was no cardiac or pulmonary disease (other than emphysema, bronchitis, bronchiectasis, or asthma) likely to affect pulmonary function.

Roentgenograms of the chest in posteroanterior and lateral projection were available for all but three patients, who had only single roentgenograms in anteroposterior projection and in whom all parameters except overinflation could be evaluated. In addition, full lung tomograms obtained by a technique previously described[1876] were available in approximately half the cases and were included in the survey. These roentgenograms, together with chest roentgenograms of a similar number of necropsied patients (some with no chest disease and others with various pulmonary diseases), were given code numbers, randomized, and assessed by one of the authors on two occasions without knowledge of the function test or clinical or pathologic findings.

Four indices were assessed:

1. The degree of overinflation was graded on

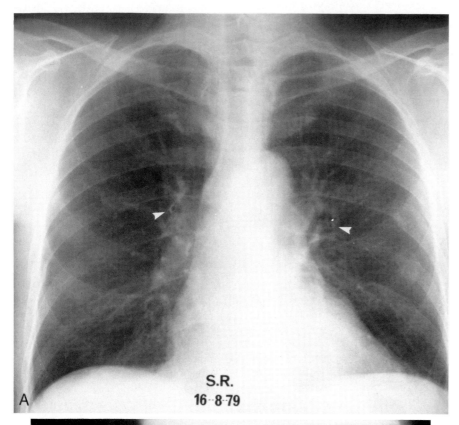

S.R.
16-8-79

A

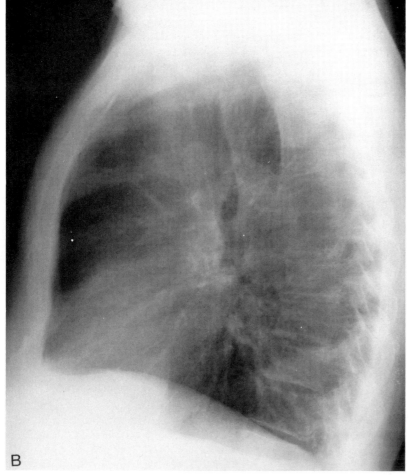

B

Figure 11–61. Chronic Bronchitis.
Posteroanterior *(A)* and lateral *(B)* chest roentgenograms reveal thickened bronchial walls viewed end-on in the right and left upper lobes *(arrowheads)*. Lung volume, vasculature, and cardiac size are normal. These features are compatible with chronic bronchitis.

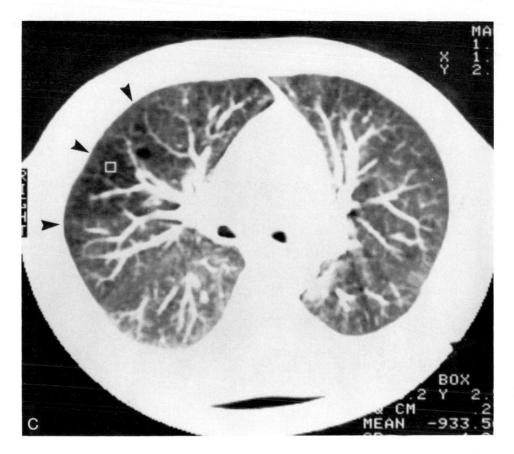

Figure 11–61. *Continued.* A CT scan through the upper lobes *(C)* is essentially normal except for a small area of oligemia in the anterolateral part of the right upper lobe *(arrowheads)*, suggesting a focal area of emphysema. The cursor box in the oligemic area revealed a CT density of −933 Hounsfield units (HU), some 90 HU lower than normal. The patient is a 58-year-old man with a 15-year history of chronic productive cough.

a scale of 0 to 4+ using the criteria of depression and flattening of the diaphragmatic domes, and increase in the depth of the retrosternal airspace as judged by the distance from the sternum to the shadow of the ascending aorta and by the point at which the heart shadow separated from the sternum.

2. The state of the peripheral vascular markings was recorded as normal, diminished, or accentuated.

3. Pulmonary arterial hypertension was determined by the single criterion of enlargement of the hilar pulmonary arteries.

4. Right ventricular enlargement was determined on the somewhat tenuous criteria of increased width of the cardiac silhouette, elevation of the apex of the heart, bulging of the anterior cardiac contour, and prominence of the main pulmonary artery segment.

A final opinion of whether there was roentgenologic evidence of emphysema was based on these four parameters.

As shown in Table 11–3, the morphologic appearance was normal in five of the 61 patients. Two patients had asthma, five bronchiectasis, and the other 49 had emphysema. The severity of the disease morphologically, measured by a modification of the Dunnill stratified random point count method,[1877, 1878] ranged from grade I to grade V, and the patients were grouped accordingly.

Table 11–3. Roentgenologic Findings in 61 Patients*

MORPHOLOGIC DIAGNOSIS		NUMBER	OVERINFLATION†	ARTERIAL HYPERTENSION	RIGHT VENTRICULAR HYPERTROPHY	EMPHYSEMA‡
No emphysema		5	0.4	0/5	0/5	0/5
Emphysema group	I	10	0.8	2/10	1/10	4/10
	II	7	1.6	3/6	2/5	4/7
	III	12	2.1	4/12	2/12	9/11
	IV	9	2.3	5/9	4/9	9/9
	V	11	3.0	9/11	9/11	11/11
Asthma		2	2.5	0/2	0/2	0/2
Bronchiectasis		5	1.8	3/4	3/4	3/4

*Modified slightly from Thurlbeck et al.[1875]
†Overinflation was estimated on a 0 to 4+ scale.
‡Diagnosis of emphysema includes both the arterial deficiency (AD) and increased markings (IM) patterns.

The roentgenographic appearance of *overinflation* correlated well with the severity of the emphysema, there being a steady increment throughout the group. It is of some interest that a highly significant relationship was found between the degree of overinflation assessed roentgenologically and values for TLC and RV obtained on pulmonary function testing. *Pulmonary hypertension* was absent in the patients without emphysema; it was thought to be present in one fifth of group I, in all but two patients in group V, and in roughly equal numbers totaling about half the patients in groups II, III, and IV. *Right ventricular hypertrophy* was absent in all patients without emphysema and present in one of ten patients in group I, in nearly all in group V, and in intermediate numbers in the other three groups.

Two different roentgenographic patterns of altered pulmonary vascularity were recognized and were designated "arterial deficiency" (AD) and "increased markings" (IM). AD represented peripheral vascular deficiency (oligemia), in most cases associated with severe overinflation, and IM indicated increased prominence of the vascular markings, almost invariably with milder overinflation. In the latter group, pulmonary arterial hypertension was evident in the great majority and cor pulmonale in many.

On the basis of these findings, the following correlations were established. None of the patients without emphysema was diagnosed as having the disease, and all patients in groups IV and V were diagnosed correctly. About half the patients in groups I and II and all but two in group III were considered to have the disease. It was thus apparent from this study that the roentgenologic diagnosis of emphysema is reasonably precise *provided that the disease is at least moderately advanced and that both the "arterial deficiency" and "increased markings" patterns are recognized.*

The "Arterial Deficiency" Pattern of Emphysema

The roentgenologic signs of the "arterial deficiency" (AD) pattern of emphysema make up the classic triad of overinflation, pulmonary oligemia, and bullae (*see* Fig. 11–63).

OVERINFLATION

Characteristically, the overinflation was of severe degree, usually 4+ and never less than 3+ (assessed on a scale of 0 to 4+). Regardless of which definition of emphysema is used, distention of distal air sacs beyond their normal size is a fundamental derangement. It is obvious, therefore, that pulmonary overinflation must be a major roentgenologic criterion although for reasons that we do not fully understand, overinflation can be minimal or absent altogether in occasional patients with established emphysema (Fig. 11–62). In addition, since overinflation is an integral part of certain other diseases, notably spasmodic asthma, this sign by itself is insufficient for definitive diagnosis unless the possibility of asthma can be excluded on the basis of history.

Probably the most dependable single piece of evidence of pulmonary overinflation is *flattening* of the diaphragmatic domes (Fig. 11–63). In the careful roentgenologic-pathologic correlative study by Nicklaus and his colleagues,[1879] of the five roentgenologic criteria employed, diaphragmatic flattening was the most accurate indicator of the presence of morphologic emphysema and gave rise to the least intra- and interobserver variation. As pointed out in Chapter 1, it is important to realize that the level of the diaphragm in relation to the rib cage may be misleading, since in normal subjects the diaphragmatic domes are usually depressed to the level of the eleventh rib posteriorly at full inspiration, a point below which it is uncommon to see the diaphragm even in advanced emphysema. Flattening of the domes, however, is a frequent although not invariable sign of significant emphysema, particularly of panacinar type; for example, Simon and his colleagues[1880] found that an occasional patient with severe airflow obstruction and a large TLC can show a normal position and configuration of the diaphragm roentgenographically. We find that if the configuration of the diaphragm is concave superiorly, the presence of emphysema is virtually certain, at least in adults (Fig. 11–63). (Severe overinflation of the lungs in children—from acute bronchiolitis, for example—may result in sufficient depression of the diaphragm to show a concave configuration superiorly.) Other traditional signs of overinflation include increase in the width of the retrosternal airspace (judged by the distance from the sternum to the shadow of the ascending aorta and by the point at which the heart shadow separates from the sternum), anterior bowing of the sternum, accentuation of the thoracic kyphosis, and horizontally inclined, widely spaced ribs.

However, the study by Thomson and his colleagues[1881] cast considerable doubt on the value of these signs in the assessment of overinflation. These authors reported a plethysmographic and roentgenographic study of 42 healthy volunteers with no known pulmonary disease and 24 patients with emphysema. Twenty-three measurements from posteroanterior and lateral roentgenograms were subjected to discriminant and regression analysis to discover which variables best distinguished normal from overinflated lungs. It was found that the best discriminant was the sum of the convexity of the right hemidiaphragm measured in both projections (determined by the distance from its secant to its highest point), a conclusion that is in accord with the observation that diaphragmatic flattening is the most reliable indicator of emphysema. In this study it was shown that some commonly used roent-

Text continued on page 2125

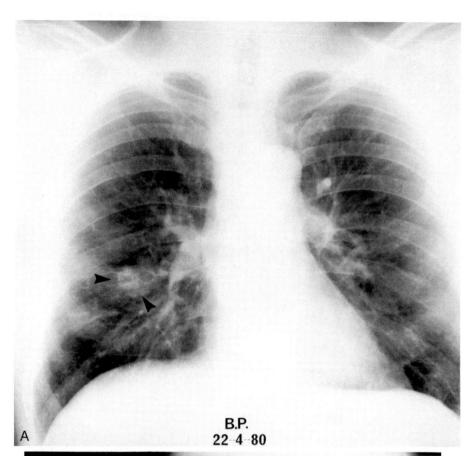

B.P.
22-4-80

A

Figure 11–62. Diffuse Emphysema Associated with Only Mild Overinflation. Posteroanterior *(A)* and lateral *(B)* chest roentgenograms reveal a mass *(arrowheads)* in the lateral segment of the middle lobe, subsequently proven to be a primary adenocarcinoma. Lung volume is only mildly increased as evidenced by the lateral projection. Apart from focal areas of oligemia (e.g., the right base and right upper lobe) and a curvilinear displacement of some vessels, the pulmonary vasculature is within normal limits.

Illustration continued on following page

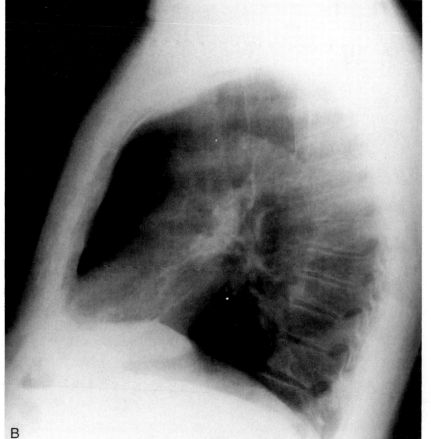

B

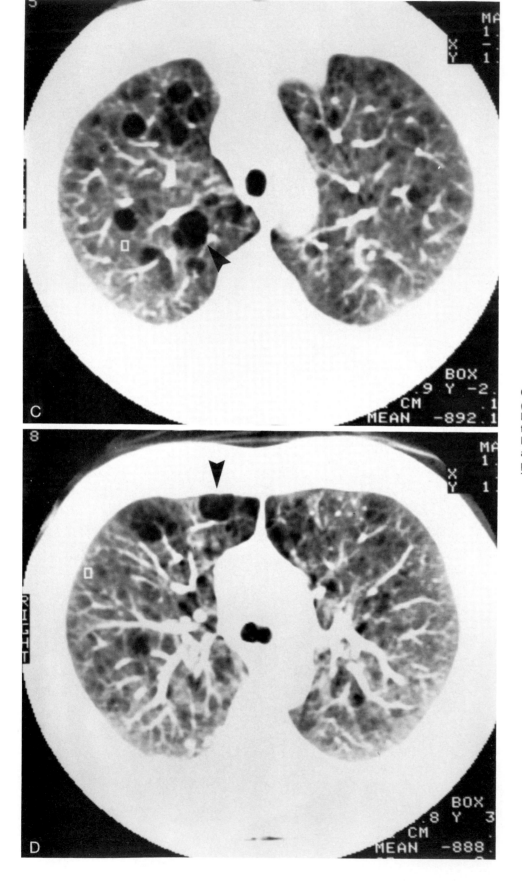

Figure 11–62. *Continued.* CT scans through the upper lobes *(C)*, hila *(D and E)*, and lower lobes *(F)* reveal several areas of typical emphysema (e.g., anterior lung zones in *E*), in some foci appearing as multiple central and peripheral bullae *(arrowheads)*. The patient is a 60-year-old man.

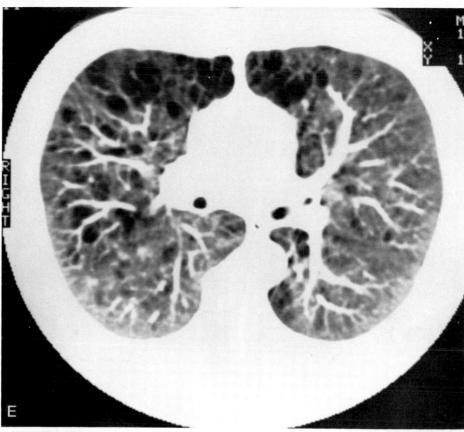

Figure 11–62 *Continued*

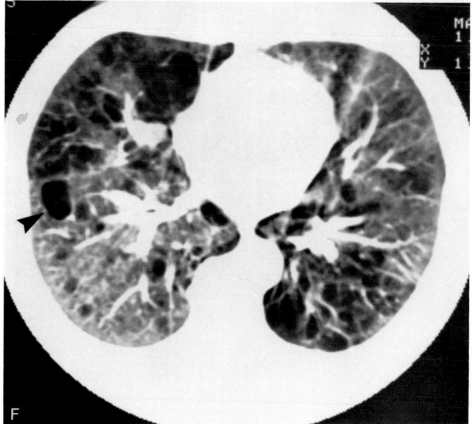

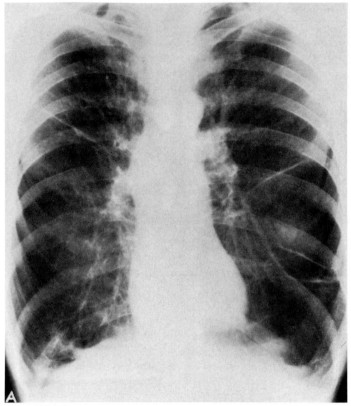

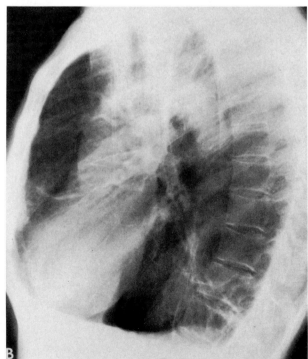

Figure 11–63. "Arterial Deficiency" (AD) Emphysema Associated with Bullae. Posteroanterior *(A)* and lateral *(B)* roentgenograms of a 43-year-old woman reveal severe overinflation of both lungs. The diaphragm is low and its superior surface concave. Note the prominent costophrenic muscle slips. The retrosternal airspace is deepened. The peripheral vasculature of the lungs is severely diminished, but, in contrast to the case illustrated in Figure 11–69, there is no evidence of pulmonary arterial hypertension. (It is probable that the upper lung zones are less severely involved than the lower, permitting redistribution of blood flow and a lack of any tendency for the development of hypertension.) Numerous bullae are present in both lower lung zones, particularly the left.

genologic criteria of pulmonary overinflation, such as the anterior rib count and the distance from the ascending aorta to the sternum, were poor discriminants of normal and overinflated lungs. By the authors' admission, the results of this study must be regarded as preliminary, and until more concrete data are provided it should be assumed that the roentgenographic assessment of overinflation other than that of severe degree is potentially inaccurate. By contrast with these results, in the study carried out by Nicklaus and coworkers,[1879] diaphragmatic flattening had a slight advantage over enlargement of the retrosternal space in terms of correctness of diagnosis and reproducibility. Simon and his coworkers[1880] found that the width of the retrosternal space had to be 4.5 cm or greater before it could be considered a reliable indicator of severe airway obstruction, and further, that when the space was this deep, the diaphragm was usually low and flat and the lungs oligemic.

Another criterion for pulmonary overinflation has been provided by Burki[1882] on the basis of the presence or absence of airflow *obstruction* (defined as FEV_1 at or below 70 per cent of the FVC). Of 189 patients referred to his laboratory for pulmonary function tests, 132 fulfilled this definition; correlating this finding with the changes on posteroanterior chest roentgenograms, he contended that the most obvious and simplest sign of the presence of airflow obstruction *(sic)* was a level of the right hemidiaphragm at or below the anterior end of the seventh rib (specificity 97 per cent). However, as pointed out by Pratt,[1883] Burki's results did not take into consideration the sensitivity of his criterion, which amounted to about 21 per cent (a false-negative rate of approximately 79 per cent). Pratt concluded that whereas chest roentgenograms provide useful information for the presence or absence of emphysema, they cannot reliably detect COPD.

In another study in which measurements from conventional chest roentgenograms in posteroanterior and lateral projection were compared with pulmonary function test values, Reich and his colleagues[1884] carried out statistical correlations in 104 men and found that two roentgenographic measurements were significantly correlated with abnormal function test values:

1. When the height of the arch of the right hemidiaphragm in lateral projection was 2.6 cm or less, it identified 67.7 per cent of all patients with abnormal pulmonary function tests and 78.3 per cent of patients with moderately or severely abnormal pulmonary function tests.

2. When the height of the right lung from the apex to the highest point on the right hemidiaphragm was 29.9 cm or more, it identified 69.8 per cent of all patients with abnormal pulmonary function tests and 79.7 per cent of patients with moderately to severely abnormal pulmonary function tests.

Although the authors use the term chronic obstructive pulmonary disease in their paper, we can assume that they were in fact evaluating the presence or absence of overinflation and thus of emphysema.

In addition to these static changes observed on standard posteroanterior and lateral roentgenograms exposed at TLC, air trapping constitutes an important sign in the assessment of patients with emphysema. Trapping may be visible fluoroscopically during deep respiration or on roentgenograms exposed at TLC and RV. With such procedures, diaphragmatic excursion may be seen to be restricted to one interspace or less (normally it occurs over two or three interspaces), and the normal reduction in lung translucency during expiration may be barely discernible. Limitation of diaphragmatic excursion provides convincing evidence for the presence of air trapping but is only an indirect indication of overinflation.

Roentgenographic techniques have been devised for the determination of lung volumes. The procedure originally described by Barnhard and his colleagues[1885] in 1960 produced results that correlated well with inert gas dilution techniques in healthy subjects and to a lesser degree in patients with emphysema. Using the same technique, Loyd and his colleagues[1886] found close correlation of roentgenographic measurements of TLC and those obtained in the body plethysmograph. In fact, the results obtained by the roentgenographic method were more accurate than were inert gas dilution techniques in the assessment of TLC in patients with emphysema. Glenn and Greene[1887] have developed a semiautomatic roentgenographic method utilizing a position transducer and a small computer that reduces the time for each determination to 1 minute; agreement with manual calculations in 80 controls and 80 patients with airways disease was excellent (average correlation coefficient, 0.9872). Although these special techniques are of interest and may be of value in selected cases, the information they provide does not appear to warrant their general use.

Patients in status asthmaticus may manifest severe overinflation of the lungs and roentgenologic changes indistinguishable from those seen in emphysema except for oligemia; some even show a concave configuration of the upper surface of the diaphragm (see Fig. 11–33, page 2063). Some authors have pointed out the possibility of confusing the "aged chest" with emphysema.[1888, 1889] In elderly persons the kyphotic curvature of the thoracic spine is greatly increased and excursion of the diaphragm is said to be reduced.[1888] However, in an analysis of chest roentgenograms of elderly patients, Simon[1890] found that the only constant roentgenographic abnormality was a loss of calcium in the bones. He concluded that air trapping and overinflation in the elderly are attributable to emphysema despite the rarity of this disease in persons over 75 years of age.

The development of left-sided heart failure in emphysematous patients with roentgenographic evidence of overinflation gives rise to a curious change in the chest roentgenogram. In addition to the usual evidence of interstitial pulmonary edema, the signs of overinflation may diminish or disappear altogether.[1874, 1891, 1892] Since roentgenologic signs of emphysema, particularly oligemia, are often more apparent in some lung zones than in others (lower lung zones are affected predominantly in many cases of emphysema), interstitial edema will be evident in those zones receiving the major blood flow; as a consequence, the edema is "inappropriately" distributed. Milne and Bass[1892] also found that left-sided heart failure has a marked effect on lung function by concealing evidence of overinflation and, in some cases, by improving diffusing capacity and flow rates.

ALTERATION IN PULMONARY VASCULATURE (OLIGEMIA)

Diminution in the caliber of the pulmonary vessels, with increased rapidity of tapering distally, is regarded by several investigators[1869, 1893–1896] as the most reliable roentgenologic sign of emphysema. However, in the study conducted by Nicklaus and his colleagues,[1879] attenuation of the pulmonary vasculature was recognized in a relatively small proportion of patients with moderate and severe emphysema and, as a sign of emphysema, yielded a fair number of false-positive diagnoses and showed poor intraobserver and interobserver reproducibility. In our experience, however, diminution of the peripheral vasculature is a sign of great value in differentiating emphysema from other diseases in which hyperinflation is an integral part, notably spasmodic asthma. This differentiation is particularly accurate if full lung tomography is employed in addition to standard roentgenograms of the chest.[1876, 1891, 1897] Of equal or greater importance in the identification of emphysema, demonstrable on both conventional roentgenograms and full-lung tomograms, are certain other vascular abnormalities, including amputation, side branch obliteration, and curvilinear displacement, the last-named serving to indicate the presence of otherwise invisible emphysematous spaces. Like others,[1898–1900] we have performed pulmonary angiography to assess fully the state of the pulmonary vascular tree. Although undoubtedly the contrast medium produces better visualization of the lung vasculature, we consider that this procedure provides little more information than can be deduced from full lung tomograms. It is perhaps significant that Nicklaus and his associates[1879] made their evaluation (intentionally) on the basis of standard chest roentgenograms without the benefit of tomography. Simon[1901] has emphasized the value of the "marker vessel" in the assessment of vascular loss in emphysema (Fig. 11–64). It is common for blood to be diverted from more severely affected zones to those least affected, producing dilatation of segmental vessels in either upper or lower zones. We agree that identification of marker vessels can be of assistance in diagnosis in some cases, but their presence was not specifically recorded in Thurlbeck and coworkers' study.[1875]

In a 1973 roentgenologic-physiologic study of 101 patients with chronic airflow obstruction, Simon and his colleagues[1880] found that when the roentgenogram showed widespread vascular attenuation as well as overinflation, the impairment in FEV_1 and other tests of pulmonary function was considerably more severe than when there was evidence of overinflation alone. Severe reduction in diffusing capacity was usually associated with changes in the pulmonary vessels. These observations were confirmed in a more recent study of 61 patients with chronic airflow obstruction on whom measurements of the diameter of midzonal pulmonary vessels on conventional chest roentgenograms were compared with values for diffusing capacity:[1902] the mean diameters of the vessels were 1.8 mm (0.4 mm SD) in the upper zone, 2.0 mm (0.4 mm SD) in the midzone, and 2.4 mm (0.4 mm SD) in the lower zone. A significant linear association ($p < 0.001$) was found to exist between the mean diameter of all vessels and the diffusing capacity of the lung.

From their study, Simon and his colleagues[1880] concluded that the radiologic diagnosis of widespread emphysema can be made with confidence only when there is attenuation of pulmonary vessels as well as evidence of overinflation. We feel that this conclusion is a bit conservative. If the presence of overinflation can be regarded as convincing evidence of loss of elastic recoil *in the absence of clinical evidence of asthma*, then this sign by itself should permit a confident diagnosis of emphysema. The *additional* finding of oligemia, either local or general, might then be construed as evidence of *severity* of the disease rather than simply of its presence.

In our experience, emphysema occurs more often in local form than is usually recognized. In one series, fully half of the 26 cases had peripheral vascular deficiency localized to one or more areas of both lungs, the vasculature in the remaining portions being normal or of increased caliber.[1876] In this series the lower lung zones were most predominantly involved (in ten of the 26 patients), although we have observed various patterns of localization to the upper lung zones, to one or two lobes of one lung (Fig. 11–65), or to different lobes in the two lungs, an irregularity of distribution that has been noted by others.[1903] A predominantly "medullary" pattern can also be seen occasionally (Fig. 11–66). The type of emphysema associated with alpha₁ PI deficiency (*see* page 2163) usually predominantly involves the lower lobes, with relatively normal vasculature in upper lung zones (Fig. 11–67).[1618, 1904, 1905] However, such anatomic predilection also is found in an appreciable number of patients with normal alpha₁ PI values.[1906] After excluding patients with

Text continued on page 2132

Figure 11–64. Severe Local Emphysema. A conventional posteroanterior chest roentgenogram *(A)* demonstrates marked oligemia and overinflation of the right lung and base of the left lower lobe. The appearance of the right lung could conceivably be caused by a giant bulla. The vessels in the upper two thirds of the left lung are dilated, indicating that this parenchyma is relatively devoid of emphysema. There is enlargement of the left hilum, whereas the right hilum is small and displaced inferiorly. A CT scan *(B)* through the upper lobes at the level of the azygos vein arch (AV) shows severe overinflation and oligemia of the right lower lobe (RL); note that thin attenuated vessels can be identified throughout the distended lobe, indicating diffuse emphysema rather than a bulla. Similar but much less pronounced changes are present in the left lower lobe (LL). The right upper lobe (RU) is compressed and displaced anteromedially. The vasculature in the left upper lobe (LU) is dilated and there is a diffuse increase in CT density of the parenchyma, resulting in complete effacement of the corticomedullary distinction.

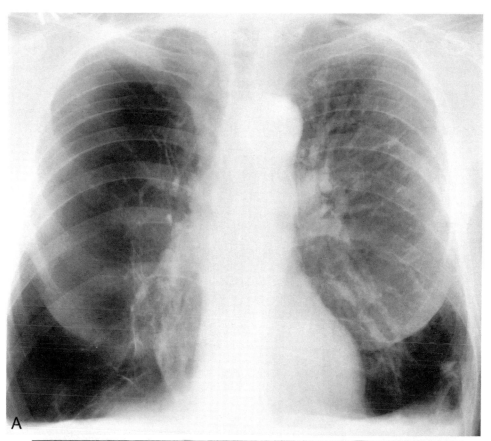

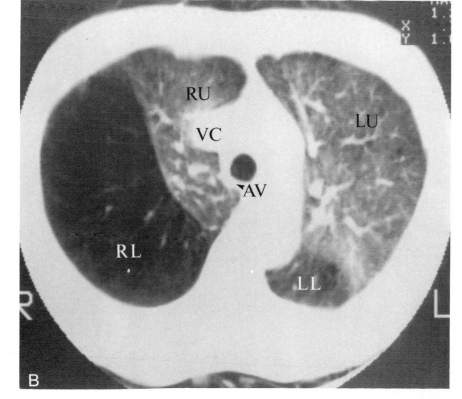

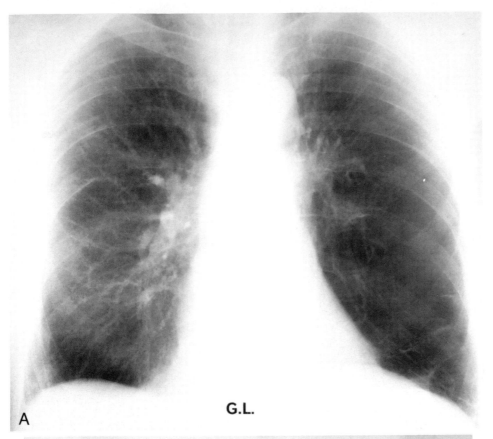

G.L.

A

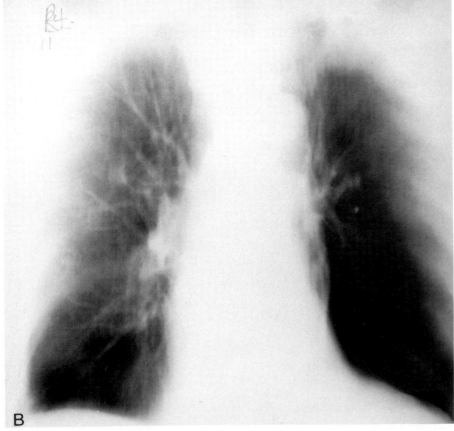

B

Figure 11–65. Emphysema: Unilateral Predominance. A posteroanterior chest roentgenogram *(A)* shows asymmetric transradiancy of the lungs, the left being more lucent than the right. Both lungs are hyperinflated. The left lung is severely oligemic as is the basal portion of the right lung. A full lung tomogram *(B)* confirms the asymmetric pattern of emphysema; note the larger vessels and background haze in the mid and upper zones of the right lung, signifying less severe emphysema. The patient is a 60-year-old man with a long history of cigarette use.

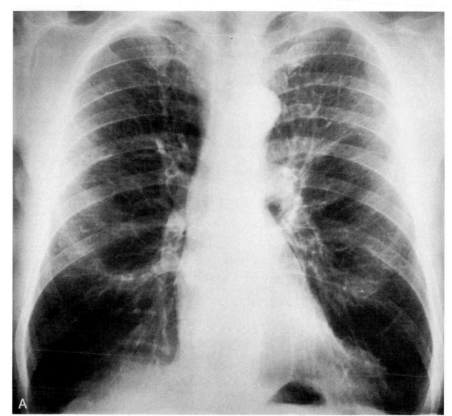

Figure 11–66. Diffuse Emphysema: "Medullary" Predominance. Posteroanterior *(A)* and lateral *(B)* chest roentgenograms show thickened bronchial walls, marked overinflation, and bilateral lower and right upper zonal oligemia. The findings are indicative of diffuse emphysema with lower lobe predominance.

Illustration continued on following page

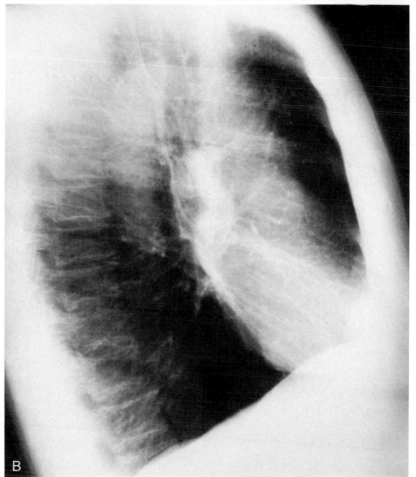

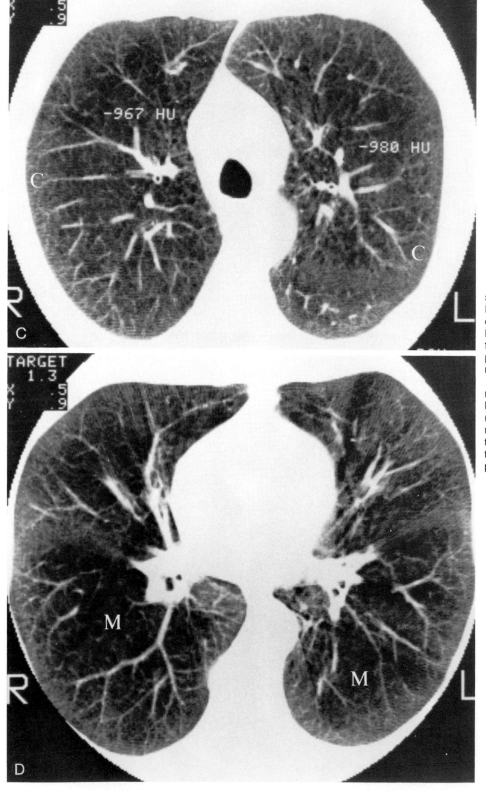

Figure 11–66. *Continued.* CT scans through the upper *(C)* and lower *(D)* lobes reveal diffuse low CT-density areas in the upper and lower lobes that is almost exclusively confined to the central (medullary [M]) portion of the lungs (cursor box measurements recorded values of −967 and −980 Hounsfield units, respectively, in the right and left lungs). Note the normal peripheral (cortical, C) vascularity that surrounds the abnormal lung. The patient is a 66-year-old man with a 10- to 15-year history of worsening dyspnea.

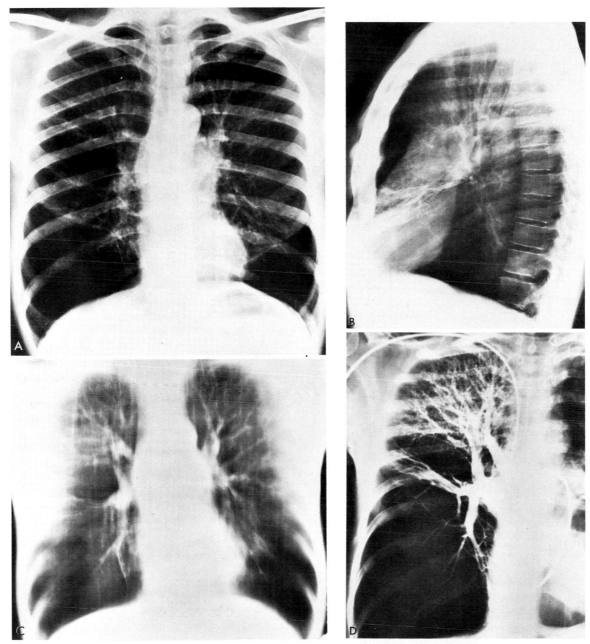

Figure 11–67. Emphysema Caused by Alpha₁-Antitrypsin Deficiency. A 47-year-old woman had noted increasing shortness of breath on exertion over the past few years. Roentgenograms of the chest in posteroanterior *(A)* and lateral *(B)* projections reveal marked overinflation of both lungs. The lower half of both lungs shows sparse vasculature and the vessels to the upper zones are more prominent than normal, indicating redistribution of flow. The vascular changes are particularly well seen on a full lung tomogram *(C)* and a pulmonary angiogram *(D)*.

alpha$_1$ PI deficiency, Martelli and associates[1907] correlated clinical and physiologic findings in cases manifesting predominantly upper and lower zone disease. They found that chronic bronchitis occurred with equal frequency in the two groups but that on average it had its onset about 10 years earlier in patients with lower zone oligemia. The group with lower lobe disease also manifested more severe airflow obstruction and more severe blood gas abnormalities. In contrast to patients with predominantly lower zone disease, a few patients with upper lobe emphysema were free from exertional dyspnea.

Xenon-133 studies of patients with pulmonary emphysema have confirmed the observation that destructive lung disease frequently is local rather than general[1908] and have shown excellent correlation with tomographic evaluation of regional perfusion distribution and quantitation.[1908–1910] In fact, some authors[1911, 1912] believe that ventilation-perfusion lung imaging is a more sensitive indicator of early COPD than are pulmonary function tests, ventilation being studied by radioaerosol and perfusion by either Xe or radioactive macroaggregated albumin.[1913] Levant and his colleagues[1914] carried out a comparative study in which the relative contributions of tomography, angiography, and radioactive isotopic techniques in the assessment of the microvascular circulation were compared. In general, the degree of tomographic "grayness" as a measure of microvascular circulation correlated well with angiographic microvascular blush in all lung zones and with radioactive xenon perfusion indices in severely affected lung zones. We find the estimation of tomographic "grayness" of value in estimating the extent of lung destruction in local emphysema, particularly when diminution of the peripheral vasculature is equivocal.

Computed tomography has also been found to be an accurate method of identifying zones of oligemia in patients with emphysema (Fig. 11–68): in a CT study of 53 patients with obstructive airway disease, Goddard and his colleagues[1915] found that alteration in the configuration of the pulmonary vasculature was manifested in three ways—pruning of small branches resulting in a simplified vascular tree with fewer orders of branching, distortion of blood vessels around areas of low attenuation value, and enlargement of the main pulmonary arteries. Areas of low attenuation value that were detected visually as ill-defined or well-defined regions of low density were considered to represent bullae.

In a more recent study in which CT was correlated with pulmonary function tests and conventional chest roentgenograms in 60 patients, Sanders and her colleagues[2759] found that CT was as sensitive as function tests and more sensitive than conventional roentgenograms in detecting emphysema. There was some evidence that CT might be more sensitive than function tests in the detection of mild emphysema. Others have also emphasized the value of high-resolution CT of the lungs in the evaluation of centrilobular emphysema.[1916–1918] However, CT is relatively insensitive in the detection of mild emphysema because most centriacinar and panacinar lesions less than 5 mm cannot be identified.[2795]

Pulmonary arterial hypertension secondary to emphysema usually is easily recognizable, not by a deficiency in the peripheral vasculature alone but with the additional finding of an increase in the size of the hilar pulmonary arteries. In cases in which previous films are available for comparison, such increase in size should be readily apparent; when no previous films exist, a diameter of the right interlobar artery exceeding 16.0 mm should be regarded as convincing evidence of pulmonary arterial hypertension. As noted above, peripheral arterial deficiency often is localized to certain areas of the lungs, vessels elsewhere being of normal or even increased caliber. In such cases usually the hilar arteries are of normal size, suggesting that the relatively uninvolved portions of the lungs are the sites of redistribution of blood flow, thus—at least temporarily—delaying the development of pulmonary arterial hypertension. In cases of general arterial deficiency when redistribution of blood flow to normal zones is impossible, the development of hypertension is evidenced by an increase in the size of the hilar arteries and a greater discrepancy in the caliber of central and peripheral vessels (Fig. 11–69). Tapering of arteries distally may be so striking as to constitute sufficient evidence of cor pulmonale despite a small cardiac size. It is well recognized that cor pulmonale cannot be appreciated in the majority of cases of emphysema unless cardiac failure has developed, since the heart shadow typically is long and narrow.[1874, 1893]

In fact, from a study of a large number of Mayo Veterans Hospital patients between the ages of 41 and 83, Wigh[1919] found that the probability of an individual without emphysema having a cardiothoracic ratio of 38 per cent or less was under 1 per cent; he considered this figure to constitute "microcardia," a condition that he feels should make one strongly suspect the presence of subclinical emphysema, even as an isolated sign. Despite Wigh's observation, it is noteworthy that in some cases of emphysema, notably of the "increased markings" variety (see farther on), evidence of cardiac enlargement and cor pulmonale may be convincing, particularly when serial roentgenograms are available for comparison.

Only very seldom is one able to observe the development of emphysema on serial roentgenograms over a period of years; we have seen only two patients in whom such changes were demonstrated convincingly.

BULLAE

Bullae are local, air-containing cystic spaces within the lung, ranging from 1 cm in diameter up

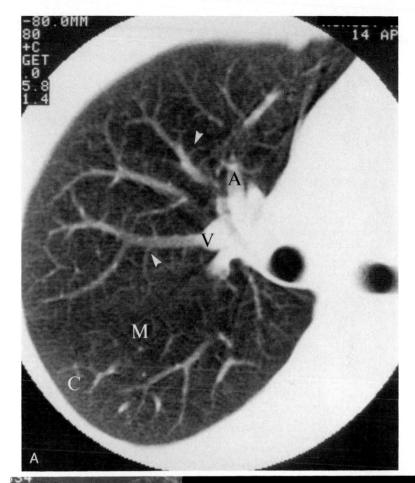

Figure 11–68. High-Resolution CT in Distinguishing Normal from Emphysematous Lung. A detail view of the right lung at the level of the carina from a high-resolution CT scan (A) is normal. Note the orderly regular and irregular dichotomous branching pattern of the arteries (A) and veins (V). Right angle branching (arrowheads) is termed "monopodial branching" and is strong evidence in favor of a normal vasculature. The peripheral cortex (C) possesses slightly higher CT density and is easily separated from the lower CT density of the medulla (M). A detail view from a high-resolution CT scan through the right lower lobe of a patient with emphysema (B) shows increased vessel tapering (1), increased branching angle (2), side branch obliteration (3), low-density cystic areas (4), and curvilinear vascular displacement (5), largely confined to the medulla. The cortex (C) has been largely spared of emphysema, creating a positive stripe sign. CT attenuation values in the medulla are abnormally low (−960 Hounsfield units). The patient is a middle-aged man with chronic dyspnea and nonproductive cough.

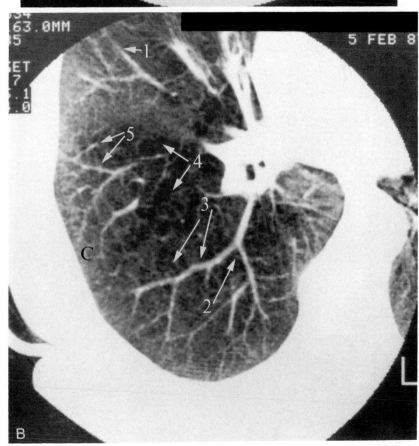

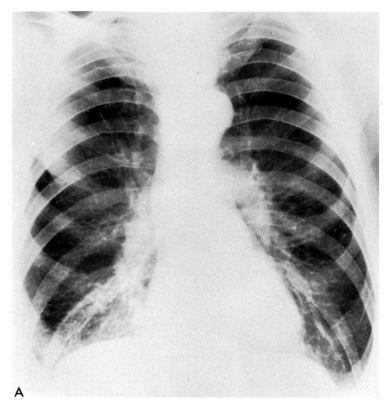

A

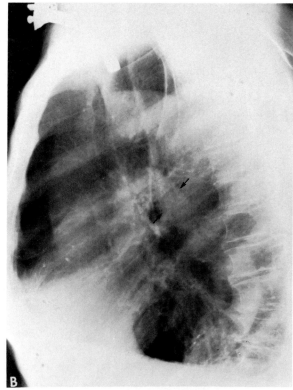

B

Figure 11–69. "Arterial Deficiency" (AD) Emphysema with Pulmonary Arterial Hypertension. Posteroanterior (A) and lateral (B) roentgenograms reveal severe overinflation of both lungs as evidenced by marked flattening of the diaphragm (seen to best advantage in lateral projection) and increase in the depth of the retrosternal airspace. The lungs generally are oligemic, arterial deficiency being more apparent in the upper two-thirds than in the bases. The hilar pulmonary arteries are moderately enlarged and taper rapidly distally. In lateral projection, note the shadow of the dilated descending branch of the left pulmonary artery (arrow). Despite the evidence of severe pulmonary arterial hypertension, the heart is only slightly enlarged. The patient is a 71-year-old man severely incapacitated by long-standing emphysema.

to the volume of a whole hemithorax. They may be single or multiple. Their walls are usually of no more than hairline thickness, so that it may be difficult to distinguish them from uninvolved parenchyma. In fact, Laws and Heard[1893] showed that frequently large bullae may be observed pathologically that are quite invisible roentgenologically, even in retrospect; such bullae were situated anteriorly or posteriorly (where their presence was masked by normal lung), or in the subpleural zone (where the absence of visible blood vessels prevented appreciation of vascular distortion).

Although bullae may occur in the absence of diffuse centrilobular or panlobular emphysema, their identification in a patient with other roentgenographic signs of pulmonary emphysema is of diagnostic value.[1874] When they occur as part of general panlobular or centrilobular emphysema, the diagnosis of bullous emphysema is only semantic; as pointed out by Bates and Christie,[2796] cystic spaces up to 1 cm in diameter are common in severe panlobular emphysema and whether they should be termed bullae or merely large emphysematous spaces is a matter of preference.

The "Increased Markings" Pattern of Emphysema

The roentgenographic appearance of "IM emphysema" is the antithesis of the AD pattern (Fig. 11–70). Instead of the vascular markings being attenuated and diminished in caliber as in Figure 11–71, they are more prominent than normal and tend to be irregular in contour and indistinct in definition. Thus, in contrast to the exceptionally clear lungs characteristic of "AD emphysema," the appearance is that of the "dirty chest" suggestive of some cases of severe chronic bronchitis. Overinflation seldom is present to the degree seen in AD disease and, in the majority of cases, is no more than slight or moderate. Pulmonary arterial hypertension (as evidenced by enlargement of the hilar pulmonary arteries) is invariable and in many cases is associated with cardiac enlargement (cor pulmonale); in fact, cardiac enlargement is a much more frequent feature of IM than of AD disease. Bullae seldom are seen. CT is sometimes capable of revealing abnormal vascular patterns, including sinuosity and tortuosity, amputation, side branch obliteration, increased branching angle, and curvilinear displacement (Fig. 11–72).

Significance of "Arterial Deficiency" and "Increased Markings" Patterns and Their Relationship to Panlobular and Centrilobular Emphysema

As pointed out by Thurlbeck and his colleagues[1875] in their report of 61 patients, the increased markings pattern of obstructive airway disease has complex connotations. However, their

study revealed that disregard of this pattern would result in lack of roentgenologic recognition of emphysema in a significant proportion of patients in whom severe disease would be diagnosed at necropsy. Prevalence of the AD and IM patterns was roughly similar in patients with severe emphysema, and it is clear that there is no absolute relationship to one type of morphologic disease (Fig. 11–73). However, of the 11 patients with the IM pattern, seven had CLE and only one had PLE (all had chronic bronchitis); and of the 20 patients with the AD pattern, only four had CLE, six had PLE, and the remainder were mixed. Frequency of the IM pattern appeared to increase with severity of the emphysema. In groups IV and V the IM pattern was seen in seven cases, classic AD in eight, and a mixed pattern in five. Also, pulmonary arterial hypertension and cor pulmonale were more likely to develop in association with the IM than with the AD pattern. Thus, although the relationships are by no means definitive, and the designations represent the two ends of a wide spectrum, there is some indication that *patients who manifest the arterial deficiency pattern roentgenographically have panlobular emphysema morphologically and that those who show the increased markings pattern have centrilobular emphysema.* Extending this relationship to the clinical presentation and employing the terms coined by Dornhorst,[1920] patients with the AD pattern present as "pink puffers" and those with the IM pattern as "blue bloaters." Supporting the relationship between the AD pattern and PLE is the observation that patients with either Swyer-James syndrome or alpha$_1$-antitrypsin deficiency manifest an arterial deficiency pattern roentgenographically and have panlobular emphysema morphologically.[1921, 1922]

Despite the similarity between the "dirty chest" appearance of chronic bronchitis and the classic appearance of the IM pattern with attendant pulmonary arterial hypertension and cor pulmonale, we have only rarely seen a transition from one to the other in our patients (Fig. 11–74). It is conceivable that the IM pattern is due, at least in part, to the "inflammatory changes" described by Burrows and associates[1923] or the "recurrent bronchopneumonitis" reported by Milne and Bass[1924] based on pathologic evidence provided by Reid.[1925, 1926] Their roentgenologic criteria for the diagnosis of "recurrent bronchopneumonitis" include tortuosity, marginal blurring and segmentation of the vasculature, enlargement of the central arteries, patchy interstitial fibrosis, and loss of vascular lability. The irregularity and slight tortuosity of the peripheral pulmonary vessels are stated to be affected by contiguous areas of fibrosis and by arteriolar endarteritis obliterans. These changes (which the authors state occur predominantly at the lung bases) may be associated with both hypoventilation and hypoperfusion, with the result that blood flow is diverted from these areas to upper lung zones. It appears probable that the "recurrent bronchopneumonitis"

Text continued on page 2143

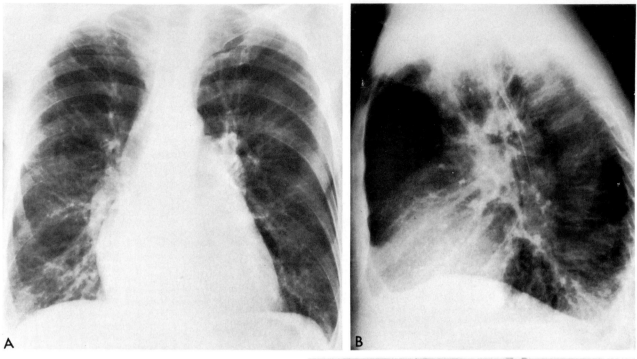

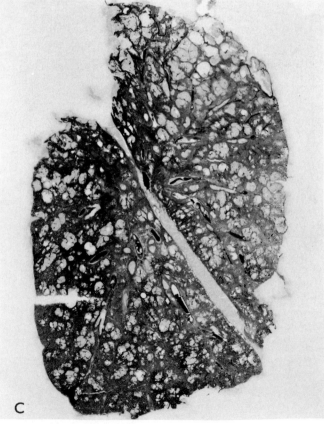

Figure 11–70. "Increased Markings" (IM) Emphysema. Roentgenograms of the chest in posteroanterior *(A)* and lateral *(B)* projections reveal only slightly increased volume (note the deep retrosternal airspace). The vascular markings throughout the lungs are prominent except in the subapical zones, where there appears to be local vascular deficiency. The heart is moderately enlarged (consistent with right ventricular enlargement) and the hilar pulmonary arteries dilated, indicating the presence of pulmonary arterial hypertension. At necropsy, the lungs were found to be extensively involved by emphysema, which was almost purely centrilobular in type (as revealed on a paper-mounted section of lung in *C).*

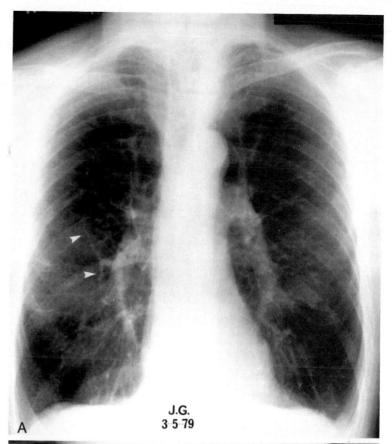

J.G.
3·5·79

Figure 11–71. Diffuse Emphysema: The "Arterial Deficiency" Pattern. Posteroanterior *(A)* and lateral *(B)* chest roentgenograms reveal typical features of diffuse, severe emphysema including marked overinflation, widespread oligemia, and vascular abnormalities consisting of increased attenuation, amputation, side branch obliteration, and curvilinear displacement *(arrowheads)*. The last-named indicates the presence of an otherwise invisible bulla. Although heart size is normal, enlargement of the hilar arteries is consistent with the presence of precapillary hypertension.

Illustration continued on following page

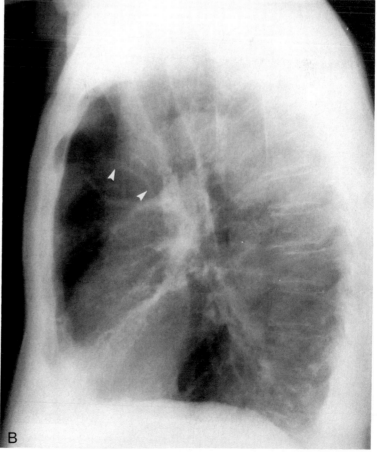

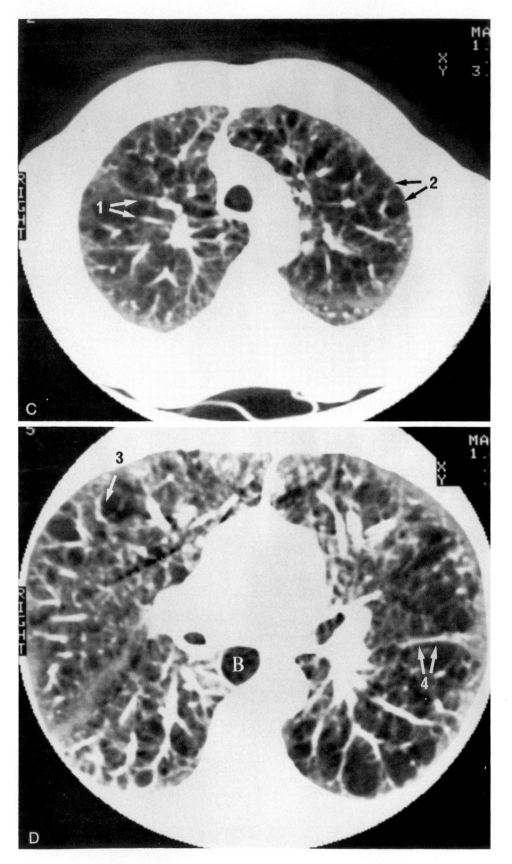

Figure 11–71. *Continued.* CT scans through the upper lobes *(C)* and mid-lung zones *(D)* demonstrate attenuated and amputated vessels *(1)*, cystic emphysematous spaces *(2)*, curvilinear displacement *(3)*, and side branch obliteration *(4)*. A bulla (B) is present in the azygoesopheageal recess. The patient is a 60-year-old man.

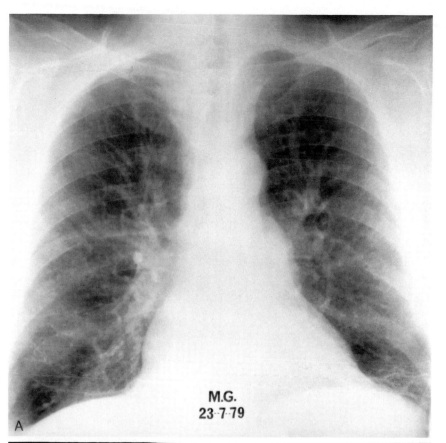

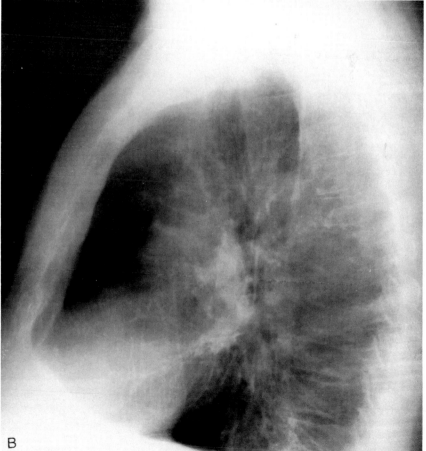

Figure 11–72. Diffuse Emphysema: The "Increased Markings" Pattern. Posteroanterior *(A)* and lateral *(B)* chest roentgenograms reveal moderate overinflation, bilateral upper zonal oligemia, and bronchial wall thickening. Mid and lower lung vessels are more prominent than normal, and the enlarged cardiac silhouette possesses a configuration consistent with cor pulmonale.

Illustration continued on following page

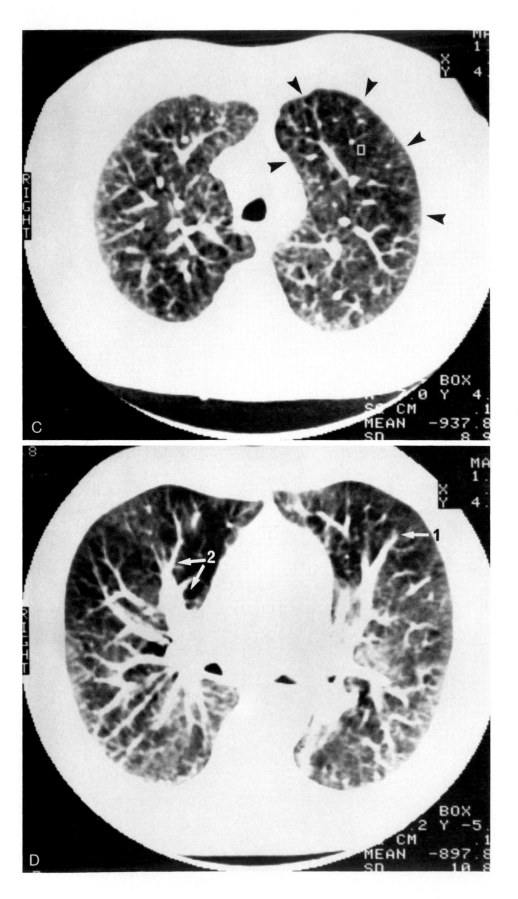

Figure 11–72. *Continued.* CT scans through the upper lobes *(C)*, hila *(D)*, and lower lobes *(E)* show dilated central and midlung vessels. Low-density oligemic areas are rather sparse *(between arrowheads)*, and some vessels appear amputated *(1)*, attenuated *(2)*, or displaced *(3)*. The cursor box in the right lower lobe shows an abnormally low CT density (−938 Hounsfield units). The patient is a 55-year-old-man with chronic cough and dyspnea.

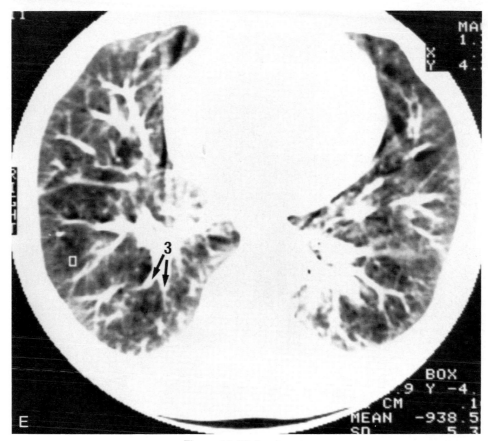

Figure 11–72 *Continued*

Radiologic	EMPHYSEMA GROUP						Bronch-	Asthma
Diagnosis	O	I	II	III	IV	V	iectasis	
No Emphysema	OOOO O	MMMP CC	UCC	CC			M	OO
AD		MPC	MU	MMMP PPC	MUC	MMPP C	M	
AD/IM				M	MPCC	M		
IM		M	CC	P	CC	MUCC C	PC	
?IM				P				

Figure 11–73. The Roentgenologic Diagnosis of Emphysema Compared with the Severity and Type of Disease Found Morphologically. AD = arterial deficiency pattern; IM = increased markings pattern; AD/IM = mixed pattern; ? — doubtful; C = centrilobular emphysema; P = panlobular emphysema; M = mixed emphysema; U = unclassified emphysema; O = no emphysema. (Reprinted from Thurlbeck WM, Henderson JA, Fraser RG, Bates DV: Medicine *49*:81, 1970, with permission of the authors and editor.)

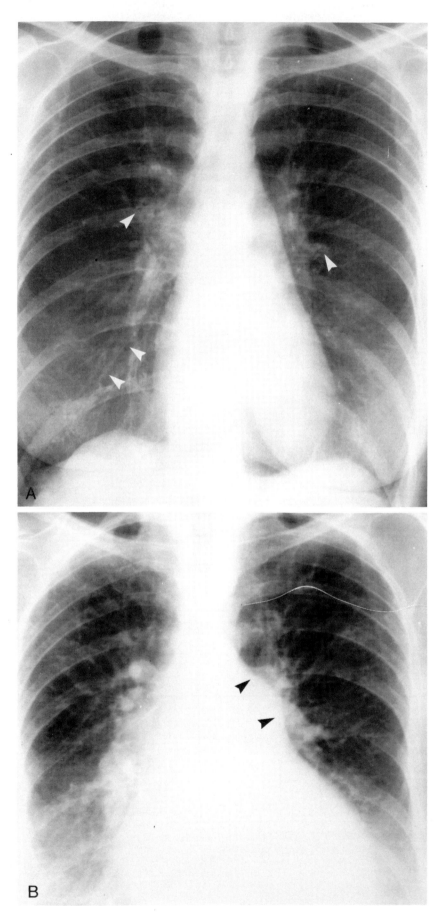

Figure 11-74. Diffuse Emphysema: Progression to Biventricular Failure. A posteroanterior chest roentgenogram *(A)* shows moderate to severe overinflation, bronchial wall thickening *(arrowheads)*, and diffuse oligemia. Hilar pulmonary arteries are borderline normal in size. These features indicate the presence of chronic bronchitis and emphysema. Nine years later, a posteroanterior roentgenogram *(B)* demonstrates marked nonspecific cardiomegaly. The main pulmonary artery *(arrowheads)* and hilar arteries have become markedly dilated as a result of pulmonary arterial hypertension and there has developed diffuse interstitial pulmonary edema. The combination is virtually diagnostic of biventricular decompensation, presumably secondary to severe chronic bronchitis and emphysema. The patient is a 60-year-old woman.

of Milne and Bass is equivalent to IM emphysema, although there is some question in our minds as to whether the roentgenographic pattern can be attributed to the specific pathologic changes they describe.

Other possibilities have been suggested as the morphologic basis for this pattern. In a review of the roentgenographic features of chronic obstructive pulmonary disease, Heitzman and his colleagues[1927, 1928] describe and illustrate a patient who showed a typical IM roentgenographic pattern during life and whose lung at necropsy revealed gross bronchial dilatation and a pulmonary arterial tree whose branches were of large caliber out to the periphery of the lung. They speculate that one or both of these abnormalities could have contributed to the prominence of lung markings, and this explanation appears perfectly valid in this patient. However, since bronchiectasis was not a prominent feature of most of the cases with the IM pattern described by Thurlbeck and associates,[1875] it might be concluded that the vascular nature of the shadows would be the more likely explanation in that group. In fact, Scarrow[1898] has documented dilatation of intrapulmonary branches of the pulmonary artery in some cases of chronic obstructive pulmonary disease.[1929] An alternative—or perhaps additional—explanation for the IM pattern exists in the possibility of cardiac decompensation and pulmonary edema. Since publication of Thurlbeck and associates' correlative study in 1970,[1875] we have seen a few patients in whom the severity of the typical IM pattern appeared to lessen with bed rest and therapy directed toward cardiac decompensation. This suggests that interstitial pulmonary edema might have contributed to the prominence of bronchovascular markings, although specific evidence of interstitial pulmonary edema—such as septal lines—was observed in few of these cases. Despite this improvement, however, lung markings never returned to normal and the pattern did not change to the AD type. It is possible that these patients had left-sided cardiac decompensation resulting from chronic hypoxemia or unrelated cardiac disease, but it is not known whether pulmonary venous hypertension or interstitial edema contributed to the increased markings pattern.

Accuracy of the Roentgenologic Diagnosis of Emphysema

As there is no unanimity about the diagnostic criteria for emphysema during life, we must rely on studies that relate emphysema identified at necropsy to roentgenographic appearances.[1834, 1875, 1893, 1930–1932] All such reports agree that whatever the criteria used, severe morphologic emphysema is usually diagnosed roentgenologically and normal or mildly affected lungs are usually considered free of the disease. In the study by Nicklaus and his colleagues,[1834] overinflation was the most accurate indicator of emphysema, whereas alteration in the peripheral vasculature—a sign considered of great importance and accuracy in several other roentgenologic-pathologic studies including our own—was observed in a relatively low proportion of patients with moderate or severe emphysema. By contrast, in the series by Thurlbeck and colleagues,[1875] the use of only the overinflation criterion would have resulted in a false-positive diagnosis in two cases and failure to distinguish asthma from emphysema in two others. Unfortunately, patients with asthma were excluded from some of the earlier reported studies; if they had been included, some false diagnoses of emphysema might have been made.

Perhaps the definitive study on the accuracy of the roentgenologic diagnosis of emphysema was carried out by Thurlbeck and Simon,[1933] who performed a roentgenologic-pathologic correlative study of 696 patients from whose lungs paper-mounted, whole-lung sections were available; however, only about 250 of these could be thoroughly evaluated because of unsatisfactory roentgenograms. The major roentgenographic criterion employed for the presence of emphysema was arterial deficiency, although other signs, including diaphragm level and the depth of the retrosternal space, were also used as ancillary features. Only occasionally were patients without emphysema or with mild emphysema thought to have the disease based on roentgenologic evidence. Of the patients with moderately severe and severe emphysema, 41 per cent were diagnosed as having the disease, as were two thirds of those with the most severe grade of emphysema. Centrilobular disease was usually present when emphysema was diagnosed roentgenologically in upper lung zones, as was panacinar disease when emphysema was diagnosed in lower zones. No combination of roentgenologic variables, including those generally accepted as indicating overinflation, was found that recognized emphysema better than the subjective diagnosis of the disease based on arterial deficiency.

On the strength of his belief that conventional chest roentgenograms can be reliably interpreted both for diagnosis and for exclusion of pulmonary emphysema,[1934] Pratt has taken issue with the conclusions reached by Thurlbeck and Simon,[1935] pointing out that the emphasis placed on arterial deficiency as the single criterion for the diagnosis of emphysema gave short shrift to the importance of pulmonary overinflation. In addition, he criticized the method by which the presence or absence of overinflation was estimated (simple measurement of diaphragm level and retrosternal space) rather than including diaphragmatic configuration, as has been customary in several previous studies. We are inclined to agree with Pratt's views that despite the somewhat discouraging results obtained by Thurlbeck and Simon, the roentgenologic diagnosis of emphysema can be made with a high degree of confidence in the presence of moderate or advanced disease.

It should be borne in mind that roentgenography may reveal emphysema that is not apparent clinically. For example, Sutinen and his associates[1930] recognized 13 of 19 patients with morphologically proven emphysema that had not been diagnosed clinically and whose lungs did not show evidence of gross expiratory airway obstruction during postmortem pulmonary function testing.

It is apparent from the Thurlbeck study of 61 patients[1875] that the roentgenologic diagnosis of emphysema is reasonably precise *provided that both IM and AD patterns are recognized.* None of the seven patients without emphysema was diagnosed as having the disease, and all who had more than 15 units of emphysema (groups IV and V) were recognized roentgenologically. Of the 28 patients in the intermediate groups I, II, and III, 17 (60 per cent) were recognized by our roentgenologic criteria as having emphysema. Why the diagnosis was not made in the remaining 40 per cent is not clear; possibly it was related to the lack of convincing evidence of pulmonary arterial hypertension, since such evidence constitutes an important criterion in the diagnosis of emphysema of the IM type.

In summary, the roentgenologic signs of morphologically proven emphysema consist of two distinctly different patterns, "arterial deficiency" and "increased markings." Provided that both patterns are recognized, the roentgenologic diagnosis of emphysema is highly accurate in cases of severe disease and reasonably precise in those of less severity. If only the traditional roentgenologic criteria of emphysema are recognized—general pulmonary overinflation and pulmonary oligemia—many patients with severe emphysema will not be recognized, including those with clear-cut evidence of pulmonary hypertension and cor pulmonale.

The terms "emphysema" and "chronic bronchitis" mean different things to different people. For example, Fletcher and his colleagues[1936] found an almost identical spectrum of diseases in an "emphysema clinic" in Chicago and a "chronic bronchitic" clinic in London. The euphemistic terms "pink puffer" and "blue bloater" applied by Dornhorst[1920] to patients, who manifest predominantly emphysematous and chronic bronchitic characteristics, respectively, describe two ends of a spectrum between which are the majority of patients, who manifest elements of both. If the selection of a therapeutic regimen depends in part on the categorization of a patient into one or other of these two types, as has been suggested,[1937] the radiologist should recognize changes appropriate to each type and describe them in a manner clearly understood not only by the referring physician but by his radiologist-colleagues.

The confusion existing in the radiologic literature derives not from the "classic" picture of emphysema—marked pulmonary overinflation and oligemia—but from the picture designated as the IM pattern of disease. Evidence that the classic pattern is caused by morphologic emphysema is undisputed and it is appropriate for the radiologist to make the diagnosis of *emphysema* in the presence of such findings.[1938] In the case of the IM pattern, however, the position is not nearly as clear-cut. Whether or not the pathophysiology of this disease is related to the presence of emphysema is disputable. Reid[1939–1941] has stated that CLE is not associated with roentgenologic abnormality, whereas others, including ourselves, have found the contrary,[1834, 1875, 1893, 1930–1932] *a discrepancy due to differences in morphologic rather than roentgenologic interpretation.* It is almost certain that patients categorized by us as having the IM pattern are similar or identical to the British "chronic bronchitic with cardiac decompensation."[1875] Which label one wishes to place on this roentgenographic pattern of disease is probably more of semantic than of practical importance, although logically it must be differentiated from the classic AD pattern. Its morphologic and physiologic characteristics require clarification by the pathologist and physiologist and need not engender dispute among radiologists, a point of view with which Simon[1901] enthusiastically concurs. Since there is a general agreement that *all* patients with this clinical and roentgenologic characterization are severe chronic bronchitics,[1875, 1901] it is recommended that this roentgenographic pattern of obstructive airway disease be designated "the chronic bronchitic pattern with arterial hypertension."

Airway Dynamics in Obstructive Airway Disease

It has been established that the morphologic common denominator of obstructive airway disease is organic obstruction of small airways and that extensive involvement may cause no detectable change in total airway resistance. In the seven excised lungs with various grades of emphysema studied bronchographically and morphologically by Hogg and his colleagues,[1799] the small bronchi and bronchioles were extensively inflamed and were partially or totally occluded by mucous plugs (both potentially reversible). The fixed obstructions consisted of distorted and narrowed small airways with fibrous obliteration (irreversible changes). Determination of the pathogenesis of these extensive morphologic abnormalities may lie in a study of the means by which the lung rids itself of mucus. In the normal lung, mucus is swept up the tracheobronchial tree by ciliary action; cough is a reserve mechanism that operates only when mucus production increases and overwhelms the capacity of cilia to remove it (as in acute bronchitis) or when ciliary function is impaired (as in heavy smokers). In chronic bronchitis, both situations pertain and cough becomes essential for clearance of mucus. Since impairment of the cough mechanism results in the retention of secretions, if a mechanism impairing the effectiveness of cough could be demonstrated, a hypothesis for the development of obstructive disease in small airways might be proposed. Such a possibility exists in the area of bronchial dynamics.

It has long been known that in normal subjects an airflow obstruction that is absent during inspiration develops during forced expiration; this is caused by airway compression when pleural exceeds atmospheric pressure.[1942-1950] In certain pulmonary diseases, notably emphysema, this expiratory obstruction is much more marked and, in fact, may cause severe respiratory disability and even fatal impairment of ventilation. Attempts to locate the site of obstruction,[1787, 1788, 1951-1953] using measurements of bronchial pressure, with and without roentgenographic measurements of bronchial caliber, have suggested a mechanism of obstruction.

It has been recognized for many years, both roentgenologically and bronchoscopically, that the proximal large bronchi collapse disproportionately during forced expiration and cough in patients with obstructive airway disease, particularly emphysema,[1955-1957] and it has been suggested that this collapse may represent the pathogenetic mechanism of expiratory airway obstruction in these diseases. These changes were quantified in a cinebronchographic study of ten normal subjects and 22 patients with obstructive airway disease (five with spasmodic asthma, nine with chronic bronchitis, and eight with emphysema).[1951] The maximal inspiratory and minimal expiratory calibers of five divisions of the right bronchial tree (or four of the left) were measured during quiet respiration and during forced expiration and coughing. In the normal subjects, the calibers of all bronchi reduced roughly equally during coughing, from a maximum at the height of

inspiration to a minimum at the end of expiration (Fig. 11–75). By contrast, in the patients with chronic bronchitis or emphysema forced expiration caused a disproportionate collapse of the large proximal bronchi, particularly the main bronchi of the lower lobes. Caliber reduction averaged 67 per cent compared with 49 per cent in the normal subjects (Figs. 11–76 and 11–77). At the moment that a lower lobe bronchus collapsed, the segmental and subsegmental airways distal to the collapsing segment responded in one of two ways: in some patients the reduction was roughly normal, averaging 60 per cent of maximal inspiratory caliber, but in others it amounted to little more than 40 per cent. The significance of this different response of the segmental and subsegmental bronchi will become clear later.

At about the same time, in a study of six normal subjects and 14 patients (seven with emphysema, two with chronic bronchitis, and five with asthma), Macklem and Wilson[1788] had determined the pressure drop down the bronchial tree from direct measurements of esophageal and bronchial pressures (Fig. 11–78). In the normal subjects, pressure decreased regularly from alveolus to mouth, as down an unobstructed tube. In the patients with chronic bronchitis or emphysema, however, there was a large pressure drop across the lobar bronchus indicating obstruction at that point. Since expiratory obstruction produced by the lower lobe bronchus had been demonstrated independently by cinefluorographic and manometric studies, simultaneous cinebronchography and manometry were necessary to integrate the findings by the two techniques.

Figure 11–79 depicts simultaneous measurements of bronchial pressures and dimensions in a

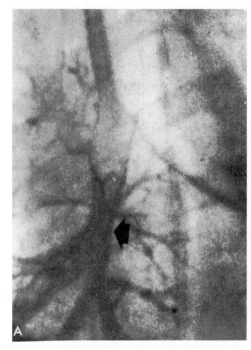
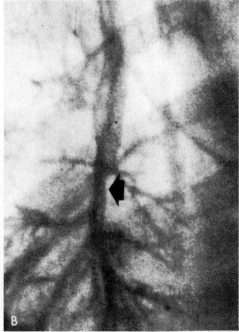

Figure 11–75. Bronchial Dynamics in a Normal Subject. Selected frames from cinestrips of a right bronchogram of a normal subject. The frame on the left (A) shows maximal caliber on full inspiration and that on the right (B) minimal caliber on forced expiration. The lower lobe bronchus is indicated by arrows. Note the roughly proportional reduction in caliber of all airways on expiration. Compare with Figures 11–76 and 11–77. (Reprinted from Fraser RG, Macklem PT: Frontiers of Pulmonary Radiology. New York, Grune & Stratton, Inc, 1969, p 76, with permission of the authors and publishers.)

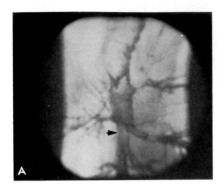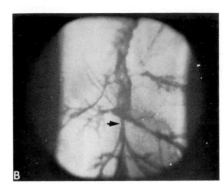

Figure 11–76. Bronchial Dynamics in Chronic Bronchitis. Selected frames from a cinebronchographic study of the right bronchial tree of a patient with chronic bronchitis show a normal appearance of the major bronchi at TLC *(A)*. During forced expiration *(B)*, the lower lobe bronchus *(arrow)* collapsed, its minimal diameter being approximately 15 per cent of the caliber at full inspiration. This disproportionate collapse resulted in air trapping distally.

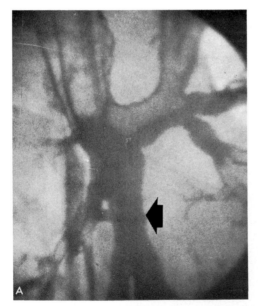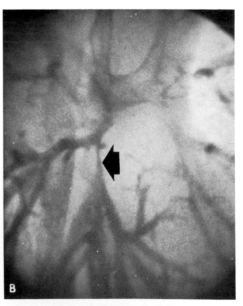

Figure 11–77. Bronchial Dynamics in Emphysema. Selected frames from a cinebronchogram of a patient with advanced emphysema reveal a normal configuration and caliber of the central bronchi at total lung capacity *(A)*. During forced expiration *(B)*, the lower lobe bronchus *(arrow)* collapsed abruptly, reducing its caliber from 11 to 1.5 mm. (Reprinted from Fraser RG, Macklem PT: Frontiers of Pulmonary Radiology. New York, Grune & Stratton, Inc, 1969, p 76, with permission of the authors and publishers.)

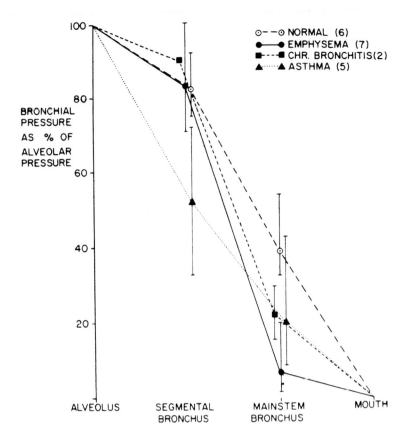

Figure 11–78. Pressure Drop Down the Bronchial Tree. The mean pressure drop down various segments of the bronchial tree from the alveolus to the mouth of six normal subjects, seven patients with emphysema, two with chronic bronchitis, and five with asthma. See text for description. (Reprinted from Fraser RG, Macklem PT: Frontiers of Pulmonary Radiology. New York, Grune & Stratton, Inc, 1969, p 76, with permission of the authors and publishers.)

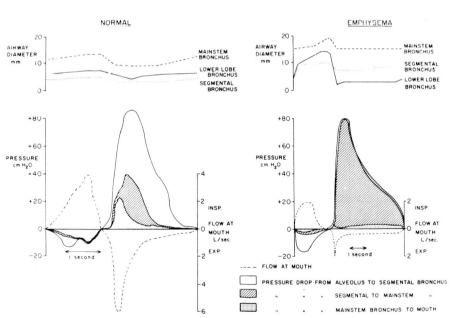

Figure 11–79. Simultaneous Measurements of Bronchial Pressures and Dimensions in a Normal Subject (Left) and a Patient with Emphysema (Right). Alveolar pressure, bronchial pressure, flow at the mouth, and airway diameters in a normal subject and a patient with emphysema during a single forced inspiration and expiration. These tracings were obtained with two bronchial pressure catheters in place, one immediately proximal and one immediately distal to the lower lobe bronchus. The two lower graphs show recordings of flow at the mouth *(dotted line)*, alveolar pressure, and the two bronchial pressures during inspiration and during forced expiration. Simultaneous measurements of bronchial diameters of the mainstem, lower lobe, and segmental bronchi are shown above. The clear area represents decrease in pressure from the alveolus to the segmental bronchus; the shaded area is the decrease from the segmental bronchus through the lower lobe bronchus to the mainstem bronchus; and the dotted area is the increase in pressure from the mainstem bronchus to the mouth. See text for description. (Reprinted from Fraser RG, Macklem PT: Frontiers of Pulmonary Radiology. New York, Grune & Stratton, Inc, 1969, p 76, with permission of the authors and publishers.)

normal subject and in a patient with emphysema during a single forced inspiration and expiration. Several alterations are apparent in the recordings of the emphysema patient:

1. Flows are much less, even though the pressure producing the flow (alveolar pressure) is almost the same as in the normal subject; thus resistance is much greater.

2. The lower lobe bronchus collapses so markedly during forced expiration that its caliber becomes less than that of the distal segmental bronchi; thus the lower lobe bronchus appears to constitute a discrete obstruction.

3. The lower lobe bronchus collapses simultaneously with an abrupt change in the expiratory flow curve from acceleration to deceleration.

4. The decrease in pressure across the lower lobe bronchus during expiration amounts to almost the total pressure drop from alveolus to mouth, whereas in the normal subject it represents only a relatively small proportion.

5. During inspiration, as the bronchial tree dilates, the lower lobe bronchus no longer obstructs flow and all obstruction is in the small airways.

We can conclude that this patient has two levels of obstruction—one in the small airways and the other in the lower lobe bronchus, the latter being present only during forced expiration under circumstances of dynamic compression. Similar studies in nine patients with chronic bronchitis and emphysema have confirmed the two levels of obstruction. The one in the small airways is relatively fixed, being present during inspiration and expiration and affected very little by changes in lung volume. Obstruction in the large airways, which is highly variable, is present only during expiration and is markedly increased by reduction in lung volume. In five of the nine patients expiratory flow was limited by large airway obstruction, in two by small airway obstruction, and in the other two simultaneously by both large and small airways. In these three groups of patients, the response of mainstem, intermediate, and lower lobe bronchi did not differ significantly but the reactions of the segmental and subsegmental bronchi differed markedly. When the small airways limited or participated in limiting flow, the reduction in caliber of segmental bronchi averaged 62.5 per cent; when lobar bronchi were flow-limiting, however, reduction averaged only 41 per cent, suggesting more severe impairment of the cough mechanism.

In summary, segments that limit flow, whether large or small airways, or both, can be identified by assessment of the dynamic activity of the tracheobronchial tree cinebronchographically. The caliber of segmental bronchi changes only slightly when flow is limited by the lobar bronchus, but narrows significantly when the small airways limit flow.

These findings provide clues to the cause of large airway collapse in chronic bronchitis and emphysema. Airway caliber is dependent upon two factors—the difference between the pressure inside and outside the airway and the structural stability or compliance of its walls. In patients with bronchitis or emphysema, the lobar bronchi are abnormally compliant or compressible, suggesting an anatomic defect in the walls. In fact, Wright[1954] described pathologic changes in the bronchi of patients with emphysema that suggested an increase in their compliance, although the major changes he reported were in segmental airways. Thurlbeck and his colleagues[1784] quantified the bronchial cartilage of 19 patients with various degrees of anatomic emphysema, mucous gland hyperplasia, and clinical chronic bronchitis. Like Wright[1954] and Maisel and associates,[1785, 1786] they reported that the most severe cartilage atrophy had occurred in the segmental and subsegmental bronchi of the emphysematous lungs. Furthermore, the proportion of bronchial cartilage in lungs of patients with more than one unit of emphysema was less than in comparable bronchi of subjects with only trace amounts or no emphysema, in whom the proportions were within normal limits. In general, these changes were more apparent in the lower than the upper lobe. The Reid index of each patient's lungs, assessed as below or above 0.46, did not reflect the amount of bronchial wall cartilage or show a group relationship. Thus, this study showed that bronchial cartilage diminishes in COPD and that the diminution is associated primarily with anatomic emphysema rather than chronic bronchitis. However, as discussed previously (see page 2105), not all studies have found evidence of cartilage abnormality in COPD.[1779, 1789, 1790]

Of perhaps even greater importance in the present context is the observation that cartilage reduction was statistically significant only in the segmental and subsegmental orders of bronchi in the lower lobe. Although reduction was observed in the lower lobe bronchus itself, this loss did not reach statistical significance. Therefore, these findings do not confirm our suspicion that an anatomic defect in the wall of the lower lobe bronchus creates an increase in compliance that, together with other factors, permits disproportionate collapse during expiration. However, as Thurlbeck and his associates[1784] pointed out, their series was small and did not include any patients with severe emphysema; study of a larger series or one with more severely emphysematous patients might show significant differences in the main bronchi.

SIGNIFICANCE OF CHANGES IN AIRWAY DYNAMICS

Studies by Mead and his coworkers[1950] have indicated that the gross reduction in maximal expiratory flow in emphysema is due primarily to two factors—organic obstruction of the small airways and loss of elastic recoil. Thus disproportionate large airway collapse plays only a secondary role. What, then, is the significance of this finding?

Earlier we described a hypothetical situation, a case of chronic bronchitis with both increased mucus production and impaired ciliary activity, a combination the lungs could handle only by bringing the cough mechanism into play. However, if the cough mechanism was impaired—as in lobar bronchial collapse—the retention of secretions would be inevitable. It has been suggested[1953] that such retention could lead to the small airways disease described by Hogg and his associates[1799] in emphysematous lungs. Trapped mucus spreads into the bronchioles, plugs them, and produces extensive obstruction that could conceivably result in recurrent inflammation, scarring, and irreversible obliteration. An additional factor of potential significance, suggested by Macklem and associates[1958] and by Green,[1959] is the effect of mucus on small airway surface tension. The mucous lining diminishes the effect of surfactant, thereby increasing surface tension and permitting small airway instability, premature closure, and air trapping. Thus, the expiratory obstruction in small airways characteristic of hypersecretory states may be caused as much by dynamic factors as by organic narrowing.

It has been postulated[1953] that the following chain of events may constitute the pathogenesis of chronic obstructive airway disease:

1. Ciliary paralysis associated with increased mucus production leads to chronic cough.

2. Disproportionate collapse of large airways limits the effectiveness of cough leading to the retention of secretions.

3. Retention of secretions results in mucous plugging, recurrent episodes of bronchiolitis, and eventual fibrous obliteration—"small airway disease." An additional factor, replacement of the normal surfactant lining of small airways by mucus, leads to instability, premature closure, and air trapping.

CLINICAL MANIFESTATIONS

Patients with COPD complain of cough, expectoration, and dyspnea. In over 75 per cent of cases, either cough antedates the onset of dyspnea or the two symptoms appear simultaneously; shortness of breath preceded the onset of cough in only 22 per cent of the 175 patients studied by Burrows and his associates.[1960] The majority of patients who complain of cough and expectoration have mucoid sputum, only periodically yellow or green. Hemoptysis is very uncommon, and its presence should stimulate a careful search for other causes. In temperate climates most patients attest to an increased frequency of respiratory infections during the winter, and such episodes may increase the severity of dyspnea. Most patients are heavy smokers;[1961, 1962] however, in individual patients the number of years of smoking may not correlate with the amount and duration of coughing and expectoration[1962] or with the degree of pulmonary dysfunction.[1961]

When COPD is mild or moderate in severity, dyspnea occurs only on exertion; as the disease worsens, however, shortness of breath is precipitated by less and less effort and in the terminal stages is present at rest. In patients with severe COPD, dyspnea can be influenced by posture; in one study, patients with FEV_1 values of less than 20 per cent of those predicted were more short of breath when they were standing or sitting erect than when they were supine or sitting leaning forward. The influence of posture on the mechanical advantage of the diaphragm and the intercostal inspiratory muscles is the likely explanation for this effect.[1963] Dyspnea induced by the upright posture and relieved by recumbency is termed "platypnea" and can also occur after pneumonectomy or following pulmonary emboli.[1964] In these latter conditions, platypnea may be associated with orthodeoxia (a decrease in arterial saturation produced by the upright posture).[1964] Conversely, patients with COPD may complain of orthopnea (increased dyspnea in the supine posture) in which circumstances accompanying left heart failure should be excluded. The assumption of the recumbent posture can be associated with either an improvement or deterioration in arterial Po_2, and there are no clinical or physiologic features that allow a prediction as to which response will occur in an individual patient.[1965] In normal subjects in the decubitus position, the majority of ventilation goes to the dependent lung; in some patients with COPD, however, ventilation is predominantly distributed to the nondependent lung,[1966] presumably because of airway closure in the dependent lung.

The dyspnea of COPD is not closely related to abnormalities of arterial blood gases, a dissociation that is highlighted by the clinical differentiation of patients with COPD into "pink puffers" and "blue bloaters."[1920, 1967] A "pink puffer," or type A patient, tends to be thinner, does not have cor pulmonale or right heart failure, is relatively well oxygenated, does not have hypercapnia, but complains of severe dyspnea. A "blue bloater," or type B patient, has peripheral edema caused by right heart failure and has more severe hypoxemia and hypercapnia but less dyspnea. Although the great majority of patients with COPD cannot be placed precisely into one of these categories, the concept that there is a spectrum of clinical presentations is valuable. The physiologic and clinical responses to a given degree of airflow obstruction differ between individuals, part of the variation probably being the result of differences in the responsiveness of the respiratory center to hypoxia and hypercapnia. There is an extremely wide range of responsiveness to hypoxia and hypercapnia in the general population (see page 439), and it is likely that in individuals with a well-developed ventilatory responsiveness blood gases will be preserved at the expense of increased respiratory effort when disease does develop; conversely, those with relatively blunted respiratory center responsiveness may hypoventilate, thus allowing P_{O_2} to fall further and P_{CO_2} to rise higher.

Over a period of years, most patients with COPD experience slow but inexorable worsening of symptoms and progressive impairment of pulmonary function, although this progression is not inevitable. One hundred forty-nine working Canadian Armed Forces veterans who were considered to have COPD on the basis of the British Medical Research Council (BMRC) questionnaire and periodic clinical and physiologic assessment showed a mean rate of change in pulmonary function over a 10-year period that was not much greater than the rate predicted from normal age regressions.[1968] The patients who showed deterioration in lung function were heavy smokers at the beginning of the study and continued to smoke heavily during the 10-year period. Follow-up studies of patients seeking medical help may not accurately reflect the prognosis of COPD in the general population;[1969, 1970] however, when ventilatory impairment becomes sufficiently severe to result in dyspnea, progression to severe disability can be expected within 6 to 10 years.[1969, 1971] In addition, although a gradual decline terminating in respiratory failure and death seems virtually inevitable once the patient with COPD seeks medical aid because of dyspnea, life span has been greatly prolonged with modern therapy. In one study,[1972] 64 patients with hypercapnia survived for a period of 2 to 15 years. When disease is this far advanced, repeated episodes of "acute-on-chronic" respiratory failure may occur; 70 to 75 per cent of these patients survive such crises,[1973, 1974] although 50 per cent die within 1 year[1973] and 70 per cent within 2 years of the initial episode.[1974]

When cor pulmonale develops, the prognosis is extremely poor, although therapeutic innovations have brought about some improvements in recent years. In 1954, one third of patients died during the first episode of right-sided heart failure; of the remainder, the mean interval from the time of the first attack to death was 18 months. By contrast, between 1967 and 1969, the mean survival time of patients with similar disease was 30.8 months.[1975] In the state of Colorado, the mortality ratio standardized for age rises with increasing altitude, presumably because the lower barometric pressure induces more severe hypoxemia.[1976]

Long-term supplemental oxygen increases the survival time of patients with advanced COPD.[1977, 1978] The beneficial effect of O_2 is proportional to the hours per day it is used; in one study, for example, patients treated for 19 hours or more survived significantly longer than those treated for 12 or 15 hours per day.[1977] The exact mechanism by which O_2 therapy prolongs survival is not clear; in one study,[1979] lung function did not show improvement in the patients who received oxygen and pulmonary artery pressure did not decrease significantly, although the increase in pulmonary artery pressure was less than would have been expected without O_2.

Prevention of severe oxygen desaturation during sleep may decrease cardiac irritability, a possible contributing factor to the beneficial effects of oxygen.[1980]

Despite the foregoing, the use of uncontrolled oxygen therapy for respiratory failure in patients with severe COPD can cause serious complications: a high concentration of inspired alveolar oxygen can cause worsening of hypercapnia by (1) interfering with hypoxic vasoconstriction, (2) increasing "physiologic" dead space, and (3) depressing minute ventilation.[1981, 1982] An abrupt and sometimes catastrophic rise in P_{CO_2} can result in coma and death.[1983–1985]

Secondary polycythemia develops in some hypoxemic patients with COPD. Among individuals with similar degrees of hypoxemia, hemoglobin and hematocrit levels tend to be normal or low in patients with COPD who live at sea level[1986] whereas levels in otherwise normal subjects who live at high altitudes tend to be elevated; however, in some patients in the former group an increased red cell volume is masked by a proportional increase in plasma volume. In such circumstances, demonstration of the absolute degree of polycythemia requires direct measurement of blood volume.[1987, 1988] Increased carboxyhemoglobin levels can also contribute to the development of polycythemia. In one study of 47 patients with hypoxemia (mean Pa_{O_2} = 52), the increased red blood cell mass correlated with carboxyhemoglobin levels; oxygen therapy corrected the polycythemia only in those patients who discontinued smoking and thus diminished their carboxyhemoglobin levels.[1989]

In some patients with COPD and chronic hypoxemia, the red cell mass fails to increase.[1988] In one study, this failure could not be attributed to decreased erythropoietin production and was assumed to be the result of a bone marrow defect.[1988] A delay in complete incorporation of radioactive iron into the erythocytes of patients with COPD has been found to be proportional to their degree of hypoxemia;[1987] since parenterally administered iron increases the red cell mass,[1990] it is possible that the physiologic response to lack of oxygen may be limited by the availability of iron for hemoglobin synthesis. In patients with COPD who have secondary polycythemia, nocturnal arterial oxygen desaturation is more severe than in similarly obstructed patients with identical daytime arterial P_{O_2} values but without polycythemia.[1991] Administration of continuous oxygen to patients with polycythemia results in a decrease in hematocrit values;[1992] similarly, a decrease in the hematocrit level following venisection is associated with an improvement in arterial blood gas values.[1993]

As might be expected, patients with COPD are quite susceptible to postoperative atelectasis after upper abdominal or thoracic surgery,[1994] especially when they are treated with analgesics and high concentrations of supplemental O_2. Although spontaneous pneumothorax is an uncommon complication of COPD, it may have serious consequences because it tends to occur in patients who have little respiratory reserve. In a review of 22,000 patients with COPD at the Mayo Clinic, 95 instances of pneumothorax were found, affecting 57 patients; ten of the episodes proved fatal.[1995] Air travel can be associated with significant arterial oxygen desaturation in patients with COPD;[1996] cabin pressure in commercial jet airliners is maintained between 560 and 690 mm Hg, which is equivalent to the barometric pressure at altitudes between 900 and 2,400 meters.[1996]

Pulmonary embolism in patients with COPD may be a particularly difficult diagnosis to make, yet it represents a significant risk in these relatively inactive patients who are already hypoxemic and may have pulmonary hypertension. One of the most valuable aids in the diagnosis of pulmonary emboli—ventilation/perfusion scintigraphy—becomes relatively insensitive in the presence of COPD. Clues to the diagnosis include relative hypocapnia in a previously hypercapnic patient, hypoxemia and right heart failure out of proportion to the degree of airflow obstruction, and the development of increased dyspnea and rapid shallow breathing.[1997, 1998] The same features also suggest the possibility of superimposed left ventricular failure, the presence of which can be difficult to detect by conventional methods.

Patients with advanced COPD tend to be somatically depleted, body weight being decreased in proportion to the ideal.[1999] The decreased body weight is related to the severity of obstruction and blood gas abnormalities and appears to be attributable to both increased caloric use and decreased caloric intake.[2000–2002] Nutritional supplements in malnourished patients with COPD can increase body weight and inspiratory muscle strength but do not improve ventilation.[2003]

Hypoventilation may also occur following attempts to restore the acid-base balance to normal by the administration of bicarbonate or the carbon dioxide buffer, trihydroxymethylaminomethane (THAM).[2004, 2005] A less frequent but often fatal complication of prolonged artificial ventilation of patients with respiratory failure is a syndrome characterized by tachypnea, hypotension, anxiety, confusion, asterixis, myoclonic seizures, coma, and fever.[2006–2009] Such patients become completely dependent upon the respirator and in many cases attempts to promote return to spontaneous breathing are of no avail. It has been postulated that this complication results from too rapid correction of respiratory acidosis, the development of alkalosis leading to a drastic decrease in cerebral circulation.[1985, 2006, 2009] It has been reported in some patients following removal of oxygen therapy after initial rapid overcorrection of respiratory acidosis by artificial ventilation;[2006] such a combination of effects inevitably results in severe cerebral anoxia.

Patients with COPD manifest impaired water handling and electrolyte exchange.[2010, 2011] In one study,[2010] patients with chronic airway obstruction who received a standard water load excreted only half the amount excreted by normal controls over a 4-hour period; the percentage of load passed and the arterial PCO_2 showed a significant inverse correlation. Renal excretion is impaired during respiratory failure and usually improves during recovery. In a study of the effects of hypoxia, hyperoxia, and hypercapnia on patients in respiratory failure, Kilburn and Dowell[2012] showed that when arterial blood oxygen tension was raised, urine flow and kidney function decreased, and when PaO_2 was lowered, renal function improved. However, function decreased abruptly when hypoxia became severe (PaO_2 below 40 mm Hg). The level of $PaCO_2$ had no measurable effect until it reached 65 mm Hg, at which point renal function abruptly decreased. The results of this study represent the response of the kidney to blood gas changes over relatively short periods of time, and it is questionable whether they can be extrapolated to more protracted exposures in patients with respiratory failure.[2013]

Potassium depletion can be a major complication of both acute[1985] and chronic[2014] respiratory failure. Potassium tends to move from tissue cells to plasma, and although serum potassium values may be normal, total exchangeable potassium may be greatly reduced.[2014] Diuretics and corticosteroid therapy may add to the deficiency, and when elimination of carbon dioxide is excessive, hypokalemic hypochloremic alkalosis may develop. Turino and associates[2015] have demonstrated an association between induced abrupt reductions in PCO_2 and renal potassium loss. Depending on the circumstances, this may lead to potassium depletion.

Physical Signs

In many patients with chronic cough and expectoration, physical examination of the chest reveals no abnormalities, at least during quiet breathing. At maximal expiration or during rapid, deep breathing, however, expiratory wheezes are audible in most cases.[2016] In one study of 83 patients with COPD,[2017] the presence of wheeze did not relate to the severity of obstruction, so that the significance of this physical finding during forced expiration is dubious; however, during quiet expiration wheeze did correlate with a decrease in FEV_1 and with the magnitude of response to bronchodilators. Rhonchi usually are more numerous in the patient with COPD who complains of shortness of breath on exertion, and commonly they are present during both inspiration and expiration.

When emphysema becomes widespread it gives rise to physical signs attributable to the combination of airway obstruction, bullae, and pulmonary overinflation. The most characteristic of these additional signs is decreased intensity of breath sounds, usually described incorrectly as a reduction in "air entry." Expiration becomes prolonged; this can be timed while listening through a stethoscope placed over the trachea from a position of full inspiration with the mouth wide open. Whereas expiration takes less than 4 seconds in normal subjects, it may take several times this in patients with emphysema.[1962, 2018] Loss of parenchymal elasticity results in wide fluctuations in intrapleural pressure that may be manifested clinically by intercostal and supraclavicular indrawing during inspiration and jugular venous filling during expiration.

When lung volumes are markedly increased and the thoracic cage is fixed in an inspiratory position, the physical signs are characteristic: the chest becomes barrel-shaped, and the thoracic kyphosis may be considerably increased; the shoulders are raised, and the chest tends to move *en bloc*, often with contraction of the accessory muscles of respiration in the neck.[2019] Campbell[2018] described decrease in length of that part of the trachea that is palpable above the sternal notch in such patients; he noted "tracheal descent" during inspiration and ascribed it to downward pull of the depressed diaphragm and to overinflation of the lungs. Depression of the diaphragm is believed to be responsible for a paradoxical movement of the lower thoracic costal margins during inspiration; known as Hoover's sign, it consists of an inward pulling of the costal cartilages from the flattened diaphragm.[2020] When anterior and posterior movements of the chest and abdomen are recorded separately on electromagnetic ventilation monitors, asynchronous breathing movements can be detected in some patients with advanced COPD and represent an extremely poor prognostic sign.[2021, 2022] Paradoxical abdominal motion at rest is a sign of inspiratory muscle fatigue or recruitment of expiratory muscles and is seen only with severe end-stage disease. Pulmonary overinflation may be evidenced by increased resonance of the percussion note, although this may be difficult to evaluate in obese or muscular patients. Separation of the heart from the anterior chest wall by overinflated lung results in varying degrees of faintness of heart sounds; in some cases, auscultation of the heart can be performed satisfactorily only when the stethoscope is placed over the epigastrium. Godfrey and associates[2023] attempted to correlate the many physical signs seen in patients with COPD with airway conductance and found that the only sign that was a direct reflection of the obstruction was the forced expiratory time.

Other physical signs found commonly in patients with chronic obstructive pulmonary disease include emaciation[2024] and inguinal hernias. Weight loss occurs particularly in patients with severe dyspnea. In our experience, inguinal hernias are present in almost 50 per cent of patients with chronic obstructive pulmonary disease and are usually attributed to stress from repeated coughing.

Respiratory Muscles

Inspiratory muscle fatigue may be the final common pathway that causes ventilatory failure in patients with COPD. A number of factors can influence respiratory muscle performance in these patients:

1. The inspiratory muscles must work against increased resistive loads as a result of increased pulmonary resistance.

2. The inspiratory muscles are at a mechanical disadvantage because of pulmonary hyperinflation; in the presence of hyperinflation, the muscle fibers of the diaphragm and other inspiratory muscles become shorter than the optimal length at which overlap of actin and myosin filaments permits maximal force generation for a given neural input and oxygen consumption.

3. By changing the geometry of the thoracic cage and its relationship to the inspiratory muscles, hyperinflation adds to the inefficient action of the muscles.

4. Patients tend to be relatively malnourished, a condition that along with chronic hypoxemia can impair inspiratory muscle strength and endurance.

5. With the development of cor pulmonale and right ventricular failure, cardiac output decreases, creating the potential for inadequate inspiratory muscle blood flow to meet increased demands.

Theoretically, it might be expected that patients with COPD would develop hypertrophy and increased strength of the inspiratory muscles, since these are continuously working against an increased impedance. In fact, the data support the opposite outcome—respiratory muscles undergo atrophy. At autopsy, diaphragmatic weight of patients with emphysema is decreased rather than increased.[2025] Part of this decrease may be the result of general malnutrition, since in the general population body weight is significantly related to diaphragmatic weight at autopsy; however, in patients with emphysema, the decrease in diaphragmatic weight is out of proportion to the decrease in body weight.[2025]

The morphometry of individual muscle fibers from various respiratory muscles has been studied in patients with COPD who were having lung resection for pulmonary carcinoma.[2026, 2027] When compared with normal subjects, patients had atrophy of type 1 and 2 muscle fibers in the costal portion of the diaphragm[2026] and the intercostal muscles; muscle fiber atrophy was significantly related to the severity of preoperative airflow obstruction and to body weight as a per cent predicted ideal body weight.[2026, 2027] In addition, there was a lower level of oxidative enzymes in the diaphragm of patients with COPD.[2028] In hamsters with elastase-induced emphysema, the diaphragm shortens because of loss of sarcomeres; however, it also thickens, so that total diaphragmatic weight and strength are unchanged.[2029, 2030]

Inspiratory muscle strength can be assessed by

measuring maximal inspiratory mouth pressure (PI Max), and the diaphragm itself can be specifically assessed by measuring maximal transdiaphragmatic pressure (Pdi Max). In children with obstructive pulmonary disease (mainly cystic fibrosis), PI Max is decreased when measured at FRC, an effect that is caused mainly by the mechanical disadvantage resulting from hyperinflation because performance of the test at predicted normal FRC produces normal results.[2031] In adults with COPD, however, the decrease in strength appears to be more than can be accounted for by the mechanical disadvantage alone.[2032]

The decreased inspiratory strength and increased load put the inspiratory muscles of patients with COPD at risk of developing fatigue, defined as the inability of a muscle to generate the maximal force of which it is capable, despite maximal effort. In most skeletal muscles, fatigue develops when a muscle is used repetitively to generate greater than 15 to 20 per cent of its maximal force. The respiratory muscles are relatively fatigue-resistant, since with each breath they can develop up to 40 per cent of their maximal force (PI/PI Max = 40 per cent) virtually indefinitely.[2033] However, when pressures in excess of 40 per cent of maximal are generated with each breath, fatigue eventually develops; the greater the percentage of maximum generated with each breath, the faster the onset of fatigue. The development of fatigue can also be altered by the breathing pattern; the longer the inspiratory phase of the respiratory cycle (duty cycle), the lower the pressure that can be generated indefinitely. The development of inspiratory muscle fatigue can be predicted by measuring the tension-time index, which is the product of the duty cycle (inspiratory time/total respiratory cycle time $-T_I/T_{Tot}$) and the inspiratory pressure (PI) as a percentage of the maximal inspiratory pressure (PI/PI Max); a tension-time index greater than 0.15 will result in fatigue. Patients with COPD breathe with a higher than normal tension-time index, both because Pi is increased secondary to the increased impedance of the lung and PI Max is decreased as a result of muscle atrophy and mechanical disadvantage. In one study of 20 patients with COPD, the tension-time index of the diaphragm during tidal breathing at rest averaged 0.05 (range 0.01 to 0.12); when the tension-time index was increased to more than 0.15 by prolonging the inspiratory duration, EMG indicators of diaphragmatic fatigue developed. Although the tension-time index may not be above the critical value of 0.15 during resting tidal breathing, the reserve for increase in force generation is reduced in patients with COPD (three-fold) compared with normal subjects (eight-fold).[2034] Besides tension and duty cycle, the work performed by the inspiratory muscles is also a determinant of fatigue; for the same tension and duty cycle, a muscle that contracts and shortens consumes more oxygen than the same muscle contracting isometrically.[2756, 2757]

The diagnosis of respiratory muscle fatigue in patients with COPD can be made by showing an inability to generate previously achievable pressures with voluntary contraction or with bilateral phrenic nerve stimulation.[2035] In addition, there is a shift in the frequency distribution of the EMG signals in a muscle that is performing potentially fatiguing tasks.[2033]

In patients with COPD, inspiratory muscle fatigue develops during exercise[2036, 2037] and, unlike in normal subjects, is probably a major determinant of maximal exercise performance. The fatigue can be delayed and exercise endurance increased by the administration of supplemental oxygen. The beneficial effect of O_2 is chiefly the result of a decrease in ventilation at any level of exercise, but it may also derive from a direct effect on muscle performance.[2036] In patients with COPD, inspiratory muscle strength and endurance can be improved by specific training programs;[2038, 2039] in addition, their capacity to exercise can be augmented.[2040, 2041] These studies suggest that despite the increased impedance to breathing, inspiratory muscle weakness and atrophy may develop in some patients as a result of relative disuse. It is possible that dyspnea causes some patients to avoid exercise with resulting respiratory muscle deconditioning, thus initiating a vicious circle. Theophylline therapy results in a prolonged increase in inspiratory muscle strength and endurance in patients with COPD.

Although muscle fatigue is usually considered to be an unsteady state, the concept of chronic respiratory muscle fatigue has been suggested in patients with COPD. The basis for the suggestion has derived from studies that have shown an improvement in muscle and lung function and a decrease in dyspnea in hypercapnic patients by resting respiratory muscles with ventilatory support overnight.[2033] If chronic inspiratory muscle fatigue does exist, patients with COPD would not derive benefit from inspiratory muscle training. It remains to be determined which patients with COPD should be treated with inspiratory muscle training and which should be rested.

Pulmonary Hemodynamics and Cardiac Function

Pulmonary arterial hypertension, right ventricular hypertrophy (cor pulmonale), and right ventricular failure are serious complications of severe obstructive pulmonary disease. Pulmonary hypertension is caused in part by hypoxic vasoconstriction of the muscular pulmonary arteries, but a loss of pulmonary capillary bed, a decrease of pulmonary vascular compliance,[2042] and intimal and medial hypertrophy also contribute to the increased vascular resistance. With mild-to-moderate grades of COPD (FEV_1 of 40 to 80 per cent predicted), the pulmonary artery pressure (P_{Pa}) is usually normal at rest but increases with moderate exercise.)[1860] In the presence of severe COPD ($FEV_1 < 40$ per cent predicted), pulmonary hypertension is usually present at rest (mean $P_{Pa} > 20$ mm Hg) and undergoes a disproportionate increase with mild exercise;[2043, 2044] its severity correlates with the degree of arterial desaturation and arterial P_{CO_2}.[2045]

Exacerbations of COPD are associated with acute worsening of pulmonary hypertension but the P_{Pa} usually returns to pre-exacerbation levels with treatment.[2045, 2046] During exacerbations, the pulmonary hypertension is relatively refractory to correction of hypoxemia, suggesting that mechanisms other than hypoxic vasoconstriction are important in this setting.[2047] Pulmonary artery pressure can also increase acutely during the episodes of hypoxemia that occur during sleep, and it has been suggested that recurrent nocturnal pulmonary hypertension can eventually result in pathologic changes in pulmonary vessels and fixed hypertension.[2048, 2049] Oral and parenteral smooth muscle–relaxing drugs cause a decrease in P_{Pa} but not to normal levels.[2050, 2051] A new therapeutic agent, almitrine, improves arterial blood gases in patients with COPD by stimulating ventilation and enhancing hypoxic vasoconstriction;[2052] the latter results in an improvement in PaO_2 out of proportion to the increase in ventilation but also causes an increase in P_{Pa}.[2053]

In the absence of therapy, the pulmonary hypertension in patients with COPD progresses slowly but inexorably,[2046] the increase in P_{Pa} over time correlating with a decrease in FEV_1 and PaO_2;[2054, 2055] this increase in P_{Pa} can be prevented by chronic oxygen therapy.[2056, 2057] In one study, 16 patients with severe COPD ($FEV_1 = 0.9$ liter) were followed for 47 months prior to and 31 months after the institution of long-term oxygen therapy: during the period before O_2 therapy, mean P_{Pa} increased from 23 to 28 mm Hg and PaO_2 decreased from 59 to 50 mm Hg; during the 31 months following the institution of O_2 therapy, P_{Pa} decreased from 28 to 24 mm Hg and PaO_2 remained stable at 50 mm Hg (all measurements were made during breathing of room air). Nocturnal oxygen therapy may be particularly beneficial in preventing the progression of pulmonary hypertension.[2058] In patients with COPD, the long-term response of the pulmonary vasculature to the breathing of an enriched oxygen mixture can be predicted by measuring changes in pulmonary artery pressure during a 24-hour period of oxygen administration. In one study, 25 of 43 patients with COPD showed a decrease greater than 5 mm Hg in P_{Pa} after breathing 28 per cent oxygen for 24 hours; these individuals showed significantly improved survival after 1, 2, and 3 years of chronic low-flow oxygen therapy in comparison with those who did not show an acute decrease in pulmonary artery pressure.[2059]

Although there is a relationship between arterial desaturation and pulmonary hypertension, there is also significant interindividual variation. Patients with COPD can be divided into two groups on the basis of the change in the ratio of physiologic dead space to tidal volume (V_T/V_D)[2060] and their pulmonary arterial pressure during oxygen breathing.[2061] Approximately two thirds of patients show an increase in dead space while breathing oxygen, and it has been suggested that these individuals respond to hypoxemia with pulmonary vasoconstriction; when oxygen is administered, hypoxic vasoconstriction is abolished and blood flow to poorly ventilated areas of the lungs increases, with a resultant increase in V_T/V_D. In other words, in "vascular responders," perfusion remains relatively well matched to ventilation, and blood gas tensions are preserved at the expense of an increase in pulmonary vascular resistance and an increased load on the right side of the heart. By contrast, hypoxic vasoconstriction and pulmonary hypertension do not develop in "vascular nonresponders," although for a given degree of pulmonary disease blood gas values in this group are worse. Vascular nonresponsiveness can have a beneficial effect on patient survival, suggesting that it is not the abnormal blood gas level *per se* but the host response to the hypoxemia that is detrimental to survival.[1769]

Because pulmonary arterial pressure is such a valuable measurement and a good predictor of prognosis in patients with COPD, a number of attempts have been made to develop noninvasive methods to estimate it. Echocardiographic estimates of systolic and diastolic pulmonary artery diameter[2062] and the time interval between tricuspid valve closure and pulmonic valve opening[2063] have both been shown to correlate with P_{Pa}.

Prolonged pulmonary hypertension causes right ventricular hypertrophy and ultimately right ventricular failure. Right ventricular hypertrophy can be diagnosed by electrocardiography and echocardiography. The electrocardiogram (ECG) may be perfectly normal in patients with COPD despite the development of increased pulmonary vascular resistance on exercise; however, as airway obstruction becomes more severe, signs of right axis deviation develop, with large S waves and diphasic T waves over the left precordium beyond the V_2 position. These changes correlate best with total pulmonary vascular resistance.[2064] With decreasing FEV_1/FVC ratios, there is an increased frequency of P waves greater than 2.0 mm, P axis greater than +75 degrees, S waves greater than 5 mm in V_5 and V_6, and QRS axis greater than +75 degrees.[2065] An R/S ratio of less than 1.0 in lead V_6 is also good evidence for right ventricular hypertrophy. In a study of 71 patients in whom ECG changes during life were correlated with right ventricular mass at autopsy,[2066] 30 had definite and three probable right ventricular hypertrophy, 20 had normal ventricular weight, and 18 had left ventricular hypertrophy. Four criteria were found to be the most reliable indicators of right ventricular hypertrophy: S_1, Q_3 pattern, right axis deviation (≥ 110), S_1, S_2, S_3 pattern, and an RS ratio in $V_6 \leq 1.0$.[2066]

Right ventricular function can be assessed by measuring right ventricular ejection fraction with single-pass[2067] or gated equilibration radionuclide techniques.[2068] The normal right ventricle ejects approximately 55 per cent of its end-diastolic blood volume with each cardiac contraction. Severe COPD is associated with a significant decrease in right ventricular ejection fraction,[2068, 2069] a close relationship existing between the increase in pulmonary artery pressure and the decrease in ejection fraction.[2070] In patients with COPD, exercise does not normally increase right ventricular ejection fraction[2071] although in one study it was shown that exercise with supplemental oxygen was associated with improved right ventricular function.[2067] Echocardiographic studies of right ventricular cavity size and muscle thickness suggest that dilatation precedes hypertrophy in the development of cor pulmonale.[2072] In a study of 15 patients with COPD, Yamaoka and associates showed that the assessment of right ventricular function with myocardial perfusion single-photon emission computerized tomography (SPECT) using thallium-201 was complementary to the measurement of right ventricular ejection fraction in the identification of the presence of cor pulmonale.[2073]

Most studies show that left ventricular function as assessed by ejection fraction is relatively normal in patients with COPD, although dysfunction may be observed when cor pulmonale and right ventricular failure have developed.[2068, 2069, 2074] As right ventricular hypertrophy increases, the septal wall between the ventricles thickens; coupled with right ventricular dilatation and leftward shift of the septum, this may decrease the diastolic compliance of the left ventricle.[2075, 2076] The reduced left ventricular compliance may explain the results of studies that have reported mild elevation in pulmonary arterial wedge pressure and left ventricular end-diastolic pressure in some patients with COPD.[1860] However, measurement of pulmonary arterial wedge pressure may not be a reliable indicator of left ventricular end-diastolic pressure in patients with COPD; this is certainly the case if the catheter is wedged in an area of Zone II blood flow conditions, but even in Zone III the pulmonary artery wedge pressure may overestimate end-diastolic pressure. In some patients with COPD, left ventricular hypertrophy is found at necropsy[2077] but in most it is attributable to hypertensive or arteriosclerotic heart disease.[2078]

Chronic cor pulmonale may be associated with cardiac arrhythmias, as was the case in 33 of 70 patients in one series[2079] and in 47 of 102 patients in another.[2080] In another study of 35 hospitalized patients whose ECGs were recorded continuously for 72 hours, arrhythmias were identified in 89 per cent, 57 per cent of them being sufficiently severe to require therapy.[2081] Supraventricular arrhythmias were found to be slightly more common than ventricular, the most frequent being atrial and multifocal tachycardia; ventricular arrhythmias were often preceded by premature ventricular contractions or supraventricular arrhythmias and were associated with a poor prognosis. Seventy per cent of the patients with ventricular arrhythmia died during their hospital stay, and none survived to the end of the 2.5-year study period.

Prognosis is significantly related to the pulmonary hemodynamic and right ventricular consequences of COPD.[2082] Burrows and coworkers[2083] evaluated the cardiovascular function of 50 patients with COPD by catheterization when their condition was stable and showed that survival was inversely related to pulmonary vascular resistance. They described two different patterns of cardiovascular abnormality in patients with high vascular resistance: one consisted of low cardiac output, relatively normal blood gas levels, and near-normal resting pulmonary arterial pressure—an "emphysematous" type of COPD; the other pattern was a well-maintained cardiac output with more severe pulmonary hypertension and blood gas abnormalities—a group judged clinically to have a predominant "bronchitic" type of disease. It was found that patients in the first group were unlikely to be diagnosed clinically as having cor pulmonale, since cardiomegaly, chronic congestive heart failure, and ECG evidence of right ventricular hypertrophy were relatively infrequent; by contrast, patients in the second group more regularly presented with the classic clinical and ECG features of pulmonary heart disease.

In a long-term follow-up study of 175 patients with COPD, Weitzenblum found that pulmonary arterial pressure, FEV_1, and $PaCO_2$ were equally effective in predicting survival.[2084] If P_{Pa} was less than 20 mm Hg at the beginning of the study, 5-year survival averaged 72 per cent compared with 49 per cent for patients in whom the P_{Pa} was greater than 20; PCO_2 levels above 45 mm Hg were associated with 45 per cent 5-year survival, whereas 70 per cent of patients with a PCO_2 in the normal range survived 5 years.[2084] Age, initial FEV_1, and the presence of cor pulmonale were the best predictors of mortality in a 15-year follow-up study of 200 American patients with COPD.[2085]

In other longitudinal studies, the yearly increase in P_{Pa} and pulmonary vascular resistance, the absence of an increase in PaO_2 with exercise, and the presence of electrocardiographic evidence of right ventricular hypertrophy also were predictive of decreased survival in patients with COPD.[2086–2089]

PULMONARY FUNCTION

Although the basic pathophysiologic processes that contribute to the development of COPD (parenchymal dissolution and airway narrowing) are different, the functional abnormalities that they cause are similar. Although certain function tests help to predict which pathologic process is predominant in an individual patient, the most important applications of pulmonary function tests lie in detecting the presence of disease (preferably at an early stage) and in following its progression. Although symptomatic COPD develops in only a small proportion of smokers, these individuals can be identified long before the development of symptoms because the disease follows an insidiously progressive course for years prior to clinical presentation.[1969] Smoking cessation in such subjects results in some functional improvement but, more important, causes a normalization in the rate of age-related decline of lung function.[2090] Thus, COPD can be prevented, but only if it is recognized at an early stage by pulmonary function testing. In addition to aiding in the recognition of disease, pulmonary function studies help to quantify the degree of functional impairment in individual subjects and are useful in research studies of the natural history and pathogenesis of COPD.

Small Airway Tests

The demonstration by Hogg and his colleagues in 1968 that airways smaller than 3 mm in internal diameter were the most important site of increase in resistance in the lungs of patients with established airway disease[1799] led to the development of tests to detect abnormalities of small airway function.[2091–2093] It was reasoned that a test that could detect abnormal function in the airways prior to the onset of a decrease in FEV_1 would allow the identification of a small subset of smokers who had preclinical COPD and were therefore at risk for the development of symptomatic disease. Intensive smoking cessation campaigns directed at such individuals would have an important preventative effect. The so-called small airway tests that were developed include the frequency dependence of dynamic compliance (Cdyn), the single-breath nitrogen washout (ΔN_2/liter, closing volume and closing capacity), the density dependence of maximal expiratory flow, and flows at low lung volumes (FEF_{25-75}, $\dot{V}max_{50}$, $\dot{V}max_{25}$).

Frequency dependence of Cdyn is a decrease in compliance with increasing frequency of breathing. In normal individuals, dynamic compliance remains constant as frequency increases up to 60 to 90 breaths/minute. Cdyn will decrease with frequency only if there are substantially different time constants in peripheral parallel lung units. In the presence of patchy small airway narrowing, Cdyn would be expected to decrease with increasing respiratory frequency; in fact, some smokers without a significant decrease in maximal expiratory flow do show frequency dependence of Cdyn.[2094] Measurement of Cdyn is technically difficult because it requires

placement of an esophageal balloon and the test has not been employed in any of the screening studies.

Because it is the "small airways" that close at low lung volumes,[2095] the *single-breath nitrogen washout* (closing volume) is theoretically an attractive test for the detection of early abnormalities in COPD. The single-breath test also gives a measure of the evenness of lung emptying. The slope of the alveolar plateau (phase 3) would be flat if all lung units emptied homogeneously; sequential emptying of units would occur if there were regional differences in small airway resistance and airspace compliance. Both closing volume and the slope of phase 3 are abnormal in some smokers,[2091] and these derangements of function correlate with pathologic abnormalities in the membranous and respiratory bronchioles.[1800, 2096] The tests of "small airway" function may be abnormal even when the decrease in maximal expiratory flow is caused by loss of lung elasticity.[2097]

Density dependence of maximal expiratory flow should theoretically provide information about the flow regimen at the site of flow limitation. Because the equal pressure point moves from large to small airways with increased peripheral airway resistance, the density dependence of maximal flow should decrease if the flow-limiting segments also move peripherally where flow tends to be relatively laminar rather than turbulent. In practice, the density dependence of maximal expiratory flow has not proved to be an effective screening test nor does it appear to relate to pathologic abnormalities in small airways.[2758] In patients with established COPD and definite bronchiolar pathology, density dependence may be preserved, probably because flow-limiting segments remain in central airways despite the increase in peripheral resistance.

A similar explanation can be given for the reason why flows at low lung volumes should reflect small airway narrowing. During most of the FEV_1 maneuver, flow either is not limited or is limited at choke points in central airways. Since the equal pressure point and choke points move outward in the lung at low lung volumes, flow at these volumes ($\dot{V}max_{50}$, $\dot{V}max_{25}$, FEF_{25-75}) is influenced to a greater extent by narrowing at these sites.

The basic premise behind the hypothesis that small airway tests will predict later decline in FEV_1 is that they are more sensitive than simple spirometry, but there is now considerable evidence that this is incorrect. Small airway resistance probably contributes more to total pulmonary resistance than was originally believed (50 per cent rather than 10 to 20 per cent).[2098] It has been shown that changes in FEV_1 and FEV_1/FVC parallel those in the small airway tests,[2099–2101] and although the absolute changes in FEV_1 may be less than those in the small airway tests, they are of equal or greater significance since the coefficients of variation of FEV_1 and FVC are much smaller. Alteration in the forced expiratory spirogram occurs in young smokers and probably reflects those at risk.[2102] Because spirometry is easier and cheaper to perform, it will probably remain the most valuable test in the clinical management and epidemiologic investigation of patients with COPD.[2103] The results of longitudinal studies of small airway tests and the rate of decline in lung function are in conflict.[2104, 2105]

Maximal Expiratory Flow

A decrease in maximal expiratory flow is the diagnostic hallmark of COPD. Expiratory flow can be measured as peak flow (PEFR), flow in the first second of a forced vital capacity maneuver (FEV_1), average flow over the middle half of the forced expired volume (FEF_{25-75} or maximal mid-expiratory flow rate—MMEF), or instantaneous flow rates at different percentages of the forced vital capacity ($\dot{V}max_{50}$, $\dot{V}max_{25}$). All of these measures of flow decrease with the development of COPD. The FEV_1 has the advantage of being most reproducible in a given individual and there is little evidence that FEF_{25-75}, or $\dot{V}max_{50}$, or $\dot{V}max_{25}$, is more sensitive in detecting the early stages of the disease.[2106, 2107] There is a wide range of values within the normal population for these tests of flow, but the range is narrowed by expressing forced expiratory flow as a percentage of forced vital capacity (FEV_1/FVC per cent).

Examination of a flow-volume curve provides additional information in a patient with airflow obstruction. If the decreased flow is caused by upper airway obstruction, the shape of the expiratory and/or inspiratory curve will be characteristic (see page 1979). It has been suggested that the shape of the expiratory flow-volume curve can be helpful in determining whether the obstruction is caused by emphysema or asthma,[2108] but the evidence supporting this claim does not have much merit. The ratio of forced expiratory flow to forced inspiratory flow at isovolume has also been suggested as a test to distinguish emphysema from diseases that cause intrinsic airway narrowing, the hypothesis being that patients with emphysema will show disproportionate expiratory obstruction as a result of dynamic collapse of the airways.[2109]

With the development of obstructive pulmonary disease, forced expiratory flow decreases over the entire vital capacity range and the effort-independent portion of the curve becomes more curvilinear than normal and is convex (lowered toward the volume axis) (Fig. 11–80).[2110] The relative contribution of loss of elastic recoil and increased resistance to flow through airways upstream from the flow-limiting segments can be determined by plotting maximal flow against static recoil pressure. The slope of this relationship represents upstream conductance. If a decrease in flow is related entirely to loss of elasticity, the slope of the maximal flow static recoil plot will be normal; however, when airway

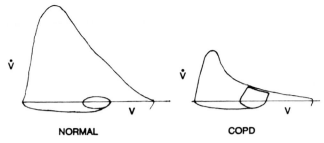

Figure 11–80. Flow-Volume Curve in a Normal Subject and a Patient with Severe Chronic Obstructive Pulmonary Disease (COPD). A normal tidal flow-volume ($\dot{V}$-V) loop and a complete maximal expiratory flow-volume curve show that during tidal breathing the patient with COPD achieves maximal expiratory flow. There is considerable reserve for increased expiratory flow in the normal subject.

narrowing is the cause, the slope is decreased (increased upstream resistance). In most patients with COPD, the loss of flow is related to a combination of loss of recoil and airway narrowing.[2109, 2111]

As discussed above, the density dependence of maximal expiratory flow has been suggested as a test to determine the site of flow limitation and to identify early small airway obstruction. However, the test has a large coefficient of variation when repeated on the same subject;[2112] in addition, animal studies have questioned the usefulness of density dependence in identifying the site of flow limitation.[2113, 2114]

Patients with COPD can show a substantial increase in forced expiratory flow following inhalation of a bronchodilator. In a 3-year follow-up study of patients with established COPD, the mean increase in FEV_1 with inhaled beta-adrenergic agonist was 15 per cent; over 30 per cent of patients showed an increase greater than 20 per cent.[2115] Although the percentage increase in FEV_1 was substantial, the absolute increase was small (0.15 liter or 5 per cent of predicted normal); the percentage increase in FEV_1 was inversely related to the initial FEV_1 as a percentage of predicted. In other words, patients in whom the airflow obstruction was more severe showed a greater percentage increase in FEV_1 than in those who were less obstructed. This is mainly a mathematical artefact, however, because the *absolute* increase in FEV_1 was less in patients with the worst airflow obstruction. This important study[2115] showed that patients with asthma or COPD cannot be easily distinguished by their response to inhaled bronchodilator, especially if the response is measured as a relative change in flow. Some patients with COPD also show substantial improvement in function following a course of oral corticosteroid therapy,[2116] and like asthmatic patients can show substantial diurnal variation in expiratory flow[2117, 2118] and a decrease in expiratory flow rates coincident with propranolol therapy.[2119]

In eight nonallergic patients with COPD, the circadian change in FEV_1 was 27 ± 2 per cent compared with 7 ± 1 per cent in eight age- and-sex-matched control subjects.[2120] The lowest values were recorded at night; in the patients, these values were associated with evidence of increased vagal tone and decreased catecholamine secretion, suggesting that an imbalance in autonomic nervous system activity may cause the nocturnal dyspnea experienced by these patients.

Middle-aged smokers with relatively normal expiratory flow can exhibit substantial abnormalities of the distribution of inspired gas[2121, 2122] although the significance of the maldistribution in terms of the progression of obstruction is unknown. Some studies have shown that ventilation maldistribution correlates with tests of small airway function,[2121] whereas others have shown poor correlation.[2122]

Patients with COPD show increased airway and pulmonary resistance.[2123, 2124] Airway resistance can increase paradoxically following a deep inspiration although to a lesser degree than in asthmatics.[2123] The forced oscillation technique allows the measurement of resistance over a wide range of frequencies. An increased frequency dependence of resistance in the 8- to 24-Hz range measured by maximal expiratory flow rates has been reported in patients with mild airflow obstruction.[2125] Theoretically, it would be expected that the increase in pulmonary resistance in patients with COPD would be associated with a decrease in the density dependence of resistance because the site of increased resistance is small airways. However, a study of 40 patients with mild-to-moderate COPD did not show a decrease in the density dependence of resistance in subjects with increased resistance.[2124] A concomitant narrowing of the upper airway could explain these results. Higenbottom[2126] has shown that there is both inspiratory and expiratory narrowing of the larynx in patients with COPD and that the narrowing correlates with severity of lower airway obstruction as measured by FEV_1. Because the flow regimen across the larynx is density-dependent, the increased upper airway resistance could mask a decrease in density dependence of lower airway resistance.

Lung Volumes

The initial alteration in lung volumes in patients with COPD is an increase in RV.[2127] As the disease worsens, RV increases further and encroaches on VC; FRC and TLC also increase.

The early change in RV is probably related to premature airway closure at the lung bases as has been demonstrated in otherwise asymptomatic young (24 years of age) smokers.[2128] In normal subjects and patients with mild COPD, there is no difference between the slow and the forced VC; when obstruction becomes more severe, the FVC can decrease disproportionately,[2129] perhaps as a result of dynamic compression and closure of airways. Vital capacity can decrease substantially in patients with COPD when they assume the supine posture, amounting to a mean of 11.2 per cent in 30 patients in one study.[2117]

The increase in FRC is caused by at least two mechanisms.

1. In normal subjects, FRC is determined by the balance between the static outward recoil of the chest wall and the static inward recoil of the lung. With the development of COPD, there can be loss of lung elasticity such that the volume at equilibration increases towards the relaxed position of the chest wall (about 70 per cent TLC). However, the increase in FRC is often greater than can be explained by this passive hyperinflation.

2. The increase is also caused by dynamic hyperinflation secondary to an increased expiratory resistance and prolonged expiratory phase.[2128, 2130] Patients with COPD may expire along their maximal expiratory flow-volume curve and inspire prior to complete lung emptying (see Fig. 11–78), resulting in the onset of the next inspiration while alveolar pressure is still positive.[2130, 2131] This phenomenon, which has been called "auto-PEEP" or "intrinsic PEEP," has a number of important physiologic consequences. The increased intrathoracic pressure can adversely affect venous return to the right side of the heart and the hyperinflation puts the inspiratory muscles at a mechanical disadvantage and at a shorter length on their length-tension curve. On the positive side, the hyperinflation dilates intraparenchymal airways and decreases the resistive work of breathing.

Although the prolonged expiration and "intrinsic PEEP" are caused primarily by increased resistance in the lower tracheobronchial tree, there is some evidence that glottic narrowing might also contribute. As mentioned earlier, glottic narrowing occurs on expiration in patients with COPD[2126] and expiratory resistive loading results in active laryngeal narrowing in normal subjects.[2132] Glottic narrowing during expiration may be analogous to pursed lip-breathing, acting to control expiratory flow and prevent lower airway collapse. When normal subjects change from an erect or sitting to supine or lateral decubitus position, FRC decreases by 30 and 17 per cent, respectively; but when patients with COPD change position, there occurs no change in FRC.[2133]

Total lung capacity is determined by the balance between the ability of the inspiratory muscles to shorten and the inward recoil of lung and chest wall. The increase in TLC in patients with COPD is thought to be caused by a decrease in the inward elastic recoil of the lung. It is possible that adaptive changes may occur in the inspiratory muscles as a consequence of chronic hyperinflation, which would allow greater shortening. Such an adaptive response to chronic hyperinflation has been demonstrated in the diaphragm of hamsters with experimental emphysema;[2134] the entire diaphragm shortened as a result of a drop-out of sarcomeres, resulting in a relative preservation of the length-tension advantage of individual sarcomeres.

Although it is clear that TLC increases with the development of COPD, the magnitude of the increase is controversial. The two most frequently employed methods to determine TLC—helium dilution and body plethysmography—are both subject to error in patients with COPD: the helium dilution technique tends to underestimate thoracic gas volume to the extent that inspired gas fails to equilibrate with intrathoracic gas beyond obstructed airways;[2135, 2136] by contrast, the plethysmographic technique tends to overestimate thoracic gas volume because changes in mouth pressure during panting may be less than the simultaneous changes in the alveolar pressure.[2137] Esophageal pressure more accurately reflects alveolar pressure and gives a closer estimate of true TLC.[2135, 2138] Since the underestimation of the measurements of Palv by Pmouth is frequency-dependent, the simplest way to overcome the potential error in the plethysmographic measurement of TLC is to limit the panting frequency to 1 Hz or less;[2139, 2140] with this precaution, the plethysmographic method provides the most accurate measurements.

The changes in lung distensibility that occur in COPD are reflected not only by an increase in TLC but also by an alteration in the pulmonary pressure-volume curve. The maximal elastic recoil pressure at TLC and recoil pressures at various percentages of TLC decrease with increasing age,[2141–2143] but in smokers the decrease is accelerated.[2144, 2145] Unfortunately, there is a large range of "normal" values for absolute elastic recoil pressures, creating difficulty in designating abnormality in an individual subject. A narrower range of "normality" can be achieved by describing the entire pressure-volume curve of the lungs with an exponential equation:

$$V = A - Be^{-kp}$$

where V = lung volume, A = theoretical maximal lung volume at infinite transpulmonary pressure, P = transpulmonary pressure, and K is a constant that describes the shape of the exponential relationship between pressure and volume.[2141]

As discussed in Chapter 3 (see page 433), an increase in K reflects a loss of lung recoil and a shift in the pressure-volume curve upward and to the left. K increases with age in nonsmoking men and women,[2141] and the increase is greater in smokers.[2144] Although in some studies, K has been correlated with the presence of emphysema,[1857, 2146] it probably more accurately reflects the mean size of the airspaces that contribute to expired volume.[1856] In smokers with no emphysema, an increase in K correlates with an increase in TLC and a decrease in diffusing capacity–alveolar volume.[2144, 2147] In one study of postmortem lungs, it was shown that K correlated with ΔN_2/liter, suggesting that it reflects not only increased lung distensibility but also an increased variation in the distensibility of different lung units.[2148]

Although surface forces are the main contributor to the shape of the pressure-volume curve, there is evidence that parenchymal smooth muscle contraction can also affect recoil. Inhalation of a beta$_2$-agonist results in a leftward shift of the pressure-volume curve (>1.5 cm H_2O);[2149] acute smoking cessation causes a similar decrease in recoil pressure without a decrease in maximal expiratory flow, suggesting that smoke causes contraction of parenchymal and airway smooth muscle.[2150]

Arterial Blood Gases

Arterial blood gas tensions are commonly disturbed in patients with COPD; the more severe the disease, the more frequent the hypoxemia and hypercapnia.[1875] The arterial hypoxemia is a result of alveolar hypoventilation and ventilation-perfusion mismatching. On the basis of the multiple inert gas technique, three patterns of ventilation-perfusion mismatch have been recognized:[2151, 2152]

1. In about 50 per cent of patients, there is an increase in ventilation to high $\dot{V}A/\dot{Q}$ areas with no shunt or to low $\dot{V}A/\dot{Q}$ regions.

2. In 20 per cent of patients, there is an increase in perfusion to low $\dot{V}A/\dot{Q}$ regions with no shunt or to high $\dot{V}A/\dot{Q}$ regions.

3. In the remaining 30 per cent, there is an increase in both the high and low $\dot{V}A/\dot{Q}$ regions.

Wagner and associates[2151] have suggested that the high $\dot{V}A/\dot{Q}$ regions represent areas in which elastolysis has caused high compliance but in which perfusion is low as a result of capillary bed destruction. They found that this pattern of gas exchange is more common in the type A ("pink puffer") variation of COPD patient; the low $\dot{V}A/\dot{Q}$ regions, they suggest, are units with obstructed airways that are ventilated via collateral channels. The patients with an increase in the low $\dot{V}A/\dot{Q}$ regions tended to be the type B ("blue bloater") variant of COPD patient.[2151] Intrapulmonary right-to-left shunt and diffusion impairment do not contribute to the gas exchange abnormalities in COPD patients at rest.[2151, 2152]

The uneven distribution of inspired gas can be demonstrated by the single-breath oxygen test,[2153] the multiple-breath nitrogen washout,[2154] or the closed-circuit helium method (which is also used to measure FRC and RV).[2155, 2156] The time taken for the inhaled helium to be equilibrated in the lung is termed the *mixing efficiency*. In the early stages of COPD, mixing efficiency may be normal as measured by the helium technique, although more refined techniques, particularly those using radioactive xenon, frequently show regional inequalities of ventilation and perfusion.[2157–2159] Disturbances in the $\dot{V}A/\dot{Q}$ ratios can also be detected by measurement of the physiologic dead space or the ratio of dead space to tidal volume.[2160–2162]

In COPD of mild-to-moderate severity, hypoxemia exists without hypercapnia. The $\dot{V}A/\dot{Q}$ inequality impairs both the uptake of O_2 and the elimination of CO_2, but the tendency for elevation of $PaCO_2$ is overcome by an increase in alveolar ventilation to well-perfused units; however, the increase in ventilation cannot correct the hypoxemia because of the alinear shape of the O_2 dissociation curve (*see* page 134). When COPD becomes severe, CO_2 retention eventually occurs as total alveolar ventilation decreases and is accompanied by more severe hypoxemia. The relative contributions of $\dot{V}A/\dot{Q}$ mismatch and alveolar hypoventilation to the observed hypoxemia can be determined by calculating the $P(A - a)O_2$ (*see* page 136). The strong correlation between decreased PO_2 and increased PCO_2 in patients with COPD suggests that alveolar hypoventilation contributes significantly to the hypoxemia.[1332] An increase in arterial $PaCO_2$ does not occur until the FEV_1 is less than approximately 1.2 liters. The presence of hypercapnia in a patient with an FEV_1 greater than 1.5 liters should alert one to the possibility of central hypoventilation.

The hypoxemia of COPD is easily corrected by increasing the concentration of inspired oxygen; however, such an increase also causes a variable increase in arterial PCO_2, both in the stable state[1981] and especially during acute episodes of ventilatory respiratory failure.[1982, 2163] The administration of supplemental oxygen causes a decrease in minute ventilation ($\dot{V}E$), and until recently it was assumed that the rise in PCO_2 was secondary to this decrease. The accepted dogma has been that patients with COPD and chronic CO_2 retention have depressed ventilatory drive in response to CO_2 and rely on hypoxic stimulation to maintain a given level of ventilation; administration of supplemental O_2 decreases the hypoxic drive, resulting in a further decrease in $\dot{V}E$ and hypercapnia. However, the results of recent studies have challenged this mechanism as the cause of hyperoxia-induced hypercapnia.[1981, 1982, 2164] Although supplemental oxygen results in a decrease in $\dot{V}E$ in some patients with COPD, the effect is transient whereas the increase in $PaCO_2$ is persistent. The explanation is that oxygen administration worsens the matching of ventilation and perfusion, increases VD/VT, and causes a decrease in *alveolar* ventilation for a given $\dot{V}E$. Oxygen disturbs the $\dot{V}A/\dot{Q}$ match by increasing the perfusion to poorly ventilated lung regions, presumably by blocking hypoxic vasoconstriction in these areas.[2164, 2165]

During exacerbations of COPD, blood gas tensions deteriorate.[240] Although viral or bacterial respiratory tract infections are frequently implicated as the cause of episodes of deterioration, this cannot be proven in many instances. Exacerbations are frequently associated with right-sided heart failure and fluid overload, which could in themselves impair arterial blood gas tensions. Cardiac output can influence arterial blood gases by changing the mixed venous tensions of O_2 and CO_2. Given a certain disturbance of $\dot{V}A/\dot{Q}$ matching and certain metabolic rate, mixed venous PO_2 will fall and mixed venous PCO_2 will rise as cardiac output decreases.

The changes in mixed venous gas tensions will be reflected in arterial gas tensions. The development of right-sided heart failure and decreased cardiac output will therefore worsen arterial blood gas levels, other things being equal.[2166] The fluid retention associated with episodes of right-sided heart failure could also contribute to worsening gas exchange by causing mild interstitial pulmonary edema and more severe $\dot{V}A/\dot{Q}$ mismatch.[240, 2167] Although hypercapnea does not develop in patients with COPD until the FEV_1 has fallen to below approximately 1.2 liters, the relationship between FEV_1 and $PaCO_2$ below that threshold is poor;[2168, 2169] for example, patients with an FEV_1 of 0.6 liters can have either a normal PCO_2 or chronic hypercapnia. Stable patients with chronic hypercapnia can reduce arterial PCO_2 to normal levels by voluntary hyperventilation.

Genetic differences in respiratory drive are a major contributor to the variable response to airway obstruction. The adult offspring of patients with COPD and hypercapnia show depressed ventilatory responses to hypoxia and hypercapnia in comparison to those in the offspring of equally obstructed patients without hypercapnia.[2170–2172] Patients with COPD and hypercapnia also show an abnormally small increase in minute ventilation when exposed to hypoxic or hypercapnic gas mixtures; however this cannot be interpreted as decreased drive because it could be explained by increased respiratory system impedance (increased resistance and decreased dynamic compliance) in the presence of normal drive. The measurement of P0.1 during a hypoxic or hypercapnic challenge provides a better estimate of drive.[2173] P0.1 is the mouth pressure achieved after 0.1 second of an occluded inspiratory effort; since there is no flow or volume change during the obstructed breath, the pressure is not influenced by the mechanics of the respiratory system, although it is influenced by the mechanical advantage of the inspiratory muscles. Because the patient does not realize that the breath has been obstructed within the 0.1-second period, voluntary response to the stimulus is also not a problem. Another way to test central respiratory drive in obstructed patients is to correct the ventilatory response to hypoxia and hypercapnia by taking into account the maximal voluntary ventilation.[2174]

When respiratory drive is assessed using the P0.1 or the corrected ventilatory response, patients with COPD and CO_2 retention still exhibit decreased drive in comparison to normal subjects.[2175, 2176] This is in contrast to asthmatic subjects, who have increased drive. It is likely that the hypoventilation is related partly to genetic factors that influence ventilatory control and partly to an acquired tolerance to the stimulatory effects of hypoxia and hypercapnia.[2176] Although it has been suggested that endogenous endorphin secretion could depress drive and mediate the tolerance to elevated PCO_2, the results of experiments designed to test this hypothesis have been disappointing.[2177–2179] In addition, increased buffering capacity of the cerebrospinal fluid does not account for the depressed ventilatory response to CO_2.[2180] Patients with COPD and hypercapnia may have impaired load detection: when eight patients with COPD were challenged with an external resistive-load or methacholine-induced bronchoconstriction, the resulting decrease in tidal volume and increase in PCO_2 were related to the acuity with which they could perceive changes in intrathoracic pressure.[2181]

COPD patients with hypercapnia also appear to have an altered ventilatory pattern that may contribute to the CO_2 retention,[2168, 2169, 2182] respiratory rates being more rapid and tidal volumes smaller than in equally obstructed patients without hypercapnia. Although this pattern of rapid shallow breathing does not decrease minute ventilation, since dead space remains constant and VT decreases, the ratio VD/VT increases, resulting in a decrease in alveolar ventilation. This inefficient breathing pattern may be caused in part by excessive stimulation of respiratory epithelial irritant receptors. Rapid shallow breathing is also stimulated by inhalation of histamine and methacholine,[2183, 2184] and inhalation of an aerosol of local anesthetic causes an increase in VT and decrease in respiratory frequency in these patients.[2185, 2186] Rapid shallow breathing occurs in COPD patients during acute-on-chronic hypercapnic exacerbations of their airflow obstruction,[2173] and it is possible that airway inflammation and inflammatory mediator release during the acute episode stimulate irritant receptors, thus altering the ventilatory pattern and contributing to the abnormalities of arterial blood gases. It is also possible that respiratory muscle fatigue contributes to the altered breathing pattern. The ability to recognize and respond to added resistive and elastic loads is impaired in patients with COPD, a fault that may be related to endorphins, since naloxone increases the compensatory response to added resistance.[2177, 2187]

The depressed ventilatory response to hypoxia and hypercapnia in COPD does not improve with prolonged home treatment with oxygen,[2188] and although it has an adverse effect on arterial blood gas tensions, it may have a beneficial effect by decreasing dyspnea; the dyspnea experienced by patients with COPD is caused not by the alteration in blood gas tensions but by the inappropriate effort needed to maintain ventilation.[2189]

Sleep has profound effects on ventilatory control and arterial blood gases in patients with COPD and is frequently associated with a worsening of hypoxemia and hypercapnia.[2190, 2191] Since PaO_2 values fall onto the steep portion of the O_2 dissociation curve, the decrease in arterial saturation may be considerable. Patients with COPD have poor-quality sleep as a result of decreased total sleep time, increased sleep stage shifts, and increased arousal frequency.[2192, 2193] If patients are not selected on the basis of increased daytime somnolence,[2194] the frequency of apneic episodes is not increased in comparison to that of the normal population.[2192, 2194] However, despite the lack of frank apneas, patients manifest episodic arterial desaturation during sleep, episodes of decreased saturation being more severe in patients categorized as blue bloaters than as pink puffers.[2194] The desaturation is also more severe during REM sleep than during slow-wave sleep[2195] and appears to be related to periods of hypoventilation or "hypopneas." In fact, REM sleep can be divided into two stages: (1) so-called *phasic* REM, during which there is rapid eye movement, myoclonic twitches, and an alteration in breathing pattern, and (2) *tonic* REM, during which there is generalized muscular atonia. George and colleagues[2196] have shown that the most significant desaturation occurs in association with the altered breathing pattern at the onset of phasic REM.

A more severe desaturation probably develops in blue bloaters because they are more hypoxic to begin with and because any additional hypoventilation moves them onto the steep descending portion of the O_2 dissociation curve.[2194] It has been suggested that sleep desaturation is a factor that predisposes patients to the development of a clinical picture of blue bloating,[2197] but it is more likely than the excessive nocturnal desaturation is secondary to the pre-existing hypoventilation. The association of hypercapnia during the day and oxygen desaturation during sleep was examined in the patients with COPD who were followed in a nocturnal oxygen therapy trial.[2198] It was found that individuals with a higher daytime arterial PCO_2 developed nocturnal oxygen desaturation that was significantly worse than in those with normal daytime arterial PCO_2, even though the two groups showed similar values for FEV_1.

The effect on sleep quality of oxygen administration is controversial; in one study, it was shown that O_2 therapy improved sleep quality[2193] but in another study of 24 patients with COPD, Fleetham and associates[2192] found no improvement in arousals or in total sleep time despite correction of desaturation with oxygen. The latter investigators have suggested that it may be the increased arterial PCO_2 that disturbs sleep in these individuals; in another study of patients with severe but stable COPD, supplemental O_2 did not significantly increase nocturnal CO_2.[2199] The hypocapnic episodes during sleep could be caused by decreased central ventilatory drive or by increased respiratory system impedance: in a study in which respiratory effort was assessed by measuring intrathoracic esophageal pressure swings during hypopnea, in approximately half of the patients the swings were decreased and in the other half increased.[2200] In fact, individual patients can manifest hypopneic episodes during both increased and decreased pressure swings.[2201] The magnitude of sleep desaturation is inversely related to daytime arterial saturation and to the ventilatory response to hypoxia and hypercapnia during wakefulness.[2202] Medroxyprogesterone therapy improves daytime blood gases in some patients but does not reduce the incidence of hypopneas or nocturnal desaturation.[2203] Episodes of nocturnal desaturation are associated with a worsening of pulmonary hypertension, and although nocturnal O_2 administration does not prevent hypopnea, it does block the pulmonary vascular response.[2204]

The administration of aerosol or intravenous bronchodilators may be followed by changes in ventilation-perfusion matching in patients with COPD.[2205–2207] The change in PaO_2 varies from patient to patient, depending on the bronchodilator used, its dose and method of administration, and the length of time elapsed between its administration and the measurement of arterial blood gases.[2205] Arterial PO_2 usually falls in response to aerosolized beta-adrenergic drugs.[2207, 2208]

Exercise can also influence arterial blood gas tensions; in some patients, exercise induces pronounced arterial desaturation and hypercapnia whereas in others gas exchange is improved.[2209–2211] Patients in whom desaturation occurs during exercise have significantly worse airflow obstruction, a lower diffusing capacity,[2212] a higher V_D/V_T, and a lower V_T.[2213, 2214] Supplemental O_2 improves maximal work performance and endurance in patients with COPD,[2215, 2216] mainly by decreasing the level of ventilation for any given workload[2217] but also possibly by causing bronchodilatation and a decrease in airway resistance.[2215] A large carbohydrate meal immediately before exercise decreases exercise capacity by transiently increasing CO_2 production.[2218, 2219] Metabolism of carbohydrate occurs with a respiratory quotient of 1.0 (one molecule of CO_2 produced for each molecule of O_2 consumed), whereas fat and protein metabolism produces less CO_2 for a similar caloric output (respiratory quotients of 0.8 and 0.7, respectively). However, this phenomenon is rarely of clinical importance unless a patient with fixed ventilation (ventilatory support) is given a large carbohydrate load.

During exercise, patients with COPD show a normal relationship between cardiac output and total body oxygen consumption,[2220] suggesting that circulatory factors do not contribute to exercise limitation; in fact, such limitation is chiefly related to a diminished ventilatory capacity. The ventilatory requirement for any given work output is also increased because the wasted ventilation fraction of each breath is larger (increased V_D/V_T) and since the O_2 uptake per breath is decreased because of hypoxemia.[2221] In addition, the high O_2 consumption by respiratory muscles working against abnormal loads may divert O_2 away from other exercising muscles.[2220]

Even during maximal exercise, normal subjects do not achieve the level of ventilation of which they are capable, leaving considerable ventilatory reserve. By contrast, patients with COPD usually stop exercising when they reach their maximal achieva-

ble ventilation, a state that is best predicted in the laboratory from a combination of FEV_1 and inspiratory muscle strength.[2222] The symptom that stops patients with COPD from exercising further is dyspnea, a sensation that probably originates in respiratory muscle afferent receptors. Dyspnea is related to the ratio of the force-generating and force-shortening ability of inspiratory muscles to the force and shortening required for a given ventilatory level. Dyspnea can occur because the force-generating ability is reduced (respiratory muscle weakness), because the force requirements of ventilation are increased (increased impedance), or as a result of a combination of these factors. In COPD, the force requirements are increased because of increased airway resistance and the force-generating ability is decreased because of hyperinflation and (in severe disease) malnutrition.[2223] During exercise, patients with severe COPD can manifest paradoxical motion of the rib cage and abdomen[2224] and can recruit expiratory muscles;[2225] abdominal expiratory muscle contraction can passively stretch the relaxed diaphragm during exhalation, and the subsequent sudden relaxation of those muscles allows a passive inspiratory diaphragmatic movement.[2225]

Measurement of arterial pH, hydrogen ion concentration, and bicarbonate provides important information about the acid-base status of patients with COPD. When an excess of CO_2 is compensated for by an increase in bicarbonate, there is clear indication that the respiratory failure is not of "acute" onset; such patients show a greater efficiency in buffering acute changes in levels of CO_2.[2226] An arterial pH within or above the normal range is unusual in uncomplicated respiratory acidosis and suggests the possibility of concomitant metabolic alkalosis, usually secondary to diuretic usage. Alternatively, during acute exacerbations of COPD, there may be "relative hyperventilation," the PCO_2 decreasing as a result of increased drive but not reaching normal levels. Such an "acute respiratory alkalosis" superimposed on chronic respiratory acidosis could mimic "overcompensated respiratory acidosis."

An elevated PCO_2 associated with a normal or only slightly raised bicarbonate level indicates that the hypoventilation and respiratory acidosis are of recent onset. However, this conclusion is not justified if there is coexisting metabolic acidosis that has depressed the bicarbonate level. Even with the most severe hypoxemia, anaerobic metabolism does not result in the formation of lactic acid and metabolic acidosis unless there is an associated systemic circulatory disorder that causes inadequate tissue perfusion.[2227] In any assessment of arterial blood gas abnormalities and their relationship to neurologic symptoms and signs, it must be remembered that gas tensions and acid-base balance in the cerebrospinal fluid are different from those in the arterial blood and perhaps more correctly reflect the environment of the respiratory center.[2228, 2229]

Diffusing Capacity

The single-breath diffusing capacity of individuals who smoke cigarettes is lower than that of age-matched nonsmoking controls, even in the absence of other evidence of lung dysfunction. Part of the decrease is caused by elevated blood carboxyhemoglobin levels, but even after correction for the back pressure of CO, smoking subjects have lower values of $DL_{CO}SB$.[2230] The $DL_{CO}SB$ increases when normal subjects assume the supine from the sitting position, presumably because pulmonary capillary blood volume increases; by contrast, such a change in posture by cigarette smokers does not cause the same increase in diffusing capacity, suggesting the possibility of impaired pulmonary vascular distensibility.[2230]

The single-breath diffusing capacity can be overestimated in patients with advanced COPD:[1323] standard techniques to measure $DL_{CO}SB$ assume that the CO uptake occurs only during the breath-hold time, but in fact CO is taken up during the inspiratory and expiratory phases of the test also; since patients with COPD have prolonged inspiratory and expiratory times, more CO can be absorbed and $DL_{CO}SB$ overestimated. A new method to calculate $DL_{CO}SB$ to include CO uptake during inspiration and expiration would obviously correct this problem.[1323]

The diffusing capacity measured by both the single-breath and the steady-state CO methods is usually reduced in patients with COPD. There is reasonably close correlation between severely reduced diffusing capacity during life and the finding of extensive morphologic emphysema at necropsy.[1875] Even patients with relatively normal lung volumes and airway resistance have been shown to have significantly reduced $DL_{CO}SB$, a reduction that has correlated with the extent of emphysema found in lobectomy specimens. Some authors consider the diffusing capacity to be of differential diagnostic value in patients with COPD, reduction indicating emphysema and normal values indicating primary intrinsic airway narrowing.[1923, 2231] However, it should be appreciated that morphologic emphysema of mild to moderate severity can be observed at necropsy in patients who had normal diffusing capacity during life.[1875, 2146] The reduction in diffusing capacity in COPD is generally considered to be caused by both a decrease in the membrane component and a mismatch of ventilation and perfusion. It is probable, however, that there are other contributing factors, including reduction in capillary volume and perhaps limitation of diffusion in the gas phase of the "air pools" typical of emphysema.[2232, 2233]

Effect of Smoking Cessation on Lung Function

Smoking cessation results in acute decrease in lung elastic recoil[2234, 2235] but a sustained increase in maximal flow and volumes.[2235, 2236] Although the improvement in function is slight and rarely returns to predicted normal, smoking cessation also decreases the annual rate of decline in lung function.[2237, 2238] The improvement in flow rates and tests of small airway function (closing capacity and ΔN_2/liter) begin as early as 1 week following cessation and continue for 6 to 8 months.[2236, 2239] Nonspecific airway responsiveness to inhaled methacholine, which may be slightly increased in smokers, also returns toward normal with cessation of smoking.[2239]

ALPHA₁ PROTEASE INHIBITOR DEFICIENCY (ALPHA₁-ANTITRYPSIN DEFICIENCY)

Alpha₁-antitrypsin deficiency was first described by Eriksson in 1964.[1615] He observed that patients with flat alpha₁ globulin peaks on electrophoresis possessed approximately 15 to 30 per cent of normal serum trypsin inhibitory capacity and that members of the families of these individuals had normal values, intermediate levels (50 to 80 per cent of normal activity), or less than 30 per cent of normal activity and were therefore homozygotes. All the offspring of homozygotes exhibited intermediate deficiency states. He estimated that 4.7 per cent of the population were heterozygotes and only 0.06 per cent homozygotes and that in only 1 per cent of patients with emphysema did the disease develop because of alpha₁-antitrypsin deficiency. Many investigators have subsequently confirmed that a heritable disorder characterized by very low levels of serum antitrypsin activity is associated with a high familial incidence of COPD and emphysema. This unanimity of opinion became evident by 1972, when experts in the field gathered together for a symposium on pulmonary emphysema and proteolysis.[2240]

Approximately 90 per cent of the antiproteolytic activity in serum is associated with the alpha₁ globulin fraction and only 10 per cent with alpha₂ globulin.[1922] The initial studies used trypsin as the proteolytic enzyme; as a result, the inhibitor in the alpha₁ band became known as alpha₁-antitrypsin. In fact, this substance is able to inhibit a wide variety of proteases and is therefore more correctly termed alpha₁ protease inhibitor, alpha₁ proteinase inhibitor, or alpha₁ antiprotease. In this text, we will refer to it as alpha₁ protease inhibitor (alpha₁ PI) and to the deficiency as alpha₁ PI deficiency.

Human plasma contains six proteolytic inhibitors, the predominant one being alpha₁ PI.[2241] Proteolytic inhibitors have a regulatory function in the equilibrium between coagulation and fibrinolysis and in the liberation of kinins. Alpha₁ PI has been shown to inhibit a number of proteolytic enzymes, including trypsin, chymotrypsin, elastase, collagenase, urokinase, plasmin, thrombin, kallikrein, and leukocytic and bacterial proteases.[1617, 2240, 2242] Protease inhibitors with similar properties are present in the plasma of various animals, including primates, guinea pigs,[2243] cattle,[2244] rabbits,[2245] and rats.[2246]

Methods for the detection of alpha$_1$ PI were reviewed by an *ad hoc* committee at a Symposium on Pulmonary Emphysema and Proteolysis.[2240] Quantitative analysis requires measurement of inhibitory capacity or determination by immunodiffusion of the amount of alpha$_1$ PI in the serum.[2247, 2248] Because alpha$_1$ PI can be inactivated without changing its immunologic characteristics, a measure of inhibitory capacity is more accurate. The ratio of active to total immunoreactive inhibitor gives an estimate of inactivation. Deficiency of alpha$_1$ PI in homozygotes can be detected by serum electrophoresis when the alpha$_1$ globulin fraction is 0.2 gm/dl or less, but this method is not reliable in screening for heterozygotes.[1922] Serum trypsin inhibitory capacity is 0.85 units or more in normal subjects, 0.4 to 0.85 units in heterozygotes (an intermediate range), and less than 0.4 units in homozygotes with severe deficiency. Employing immunodiffusion, values for serum concentration of alpha$_1$ PI are 200 mg/dl in normal subjects, 60 to 199 mg/dl in patients with intermediate deficiency, and less than 60 mg/dl in those with severe deficiency.[1922] However, because of the well-documented overlap of serum concentrations of alpha$_1$ PI, particularly between normal subjects and patients in the intermediate range, there is general agreement that protease inhibitor (Pi) phenotyping is necessary for the recognition of heterozygotes.[2247, 2251, 2252]

Alpha$_1$ PI is an acute phase-reactant protein the serum levels of which may rise in the presence of inflammation (infectious or noninfectious), pregnancy, malignant disease, following the administration of estrogens,[1922, 2243, 2249] or postoperatively. Serum levels are also higher in homozygotes who are cigarette smokers or who are exposed to high concentrations of dust.[2253] In any of these circumstances, heterozygotes may show an increase in serum concentration of alpha$_1$ PI to low normal values; similarly, severe infections in homozygotes may occasionally elevate values to intermediate levels.[2249] In certain infections, notably those caused by some species of *Pseudomonas* and by *Proteus mirabilis*, an alpha$_1$ PI inactivator is produced that permits uninhibited destruction of lung tissue by proteolytic enzymes.[2250] At the other extreme, *S. pneumoniae* contains a potent inhibitor of elastase, a fact that may explain the lack of lung destruction with this infection despite the presence of enormous numbers of activated neutrophils.[1682]

Pi PHENOTYPES

In his original investigations, Eriksson[1615] showed that alpha$_1$ PI levels in deficient patients (homozygotes) were about 20 per cent of normal, whereas levels in carriers (heterozygotes) were about 60 per cent of normal. Subsequent studies in families of patients with alpha$_1$ PI deficiency indicated that this distribution cannot be explained on the basis of one recessive and one dominant gene but is compatible with an autosomal recessive disorder with two concomitant genes, one contributing about 50 per cent and the other about 10 per cent of the total alpha$_1$ PI concentration. This theory readily explains the trimodal distribution of alpha$_1$-antitrypsin concentrations.

1. Deficient subjects possess two genes, each of which is responsible for 10 per cent of normal concentration, for a total of 20 per cent.

2. Carriers possess one deficient (10 per cent) and one normal (50 per cent) gene, for a total of 60 per cent of normal concentration.

3. Normal subjects possess two normal genes, each of which contributes 50 per cent, for a total of 100 per cent alpha$_1$ PI concentration.[2254]

On the basis of their mobility on acid-starch gel and antigen-antibody electrophoresis,[2254, 2255] approximately 25 molecular variants of alpha$_1$ PI have been described.[2256] By far the commonest codominant allele determining structure and serum concentrations of alpha$_1$ PI is the gene Pi^M, which, in its homozygous state (MM), has been found in over 90 per cent of the population of Oslo and St. Louis,[2257, 2258] in 88.4 per cent of New York State inhabitants,[2259] in 86.5 per cent of the population of northern Ireland,[2260] and in 87 per cent of individuals in Montreal.[2261] Pi^{MM} is associated with normal quantitative determinations of alpha$_1$ PI. Other alleles, designated Pi^S, Pi^F, Pi^I, Pi^X, Pi^P, Pi^Z, and so on, occur far less frequently in homozygous or heterozygous forms. In most series the major antiprotease variants reported have been MS, MZ, FM, IM, SS, SZ, and ZZ, ranging from 6 per cent to less than 0.1 per cent.[2258–2260]

Pi^{ZZ} PHENOTYPE

The gene Pi^Z in the homozygous state (ZZ) is associated with an increased frequency of pulmonary emphysema. This phenotype also is associated with the lowest serum concentration of alpha$_1$ PI and the lowest total serum antiprotease activity (amounting to only 20 per cent of normal).[2262] It has been found only once in every 1,500 to 5,000 live births[2263–2265] and is identified in 1 to 10 per cent of patients with clinically diagnosed emphysema and in a considerably higher percentage of patients less than 45 years of age whose chest roentgenograms manifest a predominantly basal distribution of disease.[1906, 2264, 2266, 2267] It has been estimated that patients with homozygous alpha$_1$ PI deficiency have a 50 per cent[2268] to 80 per cent[2269] chance of developing emphysema.

Cigarette smoking plays an important additional role in the production of emphysema in patients with alpha$_1$ PI deficiency.[2270] Symptoms of dyspnea and evidence of airflow obstruction bring smokers with alpha$_1$ PI deficiency to medical attention in the third and fourth decades of life, whereas nonsmokers may not present until the sixth or seventh decade.[2271, 2272, 2797] However, there is wide variablility in the degree of dysfunction in smokers and nonsmokers of the same age: in one 13-year follow-up study of 69 Pi^{ZZ} individuals, the rate of decrease in FEV_1 was 80 ml/year for nonsmokers and 317 ml/year for smokers.[2272] Despite this, advanced disease has been described in nonsmokers[2273] and in children.[2274] Pathologically, the emphysema is invariably panacinar in type and usually is more pronounced in the lower lobes.[2275] Some studies have suggested characteristic physiologic findings (*see* farther on).

It is believed that the abnormal gene for alpha$_1$ PI deficiency derives from northern and central European countries. Mittman[2276] and Fagerhol[1628] found low antitrypsin levels in up to 10 per cent of subjects with northern, central, or western European background. All Italians tested had normal antiprotease values and only about 2 per cent of Jews, Mexican Americans, and blacks were deficient. Phenotyping of 2,285 blood donors in St. Louis revealed the major antiprotease variants only 40 per cent as often in blacks as in the balance of the study group.[2258] A California study of 1,841 high school students detected heterozygous and homozygous deficiency states in 3.04 per cent of white subjects but in none of 461 subjects of Mexican origin or of other races.[2277] Prevalence studies of phenotypic types must be interpreted with care. In Tucson, Arizona, a prevalence rate for severe deficiency (Pi^{ZZ} or Pi^{SZ}) of 1/368 was found in 2,944 subjects.[1617] Knowing the prevalence of ZZ and SZ phenotypes in the American population at large, a rate of 1 in 676 would have been predicted in white Americans. This discrepancy suggests that patients with severe deficiency may move to Arizona.

Alpha$_1$ PI is a glycoprotein synthesized in the liver and released into the serum, presumably in sufficient quantity to neutralize circulating proteolytic enzymes and thus prevent tissue damage. The Pi^{ZZ} variant has a polypeptide core similar to that in the normal type Pi^{MM}; however, it is deficient in the carbohydrate component, sialic acid,[1617, 2278] and its secretion is blocked in hepatocytes.[2278–2280] The Pi^{ZZ} antiprotease has a lysine substituted for the normal glutamic acid at the 342 position. The glutamic acid residue is the site of sialic acid attachment, and it is the failure of sialization that causes the defective secretion. In Pi^{SS} phenotypes, a valine residue replaces glutamic acid.[888, 1617] Interestingly, the development of emphysema has been described in the recessively inherited disorder of sialic acid metabolism called *Salla disease*.[2281] The exact pathogenic mechanism for the development of severe emphysema in this rare defect and its possible association with alpha$_1$ antiprotease deficiency remain unclear.

In Pi^{ZZ} homozygotes, globular, PAS-positive diastase-resistant intracytoplasmic inclusion bodies can be identified within hepatocytes.[2278–2280] The main component of this inclusion material has been shown to be a protein of approximately the same molecular size as serum alpha$_1$ PI with similar immunologic properties.[2282] However, chemical analysis has revealed a total absence of sialic acid.[2278, 2282]

An association between alpha$_1$ PI deficiency and liver disease was first recognized by Sharp and associates in 1968.[2283] Cholestasis, hepatitis, cirrhosis, and severe deficiency of antiprotease (Pi^{ZZ}) is a rare combination, in contrast with the more common types of hepatic disease such as primary biliary cirrhosis and the cirrhosis associated with chronic active hepatitis. In the latter, high levels of antiproteolytic enzyme are found in the serum, presumably reflecting the inflammatory process.[2284] Recent studies have confirmed a significant association between alpha$_1$ PI deficiency and neonatal hepatitis.[2285, 2286] Infants may die from cirrhosis.[2274, 2287, 2288] Occasionally, cirrhosis and panlobular emphysema are found together in children with the Pi^{ZZ} phenotype.[2274] Liver cirrhosis also occurs in alpha$_1$ PI–deficient adults, usually in combination with emphysema.[2287, 2289–2294] Several reports have suggested that deficiency of the Pi^Z genotype may also be associated with an increased incidence of hepatomas.[2289, 2294–2296] As with COPD (*see* farther on), opinions differ as to whether patients with other variants of alpha$_1$ PI deficiency, particularly Pi^Z heterozygotes, are more susceptible to liver disease; however, there are several reports of liver cirrhosis in patients with the MZ phenotype[2294, 2297] and one in a patient with Pi^{SZ} phenotype.[2298] Despite these observations, some studies of population groups[2284, 2299] suggest that the simultaneous presence of these two rather infrequently occurring conditions (Pi^Z heterozygosity and hepatic cirrhosis) does not indicate a causal relationship but is fortuitous. In addition, many patients with severe alpha$_1$ PI deficiency do not develop liver disease, suggesting that other factors may be operative. For example, Australia antigen or antibody has been said to be present in several patients with this form of hepatitis.[2261, 2285]

Individual reports have appeared of patients who have demonstrated deficiency of alpha$_1$ PI associated with emphysema, cirrhosis, intestinal mucosal atrophy,[2300] pancreatic fibrosis,[2301] and severe panniculitis (Weber-Christian disease).[2302] The diagnosis of alpha$_1$ PI deficiency can be made prenatally by obtaining fetal blood at fetoscopy or (more safely) by direct genetic examination of cultured amniotic fluid cells.[2303]

Other Pi Variants

In addition to the Pi^Z genotype, a number of other variants that may be associated with subnormal levels of antiprotease are detectable by serum electrophoresis on acid-starch gels and antigen-antibody crossed electrophoresis. Heterozygotes with Pi^M genotype, when combined with Pi^Z (MZ) and Pi^S (MS), may show alpha$_1$ PI activity and concentration in the intermediate or low normal range. Lieberman and associates[2255] determined that 15 per cent of MZ heterozygotes and 60 to 80 per cent of MS heterozygotes can be recognized only by phenotyping. Most patients with variants of the normal Pi^{MM} phenotype manifest only intermediate deficiency of alpha$_1$ PI, and it is highly questionable whether they have an increased susceptibility to emphysema (*see* risk factors above). Rarely, emphysema with alpha$_1$ PI deficiency is described in patients showing Pi variants other than Pi^{ZZ}; the heterozygous Pi^{SZ} phenotype has been associated with alpha$_1$ PI levels as low as those seen in Pi^{ZZ} patients.[1628] In one study of 25 Pi^{SZ} patients, emphysema was present only in those who smoked.[2305]

A genotype designated as Pi^M Duarte[2304] and a "null gene" for alpha$_1$ PI[2798] have been described, both of which lead to severe deficiency when in the homozygous state. In contrast to the Z variant, the M Duarte variant has normal mobility on acid-starch electrophoresis and hence, in the heterozygous state with the normal M form, cannot be distinguished by phenotyping procedures. Similarly, when intermediate antiprotease deficiency is found in the presence of a normal phenotypic pattern, the possibility must be considered that the patient has inherited a null gene for alpha$_1$ PI synthesis. A family has been described in which a "null gene" has been associated with a normal phenotypic pattern and with intermediate quantitative levels of alpha$_1$ PI somewhat lower than those customarily seen in the MZ heterozygotes.[2306] Rare cases have been described in which serum alpha$_1$ PI has been completely absent ("null" homozygotes) accompanied by an absence of liver globules, a combination that may represent complete deletion of the gene for alpha$_1$ PI synthesis.[1617] Severe emphysema develops more rapidly in these patients than in those with Pi^{ZZ}, suggesting that even 20 per cent of the normal plasma concentration of alpha$_1$ protease can provide some protection to the lungs.[2281]

The vast majority of patients who develop symptomatic COPD and emphysema have the normal Pi^{MM} genotype and normal levels of alpha$_1$ PI. There are subtypes of the Pi^{MM} phenotype (M$_1$, M$_2$, M$_3$, and combinations) that can be recognized with isoelectric focusing, and it has been suggested that M$_1$M$_2$ and M$_2$M$_2$ types exhibit a higher incidence of COPD.[2307] With the exception of the M Duarte variant, in which liver cells possess identical diastase-resistant, PAS-positive globules,[2304] patients with other Pi variants do not have intracytoplasmic PAS-staining globules in their hepatocytes. The mechanism or mechanisms responsible for reduced alpha$_1$ PI serum concentration in patients with variants other than Pi^{ZZ} are unknown, although Lieberman and his group[2279, 2308, 2309] have shown that the alpha$_1$ PI of these genetic mutants possesses increased lability and shows a "double-ring" antigen-antibody precipitation pattern on radial immunodiffusion assay, while only one line is created by the sera from M phenotypes. The second line is believed to represent antibody response to spontaneous degradation of variant alpha$_1$-antitrypsin proteins *in vivo*. Serum from MM homozygotes may also show a double ring after prolonged incubation or when concentrated fivefold. This phenomenon of altered antigenicity has been proposed as a screening test for alpha$_1$-antitrypsin variants.[2309]

Clinical Manifestations in Severe Alpha$_1$ Protease Inhibitor Deficiency

In the vast majority of smokers with COPD, airway obstruction relates to a combination of loss of lung elasticity and airway narrowing, but it is difficult to separate the relative contribution of each of these mechanisms in individual subjects. The existence of nonsmoking patients with severe antiprotease deficiency should permit the study of a pure form of elastolytic lung injury unadulterated by the airway inflammation and narrowing associated with cigarette smoke. Studies of asymptomatic individuals with severe alpha$_1$ PI deficiency have revealed a pattern that is believed to represent early emphysema,[2310–2312] the major abnormalities being a loss of lung elastic recoil and a redistribution of blood flow characterized by a loss of the normal perfusion gradient from apex to base. At this stage, the patient may show hyperinflation without evidence of airway obstruction, at least as measured by routine methods.

When symptoms develop in patients with phenotype Pi^{ZZ}, pulmonary function testing reveals a decreased FEV_1, FEV_1/FVC, and DL_{CO}/VA, and there is roentgenographic evidence of lower lobe emphysema.[2799] The relative contribution of loss of lung recoil and airway narrowing to decreased expiratory flow can be determined by plotting maximal flow against recoil pressure at isovolume points (Fig. 11–81). In most patients with homozygous alpha$_1$ PI deficiency, the decreased flow can be attributed to loss of elasticity; in some, however, there also appears to be an element of increased upstream resistance.[2303] When symptoms are severe, the disturbances of pulmonary function are similar to those of "ordinary" emphysema.[2313] Of some interest is the fact that the incidence of chronic cough and sputum production is increased in patients with alpha$_1$ PI deficiency irrespective of their smoking history,[2271, 2314] a clinical manifestation that could be related to an increased susceptibility to pulmonary infection; in fact, in one report, three patients with severe alpha$_1$ PI deficiency presented with bronchiectasis.[2303]

BULLOUS DISEASE OF THE LUNGS

Considerable semantic confusion surrounds this diagnosis, chiefly because the words "bulla," "cyst," and "bleb" tend to be used interchangeably.

Figure 11–81. Maximal Flow–Static Recoil Plots in Four Patients with Alpha₁-Protease Inhibitor Deficiency. Maximal expiratory flow can be limited because of a decrease in lung elastic recoil or an increase in upstream resistance. In patients with relatively pure emphysema, such as occurs in alpha₁-protease inhibitor deficiency, maximal expiratory flow is limited primarily by a loss of lung elastic recoil. This can be appreciated by plotting maximal flow expressed as per cent predicted vital capacity per second versus lung elastic recoil derived from a static pressure-volume curve of the lung. In this diagram, plots from four patients with homozygous deficiency show that the slope of the maximal flow-recoil plot is normal and that maximal flow is limited because of a loss of recoil.

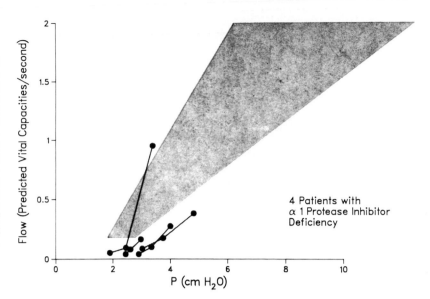

The word "cyst" mostly is used to describe the congenital variety of bronchial or bronchogenic cyst and also to describe the thin-walled space that sometimes remains as a residuum of a lung abscess, particularly one of staphylococcal etiology. Bronchial cysts commonly are lined by recognizable respiratory epithelium unless they have become infected, in which circumstance the wall may be composed solely of fibrous tissue. The word "bleb" usually connotes a collection of air within the layers of visceral pleura; this lesion is often associated with the development of spontaneous pneumothorax. A "bulla" is an air-filled, thin-walled space within the lung usually considered to result from destruction of alveolar tissue. The CIBA symposium report of 1959[1423] recommended use of the term for spaces greater than 1 cm in diameter in the distended state. The walls of bullae are formed by pleura, connective tissue septa, or compressed lung parenchyma; the character of the wall depends on the site of the bulla. The word "pneumatocele" is sometimes used as a synonym for bulla but incorrectly: in our opinion, use of this word should be restricted to a thin-walled, gas-filled space within the lung that develops in association with acute pneumonia, most commonly of staphylococcal etiology and almost invariably transient (*see* Fig. 4–107, page 612).

It is useful and traditional to divide patients with bullous disease of the lungs into two groups—those with COPD and those judged to have normal pulmonary parenchyma between the bullae and who thus are free of airway obstruction (primary bullous disease).[2316–2320]

Pathologic Characteristics

As indicated above, bullae occur both singly and in multiples, either in otherwise normal lung or as part of generalized emphysema. Reid[1925] divided them into three morphologic types.

Type 1 bullae originate in a subpleural location or in the vicinity of parenchymal scars. They are commonly located in the apex of an upper lobe or along the costophrenic rim of the middle lobe and lingula. Each bulla characteristically has a narrow neck and usually contains only gas, without evidence of alveolar remnants or blood vessels. When seen in an excised lung, a bulla appears as a variably sized, spherical sac projecting above the pleural surface (Fig. 11–82); of necessity, it extends into the contiguous lung *in vivo*, compressing the parenchyma and causing passive atelectasis. Occasionally, the bulla can become enormous, displacing the mediastinum into the contralateral hemithorax and interfering with the function of the opposite lung. They can also be multiple, extending in rows beneath the pleura and in some cases coalescing to form large airspaces that may be visible roentgenographically. It is possible that this type is related pathogenetically to paraseptal emphysema.[2317, 2318]

Type 2 bullae are also superficial in location but have a very broad neck. They may occur anywhere over the lung surface, but most often develop over the anterior edge of the upper and middle lobes and over the diaphragmatic surface. In contrast to type 1 bullae, this variety characteristically contains blood vessels and strands of partially destroyed lung, indicating that it probably represents a localized exaggeration of generalized emphysema.

Type 3 bullae lie deep within the lung substance but are otherwise similar to the type 2 variety, commonly containing strands of emphysematous lung and intact blood vessels. They appear to affect both upper and lower lobes equally. Although a type 3 bulla usually represents an exaggerated form of generalized emphysema, it occasionally develops in its absence, in which case it probably represents the residuum of a lung abscess (and thus can more appropriately be termed a cyst).

Although any of the three types can rupture and cause pneumothorax, the most common to do

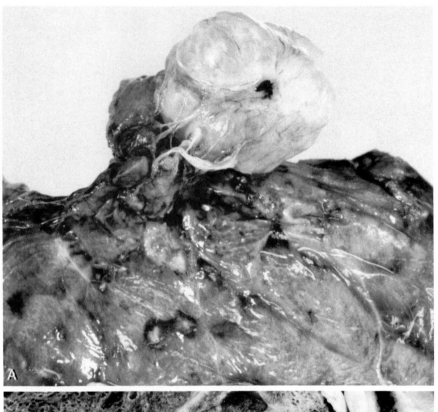

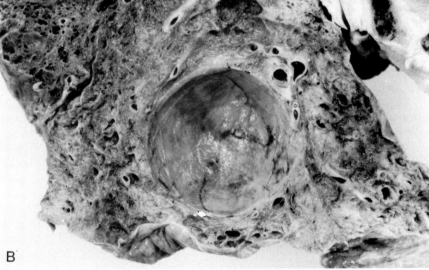

Figure 11–82. Bullae. *A*, A discrete narrow-necked bulla is present on the apical aspect of the upper lobe. *B*, The basal portion of the lower lobe from another patient shows a spherical, smooth-walled bulla projecting into the lung parenchyma (the other half of the bulla extended to the lateral pleural surface). The remainder of the lung parenchyma shows moderate emphysema.

so is type 2; in one study, of 54 resected bullae associated with spontaneous pneumothorax, 65 per cent were of this type.[2321]

Roentgenographic Manifestations

The diagnosis of bullous disease of the lungs depends upon roentgenologic identification of local, thin-walled, sharply demarcated areas of avascularity (Fig. 11–83). The walls are characteristically apparent as hairline shadows, but since the air cysts are most often at or near the lung surface, usually only a portion of the wall is visible. Location within the substance of the lung renders identification

much more difficult, and even peripheral bullae may be extremely difficult to identify. This was shown by Laws and Heard,[1893] who found many more bullae at necropsy than had been detected roentgenologically. Since the bullae trap air during expiration, they may be identified on roentgenograms exposed at RV and yet be barely or not at all visible on those exposed at TLC. In fact, bullae may undergo an increase in size during expiration, probably as a result of collateral air drift and their increased compliance compared with contiguous lung parenchyma.

Bullae develop much more commonly in the upper lobes than elsewhere in the lungs, particu-

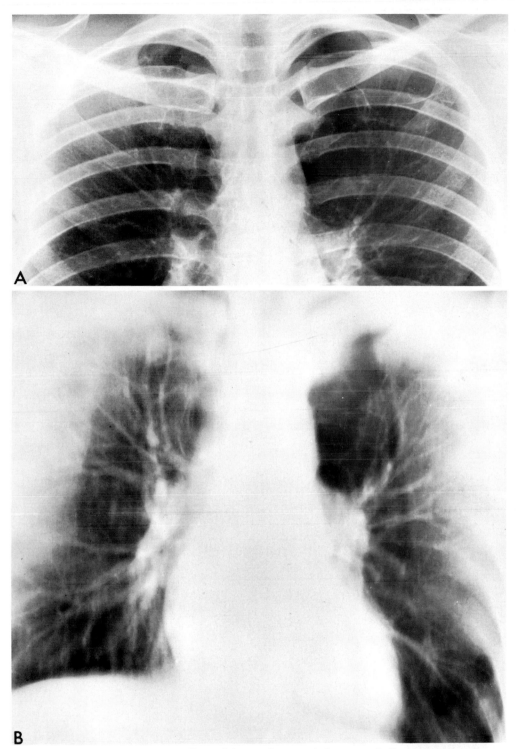

Figure 11–83. Multiple Bullae in Otherwise Normal Lung. A view of the upper half of the thorax from a posteroanterior roentgenogram *(A)* reveals numerous curved hairline shadows in the upper portion of the left lung representing the walls of multiple large bullae. A single bulla is present in the right paramediastinal area. An anteroposterior tomogram *(B)* demonstrates a normal distribution and caliber of the pulmonary vessels bilaterally, except for the avascular bullae.

larly in asymptomatic patients (Fig. 11–83); in such circumstances they can probably be regarded as an exaggerated form of "paraseptal" emphysema.[2317, 2318] However, in a study of a large number of patients with widespread emphysema, Reid[1925] found only a slight predilection by bullae for the upper lobes.

Tomography, both conventional and computed, may provide greatly improved visibility of a bulla already identified and may reveal bullae not even suspected on plain roentgenograms (Fig. 11–84).[2322] Similarly, tomography may be useful in the assessment of the vasculature throughout the lungs, particularly in establishing whether the bullae are

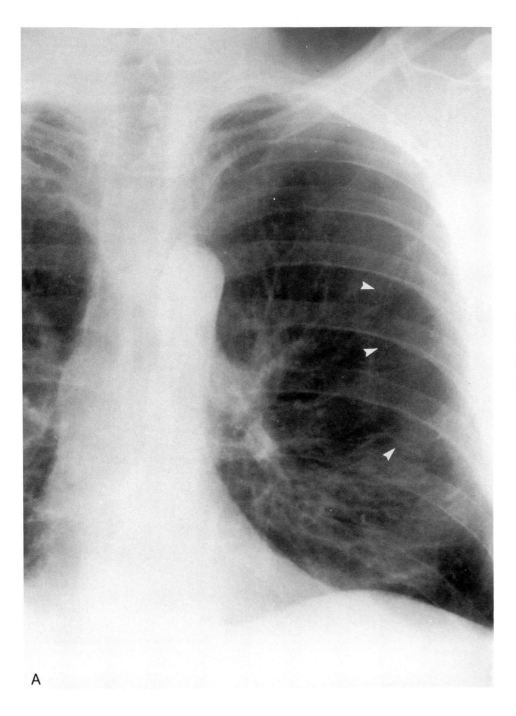

Figure 11–84. Bullae and Paraseptal Emphysema. A detail view of the left lung from a posteroanterior chest roentgenogram *(A)* shows curvilinear hairline-thick subpleural opacities *(arrowheads)* in the middle and upper parts of the lung. There is no evidence of pulmonary overinflation or generalized oligemia.

A

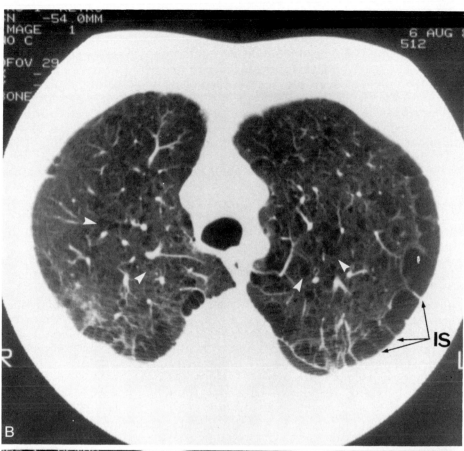

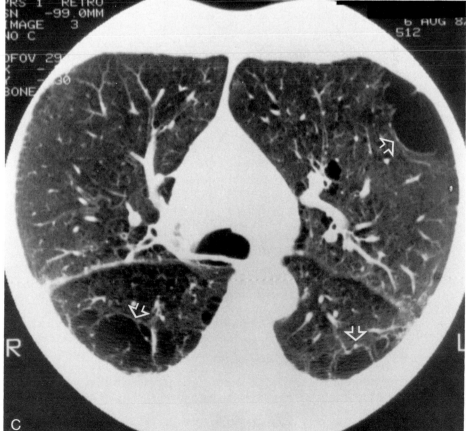

Figure 11–84. *Continued.* High-resolution CT scans through the midtrachea *(B)* and carina *(C)* show multiple small cystic spaces *(arrowheads)* widely dispersed throughout the upper lobes. Additionally, there are a number of larger bullae *(open arrows)* in the subpleural parenchyma of the upper and lower lobes; on the left, interlobular septa (IS) partition the cystic areas into prominent arcades. These latter findings are characteristic of paraseptal emphysema. The patient is a middle-aged man with mild dyspnea.

part of general emphysema or merely local abnormalities in otherwise normal lungs (see Fig. 11–83). In the former instance the peripheral vasculature is narrow and attenuated, and in the latter the vessels between the bullae appear normal although perhaps somewhat displaced and distorted by the contiguous air sacs. Computed tomography is particularly valuable in defining the anatomy of bullae and in determining the extent of emphysema or parenchymal compression of adjacent lung tissue.[2323] The volume of bullae can also be measured at total lung capacity and residual volume on CT scans. Studies of 43 patients showed that bullae contribute little to expired lung volume; the RV/TLC ratio of the bullae averaged approximately 90 per cent whereas the total lung RV/TLC ratio was approximately 60 per cent.[2323]

Angiography may be of value in the preoperative assessment of patients with bullous disease.[2317, 2319, 2324] Perfusion-ventilation lung scanning is considered by some[2325, 2326] to be useful in the assessment of bullous disease prior to resection, but it is doubtful if this technique contributes information not readily obtainable from a plain chest roentgenogram and tomogram.[2327] Although bronchography may aid in determining the amount of lung parenchyma lost and in identifying the precise location of a bulla,[1925] we consider that this procedure is seldom indicated.

Rarely, bullae disappear as a result of secondary infection[2317, 2319, 2328, 2329] or because of inflammatory stenosis of the supply airway. In the majority of cases, however, they enlarge progressively (Fig. 11–85). Boushy and colleagues[2317] studied a group of 49 patients with bullous disease for whom serial roentgenograms over a period ranging from 1 to more than 10 years were available. They found a consistent tendency for the lesions to enlarge, although the rate of enlargement was not predictable. Some increased slowly and continuously, whereas others remained constant in size for several years and then, for no obvious reason, enlarged. In many cases bullous disease was apparent roentgenographically for many years before the onset of symptoms; this has been our experience also.

Infection of a bulla usually is manifested roentgenographically by a fluid level within the air sac,[2319, 2328, 2329] with or without some degree of pneumonitis in the surrounding lung parenchyma. Fluid accumulation in a bulla occasionally may be caused by hemorrhage,[2330] a complication that may be suspected when there is an accompanying drop in hemoglobin level; rarely, hemorrhage may be so massive as to require emergency surgery.[2331] Since bullous disease commonly does not produce any symptoms, its presence may become evident only when chest roentgenography is carried out during investigation of acute lower respiratory tract infection. In such circumstances, the roentgenographic appearance may be misinterpreted as a lung cavity secondary to abscess formation, but differentiation

is aided by the fact that most patients with infected bullae are much less ill than those with acute lung abscess. Also, most infected bullae have much thinner walls (Fig. 11–86), are surrounded by lesser degrees of pneumonitis, and usually contain much less fluid than cavitated lung abscesses.[2332–2334] Complete clearing of fluid from infected bullae may be protracted, averaging about 6 weeks.[2336] Bullous disease can also be confused with neonatal lobar overinflation in infants, with cystic adenomatoid malformation in infants and children, and with bronchial cysts in adults.[2337, 2338]

Spontaneous pneumothorax commonly occurs in association with small blebs or bullae affecting the lung apices. Rarely, pneumothorax may be associated with large bullae involving the lower lobes.[2335] When spontaneous pneumothorax develops in patients with peripheral lung bullae, the air sacs may be much more easily identified when the lung is collapsed than when it is fully inflated; this improved visibility results from the tendency of bullae to remain air-containing while surrounding lung collapses. Sometimes the presence of spontaneous pneumothorax can be exceedingly difficult to recognize when large bullae occupy much of the volume of one lung (Fig. 11–87); in such circumstances, it has been shown that CT can be of value in confirming its presence or absence (see Fig. 11–64, page 2127).[2339]

Clinical Manifestations

Primary bullous disease characteristically occasions no symptoms or signs. A familial occurrence has been reported.[2335, 2340] The incidence of bullae is increased in patients with Marfan's syndrome[2341] and Ehlers-Danlos syndrome.[2342] Usually there is minimal abnormality in pulmonary function. The VC usually is within normal range, although FRC and RV may be increased, especially if they are measured by the body plethysmograph. (Since the small necks of many bullae permit very slow distribution of inspired gas, results obtained with inert gas washout techniques may be misleading.) Mixing efficiency may be severely impaired. Flow rates and diffusing capacity are normal or near normal, although diffusion may be affected if adjacent lung parenchyma is severely compressed. Blood gas values typically are normal at rest but may reveal evidence of hypoxemia during exercise.[2318, 2319] Bronchospirometry in patients with unilateral bullae shows decreased VC and minute volume of ventilation in the involved lung,[2343] but the most striking interlung difference occurs in the distribution of inert gas, which is impaired on the affected side as a result of poor ventilation of the bullae.[2317] Bullae rarely contribute significantly to dead space ventilation because they are so poorly ventilated.[2327] However, they permit relaxation of surrounding normal lung and thus reduce elastic recoil pressure. In primary bullous disease, airway resistance usually

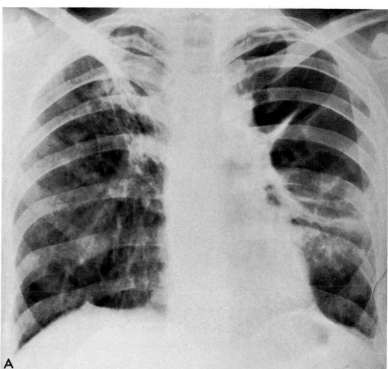

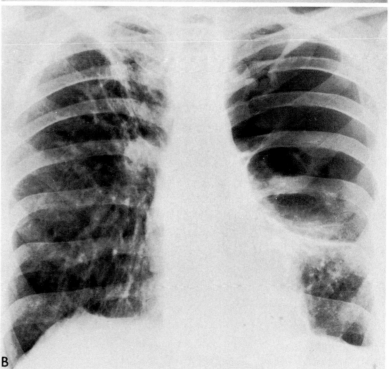

Figure 11–85. Progressive Enlargement of Bullae. A posteroanterior roentgenogram *(A)* reveals a large bulla occupying the upper half of the left lung. The extensive bilateral parenchymal disease is due to chronic fibrocaseous tuberculosis. Approximately 1 year later *(B)*, the bulla has increased considerably in size. (Courtesy of Montreal Chest Hospital Center.)

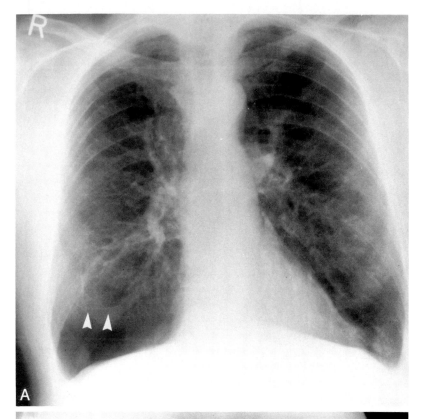

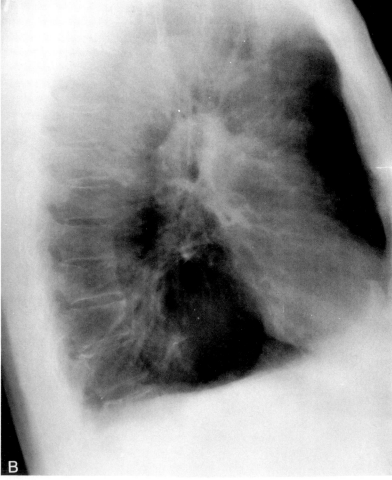

Figure 11–86. Infected Bullae. Posteroanterior *(A)* and lateral *(B)* chest roentgenograms reveal typical features of diffuse emphysema. In addition, the supradiaphragmatic portion of the right lower lobe is severely oligemic, and there is displacement of vessels upwards, backwards, and laterally by one or more large bullae; a faint curvilinear opacity may represent the wall of a bulla *(arrowheads)*.

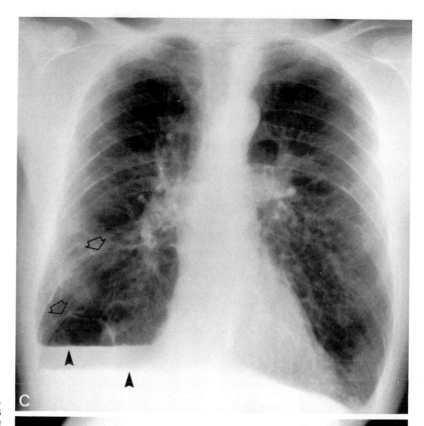

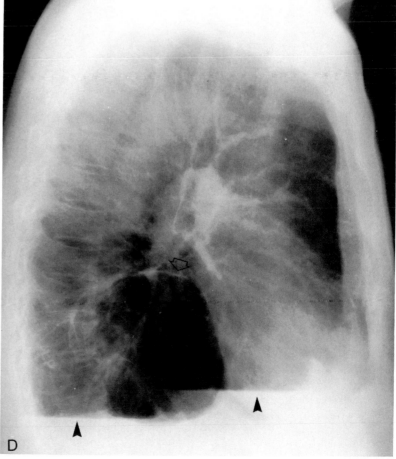

Figure 11–86. *Continued.* Three months later, posteroanterior *(C)* and lateral *(D)* roentgenograms reveal two long fluid levels *(arrowheads)* in adjacent bullae. Note that the walls of the bullae are more clearly outlined *(open arrows)*, presumably as a result of thickening of adjacent tissue by inflammatory cells, edema, and fibrovascular tissue. The fluid levels regressed very slowly over a period of 6 weeks.

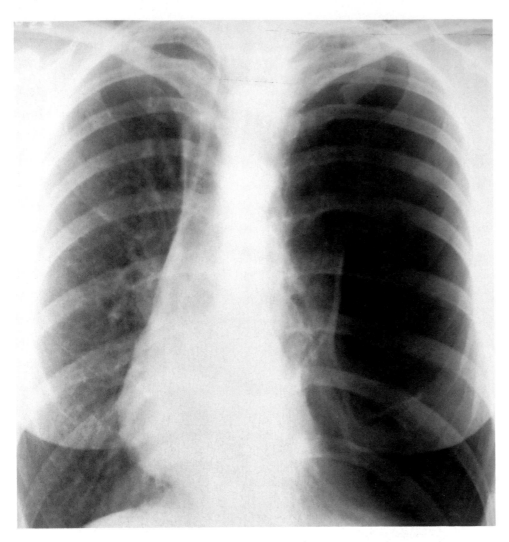

Figure 11–87. A Huge Bulla Simulating Pneumothorax. A posteroanterior chest roentgenogram demonstrates a severely overinflated and almost totally oligemic left hemithorax. A small amount of distorted and compressed left lung parenchyma is situated contiguous with the heart border. The mediastinum is displaced to the right. The vasculature of the right lung is within normal limits. With almost any diagnostic procedure, including conventional roentgenography, the distinction between a huge bulla and a large pneumothorax is extremely difficult if not impossible to make. In this patient, however, previous roentgenograms extending over a period of several years were virtually identical, thereby providing reasonably convincing evidence that the cause of the abnormality was a bulla. The patient is an essentially asymptomatic middle-aged woman.

is found to be within normal limits at high lung volumes but may be increased at low lung volumes as a result of the reduction in elastic recoil.[2344] The rationale for bullectomy lies in the potential for healthy lung to expand and fill the space occupied by the bullae and in the expected increase in elastic recoil pressure that reduces the tendency for airways to collapse on expiration.[2345] In the great majority of patients with primary bullous disease, there is no clinical disability and hence surgery is not indicated. However, when bullae are large, their surgical removal may become necessary; in such cases, pulmonary function studies carried out before and after surgery have revealed significant improvement.[2318, 2319, 2325, 2346]

Sometimes patients complain of dyspnea on exertion[2320, 2347] or (rarely) present clinically with severe pulmonary insufficiency and cor pulmonale.[2348] It should be kept in mind that patients with primary bullous disease also may have chronic bronchitis. Stone and his associates[2319] described this association in a group of young patients with chronic productive cough, who, on the basis of physiologic testing, were thought to have primary

bullous disease rather than bullae associated with general obstructive emphysema. As discussed previously, a bulla occasionally ruptures and causes pneumothorax; enlargement as a result of decreased ambient pressure in an airliner can cause air emboli and sudden death.[2349]

Bullae associated with chronic obstructive pulmonary disease show little difference clinically or functionally from chronic obstructive pulmonary disease without bullae. Pulmonary function studies reveal decrease in the VC, increase in FRC and RV (the TLC may be increased, normal, or decreased), impaired mixing efficiency, reduction in flow rates, decreased diffusing capacity at rest and during exercise, and usually hypoxemia and hypercarbia. In one study,[2318] cardiac catheterization in such patients revealed a rise in pulmonary arterial pressure on exercise in all cases. This contrasts with the findings in primary bullous disease, in which normal pulmonary arterial pressures have been recorded at rest and during exercise. In this group, surgical intervention is not nearly as successful as in patients with primary bullous disease, although some patients improve clinically and show better gas exchange and lung elastic recoil postoperatively,[2326, 2327, 2343, 2345] particularly when the bullae are large.[2326, 2350]

UNILATERAL OR LOBAR EMPHYSEMA (SWYER-JAMES OR MACLEOD'S SYNDROME)

Unilateral or lobar emphysema (unilateral hyperlucent lung) is one of the very few "diseases" whose name derives entirely from the manifestations it produces roentgenographically—a state in which the density of one lung (sometimes only one lobe) is markedly less than the density of the other. The condition was originally described by Swyer and James[2351] in 1953 in a 6-year-old boy who underwent pneumonectomy; nine more cases were described by Macleod[2352] in 1954 under the title "Abnormal Transradiancy of One Lung."

Unfortunately, use of the term "unilateral hyperlucent lung" has directed attention to a single roentgenographic feature of a disease whose potentialities and modes of expression are varied. For example, the condition does not always affect just one lung to the total exclusion of the other. It may occur in various anatomic distributions, including one lobe, two lobes in the right lung, and the lower lobe of one lung and the upper lobe of the other. In addition, undoubtedly some patients who present in adulthood with chronic obstructive pulmonary disease, shown roentgenologically and physiologically to be local emphysema (for example, disease localized to both upper lobes), clearly represent examples of this disease pathogenetically. We have seen at least one such example in a 49-year-old woman in whom bilateral upper lobe emphysema was discovered several years after she had a protracted lower respiratory illness whose roentgenographic pattern suggested interstitial viral pneumonitis. Finally, it should also be remembered that other disease entities, such as proximal interruption of a pulmonary artery and massive thromboembolism, can lead to increased transradiancy of one lung. The assumption that this roentgenologic pattern is synonymous with Swyer-James syndrome has led to considerable confusion in published reports.[2353] For these reasons, we prefer to use the designation "unilateral or lobar emphysema" or, better, the eponymous term Swyer-James syndrome.

Pathogenesis and Pathologic Characteristics

There have been few descriptions of the pathologic characteristics of Swyer-James syndrome. Specimens that have been examined have shown bronchitis, bronchiectasis, bronchiolitis, bronchiolitis obliterans, and a variable degree of destruction of lung parenchyma.[2351, 2354–2356] Focal anthracosis,

which is almost invariable in adult lungs with proximal acinar emphysema, is typically absent in the Swyer-James syndrome, probably because of the young age at which the condition is usually acquired (see farther on) and of the reduction in ventilation that characterizes the disease.

This morphologic appearance lends support to the conclusion that in the majority of cases the disease is caused by bronchial and bronchiolar infection, probably of viral origin. In many cases, the disease is recognized (or at least suspected) in childhood when chest roentgenography is carried out in the investigation of repeated respiratory infections. In others, the condition does not become apparent until adulthood on the basis of a screening chest roentgenogram of a completely asymptomatic patient. Inquiry in these cases often reveals a history of acute lower respiratory tract infection, generally during childhood.[1931, 2357–2359] Peters and colleagues[2360] have described a child in whom a baseline normal chest roentgenogram was obtained shortly before the development of an adenoviral pneumonia; following resolution of the pneumonia, the affected lung was hyperlucent and on subsequent follow-up was of reduced volume and exhibited gas trapping and bronchographic evidence of bronchiectasis. A report by MacPherson and Gold[2361] of six children with unilateral or lobar emphysema whose previous history showed definite or highly suggestive evidence of adenoviral pneumonia suggests that this organism is the responsible agent in the majority of cases (see Fig. 11–89). It seems likely, therefore, that in most cases the condition begins as an acute bronchiolitis that in turn causes obliteration of small airways; the peripheral parenchyma is largely unaffected, being ventilated by collateral air drift with resulting air trapping; ultimately destructive changes characteristic of emphysema may occur.[2362] The pathogenesis of the latter process is unclear; it is conceivable that in some cases infection could persist after the acute viral infection, with consequent elastolysis from phagocytic proteases.

Although most cases appear to be related to viral infection, we have seen a patient with typical Swyer-James syndrome associated with hypoplasia of the ipsilateral breast and chest wall muscles, suggesting that some cases may represent a developmental anomaly (Fig. 11–88).[2363]

Roentgenographic Manifestations

The roentgenographic manifestations usually are easily recognized and are virtually pathognomonic. A posteroanterior roentgenogram of the chest exposed at TLC reveals a remarkable difference in the radiolucency of the two lungs (or of the lobes), caused *not* by a relative increase in air in the affected lung but by decreased perfusion (Fig. 11–88). The peripheral pulmonary markings are diminutive, indicating severe narrowing and atten-

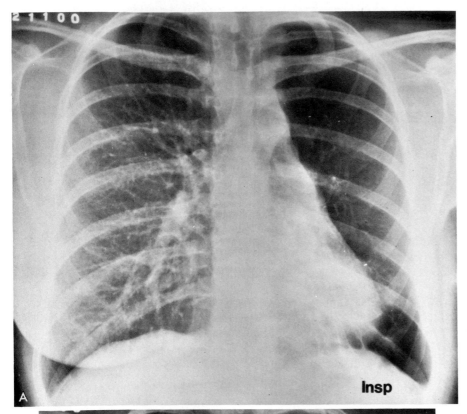

Insp

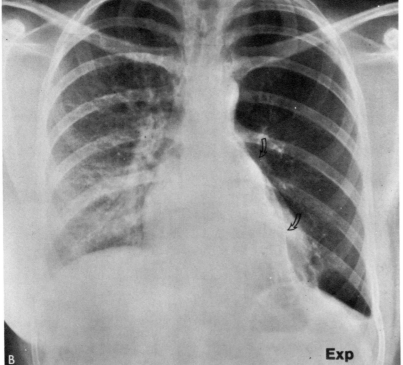

Exp

Figure 11–88. Swyer-James Syndrome Associated with Absence of the Ipsilateral Breast. Posteroanterior roentgenograms at inspiration *(A)* and expiration *(B)* reveal marked oligemia of the left lung and severe air trapping on expiration. A left breast shadow is not visualized nor was breast tissue apparent on physical examination. The left lower lobe shows a severe degree of loss of volume *(open arrows* in *B)* and the left hilum is diminutive.

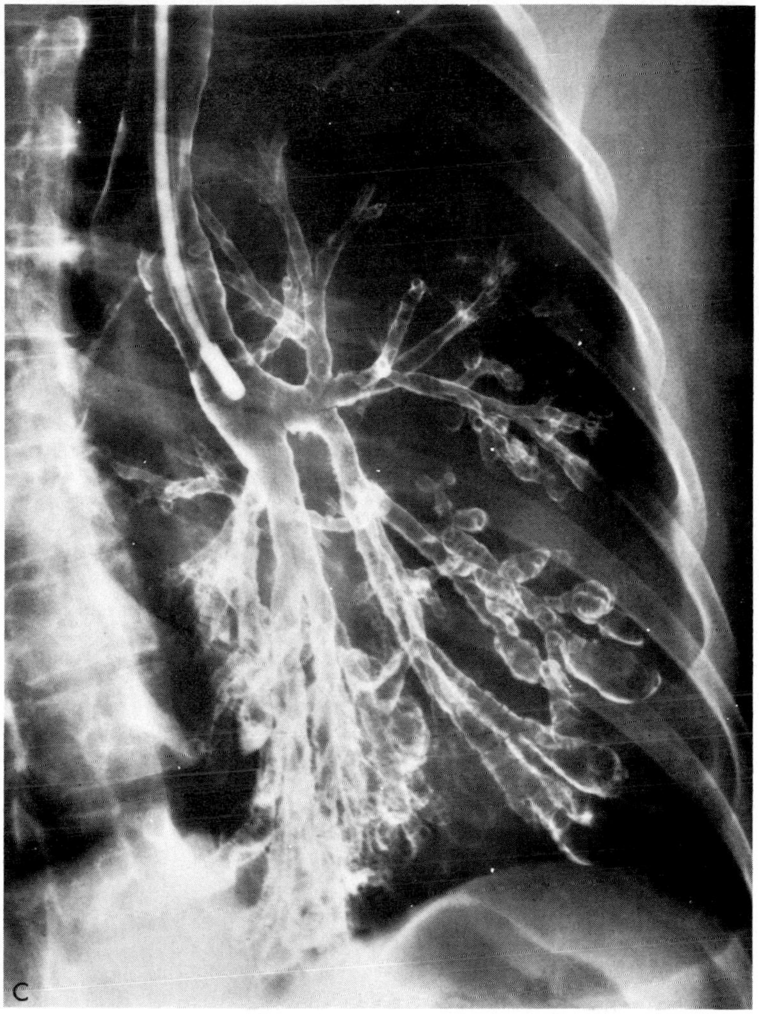

Figure 11–88. *Continued.* A left bronchogram *(C)* reveals bronchiectasis of all segments, those in the lower lobe being the most severely involved and thus accounting for the loss of volume. All bronchial segments terminate abruptly in a configuration characteristic of obliterative bronchiolitis. Whether a relationship exists between the left-sided emphysema and congenital absence of the left breast is not known. This young woman complained of chronic cough productive of mucopurulent sputum. (Courtesy of Montreal Chest Hospital Center.)

uation of the vessels. The ipsilateral hilum also is diminutive but is *present*, a feature of great value in the differentiation from proximal interruption of a pulmonary artery (pulmonary artery agenesis). In roentgenograms exposed at TLC, the volume of the affected lung (or lobe) either is comparable to that of the normal contralateral lung or is reduced (Fig. 11–89); volume is seldom if ever increased. The volume of the affected lung depends almost entirely on the age of the patient at the time of the infectious insult. The younger the patient at the time of the pneumonia, the smaller the fully developed lung, since the insult retards further maturation.[2354, 2363] However, the volume probably relates also, in part, to the presence of focal atelectasis and fibrosis as well as emphysema.[2362] Should the original viral pneumonia affect both lungs more or less diffusely, the result can be devastating, consisting of what is essentially diffuse emphysema (Fig. 11–90).

One of the characteristic roentgenologic features of unilateral or lobar emphysema—in fact, a *sine qua non* for diagnosis—is the presence of air trapping during expiration (*see* Fig. 11–88). This indicates the presence of airway obstruction and is

of absolute value in differentiation from other conditions that may give rise to unilateral or lobar translucency. Since the contralateral lung is normal, expiration (particularly if rapid) causes the mediastinum to swing abruptly toward the normal lung, and excursion of the hemidiaphragms is markedly asymmetric, being severely diminished on the affected side. Roentgenograms exposed at RV also accentuate the disparity in radiolucency of the two lungs, the density of the normal lung being much greater. This is not only because the normal lung contains less air but, perhaps more importantly, because its blood flow is virtually the total output of the right ventricle. For some reason that is enigmatic, of all the cases of Swyer-James syndrome that we have seen (and there have been many), only two have been right-sided.

Pulmonary angiography outlines clearly the diminutive hilar vessels on the affected side and the much narrowed, attenuated arteries coursing through the radiolucent lung (Fig. 11–91). However, we feel that only seldom is angiography indicated in the investigation of these patients; the roentgenologic signs are almost pathognomonic and require no embellishment (however, *see* below under

Text continued on page 2185

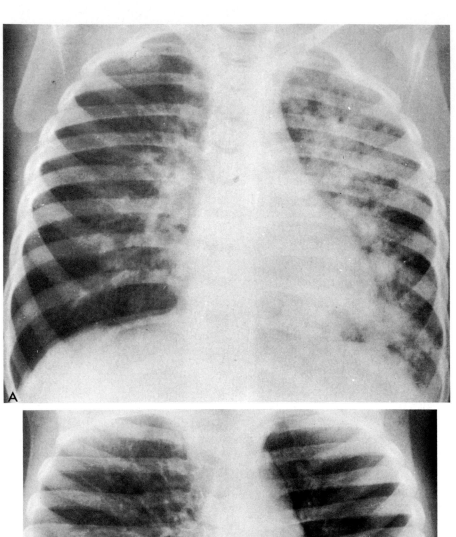

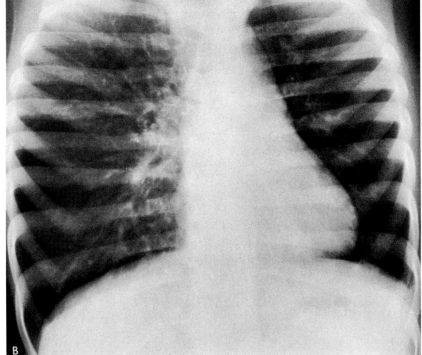

Figure 11–89. *See legend on opposite page.*

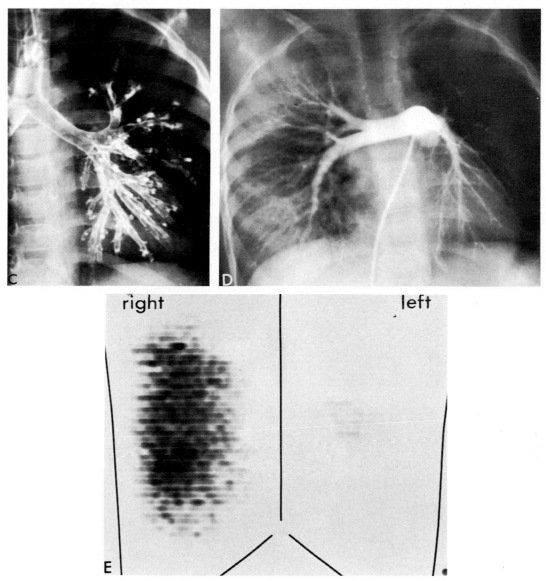

Figure 11–89. Unilateral Emphysema (Swyer-James Syndrome). This girl was first seen at the Winnipeg Children's Hospital at the age of 17 months with a history of recent onset of cough and fever; the white blood cell count was normal, but a differential count showed a relative lymphocytosis. A chest roentgenogram *(A)* revealed diffuse patchy pneumonia of the left lung and medial third of the right lung. The etiology was not established at that time, although several months later titers of 1:32 to adenovirus were found on two consecutive occasions, suggesting that this may have been the responsible organism. During the subsequent 3 years, the child developed chronic adhesive atelectasis of the left lower lobe *(see* Figure 4–23, page 491), which eventually expanded spontaneously. Three-and-a-half years after the initial episode, a chest roentgenogram *(B)* revealed marked asymmetry in density of the two lungs, the left being relatively radiolucent and showing a sparsity of vascular markings. The left lung is considerably smaller than the right. A left bronchogram *(C)* demonstrated general slight dilatation of all segmental bronchi, each bronchus terminating abruptly in a squared or truncated ending. The appearance is highly suggestive of obliterative bronchiolitis and mild cylindrical bronchiectasis. A pulmonary angiogram *(D)* revealed marked disparity in the perfusion of the two lungs, most of the contrast medium passing to the right lung; the vessels throughout the left lung are thin and attenuated. It is of considerable interest that the medial third of the right lung shows an oligemia similar to that throughout the left lung, probably reflecting the anatomic distribution of the acute pneumonia originally observed in *A*. During cardiac catheterization, the left atrium was entered through a patent foramen ovale and samples of blood obtained from the right and left pulmonary veins; that from the left lung showed a significant reduction in oxygen saturation. Pulmonary arterial pressures were normal. A pulmonary scan *(E)* shows to excellent advantage the disparity in perfusion of the two lungs. (Courtesy of Dr. R. I. Macpherson.)

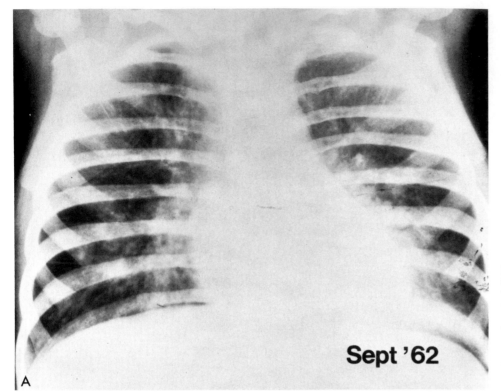

Sept '62

A

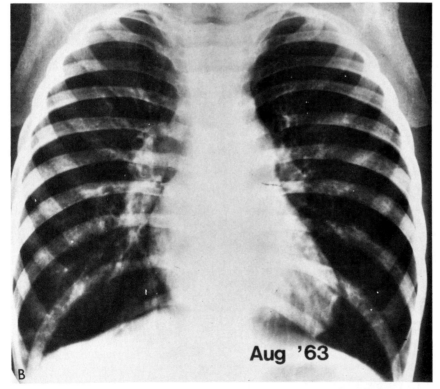

Aug '63

B

Figure 11–90. Diffuse "Emphysema" (Bronchiolitis Obliterans) in a Young Girl. This 1½-year-old girl was admitted to the hospital with an acute respiratory illness that progressed to respiratory failure requiring intermittent positive pressure ventilation. A roentgenogram on admission revealed (A) widespread pulmonary disease more evident in the lower lung zones and consistent with (but in no way diagnostic of) acute viral pneumonia. Viral antibody titers were not measured, although repeated sputum cultures revealed no evidence of bacterial infection. Following recovery from her acute illness, she manifested shortness of breath on mild exertion. A roentgenogram approximately 1 year after the acute episode (B) revealed marked overinflation.

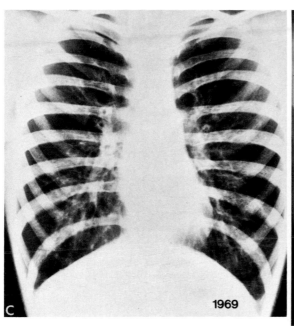

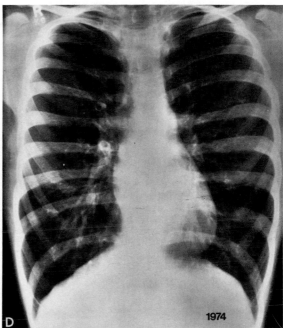

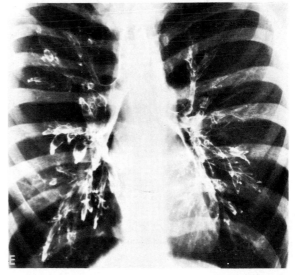

Figure 11–90. *Continued.* By the time the child was 8 years of age *(C)*, the overinflation had become more marked and diffuse peripheral oligemia consistent with a diagnosis of diffuse emphysema had developed. By age 13, she suffered from chronic cough productive each day of 10 to 15 ml of mucopurulent sputum and from breathlessness on mild exertion. A roentgenogram of her chest *(D)* again revealed severe overinflation and peripheral oligemia. Pulmonary function studies showed severe airway obstruction (FEV_1 0.53 l, predicted 2.70; FVC 1.40, predicted 3.00; FEV_1/FVC 38 per cent, predicted 90; MMFR 0.23, predicted 3.50), marked increase in lung volumes (RV 4.19, predicted 0.84; FRC 4.57, predicted 1.67), and a severe reduction in carbon monoxide diffusion both at rest ($DlCO$ 4.9, predicted 17.5) and on exercise. These results were interpreted as being consistent with a clinical diagnosis of emphysema. A bronchogram *(E)* showed moderate uniform dilatation of all segmental and subsegmental bronchi of both lungs, with abrupt, conical termination of all segments distally. There was no opacification of peripheral branches of the airway system. The airway obstruction was unresponsive to oral and inhaled bronchodilators or corticosteroid therapy. (Courtesy of Drs. J. S. D. McEvoy and Richard Slaughter, The Prince Charles Hospital, Brisbane, Australia.)

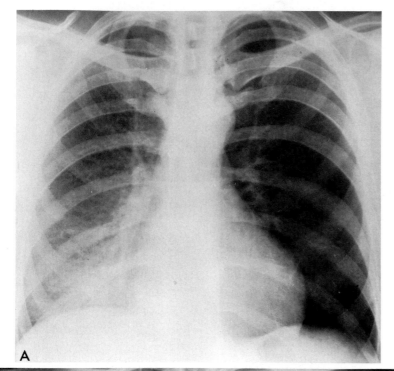

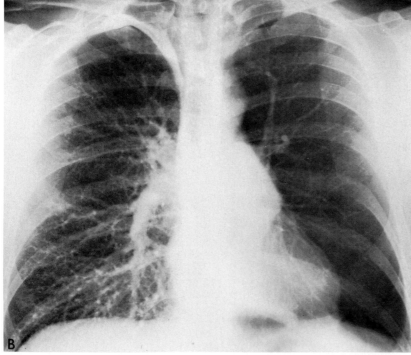

Figure 11–91. Unilateral Emphysema: Angiographic and Bronchographic Manifestations. A posteroanterior roentgenogram *(A)* reveals the typical appearance of unilateral hyperlucent lung. A pulmonary angiogram *(B)* shows to excellent advantage the marked disparity in perfusion of the two lungs, vessels on the left being narrow and attenuated. A left bronchogram *(C)* demonstrates irregular dilatation of all visualized segmental bronchi in the form of "varicose" bronchiectasis; all bronchi terminate in squared or tapered endings and there is a notable absence of filling of peripheral bronchiolar radicles. This 34-year-old man complained of paroxysmal attacks of dyspnea over a period of several years.

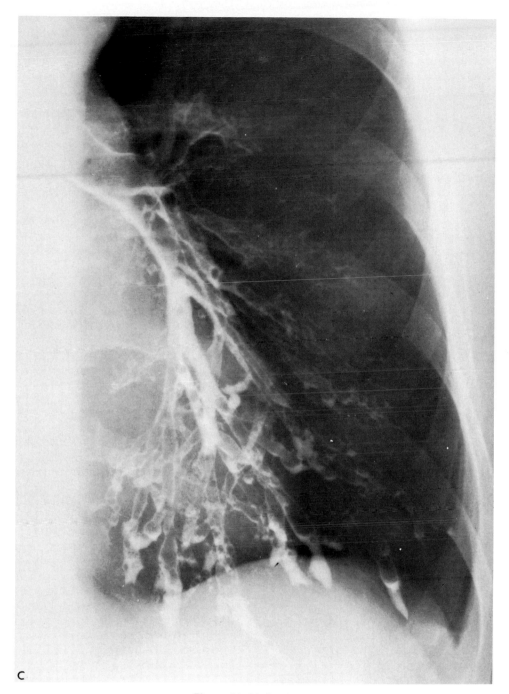

C

Figure 11–91 *Continued*

differential diagnosis). Houk and colleagues[2358] pointed out that unless the contrast medium is injected directly into the affected pulmonary artery, this vessel may not be opacified, creating the erroneous impression that the abnormality may represent proximal interruption of the pulmonary artery. Pulmonary arteriography is seldom indicated in the investigation of these patients, but a perfusion lung scan may provide useful information in selected cases and is less hazardous.[2364] In a review of 607 perfusion lung scans performed over a 1-year period, White and his colleagues[2361] found that only

13 revealed total absence of perfusion of one lung. Only one of these was associated with the Swyer-James syndrome, the remainder being the result of pulmonary embolism (three cases), parenchymal lung disease (three), pulmonary carcinoma (three), congenital heart disease (two), and pneumonectomy (one). Radionuclide $\dot{V}/\dot{Q}$ scans may reveal additional areas of involvement, as in a patient reported by Daniel and associates[2366] in whom an area of diminished perfusion was detected in the contralateral lung which did not appear hyperlucent on a conventional chest roentgenogram. O'Dell and his

associates[2365] recommend ventilation-perfusion lung imaging as preferable to perfusion scanning alone, since the latter does not exclude purely vascular abnormalities such as pulmonary embolism. However, we feel that such difficulty should seldom arise if there is adequate correlation with roentgenographic and clinical presentations. Selective bronchial arteriography and bronchial arterial lung scans have revealed extensive hypervascularity and increased perfusion of the hyperlucent lung.[2367]

In the majority of patients, bronchography reveals a characteristic deformity of the bronchial tree. The segmental bronchi are irregularly dilated and end abruptly in squared or tapered terminations in the vicinity of the fifth- or sixth-generation divisions (see Figs. 11–88 and 11–91). The "broken bough" appearance seen in other forms of bronchiectasis may be present.[2354] Filling of peripheral bronchiolar radicals is notable by its absence, even with repeated deep respirations.[2351, 2356, 2358, 2363] Cinebronchographic examination of the patient illustrated in Figure 11–91 revealed disproportionate collapse of the lower lobe bronchus on forced expiration and cough, reduction in caliber being from 11 mm at TLC to 1.5 mm at RV.

In differential diagnosis, a number of conditions can create a similar roentgenographic appearance, but in only one does a serious potential difficulty exist. A partly obstructing lesion situated within a main bronchus can create a triad of roentgenographic signs that are indistinguishable from those in Swyer-James syndrome—a smaller than normal lung volume, air trapping on expiration, and diffuse oligemia as a result of hypoxic vasoconstriction (Fig. 11–92). As a consequence, in any patient presenting with these signs, the presence of a lesion within the ipsilateral main bronchus must be excluded before a diagnosis of Swyer-James syndrome is accepted; the easiest way to accomplish this is by bronchoscopy although linear or computed tomography is probably just as effective in accomplishing this task. Other conditions that give rise to unilateral or lobar radiolucency, such as proximal interruption of a pulmonary artery, hypogenetic lung syndrome, and obstruction of a main pulmonary artery or one of its branches from thromboembolic disease, are readily differentiated by the absence of air trapping during expiration and by other roentgenologic signs that characterize these conditions.

In one study,[2368] the data obtained from a series of 40 consecutive patients with chronic unilateral hyperlucent lung were analyzed to determine the etiology; cases of acute pulmonary embolism were excluded. Etiologies included the Swyer-James syndrome in 18 patients (45 per cent), unilateral bullous emphysema in eight (20 per cent), congenital hypoplastic pulmonary artery in four (10 per cent), previous massive pulmonary embolism in four (10 per cent), a partly obstructing pulmonary carcinoma in three (7.5 per cent), the late sequelae of radiation therapy in two (5 per cent), and a benign intrabron-

chial neoplasm in one (2.5 per cent). On the basis of a scoring system for reduction in pulmonary vasculature, patients with the Swyer-James syndrome were found to have the most significant oligemia whereas those with bronchial carcinoma had the least.

Clinical Manifestations

Clinically, the presentation is highly variable. Some patients are completely asymptomatic,[2359, 2369] some complain of dyspnea on exertion,[2357, 2363, 2370] and others present with a history of repeated lower respiratory tract infections.[2351, 2363] Physical examination reveals restriction of chest expansion on the affected side, associated with diminished breath sounds, relative hyperresonance, and sometimes scattered rales.[2351, 2371]

Pulmonary function test values are as might be anticipated with destruction of virtually half the functioning parenchyma of both lungs. There is reduction in VC and to a lesser extent in expiratory flow; mixing efficiency as measured by helium or another inert gas usually is greatly reduced as a consequence of the slow movement of gas into the emphysematous lung. Diffusing capacity measured by the steady-state method usually is reduced but may be normal with the single-breath method, since breath-holding permits time for more uniform gas distribution. Blood gas concentrations usually are normal but may fall during exercise. Bronchospirometry reveals reduction in ventilation by as much as 90 per cent on the affected side, oxygen uptake being reduced to as low as 5 per cent of normal.[2370, 2372] Cases of unilateral hyperlucent lung associated with hypoxemia, polycythemia, pulmonary hypertension, and cor pulmonale, such as those reported by Llamas,[2373] probably are the result of the subsequent development of COPD (with or without emphysema) in the contralateral lung. Mont and associates[2374] have described a patient with Swyer-James syndrome who developed Goodpasture's syndrome; pulmonary hemorrhage occurred exclusively on the side of the normal lung, the hyperlucent lung being unaffected.

BRONCHIECTASIS

Bronchiectasis is defined as irreversible abnormal dilatation of the bronchial tree. As a pathologic abnormality, it is common and occurs in a variety of conditions in both surgical and autopsy specimens (Table 11–4). As a clinically significant affliction, however, it has decreased considerably in importance since the advent of antibiotic therapy, at least in industrialized societies.[2375] Thus, although its precise incidence in the population as a whole or even in a general hospital population is not known, its frequency as a disease requiring surgical resection has greatly decreased.[2376] It is probable

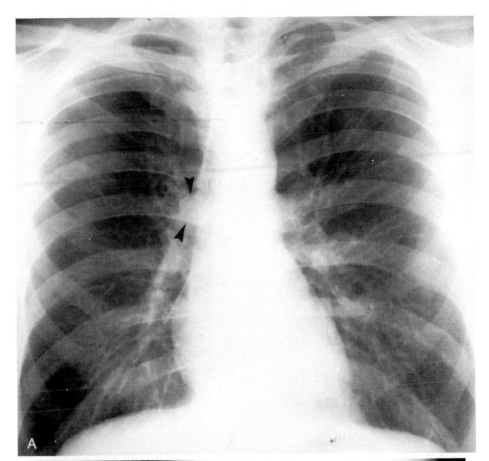

Figure 11–92. Unilateral Hyperlucency Caused by a Partly Obstructing Endobronchial Mass. Posteroanterior *(A)* and lateral *(B)* chest roentgenograms reveal diffuse oligemia of the right lung, more marked in the upper lobe. The right hilum is considerably smaller than the left, reflecting reduced perfusion. Note that the volume of the right lung is smaller than the left. Although these findings are consistent with a diagnosis of Swyer-James syndrome, the presence of an endobronchial mass *(arrowheads)* in the right main and upper lobe bronchi renders this presumptive diagnosis inappropriate and mandates further investigation.

Illustration continued on following page

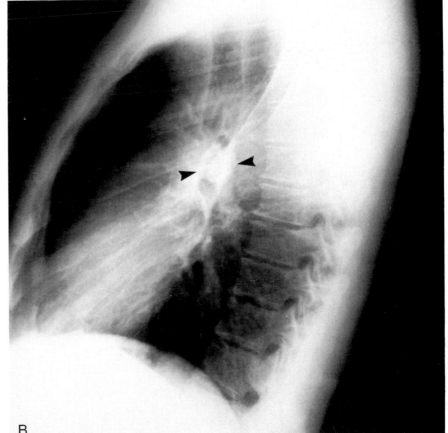

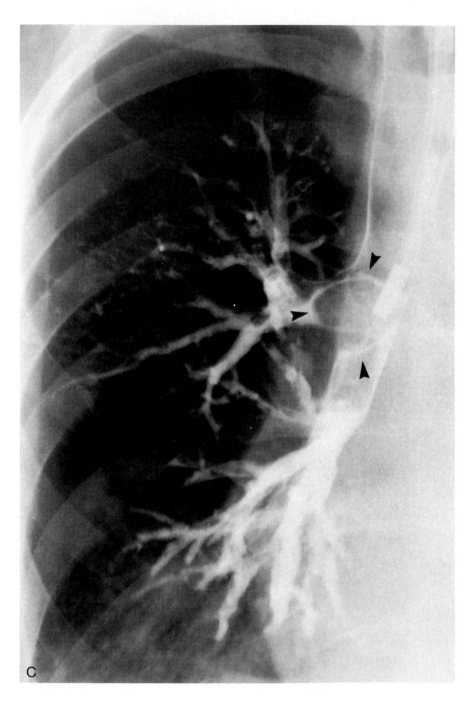

Figure 11–92. *Continued.* In this instance, a right bronchogram *(C)* was performed (conventional or computed tomography [CT] would have been preferred) and disclosed an ovoid intraluminal mass *(arrowheads)* in the right main and upper lobe bronchi. The basal bronchi of the lower lobe show varicose bronchiectasis. Surgical removal of the lesion confirmed a bilobed (dumbell-shaped) carcinoid tumor. The patient is a young man with complaints of a chronic cough, occasionally accompanied by hemoptysis. (Courtesy of Dr. William Brown, Regina General Hospital, Regina, Saskatchewan.)

Table 11–4. Classification of Bronchiectasis

GENERAL CATEGORY	DISEASE EXAMPLES
Congenital abnormality in bronchial structure	Absent or defective cartilage, intraluminal webs
Dyskinetic cilia syndrome	
Cystic fibrosis	
Deficiency in host defense	Agammaglobulinemia, chronic granulomatous disease of childhood, etc.
Immunologic abnormality	Allergic bronchopulmonary aspergillosis
Postinfectious bronchitis	Classic bronchiectasis secondary to measles or pertussis pneumonia
	Swyer-James syndrome
Post-toxic bronchitis	Ammonia inhalation, gastric acid aspiration, etc.
Acquired bronchial obstruction	Intraluminal obstruction by neoplasm, aspirated foreign body, broncholiths
	Compression by lymph nodes (neoplasms, tuberculosis, etc.)
Parenchymal fibrosis	Tuberculosis, sarcoidosis, etc.
Chronic obstructive pulmonary disease	Emphysema

that the most important cause of clinically significant bronchiectasis in North America and Europe today is cystic fibrosis; in other areas of the world without a large white population, especially nonindustrialized societies where the incidence of serious childhood infection is still appreciable, postinfective bronchiectasis is probably still of great significance. The subject of bronchiectasis has been reviewed by Barker and Bordona.[2377]

Pathogenesis

Some of the conditions associated with bronchiectasis, such as cystic fibrosis and the dyskinetic cilia syndrome, are characterized by abnormal mucociliary clearance. In such cases, it is possible that this deficiency leads to local airway colonization by various microorganisms and that the chronic inflammatory reaction to them results in turn in progressive bronchial wall damage and dilatation; this can cause even greater deficiency of mucociliary clearance, establishing a vicious circle and ever increasing bronchiectasis.[2379] A disturbance in mucociliary clearance may also be important in causing the bronchiectasis associated with bronchial obstruction, although it is likely that retained secretions themselves also cause some degree of airway dilatation.[2378] By predisposing to bronchial wall infection or colonization, immunologic deficiency states such as agammaglobulinemia (*see* Fig. 7–29, page 1252) and chronic granulomatous disease of childhood may act by the same mechanism as impaired mucociliary clearance. Cole[2379] has suggested that postinfective bronchiectasis secondary to childhood measles and pertussis pneumonia is caused by a similar vicious circle, although the precise form of

bronchial wall damage that causes an increased susceptibility to colonization in these patients is not clear. The bronchiectasis that develops following the inhalation of various fumes or gases such as ammonia[2380] or following aspiration of liquid gastric contents (especially in heroin addicts)[2381, 2382] probably occurs by a similar mechanism. Perhaps in the same category is the bronchiectasis that almost invariably accompanies unilateral or lobar emphysema (Swyer-James[2351] or MacLeod's[2352] syndrome), the pathogenesis almost certainly relating to acute bronchiolitis in infancy or childhood. We are of the opinion that most, if not all, cases of so-called hypoplasia of the pulmonary artery associated with bronchiectasis[2383] are acquired rather than congenital and possess a pathogenesis similar or identical to that of Swyer-James syndrome.

Of a somewhat different pathogenesis is the bronchiectasis that occurs in patients with chronic upper lobe tuberculosis and some interstitial lung diseases such as sarcoidosis. In these conditions, the parenchyma appears to be the primary site of disease, replacement of alveoli by fibrous tissue resulting in parenchymal retraction and secondary bronchial dilatation.

Patients with chronic bronchitis also may show permanent, although typically slight, dilatation of the bronchial tree. In these individuals, however, the dilatation is general, whereas in bronchiectasis it is more often local.

Pathologic Characteristics

The definitive description of the pathologic findings and the pathologic-roentgenographic correlation of bronchiectasis was reported by Lynne Reid[2384] in 1950. By correlating the pathologic and bronchographic findings in 45 lobes removed because of bronchiectasis, this author classified the disease into three groups, using the criteria of severity of bronchial dilatation and degree of bronchial and bronchiolar obliteration.

Group I: Cylindrical Bronchiectasis. The bronchi were of regular outline and not greatly increased in diameter distally; their lumens ended squarely and abruptly (Fig. 11–93). Although patent anatomically, the smaller bronchi and bronchioles were plugged with thick, yellow, purulent material and did not fill with bronchographic contrast medium. The number of subdivisions of the bronchial tree from the main bronchus to the periphery was considered to be within normal limits (16 subdivisions compared with 17 to 20 normally).

Group II: Varicose Bronchiectasis. The degree of dilatation was somewhat greater than in Group I. Local constrictions caused an irregularity of outline that resembled varicose veins (*see* Fig. 11–96). This irregularity and bulbous termination of bronchi were the cardinal features in this group, in contrast to the regular outline and abrupt termination seen in Group I. There was much more

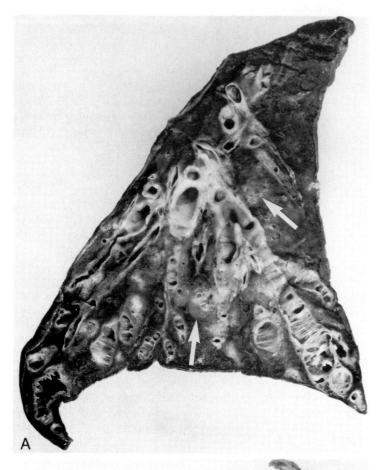

A

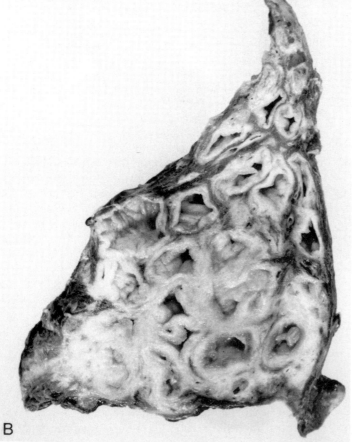

B

Figure 11–93. Bronchiectasis. Illustrated are the cut sections of lower lobes from two patients with bronchiectasis, that in *A* showing mild ("cylindrical") bronchiectasis and that in *B*, severe ("saccular" or "cystic") bronchiectasis. Although much of the parenchyma in *A* is normal, focal areas of organizing or organized pneumonia are apparent *(arrows)*. This process is advanced in *B*, there being almost no evidence of residual normal parenchyma.

Figure 11–94. Bronchiectasis. A histologic section of bronchiectatic lung *(A)* shows bronchial dilatation, atelectasis, and parenchymal fibrosis and chronic inflammation. An *arrow* points to a tumorlet. Another histologic section *(B)* reveals a bronchus with a somewhat irregular contour whose wall shows mural fibrosis and chronic inflammation, focally with lymphoid follicle formation. The adjacent parenchyma shows fibrosis and patchy inflammation. (*A*, × 10; *B*, × 30.)

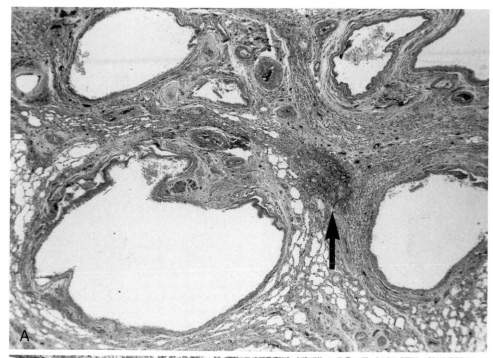

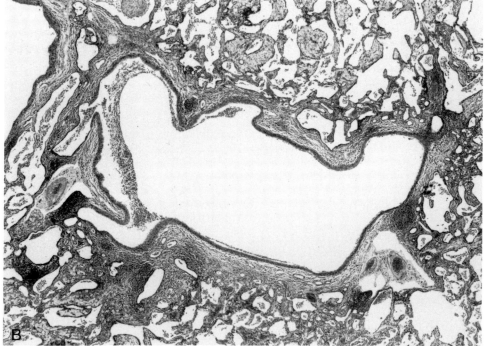

obliteration of peripheral bronchial lumens than in Group I, some bronchi terminating abruptly in a bed of fibrous tissue that continued as a discrete cord of tissue toward the periphery of the lung. The average number of patent bronchial subdivisions was four bronchographically, 6.5 macroscopically, and eight microscopically (compared with 17 to 20 normally).

Group III: Saccular (Cystic) Bronchiectasis. Bronchial dilatation increased progressively toward the periphery (Fig. 11–93). The bronchi had a ballooned outline, and the maximum number of subdivisions that could be counted by any technique was five. No remnants of the peripheral bronchial tree could be shown to be directly continuous with the dilated bronchi. It is of great interest that, despite the fact that only five subdivisions of the bronchial tree could be counted, the cysts or saccules were situated immediately deep to the pleura. Thus it is erroneous to consider one form of bronchiectasis as involving the smaller bronchi and another the larger bronchi (except in mucoid impaction); the position of a diseased bronchus can be determined accurately only by counting from the hilum.

Bronchiectasis often varies considerably in severity between different lobes and even between different segments in the same lobe. The intervening pulmonary parenchyma may be normal but often shows multifocal areas of organizing or organized pneumonia, reflecting the frequent bouts of infection experienced by these patients; in some cases, bronchial dilatation and parenchymal fibrosis can result in a completely functionless lobe (Fig. 11–93B).

Microscopic changes are predictable from the gross appearance. In addition to obvious luminal dilatation, the bronchial wall is typically irregular in shape and is the site of fibrosis and chronic inflammation, frequently with lymphoid follicle formation (Fig. 11–94; see previous page).[2385] The adjacent lung parenchyma shows evidence of recent or remote pneumonia and, in some areas, atelectasis and obstructive pneumonitis. The latter is presumably related to obliteration of small airways and can sometimes be identified as small fibrous cords adjacent to pulmonary arteries.[2384] The bronchial artery circulation is typically markedly increased;[2386] bronchial wall ulceration with disruption of bronchial arteries secondary to focal infection is considered to be the pathogenesis of the hemorrhage that so often complicates the disease.

Roentgenographic Manifestations

We have found Reid's classification eminently satisfactory for roentgenologic description. Not only does it permit accurate description of the degree of bronchial deformity, but it has the added advantage of supplying fairly precise information on the amount of parenchymal destruction encountered in each group.

The plain roentgenogram reveals changes highly suggestive of bronchiectasis in the great majority of patients. In a retrospective study of 112 bronchographically proven cases of bronchiectasis, Gudbjerg[2389, 2390] found a perfectly normal chest roentgenogram in only 7.1 per cent. The typical changes on plain roentgenograms consist of the following:

1. Increase in size and loss of definition of the markings in specific segmental areas of the lungs (Fig. 11–95). Gudbjerg[2389, 2390] found this change to relate morphologically to peribronchial fibrosis and to a lesser extent to retained secretions.

2. Markings are crowded, indicating the almost invariable associated loss of volume (Fig. 11–95). Gudbjerg considered atelectasis to be caused by obstruction by secretions of peripheral rather than central bronchial radicals. In some cases of more severe disease such as varicose bronchiectasis, reduction in pulmonary artery perfusion is reflected in roentgenographic evidence of oligemia (Fig. 11–96).

3. In more advanced disease, particularly Groups II and III, cystic spaces, up to 2 cm in diameter and sometimes containing fluid levels, may be identified (Figs. 11–97 and 11–98).

4. In very severe disease there is a tendency to the formation of a rather coarse "honeycomb" pattern consisting of rarefied areas which, in contrast to the cystic spaces described in No. 3 above, do not fill with contrast medium. Histologically, Gudbjerg found these to be "emphysematous" spaces surrounded by fibrosis rather than dilated bronchi. In advanced disease, atelectasis may be complete and associated with total airlessness of a lobe (Fig. 11–99).

5. Signs of compensatory overinflation of the remainder of the lung are present in most cases (Fig. 11–98).

6. Pleural thickening is seen more commonly at thoracotomy than roentgenologically.

Bateson and Woo-Ming[2391] have described 12 patients, eight West Indian blacks and four Australian aborigines, who showed evidence of total destruction of one lung by bronchiectasis associated with a normal contralateral lung. We have seen at least one case of a similar nature. These authors also point out that while bronchiectasis is now a rare disease in developed countries it is still fairly common in developing countries. For example, they recorded over 80 cases at the University Hospital of the West Indies over a 5-year period (1965 to 1970) and 40 cases among Australian aborigines over an 18-month period in the early 1970s.

Although the plain roentgenogram may strongly suggest the diagnosis of bronchiectasis, bronchography is mandatory to establish its presence beyond question and to determine its precise extent—but only if surgery is contemplated. Bronchography should be performed only after adequate postural drainage and antibiotic therapy have

Text continued on page 2198

Figure 11–95. Cylindrical Bronchiectasis.
A posteroanterior roentgenogram *(A)* demonstrates a slight elevation of the left hemidiaphragm, chiefly in its posterior portion *(see C)*. The linear markings in the basal segments of the left lower lobe are more prominent than normal and have lost their sharp definition; they are slightly crowded. Elsewhere, the lungs appear normal. A left bronchogram in posteroanterior *(B)* and lateral *(C)* projections reveals uniform dilatation of all basal bronchi of the left lower lobe; prominent transverse striations are present in the lateral basal bronchus *(arrow)*. All bronchiectatic segments end abruptly, and there is little or no peripheral filling. The remainder of the bronchial tree is normal. In lateral projection, note the crowding of the bronchiectatic segments and the elevation of the posterior portion of the hemidiaphragm, both findings indicating moderate loss of volume. Cinefluorographic studies revealed normal bronchial dynamics. This 31-year-old man had a history of productive cough dating from an attack of whooping cough and bronchopneumonia as a child; pulmonary function studies were normal.

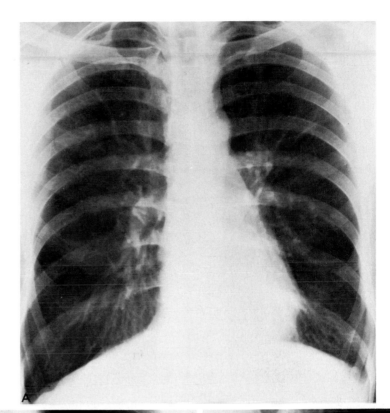

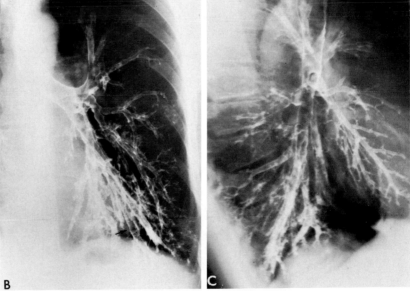

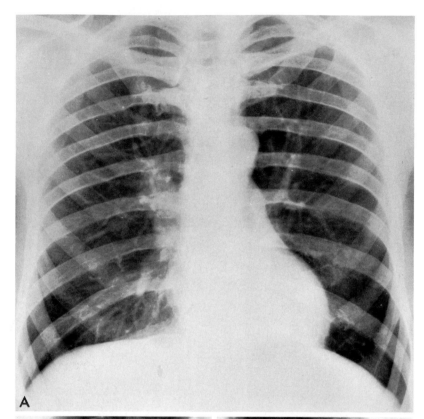

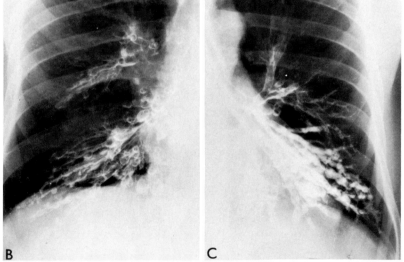

Figure 11–96. Varicose Bronchiectasis. At first glance, the posteroanterior roentgenogram *(A)* of this 38-year-old man shows no significant abnormality; however, a rather subtle change is present in the size of the vascular markings throughout the lungs, the upper lobe vessels being somewhat larger than normal and the lower lobe vessels comparatively inconspicuous. Right *(B)* and left *(C)* bronchograms reveal extensive dilatation of all basal bronchi of the lower lobes and of the right middle lobe; the dilatation is not uniform, as in Figure 11–95, but is characterized by numerous local constrictions that give the bronchi a configuration resembling varicose veins. There is a notable absence of peripheral filling. It is unusual for such extensive bronchiectasis to be associated with the inconspicuous plain roentgenographic changes depicted; it is assumed that the alteration in vascular pattern resulted from a redistribution of blood flow from the lower lobes as a result of hypoxic vasoconstriction, bronchial artery hypertrophy, and systemic-pulmonary arterial anastomoses. This patient gave a history of the accidental ingestion of camphorated oil 1 year previously and had had cough productive of "dirty" sputum ever since; it seems reasonable to postulate a cause and effect relationship between this episode and the severe bronchiectasis.

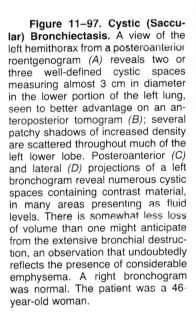

Figure 11–97. Cystic (Saccular) Bronchiectasis. A view of the left hemithorax from a posteroanterior roentgenogram *(A)* reveals two or three well-defined cystic spaces measuring almost 3 cm in diameter in the lower portion of the left lung, seen to better advantage on an anteroposterior tomogram *(B)*; several patchy shadows of increased density are scattered throughout much of the left lower lobe. Posteroanterior *(C)* and lateral *(D)* projections of a left bronchogram reveal numerous cystic spaces containing contrast material, in many areas presenting as fluid levels. There is somewhat less loss of volume than one might anticipate from the extensive bronchial destruction, an observation that undoubtedly reflects the presence of considerable emphysema. A right bronchogram was normal. The patient was a 46-year-old woman.

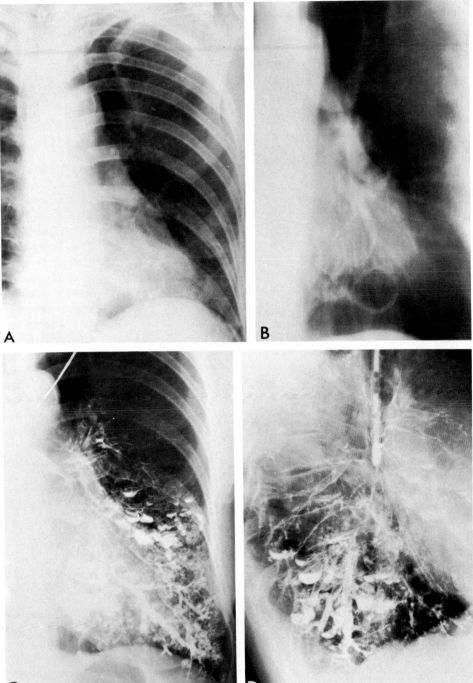

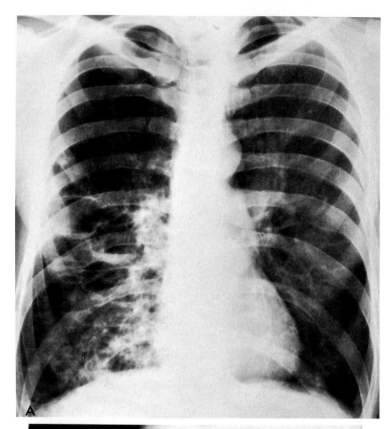

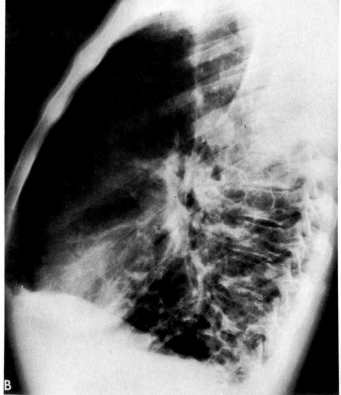

Figure 11–98. Advanced Cystic Bronchiectasis.
Posteroanterior *(A)* and lateral *(B)* roentgenograms of a 38-year-old man demonstrate extensive replacement of the right lower lobe by multiple thin-walled cysts, many of which contain air-fluid levels. The left lung is normal; the right upper and middle lobes show severe oligemia, possibly caused by emphysema. Bronchography was not performed.

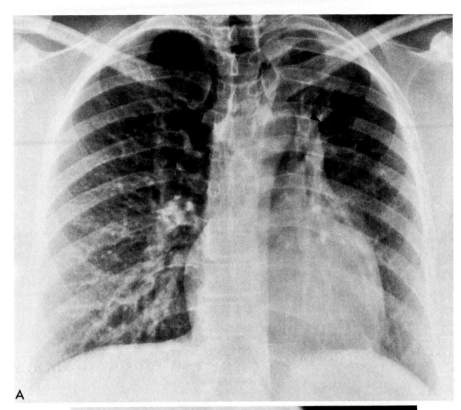

Figure 11–99. Severe Atelectasis of the Left Upper Lobe Associated with Bronchiectasis. Posteroanterior *(A)* and lateral *(B)* roentgenograms of a 30-year-old woman reveal marked loss of volume of the left upper lobe, indicated by shift of the mediastinum to the left and marked anterior displacement of the major fissure *(arrows* in *B).* In lateral projection the lobe appears airless, suggesting the possibility of an endobronchial obstructing lesion, but in posteroanterior projection a broad air-containing space is visible *(arrowheads),* which makes an endobronchial lesion most unlikely. Bronchoscopy revealed a patent left upper lobe bronchus.

Illustration continued on following page

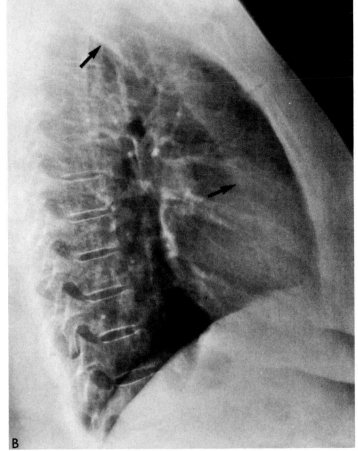

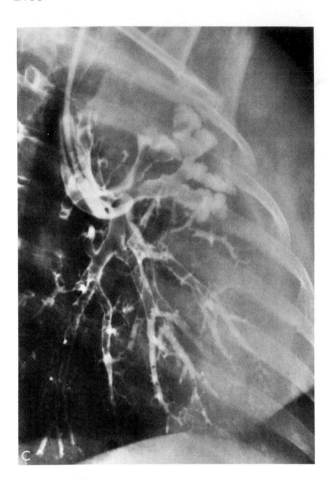

Figure 11–99. *Continued.* A left bronchogram *(C)* shows severe cystic bronchiectasis of all segments of the left upper lobe. The air-containing space in *A* represents a markedly dilated bronchus.

rendered the bronchial tree as free as possible of retained secretions. As discussed in Chapter 2, it is our policy to examine each lung at a separate sitting; this allows better visualization of each bronchial tree separately and avoids the undesirable functional side-effects of the procedure, particularly in patients with borderline pulmonary insufficiency. The bronchographic findings in the three types of bronchiectasis are as described in the section on pathology (Figs. 11–95 to 11–97 and 11–100). We wish to stress again the importance of having the patient cough vigorously after the usual postbronchographic roentgenography in three projections. The deep inspirations associated with coughing nearly always result in more complete filling of the peripheral bronchial and bronchiolar radicals than is possible with the usual techniques of bronchography. Better filling may reveal unsuspected diseased segments or may negate the suspicion of bronchiectasis on roentgenograms showing insufficient peripheral dissemination of contrast medium.

The role of CT in the diagnosis of bronchiectasis is somewhat controversial, one study having shown it to be unreliable in the detection of cylindrical and varicose changes,[2392] whereas others[2393, 2394] have shown the technique to be highly accurate (Fig. 11–101). In a study of 36 patients with clinical findings suggestive of this diagnosis, Grenier and his colleagues[2393] employed 1.5-mm section thick-

ness and 10-mm intersection spacing to compare CT findings with those of bronchography. In 15 lungs, no bronchiectasis was demonstrated on either CT scans or bronchograms; in 25 lungs, both examinations accurately indicated the presence and extent of bronchiectasis. In a more recent study in which 4-mm-thickness cuts were performed at 5-mm intervals, Joharjy and his coworkers[2394] compared the results of CT with those of bronchography in 323 segmental bronchi in 20 patients. No bronchiectasis was found in either study in 222 segmental bronchi; of the 101 segmental bronchi in which bronchiectasis was shown on bronchography, CT correctly identifed the disease in 98 segments (97 per cent); bronchography showed cystic bronchiectasis in 35 and varicose bronchiectasis in 14 segmental bronchi, all of which were correctly identified in CT. Of the 52 segmental bronchi in which cylindrical bronchiectasis was identified on bronchography, CT correctly identified these changes in 49 segments but failed to detect them in three. The authors of this paper concluded that CT with medium-thickness cuts and medium-slice intervals is 100 per cent specific for all types of bronchiectasis, 100 per cent sensitive for cystic and varicose bronchiectasis, and 94 per cent for cylindrical disease. While the results of these two studies are most impressive, we are nevertheless of the opinion that although CT can be employed with benefit to iden-

Figure 11–100. Bronchographic Features of Varicose and Cystic Bronchiectasis. A left tracheobronchogram in a shallow posterior oblique projection *(A)* reveals mildly dilated and slightly irregular bronchi that terminate four to six generations of branchings from the trachea in a squared or bulbous appearance *(arrowheads)*. The findings are those of varicose bronchiectasis. A bilateral tracheobronchogram in anteroposterior projection *(B)* demonstrates a multitude of contrast-filled cystic spaces resembling a cluster of grapes *(arrowheads)*, a characteristic feature of cystic bronchiectasis. Note that the cystic spaces appear after only two to three bronchial generations. Less severe bronchiectasis of varicose type is present in the right lower lobe *(open arrows)*.

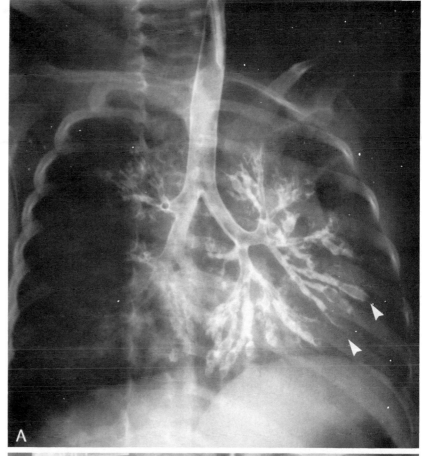

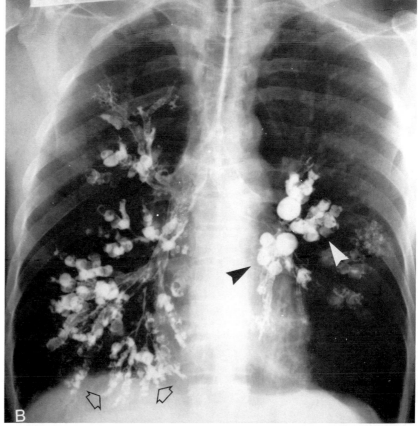

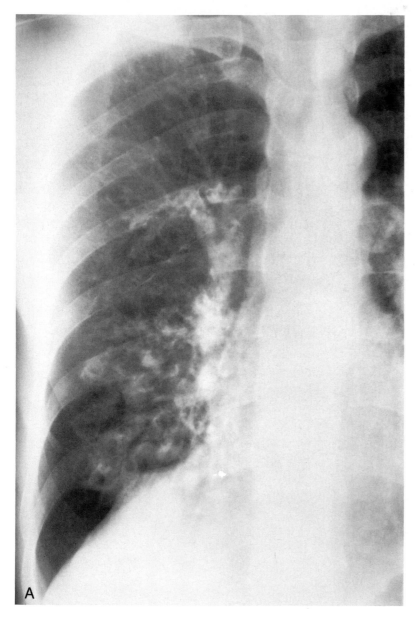

Figure 11–101. Varicose and Cystic Bronchiectasis: CT Features. A detail view of the right lung *(A)* from a posteroanterior chest roentgenogram shows multiple cystic spaces in the right lower lobe, some containing a fluid level. There is downward displacement of the major fissure, indicating loss of volume. Similar but less pronounced findings were present in the left lung (not illustrated).

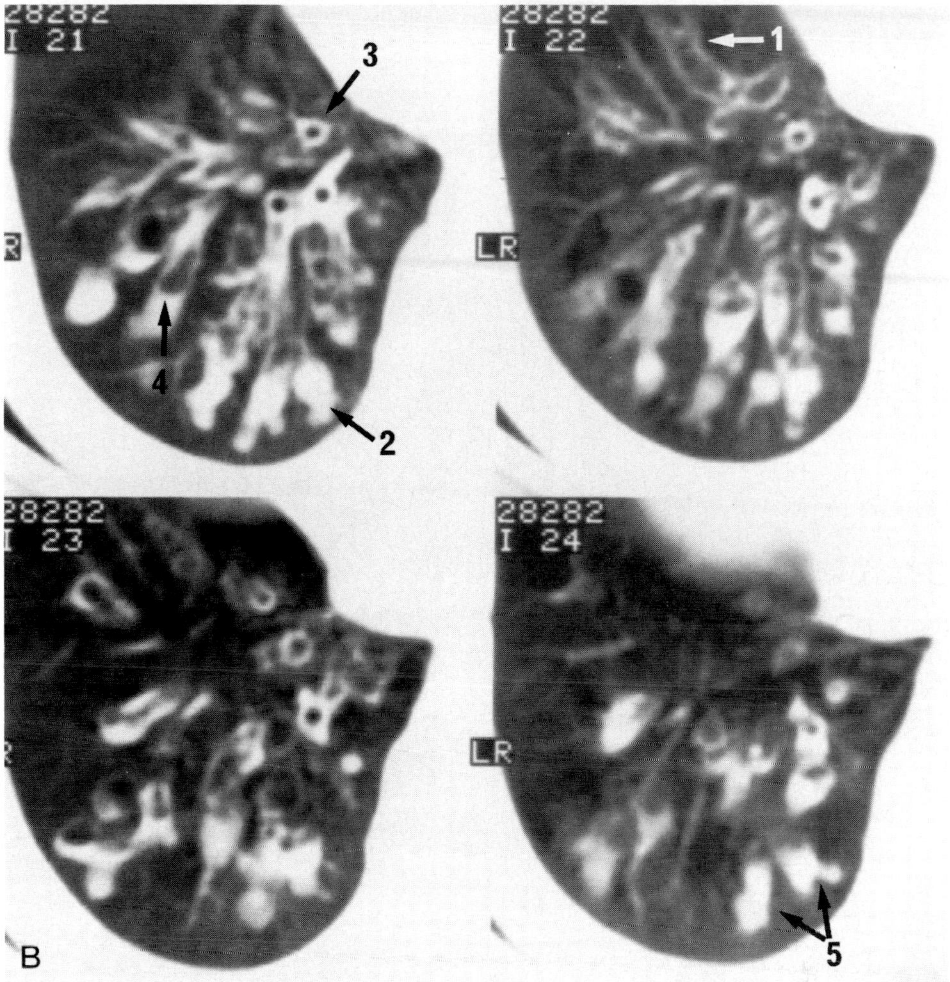

Figure 11–101. *Continued.* A sequence of CT scans 10 mm thick, with 10-mm interspacing through the right lower lobe *(B)* reveals varicose *(1)* and cystic *(2)* bronchiectasis, thickened bronchial walls *(3)*, fluid levels *(4)*, and mucoid impaction *(5)*. The patient is a 27-year-old man with a chronic cough productive of purulent sputum.

tify the disease in patients in whom it is suspected clinically, bronchography should be performed on all patients for whom surgical resection is planned. Tarver and his colleagues[2800] have drawn attention to the possibility of making a false diagnosis of bronchiectasis on CT scans because of motion artifacts.

"Reversible bronchiectasis" designates the form of bronchial dilatation that usually is a manifestation of acute pneumonia.[2395, 2396] Dilatation develops as a result of retained secretions and of the atelectasis that is an invariable accompaniment of resolving pneumonia. With complete resolution of the pneumonia the dilatation gradually disappears, although it may be as long as 3 to 4 months before the integrity of the bronchial tree is restored (Fig. 11–102). Consequently, to be on the safe side, if surgery is contemplated it is advisable to allow 4 to 6 months to elapse after acute pneumonia before performing bronchography for the assessment of bronchiectasis.

Clinical Manifestations

The main symptoms are cough and the expectoration of purulent sputum. The quantity of sputum varies with the severity of the disease, but most patients expectorate daily. Some patients become aware of purulent expectoration only after respiratory infections (which tend to be frequent). Although the level of serum protein in purulent sputum of patients with bronchiectasis is moderately increased, in one study no relationship was found between the clinical severity of bronchiectasis and the sputum levels of serum proteins.[2397] Hemoptysis occurs in about 50 per cent of older patients but is relatively rare in children. If the disease is widespread, the patient may complain of shortness of breath. In almost every case, persistent rales localized to the area of major involvement are detectable, and if the bronchiectasis is associated with significant airway obstruction, diffuse rhonchi may be heard over both lungs. Extrathoracic manifestations include finger clubbing, seen in about one third of cases,[2387] and rarely brain abscess and amyloidosis. Neuropathy has been reported;[2398] surgical resection of the affected segments results in improvement or complete cure. Four patients have been described in whom purpuric vasculitic skin lesions developed during exacerbations of bronchiectasis, associated with elevated levels of circulating immune complexes.[2399]

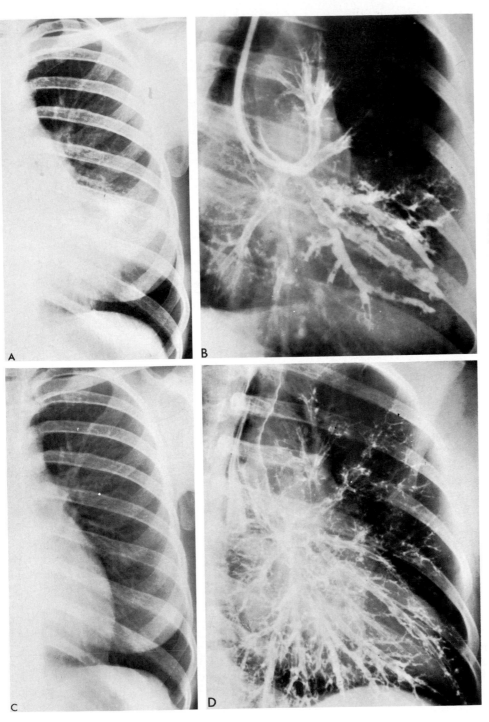

Figure 11–102. Reversible Bronchiectasis. A 26-year-old woman was admitted to the hospital for the first time with an acute pneumonia of the lingula *(A)*. During each day of her convalescence, she coughed up a cup of greenish, purulent sputum; because of this symptom, she was referred for bronchography 3 weeks after the onset of the acute pneumonia. The bronchogram *(B)* revealed moderate cylindrical and varicose bronchiectasis of both segments of the lingula. Subsequent treatment was supportive only, and her symptoms gradually diminished. One year after the acute pneumonia, a posteroanterior view of the left hemithorax *(C)* reveals a normal appearance of the left lung. Bronchography performed at this time *(D)* shows a normal bronchial tree; the lingular segments show none of the deformity observed a year previously.

Postinfective bronchiectasis is predominantly a pediatric disease, the history commonly dating from early childhood. For example, 50 per cent of a series of 116 patients gave a history indicating the onset of symptoms before the third birthday.[2387] In a majority of cases, a history of pneumonia developing as a complication of measles, whooping cough, or some other contagious disease of childhood can be elicited. Bronchiectasis is bilateral in approximately 50 per cent of patients[2387, 2388] and in the great majority involves the basal segments of the lower lobes. In only about 10 per cent of cases is the middle lobe or lingula affected without concomitant involvement of the ipsilateral lower lobe.[2388]

Pulmonary Function Studies

In our experience there is no specific pattern of pulmonary function in bronchiectasis. Patients with well-localized disease unassociated with chronic bronchitis suffer little or no functional impairment. However, with appropriate testing, such patients may show generalized disease of small airways,[2381] a well-recognized pathologic finding in this disease.[2400] In the presence of appreciable atelectasis, the abnormality of function may be restrictive, with decrease in the VC and FRC. In more diffuse disease, as reported by Cherniak and his coworkers,[2101] the pattern is more like that of obstructive disease, with proportionally greater decrease in the timed VC and, in many cases, impairment of mixing, increase in the FRC, and reduction of diffusing capacity. Part of the airway obstruction is reversible; in one study of 14 patients with diffuse bronchiectasis, a mean increase of 16 per cent in FEV_1 occurred following the administration of beta-agonist bronchodilators. A small percentage of patients with diffuse disease manifest the typical pattern of advanced COPD, including hypoxemia and carbon dioxide retention.

Bahous and associates measured pulmonary function and bronchial responsiveness in 50 patients with bronchiectasis, excluding individuals whose disease was secondary to tuberculosis or hypogammaglobulinemia.[2402] The predominant functional abnormality consisted of airflow obstruction unaccompanied by marked hyperinflation: values of individual tests as a percentage of predicted included mean vital capacity (83), mean residual volume (150), and diffusing capacity corrected for alveolar volume (90). In 35 of the 50 patients, FEV_1 was less than 80 per cent of predicted, and in 34 the FEV_1/FVC ratio was less than 70 per cent. Of the 29 patients in whom the FEV_1 was greater than 1.5 liters, an inhalation dose-response curve for methacholine showed that in 69 per cent the PC_{20}/FEV_1 was less than 16 mg/ml; there was a significant relationship between PC_{20} and the prechallenge FEV_1. In a study of distribution and clearance of tagged radioactive aerosol particles 2 μm in diameter in 14 patients with bronchiectasis, Lourenco and associates[2404] found that particles were deposited in central bronchi and were cleared more slowly than normal. They attributed the central deposition to increased turbulence in obstructed larger airways, permitting impaction by inertia; the impaired clearance was similar to that seen in simple bronchitis and was ascribed to damage to the mucociliary apparatus. Currie and associates[2403] have confirmed the considerable impairment in tracheobronchial clearance that occurs in patients with bronchiectasis.

Prognosis

After pulmonary resection for localized bronchiectasis, the disease commonly affects segments previously shown to be normal bronchographically,[2405] a development attributed to postoperative atelectasis or pneumonitis[2406] or to an underlying structural defect in the bronchial wall.[2407] Perhaps of a similar nature is the development of bronchiectasis in segments previously shown to be normal bronchographically in patients who have not undergone resectional surgery.[2387]

Despite the occurrence of such progressive disease, the prognosis of patients with bronchiectasis has improved considerably in this century. In a 1940 report based on a follow-up of 400 patients with the disease, Perry and King[2408] found that 92 per cent of the deaths were directly attributable to the bronchiectasis and that about 70 per cent of the patients died before the age of 40 years. By contrast, in a 1969 report of a 12-year follow-up of 62 patients with bronchiectasis, only 50 per cent of the deaths that occurred were attributed to bronchiectasis or its complications. The average age at death was 55 years, and only two patients died who were under the age of 40.[2409] In 1974, Sanders and associates[2410] reviewed the results of surgical and medical management of 393 patients with bronchiectasis who were followed over a period up to 15 years. Only 9 per cent died during this follow-up period, 60 per cent of these being patients ranging in age from 45 to 59 years. In a more recent review of the prognosis of 116 patients with bronchiectasis, Ellis and colleagues[2411] reported a mortality rate of 19 per cent during a 14-year follow-up period, the mean age at death being 54 years. Like the decrease in incidence of the disease, this significant improvement in prognosis undoubtedly can be attributed to antibiotic therapy.

DYSKINETIC CILIA SYNDROME

The syndrome of situs inversus, paranasal sinusitis, and bronchiectasis was first reported by Siewert in 1904,[2412] but acquired its eponym somewhat later after Kartagener described it in detail. Since that time, it has become clear that other abnormalities are occasionally associated with the classic triad, including transposition of the great vessels,[2413] trilocular or bilocular heart, pyloric stenosis, urethral meatus on the ventral ridge of the glans penis,[2414] and postcricoid web (Paterson-Brown-Kelly syndrome).[2415] Because of the presence of these congenital anomalies and of the familial association of the disorder in some cases,[2416] a hereditary abnormality was assumed to be the cause. The precise nature of this, however, eluded recognition until 1975, when Camner and associates described two subjects with Kartagener's syndrome who also had immotile spermatozoa and immotile cilia.[2417] These authors were the first to suggest that the immotile cilia were the underlying abnormality responsible for the classic features of the disease.

Since that time, numerous reports have appeared in the literature confirming the presence of abnormalities of ciliary structure and function in patients with the syndrome.[2418] The identification of these abnormalities as the cause of the condition initially led to the use of the more descriptive term immotile cilia syndrome in place of Kartagener's syndrome. However, it has since become clear that most patients with the disease possess cilia that do move, although the motion is abnormal and dysynchronous when examined by microphoto-oscillographic methods.[2419] In a study of patients with Kartagener's syndrome whose cilia displayed an absence of dynein arms, an absence of radial spokes, and a translocation of microtubule doublets, Rossman and her associates[2420] correlated ultrastructural defects in cilia with abnormalities in their motion. In all subjects, there was some motion when the cilia were examined microscopically, but this was invariably abnormal, ineffective, and uncoordinated; patterns of motion varied with the different structural abnormalities. Thus, they concluded that the term immotile cilia syndrome is a misnomer and suggested instead the name *dyskinetic cilia syndrome* (DCS); this term (or its synonym, *primary ciliary dyskinesia*) has now gained general acceptance. More recently, Pedersen[2421] has extended the observations of Rossman and associates by describing a variant of DCS with normal ultrastructure but "trembling" hypermotile cilia. Some investigators have even suggested that microscopic examination and quantification of the frequency and pattern of ciliary beating from mucosal biopsy specimens is a more effective means of establishing a diagnosis of DCS than is electron microscopy.[2422]

The incidence of DCS in the total white population is estimated to be one in 40,000.[2414] This is considerably lower than the figures reported for the Japanese population,[2423] a difference that has been attributed to a greater prevalence of consanguinity in marriage among the Japanese. In 1979, Waite and his associates[2424] described three Maori with abnormal ciliary ultrastructure and bronchiectasis and suggested that the high incidence of bronchiectasis in Polynesians could be related to ciliary dyskinesia. However, they have subsequently described a larger series of similar patients, and it appears that these individuals do not fit the pattern of most patients with DCS; in addition, situs inversus is not present.[2425, 2426] It has been suggested that the defects described in these patients may be acquired rather than congenital.[2427–2429]

As indicated, the etiology of DCS in most instances is believed to be a genetically determined abnormality of ciliary structure and function. The mode of inheritance is not well defined, but most studies suggest a basic autosomal recessive pattern;[2423, 2430, 2431] the variety of ultrastructural defects associated with the clinical syndrome suggests considerable genetic heterogeneity.[2432] In addition, patients have been described with classic Kartagener's syndrome and abnormal airway ciliary ultrastructure but with normal spermatozoa, indicating that discordance in phenotypic presentation can occur.[2433, 2434] Familial sterility associated with ultrastructural abnormalities of sperm but with normal respiratory ciliary structure and function has also been reported.[2435] DCS has also been reported in association with Marfan's syndrome[2436] and polysplenia,[2437] and an increased incidence of ciliary

defects has been identified in patients with retinitis pigmentosa.[2438]

The structure and function of the normal cilium are complex and have been reviewed previously (*see* Chapter 1, page 6). Briefly, each cilium contains an axoneme consisting of two central microtubules surrounded by nine peripheral pairs of microtubules. The peripheral and central microtubules are joined by radial spokes, and the peripheral microtubules connect to each other by inner and outer dynein arms; the latter are believed to be the site of energy conversion leading to ciliary movement. Ultrastructural abnormalities in each of these components have been identified in patients with DCS (Fig. 11–103); these include a lack of outer dynein arms, absent or short radial spokes,[2437] deficient central sheath, absent or defective inner dynein arms,[2438] absent central microtubules, transposition of peripheral microtubules,[2439, 2440] and supernumerary microtubules;[2441] the most common of these is a lack of dynein arms. In some patients the abnormality may be not in the cilium itself but rather in the basal apparatus.[2442] Classic Kartagener's syndrome has also been reported in patients with ultrastructurally normal cilia; in some of these individuals, disease has been attributed to abnormally long cilia[2443] whereas in others it is possible that the structural defect could develop later in life or that a functional defect can occur without morphologic abnormalities.[2444–2446]

It is important to recognize that structural defects of cilia can be acquired rather than congenital,[2447] and it has occasionally proved difficult to distinguish the two in single biopsy specimens of nasal or bronchial mucosa.[2448, 2449] Such abnormalities are not uncommon, having been described in a high proportion of smokers,[2766–2768] in individuals with chronic bronchitis and influenza or other viral infection,[2418, 2769] and in some apparently normal individuals who manifest neither acute nor chronic respiratory disease.[2768–2771] Derangements include compound cilia (showing partial or multiple complete axonemes within a single cell membrane), internalized cilia (projecting into cytoplasmic cavities in the cell apex rather than into the airway), cilia with disorganized axonemes, changes in the ciliary membrane or amount of cytoplasm, transposition of microtubules,[2768] radial spoke defects,[2768] flaccid cilia,[2418] and a variety of minor microtubular abnormalities.[2769–2771] (*See also* Chapter 1.) Despite these observations, differentiation between acquired and congenital defects should usually be straightforward if sufficient cilia are examined.[2450] Rossman and coworkers carried out a quantitative study of ciliary beat frequency, beat pattern, and ultrastructure in a large group of normal subjects, patients with atopic rhinitis, asymptomatic smokers, patients with pulmonary disease not related to DCS, and patients with DCS. About 5 per cent of the cilia from normal subjects and patients with non-DCS pulmonary disease had abnormal ciliary structure,

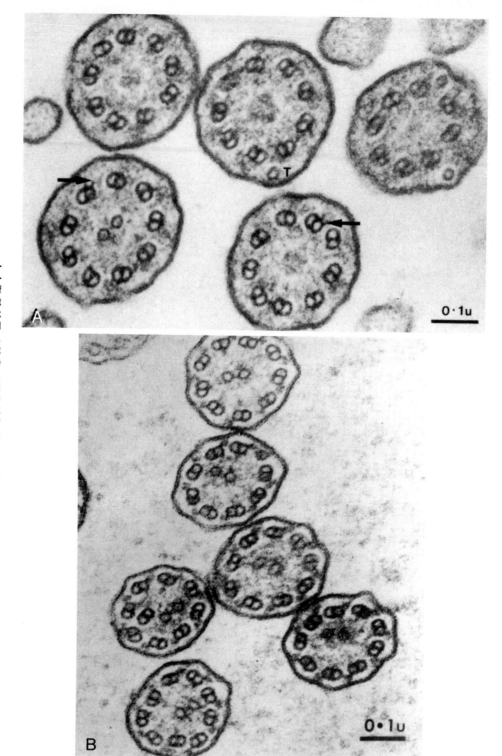

Figure 11–103. Ciliary Abnormalities in Dyskinetic Cilia Syndrome. A cross section of a group of cilia and microvilli *(A)* shows that most of the outer ciliary doublets lack dynein arms, although occasional partial arms are present *(arrows).* The central tubules are also absent in four of the cilia; supernumary single tubules (T) are occasionally present. (Original magnification, × 130,000.) (From Wakefield St J, Waite D: Am Rev Respir Dis *121*:1003, 1980.) A cross section of cilia from another patient *(B)* shows normal structure except for the absence of inner dynein arms. (Original magnification, × 100,000.) (From Neustein HG, Nickerson B, O'Neal M: Am Rev Respir Dis *122*:979, 1980.)

whereas 30 to 95 per cent of cilia from patients with DCS were structurally abnormal; beat frequency and pattern of ciliary motion were obviously different in the latter group.

The abnormalities identified in ciliary microtubular structure may represent only part of a generalized disease process. Thus, microtubules are essential for phagocytic cell motility, and leukocyte chemotaxis and phagocytosis have been reported to be mildly impaired in DCS; for example, polymorphonuclear leukocytes show an excessive rambling and circuitous movement when placed on a flat surface.[2451-2453] Although the bactericidal activity of the polymorphonuclear cells is normal, it is possible that the decreased motility and phagocytosis could contribute to the increased frequency of pulmonary infections to which these patients are subject.

The roentgenographic manifestations of DCS

have been described in detail by Nadel and her colleagues[2454] from a study of 30 patients, 15 of each sex. Ages ranged from newborn to 26 years. Except for two neonates, sinusitis and otitis were present in all patients. Roentgenographic abnormalities in the chest were present in all patients and included bronchial wall thickening, hyperinflation, segmental atelectasis or consolidation, and segmental bronchiectasis. Situs inversus was present in only half the patients (seven female, eight male) (Fig. 11–104) and obviously was not an essential part of the disorder. The authors regarded the roentgenographic abnormalities and clinical presentation to be very similar to those of cystic fibrosis, although somewhat less severe and less progressive.

Clinically, individuals with full-blown DCS have chronic rhinitis, sinusitis, otitis, chronic and recurrent infections of the airways, bronchiectasis, male sterility, corneal abnormalities, and a poor sense of smell. Situs inversus or dextrocardia is present in approximately 50 per cent of patients. Except for the last-named finding, roentgenographic features are not specific and resemble those of bronchiectasis from a variety of other causes. To make a diagnosis of the dyskinetic cilia syndrome, Afzelius[2418] recommended that patients must have signs of chronic bronchial infection and rhinitis from early childhood, combined with one or more of the following features: (1) situs inversus or dextrocardia in the patient or a sibling, (2) living but immotile spermatozoa of normal appearance, (3) tracheobronchial clearance that is absent or nearly so, and (4) cilia in a nasal or bronchial biopsy specimen that have ultrastructural defects characteristic of the syndrome. The association of otitis with the lower respiratory tract symptoms is a consistent feature and should alert one to the possibility of a ciliary defect.[2455]

The decrease in airway mucociliary clearance in patients with DCS[1662, 2456, 2457] is profound and is greater than that seen in individuals with advanced cystic fibrosis, bronchiectasis, COPD, or asthma.[1662, 2456] Despite this, severe airflow obstruction does not develop in these patients. Although such obstruction has been reported by Mossberg and associates,[1662] it was not incapacitating, suggesting to these authors that impaired mucociliary clearance may contribute to the production of obstructive airway disease but cannot be of major importance. Early in the course of the disease, patients have a pattern of functional abnormalities consistent with small airways dysfunction and increased bronchial reactivity to methacholine; however, one group of patients followed over a period to 4 to 14 years showed a remarkably stable pattern of mild obstruction.[2458, 2459]

YOUNG'S SYNDROME

Young's syndrome (obstructive azoospermia) is a condition characterized by infertility; the subject has recently been reviewed.[2460] The combination of infertility and sinopulmonary infections may suggest a diagnosis of cystic fibrosis or DCS.[2461, 2462] It has been suggested that simple obstruction is not the only cause of this syndrome because surgical correction is relatively ineffective in restoring fertility and there is a high incidence of associated bronchitis and bronchiectasis. Pavia and his associates[2463] examined lung mucociliary clearance in 14 patients with Young's syndrome and in 14 age-matched, smoking-matched control subjects; they found a significant decrease in mucociliary clearance in the patients, accompanied by slight but definite abnormalities of pulmonary function.[2463] In a review of 102 patients with obstructive azoospermia, 23 per cent were considered to have Young's syndrome.[2464] A familial disorder has been reported in men which is characterized by oligospermia, impaired spermatic motility, bronchiectasis, and normal ciliary ultrastructure.[2465]

THE SYNDROME OF YELLOW NAILS, LYMPHEDEMA, PLEURAL EFFUSION, AND BRONCHIECTASIS

The syndrome of yellow nails and lymphedema was first described by Samman and White in 1964.[2466] Later, Emerson[2467] added pleural effusion as a frequent feature of the disease. Some physicians restrict the diagnosis to patients with the triad of yellow nails, lymphedema, and pleural effusion, whereas others accept any two of these characteristics. In 1986, Nordkild and associates[2468] reviewed the reports of 97 patients described in the literature. Age at onset varies widely: for example, lymphedema can be present at birth or can become manifest at the age of 65 years; the median age *at onset* was 40 years. Eighty-nine per cent of the patients had yellow nails, 80 per cent lymphedema of varying severity, and 36 per cent pleural effusion. In 29 per cent of patients, the initial symptom was related to pleural effusion. Patients often give a history of recurrent attacks of bronchitis and may have chronic sinusitis, bronchiectasis, and recurrent pneumonia. Typically, the nails grow slowly, are yellowish-green in color, and are thickened and excessively curved from side to side; they have a tendency to become infected.[2469, 2470] Lymphedema is often mild and usually affects the lower extremities and sometimes the breasts[2471] and face.[2472] The lymphedema results from hypoplasia (sometimes atresia) of the lymphatics, defects that can be demonstrated by peripheral lymphangiography.[2469] The pleural fluid is characteristically an exudate. Light and electron microscopy shows dilatation of both visceral and parietal pleural lymphatics associated with perilymphatic inflammation; the pleural fluid characteristically contains a high percentage of lymphocytes.[2473]

Two siblings have been described who manifested signs of both the syndrome and immunologic

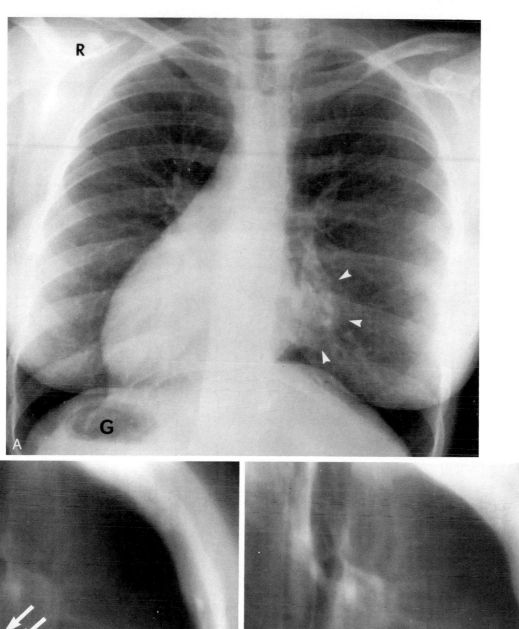

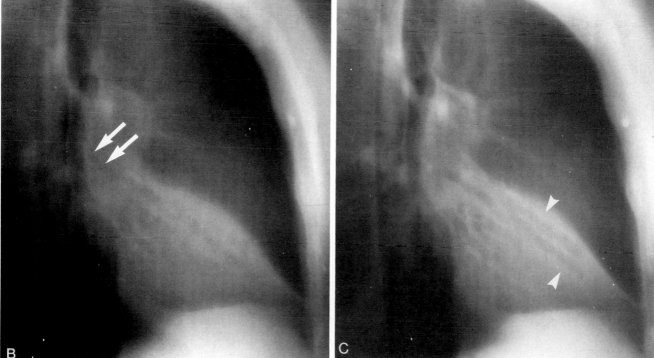

Figure 11–104. Dextrocardia, Situs Inversus, and Chronic Middle Lobe Bronchiectasis (Kartagener's Syndrome). A postero-anterior chest roentgenogram *(A)* shows dextrocardia and situs inversus; note the position of the gastric air bubble (G). The right atrial contour is effaced by an inhomogeneous triangular opacity *(arrowheads)* consistent with atelectasis. Linear tomograms through the left hilum in 55 degrees posterior oblique projection *(B and C)* reveal patency of the middle lobe bronchus *(arrows)* and air-filled bronchiectatic bronchi distally *(arrowheads)*. The patient is a 19-year-old woman with a chronic mucopurulent cough.

deficiency; however, this familial occurrence is unique among the cases reported to date.[2474] The yellow nail syndrome has been reported in association with thyroid disease (six of 97 patients), hypogammaglobulinemia in various forms (seven of 97 patients), the nephrotic syndrome, and protein-losing enteropathy.[2468, 2475] One case of obstructive sleep apnea has been reported,[2476] the authors suggesting that edema of the pharynx and palate contributed to the upper airway obstruction. Of the 12 patients reported from the Mayo Clinic,[2474] eight had recurrent pleural effusion and five bronchiectasis; in this series, the first manifestation of the syndrome was either lymphedema or yellow nails, pleural effusion appearing somewhat later in all cases. However, in two other series bronchiectasis and yellow nails were reported as developing simultaneously in three patients aged 10, 18, and 20 years, lymphedema becoming manifest somewhat later in each patient.[2471, 2477] The pathogenesis of the bronchiectasis is unknown, although it is frequently associated with sinusitis;[2474] in one patient the bronchiectasis was confined to the upper lobes.[2478]

CYSTIC FIBROSIS

Cystic fibrosis (CF) is a hereditary disease of mendelian recessive transmission also known as mucoviscidosis or cystic fibrosis of the pancreas. The fundamental abnormality consists of the production of abnormal secretions from a variety of exocrine glands, including the salivary and sweat glands and those of the pancreas, large bowel, and tracheobronchial tree. With the first description of the latter abnormalities by di Sant'Agnese in 1953,[2479] the designation cystic fibrosis became generally accepted and that of mucoviscidosis largely discarded. The major clinical manifestations are chronic obstructive pulmonary disease (found in varying degrees of severity in almost all cases) and pancreatic insufficiency (present in 80 to 90 per cent of patients).[2480, 2481] Although a family history may suggest the diagnosis, confirmation requires the demonstration of elevated levels of sodium and chloride in sweat.

Cystic fibrosis is the most common lethal genetically transmitted syndrome among white children, the estimated incidence in this group being approximately one case per 2,000 to 3,500 live births.[2482-2486] There is no sex predominance. The disease is uncommon in non-whites; its incidence among North American blacks is 1 in 17,000 and among North American Indians and Orientals 1 in 90,000.[2486] It is chiefly a disease of infants and children, although adult cases are being recognized with greater frequency.[2487-2491] In 80 per cent of cases, the diagnosis is made before the age of 5 years; in 10 per cent, the disease is not recognized until adolescence.[2486, 2492] One pedigree has been described in which three siblings had such mild disease that diagnosis was not established until ages 36, 40, and 44.[2498]

Cystic fibrosis is transmitted as an autosomal recessive trait, although there is considerable controversy as to whether a single mutant allele or two or three loci are responsible for its manifestations.[2480, 2493] A genetic study of first cousins of index cases of CF estimated a gene frequency of 0.0281, an incidence that is higher than that predicted by direct counting of cases. These results could be explained by two mutant gene loci with frequencies of 0.014,[2494] and in fact, present knowledge suggests that a patient with CF must inherit two genes to express the disease, one from each parent.[2495] Chromosomes are morphologically normal, and there is no correlation with blood groups or major HLA loci.[2486, 2496] The large variation in the severity of clinical manifestations of CF suggests that there may be genetic heterogeneity.[2497]

In the white population, approximately one in 20 individuals is heterozygous for CF. No clinical characteristics have been demonstrated that identify the heterozygotes because they do not express the disease and generally are unaware that they are carriers until they have children with CF.[2495] Each unaffected brother or sister of a patient with CF has a two-thirds chance of being a carrier. If a carrier of the gene marries another person who is heterozygous with the same gene, each pregnancy has a 25 per cent risk of resulting in a child with the disease. If one parent has no familial history of CF and the other parent has the disease, there is a 1 in 40 chance of the child's being affected.[2495] Because effective genetic counseling is dependent on identifying heterozygous carriers and on prenatal detection of affected homozygotes, considerable research has been carried out into the development of tests for these states. A number of methods have been tried to identify heterozygotes, including detection of a unique circulating protein by isoelectric focusing, detection of a lectin-like factor in the serum by hemagglutination, isolation of a CF-specific lectin from the serum by affinity chromatography, and measurement of MUGB-reactive* proteases in the plasma.[2499] None of these has been found to be sufficiently sensitive or specific to employ in a screening study. Cultured fibroblasts from CF homozygotes and heterozygotes demonstrate a leakage of certain hydrolases and a pathologic increase in intracellular alkaline phosphatase, but this too has not proved effective enough to use as a screening test.[2500] Although a 3-day loading test with sodium bromide and subsequent analysis of bromide in serum and sweat allowed correct classification of 91 per cent of known heterozygotes, an easier test with much greater precision is required before any screening program is attempted.[2501]

---

*MUGB = 4-methylumbelliferylguanidinobenzoate.

The tests that have been proposed for prenatal diagnosis are the analysis of amniotic fluid for MUGB-reactive proteases, alkaline phosphatase isoenzymes, and the proteolytic hydrolases of arginine esters.[204, 2502, 2503] Unfortunately, all of these have an unacceptably high false-positive rate and the results cannot be used in individual cases to provide counseling.

PATHOGENESIS

Despite intensive investigation, the pathogenesis and pathophysiology of the many manifestations of CF are not completely understood. This subject has been reviewed by di Sant'Agnese and Davis,[2493, 2504] and by Ceder,[2503] and the interested reader is directed to these sources for more complete coverage. The morphologic changes in affected organs are partly the result of the plugging of the ducts into which the secretions of exocrine glands are secreted. In the tracheobronchial tree, in addition to an abnormality of mucous secretion, there is considerable evidence to implicate a disturbance of water and electrolyte balance across the epithelium as well as abnormalities in autonomic nervous control. The suggestion that increased serum pancreatic enzymes may cause the lung damage seen in CF has not been supported by data.[2505]

Abnormalities of Mucoprotein Secretion and Mucociliary Clearance

The abnormal rheologic properties of exocrine gland secretions in CF and the pivotal role played by these abnormal secretions in the pathophysiology of the disease have directed considerable attention to an examination of their biochemical makeup. A number of organic substances present in exocrine secretions could play a role in the formation of the thick, tenacious material that obstructs the conducting systems. In the lung, most interest has centered around the mucous glycoproteins which are secreted in increased amounts in CF and are capable of forming visco-elastic gels. Unfortunately, many of the methods of measuring the physical properties of sputum are unreliable; in CF there is the additional complicating factor of infection, which is almost certainly a secondary phenomenon. Nasal and tracheobronchial mucous glycoproteins contain a higher than normal content of sulfate, which may be a determinant of physical properties.[2480] One study has shown that the lipid content of airway secretions is increased in CF, suggesting that this may be responsible in part for the tenacity and insolubility of the secretions and for the concomitant airway obstruction.[2506]

In patients with CF, impaired mucociliary clearance is an almost invariable feature, at least in those with detectable airflow obstruction. Indeed, abnor-malities in the secretory processes for mucus or sol-phase fluid (or both) have been implicated in the pathogenesis of the disease. However, despite extensive investigation, a specific quantitative defect of the mucus from patients with CF has not yet been identified. With the Teflon disk method, central clearance from the tracheobronchial tree was shown to be markedly depressed in 14 adult CF patients (2.6 ml/minute compared with a normal value of 20 ml/minute).[387] Most of these patients showed severe airflow obstruction, but there was no correlation between tracheal mucous velocity and abnormalities of pulmonary function. Despite the marked decrease in clearance, the rate was doubled by inhalation of terbutaline, a beta-adrenergic agonist.[2507] In another study,[2508] patients with CF were divided into groups on the basis of their tracheal mucociliary clearance rates; a substantial number of these patients had normal mucociliary clearance, and these tended to be the ones without airflow obstruction. Those with the slowest clearance also had the lowest Shwachman-Kulczycki scores, the worst blood gases, and the most severe expiratory airflow obstruction. Of some note was the observation that serum from patients with the fastest transport rates caused the most rapid ciliary dyskinesia when added to rabbit tracheal explants.[2508]

The sputum from patients with CF has been examined for its biochemical and visco-elastic characteristics. When sputum from such patients and from those with chronic bronchitis, bronchiectasis, or asthma were matched for purulence, that from the CF group was shown to have higher levels of serum glycoproteins, suggesting increased serum transudation in these patients.[383] Using a magnetic oscillatory microrheometer to study the visco-elastic properties of the sputum from CF patients, King[2509] found that there was no characteristic abnormality but that markedly purulent sputum had higher elasticity and viscosity and a lower viscosity-to-elasticity ratio. When this investigator assessed the rate of transport of mucus from patients with CF on the isolated frog palate, the rate was slightly less than would be predicted from the visco-elastic properties, suggesting the possibility of an inhibitory factor in the sputum. Despite these observations, King concluded that CF mucus is probably normal except for the effects of purulence.[2509] This conclusion is supported by a study in which the mucociliary transport rate on frog palate correlated with scores of clinical severity and evidence of superinfection.[2510]

The evidence for ciliary dysfunction rests largely on the discovery by Spock and associates of a cilio-inhibitory factor in the euglobulin fraction of the serum of patients with the disease and of the "carrier" parents.[2511, 2512] These workers observed that serum from patients with CF disorganizes the ciliary rhythm in explants of the respiratory epithelium of rabbits. Using a variety of bioassay systems requiring highly subjective interpretation, some investigators[2513] have been able to reproduce the ciliary dyskinesia. It has been postulated that the responsible ciliary factor is a component of the complement system (C3a)[2514] and that this substance may accumulate in the blood of patients with CF as a result of a deficiency of a carboxypeptidase B-like enzyme that normally inactivates C3a. Conover and associates[2514] found that the total concentration of C3a was elevated in the blood of patients with CF, although this observation was not confirmed by Lieberman,[2515] who failed to find either a deficiency of carboxypeptidase B-like activity or an elevation of C3a levels. In patients with CF, ciliary dyskinetic substances are secreted by mononuclear cells cultured in vitro. In one study, it was shown that cultured monocytes from normal subjects secrete up to six different chemotactic agents, but in CF patients levels of these substances are higher. These chemotactic agents also have ciliary dyskinetic activity.[2516] Cilio-inhibitory factor has also been reported to be produced by fibroblasts and by long-term lymphoid cell cultures in both homozygotes and heterozygotes for CF.[2480] The serum CF factor has been linked to the metachromasia displayed in tissue culture by fibroblasts from CF patients.[2517] When serum from a patient with CF is added to a rabbit ciliary explant in vitro, progressive ciliary dyskinesia develops over a 2-hour period, resulting in almost complete akinesia by the end of this time.[2512] The substance that causes the dyskinesia has not been characterized, although one study has suggested that it is a specific protein that can be detected in the serum of CF patients.[2518] One study of 46 CF patients under 24 years of age showed no correlation between the levels of serum cilia dyskinetic substance and clinical parameters, including Shwachman-Kulczycki score, symptoms, lung function, and blood gases.[2519]

The importance of the ciliary dyskinetic substance in CF serum has recently been questioned. Rutland and associates[2512] added the serum of CF patients to nasal and bronchial ciliated cells from normal subjects and patients with CF and to ciliated cells from rabbit trachea. The serum had no effect on normal or CF cilia from either location, although it inhibited the rabbit cilia, resulting in akinesia within a 2-hour period. These investigators concluded that an inhibitory factor for cilia is not the basis for the decreased mucociliary clearance in patients with CF and speculated that antibodies directed against cilia may be present in CF serum that result in decreased ciliary beat frequency in rabbits. Acquired abnormalities of cilia are not only structural but also functional: in an in vitro assay, Smallman and associates[2520] showed that sputum from patients with bronchiectasis caused a significant decrease in ciliary beat frequency; this inhibiting effect of sputum was attenuated by alpha$_1$ antiprotease inhibitor, suggesting that it was mediated via a protease. Ciliary function was also inhibited by elastase. Increased levels of elastolytic activity have been detected in the sputum of patients with bronchiectasis when it is purulent but not when it is mucoid.[2521]

The beat frequency of nasal cilia in patients with CF is normal although nasal clearance of mucus is decreased, suggesting an alteration in the coupling of cilia and mucus.[2522] Morphologically, the ultrastructure of respiratory cilia in patients with CF show nonspecific changes.[2523, 2524] In one study in which both bioassay and high-pressure liquid chromatography were employed,[2525] leukotrienes (specifically leukotrienes D and B) were demonstrated in the sputum of patients with CF, but the importance of these mediators in the mucus and sputum of these patients is speculative.

Disturbances of Autonomic Nervous Control

Patients with CF and, to a lesser extent, heterozygous carriers of the CF genes show a pattern of autonomic dysfunction similar to that which has been associated with increased nonspecific airway responsiveness in patients with asthma.[2526, 2527] There is increased responsiveness of the papillary constrictors of the eye to locally applied alpha-adrenergic (phenylepherine) and cholinergic (carbachol) agonists, and a decreased dilator response to the beta-adrenergic agonist isoproterenol.[2526] The lymphocytes and granulocytes of patients with CF and of heterozygous carriers show decreased cAMP production in response to stimulation with beta-adrenergic agonists, despite the fact that there is a normal number of beta-receptors on the cells.[2528] The decreased beta-adrenergic responsiveness is also seen in the sweat glands[2529] and submandibular glands.[2530] Normal beta-adrenergic responsiveness, measured by amylase and mucin secretion, can be restored to the excised submandibular gland tissue by the addition of a cyclic nucleotide phosphodiesterase inhibitor, suggesting that an abnormality beyond the beta-receptor, perhaps at the level of cAMP metabolism, may be at fault.[2531] Although the interpretation of studies of NSBH are difficult in patients with CF because of the airway obstruction that is usually present preceding challenge, it is possible that this autonomic abnormality contributes to the pathogenesis of the pulmonary disease.[2527]

Disturbances of Electrolyte Secretion

The abnormal secretion of electrolytes varies from one exocrine gland to another. The concentration of sodium and chloride is slightly diminished in tracheobronchial and cervical mucus. Pancreatic secretions are severely deficient in electrolytes, particularly bicarbonate. Saliva from parotid, submaxillary, and sublingual glands contains normal amounts of sodium and chloride, but the minor salivary gland secretion, like that from sweat glands, shows an excess of these electrolytes.[2480, 2504, 2532]

Submaxillary saliva has a high concentration of calcium.[2533]

The sweat of patients with CF contains elevated concentrations of sodium and chloride and, to a lesser extent, of potassium. The primary secretions in sweat glands are normally isotonic, but become hypotonic in the duct system as a result of the reabsorption of sodium in excess of water.[2480] When saliva and sweat from CF patients are perfused through the parotid duct of a rat or the duct of a normal sweat gland, reabsorption of sodium by the duct is blocked so that sodium and chloride content increases.[2534, 2535] The determination of sodium and chloride concentrations in sweat is a basic requirement for the diagnosis of cystic fibrosis (see farther on).

In 1981, Knowles and associates[2536] reported that patients with CF have a marked increase in the electrical potential difference across their nasal and tracheobronchial epithelium in vivo in comparison to normal subjects or their heterozygous relatives. This finding was not present in patients with bronchiectasis unassociated with CF. Because the drug amiloride decreased the transepithelial electrical difference in these subjects and selectively inhibited sodium transport across airway epithelium, these investigators suggested that the defect was related to excessive transmucosal transport of sodium and further speculated that this could result in dehydration of airway secretions. These results have been confirmed by others, and the abnormality has been shown to be a widespread defect of epithelial ion transport.[2537] The possibility that this abnormality of ion transport represents *the* genetic defect in CF is strengthened by studies showing that the abnormally high membrane potential is present in the cultured respiratory epithelial cells of patients with CF.[2538]

Boucher and coworkers[2539] carried out an elegant investigation in which the epithelia from nasal polyps of patients with and without CF and control subjects were studied in Ussing chambers; they found that the basal sodium absorption was increased in the tissue from the CF patients and that the addition of beta-adrenergic agonists paradoxically increased sodium absorption further without increasing chloride permeability as it does in tissue from normal or atopic subjects. The defect was not attributable to abnormal beta-receptor function because forskolin, a substance that stimulates adenyl cyclase directly, had a similar effect. The discovery of these abnormalities of ion transport in CF is exciting, not only because they suggest a possible link between a basic cellular defect and the hyperviscous exocrine secretions that are pivotal in the pathogenesis of CF but also because the defect can be modified with specific pharmacologic agents. Anderson has suggested that the altered electrolyte handling could be secondary to an underlying abnormality in prostaglandin metabolism.[2540]

The serum of patients with CF and of some heterozygous carriers contains a specific protein called "cystic fibrosis protein," which can be detected by isoelectric focusing or radioimmunoassay.[2565, 2566] This protein may be the same molecule that causes dyskinesia of rabbit cilia, and although it is not detectable with significant reliability to be used as a diagnostic test, its very presence is of considerable genetic interest. The gene for this protein has been mapped to chromosome 1, whereas the gene that is thought to be responsible for CF is in chromosome 7.[2567] The CF protein shows significant molecular homology with various calcium-binding proteins, suggesting that it may be important in the abnormal electrolyte transport that is emerging as the basic cellular defect in CF.[2567]

Host Defense and Infection

Patients with CF have an increased susceptibility to infection and possibly to asthma. The predisposition to infection is caused by bronchiectasis and that to asthma by increased permeability of the epithelial barrier. Progressive pulmonary involvement is almost invariably associated with repeated or persistent infections with *S. aureus* or *Pseudomonas aeruginosa* or both. An increase in the incidence of *Pseudomonas cepacia* colonization has been reported in CF patients; the presence of this organism is associated with more rapid deterioration.[2541, 2542] A correlation exists between the severity of the pulmonary disease and the frequency with which these bacteria are isolated.[2543]

Humoral immunologic host defense mechanisms are not impaired, and in fact immunoglobulin levels are often increased, presumably in response to chronic infection. One study[2544] has revealed hypogammaglobulin G in a number of patients under the age of 10 years with relatively mild CF, leading to the conclusion that progression of lung dysfunction may be the result of a hyperimmune response, at least in part. The administration of bacterial or viral antigen results in the development of specific humoral antibodies.[2483–2485; 2545] Although abnormalities of macrophage[2546] and lymphocyte[2547] function have been reported in CF, it is unlikely that they represent the cause of the increased susceptibility to pulmonary infection.

Local defenses against a variety of bacteria are defective because of reduced mucociliary transport. In addition, there are specific abnormalities that predispose patients with CF to infection by certain bacterial species. Serum from CF patients who are colonized by *P. aeruginosa* specifically inhibits the phagocytosis of this organism by alveolar macrophages.[2548] A similar phenomenon occurs in non-CF patients who are chronically colonized with *P. aeruginosa*.[2549] The ability of the serum from chronically colonized patients to inhibit opsonization and phagocytosis of these organisms is caused by a shift in the IgG subclasses of antibody to the lipopolysaccharide antigens of *P. aeruginosa*.[2549, 2550] Chronically colonized patients show an increase in the level of IgG$_2$ relative to the other IgG subclasses, and the "opsonic index" (the ratio of IgG$_3$ and IgG$_1$ to IgG$_2$ and IgG$_4$) is inverted, i.e., (IgG$_3$ + IgG$_1$) ÷ (IgG$_2$ + IgG$_4$) is less than 1 rather than greater than 1.[2549] May and Roberts[2551] have suggested that patients with CF are predisposed to staphylococcal infection as a result of the presence of p-hydroxyphenylacetic acid in the sputum. This substance is a metabolite of tyramine and has been shown to be excreted in abnormally high concentrations in the urine of patients with CF; it has an inhibitory effect on the phagocytosis of *S. aureus.*

Patients with CF have detectable levels of circulating immune complexes in their blood.[2552] Although the presence and level of complexes do not correlate specifically with any one clinical feature,[2552, 2553] high levels appear to be associated with a worse prognosis.[2553, 2554] In a 5-year prospective study of 139 CF patients, the presence of circulating immune complexes was associated with a 31 per cent death rate whereas in a group without detectable immune complexes, there were no deaths.[2554] It is unknown whether the elevated immune complexes are related to bacterial antibodies; however, in one study, increased serum antibodies to *P. aeruginosa* lipopolysaccharide and endotoxin A were correlated with both the level of circulating immune complexes and the degree of complement activation, and the combination was associated with a worse prognosis.[2555] Immune complex deposition may explain the episodic inflammatory arthritis that occasionally develops in patients with CF.[2556]

There is a higher incidence of atopy and asthma among patients with CF than among the general population.[2557–2559] Many patients show Type I and Type III hypersensitivity reactions to a variety of antigens, including food, bacteria, fungi, human body tissues, and other allergens.[2560] Tobin and associates[2558] measured serum IgE and IgG levels, peripheral eosinophil counts, nonspecific bronchial responsiveness, and skin test responses to a variety of allergens in 25 patients with CF and 25 age-matched controls. The patients manifested significantly higher serum IgG and IgE levels, higher eosinophil counts, and greater airway responsiveness than did the controls; 81 per cent of the CF patients showed positive skin test responses compared to 36 per cent of the normal subjects. Similarly, the patients had more atopic symptoms and 76 per cent of them had a positive family history of atopy versus 25 per cent of the controls. In another study of 100 patients with CF, 46 per cent were found to be atopic—22 per cent with asthma and 24 per cent with allergic rhinitis.[2559] Atopy and llergic symptoms are not associated with earlier age of onset, more severe symptoms, more rapid pulmonary function deterioration, or worse survival rates.[2561, 2562] The frequency with which IgE antibodies and serum precipitins to *Aspergillus* species and *Candida albicans* have been identified is higher in patients with CF than in those with bronchial asthma.[2545, 2563, 2801] Using the usual diagnostic criteria, 10 per cent of 100 CF patients were found to have allergic bronchopulmonary aspergillosis;[2559] the early skin test response was positive in 53 per cent of affected individuals and the late in 21 per cent. Serum precipitins against *A. fumigatus* were detected in 51 per cent of the 100 patients and serum IgE levels were significantly increased in 21 per cent.[2559] The increased incidence of atopy in patients with CF is not secondary to bronchiectasis itself. In a study of 23 patients in whom bronchiectasis was unrelated to CF, Murphy and associates[2564] were unable to detect an increased incidence of skin test responsiveness, eosinophilia, or elevated blood levels of IgE.

PATHOLOGIC CHARACTERISTICS

Pathologic studies of neonates or infants who have died of CF have shown essentially normal lungs. For example, in two studies of infants with CF who died of meconium ileus at birth or before 3 weeks of age, there was little or no pulmonary structural abnormality or mucous gland hypertrophy.[2568, 2569] In another investigation of infants under 4 months of age, both with and without a history of meconium ileus or pulmonary infection, no differences from control measurements were found in tracheal gland and submucosal area or in tracheal airway diameter;[2570] only tracheal gland acinar diameter was significantly increased in the CF patients compared with controls. An autopsy of an adult CF patient who had not manifested pulmonary signs clinically showed hypertrophy and hyperplasia of mucous glands and smooth muscle as well as thickening of the epithelial basement membrane;[2571] these changes are identical to those described in bronchial asthma and could have been related to the concomitant presence of this disease.

In contrast to these rather minor abnormalities, however, older patients who die of the disease invariably show pulmonary changes pathologically,[2572, 2573] including airway mucous plugging, acute and organizing pneumonitis (often with abscess formation), bronchiolar obstruction and dilatation,[2574, 2575] bronchiectasis, and focal areas of atelectasis and overinflation distal to obstructed segmental bronchi (Fig. 11–105).[2483–2485, 2576] All these changes are variable in severity and patchy in distribution; however, there is a tendency to more marked involvement of the upper lobes.[753, 2577] Focal emphysema can be present[2573] but is rarely appreciable except in patients who reach adulthood;[2574, 2578] occasionally, bullae and blebs are present.[2573] Cyst-like spaces related to bronchiectatic airways and considered pathogenetically to be analogous to pneumatoceles were found in nine of 21 patients in one series.[2573] In children and young teenagers, the small airways tend to be dilated

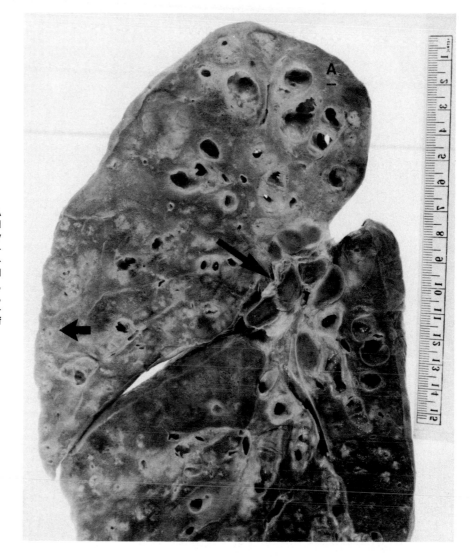

Figure 11–105. Cystic Fibrosis. A slice of the left lung from a 23-year-old man with cystic fibrosis shows variably severe bronchiectasis, worse in the apicoposterior segment (A). Extensive organizing pneumonia in the same region and multiple foci of acute bronchopneumonia, most marked in the lingula *(short arrow)*, are present. Note the hyperplastic peribronchial lymph nodes at the junction of upper and lower lobes *(long arrow)*.

although in older teenagers and adults, there is predominant small airway narrowing.[2578] The bronchial mucosa may undergo squamous metaplasia;[2576, 2579] in one family, cytologic changes interpreted as carcinoma *in situ* were identified in two affected members.[2579]

Most patients who die from cystic fibrosis manifest right ventricular hypertrophy at autopsy, identified by Ryland and Reid[2580] in 30 of 36 patients. The remaining six patients showed some degree of hypertrophy of pulmonary artery muscle unassociated with right ventricular hypertrophy. These authors found that right ventricular hypertrophy was rarely recognized clinically, presumably because the pulmonary manifestations overshadowed the cardiac ones. Smaller arteries that normally develop in postnatal life were reduced in number in all cases. These changes were most apparent in those lung zones that were most severely damaged and presumably hypoxic.[2580]

In addition to the staphylococcal and *Pseudomonas* infections that persist despite prolonged an-

tibiotic therapy,[2581–2584] botryomycosis can occasionally develop in patients with CF.[2585]

ROENTGENOGRAPHIC MANIFESTATIONS

Plain roentgenography reveals a pattern typical of extensive obstruction of medium-sized and small airways of the lungs; hyperinflation is almost invariable.[2576] The earliest change perhaps is accentuation of the linear markings, usually generalized throughout the lungs and caused by thickening of bronchial walls (Fig. 11–106). An early clue to the diagnosis may be a distinctly outlined orifice of the right upper lobe bronchus on the lateral chest roentgenogram, a feature that was identified in 90 per cent of CF patients in one study compared to 25 per cent of asthmatics and 18 per cent of normal subjects.[2587] Atelectasis may be subsegmental, segmental, or lobar (the last having been reported in 10 per cent of cases), most frequently in the right upper lobe.[2586] Curiously, lobar collapse seldom oc-

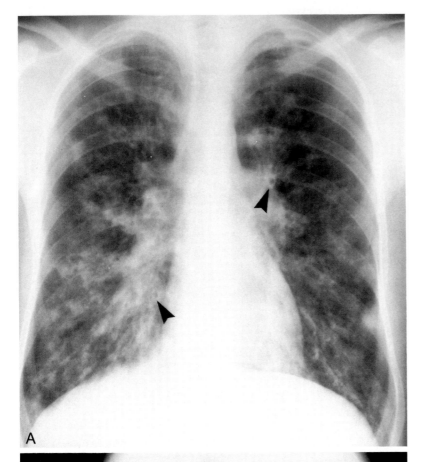

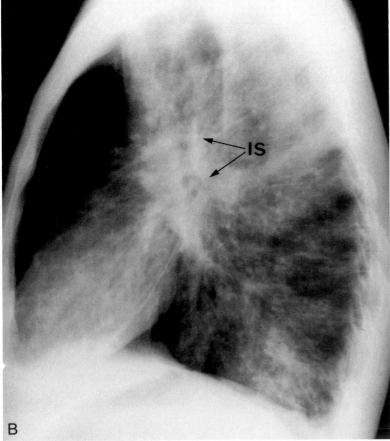

Figure 11–106. Cystic Fibrosis. Posteroanterior *(A)* and lateral *(B)* chest roentgenograms demonstrate diffuse bronchial wall thickening *(arrowheads)*, peribronchial thickening, diffuse small patchy opacities, and areas of inhomogeneous airspace consolidation. Note the remarkable thickening of the posterior wall of the bronchus intermedius (IS). The lungs are moderately overinflated. Both hila are enlarged, almost certainly as a result of lymph node enlargement rather than pulmonary arterial hypertension. The patient is a 24-year-old man.

curs in the left lung.[2592] Recurrent local pneumonitis occurs in most cases. Cylindrical and even cystic bronchiectasis and multiple small bronchiolar abscesses may be present.[2488, 2588, 2586, 2589] In a roentgenographic study of 42 adults with CF (age range, 30 to 45 years), Griscom and his colleagues found both sagittal and coronal diameters of the trachea to be significantly increased;[2590] some of the tracheas were grossly irregular in outline. Waring and his colleagues[2591] described a pattern of nodular, fingerlike shadows along the distribution of the bronchovascular bundles, strongly suggestive of the picture of mucoid impaction (Fig. 11–107). Focal areas of parenchymal overinflation are probably largely compensatory in nature, but true bullous emphysema has been reported, particularly in adults.[2593] Involvement of the lung parenchyma contiguous to the heart may create the nonspecific "shaggy heart" sign.

In their analysis of the roentgenographic features of 55 patients with CF who had passed their 17th birthday, Schwartz and Holsclaw[2594] arbitrarily graded the degree of pulmonary involvement on the basis of severity and distribution. Only seven patients were minimally affected, 30 had moderately severe changes, and 18 had advanced lesions of one or more types (including a mixed interstitial pattern, a honeycomb pattern, transient nodular opacities probably related to mucoid impaction, and hyperinflation). In this series, pulmonary complications included cor pulmonale (in 26 patients), pneumonitis (16), right-sided heart failure (six), hemorrhage (seven), pneumothorax (four), pleural effusion (two), and atelectasis (one). In a study in which MRI and conventional roentgenograms were compared for the detection of thoracic abnormalities, the former proved superior in revealing hilar and mediastinal node enlargement and in distinguishing nodes from prominent hilar vessels.[2596] CT has also been shown to reveal pathologic changes not visible on conventional chest roentgenograms, particularly mucoid impaction.[2597]

Mearns and Simon[2595] have described patterns of lung and heart growth in 76 children with CF as determined from serial roentgenograms. They found that at 6 years of age the majority of patients had a lung width larger and a heart diameter smaller than was expected. During a follow-up period averaging 7 years, a decrease in lung width occurred without a proportionate increase in lung length. In this study there were no signs, including flattening of the diaphragm, to suggest pulmonary overinflation. Cystic fibrosis has been shown to be associated with an increased incidence of pneumatosis intestinalis.[2598]

CLINICAL AND BIOCHEMICAL FINDINGS

The lack of pancreatic enzymes results in poor digestion, particularly of fat, in the small bowel, so

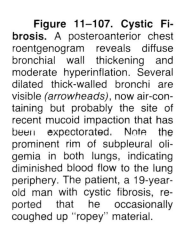

Figure 11–107. Cystic Fibrosis. A posteroanterior chest roentgenogram reveals diffuse bronchial wall thickening and moderate hyperinflation. Several dilated thick-walled bronchi are visible *(arrowheads)*, now air-containing but probably the site of recent mucoid impaction that has been expectorated. Note the prominent rim of subpleural oligemia in both lungs, indicating diminished blood flow to the lung periphery. The patient, a 19-year-old man with cystic fibrosis, reported that he occasionally coughed up "ropey" material.

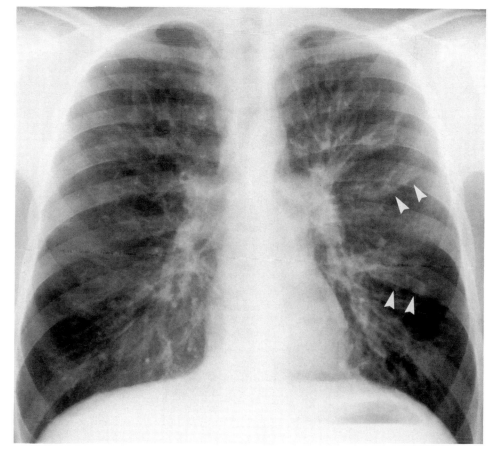

that patients characteristically have bulky, fatty stools. Approximately 10 to 20 per cent of neonates with cystic fibrosis develop intestinal obstruction as a result of meconium ileus; surgical therapy is usually required. Abnormal intestinal mucoproteins and an excess of tenacious intestinal mucus are presumably responsible for the obstruction. "Meconium ileus equivalent" is a term used to describe intestinal obstruction in patients with CF when it occurs after the neonatal period.[2599] These meconium masses tend to develop in the terminal ileum and may be discovered on routine physical examination; usually, they are mobile and nontender. The clinical presentation is of colicky abdominal pain, vomiting, and constipation. Roentgenograms of the abdomen typically show small bowel obstruction. Although the occurrence of meconium ileus in neonates is associated with a worse long-term prognosis than when it presents at a later age, successful treatment is commonly followed by prolonged survival.[2600] Intestinal obstruction in adults usually responds to intravenous fluid administration and acetylcysteine by nasogastric tube and enema.[2599] Occasionally, however, surgery is required to relieve the obstruction.[2599, 2601] In some cases of CF gastrointestinal symptoms are minimal or absent.

Involvement of the lungs usually is manifested clinically by recurrent chest infections associated with wheezing, dyspnea, productive cough, and hemoptysis. Such involvement may present clinically as simple bronchiectasis.[2602] The organisms most often responsible for pulmonary infection are *P. aeruginosa* of the mucoid and nonmucoid types, *S. aureus*, and *H. influenzae*; sputum culture shows good correlation with cultures obtained by protected endobronchial swabs.[2603] The isolation of nonfermenting gram-negative bacilli (other than *P. aeruginosa*) from the tracheobronchial tree has increased in recent years;[2542] the presence of *P. cepacia* in particular is associated with the terminal stages of the disease. The subject of pulmonary infection and antibiotic treatment in patients with CF has recently been reviewed.[878]

Occasionally, hemoptysis may be massive. In one report of 19 patients in whom blood loss was estimated at 500 ml or more, 13 were dead within 6 months of the initial episode. Many of the initial episodes were fatal; in one instance, emergency surgery was attempted but the patient died 10 days later. Hemoptysis usually occurs as a result of bronchiectasis but sometimes may be associated with bronchial artery and pulmonary artery anastomoses.[2604, 2605] Although bronchoscopy is the definitive method of identifying the bleeding site in such cases, in circumstances in which bronchoscopy cannot be performed because of continuous hemorrhage or because the severity of the lung disease precludes the use of general anesthesia, bronchial arteriography may effectively demonstrate the bleeding site and can provide a route for therapeutic embolization.

Physical findings in adult patients with CF are typical of bronchiectasis and obstructive airway disease. Coarse crackles may be localized but are often diffuse; generalized wheezing may suggest asthma. These patients are more subject to asthma than the average individual, so that it is important to measure flow rates before and after use of a bronchodilator in order to recognize a reversible component to the obstruction. Finger clubbing is a frequent sign in patients with advanced disease, and hypertrophic pulmonary osteoarthropathy has been reported.[2606] In one study of 300 patients with CF, 15 per cent complained of long bone or joint pain typical of hypertrophic pulmonary osteoarthropathy; approximately 81 per cent manifested roentgenographic evidence of periostitis.[2607] The latter group had more severe pulmonary disease. Patients with clubbing and changes in their bones have increased blood levels of prostaglandins PGE and PGF$_{2\alpha}$.[2608]

Complications include spontaneous pneumothorax, respiratory insufficiency, cor pulmonale, infertility in the male, maldigestion and malabsorption, pancreatic atrophy, cirrhosis, and rectal prolapse. Pneumothorax is common and frequently recurrent;[2609, 2610] it was observed in seven of 49 patients in one series.[2611] Open thoracotomy with pleurectomy or pleural abrasion may be required when such episodes are recurrent. Limited studies suggest that functional disturbances resulting from this operation are insignificant.[2611, 2612] In one study, quinacrine-induced pleuritis and surgery were associated with recurrence rates of 13 and 0 per cent, respectively, but intrapleural tetracycline was followed by a recurrence of pneumothorax in 86 per cent of cases.[2610]

Respiratory insufficiency and cor pulmonale develop frequently in the later stages of the disease. Ventilation-perfusion inequality is worsened by acute infectious episodes and may lead to cardiac decompensation. Hypoxemia may be corrected by breathing a high concentration of oxygen (which frequently results in a fall in pulmonary arterial pressure towards normal levels[2483–2485, 2613]) or by treatment of the infection.[2614] Eventually, however, some degree of persistent pulmonary arterial hypertension develops.

Reproductive failure in males was first described by Kaplan and his associates in 1968.[2615] A review of 25 patients over 17 years of age revealed aspermia that was shown in surgical and autopsy specimens to result from absence of the vas deferens. In a 1972 survey of 105 CF centers,[2616] normal fertility was found in only 2 to 3 per cent of affected males. Among 15 males with CF who had been married for a total of 46 years, only one offspring had been reported, whereas 18 married women with the disease had had nine children. Despite these figures, women with CF are relatively infertile, the probable cause being abnormally viscous cervical mucus. The cervical mucus of women with CF does not hydrate normally at midcycle and contains only 80 per cent water, whereas 93 to 96 per cent hydration appears to be necessary for normal sperm migration.[2617] Intrauterine insemination results in normal pregnancy. Pregnancy does not appear to have adverse effects in women with mild to moderately severe disease.[2617-2619]

Maldigestion and occasionally malabsorption may be present, particularly in children. Malnutrition and protein depletion are also consequences of recurrent pulmonary infection, which can accelerate the course of pulmonary disease.[2620, 2621] In such individuals, nocturnal intragastric feeding or oral supplementation may decrease weight loss and the incidence of pulmonary infection. Hepatic involvement includes a fatty liver and focal biliary cirrhosis. Concretions of eosinophilic mucinous material in the intrahepatic ducts are a more common complication with advancing age and can occasionally result in hepatic failure.[2480] Pancreatic involvement is reflected in recurrent attacks of acute pancreatitis and rarely is the initial presenting symptom in young adults with CF;[2622] in a small percentage of patients, the pancreatitis is associated with the subsequent development of diabetes mellitus. The incidence of symptomatic glucose intolerance is estimated to be at least 1 per cent, two or three times higher than in the general population under 25 years of age.[2480] In older patients, the incidence of diabetes may increase to 8 per cent.[2623] A curious unexplained abnormality found in a significant percentage of cases is rectal prolapse, observed in 87 (22.6 per cent) in one series of 386 patients.[2624] In fact, the prolapse was the presenting complaint in 16 of these patients and in three cases occurred 7 to 10 years before the presence of CF was recognized. Additional gastrointestinal complications include inguinal hernia and intestinal intussusception.[2625]

Corresponding with the increased longevity of patients with CF, systemic amyloidosis is becoming recognized with increasing frequency;[2626-2628] in one retrospective study, it was identified in 11 (33 per cent) of 33 patients.[2626] The spleen, liver, and kidneys are most commonly affected, the lung only rarely. In most cases, symptoms related to amyloid deposition are absent.

Sweat Testing

Although the diagnosis of cystic fibrosis may be suggested by family history, persistent respiratory disease, or clinical evidence of pancreatic insufficiency, confirmation requires a positive sweat test. Determination of electrolyte concentration in sweat is subject to considerable error, and a sufficient load of requests and an experienced technician are essential for reliable analysis. As an example of potential error, in one large CF referral center, about one-half of the patients referred with "positive sweat tests" were found on repeat analysis to have values within normal limits.[2480] Both the method of sample collection and analysis of electrolyte concentrations

are important. The screening test described by Shwachman and Gahm[2629] using a finger imprint on specially prepared agar has been abandoned. Direct-reading skin electrodes are useful only for screening. The most generally accepted method is pilocarpine iontophoresis sweat collection, with chemical analysis of ionic composition.[2630] Employing this method, a Mayo Clinic group[2631] showed a clear differentiation of normal subjects from patients with the disease, although a few (generally adults in the 40- to 70-year-old range) fell into a gray area. With this method, the amount of sweat collected should never weigh less than 50 mg and ideally should be over 100 mg. False-positive results may occur in patients with adrenal insufficiency, glucose 6-phosphate deficiency, glycogen storage disease, diabetes, hypothyroidism, nephrogenic diabetes insipidus, and ectodermal dysplasia.[2480, 2486, 2631]

Sweat electrolyte testing is not reliable in newborn infants. In children a chloride concentration of 60 mEq/liter or higher indicates the presence of CF; a value of 50 mEq/liter requires repeating. Since normal adults may have values above 60 mEq/liter, a diagnosis of CF should not be made at this level in the absence of an appropriate clinical history and unless repeated values of sodium and chloride are at or above this level.[2481, 2495] With a cut-off of 40 mmol/liter, the measurement of sweat chloride levels results in a 100 per cent sensitivity and 93 per cent specificity for the diagnosis of CF.[2632] However, the absolute level of sweat chloride does not provide a prognostic index of disease severity.[2633]

A number of recently developed techniques (including one in which sweat osmolarity can be measured on as little as 10 μL of sweat) appear promising alternatives to the gold standard.[2632, 2634] For example, nail clippings of CF patients have an increased chloride content that can be detected by x-ray microanalysis;[2635] like many other newly designed tests for CF, however, its sensitivity has not been evaluated.

The controversy over the incidence of respiratory infections and increased sweat electrolytes in heterozygous parents and siblings of CF patients seems to have been largely resolved. While there may be a slight increase in the incidence of respiratory infections in siblings,[2636] there is no convincing evidence of an increase in chronic respiratory disease in heterozygous parents.[2636-2639] Studies in which sweat electrolyte levels were determined in heterozygotes and normal subjects have revealed no significant differences.[2637, 2638] The contention that peptic ulceration is more common in the parents and siblings of cystic fibrosis patients also was not confirmed in at least two studies.[2636, 2639]

Original reports that patients with COPD possess higher than normal sweat electrolyte levels[2640-2643] have not been substantiated.[2636, 2644, 2645] Values for sodium and chloride concentrations in sweat increase with advancing age,[2631] a finding which, in addition to variations in techniques of collection and methods of qualitative testing, probably explains this misconception.

Pancreatic Function

Pancreatic insufficiency can be diagnosed by measuring the trypsin and chymotrypsin content of stool, or by the determination of bicarbonate and enzyme content of duodenal secretions obtained by intubation following stimulation with secretin and pancreozymin.[2480] The identification of increased levels of albumin in meconium[2646] and of bile acids in stool[2647] are two other tests that have proved useful, at least for some investigators. The measurement of serum immunoreactive pancreatic lipase and trypsinogen has been evaluated as a simple test of pancreatic function.[2648-2650] In one study, serum trypsinogen levels were measured in 381 patients with CF and 99 control subjects; 314 of the patients had steatorrhea documented by fecal fat balance studies, pancreatic stimulation tests, or both. In patients under the age of 2 years with steatorrhea, serum trypsinogen levels were significantly elevated, but in those over 6 years of age, malabsorption was associated with significantly lower blood levels.[2648] This age-related decline in blood enzyme levels has been confirmed by others.[2649, 2650] It is concluded that decreased blood levels are a good indicator of pancreatic insufficiency in patients over 6 years of age. Ultrasonic examination of the pancreas is effective in the detection of structural abnormalities, but these do not correlate well with the functional status.[2651, 2652] Although malabsorption of crystalline vitamin B_{12} is a feature of cystic fibrosis, it is not associated with a clinical picture of vitamin B_{12} deficiency.[2653] However, nutritional hypoalbuminemia, anemia, and edema may be the presenting symptom complex in some infants with cystic fibrosis, sometimes resulting in a misdiagnosis of milk sensitivity. This deficiency is readily corrected by the addition of a pancreatic enzyme supplement to the diet.[2654]

Pulmonary Function

Most investigators[2655-2657] have found that the various tests that measure small airway function are the most sensitive means of detecting pulmonary involvement in patients with CF. Early impairment of intrapulmonary mixing has also been reported.[2658-2660] As the disease progresses, VC diminishes and RV increases, the latter sometimes to four or five times predicted normal, with a resultant increase in total thoracic gas volume.[2657, 2661, 2662] FEV_1 values fall and CO diffusing capacity also may decrease.[2655] Patients with a low diffusing capacity tend to show arterial desaturation when they exercise.[2663] A nebulized bronchodilator produces less response in patients with CF than in those with asthma.[2664] In some patients, bronchodilators may have a detrimental effect, perhaps by increasing large airway collapsibility;[2665] as in patients with COPD, an anticholinergic bronchodilator may be more effective than a beta-adrenergic agent.[2666] In advanced cases, there may be some loss of elastic recoil, but this is usually minimal and consistent with the degree of emphysema observed at necropsy. Thus, the major factor reducing expiratory flow appears to be airway obstruction.[2667] Patients with advanced disease may also manifest abnormal collapse of large airways on expiration.[2668]

Hypoxemia is present in some cases and hypercapnia in a minority. The impairment in gas exchange has been shown to be caused equally by shunt and $\dot{V}/\dot{Q}$ inequality.[2669] Elaborate studies of respiratory center control and of the mechanics of ventilation have been reported in children.[2670] The ratio of physiologic dead space to tidal volume increases, as does the alveolar-arterial oxygen difference.[2655] In one study in which the multiple inert gas technique was used to assess the gas exchange abnormalities in six adult patients,[2671] the arterial hypoxemia was explained by shunt and areas of low ventilation-perfusion ratios. Episodes of arterial desaturation occur during sleep in patients with CF,[2672, 2673] the largest decrease occurring during REM sleep; they are associated with periods of hypoventilation rather than apnea. Part of the decrease during sleep is related to postural hypoxemia caused by a decrease in FRC in the supine position.[2672, 2674] In one group of 33 patients, the change from a sitting to a supine position caused a mean decrease in Po_2 of 6.5 ± 6.8 mm Hg accompanied by trivial changes in arterial Pco_2.[2674] Ventilatory response to inspired CO_2 is impaired in proportion to the degree of airway obstruction.[2675] The demonstration that inspiratory muscle weakness and fatigue can play a role in the respiratory failure of COPD has resulted in considerable study of inspiratory muscle strength in patients with CF.[2676-2678] Although some investigators report a decrease in respiratory muscle strength in malnourished patients,[2676] others[2677, 2678] have found normal strength despite hyperinflation and malnutrition, and have suggested that the chronic increase in the work of breathing in these patients may have a training effect.

In a follow-up study of 132 patients with CF in whom pulmonary function changes were documented over periods ranging from 4 to 7 years, Corey and associates[2679] found considerable variation in the rate of change in flow rates and FVC, the general pattern being consistent with the theory of exponential decline. During the follow-up period, the pulmonary function of 33 patients (25 per cent) remained stable or improved, possibly reflecting a mild form of pulmonary disease or efficacy of therapy. In this study, progress of the disease resulted in a rate of decline in pulmonary function values that was steeper in female than in male patients.

In an attempt to determine correlation of roentgenologic changes with pulmonary function, Reilly and his colleagues[2680] studied 69 patients with CF, employing VC, maximal mid-expiratory flow rate, diffusing capacity, and arterial blood gases as function test criteria. Dead space to tidal volume ratios were used as the index of ventilation-perfusion imbalance. Chest roentgenograms were assessed independently for air trapping, bronchial wall thickening, cyst formation, retained secretions, and extent of the disease. Overall, the correlation between abnormalities in pulmonary function and roentgenologically detectable pulmonary disease was excellent. In another correlative study designed to determine the usefulness of computer-assisted ventilation-perfusion scanning in the analysis of regional pulmonary function in patients with CF, Alderson and coworkers[2681] obtained ventilation-perfusion scintiphotographs of 25 children and adolescents aged 8 months to 17 years and compared them with chest roentgenograms. Ventilation-perfusion ratio gradients were reversed in patients with predominantly upper zone disease, and regional ventilation-perfusion ratios were uneven in distribution. The results correlated well with roentgenographic scores. The authors concluded that quantitative assessment of regional ventilation and perfusion is a useful technique for assessing severity of pulmonary disease in CF.

PROGNOSIS

As a result of improved medical care, chiefly through antibiotic therapy, life expectancy has increased dramatically over the last two decades.[2682, 2683] Whereas the survival rate for affected patients over the age of 17 years used to be approximately 5 per cent,[2684, 2685] it is now closer to 50 per cent.[2480, 2495] The prognosis for patients with CF varies in different countries; for example, in a comparative study, the death rates in England and Wales were found to be two times higher than those in Victoria, South Australia.[2686] In England and Wales, a child had an 80 per cent chance of surviving to age 9 while in Victoria there was an 80 per cent chance of surviving to age 20. The death rates in Australia were similar to those in North America, whereas those in New Zealand were closer to those in England and Wales.[2687] This regional difference has been attributed to the practice in Australia and North America of managing patients with CF in centralized specialist centers.[2686] Prognosis also relates to the age at diagnosis.[2688] The clinical course of 40 patients diagnosed as having CF by a neonatal screening test was compared with that of 56 patients born prior to the institution of the screening procedure: the average number of hospitalization days during the first two years of life was 3.9 in the former group and 27.2 days in the latter group. Although this difference is partly the result of the

earlier diagnosis of mild cases, it also relates to institution of appropriate preventative and therapeutic measures early in the course of the disease.

Doershuk and associates[2689] have used the chest roentgenogram to define patient groups and to predict survival. Based on a scale of 25 points (the highest rating being given for a perfectly normal chest roentgenogram), these authors divided their 535 patients with CF into two groups according to the roentgenographic scores designated during the first year of treatment. Patients in whom the degree of pulmonary involvement was sufficiently reversible to return to near normal, as evidenced by a score of 19 or more points, were placed in Group I. Those who showed no improvement or never achieved a score higher than 18 points were placed in Group II. Follow-up studies revealed decidedly different survival rates for the two groups: only 13 of 280 patients (5 per cent) in Group I died during an 18-year-period compared with 106 of 255 patients (41 per cent) in Group II. Undoubtedly, this improved prognosis can be explained at least partly by earlier recognition of the disease and by the detection of milder cases.

Infants with severe pancreatic insufficiency usually die of meconium ileus and children and young adults of progressive lung disease. In patients who live to the age of 18 years, subsequent survival is best predicted from clinical features.[2690] The clinical evaluation of 142 patients at age 18 was used to determine prognostic factors. The evaluation was based on the Shwachman-Kulczycki scoring system,[2691] a chest roentgenographic scoring system, pulmonary function tests, height-adjusted weight, sputum bacteriologic results, number of previous hospitalizations, age at onset of clubbing, and frequency of complications. A stepwise logistic regression analysis identified the Shwachman-Kulczycki score as the best predictor. A score of 30 to 49 predicted an average survival of 5 years beyond age 18, whereas a score of 65 to 75 predicted an additional 12 years of life. Low body weight and *P. cepacia* colonization of the tracheobronchial tree were also identified as negative prognostic indicators.[2690]

FAMILIAL DYSAUTONOMIA
(Riley-Day Syndrome)

Familial dysautonomia, which is probably the result of a biochemical, perhaps enzymatic, anomaly, is manifested by malfunction of the autonomic nervous system with consequent hypersecretion of mucous glands and obstruction of the bronchial tree. It was originally described by Riley and his colleagues in 1949[2692] and is commonly known as the Riley-Day syndrome. It is transmitted as an autosomal recessive trait and occurs almost exclusively in Jewish infants. Brunt and McKusick[2693] interviewed 172 families with a total of 210 affected children equally distributed as to sex; of 334 parents, only one (a mother) was not Jewish or did not have Jewish ancestry. Furthermore, all were of Ashkenazic stock, the great majority tracing their ancestry to an area of Eastern Europe comprising central and southern Poland, Galicia, western Ukraine, northeast Rumania, and, to a lesser extent, Lithuania.

Clinical manifestations suggest a widespread neural disturbance, better explained on a metabolic than on a primary structural basis.[2693] Much of the pathophysiology appears to result from an inability to release catecholamines. In one study,[2694] six of 26 affected patients had no detectable dopamine beta-hydroxylase (DBH) activity in their plasma, and their mothers had decreased DBH activity (DBH is the enzyme that converts dopamine to norepinephrine). However, in the same study, five of 97 normal children also showed a lack of DBH activity. More recent interest has centered around nerve growth factor (NGF), a protein that causes a striking increase in sensory and sympathetic ganglions when injected into chick embryos. When injected into a laboratory animal, antiserum to NGF causes pathologic and physiologic changes similar to those of dysautonomia. A bioassay method has been described that can measure the blood level of NGF.[2695, 2696] Using a radioimmune assay of three subunits of this substance called alpha, beta, and gamma, Siggers and associates[2695] found a threefold increase in serum antigen levels of the biologically active subunit beta NGF in patients with dysautonomia as compared with normal subjects. The groups showed similar findings with all other assays, including the bioassay method. The marked discrepancy in levels of beta NGF between antigenic and functional measurements suggested a qualitative abnormality of beta NGF in patients with dysautonomia.

The disease usually becomes manifest in infancy, and the prognosis is extremely poor. A small number of patients live into adulthood, although it appears that none has had children.[2693] Recurrent respiratory infections are common and are the most frequent direct cause of death. Some of these episodes may be caused by aspiration, since a large percentage of patients manifest swallowing difficulties.

Chest roentgenograms were stated to be abnormal in 19 of 34 patients in one series[2697] and in 13 of 20 in another.[2692] The roentgenographic picture is one of diffuse interstitial disease associated with patchy areas of pneumonia, atelectasis, and emphysema that may undergo remission and exacerbation. It is not surprising that the roentgenographic pattern resembles that of CF, since the basic cause of pulmonary abnormality in both diseases is similar. Atelectasis occurs predominantly in the right upper lobe and with less frequency in the right middle and left lower lobes.[2698] It has been emphasized that standard barium studies in the erect position may

not reveal the primary esophageal disturbance, a delay in coordinated relaxation of the upper esophageal sphincter. This abnormality accounts for tracheal aspiration and can be demonstrated satisfactorily only by cineroentgenography.[2693]

Clinically, the picture is characterized by episodes of acute respiratory difficulty with fever, cough, and shortness of breath associated with typical signs of bronchopneumonia, usually over both lungs. In their series of 210 patients, Brunt and McKusick[2693] described the following clinical features in addition to the pulmonary manifestations: absence of fungiform papillae on the tongue (100 per cent of patients), absence of overflow tears (100 per cent), vasomotor disturbances exemplified by blotching (98 per cent), abnormal sweating (97 per cent), episodic fever (92 per cent), incoordination and unsteadiness (90 per cent), swallowing difficulty, particularly in infants (85 per cent), physical retardation (78 per cent), episodic vomiting (67 per cent), breath-holding attacks (66 per cent), marked emotional instability (65 per cent), scoliosis (55 per cent), and bowel disturbances (49 per cent). Among the neurologic features, the most striking was a patchy insensitivity to pain, variable in individual patients. Intellect is unimpaired.[2693] Patients are relatively unresponsive to hypoxia and hypercarbia,[2699] presumably on the basis of a carotid body defect. One group of investigators[2700] described similar findings in an adult with amyloidosis of the carotid body under the title of "acquired dysautonomia."

Although the clinical and roentgenographic findings usually suggest the diagnosis, the lack of a flare reaction to scratch or intradermal histamine is considered by Riley and Moore[2701] to be a requirement for confirmation.

BRONCHOLITHIASIS

The term broncholithiasis is used to denote the presence of calcified or ossified material within the lumen of the tracheobronchial tree. According to Moersch and Schmidt,[2702] this material can originate in three ways: (1) by in situ calcification of aspirated foreign material that has impacted within the bronchial wall, (2) by erosion of calcified or ossified bronchial cartilage plates into the airway wall and eventual extrusion into the lumen, or (3) by similar erosion and extrusion of calcified necrotic material derived from bronchopulmonary lymph nodes. Rare cases have also been associated with calcified pleural plaques[366] and with nephrobronchial fistulas associated with nephrolithiasis.[2703] By far, the most common of all these mechanisms is that associated with long-standing necrotic foci of granulomatous lymphadenitis; any organism leading to such inflammation, e.g., M. tuberculosis, Histoplasma capsulatum, Coccidioides immitis, and a variety of others,[371] can theoretically result in broncholithiasis. In North

America, the most common agent is probably *H. capsulatum*, undoubtedly related to the high incidence of lymphadenitis in endemic areas.[372, 2704] Despite the fact that it is the most common pathogenetic mechanism, the incidence of broncholithiasis complicating granulomatous infection is undoubtedly quite low.[368]

Broncholiths are variable in size, ranging from less than 1 mm to the exceptional instance of one weighing 139 gm.[2570] They are usually quite irregular in shape and often possess multiple pointed spurs and sharp edges. Their formation has been hypothesized to be related to the repeated physical impingement of these irregular and hard foci on the bronchial wall during the respiratory cycle.[366]

The effects of broncholithiasis are variable and depend on the size and degree of calcification of the stone and its location. Broncholiths that contain relatively little calcium may disintegrate easily, and it is presumably this type that is associated with recurrent lithoptysis. By contrast, stones that are heavily calcified or ossified are less likely to break up, and can cause occlusion with distal obstructive effects, especially when situated in a smaller segmental airway (*see* Fig. 6–45, page 902).

Histologic examination of surgically excised broncholiths typically shows amorphous, necrotic material with extensive dystrophic calcification; bone is seen occasionally. Organisms can often be identified with appropriate special stains.[371, 2570] The adjacent bronchial wall is invariably inflamed and may be ulcerated. It has been suggested that focal pigmented scars in the bronchial mucosa that are occasionally found incidentally at autopsy may represent the site of a prior broncholith that had perforated the airway.[2704]

Roentgenographic findings may be entirely absent or may consist only of foci of hilar or parenchymal calcification suggestive of remote granulomatous disease. Segmental or subsegmental atelectasis may be found in relation to obstruction; focal calcification near the apparent origin of the atelectasis as viewed on conventional or computed tomograms is virtually pathognomonic of the condition. Bronchography may show the intraluminal nature of the broncholith but is seldom indicated.

The most prominent symptom is cough, which is usually nonproductive but frequently associated with hemoptysis. Less commonly, the presence of bronchial obstruction and secondary infection causes pain, chills, and fever. Although these lesions are most often solitary, a history of prior expectoration of calcified material (broncholithoptysis) is not infrequently obtained, as in 44 of 99 patients in one series.[2702] In most instances, this probably represents gradual disintegration and expectoration of a single mass of calcified material. Rarely, gradual dissolution and expectoration of a broncholith results in disappearance of symptoms caused by bronchial compression by an enlarged lymph node; this was illustrated in one patient with left vocal cord paralysis that disappeared following expectoration of calcified material.[2705]

BRONCHIOLITIS

A variety of pulmonary diseases are characterized predominantly by inflammation of membranous and respiratory bronchioles. Pathologically, this can occur as a simple bronchiolitis characterized by either an acute inflammatory exudate within the bronchiolar wall and lumen or a chronic mononuclear cell infiltrate. Either of these reactions can be associated with airway narrowing sufficient to cause clinical and functional effects. In addition, some cases of bronchiolitis are complicated by the development of intraluminal fibrosis, which can be severe enough to cause complete obliteration of the bronchiolar lumen (bronchiolitis obliterans). In the early stages, such fibrosis is manifested by plugs of loose connective tissue containing plump fibroblasts and scattered macrophages and lymphocytes; it is usually associated with epithelial destruction, although the fibrous tissue is occasionally present between the muscularis mucosa and an intact epithelium (so-called "constrictive" bronchiolitis) (*see* Fig. 7–18, page 1302). In the later stages, the airway lumen may be replaced by mature fibrous tissue.

Roentgenographic features of bronchiolitis are variable. In a study of 52 patients with bronchiolitis of varied etiology, Gosink and her associates[2706] distinguished three main patterns of disease roentgenographically: (1) nodular opacities (18 cases), (2) alveolar opacities (39 cases), and (3) hyperinflation (two cases); in several of the cases, a combination of these patterns was shown. The nodular opacities could be subdivided into (a) micronodular (nodules smaller than 5 mm in diameter), (b) discrete nodular (nodules greater than 5 mm), (c) confluent nodular (in which parenchymal consolidation was associated with a nodular pattern in less involved peripheral regions), and (d) lineonodular (a reticular pattern in addition to micronodular opacities). It is probable that the patient population described by Gosink and her colleagues contained a substantial number of patients who would now be classified as having bronchiolitis obliterans with organizing pneumonia (BOOP). The latter is characterized by patchy areas of consolidation that are usually bilateral; many cases also feature small rounded opacities, and in some cases this is the only roentgenographic abnormality.[2707, 2708]

A spectrum of clinical entities is encompassed by the term bronchiolitis.[2709, 2710] Specific details of many of the conditions are provided in appropriate sections of the book.

Fume- and Toxic Gas–Related Bronchiolitis

Acute exposure to smoke[2711] or to a high concentration of NO_2, SO_2, and a variety of other gases and fumes can cause bronchiolitis that is associated with severe airflow obstruction. Respiratory symptoms of cough and dyspnea appear minutes or hours following exposure and may be accompanied by the development of pulmonary edema within 4 to 24 hours after exposure. The pathologic changes at this stage consist mainly of necrosis of bronchiolar epithelium and the development of an acute inflammatory exudate.[2712] If patients survive this acute stage, within 2 to 5 weeks there may occur a delayed second phase characterized by increased obstruction, fever, chills, cough, dyspnea, and cyanosis[2713–2715] during which the pathologic findings are predominantly those of bronchiolitis obliterans.

Acute Infectious Bronchiolitis

Acute viral infection of the small airways most commonly causes severe illness in children under three years of age. Although it is likely that the trachea and large bronchi are also involved in the acute inflammatory process, it is the involvement of the small bronchi and bronchioles that causes the morbidity. In infants, the commonest etiologic agents are the respiratory syncytial virus (RSV), the adenoviruses (types 3, 7, and 21), rhinovirus, parainfluenza virus (type 3 especially), and, less frequently, the mumps and influenza viruses[2716–2720] and *M. pneumoniae*. In the northern hemisphere, the peak incidence of hospital admissions for RSV epidemics occurs in the winter months. RSV infection can vary in severity from upper respiratory tract infection through croup, bronchitis, bronchiolitis, and pneumonia. Approximately 1 per cent of patients with proven RSV bronchiolitis die,[2716] but in some series in which the infection has been caused by a variety of organisms, the death rate has been much higher—5.5 per cent in one series of 1,230 cases.[2721] Most of the deaths occurred in infants younger than 6 months of age with associated congenital anomalies.

Pathologically, disease is characterized by an acute bronchiolitis that usually completely resolves, resulting in the restoration of normal architecture; sometimes (particularly following adenovirus infection), bronchiolectasis, bronchiolitis obliterans, and bronchiectasis remain as sequelae (Swyer-James syndrome).[2722–2724]

Roentgenologically, severe, general overinflation of the lungs is present in nearly all cases and may be the only apparent abnormality.[2725] Other changes include widespread nodular shadows of "miliary" appearance and accentuation of lung markings, particularly in the lower lung zones (Fig. 11–108).[2726–2728] Pathologic correlation shows these patterns to be related to peribronchiolitis and to small focal areas of atelectasis and pneumonitis.[2727, 2728] Of the 1,230 infants with acute bronchiolitis reported by Heycock and Noble,[2721] 15 per cent showed local areas of parenchymal collapse roentgenographically.

A similar type of roentgenographic abnormality may be seen in adults when acute bronchiolitis develops in patients with bronchial asthma. Felson and Felson[2728] described 16 patients with spasmodic asthma in whom the development of diffuse, small, poorly defined, patchy opacities throughout the lungs was attributed to acute bronchiolitis, focal atelectasis, and pneumonitis; in most cases the roentgenographic picture cleared within a few days.

The *clinical manifestations* typically begin with symptoms of an upper respiratory tract infection, which is followed 2 to 3 days later by the abrupt onset of dyspnea, tachypnea (respiratory rates between 50 and 80), fever, cyanosis, and often severe prostration. Physical signs include widespread low- and high-pitched rhonchi, fine and coarse crackles, and evidence of hyperinflation. In infants in previous good health, the usual course of the disease consists of 2 or 3 days of severe symptoms followed by progressive recovery. Two to 5 per cent of hospitalized infants develop severe gas exchange abnormalities and ventilatory respiratory failure.

The relationship between bronchiolitis and the subsequent development of asthma is unclear, some reports suggesting that as many as 50 per cent of children with bronchiolitis during infancy develop recurrent wheezing and asthma. It is possible that in susceptible individuals, either the bronchiolitis precipitates the onset of asthma or what is diagnosed as bronchiolitis is in fact the first attack of asthma.[2716] Whatever the relationship, there is evidence that disease in small airways during infancy can cause chronic problems that may last a lifetime. Seventy-five per cent of patients with viral bronchitis have abnormalities of lung function that persist for 10 years. Although the adenoviruses cause less than 5 per cent of cases of bronchiolitis in the United States, they can produce severe and often fatal disease; Polynesian and Canadian Indian and Metis children are particularly susceptible to infection with these organisms.[2716]

Adults are probably infected with respiratory tract viruses as often as infants, but in otherwise healthy individuals the consequences of infection are much less severe; however, extensive inflammation of the small bronchioles can be a potentially fatal complication.[2729] Adults may be spared the severe symptoms characteristic of the infection in infants because their small airways contribute less to total pulmonary resistance;[2730] in a morphologic-physiologic correlative study, Hogg and his colleagues showed that the conductance of the peripheral airways of children under 5 years of age is normally low, making them particularly susceptible to bronchiolar infection.[2730]

Bronchiolitis Associated with Connective Tissue Disease

Bronchiolitis, with or without bronchiolitis obliterans, is an occasional complication of a number of connective tissue diseases, particularly rheu-

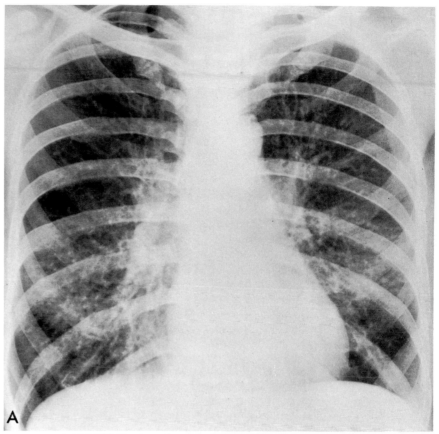

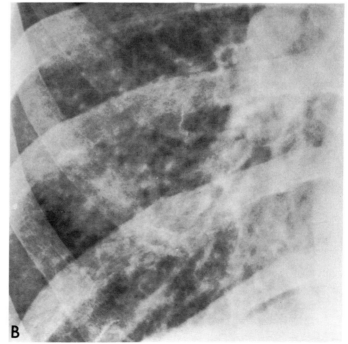

Figure 11–108. Acute Bronchiolitis in the Adult. A posteroanterior roentgenogram *(A)* shows an extensive coarse reticulonodular pattern throughout both lungs associated with moderate pulmonary overinflation. The pattern is well seen in a magnified view of the lower portion of the right lung *(B)*. This 70-year-old man was admitted to the hospital with an acute respiratory illness; pulmonary function studies revealed changes consistent with extensive obstruction of small airways. Proven *Mycoplasma* infection.

matoid disease.[2731–2737] Lung function tests show severe obstruction unassociated with evidence of loss of lung recoil or impaired diffusion.[2738, 2739] The association between rheumatoid disease and bronchiolitis is discussed in detail in Chapter 7 (*see* page 1219).

Bronchiolitis Obliterans Associated with Organ Transplantation

In 1982, severe progressive bronchiolitis obliterans was reported following bone marrow transplantation,[2740] and since that time a number of additional cases have been described in bone marrow recipients.[2741, 2742] More recently, a high incidence of bronchiolitis obliterans has been reported following heart-lung transplantation.[2803] The bronchiolitis can become manifest months following successful transplantation and is associated with progressive dyspnea that may be very severe; the development of respiratory failure may indicate the need for retransplantation. Bronchiolitis has not been reported following single lung transplantation. The pathogenesis of the bronchiolitis is unknown but is presumably related to a chronic immunologic manifestation of tissue incompatibility. This subject is discussed in greater detail on pages 1301 and 1303.

Idiopathic Bronchiolitis with and without Organizing Pneumonia

Although in many patients bronchiolitis occurs in association with a specific disease entity or possesses a specific etiology, there are also instances in which no underlying cause can be identified (Fig. 11–109). This idiopathic variety can occur with or without organizing pneumonia. In its presence, the abnormality has been termed bronchiolitis obliterans with organizing pneumonia, commonly known by the acronym BOOP.[2743] Epler and associates[2743] consider BOOP a clinically distinct entity with a characteristic roentgenographic and pathologic pattern. From a retrospective analysis of 2,500 open lung biopsy specimens obtained for the diagnosis of diffuse lung disease, they identified 67 adults in whom bronchiolitis obliterans was a prominent feature of the pathology. In 57 (85 per cent) of these patients, the bronchiolitis obliterans was associated with organizing pneumonia and in 50 of these there was no apparent cause or underlying disorder. Since the roentgenographic appearance suggests interstitial lung disease and pulmonary function studies reveal a restrictive rather than an obstructive derangement, BOOP is often confused with other forms of interstitial pneumonia rather than with the obstructive airway syndromes.

Pathologically, BOOP is characteristically distributed in a patchy fashion throughout the lung. Plugs of loose fibroblastic connective tissue can be identified principally within respiratory bronchioles and alveolar ducts (Fig. 11–110). The parenchyma adjacent to the affected bronchioles shows obliteration of alveolar airspaces, interstitial fibrosis, and chronic inflammation. Ultrastructural features have been described by Myers and Katzenstein[2802] and suggest that the condition results from acute epithelial injury localized to the bronchiolar and peribronchiolar epithelium.

BOOP usually presents as a subacute illness whose duration of symptoms prior to diagnosis ranges from 3 to 6 months.[2707, 2743] The most common symptoms are cough (90 per cent), dyspnea (80 per cent), fever (60 per cent), sputum expectoration, malaise, and weight loss (50 per cent). Crackles are audible on auscultation in 75 per cent of cases, but clubbing is not observed. The great majority of patients with BOOP show restrictive disease and gas exchange impairment.[2707, 2743] The presence of such marked bronchiolar pathology without airflow obstruction is confusing. It is probable that the lung units subtended by the diseased small airways are completely nonfunctional because of the airway obstruction and distal pneumonitis; these units contribute nothing to lung emptying, whereas functioning airways are those that are not obstructed.[2707] Systemic corticosteroid therapy has a salutory effect in patients with BOOP, and in many the clinical and roentgenologic signs of disease completely remit.[2707, 2743] By contrast, patients with bronchiolitis obliterans associated with the inhalation of toxic fumes, rheumatoid disease, or organ transplantation show little or no response to corticosteroid therapy.

The relationship of bronchiolitis obliterans and BOOP to the syndrome of small airway obstruction described by Macklem and his colleagues[2744] is unclear. These authors described seven patients with severe airflow obstruction, roentgenographic evidence of a widespread medium-to-coarse reticular pattern, and pathologic features of inflammatory narrowing, mucous plugging, and fibrous obliteration of membranous bronchioles; however, the polypoid intraluminal lesions described above were not observed.

Diffuse Panbronchiolitis

Diffuse panbronchiolitis is a disease of unknown etiology and pathogenesis characterized by chronic inflammation of respiratory bronchioles with secondary obstructive effects. It has been recognized almost exclusively in Japan; a survey in that nation between 1978 and 1980 collected more than 1,000 probable cases, of which 82 were confirmed pathologically.[2745] By contrast, the disease is almost unheard of in Europe and North America, although it has been hypothesized that some cases documented as small airway disease or bronchiolitis obliterans in reality represent this entity.[2745]

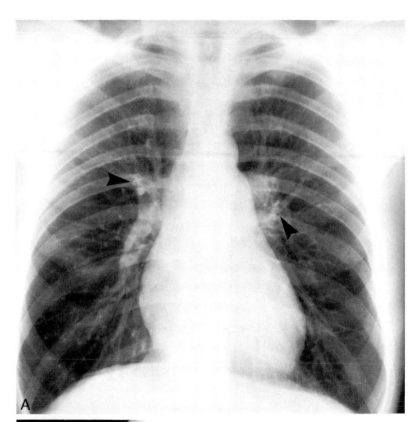

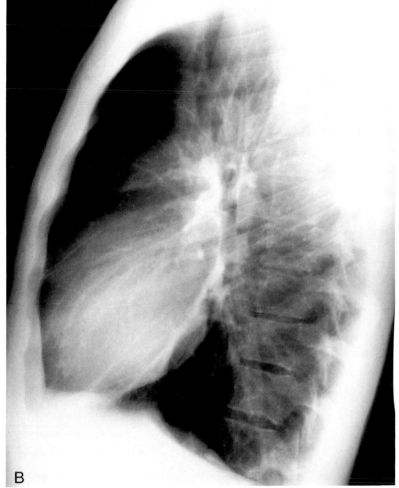

Figure 11–109. "Constrictive" Bronchiolitis Obliterans of Unknown Etiology. Posteroanterior *(A)* and lateral *(B)* chest roentgenograms reveal marked pulmonary overinflation. The vasculature in lower lung zones appears somewhat attenuated and in upper lung zones more prominent than normal, indicating recruitment. When these changes are considered in conjunction with prominence of the main pulmonary artery and probable right ventricular enlargement, the findings are consistent with pulmonary arterial hypertension. Bronchial walls are thickened *(arrowheads)*, and some bronchi seem narrow in comparison with the diameter of their companion arteries.

Illustration continued on following page

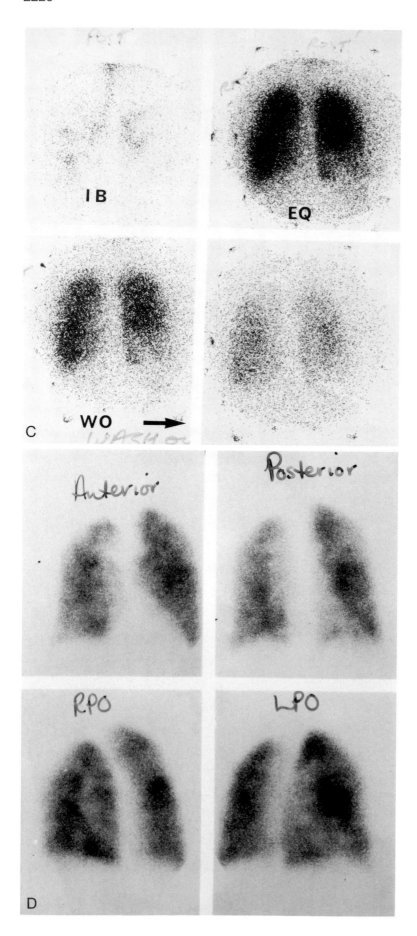

Figure 11–109. *Continued*. Ventilation *(C)* and perfusion *(D)* radionuclide scintigrams show multiple central and peripheral ill-defined perfusion deficits in both lungs; the latter are both matching and mismatching with the ventilation images. Air trapping is present on the washout images.

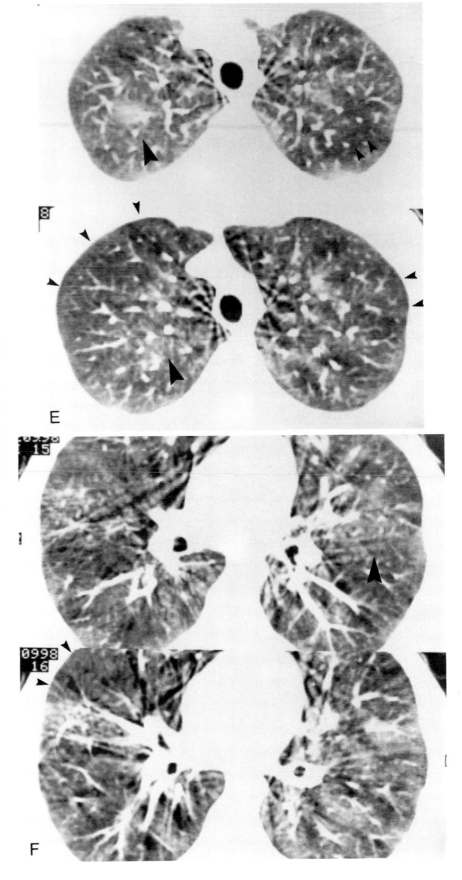

Figure 11–109. *Continued.* CT scans at two levels in the upper lobes *(E)* and lower lobes *(F)* reveal multiple, alternating, poorly defined areas of oligemia *(small arrowheads)* and pleonemia *(large arrowheads)*. At autopsy, the walls of small bronchi and bronchioles were markedly thickened and their lumens severely compromised as a result of hypertrophy of the muscularis mucosa and submucosal and peribronchial fibrosis. Severe intimal and medial hyperplasia was present in the arterioles, indicative of precapillary hypertension. The patient is a young man who presented with progressive dyspnea and right-sided heart failure.

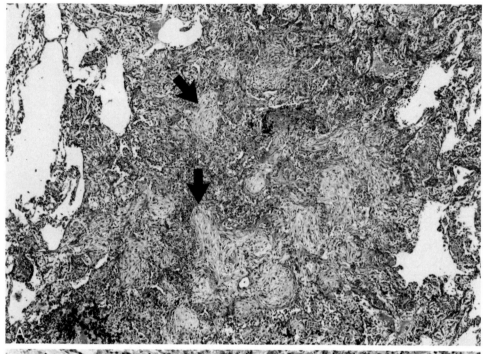

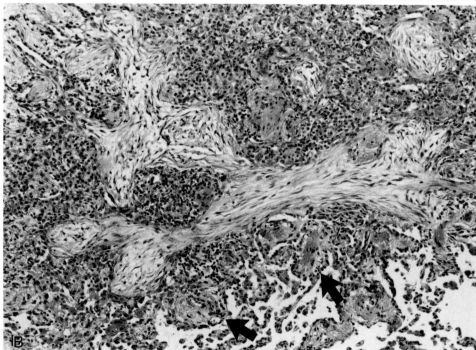

Figure 11–110. Bronchiolitis Obliterans with Organizing Pneumonia. A histologic section of lung parenchyma *(A)* shows a poorly defined focus of chronic inflammation associated with numerous small foci of loose connective tissue *(arrows)*. A magnified view of similar disease from another area *(B)* shows branching of the connective tissue plugs, implying that they are present in the lumens of alveolar ducts and respiratory bronchioles. The interstitial nature of the chronic inflammatory infiltrate is apparent at the junction with normal lung *(arrow)*. *(A,* × 40; *B,* × 100.)

Pathologically,[2745, 2746] diffuse panbronchiolitis is characterized by thickening of the walls of terminal and respiratory bronchioles by lymphocytes, plasma cells, and histiocytes; the infiltrate is often fairly well limited to this site, although it can extend into adjacent parenchyma. Intraluminal fibrosis may be present[2746] and, in combination with the mural infiltrate, results in significant airway narrowing. Apart from hyperinflation and the accumulation of lipid-laden macrophages, distal alveolar ducts and lung parenchyma are usually normal.

The changes are more or less diffuse throughout the lungs resulting in roentgenographic evidence of a disseminated nodular pattern with lower zonal predominance.[2745] Evidence of hyperinflation is also present. Akira and associates[2747] have described the findings in 20 patients as revealed by high-resolution CT. Four types of opacities were identified: (1) small nodules around the end of bronchovascular branchings, (2) small nodules in the centrilobular area connected with small branching linear opacities, (3) nodules accompanied by small ductal opacities connected to proximal bronchovascular bundles, and (4) large cystic opacities accompanied by dilated proximal bronchi. The authors concluded that these CT findings accurately reflected the clinical stages and pathologic manifestations of diffuse panbronchiolitis.

Most patients are between 30 and 60 years of age; the male to female ratio is approximately 2 to 1.[2745] The chief clinical manifestations are dyspnea on exertion and cough, often with sputum production. Sinusitis is common.[2745, 2746] Progression of disease appears to be common and is sometimes accompanied by respiratory failure. In the late stages, sputum culture often reveals the presence of microorganisms, especially *P. aeruginosa*, suggesting the development of airway colonization. Pulmonary function tests show marked obstructive and mild restrictive impairment. Arterial hypoxemia is common.[2746]

REFERENCES

1. Proctor DF: All that wheezes. Am Rev Respir Dis *127*:261, 1983.
2. Bass JW, Steele RW, Wiebe RA: Acute epiglottis. A surgical emergency. JAMA *229*:671, 1974.
3. Wanner A, Cutchavaree A: Early recognition of upper airway obstruction following smoke inhalation. Am Rev Respir Dis *108*:1421, 1973.
4. Capitanio MA, Kirkpatrick JA: Obstructions of the upper airway in children as reflected on the chest radiograph. Radiology *107*:159, 1973.
5. Evans AS: Clinical syndromes in adults caused by respiratory infections. Med Clin North Am *51*:803, 1967.
6. Editorial: Upper respiratory tract infections. Br Med J *3*:101, 1971.
7. Hobson D: Acute respiratory virus infections. Br Med J *2*:229, 1973.
8. Hable KA, O'Connell EJ, Herrmann EC Jr: Group B coxsackieviruses as respiratory viruses. Mayo Clin Proc *45*:170, 1970.
9. Hawley HB, Morin DP, Geraghty ME, et al: Coxsackievirus B epidemic at a boys' summer camp. Isolation of a virus from swimming water. JAMA *26*:33, 1973.
10. Han BK, Dunbar JS, Striker TW: Membranous laryngotracheo-bronchitis (membranous croup). Am J Roentgenol *133*:53, 1979.
11. Schabel SI, Katzberg RW, Burgener FA: Acute inflammation of epiglottis and supraglottic structures in adults. Radiology *122*:601, 1977.
12. Ossoff RH, Wolff AP: Acute epiglottitis in adults. JAMA *244*:2639, 1980.
13. Shackelford GD, Siegel MJ, McAlister WH: Subglottic edema in acute epiglottitis in children. Am J Roentgenol *131*:603, 1978.
14. Connor JD: Evidence for an etiologic role of adenoviral infection in pertussis syndrome. N Engl J Med *283*:390, 1970.
15. Connor JD: Communication in answer to a letter re: Pertussis syndrome. N Engl J Med *283*:1174, 1970.
16. Weissler MC, Fried MP, Kelly JH: Laryngopyocele as a cause of airway obstruction. Laryngoscope *95*:1348, 1985.
17. Sheffer AL: Urticaria and angioedema. Pediatr Clin North Am *22*:193, 1975.
18. Michel RG, Hudson WR, Pope TH: Angioneurotic edema. A review of modern concepts. Arch Otolargyngol *101*:544, 1975.
19. Frank MM, Gelfand JA, Atkinson JP: Hereditary angioedema: The clinical syndrome and its management. Ann Intern Med *84*:580, 1976.
20. Cahalane M, Demling RH: Early respiratory abnormalities from smoke inhalation. JAMA *251*:771, 1984.
21. Haponik EF, Munster AM, Wise RA, et al: Upper airway function in burn patients—correlation of flow-volume curves and nasopharyngoscopy. Am Rev Respir Dis *129*:251, 1984.
22. Colice GL, Munster AM, Haponik EF: Tracheal stenosis complicating cutaneous burns: an underestimated problem. Am Rev Respir Dis *134*:1315, 1986.
23. Waymack JP, Law E, Park R, et al: Acute upper airway obstruction in the postburn period. Arch Surg, *120*:1042, 1985.
24. Hayden CK Jr, Swischuk LE: Retropharyngeal edema, airway obstruction and caval thrombosis. Am J Roentgenol *138*:757, 1982.
25. Hawke M, Kwok P: Acute inflammatory edema of the uvula (uvulitis) as a cause of respiratory distress: a case report. J Otolaryngol *16*:188, 1987.
26. Eshagby B, Loeb HS, Miller SE, et al: Mediastinal and retropharyngeal hemorrhage. A complication of cardiac catheterization. JAMA *226*:427, 1973.
27. Morris P, Shaw EA: Acute upper respiratory tract obstruction complicating childhood leukemia. Br Med J *2*:703, 1974.
28. Genovesi MG, Simmons DH: Airway obstruction due to spontaneous retropharyngeal hemorrhage. Chest *68*:840, 1975.
29. Duong TC, Burtch GD, Shatney CH: Upper-airway obstruction as a complication of oral anticoagulation therapy. Crit Care Med *14*:830, 1986.
30. Waldron J, Youngs RP: Respiratory arrest produced by anticoagulant-induced haemorrhage into parapharyngeal space. J Laryngol Otol *100*:857, 1986.
31. Mackenzie JW, Jellicoe JA: Acute upper airway obstruction. Spontaneous retropharyngeal haematoma in a patient with polycythaemia rubra vera. Anaesthesia *41*:57, 1986.
32. Brooks JW: Foreign bodies in the air and food passages. Ann Surg *175*:720, 1972.
33. Mearns AJ, England RM: Dissolving foreign bodies in the trachea and bronchus. Thorax *30*:461, 1975.
34. Givan DC, Scott PH, Eigen H, et al: Achalasia and tracheal obstruction in a child. Eur J Respir Dis *66*:70, 1985.
35. Handler SD, Beaugard ME, Canalis RF, et al: Unsuspected esophageal foreign bodies in adults with upper airways obstruction. Chest *80*:234, 1981.
36. Twigg HL, Buckley CE: Complications of endotracheal intubation. Am J Roentgenol *109*:452, 1970.
37. Bergström J: Intubation and tracheotomy in barbiturate poisoning. Int Anesthesiol Clin *4*:323, 1966.
38. Conrardy PA, Goodman LR, Laing F, et al: Alteration of endotracheal tube position—flexion and extension of the neck. Crit Care Med *4*:7, 1976.
39. Goodman LR, Conrardy PA, Laing F, et al: Radiographic evaluation of endotracheal tube position. Am J Roentgenol *127*:433, 1976.
40. Todres ID, deBros F, Kramer SS, et al: Endotracheal tube displacement in the newborn infant. J Pediatr *89*:126, 1976.
41. Martin KW, McAlister WH: Intratracheal thymus: a rare cause of airway obstruction. AJR *149*:1217, 1987.
42. Thompson JW, Ahmed AR, Dudley JP: Epidermolysis bullosa dystrophica of the larynx and trachea. Acute airway obstruction. Ann Otol *89*:428, 1980.
43. Kryger M, Bode F, Antic R, et al: Diagnosis of obstruction of the upper and central airways. Am J Med *61*:85, 1976.
44. Empey DW: Assessment of upper airways obstruction. Br Med J *3*:503, 1972.
45. Miller RD, Hyatt RE: Obstructing lesions of the larynx and trachea: Clinical and physiologic characteristics. Mayo Clin Proc *44*:145, 1969.
46. Bass H: The flow volume loop: Normal standards and abnormalities in chronic obstructive pulmonary disease. Chest *63*:171, 1973.
47. Al-Bazzaz P, Grillo H, Kazemi H: Response to exercise in upper airway obstruction. Am Rev Respir Dis *111*:631, 1975.
48. Gibson GJ, Pride NB, Empey DW: The role of inspiratory dynamic compression in upper airway obstruction. Am Rev Respir Dis *108*:1352, 1973.
49. Shim C, Corro P, Park SS, et al: Pulmonary function studies in patients with upper airway obstruction. Am Rev Respir Dis *106*:233, 1972.
50. Spivey CG Jr, Walsh RE, Perez-Guerra F, et al: Central airway obstruction. Report of seven cases. JAMA *226*:1186, 1973.
51. Wittenborg MH, Gyepes MT, Crocker D: Tracheal dynamics in infants with respiratory disease, stridor, and collapsing trachea. Radiology *88*:653, 1967.
52. Moreno R, Taylor R, Müller N, et al: *In vivo* human tracheal pressure-area curves using computerized tomographic scans. Am Rev Respir Dis *134*:585, 1986.
53. Brown IG, Maclean PA, Webster PM, et al: Lung volume dependence of esophageal pressure in the neck. J Appl Physiol *59*:1849, 1985.
54. Gamsu G, Borson DB, Webb WR, et al: Structure and function and tracheal stenosis. Am Rev Respir Dis *121*:519, 1980.
55. Vincken W, Dollfuss RE, Cosio MG: Upper airway dysfunction detected by respiratory flow oscillations. Eur J Respir Dis *68*:50, 1986.
56. Vincken W, Cosio MG: Flow oscillations on the flow-volume loop: A nonspecific indicator of upper airway dysfunction. Bull Eur Physiopathol Respir *21*:559, 1985.
57. Strieder DJ, Goodman ML: Cough and wheezing with radiologic abnormality involving the trachea. N Engl J Med *293*:866, 1975.
58. Clark TJH: Inspiratory obstruction. Br Med J *3*:682, 1970.
59. Paré PD, Donevan RD, Nelems JM, et al: Clues to unrecognized upper airway obstruction: a case report. Can Med Assoc J *127*:39, 1982.
60. Miller RD, Hyatt RE: Evaluation of obstructing lesions of the trachea and larynx by flow-volume loops. Am Rev Respir Dis *108*:475, 1973.
61. Sackner MA: Physiologic features of upper airway obstruction. Chest *62*:414, 1972.
62. Lavelle TF Jr, Rotman HH, Weg JG, et al: Isoflow-volume curves in the diagnosis of upper airway obstruction. Am Rev Respir Dis *117*:845, 1978.
63. Houston HW, Payne WS, Harrison EG Jr, et al: Primary cancers of the trachea. Arch Surg *99*:132, 1969.
64. Gamsu G, Webb WR: Computed tomography of the trachea: normal and abnormal. Am J Roentgenol *139*:321, 1982.

65. Kittredge RD: Computed tomography of the trachea: A review. J Comput Tomogr 5:44, 1981.
66. Stitik FP, Bartelt D, James AE Jr, et al: Tantalum tracheography in upper airway obstruction: 100 experiences in adults. Am J Roentgenol 130:35, 1978.
67. Ell SR, Jolles H, Galvin JR: Cine CT demonstration of nonfixed upper airway obstruction. AJR 146:669, 1986.
68. Capitanio MA, Kirkpatrick JA: Obstructions of the upper airway in children as reflected on the chest radiograph. Radiology 107:159, 1973.
69. Ingram RH, Bishop JB: Ventilatory response to carbon dioxide after removal of chronic upper airway obstruction. Am Rev Respir Dis 102:645, 1970.
70. Massumi RA, Sarin RK, Pooya N, et al: Tonsillar hypertrophy, airway obstruction, alveolar hypoventilation, and cor pulmonale in twin brothers. Dis Chest 55:110, 1969.
71. Krumholz RA, Manfredi F, Weg JG, et al: Needle biopsy of the lung. Report on its use in 112 patients and review of the literature. Ann Intern Med 65:293, 1966.
72. Bland JW Jr, Edwards FK, Brinsfield D: Pulmonary hypertension and congestive heart failure in children with chronic upper airway obstruction. Am J Cardiol 23:830, 1969.
73. Djalilian M, Kern EB, Brown HA, et al: Hypoventilation secondary to chronic upper airway obstruction in childhood. Mayo Clin Proc 50:11, 1975.
74. Clairmont AA, Hart NJ, Rooker DT, et al: Upper airway obstruction and ventricular septal defect. JAMA 233:813, 1975.
75. Lyons HA: Another curse of Ondine. Chest 59:590, 1971.
76. Levy AM, Tabakin BS, Hanson JS, et al: Hypertrophied adenoids causing pulmonary hypertension and severe congestive heart failure. N Engl J Med 277:506, 1967.
77. Walsh RE, Michaelson ED, Harkleroad LE, et al: Upper airway obstruction in obese patients with sleep disturbance and somnolence. Ann Intern Med 76:185, 1972.
78. Dowell AR, Sieker HO, Schwartzman R: Atypical periodic respiration in an obese patient. Arch Intern Med 120:591, 1967.
79. Gastaut H, Tassinari CA, Duron B: Étude polygraphique des manifestations épisodiques (hypniques et respiratoires), diurnes et du syndrome de Pickwick. Rev Neurol (Paris) 112:568, 1965.
80. Kryger M, Quesney LF, Holder D, et al: The sleep deprivation syndrome of the obese patient. A problem of periodic nocturnal upper airway obstruction. Am J Med 56:531, 1974.
81. Brancatisano A, Engel LAV: Role of the upper airway in the control of respiratory flow and lung volume in humans. In Mathew OP, Sant 'Ambrogio G (eds): Respiratory Function of the Upper Airway. New York, Marcel Dekker, 1988.
82. Rotman HH, Lisa HP, Weg JG: Diagnosis of upper airway obstruction by pulmonary function testing. Chest 68:796, 1975.
83. Cormier Y, Kashima H, Summer W, et al: Upper airways obstruction with bilateral vocal cord paralysis. Chest 75:423, 1979.
84. Vincken W, Elleker G, Cosio MG: Detection of upper airway muscle involvement in neuromuscular disorders using the flow-volume loop. Chest 90:52, 1986.
85. Caffey J: Pediatric X-ray Diagnosis, 6th ed, Vol 1. Chicago, Year Book Medical Publishers, Inc, 1972, p 235.
86. Holinger LD, Tansek KM, Tucker GF: Cleft larynx with airway obstruction. Ann Otol Rhinol Laryngol 94:622, 1985.
87. Williams JL, Capitanio MA, Turtz MG: Vocal cord paralysis: Radiologic observations in 21 infants and young children. Am J Roentgenol 128:649, 1977.
88. Kanner RE: Bilateral vocal cord paralysis for 26 years with respiratory failure. Chest 84:304, 1983.
89. Bogaard JM, Pauw KH, Stam H, et al: Interpretation of changes in spirographic and flow-volume variables after operative treatment in bilateral vocal cord paralysis. Eur Soc Clin Respir Physiol 21:131, 1985.
90. Cormier Y, Kashima H, Summer W, et al: Airflow in unilateral vocal cord paralysis before and after Teflon injection. Thorax 33:57, 1978.
91. Rodenstein DO, Francis D, Stanescu DC: Emotional laryngeal wheezing—a new syndrome. Am Rev Respir Dis 127:354, 1983.
92. Macklem PT, Wang KP, Summer WR: Upper airway obstruction in asthma. Johns Hopkins Med 147:233, 1980.
93. Collett PW, Brancatisano T, Engel LA: Spasmodic croup in the adult. Am Rev Respir Dis 127:500, 1983.
94. Wood RP, Jafek BW, Cherniack RM: Laryngeal dysfunction and pulmonary disorder. Otolaryngol Head Neck Surg 94:374, 1986.
95. Lisboa C, Jardim J, Angus E, et al: Is extrathoracic airway obstruction important in asthma? Am Rev Respir Dis 122:115, 1980.
96. Higenbottam T: Narrowing of glottis opening in humans associated with experimentally induced bronchoconstriction. J Appl Physiol Respir Environ 49:403, 1980.
97. Collett PW, Brancatisano T, Engel LA: Changes in the glottic aperture during bronchial asthma. Am Rev Respir Dis 128:719, 1983.
98. Campbell AH, Imberger H, Jones M: Increased upper airway resistance in patients with airway narrowing. Br J Dis Chest 70:58, 1976.
99. Higenbottam T, Payne J: Glottis narrowing in lung disease. Am Rev Respir Dis 125:746, 1982.
100. Smaldone GC, Smith PL: Location of flow-limiting segments via airway catheters near residual volume in humans. J Appl Physiol 59:502, 1985.
101. Wilson TA, Hyatt RE, Rodarte JR, et al: The mechanisms that limit expiratory flow. Lung 158:193, 1980.
102. Osmanliev D, Bowley N, Hunter DM, et al: Relation between tracheal size and forced expiratory volume in one second in young men. Am Rev Respir Dis 126:179, 1982.
103. Montner P, Miller A, Calhoun F, et al: Tracheal diameter as a predictor of pulmonary function. Lung 162:115, 1984.
104. Gibellino F, Osmanliev DP, Watson A, et al: Increase in tracheal size with age—implications for maximal expiratory flow. Am Rev Respir Dis 132:784, 1985.
105. Griscom N, Wohl ME: Dimensions of the growing trachea related to body height, length, anteroposterior and transverse diameters, cross-sectional area, and volume in subjects younger than 20 years of age. Am Rev Respir Dis 131:840, 1985.
106. Breatnach E, Abbott GC, Fraser RG: Dimensions of the normal human trachea. AJR 141:903, 1984.
107. Dixon TC, Sando MJW, Bolton JM, et al: A report of 342 cases of prolonged endotracheal intubation. Med J Aust 2:529, 1968.
108. Pearson FG, Goldberg M, da Silva AJ: Tracheal stenosis complicating tracheostomy with cuffed tubes. Clinical experience and observations from a prospective study. Arch Surg 97:380, 1968.
109. Hemmingsson A, Lindgren PG: Roentgenologic examination of tracheal stenosis. Acta Radiol Diagn 19:753, 1978.
110. James AE Jr, MacMillian AS Jr, Eaton SB, et al: Roentgenology of tracheal stenosis resulting from cuffed tracheostomy tubes. Am J Roentgenol 109:455, 1970.
111. MacMillan AS, James AE Jr, Stitik FP, et al: Radiological evaluation of post-tracheostomy lesions. Thorax 26:696, 1971.
112. Klainer AS, Turndorf H, Wu W-H, et al: Surface alterations due to endotracheal intubation. Am J Med 58:674, 1975.
113. Goldberg M, Pearson FG: Pathogenesis of tracheal stenosis following tracheostomy with a cuffed tube—an experimental study in dogs. Thorax 27:678, 1972.
114. Leverment JN, Pearson FG, Fae S: Tracheal size following tracheostomy with cuffed tracheostomy tubes: An experimental study. Thorax 30:271, 1975.
115. Harley HRS: Laryngotracheal obstruction complicating tracheostomy or endotracheal intubation with assisted respiration: A critical review. Thorax 26:493, 1971.
116. Silva LU, Wood GJ: Tracheomalacia from excessive cuff pressure of an endotracheal tube. King Faisal Specialist Hosp Med 4:201, 1984.
117. Grillo HC: The management of tracheal stenosis following assisted respiration. J Thor Cardiovasc Surg 57:52, 1969.
118. Grillo HC: Surgical approaches to the trachea. Surg Gynecol Obstet 129:347, 1969.
119. Peison B, Williams MC: Primary carcinoma of trachea metastatic to heart. Chest 64:362, 1973.
120. Hadju SI, Huvos AG, Goodner JT, et al: Carcinoma of the trachea. Clinicopathologic study of 41 cases. Cancer 25:1448, 1970.
121. McCafferty GJ, Parker LS, Suggit SC: Primary malignant disease of the trachea. J Laryngol Otol 78:441, 1964.
122. Garces M, Tsai E, Marsan RE: Endotracheal metastasis. Chest 65:350, 1974.
123. Johnstone RE, Brooks SM: Upper airway obstruction after extubation. JAMA 218:92, 1971.
124. Hakimi M, Pai RP, Fine G, et al: Fibrous histiocytoma of the trachea. Chest 68:367, 1975.
125. Pollak ER, Naunheim KS, Little AG: Fibromyxoma of the trachea. A review of benign tracheal tumors. Arch Pathol Lab Med 109:926, 1985.
126. Slasky BS, Hardesty RL, Wilson S: Tracheal chondrosarcoma with an overview of other tumors of the trachea. J Comput Tomogr 9:225, 1985.
127. Baydur A, Gottlieb LS: Adenoid cystic carcinoma (cylindroma) of the trachea masquerading as asthma. JAMA 234:829, 1975.
128. Cleveland RH, Nice CM Jr, Ziskind J: Primary adenoid cystic carcinoma (cylindroma) of the trachea. Radiology 122:597, 1977.
129. Mackenzie CF, McAslan TC, Shin B, et al: The shape of the human adult trachea. Anesthesiology 49:48, 1978.
130. deKock MA: Functional anatomy of the trachea and main bronchi. In deKock MA, Nadel JA, Levis CM (eds): Mechanisms of Airways Obstruction in Human Respiratory Disease. Cape Town, South African Medical Research Council, 1979.
131. Greene R, Lechner GL: "Saber-sheath" trachea: A clinical and functional study of marked coronal narrowing of the intrathoracic trachea. Radiology 115:265, 1975.

11

132. Greene R: "Saber-sheath" trachea: Relation to chronic obstructive pulmonary disease. Am J Roentgenol *130*:441, 1978.
133. Pearson CM, Kline HM, Newcomber VD: Relapsing polychondritis. N Engl J Med *263*:51, 1960.
134. Hainer JW, Hamilton GW: Aortic abnormalities in relapsing polychondritis. Report of a case with dissecting aortic aneurysm. N Engl J Med *280*:1166, 1969.
135. Dolan DL, Lemmon GB Jr, Teitelbaum SL: Relapsing polychondritis. Analytical literature review and studies on pathogenesis. Am J Med *41*:285, 1966.
136. Choplin RH, Wehunt WD, Theros EG, et al: Diffuse lesions of the trachea. Semin Roentgenol *18*:38, 1983.
137. Mohsenifar Z, Tashkin DP, Carson SA, et al: Pulmonary function in patients with relapsing polychondritis. Chest *81*:711, 1982.
138. Gibson GJ, Davis P: Respiratory complications of relapsing polychondritis. Thorax *29*:726, 1973.
139. Islam N, Ahmed Z, Alam MN, et al: Cryptogenic cirrhosis in relapsing polychondritis. Postgrad Med *59*:260, 1983.
140. Job-Deslandre C, Delrieu F, Delbarre F, et al: Relapsing polychondritis and systemic lupus erythematosus (letter). J Rheumatol *10*:666, 1983.
141. Small P, Black M, Davidman M, et al: Wegener's granulomatosis and relapsing polychondritis: a case report. J Rheumatol 7:915, 1980.
142. Dahlqvist A, Lundberg E, Östberg Y, et al: Hydralazine-induced relapsing polychondritis-like syndrome. Report of a case with severe chronic laryngeal complications. Acta Otolaryngol *96*:355, 1983.
143. Mohsenifar Z, Tashkin DP, Carson SA, et al: Pulmonary function in patients with relapsing polychondritis. Chest *81*:711, 1982.
144. Neilly JB, Winter JH, Stevenson RD, et al: Progressive tracheobronchial polychondritis: need for early diagnosis. Thorax *40*:78, 1985.
145. Dupont A, Bossuyt A, Sommers G, et al: Relapsing polychondritis: Gallium-67 uptake in recurrent lung lesions. J Nucl Med Allied Sci *27*:57, 1983.
146. Higenbottam T, Dixon J: Chrondritis associated with fatal intramural bronchial fibrosis. Thorax *34*:563, 1979.
147. Johnston RF, Green RA: Tracheobronchiomegaly. Report of five cases and demonstration of familial occurrence. Am Rev Respir Dis *91*:35, 1965.
148. Ettman IK, Keel DT Jr: Tracheal diverticulosis. Radiology *78*:187, 1962.
149. Mounier-Kuhn P: Dilatation de la trachée: Constations radiographiques et bronchoscopiques. (Tracheal dilatation: Roentgenographic and bronchographic findings.) Lyon Med *150*:106, 1932.
150. Campbell AH, Young IF: Tracheobronchial collapse, a variant of obstructive respiratory disease. Br J Dis Chest *57*:174, 1963.
151. Bateson EM, Woo-Ming M: Tracheobronchomegaly. Clin Radiol *24*:354, 1973.
152. Hunter TB, Kuhns LR, Roloff MA, et al: Tracheobronchomegaly in an 18 month old child. Am J Roentgenol *123*:687, 1975.
153. Katz I, LeVine M, Herman P: Tracheobronchomegaly. The Mounier-Kuhn syndrome. Am J Roentgenol *88*:1084, 1962.
154. Al-Mallah Z, Quantock OP: Tracheobronchomegaly. Thorax *23*:230, 1968.
155. Aaby GV, Blake HA: Tracheobronchomegaly. Ann Thorac Surg 2:64, 1966.
156. Ayres J, Rees J, Cochrane GM, et al: Hemoptysis and non-organic upper airways obstruction in a patient with previously undiagnosed Ehlers-Danlos syndrome. Br J Dis Chest *75*:309, 1981.
157. Wonderer AA, Elliot FE, Goltz RW, et al: Tracheobronchomegaly and acquired cutis laxa in child: Physiologic and immunologic studies. Pediatrics *44*:709, 1969.
158. Rindsberg S, Friedman AC, Fiel SB, et al: MRI of tracheobronchomegaly. J Can Assoc Radiol *38*:126, 1987.
159. Van Nierop MA, Wagenaar SS, Van den Bosch JM, et al: Tracheobronchopathia osteochondroplastica. Report of four cases. Eur J Respir Dis *64*:129, 1983.
160. Whitehouse G: Tracheopathia osteoplastica: Case report. Br J Radiol *41*:701, 1968.
161. Baird RB, McCartney JW: Tracheopathia osteoplastica. Thorax *21*:321, 1966.
162. Dalgaard JB: Tracheopathia chondro-osteoplastica. A case elucidating the problems concerning development and ossification of elastic cartilage. Acta Pathol Microbiol Scand *24*:118, 1947.
163. Carr T, Olsen AM: Tracheopathia osteoplastica. JAMA *155*:1563, 1954.
164. Bowen DAL: Tracheopathia osteoplastica. J Clin Pathol *12*:435, 1959.
165. Sakula A: Tracheobronchopathia osteoplastica. Its relationship to primary tracheobronchial amyloidosis. Thorax *23*:105, 1968.
166. Shuttleworth JS, Self CL, Pershing HS: Tracheopathia osteoplastica. Ann Intern Med *52*:234, 1960.
167. Alroy GG, Lichtig C, Kaftori JK: Tracheobronchopathia osteoplastica: End stage of primary lung amyloidosis? Chest *61*:465, 1972.
168. Weiss L: Isolated multiple nodular pulmonary amyloidosis. Am J Clin Pathol *33*:318, 1960.
169. Pounder DJ, Pieterse AS: Tracheopathia osteoplastica: Report of four cases. Pathology *14*:429, 1982.
170. Pounder DJ, Pieterse AS: Tracheopathia osteoplastica. A study of the minimal lesion. J Pathology *138*:235, 1982.
171. Eimind K: Tracheopathia osteoplastica. Nord Med *72*:1029, 1964.
172. Pieri J, Casalonga J: Chondromatose diffuse de la trachée et des bronches. (Diffuse chondromatosis of the trachea and bronchi.) Presse Med *65*:1933, 1957.
173. Clee MD, Anderson JM, Johnston RN, et al: Clinical aspects of tracheobronchopathia osteochondroplastica. Br J Dis Chest *77*:308, 1983.
174. Onitsuka H, Hirose N, Watanabe K, et al: Computed tomography of tracheopathia osteoplastica. Am J Roentgenol *140*:268, 1983.
175. Lundgren R, Stjernberg NL: Tracheobronchopathia osteochondroplastica—a clinical bronchoscopic and spirometric study. Chest *80*:706, 1981.
176. Secrest PG, Kendig TA, Beland AJ: Tracheobronchopathia osteochondroplastica. Am J Med *36*:815, 1964.
177. Feist JH, Johnson TH, Wilson RJ: Acquired tracheomalacia, etiology and differential diagnosis. Chest *68*:340, 1975.
178. Cogbill TH, Moore FA, Accurso FJ, et al: Primary tracheomalacia. Am Thorac Surg *35*:538, 1983.
179. Williams H, Campbell P: Generalized bronchiectasis associated with deficiency of cartilage in the bronchial tree. Arch Dis Child *35*:182, 1960.
180. Baxter JD, Dunbar JS: Tracheomalacia. Ann Otol *72*:1012, 1963.
181. Horns JW, O'Loughlin BJ: Tracheal collapse in polychondritis. Am J Roentgenol *87*:844, 1962.
182. Nuutinen J: Acquired tracheobronchomalacia. Eur J Respir Dis *63*:380, 1982.
183. Maayan C, Mogle P, Tal A, et al: Prolonged wheezing and tracheal compression caused by an aberrant right subclavian artery. Thorax *36*:793, 1981.
184. MacGillivray RG: Tracheal compression caused by aneurysms of the aortic arch. Implications for the anaesthetist. Anaesthesia *40*:270, 1985.
185. Kandora TF, Gilmore IM, Sorber JA, et al: Cricoarytenoid arthritis presenting as cardiopulmonary arrest. Ann Emerg Med *14*:700, 1985.
186. Miller A, Brown LK, Teirstein AS, et al: Stenosis of main bronchi mimicking fixed upper airway obstruction in sarcoidosis. Chest *88*:244, 1985.
187. Breuer R, Simpson GT, Rubinow A, et al: Tracheobronchial amyloidosis: treatment by carbon dioxide laser photoresection. Thorax *40*:870, 1985.
188. Karbowitz SR, Edelman LB, Nath S, et al: Spectrum of advanced upper airway obstruction due to goiters. Chest *87*:18, 1985.
189. Morewood DJ, Belchetz PE, Evans CC, et al: The extrathoracic airway in acromegaly. Clin Radiol *37*:243, 1986.
190. Solomons NB, Linton DM, Potgieter PD: Cervical osteophytes and respiratory failure. An unusual case of upper airway obstruction. S Afr Med J *71*:259, 1987.
191. Sidi J, Hadar T, Shvero J, et al: Respiratory distress due to diffuse cervical hyperostosis. Ann Otol Rhinol Laryngol *96*:178, 1987.
192. Benisch BM, Wood WG, Kroeger GB, et al: Focal muscular hyperplasia of the trachea. Arch Otolaryngol *99*:226, 1974.
193. Krieger J: Breathing during sleep in normal subjects. In Kryger MH (ed): Clinics in Chest Medicine—Sleep Disorders, Vol 6, No. 4. Philadelphia, WB Saunders Co, 1985, p 577.
194. Bülow K, Inguar D: Respiration and state of wakefullness in normals, studied by spirography, capnography and EEG. Acta Physiol Scand *51*:230, 1961.
195. Robin ED, Whaley RD, Crump CC, et al: Alveolar gas tensions, pulmonary ventilation and blood pH during physiological sleep in normal subjects. J Clin Invest *37*:981, 1958.
196. Gothe B, Altose MD, Goldman MD, et al: Effect of quiet sleep on resting and CO_2 stimulated breathing in humans. J Appl Physiol *50*:724, 1981.
197. Lopes JM, Tabachnik E, Müller NL, et al: Total airway resistance and respiratory muscle activity during sleep. J Appl Physiol *54*:773, 1983.
198. Hudgel DW, Martin RJ, Johnson B, et al: Mechanics of the respiratory system and breathing pattern during sleep in normal humans. J Appl Physiol *56*:133, 1984.
199. Douglas NJ: Control of ventilation during sleep. In Kryger MH (ed): Clinics in Chest Medicine—Sleep Disorders, Vol 6, No 4. Philadelphia, WB Saunders Co, 1985, p 563.
200. Phillipson EA, Sullivan CE: Arousal: The forgotten response to respiratory stimuli. Am Rev Respir Dis *118*:896, 1978.
201. Berthon-Jones M, Sullivan CE: Ventilatory and arousal responses to hypoxia in sleeping humans. Am Rev Respir Dis *125*:632, 1982.

202. Berthon-Jones N, Sullivan CE: Ventilation and arousal responses to hypercapnia in normal sleeping adults. J Appl Physiol 57:59, 1984.

203. West P, Kryger MH: Sleep and respiration: Terminology and methodology. In Kryger MH (ed): Clinics in Chest Medicine—Sleep Disorders. Vol 6, No 4. Philadelphia, WB Saunders Co, 1985, p 691.

204. Fletcher EC: History, techniques and definitions in sleep-related respiratory disorders. In Fletcher EC (ed): Abnormalities of Respiration During Sleep. Orlando, Grune and Stratton, 1986, p 1.

205. Friede H, Lopata M, Fisher E, et al: Cardiorespiratory disease associated with Hallermann-Streiff syndrome: analysis of craniofacial morphology by cephalometric roentgenograms. J Craniofac Genet Dev Biol [Suppl] 1:189, 1985.

206. Coccagna G, Martinelli P, Zucconi M, et al: Sleep-related respiratory and haemodynamic changes in Shy-Drager syndrome: A case report. J Neurol 232:310, 1985.

207. Tan ET, Lambie DS, Johnson RH, et al: Sleep apnoea in alcoholic patients after withdrawal. Clin Sci 69:655, 1985.

208. Hoffstein V, Taylor R: Rapid development of obstructive sleep apnea following hemidiaphragmatic and unilateral vocal cord paralysis as a complication of mediastinal surgery. Chest 88:145, 1985.

209. King M, Gleeson M, Rees J: Obstructive sleep apnoea and tonsillar lymphoma. Br Med J 294:1605, 1987.

210. Alving J, Højer-Pedersen E, Schlichting J, et al: Obstructive sleep apnea syndrome caused by oral cyst: A case report. Acta Neurol Scand 71:408, 1985.

211. Stafford N, Youngs R, Waldron J, et al: Obstructive sleep apnoea in association with retrosternal goitre and acromegaly. J Laryngol Otol 100:861, 1986.

212. Commiskey J, Williams TC, Krumpe PE, et al: The detection and quantification of sleep apnea by tracheal sound recordings. Am Rev Respir Dis 126:221, 1982.

213. Steyer BJ, Quan SF, Morgan WJ: Polysomnography scoring for sleep apnea—use of a sampling method. Am Rev Respir Dis 131:592, 1985.

214. Riedy RM, Hulsey R, Bachus BF, et al: Sleep apnea syndrome—practical diagnostic method. Chest 75:81, 1979.

215. Gyulay S, Gould D, Sawyer B, et al: Evaluation of a microprocessor-based portable home monitoring system to measure breathing during sleep. Sleep 10:130, 1987.

216. Carskadon MA, Dement WC, Mitler MM, et al: Guidelines for the multiple sleep latency test (MSLT): A standard measure of sleepiness. Sleep 9:519, 1986.

217. Findlay LJ, Wilhoit SC, Suratt PM: Apnea duration and hypoxemia during REM sleep in patients with obstructive sleep apnea. Chest 87:432, 1985.

218. Parisi RA, Croce SA, Edelman NH, et al: Obstructive sleep apnea following bilateral carotid body resection. Chest 91:922, 1987.

219. Sullivan CE, Issa FG: Obstructive sleep apnea. In Kryger MH (ed): Clinics in Chest Medicine—Sleep Disorders. Vol 6, No 4. Philadelphia, WB Saunders Co, 1985, p 633.

220. Spier S, Rivlin J, Rowe RD, et al: Sleep in Pierre Robin syndrome. Chest 90:711, 1986.

221. Kuna ST, Remmers JE: Pathophysiology and mechanisms of sleep apnea. In Fletcher EC (ed): Abnormalities of Respiration during Sleep. Orlando, Grune and Stratton, 1986, p 63.

222. Zwillich CW, Picket C, Hanson FN, et al: Disturbed sleep and prolonged apnea during nasal obstruction in normal men. Am Rev Respir Dis 124:158, 1981.

223. Rajagopal KR, Bennett LL, Dillard TA, et al: Overnight nasal CPAP improves hypersomnolence in sleep apnea. Chest 90:172, 1986.

224. White DP, Cadieux RJ, Lombard RM: The effects of nasal anesthesia on breathing during sleep. Am Rev Respir Dis 132:972, 1985.

225. McNicholas WT, Coffey M, McDonnell T, et al: Upper airway obstruction during sleep in normal subjects after selective topical oropharyngeal anesthesia. Am Rev Respir Dis 135:1316, 1987.

226. Felman AH, Loughlin GM, Leftridge CA Jr, et al: Upper airway obstruction during sleep in children. Am J Roentgenol 133:213, 1979.

227. Lowe AA, Gionhaku N, Takeuchi K, et al: Three dimensional C.T. reconstructions of tongue and airway in adult subjects with obstructive sleep apnea. Am J Orthod Dentofacial Orthop 90:364, 1986.

228. Hannam A, Wood W, Fache S, et al: MR imaging and graphic reconstruction in the orofacial region. J Comput Assist Tomogr. In press.

229. Jamieson A, Guilleminault C, Partinen M, et al: Obstructive sleep apneic patients have craniomandibular abnormalities. Sleep 9:469, 1986.

230. Sturani C, Barrot-Cortez E, Papiris S, et al: Respiratory flutter during carbon dioxide rebreathing in patients with obstructive sleep apnea syndrome. Eur J Respir Dis 69:75, 1986.

231. Haponik EF, Bleecker ER, Allen RP, et al: Abnormal inspiratory flow-volume curves in patients with sleep-disordered breathing. Am Rev Respir Dis 124:571, 1981.

232. Shore ET, Millman RP: Abnormalities in the flow-volume loop in obstructive sleep apnea sitting and supine. Thorax 39:775, 1984.

233. Tammelin BR, Wilson AF, Borowiecki BD, et al: Flow-volume curves reflect pharyngeal airway abnormalities in sleep apnea syndrome. Am Rev Respir Dis 128:712, 1983.

234. Skatrud JB, Dempsey JA: Airway resistance and respiratory muscle function in snorers during NREM sleep. J Appl Physiol 59:328, 1985.

235. Issa FG, Sullivan CE: Arousal and breathing responses to airway occlusion in healthy sleeping adults. J Appl Physiol 55:1113, 1983.

236. Issa FG, Sullivan CE: Upper airway closing pressures in snorers. J Appl Physiol 57:528, 1984.

237. Issa FG, Sullivan CE: Upper airway closing pressures in obstructive sleep apnea. J Appl Physiol 57:520, 1984.

238. Brown I, Bradley TD, Phillipson E, et al: Pharyngeal compliance in snoring subjects with and without obstructive sleep apnea. Am Rev Respir Dis 132:211, 1985.

239. Bradley TD, Brown IG, Grossman RF, et al: Pharyngeal size in snorers, nonsnorers, and patients with obstructive sleep apnea. N Engl J Med 315:1327, 1986.

240. Gertz I: Blood volume and arterial blood gases in patients with chronic obstructive lung disease during and after acute respiratory failure. Scand J Respir Dis 60:6, 1979.

241. Reed WR, Roberts JL, Thach BT: Factors influencing regional patency and configuration of the human infant upper airway. J Appl Physiol 58:635, 1985.

242. Suratt PM, McTier RF, Wilhoit SC: Collapsibility of the nasopharyngeal airway in obstructive sleep apnea. Am Rev Respir Dis 132:967, 1985.

243. Hudgel DW: Variable site of airway narrowing among obstructive sleep apnea patients. J Appl Physiol 61:1403, 1986.

244. Strohl KP, Hensley MJ, Hallett M, et al: Activation of upper airway muscles before onset of inspiration in normal humans. J Appl Physiol 49:638, 1980.

245. Surratt PM, McTier R, Wilhoit SC: Alae nasi electromyographic activity and timing in obstructive sleep apnea. J Appl Physiol 58:1252, 1985.

246. Onal E, Lopata M, O'Connor T: Pathogenesis of apneas in hypersomnia-sleep apnea syndrome. Am Rev Respir Dis 125:167, 1982.

247. Warner G, Skatrud JB, Dempsey JA: Effect of hypoxia-induced periodic breathing on upper airway obstruction during sleep. J Appl Physiol 62:2201, 1987.

248. Inghar DH, Gee JBL: Pathophysiology and treatment of sleep apnea. Annu Rev Med 36:369, 1985.

249. Onal E, Burrows DL, Hart RH, et al: Induction of periodic breathing during sleep causes upper airway obstruction in humans. J Appl Physiol 61:1438, 1986.

250. Alex CG, Onal E, Lopata M: Upper airway occlusion during sleep in patients with Cheyne-Stokes respiration. Am Rev Respir Dis 133:42, 1986.

251. Parisi RA, Neubauer JA, Frank M, et al: Correlation between genioglossal and diaphragmatic responses to hypercapnia in sleeping goats. Am Rev Respir Dis 131:A295, 1985.

252. Weiner D, Mitra J, Salamone J, et al: Effect of chemical stimuli on nerves supplying upper airway muscles. J Appl Physiol 52:530, 1982.

253. Onal E, Lopata N, O'Connor T: Diaphragmatic and genioglossal electromyogram responses to isocapnic hypoxia in humans. Am Rev Respir Dis 124:215, 1981.

254. Dolly FR, Block AJ: Effect of flurazepam on sleep-disordered breathing and nocturnal oxygen desaturation in asymptomatic subjects. Am J Med 73:239, 1982.

255. Taasan VC, Block AJ, Boysen PG, et al: Alcohol increases sleep apnea and oxygen desaturation in asymptomatic men. Am J Med 71:240, 1981.

256. Bonora M, Shields GI, Knuth SL, et al: Selective depression by ethanol of upper airway respiratory motor activity in cats. Am Rev Respir Dis 130:156, 1984.

257. Remmers JE: Obstructive sleep apnea—a common disorder exacerbated by alcohol (editorial.) Am Rev Respir Dis 130:153, 1984.

258. Leiter J, Knuth S, Krol R, et al: The effect of diazepam on genioglossal muscle activity in normal human subjects. Am Rev Respir Dis 132:216, 1985.

259. Strohl KP, Saunders NA, Feldman NT, et al: Obstructive sleep apnea in family members. N Engl J Med 299:969, 1978.

260. Martin RJ, Sanders MH, Gray BA, et al: Acute and long-term ventilatory effects of hyperoxia in the adult sleep apnea syndrome. Am Rev Respir Dis 125:175, 1982.

261. Leiter JC, Knuth SL, Bartlett D: The effect of sleep deprivation on activity on the genioglossus muscle in man. Am Rev Respir Dis 132:1242, 1985.

11

262. Rajagopal KR, Abbrecht PH, Tellis CJ: Control of breathing in obstructive sleep apnea. Chest 85:174, 1984.

263. Hyland RH, Hutcheon MA, Perl A, et al: Upper airway occlusion induced by diaphragm pacing for primary alveolar hypoventilation—implications for the pathogenesis of obstructive sleep apnea. Am Rev Respir Dis 124:180, 1981.

264. Leiter JC, Knuth SL, Bartlett D Jr: The effect of sleep deprivation on activity of the genioglossus muscle. Am Rev Respir Dis 132:1242, 1985.

265. Onal E, Leech JA, Lopata M: Dynamics of respiratory drive and pressure during NREM sleep in patients with occlusive apneas. J Appl Physiol 58:1971, 1985.

266. Iber C, Davies SF, Chapman RC, et al: A possible mechanism for mixed apnea in obstructive sleep apnea. Chest 89:800, 1986.

267. Bonora M, Shields G, Knuth S, et al: Selective depression by ethanol of upper airway respiratory motor activity in cats. Am Rev Respir Dis 130:156, 1984.

268. Hwang J, St. John W, Bartlett D: Respiratory-related hypoglossal nerve activity influence of anesthetics. J Appl Physiol 55:785, 1983.

269. Robinson RW, Zwillich CW, Bixler EO, et al: Effects of oral narcotics on sleep-disordered breathing in healthy adults. Chest 91:197, 1987.

270. Vincken W, Guilleminault C, Silvestri L, et al: Inspiratory muscle activity as a trigger causing the airways to open in obstructive sleep apnea. Am Rev Respir Dis 135:372, 1987.

271. Guilleminault C, Dement WC: Sleep apnea syndromes and related sleep disorders. In Williams RL, Karacon I (eds): Sleep Disorders: Diagnosis and Treatment. New York, Wiley, 1978, p 11.

272. Guilleminault C, van den Hoed J, Mitler MM: Clinical overview of the sleep apnea syndromes. In Guilleminault C, Dement WC (eds): Sleep Apnea Syndromes. New York, Alan R. Liss, 1978, p 1.

273. Lavie P: Sleep apnea in industrial workers. In Guilleminault C, Lugaresi E (eds): Sleep/Wake Disorders: Natural History, Epidemiology, and Long-Term Evolution. New York, Raven Press, 1983, p 127.

274. Berry DTR, Webb WB, Block AJ: Sleep apnea syndrome: A critical review of the apnea index as a diagnostic criterion. Chest 86:529, 1984.

275. Ancoli-Israel S, Kripke DF, Mason W, et al: Sleep apnea and periodic movements in an aging sample. J Gerontol 40:419, 1985.

276. Berry DT, Webb WB, Block AJ, et al: Sleep-disordered breathing and its concomitants in a subclinical population. Sleep 9:478, 1986.

277. Wittels EH: Obesity and hormonal factors in sleep and sleep apnea. Med Clin North Am 69:1265, 1985.

278. Robinson RW, Zwillich CW: The effect of drugs on breathing during sleep. In Kryger M (ed): Clinics in Chest Medicine—Sleep Disorders. Vol 6, No 4. Philadelphia, WB Saunders Co, 1985, pp 6, 603.

279. Sandblom RE, Matsumoto AM, Schoene RB, et al: Obstructive sleep apnea syndrome induced by testosterone administration. N Engl J Med 108:508, 1983.

280. Matsumoto AM, Sandblom RE, Schoene RB, et al: Testosterone replacement in hypogonadal men: Effects on obstructive sleep apnoea, respiratory drives, and sleep. Clin Endocrinol (Oxf) 22:713, 1985.

281. Johnson MW, Anch AM, Remmers JE: Induction of the obstructive sleep apnea syndrome in a woman by exogenous androgen administration. Am Rev Respir Dis 129:1023, 1984.

282. Brown IG, Zamel N, Hoffstein V: Pharyngeal cross-sectional area in normal men and women. J Appl Physiol 61:890, 1986.

283. White DP, Lombard RM, Cadieux RJ, et al: Pharyngeal resistance in normal humans: influence of gender, age, and obesity. J Appl Physiol 58:365, 1985.

284. Gleeson K, Zwillich CW, Braier K, et al: Breathing route during sleep. Am Rev Respir Dis 134:115, 1988.

285. Burwell CS, Robin ED, Whaley RD, et al: Extreme obesity associated with alveolar hypoventilation—a Pickwickian syndrome. Am J Med 21:811, 1956.

286. Phillipson EA: Pickwickian, obesity-hypoventilation, or Fee-Fi-Fo-Fum syndrome? Am Rev Respir Dis 121:781, 1980.

287. Harman EM, Wynne JW, Block AJ: The effect of weight loss on sleep-disordered breathing and oxygen desaturation in morbidly obese men. Chest 82:291, 1982.

288. Smith PL, Gold AR, Meyers DA, et al: Weight loss in mildly to moderately obese patients with obstructive sleep apnea. Ann Intern Med 103:850, 1985.

289. Suratt PM, McTier RE, Findley LJ, et al: Changes in breathing and the pharynx after weight loss in obstructive sleep apnea. Chest 92:631, 1987.

290. Hoffstein V, Zamel N, Phillipson EA: Lung volume dependence of pharyngeal cross-sectional area in patients with obstructive sleep apnea. Am Rev Respir Dis 130:175, 1984.

291. Harman E, Wynne JW, Block AJ, et al: Sleep-disordered breathing and oxygen desaturation in obese patients. Chest 79:256, 1981.

292. Lugaresi E, Cirignotta F, Coccagna G, et al: Some epidemiological data on snoring and cardiocirculatory disturbances. Sleep 3:221, 1980.

293. Mondini S, Zucconi M, Cirignotta F, et al: Snoring as a risk factor for cardiac and circulatory problems: An epidemiological study. In Guilleminault C, Lugaresi E (eds): Sleep/Wake Disorders: Natural History, Epidemiology, and Long-Term Evolution. New York, Raven Press, 1983, p 99.

294. Partinen M, Palomäki H: Snoring and cerebral infarction. Lancet 2(8468):1325, 1985.

295. Orr WC, Martin RJ, Imes NK, et al: Hypersomnolent and nonhypersomnolent patients with upper airway obstruction during sleep. Chest 75:418, 1979.

296. Weitzman ED: Syndrome of hypersomnia and sleep-induced apnea. Chest 75:414, 1979.

297. Sink J, Bliwise DL, Dement WC: Self-reported excessive daytime somnolence and impaired respiration in sleep. Chest 90:177, 1986.

298. Gold AR, Schwartz AR, Bleecker ER, et al: The effect of chronic nocturnal oxygen administration upon sleep apnea. Am Rev Respir Dis 134:925, 1986.

299. Kales A, Caldwell AB, Cadieux RJ, et al: Severe obstructive sleep apnea—II: Associated psychopathology and psychosocial consequences. J Chronic Dis 38:427, 1985.

300. Podszus T, Bauer W, Mayer J, et al: Sleep apnea and pulmonary hypertension. Klin Wochenschr 64:131, 1986.

301. Hudgel DW: Clinical manifestations of the sleep apnea syndrome. In Fletcher EC (ed): Abnormalities of Respiration during Sleep. Orlando, Grune & Stratton, 1986.

302. Bradley T, Rutherford R, Grossman R, et al: Role of daytime hypoxemia in the pathogenesis of right heart failure in the obstructive sleep apnea syndrome. Am Rev Respir Dis 131:835, 1985.

303. Bradley TD, Rutherford R, Lue F, et al: Role of diffuse airway obstruction in the hypercapnia of obstructive sleep apnea. Am Rev Respir Dis 134:920, 1986.

304. Jones J, Wilhoit S, Findley L, et al: Oxyhemoglobin saturation during sleep in subjects with and without the obesity-hypoventilation syndrome. Chest 88:9, 1985.

305. Rapoport DM, Garay SM, Epstein H, et al: Hypercapnia in the obstructive sleep apnea syndrome. A reevaluation of the "Pickwickian syndrome." Chest 89:627, 1986.

306. Bradley TD, Martinez D, Rutherford R, et al: Physiological determinants of nocturnal arterial oxygenation in patients with obstructive sleep apnea. J Appl Physiol 59:1364, 1985.

307. Tilkian AG, Guilleminault C, Schroeder RS, et al: Hemodynamics in sleep-induced apnea. Studies during wakefulness and sleep. Ann Intern Med 85:714, 1976.

308. Fletcher EC, De Behnke RD, Lovoi MS, et al: Undiagnosed sleep apnea in patients with essential hypertension. Ann Intern Med 103:190, 1985.

309. Kales A, Bixler ED, Cadieux RJ, et al: Sleep apneas in a hypertensive population. Lancet 2:1005, 1984.

310. Flenley DC: Sleep in chronic obstructive lung disease. In Kryger MH (ed): Symposium on Sleep Disorders. Philadelphia, WB Saunders Co, 1985.

311. Shepard JW Jr: Gas exchange and hemodynamics during sleep. Med Clin North Am 69:1243, 1985.

312. Guilleminault C: Natural history, cardiac impact, and long-term follow-up of sleep apnea syndrome. In Guilleminault C, Lugaresi E (eds): Sleep/Wake Disorders: Natural History, Epidemiology, and Long-Term Evolution. New York, Raven Press, 1983, p 107.

313. Santamaria JC, Prior JC, Fleetham JA: Reversible reproductive dysfunction in men with obstructive sleep apnea. Clin Endocrinol 28:461, 1988.

314. Kavey NB, Blitzer A, Gidro-Frank S, et al: Sleeping position and sleep apnea syndrome. Am J Otolaryngol 6:373, 1985.

315. McEvoy RD, Sharp DJ, Thornton AT: The effects of posture on obstructive sleep apnea. Am Rev Respir Dis 133:662, 1986.

316. Sullivan CE, Issa FG, Berthor-Jones M, et al: Reversal of obstructive sleep apnea by continuous positive airway pressure applied through the nose. Lancet 1:862, 1981.

317. Issa FG, Sullivan CE: Reversal of central sleep apnea using nasal CPAP. Chest 90:165, 1986.

318. Hegstrom T, Emmons LL, Hoddes E, et al: Obstructive sleep apnea syndrome: preoperative radiologic evaluation. AJR 150:67, 1988.

319. Riley R, Guilleminault C, Powell N, et al: Palatropharyngoplasty failure, cephalometric roentgenograms, and obstructive sleep apnea. Otolaryngol Head Neck Surg 93:240, 1985.

320. Katsantonis GP, Walsh JK: Somnofluoroscopy: Its role in the selection of candidates for uvulopalatopharyngoplasty. Otolaryngol Head Neck Surg 94:56, 1986.

321. Walsh JK, Katsantonis GP, Schweitzer PK, et al: Somnofluoroscopy: Cineradiographic observation of obstructive sleep apnea. Sleep 8:294, 1985.

322. Sher AE, Thorpy MJ, Shprintzen RJ, et al: Predictive value of

Muller maneuver in selection of patients for uvulopalatopharyngoplasty. Laryngoscope *95*:1483, 1985.

323. Cartwright RD: Predicting response to the tongue retaining device for sleep apnea syndrome. Arch Otolaryngol *111*:385, 1985.

324. Scadding JG: Definition and the clinical categories of asthma. *In* Clark TJH, Godfrey S (eds): Asthma, 2nd ed. London, Chapman and Hall, 1983, pp 1–11.

325. American Thoracic Society. Chronic bronchitis, asthma, and pulmonary emphysema. Am Rev Respir Dis *85*:762, 1962.

326. Mok JYQ, Simpson H: Pulmonary function in severe chronic asthma in children during apparent clinical remission. Eur J Respir Dis *64*:487, 1983.

327. Bates DV: Impairment of respiratory function in bronchial asthma. Clin Sci *11*:203, 1952.

328. Report of the Committee on Emphysema, American College of Chest Physicians: Criteria for the assessment of reversibility in airway obstruction. Chest *65*:552, 1974.

329. Frick OL, German DF, Mills J: Development of allergy in children I. Association with virus infections. J Allergy Clin Immunol *63*:228, 1979.

330. Marsh G, Meyers A, Bias B: The edipmiology and genetics of atopic allergy. N Eng J Med *305*:1551, 1981.

331. Blumenthal MN, Mendell N, Yunis E: Immunogenetics of atopic diseases. J Allergy Clin Immunol *65*:403, 1980.

332. Beer J, Osband E, McCaffrey P, et al: Abnormal histamine-induced suppressor-cell function in atopic subjects. N Eng J Med *306*:454, 1982.

333. Smith JM: Prevalence and natural history of asthma in schoolchildren. Br Med J *1*:711, 1961.

334. Beall GN, Heiner DC, Tashkin DP, et al: Asthma: New ideas about an old disease. Ann Intern Med *78*:405, 1973.

335. Falliers CJ, de A Cordosa RR, Bare HN, et al: Discordant allergic manifestation in monozygotic twins: genetic identity vs. clinical, physiologic, and biochemical differences. J Allergy *47*:207, 1971.

336. Hopp RJ, Bewtra AK, Watt GD, et al: Genetic analysis of allergic disease in twins. J Allerg Clin Immunol *73*:265, 1984.

337. Chan Yeung M, Lam S: State of ART: Occupational asthma. Am Rev Respir Dis *133*:686, 1986.

338. Sibbold B, Turner-Warwick M: Factors influencing the prevalence of asthma among first degree relatives of extrinsic and intrinsic asthmatics. Thorax *34*:332, 1979.

339. Inouye T, Tarlo S, Broder I, et al: Severity of asthma in skin test-negative and skin test-positive patients. J Allergy Clin Immunol *75*:313, 1985.

340. McFadden ER: Pathogenesis of asthma. J Allergy Clin Immunol *73*:413, 1984.

341. Williams E, McNicol KN: Prevalence, natural history, and relationship of wheezy bronchitis and asthma in children. An epidemiological study. Br Med J *4*:321, 1969.

342. Coombs RRA, Hunter A, Jonas WE, et al: Detection of IgE (IgND) specific antibody (probably reagin) to castor-bean allergen by the red-cell-linked antigen-antiglobulin reaction. Lancet *1*:1115, 1968.

343. Woolcock AJ: Worldwide differences in asthma prevalence and mortality: Why is asthma mortality so low in the U.S.A.? Chest *90*:40S, 1986.

344. Ford RM: Aetiology of asthma: A review of 11,551 cases (1958–1968). Med J Aust *1*:628, 1969.

345. Fagerberg E: Studies in bronchial asthma. A comparative examination between patients with endogeneous and exogenous bronchial asthma, respectively, with regard to age when taken ill. Acta Allergol (Kbh) *11*:327, 1957.

346. McNichol KN, Williams HE: Spectrum of asthma in children. I. Clinical and physiological components. Br Med J *4*:7, 1973.

347. Weiss ST, Tager IB, Speizer FE, et al: Persistent wheeze: Its relation to respiratory illness, cigarette smoking and level of pulmonary function in a population sample of children. Am Rev Respir Dis *131*:573, 1985.

348. Weiss ST, Tager IB, Munoz A, et al: The relationship of respiratory infection in early childhood to the occurrence of increased levels of bronchial responsiveness and atopy. Am Rev Respir Dis *131*:573, 1985.

349. Cullen KJ: Climate and chest disorders in school children. Br Med J *4*:65, 1972.

350. Cookson JB, Makoni G: Prevalence of asthma in Rhodesian Africans. Thorax *35*:833, 1980.

351. Ross I: Bronchial asthma in Malaysia. Br J Dis Chest *78*:369, 1984.

352. Editorial: IgE, parasites and allergy. Lancet *1*:894, 1976.

353. Carswell F, Meakins RH, Harland PSEG: Parasites and asthma in Tanzanian children. Lancet *2*:706, 1976.

354. Carrasco E: Epidemiologic aspects of asthma in Latin America. Chest *91*(Suppl 6):938, 1987.

355. Woolcock AJ, Colman MH, Jones MW: Atopy and bronchial reactivity in Australian and Malaysian populations. Clin Allergy *8*:155, 1978.

356. Woolcock AJ, Green W, Alpers MP: Asthma in a rural highland area of Papua New Guinea. Am Rev Respir Dis *123*:565, 1981.

357. Woolcock AJ, Dowse GK, Temple K, et al: The prevalence of asthma in the South-Fore people of Papua New Guinea. A method for field studies of bronchial reactivity. Eur J Respir Dis *64*:571, 1983.

358. Dowse GK, Smith D, Turner KJ, et al: Prevalence and features of asthma in a sample survey of urban Goroka, Papua New Guinea. Clin Allergy *15*:429, 1985.

359. Hogg JC: The pathophysiology of asthma. Chest *82*:85, 1982.

360. Leff A: Pathophysiology of asthmatic bronchoconstriction. Chest *82*:135, 1982.

361. Glynn AA, Michaels L: Bronchial biopsy in chronic bronchitis and asthma. Thorax *15*:142, 1960.

362. Laitinen LA, Heino M, Laitinen A, et al: Damage of the airway epithelium and bronchial reactivity in patients with asthma. Am Rev Respir Dis *131*:599, 1985.

363. Sanerkin NG, Evans MD: The sputum in bronchial asthma: pathognomonic patterns. J Pathol Bacteriol *89*:535, 1965.

364. Cutz E, Levison H, Cooper DM: Ultrastructure of airways in children with asthma. Histopathology *2*:407, 1978.

365. Dunnill MS: The pathology of asthma, with special reference to changes in the bronchial mucosa. J Clin Pathol *13*:27, 1960.

366. Uragoda CG: Broncholithiasis secondary to intrapleural calcification. Br Med J *2*:1635, 1966.

367. Naylor B: The shedding of the mucosa of the bronchial tree in asthma. Thorax *17*:69, 1962.

368. Schmidt HW, Clagett OT, McDonald JR: Broncholithiasis. J Thorac Surg *19*:226, 1950.

369. Sakula A: Charcot-Leyden crystals and Curschmann spirals in asthmatic sputum. Thorax *41*:503, 1986.

370. Walker KR, Fullmer CD: Progress report on study of respiratory spirals. Acta Cytol *14*:396, 1970.

371. Weed LA, Andersen HA: Etiology of broncholithiasis. Dis Chest *37*:270, 1960.

372. Straub M, Schwarz J: The healed primary complex in histoplasmosis. Am J Clin Pathol *25*:727, 1955.

373. Laitinen LA, Heino M, Laitinen A, et al: Damage of the airway epithelium and bronchial reactivity in patients with asthma. Am Rev Respir Dis *131*:599, 1985.

374. Sobonya RE: Concise clinical study. Quantitative structural alterations in long-standing allergic asthma. Am Rev Respir Dis *130*:289, 1984.

375. Martinez Hernandez A, Amenta PS: The basement membrane in pathology. Lab Invest *48*:656, 1983.

376. Shale DJ, Lane DJ, Fisher CWS, et al: Endobronchial polyp in an asthmatic subject. Thorax *38*:75, 1983.

377. Dunnill MS, Massarella GR, Anderson JA: A comparison of the quantitative anatomy of the bronchi in normal subjects, in status asthmaticus, in chronic bronchitis, and in emphysema. Thorax *24*:176, 1969.

378. Hossain S: Quantitative measurement of bronchial muscle in man with asthma. Am Rev Respir Dis *107*:99, 1973.

379. Sobonya RE: Quantitative structural alterations in long-standing allergic asthma. Am Rev Respir Dis *130*:289, 1984.

380. Guerzon M, Paré D, Michoud M, et al: The number and distribution of mast cells in monkey lungs. Am Rev Respir Dis *119*:59, 1979.

381. Connell JT: Asthmatic deaths. Role of the mast cell. JAMA *215*:769, 1971.

382. Behrens BL, Clark RAF, Feldsien DC, et al: Comparison of the histopathology of immediate and late asthmatic and cutaneous responses in a rabbit model. Chest *87*:153S, 1985.

383. Lopez-Vidriero MT, Reid L: Chemical markers of mucous and serum glycoproteins and their relation to viscosity in mucoid and purulent sputum from variuos hypersecretory diseases. Am Rev Respir Dis *117*:465, 1978.

384. Shelhamer J, Kaliner M: Editorial: Respiratory mucus production in asthma. Clin Respir Physiol *21*:301, 1985.

385. Bateman JRM, Pavia D, Sheahan NF, et al: Impaired tracheobronchial clearance in patients with mild stable asthma. Thorax *38*:463, 1983.

386. Pavis D, Bateman JRM, Sheahan NF et al: Tracheobronchial mucociliary clearance in asthma: Impairment during remission. Thorax *40*:171, 1985.

387. Wanner A: Alteration of tracheal mucociliary transport in airway disease. Effect of pharmacologic agents. Chest *80*(6 Suppl):867, 1981.

388. Wanner A: Allergic mucociliary dysfunction. J Allergy Clin Immunol *72*:347, 1983.

389. Mezey RJ, Cohn MA, Fernandez RJ, et al: Mucociliary transport in allergic patients with antigen-induced bronchospasm. Am Rev Respir Dis *118*:677, 1978.

390. Weissberger D, Oliver W, Abraham WM, et al: Impaired tracheal

11

mucus transport in allergic bronchoconstriction: effect of terbutaline pretreatment. J Allergy Clin Immunol 67:357, 1981.

391. Maurer DR, Sielczak M, Oliver W Jr, et al: Role of ciliary motility in acute allergic mucociliary dysfunction. J Appl Physiol 52:1018, 1982.

392. Ahmed T, Greenblatt DW, Birch S, et al: Abnormal mucociliary transport in allergic patients with antigen-induced bronchospasm. Role of slow-reacting substance of anaphylaxis. Am Rev Respir Dis 124:110, 1981.

393. Phipps RJ, Denas SM, Wanner A: Antigen stimulates glycoprotein secretion and alters ion fluxes in sheep trachea. J Appl Physiol 55:1593, 1983.

394. Allegra L, Abraham WM, Chapman GA, et al: Duration of mucociliary dysfunction following antigen challenge. J Appl Physiol 55:726, 1983.

395. Dulfano MJ, Luk CK: Sputum and ciliary inhibition in asthma. Thorax 37:646, 1982.

396. Agnew JE, Bateman JR, Sheahan NF, et al: Effect of oral corticosteroids on mucus clearance by cough and mucociliary transport in stable asthma. Bull Eur Physiopathol Respir 19:37, 1983.

397. Orehek J: Asthma without airway hyperreactivity: Fact or artifact? Eur J Respir Dis 63:1, 1982.

398. Dolovich J, Hargreave FE, O'Byrne P, et al: Asthma terminology: Troubles in wordland. Am Rev Respir Dis 134:1102, 1986.

399. Weiss S, Robb GP, Blumgart HL: The velocity of blood flow in health and disease as measured by the effect of histamine on the minute vessels. Am Heart J 4:664, 1929.

400. Weiss S, Robb GP, Ellis LB: The systemic effects of histamine in man with special reference to the responses of the cardiovascular system. Arch Intern Med 49:360, 1932.

401. Curry JJ: Comparative action of acetyl-beta-methyl choline and histamine on the respiratory tract in normals, patients with hay fever and subjects with bronchial asthma. J Clin Invest 26:430, 1947.

402. Tiffeneau R: L'hyperexcitabilité acétylcholinique du poumon: critère physio-pharmacodynamique de la maladie asthmatique. Presse Med 63:227, 1955.

403. Charpin J: Bronchial hyperreactivity. Bull Eur Physiol Respir 20:5, 1985.

404. Boushey HA, Holtzman MJ, Shuler JR, et al: State of the art: Bronchial hyperreactivity. Am Rev Respir Dis 121:389, 1980.

405. Simonsson BG: Airway hyperreactivity: Definition and short review. Eur J Respir Dis [Suppl] 131:9, 1983.

406. Hargreave FE (ed): Airway Reactivity—Mechanisms and Clinical Relevance. Ontario, Astra Mississauga, 1980.

407. Hargreave FE, Woolcock AJ (eds): Airway Responsiveness—Measurement and Interpretation. Ontario, Astra Mississauga, 1985.

408. Mann JS, Cushley MJ, Holgate ST: Adenosine-induced bronchoconstriction in asthma—role of parasympathetic stimulation and adrenergic inhibition. Am Rev Respir Dis 132:1, 1985.

409. Adelroth E, Morris MM, Hargreave FE, et al: Airway responsiveness to leukotrienes C4 and D4 and to methacholine in patients with asthma and normal controls. N Engl J Med 315:480, 1986.

410. Borum P: Nasal methacholine challenge—test for the measurement of nasal reactivity. J Allergy Clin Immunol 63:253, 1979.

411. Druce HM, Wright RH, Kossoff D, et al: Cholinergic nasal hyperreactivity in atopic subjects. J Allergy Clin Immunol 76:445, 1985.

412. Douglas JS, Ridgway R, Brink C: Airway responses of the guinea pig in vivo and in vitro. J Pharmacol Exp Ther 202:116, 1977.

413. Snapper JR, Drazen JM, Loring SH, et al: Distribution of pulmonary responsiveness to aerosol histamine in dogs. J Appl Physiol 44:738, 1978.

414. Habib MP, Pare PD, Engel LA: Variability of airway responses to inhaled histamine in normal subjects. J Appl Physiol 47:51, 1979.

415. Hirshman CA, Malley A, Downes H: Basenji-Greyhound dog model of asthma: Reactivity to Ascaris suum, citric acid and methaeboline. J Appl Physiol 49:953, 1980.

416. Pauwels R, Van der Straeten M, Weyne J, et al: Genetic factors in non-specific bronchial reactivity in rats. Eur J Respir Dis 66:98, 1985.

417. Simonsson BG: Airway hyperreactivity. Definition and short review. In Simonsson BG (ed): Airway hyperreactivity. Eur J Respir Dis 64(Suppl 131):9, 1983.

418. Zamel N, Leroux M, Vanderdoelen JL: Airway responses to inhaled methacholine in healthy nonsmoking twins. J Appl Physiol 56:936, 1984.

419. Halperin SA, Eggleston PA, Beasley P, et al: Exacerbation of asthma in adults during experimental rhinovirus infection. Am Rev Respir Dis 132:976, 1985.

420. Boushey HA, Holtzman MJ: Experimental airway inflammation and hyperreactivity—searching for cells and mediators. Am Rev Respir Dis 131:312, 1985.

421. Mapp CE, Polato R, Maestrelli P, et al: Time course of the increase in airway responsiveness associated with late asthmatic reactions to toluene di-isocyanate in sensitized subjects. J Allergy Clin Immunol 75:568, 1985.

422. Lam S, Wong R, Yeung M: Nonspecific bronchial reactivity in occupational asthma. J Allergy Clin Immunol 1979:613, 28.

423. Ramsdale EH, Morris MM, Roberts RS, et al: Asymptomatic bronchial hyperresponsiveness in rhinitis. J Allergy Clin Immunol 75:573, 1985.

424. Stevens VJ, Vermeire PA: Bronchial responsiveness to histamine and allergy in patients with asthma, rhinitis, cough. Eur J Respir Dis 61:203, 1980.

425. Banks DE, Barkman HW Jr, Butcher BT, et al: Absence of hyperresponsiveness to methacholine in a worker with methylene diphenyl diisocyanate (MDI)-induced asthma. Chest 89:389, 1986.

426. Staunescu DC, Frans A: Bronchial asthma without increased airway reactivity. Eur J Respir Dis 63:5, 1982.

427. Hargreave FE, Ramsdale EH, Pugsley SO: Occupational asthma without bronchial hyperresponsiveness. Am Rev Respir Dis 130:513, 1984.

428. Giffon E, Orehek J, Vervloet D, et al: Asthma without airway hyperresponsiveness to carbachol. Eur J Respir Dis 70:229, 1987.

429. Bechtel JJ, Starr T, Dantzker DR, et al: Airway hyperreactivity in patients with sarcoidosis. Am Rev Resp Dis 124:759, 1981.

430. Olafsson M, Simonsson BG, Hansson SB: Bronchial reactivity in patients with recent pulmonary sarcoidosis. Thorax 40:51, 1985.

431. Freedman PM, Ault B: Bronchial hyperreactivity to methacholine in farmers' lung disease. J Allergy Clin Immunol 67:59, 1981.

432. Mönkäre S, Haahtela T, Ikonen M, et al: Bronchial hyperreactivity to inhaled histamine in patients with farmers' lung. Lung 159:145, 1981.

433. Mönkäre S: Clinical aspects of farmer's lung: Airway reactivity, treatment and prognosis. Eur J Respir Dis 65:1, 1984.

434. Ramsdell JW, Nachtwey FJ, Moser KM, et al: Bronchial hyperreactivity in chronic obstructive bronchitis. Am Rev Respir Dis 126:829, 1982.

435. Yan K, Salome CM, Woolcock AJ, et al: Prevalence and nature of bronchial hyperresponsiveness in subjects with chronic obstructive pulmonary disease. Am Rev Respir Dis 132:27, 1985.

436. Bahous A, Cartier A, Ouimet G, et al: Nonallergic bronchial hyperexcitability in chronic bronchitis. Am Rev Respir Dis 129:216, 1984.

437. Weiss ST, Tager IB, Weiss JW, et al: Airways responsiveness in a population sample of adults and children. Am Rev Respir Dis 129:898, 1984.

438. Mortagy AK, Howell JB, Waters WE: Respiratory symptoms and bronchial reactivity: Identification of a syndrome and its relation to asthma. Br Med J 293:525, 1986.

439. Woolcock AJ, Peat JK, Salome CN, et al: Prevalence of bronchial hyperresponsiveness and asthma in a rural adult population. Thorax 42:361, 1987.

440. Britton WJ, Woolcock AJ, Peat JK, et al: Prevalence of bronchial hyperresponsiveness in children: The relationship between asthma and skin reactivity to allergens in two communities. Int J Epidemiol 15:202, 1986.

441. Cockcroft DW, Berscheid BA, Murdock KY: Measurement of responsiveness to inhaled histamine using FEV_1: Comparison of PC_{20} and threshold. Thorax 38:523, 1983.

442. Malo JL, Pineau L, Cartier A, et al: Reference values of the provocative concentrations of methacholine that cause 6-per cent and 20-per cent changes in forced expiratory volume in one second in a normal population. Am Rev Respir Dis 128:8, 1983.

443. Henry RL, Mellis CM, South RT, et al: Comparison of peak expiratory flow rate and forced expiratory volume in one second in histamine challenge studies in children. Br J Dis Chest 76:167, 1982.

444. Dehaut P, Rachiele A, Martin RR, et al: Histamine dose-response curves in asthma: Reproducibility and sensitivity of different indices to assess response. Thorax 38:516, 1983.

445. Michoud MC, Ghezzo H, Amyot R: A comparison of pulmonary function tests used for bronchial challenges. Bull Eur Physiopathol Respir 18:609, 1982.

446. Madsen F, Rathlou NHH, Frolund L, et al: Short and long term reproducibility of responsiveness to inhaled histamine: Rt compared to FEV_1 as measurement of response to challenge. Eur J Respir Dis 67:193, 1985.

447. Fish JE, Ankin MG, Kelly JF, et al: Regulation of bronchomotor tone by lung inflation in asthmatic and nonasthmatic subjects. J Appl Physiol 50:1079, 1981.

448. Cockcroft DW, Killian DN, Mellon JJA, et al: Bronchial reactivity to inhaled histamine. A method and clinical survey. Clin Allergy 7:235, 1977.

449. Eiser NM: Calculation of data. Eur J Respir Dis (Suppl 131) 64:241, 1983.

450. Walters EH, Davies PH, Smith AP: Measurement of bronchial reactivity: a question of interpretation. Thorax 36:960, 1981.

451. Moreno RH, Hogg JC, Paré PD: Mechanism of airway narrowing. Am Rev Respir Dis *133*:1171, 1986.

452. Orehek J: The concept of airway "sensitivity" and "reactivity." Eur J Respir Dis (Suppl 131) *64*:27, 1983.

453. Michoud MC, Lelorier J, Amyot R: Factors modulating the individual variability of airway responsiveness to histamine. The influence of H_1 and H_2 receptors. Bull Eur Physiopath Respir *17*:807, 1981.

454. Woolcock AJ, Salome CM, Yan K: The shape of the dose-response curve to histamine in asthmatic and normal subjects. Am Rev Respir Dis *130*:71, 1984.

455. Sterk P, Daniel E, Zamel N, et al: Limited maximal airway narrowing in nonasthmatic subjects—role of neural control and prostaglandin in release. Am Rev Respir Dis *132*:865, 1985.

456. Orehek J, Gayrard P, Smith AP, et al: Airway response to carbachol in normal and asthmatic subjects. Am Rev Respir Dis *115*:937, 1977.

457. Cockcroft DW, Berscheid BA: Slope of the dose-response curve: usefulness in assessing bronchial responses to inhaled histamine. Thorax *38*:55, 1983.

458. Malo J, Cartier A, Pineau L, et al: Slope of the dose-response curve to inhaled histamine and methacholine and PC20 in subjects with symptoms of airway hyperexcitability and in normal subjects. Am Rev Respir Dis *132*:644, 1985.

459. Beaupré A, Malo JL: Histamine dose-response curves in asthma: Relevance of the distinction between PC20 and reactivity in characterising clinical state. Thorax *36*:731, 1981.

460. Bhagat RG, Grunstein MM: Comparison of responsiveness to methacholine, histamine, and exercise in subgroups of asthmatic children. Am Rev Respir Dis *129*:221, 1984.

461. Salome CM, Schoeffel RE, Woolcock AJ: Comparison of bronchial reactivity to histamine and methacholine in asthmatics. Clin Allergy *10*:541, 1980.

462. Juniper EF, Frith PA, Dunnett C, et al: Reproducibility and comparison of response to inhaled histamine and methacholine. Thorax *33*:705, 1978.

463. Juniper EF, Frith PA, Hargreave FE: Airway responsiveness to histamine and methacholine—relationship to minimum treatment to control symptoms of asthma. Thorax *36*:575, 1981.

464. Thomson NC, Roberts RE, Bandouvakis J, et al: Comparison of bronchial responses to prostaglandin-F2-alpha and methacholine. J Allergy Clin Immunol *68*:392, 1981.

465. Hargreave FE, Ryan G, Thomson NC, et al: Bronchial responsiveness to histamine or methcholine in asthma—measurement and clinical significance. J Allergy Clin Immunol *68*:347, 1981.

466. Cartier A, Malo JL, Begin P, et al: Time course of the bronchoconstriction induced by inhaled histamine and methacholine. J Appl Physiol *54*:821, 1983.

467. Lemire I, Cartier A, Malo JL, et al: Effect of sodium cromoglycate on histamine inhalation test. J Allergy Clin Immunol *73*:234, 1984.

468. Thomson NC, O'Byrne PM, Hargreave FE: Prolonged asthmatic responses to inhaled methacholine. J Allergy Clin Immunol *71*:357, 1983.

469. Ryan G, Dolovich MB, Roberts RS, et al: Standardization of inhalation provocation tests: Two techniques of aerosol generation and inhalation compared. Am Rev Respir Dis *123*:195, 1981.

470. Ruffin RE, Alpers JH, Crockett AJ, et al: Repeated histamine inhalation tests in asthmatic patients. J Allergy Clin Immunol *67*:285, 1981.

471. Ten Velde GPM, Kreukniet J: The histamine inhalation provocation test and its reproducibility. Respiration *45*:131, 1984.

472. Löwhagen O, Lindholm NB: Short-term and long-term variation in bronchial response to histamine in asthmatic patients. Eur J Respir Dis *64*:466, 1983.

473. Juniper EF, Frith PA, Hargreave FE: Long-term stability of bronchial responsiveness to histamine. Thorax *37*:288, 1982.

474. Anderson RC, Cuff MT, Frith PA, et al: Bronchial responsiveness to inhaled histamine and exercise. J Allergy Clin Immunol *63*:315, 1979.

475. O'Byrne PM, Ryan G, Morris M, et al: Asthma induced by cold air and its relation to non-specific bronchial responsiveness to methacholine. Am Rev Respir Dis *125*:281, 1982.

476. Aquilina AT: Comparison of airway reactivity induced by histamine, methacholine and isocapnic hyperventilation in normal and asthmatic subjects. Thorax *38*:766, 1983.

477. Anderson SD, Schoeffel RE, Finney M: Evaluation of ultrasonically nebulized solutions for provocation testing in patients with asthma. Thorax *38*:284, 1983.

478. Ryan G, Latimer KM, Dolovich J, et al: Bronchial responsiveness to histamine: relationship to diurnal variation of peak flow rate, improvement after bronchodilator, and airway calibre. Thorax *37*:423, 1982.

479. Khoo KT, Connolly CK: A comparison of three methods of measuring bronchiolability in asthmatics, bronchitic cigarette smokers and normal subjects. Respiration *45*:219, 1984.

480. Freedman BJ: The functional geometry of the bronchi. Bull Physiopathol Respir *8*:545, 1972.

481. Chung KF, Morgan B, Keyes SJ, et al: Histamine dose-response relationships in normal and asthmatic subjects—the importance of starting airway caliber. Am Rev Respir Dis *126*:849, 1982.

482. Tattersfield AE: Measurement of bronchial reactivity—a question of interpretation. Thorax *36*:561, 1981.

483. Hopp R, Bewtra A, Nair N, et al: The effect of age on methacholine response. J Allergy Clin Immunol *76*:609, 1985.

484. Zamel N: Threshold of airway response to inhaled methacholine in healthy men and women. J Appl Physiol *56*:129, 1984.

485. Rubinfield AR, Pain MCF: Relationship between bronchial reactivity airway caliber, and severity of asthma. Am Rev Respir Dis *115*:381, 1977.

486. Folkow B: The haemodynamic consequences of adoptive structural changes of the vessels in hypertension. Clin Sci *41*:1, 1971.

487. Chung KF, Snashall PD: Effect of prior bronchoconstriction on the airway response in normal subjects. Thorax *39*:40, 1984.

488. Ruffin RE, Dolovich MB, Wolff RK, et al: The effects of preferential deposition of histamine in the human airway. Am Rev Respir Dis *117*:485, 1978.

489. Smaldone GC, Messina MS: Flow limitation, cough, and patterns of aerosol deposition in humans. J Appl Physiol *59*:515, 1985.

490. Hounam RF, Morgan A: Particle deposition. *In* Brain JD, Proctor DF, Reid LM (eds): Respiratory Defense Mechanisms, Part I. New York, Marcel Dekker, 1977, p 125.

491. Hogg JC: Bronchial mucosal permeability and its relationship to airways hyperreactivity. J Allergy Clin Immunol *67*:421, 1981.

492. Laitinen LA, Heino M, Laitinen A, et al: Damage of the airway epithelium and bronchial reactivity in patients with asthma. Am Rev Respir Dis *131*:599, 1985.

493. Laitinen LA, Haahtela T, Kava T, et al: Non-specific bronchial reactivity and ultrastructure of the airway epithelium in patients with sarcoidosis and allergic alveolitis. *In* Simonsson BG (ed): Airway Hyperreactivity. Eur J Respir Dis *64*(Suppl 131):267, 1983.

494. Dusser DJ, Collignon MA, Stanislas-Leguern G: Respiratory clearance of 99m T_c-DTPA and pulmonary involvement in sarcoidosis. Am Rev Respir Dis *134*:493, 1986.

495. Hulbert WM, McLean T, Hogg JC: The effect of acute airway inflammation on bronchial reactivity in guinea pigs. Am Rev Respir Dis *132*:7, 1985.

496. Boucher RC, Paré PD, Hogg JC: Relationship between airway hyperreactivity and permeability in *Ascaris*-sensitive monkeys. J Allergy Clin Immunol *64*:197, 1979.

497. Elwood RK, Kennedy S, Belzberg A, et al: Respiratory mucosal permeability in asthma. Am Rev Respir Dis *128*:523, 1983.

498. O'Byrne PM, Dolovich M, Dirks R, et al: Lung epithelial permeability: relation to nonspecific airway responsiveness. J Appl Physiol *57*:77, 1984.

499. Borland C, Chamberlain A, Barber B, et al: Pulmonary epithelial permeability after inhaling saline, distilled water "fog" and cold air. Chest *87*:373, 1985.

500. Higenbottam T, Borland C, Barber B, et al: Pulmonary epithelial permeability after inhaled distilled water "fog." Chest *87*:156S, 1985.

501. Roehrs JD, Rogers WR, Johanson WG Jr: Bronchial reactivity to inhaled methacholine in cigarette-smoking baboons. J Appl Physiol *50*:754, 1981.

502. King M, Kelly S, Cosio M: Alteration of airway reactivity by mucus. Respir Physiol *62*:47, 1985.

503. Kelly L, Kolbe J, Mitzner W, et al: Bronchial blood flow affects recovery from contriction in dog lung periphery. J Appl Physiol *60*:1954, 1986.

504. Michoud MC, Paré PD, Boucher R, et al: Airway responses to histamine and methacholine in *Ascaris suum*—allergic rhesus monkeys. J Appl Physiol *45*:846, 1978.

505. Vidrukk EH, Hahn HL, Nadel JA, et al: Mechanisms by which histamine stimulates rapidly adapting receptors in dog lungs. J Appl Physiol *43*:397, 1977.

506. Palmer JBD, Cuss FM, Barnes PJ: Sensory neuropeptides and human airway function. Am Rev Respir Dis *133*:A239, 1986.

507. Lundberg JM, Saria A: Bronchial smooth muscle contraction induced by stimulation of capsaicin-sensitive sensory neurons. Acta Physiol Scand *116*:473, 1982.

508. Lundberg JM, Saria A: Capsaicin-induced desensitization of airway mucosa to cigarette smoke, mechanical, and chemical irritants. Nature *302*:251, 1983.

509. Martin JG, Collier B: Acetylcholine release from canine isolated airway is not modulated by norepinephrine. J Appl Physiol *61*:1025, 1986.

510. Tanaka DT, Grunstein MM: Effect of substance-P on neurally mediated contraction of rabbit airway smooth muscle. J Appl Physiol *60*:458, 1986.

511. Barnes PJ, Basbaum CB, Nadel JA: Auto radiographic localization

11

of autonomic receptors in airway smooth muscle: Marked differences between large and small airways. Am Rev Respir Dis 127:758, 1983.

512. Douglas NJ, Sudlow MF, Flenley DC: Effect of an inhaled atropine-like agent on normal airway function. J Appl Physiol 46:256, 1979.

513. Holtzman MJ, Sheller JR, Dimeo MA, et al: Effect of ganglionic blockade on bronchial reactivity in atopic subjects. Am Rev Respir Dis 122:17, 1980.

514. Sheppard D, Epstein J, Skoogh BE, et al: Variable inhibition of histamine-induced bronchoconstriction by atropine in subjects with asthma. J Allergy Clin Immunol 73:82, 1984.

515. O'Byrne PM, Thomson NC, Latimer KM, et al: The effect of inhaled hexamethonium bromide and atropine sulphate on airway responsiveness to histamine. J Allergy Clin Immunol 76:97, 1985.

516. Kallenbach JM, Webster T, Dowdeswell R, et al: Reflex heart rate control in asthma: Evidence of parasympathetic overactivity. Chest 87:644, 1985.

517. Sturani C, Sturani A, Tosi I: Parasympathetic activity assessed by diving reflex and by airway response to methacholine in bronchial asthma and rhinitis. Respiration 48:321, 1985.

518. Boulet LP, Latimer KM, Roberts RS, et al: The effects of atropine on allergen-induced increases in bronchial responsiveness to histamine. Am Rev Respir Dis 130:368, 1984.

519. Richardson JB: Nerve supply to the lungs. Am Rev Respir Dis 119:785, 1979.

520. Carstairs JR, Nimmo AJ, Barnes PJ: Auto-radiographic visualization of beta-adrenoceptor subtypes in human lung. Am Rev Respir Dis 132:541, 1985.

521. Carstairs JR, Nimmo AJ, Barnes PJ: Auto-radiographic localization of beta-adrenoceptors in human lung. Eur J Pharmacol 105:189, 1984.

522. Szentivanyi A: The beta-adrenergic theory of the atopic abnormality in bronchial asthma. J Allergy 42:203, 1968.

523. Shelhamer JH, Marom Z, Kaliner M: Abnormal beta-adrenergic responsiveness in allergic subjects. 2. The role of selective beta 2-adrenergic hyporeactivity. J Allergy Clin Immunol 71:57, 1983.

524. Parker CW, Smith JW: Alterations in cyclic adenosine monophosphate metabolism in human bronchial asthma. I: Leukocyte responsiveness to beta-adrenergic agents. J Clin Invest 52:48, 1973.

525. Brooks SM, McGowan K, Altenau P: Relationship between beta-adrenergic binding in lymphocyte and severity of disease in asthma. Chest 75:232, 1979.

526. Kariman K: Beta-adrenergic receptor binding in lymphocytes from patients with asthma. Lung 158:41, 1980.

527. Brooks SM, McGowan K, Bernstein IL: et al: Relationship between numbers of beta-adreneregic receptors in lymphocytes and disease severity in asthma. J Allergy Clin Immunol 63:401, 1979.

528. Goldie RG, Spina D, Henry PJ, et al: In vitro responsiveness of human asthmatic bronchus to carbachol, histamine, beta-adrenoceptor agonists and theophylline. Br J Clin Pharmacol 22:669, 1986.

529. Galant SP, Duriseti L, Underwood S, et al: Decreased beta-adrenergic receptors on polymorphonuclear leukocytes after adrenergic therapy. N Engl J Med 299:933, 1978.

530. Galant SP, Duriseti L, Underwood S, et al: Beta-adrenergic receptors of polymorphonuclear particulates in bronchial asthma. J Clin Invest 65:577, 1980.

531. Busse WW, Bush RK, Cooper W: Granulocyte response in vitro to isoproterenol, histamine, and prostaglandin E₁ during treatment with beta-adrenergic aerosols in asthma. Am Rev Respir Dis 120:377, 1979.

532. Conolly ME, Tashkin DP, Hui KKP, et al: Selective subsensitization of beta-adrenergic receptors in central airways of asthmatics and normal subjects during long-term therapy with inhaled Salbutamol. J Allergy Clin Immunol 70:423, 1982.

533. Tashkin DP, Conolly ME, Deutsch RI, et al: Subsensitization of beta-adrenoceptors in airways and lymphocytes of healthy and asthmatic subjects. Am Rev Respir Dis 125:185, 1982.

534. Guillot C, Fornaris M, Badier M, et al: Spontaneous and provoked resistance to isoproterenol in isolated human bronchi. J Allergy Clin Immunol 74:713, 1984.

535. Bruynzeel PLB: Changes in the β-adrenergic system due to β-adrenergic therapy: clinical consequences. Eur J Respir Dis (Suppl 65) 135:62, 1984.

536. Meurs H, Köeter GH, de Vries K, et al: Dynamics of the lymphocyte beta-adrenoceptor system in patients with allergic bronchial asthma. Eur J Respir Dis (Suppl 65) 135:47, 1984.

537. Meurs H, Köeter GH, de Vries K, et al: The β-adrenergic system and allergic bronchial asthma changes in lymphocyte beta-adrenergic receptor number and adenylate cyclase activity after an allergen-induced asthmatic attack. J Allergy Clin Immunol 70:272, 1982.

538. Davis PB, Simpson DM, Paget GL, et al: Beta-adrenergic responses in drug-free subjects with asthma. J Allergy Clin Immunol 77:871, 1986.

539. Fraser CM, Venter JC: Autoantibodies to beta 2-adrenergic receptors and allergic respiratory disease. Surv Immunol Res 1:365, 1982.

540. Blecher M, Lewis S, Hicks JM, et al: Beta-blocking autoantibodies in pediatric bronchial asthma. J Allergy Clin Immunol 74:246, 1984.

541. Basran GS, Ball AJ, Hanson JM, et al: Circulating β-adrenoceptor blocking factors in asthma. Eur J Respir Dis (Suppl 65) 135:226, 1984.

542. Kiyingi KS, Anderson SD, Temple DM, et al: Beta-adrenoceptor blockade with propranolol and bronchial responsiveness to a number of bronchial provocation tests in non-asthmatic subjects. Eur J Respir Dis 66:256, 1985.

543. Zaid G, Beall GN: Bronchial response to beta-adrenergic blockade. N Engl J Med 275:580, 1966.

544. Orehek J, Gayrard P, Grimaud C, et al: Effect of beta-adrenergic blockade on bronchial sensitivity to inhaled acetylcholine in normal subjects. J Allergy Clin Immunol 55:164, 1975.

545. Kiyingi KS, Anderson SD, Temple DM, et al: Beta-adrenoceptor blockade with propranolol and bronchial responsiveness to a number of bronchial provocation tests in non-asthmatic subjects. Eur J Respir Dis 66:256, 1985.

546. Langer I: The bronchoconstrictor action of propranolol aerosol in asthmatic subjects. J Physiol (Lond) 190:41, 1967.

547. Grieco MH, Pierson RN: Mechanism of bronchoconstriction due to beta-adrenergic blockade. J Allergy Clin Immunol 48:143, 1971.

548. Richardson PS, Sterling GM: Effects of beta-adrenergic receptor blockade on airway conductance and lung volume in normal and asthmatic subjects. Br Med J 3:143, 1969.

549. Barnes PJ: Endogenous plasma adrenaline in asthma. Eur J Respir Dis 64:559, 1983.

550. Warren JB, Keynes RJ, Brown MJ, et al: Blunted sympathoadrenal response to exercise in asthmatic subjects. Br J Dis Chest 76:147, 1982.

551. Barnes PJ, Brown MJ, Silverman M, et al: Circulating catecholamines in exercise and hyperventilation-induced asthma. Thorax 36:435, 1981.

552. Sands MF, Douglas FL, Green J, et al: Homeostatic regulation of bronchomotor tone by sympathetic activation during bronchoconstriction in normal and asthmatic humans. Am Rev Respir Dis 132:993, 1985.

553. Barnes PJ: Adrenergic receptors of normal and asthmatic airways. Eur J Respir Dis (Suppl 65) 135:62, 1984.

554. Kneussl MP, Richardson JB: Alpha-adrenergic receptors in human and canine tracheal and bronchial smooth muscle. J Appl Physiol 45:307, 1978.

555. Thomson NC, Daniel EE, Hargreave FE: Role of smooth muscle alpha-1-receptors in nonspecific bronchial responsiveness in asthma. Am Rev Respir Dis 126:521, 1982.

556. Black JL, Salome CM, Yan N, et al: Comparison between airways response to an alpha adrenoceptor and histamine in asthmatic and non-asthmatic subjects. Br J Clin Pharmacol 14:464, 1982.

557. Black JL, Salome C, Yan N, et al: The action of prazosin and propylene glycol on methoxamine-induced bronchoconstriction in asthmatic subjects. Br J Clin Pharmacol 18:349, 1984.

558. Black J, Vincenc K, Salome C: Inhibition of methoxamine-induced bronchoconstriction by ipratropium bromide and disodium cromoglycate in asthmatic subjects. Br J Clin Pharmacol 20:41, 1985.

559. Henderson WR, Shelhamer JH, Reingold DB, et al: Alpha-adrenergic hyperresponsiveness in asthma: Analysis of vascular and pupillary responses. N Engl J Med 300:642, 1979.

560. Davis PB: Pupillary responses and airway reactivity in asthma. J Allergy Clin Immunol 77:667, 1986.

561. Utting JA: Alpha-adrenergic blockade in severe asthma. Br J Dis Chest 73:317, 1979.

562. Jenkins C, Breslin ABX, Marlin GE: The role of alpha-adrenoceptors and beta-adrenoceptors in airway hyperresponsiveness to histamine. J Allergy Clin Immunol 75:364, 1985.

563. Barnes PJ, Wilson NM, Vickers H: Prazosin, an alpha-1-adrenoceptor antagonist, partially inhibits exercise-induced asthma. J Allergy Clin Immunol 68:411, 1981.

564. Walden SM, Bleecker ER, Chahal K, et al: Effect of alpha-adrenergic blockade on exercise-induced asthma and conditioned cold air. Am Rev Respir Dis 130:357, 1984.

565. Crema A, del Tacca M, Frigo GM, et al: Presence of a non-adrenergic inhibitory system in the human colon. Gut 9:633, 1968.

566. Frigo GM, del Tacca M, Lecchini S, et al: Some observations on the intrinsic nervous mechanism in Hirschsprung's disease. Gut 14:35, 1973.

567. Coburn RF, Tomita T: Evidence for non-adrenergic inhibitory nerves in the guinea pig trachealis muscle. Am J Physiol 224:1072, 1973.

568. Richardson JB, Beland J: Nonadrenergic inhibitory nerves in human airways. J Appl Physiol 41:764, 1976.

569. Davis C, Kannan MS, Jones TR, et al: Control of human airway smooth muscle: in vitro studies. J Appl Physiol 53:1080, 1982.

570. Aizawa H, Matsuzaki Y, Ishibashi M, et al: A possible role of nonadrenergic inhibitory nervous system in airway hyperreactivity. Respir Physiol 50:187, 1982.

571. Matsumoto N, Inoue H, Ichinose M, et al: Effective sites by sympathetic beta-adrenergic and vagal nonadrenergic inhibitory stimulation in constricted airways. Am Rev Respir Dis 132:1113, 1985.

572. Taylor SM, Paré PD, Armour CL, et al: Airway reactivity in chronic obstructive pulmonary disease—failure of in vivo methacholine responsiveness to correlate with cholinergic, adrenergic, or non-adrenergic responses in vitro. Am Rev Respir Dis 132:30, 1985.

573. Taylor SM, Paré PD, Schellenberg R: Cholinergic and nonadrenergic mechanisms in human and guinea pig airways. J Appl Physiol 56:958, 1984.

574. Michoud MC, Amyot R, Jeanneret-Grosjean A, et al: Reflex decrease of histamine-induced bronchoconstriction after laryngeal stimulation in humans. Am Rev Respir Dis 136:618, 1987.

575. Diamond L, Szarek JL, Gillespie MN, et al: In vivo bronchodilator activity of vasoactive intestinal peptide in the cat. Am Rev Respir Dis 28:827, 1983.

576. Barnes PJ, Dixon CMS: The effect of inhaled vasoactive intestinal peptide on bronchial reactivity to histamine in humans. Am Rev Respir Dis 130:162, 1984.

577. Barnes PJ: The third nervous system in the lung: Physiology and clinical perspectives (editorial). Thorax 39:561, 1984.

578. Eiser NM: Hyperreactivity. Its relationship to histamine receptors. Eur J Respir Dis (Suppl 131) 64:99, 1983.

579. Smith AP, Dunlop LS: In vitro evidence of H₂ receptors in human bronchus and their role in allergic bronchospasm. Br J Dis Chest 74:314, 1980.

580. Thomson NC, Kerr JW: Effect of inhaled H₁ and H₂ receptor antagonists in normal and asthmatic subjects. Thorax 35:428, 1980.

581. White J, Smith AP, Leopold D, et al: Effects of H₂ antagonists in asthma. Br J Chest 74:315, 1980.

582. Nogrady SG, Bevan C: H₂-receptor blockade and bronchial hyperreactivity to histamine in asthma. Thorax 36:268, 1981.

583. Tashkin PD, Ungerer R, Wolfe R, et al: Effect of orally administered cimetidine on histamine- and antigen-induced bronchospasm in subjects with asthma. Am Rev Respir Dis 125:691, 1982.

584. Nathan RA, Segall N, Glover GC, et al: The effects of H₁ and H₂ antihistamines on histamine inhalation challenges in asthmatic patients. Am Rev Respir Dis 120:1251, 1979.

585. Lichtenstein LM, Gillespie E: Inhibition of histamine release by histamine controlled by H₂ receptors. Nature 244:287, 1973.

586. Kaliner M: Human lung tissue and anaphylaxis: The effects of histamine on the immunologic release of mediators. Am Rev Respir Dis 118:1015, 1978.

587. Eiser NM, Guz A, Mills J, et al: Effect of H₁ and H₂ receptor antagonists on antigen bronchial challenge. Thorax 33:534, 1978.

588. Anderson KE: Airway hyperreactivity, smooth muscle and calcium. Eur J Respir Dis (Suppl 131) 64:49, 1983.

589. Fleming WW, McPhillips JJ, Westfall DP: Post-junctional supersensitivity and subsensitivity of excitable tissue to drugs. Ergeb Physiol 68:55, 1968.

590. Barnes PJ: Calcium-channel blockers and asthma. Thorax 38:481, 1983.

591. Daniel EE, Davis C, Jones T, et al: Control of airway smooth muscle. In Hargreave FE (ed): Airway Reactivity: Mechanisms and Clinical Relevance. Ontario, Astra Mississauga, 1980, p 80.

592. Liu Y, Sasaki H, Ishii M, et al: Effect of circadian rhythm on bronchomotor tone after deep inspiration in normal and in asthmatic subjects. Am Rev Respir Dis 132:278, 1985.

593. Antonissen LA, Mitchell RW, Kroeger EA, et al: Mechanical alterations of airway smooth muscle in a canine asthmatic model. J Appl Physiol 46:681, 1979.

594. Stephens NL, Van Niekerk W: Isometric and isotonic contractions in airway smooth muscle. Can J Physiol Pharmacol 55:833, 1977.

595. Stephens NL, Kroeger E, Media JA: Force-velocity characteristics of respiratory airway smooth muscle. J Appl Physiol 26:285, 1969.

596. Stephens NL, Mitchell RW, Antonissen A, et al: Airway smooth muscle: Physiol properties and metabolism. In Hargreave FE (ed): Airway Reactivity: Mechanisms and Clinical Relevance. Ontario, Astra Mississauga, 1980, p 110.

597. Macklem PT: Bronchial hyporesponsiveness. Chest 87:158S, 1985.

598. De Kock MA: Functional anatomy of the trachea and main bronchi. In De Kock MA, Nadel JA, Lewis CM (eds): Mechanisms of Airway Obstruction in Human Respiratory Disease. Capetown, South African Medical Research Council, 1979, p 49.

599. Martin JG, Dong-Jie D, Macklem PT: Effects of lung volume on methacholine-induced bronchoconstriction in normal subjects. Am Rev Respir Dis 133:A.15, 1986.

600. Thurlbeck WM, Pun R, Toth J, et al: Bronchial cartilage in chronic obstructive lung disease. Am Rev Respir Dis 109:73, 1974.

601. Kaliner M, Bretz U, Holtaman MJ, et al: Bronchial obstruction: Some patho-physiological and clinical concepts. In Herzog H, Perruchoud AP (eds): Asthma and Bronchial Hyperreactivity. Basel, Karger, 1984, p 417.

602. Dunnill MS: The pathology of asthma with special reference to changes in the bronchial mucosa. J Clin Pathol 13:27, 1960.

603. Vincenc KS, Black JL, Yan K, et al: Comparison of in vivo and in vitro responses to histamine in human airways. Am Rev Respir Dis 128:875, 1983.

604. Armour CL, Lazar NM, Schellenberg RR, et al: A comparison of in vivo and in vitro human airway reactivity to histamine. Am Rev Respir Dis 129:907, 1984.

605. Roberts J, Raeburn D, Rodger I, et al: Comparison of in vivo airway responsiveness and in vitro smooth muscle sensitivity to methacholine in man. Thorax 39:837, 1984.

606. Roberts JA, Rodger IW, Thomson NC: Airway responsiveness to histamine in man: Effect of atropine on in vivo and in vitro comparison. Thorax 40:261, 1985.

607. Cerrina J, Le Roy Laurdie M, Labat C, et al: Comparison of human bronchial muscle responses to histamine in vivo with histamine and isoproterenol agonists in vitro. Am Rev Respir Dis 134:57, 1986.

608. Downes H, Austin DR, Hirshman CA: Comparison of in vivo and in vitro responses to histamine and methacholine in airways of dogs with and without airway hyperresponsiveness. Am Rev Respir Dis 131:A279, 1985.

609. Schellenberg RR, Duff MJ, Foster A, et al: Asthmatic bronchial reactivity in vitro. Proc Can Soc Invest 8:A202, 1985.

610. Patterson JW, Lulich KM, Golpie RG: The role of beta-adrenoceptors in bronchial hyperreactivity. In Morley J (ed): Bronchial Hyperreactivity. Sydney, Academic Press, 1982, p 19.

611. Holtzman MJ: Inflammation of the airway epithelium and the development of airway hyperresponsiveness. In Herzog H, Perruchoud AP (eds): Asthma and Bronchial Hyperreactivity. Basel, Karger, 1984, p 165.

612. Walters EH: Effect of inhibition of prostaglandin synthesis on induced bronchial hyperresponsiveness. Thorax 38:195, 1983.

613. Cockcroft DW, Ruffin RE, Dolovich J, et al: Allergen-induced increase in non-allergic bronchial reactivity. Clin Allergy 7:503, 1977.

614. Altounyan REC: Changes in histamine and atropine. responsiveness as a guide to diagnosis and evaluation of therapy in obstructive airways disease. In Pepys J, Frankland AW (eds): Disodium Cromoglycate in Allergic Airways Disease. London, Butterworths, 1970, p 47.

615. Bar-Sela S, Schleuter DP, Kitt SR, et al: Antigen-induced enhancement of bronchial reactivity. Chest 88:114, 1985.

616. Black J, Schoeffel R, Sundrum R, et al: Increased responsiveness to methacholine and histamine after challenge with ultrasonically nebulised water in asthmatic subjects. Thorax 40:427, 1985.

617. Smith CM, Anderson SD, Black JL: Methacholine responsiveness increases after ultrasonically nebulized water but not after ultrasonically nebulized hypertonic saline in patients with asthma. J Allergy Clin Immunol 79:85, 1987.

618. Cartier A, Thomson NC, Frith PA, et al: Allergen-induced increase in bronchial responsiveness to histamine—relationship to the late asthmatic response and change in airway caliber. J Allergy Clin Immunol 70:170, 1982.

619. Boulet LP, Cartier A, Thomson NC, et al: Asthma and increases in nonallergic bronchial responsiveness from seasonal pollen exposure. J Allergy Clin Immunol 71:399, 1983.

620. Machado L: Increased bronchial hypersensitivity after early and late bronchial reactions provoked by allen inhalation. Allergy 40:580, 1985.

621. Sotomayor H, Badier M, Vervloet D, et al: Seasonal increase of carbachol airway responsiveness in patients allergic to grass pollen—reversal by corticosteroids. Am Rev Respir Dis 130:56, 1984.

622. Cartier A, L'Archeveque J, Malo JL: Exposure to a sensitizing occupational agent can cause a long-lasting increase in bronchial responsiveness to histamine in the absence of significant changes in airway caliber. J Allergy Clin Immunol 78:1185, 1986.

623. Fabbri LM, Di Giacomo R, Dal Vecchio L, et al: Prednisone, indomethacin and airway responsiveness in toluene diisocyanate sensitized subjects. Bull Eur Physiopathol Respir 21:421, 1985.

624. Dolovich J, Hargreave F: The asthma syndrome—inciters, inducers and host characteristics. Thorax 36:641, 1981.

625. Gordon T, Sheppard D, McDonald DM, et al: Airway hyperresponsiveness and inflammation induced by toluene diisocyanate in guinea pigs. Am Rev Respir Dis 132:1106, 1985.

626. Marsh W, Irvin C, Murphy K, et al: Increases in airway reactivity to histamine and inflammatory cells in bronchoalveolar lavage after the late asthmatic response in an animal model. Am Rev Respir Dis 131:875, 1985.

627. Pauwels R: Mediators and non-specific bronchial hyperreactivity. Eur J Respir Dis 64:95, 1983.

11

628. Persson CGA, Szensjö E: Airway hyperreactivity and microvascular permeability to large molecules. Eur J Respir Dis (Suppl 131) 64:183, 1983.

629. Nadel JA: Inflammation and asthma. J Allergy Clin Immunol (Suppl) 73:651, 1984.

630. Seltzer J, Bigby BG, Stulbarg M, et al: O₃-induced change in bronchial reactivity to methacholine and airway inflammation in humans. J Appl Physiol 60:1321, 1986.

631. Hinson JM Jr, Hutchinson AA, Brigham KL, et al: Effects of granulocyte depletion on pulmonary responsiveness to aerosol histamine. J Appl Physiol 56:411, 1984.

632. Heaton RW, Henderson AF, Dunlop LS, et al: The influence of pretreatment with prostaglandin-F₂-alpha on bronchial sensitivity to inhaled histamine and methacholnine in normal subjects. Br J Dis Chest 78:168, 1984.

633. Fuller RW, Dixon CM, Dollery CT, et al: Prostaglandin D₂ potentiates airway responsiveness to histamine and methacholine. Am Rev Respir Dis 133:252, 1986.

634. Walters EH: Prostaglandins and the control of airways responses to histamine in normal and asthmatic subjects. Thorax 38:188, 1983.

635. Flavahan NA, Aarhus LL, Rimele TJ, et al: Respiratory epithelium inhibits bronchial smooth muscle tone. J Appl Physiol 58:834, 1985.

636. Mazzoni L, Morely J, Page CP, et al: Induction of airway hyperreactivity by platelet activating factor in the guinea pig. J Physiol 365:107, 1985.

637. Cuss FM, Dixon CM, Barnes PJ: Effects of inhaled platelet activating factor on pulmonary function and bronchial responsiveness in man. Lancet 2:189, 1986.

638. Griffin MP, Macdonald N, McFadden ER: Short-term and long-term effects of cromolyn sodium on the airway reactivity of asthmatics. J Allergy Clin Immunol 71:331, 1983.

639. Löwhagen O, Rak S: Modification of bronchial hyperreactivity after treatment with sodium cromoglycate during pollen season. J Allergy Clin Immunol 75:460, 1985.

640. Löwhagen O, Rak S: Bronchial hyperreactivity after treatment with sodium cromoglycate in atopic asthmatic patients not exposed to relevant allergens. J Allergy Clin Immunol 75:343, 1985.

641. Ryan G, Latimer KM, Juniper EF, et al: Effect of beclomethasone dipropionate on bronchial responsiveness to histamine in controlled nonsteroid-dependent astham. J Allergy Clin Immunol 75:25, 1985.

642. Easton JG: Effect of an inhaled corticosteroid on methacholine airway reactivity. J Allergy Clin Immunol 67:388, 1981.

643. Bhagat RG, Grunstein M: Effect of corticosteroids on bronchial responsiveness to methacholine in asthmatic children. Am Rev Respir Dis 131:902, 1985.

644. Svedmyr N: Airway hyperreactivity. Clinical treatment with drugs. In Simonsson BG (ed): Airway Hyperreactivity. Eur J Respir Dis (Suppl 131) 64:313, 1983.

645. Killian D, Cockcroft DW, Hargreave FE, et al: Factors in allergen induced asthma: Relevance of the intensity of the airways allergic reaction and non-specific bronchial reactivity. Clin Allergy 6:219, 1976.

646. Cockcroft DW, Ruffin RE, Frith PA, et al: Determinants of allergen-induced asthma: Dose of allergen, circulating IgE antibody concentration, and bronchial responsiveness to inhaled histamine. Am Rev Respir Dis 120:1053, 1979.

647. Neijens HJ, Degenhart HC, Raatgeep HC, et al: Study on the significance of bronchial hyperreactivity in the bronchceal obstruction after inhalation of cat dander allergen. J Allergy Clin Immunol 64:507, 1979.

648. Nathan RA, Kinsman RA, Spector SL, et al: Relationship between airways response to allergens and nonspecific bronchial reactivity. J Allergy Clin Immunol 64:491, 1979.

649. Stuckey MS, Witt CS, Schmitt LH, et al: Histamine sensitivity influences reactivity to allergens. J Allergy Clin Immunol 373:75, 1985.

650. Schlueter DP, Soto RJ, Baretta ED, et al: Airway response to hair spray in normal subjects and subjects with hyperreactive airways. Chest 75:544, 1979.

651. Smith P, Stitik F, Smith J, et al: Tantalum inhalation and airway responses. Thorax 34:486, 1979.

652. Hargreave FE, Ryan G, Thomson NC, et al: Bronchial responsiveness to histamine or methacholine in asthma: Measurement and clinical significance. Eur J Respir Dis 63:79, 1982.

653. Hargreave FE, Ramsdale H, Dolovich J: Measurement of airway responsiveness in clinical practice. In Hargreave FE, Woolcock AJ (eds): Airway Responsiveness: Measurement and Interpretation. Ontario, Astra Mississauga, 1985, p 122.

654. Corrao WM, Braman SS, Irwin RS: Chronic cough as the sole presenting manipulation of bronchial asthma. N Engl J Med 300:633, 1979.

655. Woolcock AJ: Tests of airway responsiveness in epidemiology. In Hargreave FE, Woolcock AJ (eds): Airway Responsiveness: Measurement and Interpretation. Ontario, Astra Mississauga, 1985, p 136.

656. Woolcock AJ, Yan K, Salome CM: Effect of therapy on bronchial hyperresponsiveness in the long-term management of asthma. Clin Allergy 18:165, 1988.

657. Chan-Yeung M, Lam S, Tse KS: Measurement of airway responsiveness in occupational asthma. In Hargreave FE, Woolcock AJ (eds): Airway Responsiveness: Measurement and Interpretation. Ontario, Astra Mississauga, 1985, p 129.

658. Crawford ABH, Makowska M, Engel LA: Effect of normal bronchomotor tone on static mechanical properties of the lung and ventilation distribution in man. J Appl Physiol 63:2278, 1987.

659. Detroyer A, Yernault JC, Rodenstein D: Effects of vagal blockade on lung mechanics in normal man. J Appl Physiol 46:217, 1979.

660. Williams MH Jr: Why do the airways contain smooth muscle? Lung 159:291, 1981.

661. Wide L, Bennich H, Johansson SGO: Diagnosis of allergy by an in-vitro test for allergen antibodies. Lancet 2:1105, 1967.

662. Freedman SO: New perspectives in allergic asthma. Can Med Assoc J 114:346, 1976.

663. Ishizaka K, Ishizaka T, Hornbrook MM: Physio-chemical properties of reaginic antibody. V. Correlation of reaginic activity with γ E-globulin antibody. J Immunol 97:840, 1966.

664. Turner-Warwick M: Advances in asthma: Hypersensitivity mechanisms. Br Med J 4:355, 1969.

665. Warren CPW, Tse KS: Serum and sputum immunoglobulin E levels in respiratory diseases in adults. Can Med Assoc J 110:425, 1974.

666. McNichol KN, Williams HE: Spectrum of asthma in children. 2. Allergic components Br Med J 4:12, 1973.

667. Kay AB, Bacon GD, Mercer BA, et al: Complement components and IgE in bronchial asthma. Lancet 2:916, 1974.

668. Barbee RA, Halonen M, Lebowitz M, et al: Distribution of IgE in a community population sample—correlations with age, sex, and allergen skin test reactivity. J Allergy Clin Immunol 68:106, 1981.

669. Pepys J, Hutchcroft BJ: Bronchial provocation tests in etiologic diagnosis and analysis of asthma. Am Rev Respir Dis 112:829, 1975.

670. Bryant DH: Role of IgG in human asthma. In Austen KF, Lichtenstein LM (eds): Asthma—Physiology, Immunopharmacology and Treatment, Vol. II. New York, Academic Press, 1977, p 315.

671. Barbee RA, Lebowitz MD, Thompson HC, et al: Immediate skin-test reactivity in a general population sample. Ann Intern Med 84:129, 1976.

672. Hagy GW, Settipane GA: Bronchial asthma, allergic rhinitis, and allergy skin tests among college students. J Allergy 44:323, 1969.

673. Curran WS, Goldman G: The incidence of immediately reacting allergy skin tests in a "normal" adult population. Ann Intern Med 55:777, 1961.

674. Buisseret PD: Seasonal allergic symptoms due to fungal spores. Br Med J 2:507, 1976.

675. Chatterjee J, Hargreave FE: Atmospheric pollen and fungal spores in Hamilton in 1972 estimated by the Hirst automatic volumetric spore trap. Can Med Assoc J 110:659, 1974.

676. Ordman D: Seasonal respiratory allergy in Windhoek: The pollen and fungus factors. S Afr Med J 44:250, 1970.

677. Kabe J, Aoki Y, Ishizaki T, et al: Relationship of dermal and pulmonary sensitivity to extracts of Candida albicans. Am Rev Respir Dis 104:348, 1971.

678. Pepys J, Faux JA, Longbottom JO, et al: Candida albicans precipitins in respiratory disease in man. J Allergy 41:305, 1968.

679. Rosenberg GL, Rosenthal RR, Norman PS: Inhalation challenge with ragweed pollen in ragweed-sensitive asthmatics. J Allergy Clin Immunol 71:302, 1983.

680. Salvaggio J, Aukrust L: Mold-induced asthma. J Allergy Clin Immunol 68:327, 1981.

681. Licorish K, Novey HS, Kozak P, et al: Role of alternaria and penicillium spores in the pathogenesis of asthma. J Allergy Clin Immunol 76:819, 1985.

682. Kern RA: Asthma due to sensitization to a mushroom fly (Aphiochaeta agarici). J Allergy 9:604, 1938.

683. Truitt GW: The mushroom fly as a cause of bronchial asthma. Ann Allergy 9:513, 1951.

684. Maunsell K, Wraith DG, Cunnington AM: Mites and house-dust allergy in bronchial asthma. Lancet 1:1267, 1968.

685. Leading article: Mites and asthma. Lancet 1:1295, 1968.

686. Gaddie J, Skinner C, Palmer KNV: Hyposensitization with house dust mite vaccine in bronchial asthma. Br Med J 2:561, 1976.

687. Blythe ME, Al Ubaydi F, Williams JD, et al: Study of dust mites in three Birmingham hospitals. Br Med J 1:62, 1976.

688. Brown H, Morrow, Filer JL: Role of mites in allergy to house dust. Br Med J 3:646, 1968.

689. Pepys J, Chan M, Hargreave FE: Mites and house-dust allergy. Lancet 1:1270, 1968.

690. Pauli G, Bessot JC, Hirth C, et al: Dissociation of house dust allergies—A comparison between skin tests, inhalation tests, specific IgE and basophil histamine release measurements. J Allergy Clin Immunol 63:245, 1979.

691. Parker CW: Drug therapy: Drug allergy (third of three parts). N Engl J Med 292:957, 1975.

692. Barr SE: Allergy to Hymenoptera stings. JAMA 228:718, 1974.

693. Welch H, Lewis CN, Weinstein HI, et al: Severe reactions to antibiotics: A nationwide survey. Antibiot Med Clin Ther 4:800, 1957.

694. Bernstein IL, Ausdenmoore RW: Iatrogenic bronchospasm occurring during clinical trials of a new mucolytic agent, acetylcysteine. Dis Chest 46:469, 1964.

695. Raskin P: Bronchospasm after inhalation of pancreatic dornase. Am Rev Respir Dis 98:697, 1968.

696. Miller WC, Awe R: Effect of nebulized lidocaine on reactive airways. Am Rev Respir Dis 111:739, 1975.

697. Sheffer AL, Rocklin RE, Goetzl EJ: Immunologic components of hypersensitivity reactions to cromolyn sodium. N Engl J Med 293:1220, 1975.

698. Peterson IA, Grant IWB, Crompton GK: Severe bronchoconstriction provoked by sodium cromoglycate. Br Med J 2:916, 1976.

699. Bryant DH, Pepys J: Bronchial reactions to aerosol inhalant vehicle. Br Med J 1:1319, 1976.

700. Austen KF: Current concepts: Systemic anaphylaxis in the human being. N Engl J Med 291:661, 1974.

701. Routledge RC, De Kretser DMH, Wadsworth LD: Severe anaphylaxis due to passive sensitization by donor blood. Br Med J 1:434, 1976.

702. Ramirez MA: Horse asthma following blood transfusion. Report of a case. JAMA 73:984, 1919.

703. Lewis PJ, Austen KF: Fatal systemic anaphylaxis in man. N Engl J Med 270:597, 1964.

704. Hanashiro PK, Weil MH: Anaphylactic shock in man. Report of two cases with detailed hemodynamic and metabolic studies. Arch Intern Med 119:129, 1967.

705. Hendrick DJ, Davies RJ, D'Souza MF, et al: An analysis of skin prick test reactions in 656 asthmatic patients. Thorax 30:2, 1975.

706. Gaspary EA, Feinmann EL, Field EJ: Lymphocyte sensitization in asthma with special reference to nature and identity of intrinsic form. Br Med J 1:19, 1973.

707. Enerbäck L, Pipkorn U, Granerus G: Intraepithelial migration of nasal mucosal mast cells in hay fever. Int Arch Allergy Appl Immunol 80:44, 1986.

708. Kawabori S, Okuda M, Unno T, et al: Dynamics of mast cell degranulation in human allergic nasal epithelium after provocation with allergen. Clin Allergy 15:509, 1985.

709. Cockcroft DW, Hoeppner VH, Werner GD: Recurrent nocturnal asthma after bronchoprovocation with western red cedar sawdust: Association with acute increases in nonallergic bronchial responsiveness. Clin Allergy 14:61, 1984.

710. Wanner A, Russi E, Brodnan J, et al: Prolonged bronchial obstruction after a single antigen challenge in ragweed asthma. J Allergy Clin Immunol 76:177, 1985.

711. Kaliner M: Hypotheses on the contribution of late-phase allergic responses to the understanding and treatment of allergic disease. J Allergy Clin Immunol 73:311, 1984.

712. Durham SR, Lee TH, Cromwell O, et al: Immunologic studies in allergen-induced late-phase asthmatic reactions. J Allergy Clin Immunol 74:49, 1984.

713. Machado L, Stålenheim G, Malmberg P: Early and late allergic bronchial reactions: Physiological characteristics. Clin Allergy 16:111, 1986.

714. Gleich GJ: The late phase of the immunoglobulin-E-mediated reaction—a link between anaphylaxis and common allergic disease. J Allergy Clin Immunol 70:160, 1982.

715. Lam S, LeRiche J, Phillips D, et al: Cellular and protein changes in bronchial lavage fluid after late asthmatic reaction in patients with red cedar asthma. J Allergy Clin Immunol 80:44, 1987.

716. Hogg JC: The pathology of asthma. Chest 87:152S, 1985.

717. Widdicombe JG: Reflex control of tracheobronchial smooth muscle in experimental and human asthma. In Austen KF, Lichtenstein LM (eds): Asthma—Physiology, Immunopharmacology and Treatment, Vol II. New York, Academic Press, 1977, p 225.

718. Allen DH, Mathison DA, Wagner PD, et al: Mediator release during allergen-induced bronchconstriction in asthmatic subjects. Chest 75:235, 1979.

719. Chiesa A, Dain D, Meyers GL, et al: Histamine release during antigen inhalation in experimental asthma in dogs. Am Rev Respir Dis 111:148, 1975.

720. Kang B, Townley RG, Lee CK, et al: Bronchial reactivity to histamine before and after sodium cromoglycate in bronchial asthma. Br Med J 1:867, 1976.

721. Laitinen LA, Empey DW, Poppius R, et al: Effects of intravenous histamine on static lung compliance and airway resistance in normal man. Am Rev Respir Dis 114:291, 1976.

722. Bleecker ER, Cotton DJ, Fischer SP, et al: The mechanism of rapid, shallow breathing after inhaling histamine aerosol in exercising dogs. Am Rev Respir Dis 114:909, 1976.

723. Guz A: Control of ventilation in man with special reference to abnormalities in asthma. In Austen KF, Lichtenstein LM (eds): Asthma—Physiology, Immunopharmacology and Treatment, Vol II. New York, Academic Press, 1977, p 211.

724. Kaliner M: Human lung tissue and anaphylaxis: The effects of histamine on the immunologic release of mediators. Am Rev Respir Dis 118:1015, 1978.

725. Platshon LF, Kaliner M: The effects of immunologic release of histamine upon human lung cyclic nucleotide levels and prostaglandin generation. J Clin Invest 62:1113, 1979.

726. Long WM, Sprung CL, El Fawal H, et al: Effects of histamine on bronchial artery blood flow and bronchomotor tone. J Appl Physiol 59:254, 1985.

727. White J, Eiser NM: The role of histamine and its receptors in the pathogenesis of asthma. Br J Dis Chest 77:215, 1983.

728. Popa VT: Effect of an H_1 blocker, chlorpheniramine, on inhalation tests with histamine and allergen in allergic asthma. Chest 78:442, 1980.

729. O'Driscoll BRC, Lee TH, Cromwell O, et al: Immunologic release of neutrophil chemotactic activity from human lung tissue. J Allergy Clin Immunol 72:695, 1983.

730. Aitkins PC, Norman ME, Zweiman B: Antigen-induced neutrophil chemotactic activity in man—correlation with bronchospasm and inhibition by disodium cromoglycate. J Allergy Clin Immunol 62:149, 1978.

731. Nagy L: Serum neutrophil chemotactic activity and leukocyte count after house dust induced bronchospasm. Eur J Respir Dis 62.198, 1981

732. Nagy L, Lee TH, Kay AB: Neutrophil chemotactic activity in antigen-induced late asthmatic reactions. N Engl J Med 306:497, 1982.

733. Metzger WJ, Richerson HB, Wasserman SI: Generation and partial characterization of eosinophil chemotactic activity and neutrophil chemotactic activity during early and late-phase asthmatic response. J Allergy Clin 78:282, 1986.

734. Lee TH, Kay AB: Bronchial asthma and the neutrophil chemotactic factor. Clin Allergy 12:39, 1982.

735. Durham SR, Carroll M, Walsh GM, et al: Leukocyte activation in allergen-induced late-phase asthmatic reactions. N Engl J Med 311:1398, 1984.

736. Kay AB: Basic mechanisms in allergic asthma. Eur J Respir Dis 63:9, 1982.

737. Wasserman SI, Center DM: The relevance of neutrophil chemotactic factors to allergic disease. J Allergy Clin Immunol 64:231, 1979.

738. Morley J, Sanjar S, Page C: The platelet in asthma. Lancet 2:1142, 1984.

739. Basran GS, Page CP, Paul W, et al: Platelet-activating factor: A possible mediator of the dual response to allergen? Clin Allergy 14:75, 1984.

740. Ind P, Peters A, Malik F, et al: Pulmonary platelet kinetics in asthma. Thorax 40:412, 1985.

741. Taytard A, Guenard H, Vuillemin L, et al: Platelet kinetics in stable atopic asthmatic patients. Am Rev Respir Dis 134:983, 1986.

742. Taytard A, Guenard H, Vuillemin L, et al: Platelet kinetics in stable atopic asthmatic patients. Am Rev Respir Dis 134:983, 1986.

743. Newball HH, Berninger RW, Talamo RC, et al: Anaphylactic release of a basophil kallikrein-like activity. 1. Purification and characterization. J Clin Invest 64:457, 1979.

744. Newball HH, Talamo RC, Lichtenstein LM: Anaphylactic release of a basophil kallikrein-like activity: A mediator of immediate hypersensitivity reactions. J Clin Invest 64:466, 1979.

745. Fuller RW, Dixon CM, Cuss FM, et al: Bradykinin-induced bronchoconstriction in humans. Mode of action. Am Rev Respir Dis 135:176, 1987.

746. Walters EH, Davies BH: Dual effect of prostaglandin E_2 on normal airways smooth muscle in vivo. Thorax 37:918, 1982.

747. Mathé AA, Hedqvist P: Effect of prostaglandins F_2 alpha and E_2 on airway conductance in healthy subjects and asthmatic patients. Am Rev Respir Dis 111:313, 1975.

748. Cuthbert MF: Effect on airways resistance of prostaglandin E_1 given by aerosol to healthy and asthmatic volunteers. Br Med J 4:723, 1969.

749. Smith AP, Cuthbert MF: Antagonistic action of aerosols of prostaglandins $F_2\alpha$ and E_2 on bronchial muscle tone in man. Br Med J 3:212, 1972.

750. Mathé AA, Hedqvist P, Holmgren A, et al: Bronchial hyperreactivity to prostaglandin $F_2\alpha$ and histamine in patients with asthma. Br Med J 1:193, 1973.

11

751. Fish HE, Newball HH, Norman PS, et al: Novel effects of PGF₂ on airway function in asthmatic subjects. J Appl Physiol 54:105, 1983.
752. Fish JE, Jameson LS, Albright A, et al: Modulation of the bronchomotor effects of chemical mediators by prostaglandin-F₂-alpha in asthmatic subjects. Am Rev Respir Dis 130:571, 1985.
753. Newball HH, Keiser HR, Lenfant C: Prostaglandin F-2-alpha functions as a local hormone on human airways. Respir Physiol 41:183, 1980.
754. Weir EK, Greer BE, Smith SC, et al: Bronchoconstriction and pulmonary hypertension during abortion induced by 15-methylprostaglandin F₂-alpha and histamine in patients with asthma. Am J Med 60:556, 1976.
755. Hardy CC, Robinson C, Tattersfield AE, et al: The bronchoconstrictor effect of inhaled prostaglandin D₂ in normal and asthmatic men. N Engl J Med 311:209, 1984.
756. Austen KF, Orange RP: Bronchial asthma: The possible role of the chemical mediators of immediate hypersensitivity in the pathogenesis of subacute chronic disease. Am Rev Respir Dis 112:423, 1975.
757. Green K, Hedqvist P, Svanborg N: Increased plasma levels of 15-keto-13,14-dihydro-prostaglandin F₂α after allergen-provoked asthma in man. Lancet 2:1419, 1974.
758. Patel KR: Atropine, sodium cromoglycate, and thymoxamine in PGF₂α-induced bronchoconstriction in extrinsic asthma. Br Med J 2:360, 1975.
759. Fish JE, Ankin MG, Adkinson NF, et al: Indomethacin modification of immediate-type immunologic airway responses in allergic asthmatic and non-asthmatic subjects: evidence for altered arachidonic acid metabolism in asthma. Am Rev Respir Dis 123:609, 1981.
760. Parker CW: Aspirin-sensitive asthma. In Lichtenstein LM, Austen KF (eds): Asthma—Physiology, Immunopharmacology and Treatment, Vol II. New York, Academic Press, 1977, p 301.
761. Szczeklik A, Grylglewski RJ, Czerniawska-Mysik G: Relationship of inhibition of prostaglandin biosynthesis by analgesics to asthma attacks in aspirin-sensitive patients. Br Med J 1:67, 1975.
762. Robinson C, Holgate S: New perspectives on the putative role of eicosanoids in airway hyperresponsiveness. J Allergy Clin Immunol 76:140, 1985.
763. Lewis RA, Robin JL: Arachidonic acid derivatives as mediators of asthma. J Allergy Clin Immunol 76:259, 1985.
764. Lewis RA: A presumptive role for leukotrienes in obstructive airways diseases. Chest 88:98S, 1985.
765. Creticos PS, Peters SP, Adkinson NF Jr, et al: Peptide leukotriene release after antigen challenge in patients sensitive to ragweed. N Engl J Med 310:1626, 1984.
766. MacGlashan DW, Schleimer RP, Peters SP, et al: Generation of leukotrienes by purified human lung mast cells. J Clin Invest 70:747, 1982.
767. Delehunt JC, Perruchoud AP, Yerger L, et al: The role of slow-reacting substance of anaphylaxis in the late bronchial response after antigen challenge in allergic sheep. Am Rev Respir Dis 130:748, 1984.
768. Smith LJ, Greenberger PA, Patterson R, et al: The effect of inhaled leukotriene-D₄ in humans. Am Rev Respir Dis 131:368, 1985.
769. Griffin M, Weiss JW, Leitch AG, et al: Effects of leukotriene D on the airways in asthma. N Engl J Med 308:436, 1983.
770. Barnes NC, Piper PJ, Costello JF: Comparative effects of inhaled leukotriene C₄ and histamine in normal human subjects. Thorax 39:500, 1984.
771. Glovsky MM, Nagata S, Schellenberg RR, et al: Are products of complement activation C₃a and C₅a relevant factors in bronchial asthma? Chest 87:169S, 1985.
772. Stevens WJ, Bridts CH: IgG-containing and IgE-containing circulating immune complexes in patients with asthma and rhinitis. J Allergy Clin Immunol 73:276, 1984.
773. Stewart RM, Weir EK, Montgomery MR, et al: Hydrogen peroxide contracts airway smooth muscle: A possible endogenous mechanism. Respir Physiol 45:333, 1981.
774. Fuller RW, Dixon CMS, Barnes PJ: Bronchconstrictor response to inhaled capsaicin in humans. J Appl Physiol 58:1080, 1985.
775. Findlay SR, Lichtenstein LM: Basophil "releasability" in patients with asthma. Am Rev Respir Dis 122:53, 1980.
776. Gaddy JN, Busse WW: Enhanced IgE-dependent basophil histamine release and airway reactivity in asthma. Am Rev Respir Dis 134:969, 1986.
777. Joseph M, Tonnel AB, Jorfier G, et al: Involvement of immunoglobulin E in the secretory processes of alveolar macrophages from asthmatic subjects. J Clin Invest 71:221, 1983.
778. Aubas P, Cosso B, Godard P, et al: Decreased suppressor cell activity of alveolar macrophages in bronchial asthma. Am Rev Respir Dis 130:875, 1984.
779. Arnoux B, Joseph M, Simoes MH, et al: Antigenic release of pafacether and beta-glucuronidase from alveolar macrophages of asthmatics. Bull Eur Physiopathol Respir 23:119, 1987.
780. Schulman ES, Liu MC, Proud D, et al: Human lung macrophages induce histamine release from basophils and mast cells. Am Rev Respir Dis 131:230, 1985.
781. Martin TR, Altman LC, Albert RK, et al: Leukotriene-B₄ production by the human alveolar macrophage—A potential mechanism for amplifying inflammation in the lung. Am Rev Respir Dis 129:106, 1984.
782. Dahl R, Venge P: Role of the eosinophil in bronchial asthma. Eur J Respir Dis 63:23, 1982.
783. Dahl R, Venge P, Olsson I: Variations of blood eosinophils and eosinophil cationic protein in serum in patients with bronchial asthma, studies during inhalation challenge test. Allergy 33:211, 1978.
784. Ayars GH, Altman LC, Gleich GJ: Eosinophil and eosinophil granule-mediated pneumocyte injury. J Allergy Clin Immunol 76:595, 1985.
785. Taniguchi WJ, Mita W, Saito H: Increased generation of leukotriene C₄ from eosinophils in asthmatic patients. Allergy 40:571, 1985.
786. Godard P, Chaintreuil J, Damon M, et al: Functional assessment of alveolar macrophages—comparison of cells from asthmatics and normal subjects. J Allergy Clin Immunol 70:88, 1982.
787. Frigas E, Loegering DA, Solley GO, et al: Elevated levels of the eosinophil granule major basic protein in the sputum of patients with bronchial asthma. Mayo Clin Proc 56:345, 1981.
788. Diaz P, Galleguillos FR, Gonzalez MC, et al: Bronchoalveolar lavage in asthma—the effect of disodium cromoglycate (Cromolyn) on leukocyte counts, immunoglobulins, and complement. J Allergy Clin Immunol 74:41, 1984.
789. Fukuda T, Dunnette SL, Reed CE, et al: Increased numbers of hypodense eosinophils in the blood of patients with bronchial asthma. Am Rev Respir Dis 132:981, 1985.
790. Gin W, Kay AB: The effect of corticosteroids on monocyte and neutrophil activation in bronchial asthma. J Allergy Clin Immunol 76:675, 1985.
791. Neijens H, Raatgeep R, Degenhart H, et al: Altered leukocyte response in relation to the basic abnormality in children with asthma and bronchial hyperresponsiveness. Am Rev Respir Dis 130:744, 1984.
792. Carroll MP, Durham SR, Walsh G, et al: Activation of neutrophils and monocytes after allergen-induced and histamine-induced bronchoconstriction. J Allergy Clin Immunol 75:290, 1985.
793. Summary and recommendations of a workshop on the investigative use of fiberoptic bronchoscopy and bronchoalveolar lavage in asthmatics. Am Rev Respir Dis 132:180, 1985.
794. Metzger WJ, Richarson HB, Worden K, et al: Bronchoalveolar lavage of allergic asthmatic patients following allergen broncho-provocation. Chest 89:477, 1986.
795. Lam S, Leriche JC, Kijek K, et al: Effect of bronchial lavage volume on cellular and protein recovery. Chest 88:856, 1985.
796. Metzger WJ, Zavala D, Richerson HB, et al: Local allergen challenge and bronchoalveolar lavage of allergic asthmatic lungs. Description of the model and local airway inflammation. Am Rev Respir Dis 135:433, 1987.
797. Valenti S, Crimi E, Brusasco V: Bronchial provocation tests with RAST-standardized allergens and dosimetric technique. Respiration 48:97, 1985.
798. Mjörndal TO, Chesrown SE, Frey MJ, et al: Effect of beta-adrenergic stimulation on experimental canine anaphylaxis in vivo. J Allergy Clin Immunol 71:62, 1983.
799. Howarth PH, Durham SR, Lee TH, et al: Influence of albuterol, cromolyn sodium and ipratropium bromide on the airway and circulating mediator responses to allergen bronchial provocation in asthma. Am Rev Respir Dis 132:986, 1985.
800. Schleimer RP, Schulman ES, MacGlashan DW, et al: Effects of dexamethasone on mediator release from human lung fragments and purified human lung mast cells. J Clin Invest 71:1830, 1983.
801. Borum P, Mygind N: Inhibition of the immediate allergic reaction in the nose by the beta-2 adrenostimulant fenoterol. J Allergy Clin Immunol 66:25, 1980.
802. Spector SL: Effect of a selective beta-2 adrenergic agonist and theophylline on skin test reactivity and cardiovascular parameters. J Allergy Clin Immunol 64:23, 1979.
803. Imbeau SA, Harruff R, Hirscher M, et al: Terbutaline's effects on the allergy skin test. J Allergy Clin Immunol 62:193, 1978.
804. Eggleston PA, Kagey-Sobotka A, Schleimer RP, et al: Interaction between hyperosmolar and IgE-mediated histamine release from basophil and mast cells. Am Rev Respir Dis 130:86, 1984.
805. Anderson SD: Exercise induced asthma. In Allergy: Principles and Practice. St. Louis, CV Mosby, 1986.
806. Lockhart A, Régnard J, Dessanges JF, et al: State of the art: Exercise and hyperventilation induced asthma. Bull Eur Physiopathol Res 21:399, 1985.
807. Schachter EN, Kreisman H, Littner M, et al: Airway responses to exercise in mild asthmatics. J Allergy Clin Immunol 61:390, 1978.

808. Hasegawa M, Kabasawa Y, Ohki M, et al: Exercise-induced change of nasal resistance in asthmatic children. Otolaryngol Head Neck Surg 93:772, 1985.

809. Voy RO: The U.S. Olympic Committee experience with exercise-induced bronchospasm, 1984. Med Sci Sports Exerc 18:328, 1986.

810. Weiler JM, Metzger WJ, Donnelly AL, et al: Prevalence of bronchial hyperresponsiveness in highly trained athletes. Chest 90:23, 1986.

811. Mansfield L, McDonnell J, Morgan W, et al: Airway response in asthmatic children during and after exercise. Respiration 38:135, 1979.

812. Stirling DR, Cotton DJ, Graham BL, et al: Characteristics of airway tone during exercise in patients with asthma. J Appl Physiol 54:934, 1983.

813. Warren JB, Jennings SJ, Clark TJH: Effect of adrenergic and vagal blockade on the normal human airway response to exercise. Clin Sci 66:79, 1984.

814. König P, Godfrey S: Prevalence of exercise-induced bronchial lability in families of children with asthma. Arch Dis Child 48:513, 1973.

815. Lee TH, Anderson SD: Editorial: Heterogeneity of mechanisms in exercise induced asthma. Thorax 40:481, 1985.

816. McFadden ER, Soter NA, Ingram RH: Magnitude and site of airway response to exercise in asthmatics in relation to arterial histamine levels. J Allergy Clin Immunol 66:472, 1980.

817. Neijens HJ, Gargani G, Kralingen A, et al: Central versus peripheral airway obstruction in bronchial responsiveness due to exercise. Eur J Respir Dis 63:105, 1982.

818. McFadden ER Jr, Ingram RH Jr: Large and small airway effects with exercise and other bronchoconstrictor stimuli. Eur J Respir Dis 63:99, 1982.

819. Spiro SG, Bierman CW, Petheram IS: Reproducibility of flow rates measured with low density gas mixtures in exercise-induced bronchospasm. Thorax 36:852, 1981.

820. Chen WY, Horton DJ, Souhrada JF: Respiratory heat and water loss and exercise-induced asthma. Physiologist 19:152, 1976.

821. Chen WY, Horton DJ: Heat and water loss from the airways and exercise induced asthma. Respiration 34:305, 1977.

822. Strauss RH, McFadden ER, Ingram RH: Enhancement of exercise induced asthma by cold air. N Engl J Med 297:743, 1977.

823. Strauss RH, McFadden ER, Ingram RH, et al: Influence of heat and humidity on airway obstruction induced by exercise in asthma. J Clin Invest 61:433, 1978.

824. Deal EC Jr, McFadden ER Jr, Ingram RH Jr, et al: Role of respiratory heat exchange in production of exercise-induced asthma. J Appl Physiol 46:467, 1979.

825. Deal EC, McFadden ER, Ingram RH, et al: Hyperpnea and heat flux: Initial reaction sequence in exercise-induced asthma. J Appl Physiol 46:476, 1979.

826. Zeballos RJ, Shturman-Ellstein R, McNally JF Jr, et al: The role of hyperventilation in exercise-induced bronchoconstriction. Am Rev Respir Dis 118:877, 1978.

827. Tweeddale PM, Godden DJ, Grant IWB: Hyperventilation or exercise to induce asthma? Thorax 36:596, 1981.

828. Smith CM, Anderson SD: Hyperosmolarity as the stimulus to asthma induced by hyperventilation? J Allergy Clin Immunol 77:729, 1986.

829. Kivity S, Souhrada JP, Melzer E: A dose-response-like relationship between minute ventilation and exercise-induced bronchoconstriction in young asthmatic patients. Eur J Respir Dis 61:342, 1980.

830. Mahler DA, Loke J: Lung function after marathon running at warm and cold ambient temperatures. Am Rev Respir Dis 124:154, 1981.

831. McFadden ER, Ingram RH: Exercise-induced airway obstruction. Annu Rev Physiol 45:453, 1983.

832. McFadden ER, Denison DM, Waller JF, et al: Direct recordings of the temperatures in the tracheobronchial tree in normal man. J Clin Invest 69:700, 1982.

833. Baile EM, Dahlby RW, Wiggs BR, et al: Role of tracheal and bronchial circulation in respiratory heat exchange. J Appl Physiol 58:217, 1985.

834. McFadden ER Jr: Respiratory heat and water exchange: Physiological and clinical implications. J Appl Physiol 54:331, 1983.

835. Deal EC, McFadden ER, Ingram RH Jr, et al: Esophageal temperature during exercise in asthmatic and nonasthmatic subjects. J Appl Physiol 46:484, 1979.

836. McFadden ER Jr, Pichurko BM, Bowman HF, et al: Thermal mapping of the airways in humans. J Appl Physiol 58:564, 1985.

837. McFadden ER, Ingram RJ Jr: Exercise-induced asthma: Observations on the initiating stimulus. N Engl J Med 301:763, 1979.

838. Anderson SD, Shoeffel RE, Follet R, et al: Sensitivity to heat and water loss at rest and during exercise in asthmatic patients. Eur J Respir Dis 63:459, 1982.

839. Shturman-Ellstein R, Zeballos RJ, Buckley JM, et al: The beneficial effect of nasal breathing on exercise-induced bronchoconstriction. Am Rev Respir Dis 118:65, 1978.

840. Griffin MP, McFadden ER, Ingram RH: Airway cooling in asthmatic and nonasthmatic subjects during nasal and oral breathing. J Allergy Clin Immunol 69:354, 1982.

841. Anderson SD: Is there a unifying hypothesis for exercise-induced asthma. J Allergy Clin Immunol 73(Suppl):660, 1984.

842. Hahn A, Anderson SD, Norton AR, et al: A reinterpretation of the effect of temperature and water content of the inspired air in exercise-induced asthma. Am Rev Respir Dis 130:575, 1985.

843. Sheppard D, Eschenbacher WL: Respiratory water loss as a stimulus to exercise-induced bronchoconstriction. J Allergy Clin Immunol 73(Suppl):640, 1984.

844. Eschenbacher W, Sheppard D: Respiratory heat loss is not the sole stimulus for bronchoconstriction induced by isocapnic hyperpnea with dry air. Am Rev Respir Dis 131:894, 1985.

845. Foresi A, Mattoli S, Corbo GM, et al: Comparison of bronchial responses to ultrasonically nebulized distilled water, exercise, and methacholine in asthma. Chest 90:822, 1986.

846. Aitken ML, Marini JJ: Effect of heat delivery and extraction on airway conductance in normal and in asthmatic subjects. Am Rev Respir Dis 131:357, 1985.

847. Deal EC, Wasserman SI, Soter NA, et al: Evaluation of role played by mediators of immediate hypersensitivity in exercise-induced asthma. J Clin Invest 65:659, 1980.

848. Lee TH, Nagakura T, Cromwell O, et al: Neutrophil chemotactic activity and histamine in atopic and nonatopic subjects after exercise-induced asthma. Am Rev Respir Dis 129:409, 1984.

849. Anderson SD, Bye PTP, Shoeffel RE, et al: Arterial plasma histamine levels at rest, and during and after exercise in patients with asthma—effects of terbutaline aerosol. Thorax 36:259, 1981.

850. Lee TH, Brown MJ, Navy L, et al: Exercise-induced release of histamine and neutrophil chemotactic factor in atopic asthmatics. J Allergy Clin Immunol 70:73, 1982.

851. Lee TH, Nagakura T, Papageorgiou N, et al: Special problems—mediators in exercise-induced asthma. J Allergy Clin Immunol 73(Suppl):634, 1984.

852. Johnson CE, Belfield PW, Davis S, et al: Platelet activation during exercise induced asthma: Effect of prophylaxis with cromoglycate and salbutamol. Thorax 41:290, 1986.

853. Nagakura T, Lee TH, Assoufi BK, et al: Neutrophil chemotactic factor in exercise-induced and hyperventilation-induced asthma. Am Rev Respir Dis 128:294, 1983.

854. Nagy L: Serum neutrophil chemotactic activity and exercise induced asthma. Eur J Respir Dis 64:161, 1983.

855. Togias AG, Naclerio RM, Proud D, et al: Nasal challenge with cold, dry air results in release of inflammatory mediators. Possible mast cell involvement. J Clin Invest 76:1375, 1985.

856. Findlay SR, Dvorak AM, Kagey-Sobotka A, et al: Hyperosmolar triggering of histamine release from human basophils. J Clin Invest 67:1604, 1981.

857. Flint KC, Hudspith BN, Leung KBP, et al: The hyperosmolar release of histamine from bronchoalveolar mast cells and its inhibition by sodium cromoglycate. Thorax 40:717, 1985.

858. Rimmer J, Bryant DH: Effect of hypo- and hyper-osmolarity on basophil histamine release. Clin Allergy 16:221, 1986.

859. Peters SP, Naclerio RM, Togias A, et al: In vitro and in vivo model systems for the study of allergic and inflammatory disorders in man. Chest 87:162S, 1985.

860. Sheffer AL, Soter ER, McFadden ER, et al: Exercise-induced anaphylaxis—a distinct form of physical allergy. J Allergy Clin Immunol 71:311, 1983.

861. Sheffer AL, Tong AKF, Murphy GF, et al: Exercise-induced anaphylaxis—a serious form of physical allergy associated with mast cell degranulation. J Allergy Clin Immunol 75:479, 1985.

862. Kidd JM, Cohen SH, Sosman AJ, et al: Food-dependent exercise-induced anaphylaxis. J Allergy Clin Immunol 71:407, 1983.

863. Soter NA, Wasserman SI, Austen FK, et al: Release of mast-cell mediators and alterations in lung function in patients with cholinergic urticaria. N Engl J Med 302:604, 1980.

864. Kahn RC: Humidification of the airways: adequate for function and integrity? Chest 84:510.

865. Fanta CH, McFadden ER Jr, Ingram RH Jr: Effects of cromolyn sodium on the response to respiratory heat loss in normal subjects. Am Rev Respir Dis 123:161, 1981.

866. Jones RM, Horn CR, Lee DV, et al: Bronchodilator effects of disodium cromoglycate in exercise-induced bronchoconstriction. Br J Dis Chest 77:362, 1983.

867. Breslin FJ, McFadden ER, Ingram RH Jr: The effects of cromolyn sodium on the airway responses to hyperapnea and cold air in asthma. Am Rev Respir Dis 122:11, 1980.

868. McNally JF Jr, Enright P, Hirsch JE, et al: The attenuation of exercise-induced bronchoconstriction by oropharyngeal anaesthesia. Am Rev Respir Dis 119:247, 1979.

869. Enright PL, McNally JF, Souhrada JF: Effect of lidocaine on the ventilatory and airway responses to exercise in asthmatics. Am Rev Respir Dis 122:823, 1980.

11

870. Fanta H, Ingram RH Jr, McFadden ER Jr: A reassessment of the effects of oropharyngeal anaesthesia in exercise-induced asthma. Am Rev Respir Dis 122:381, 1980.

871. Griffin MP, McFadden ER, Ingram RH, et al: Controlled-analysis of the effects of inhaled lignocaine in exercise-induced asthma. Thorax 37:741, 1982.

872. Deal EC, McFadden ER Jr, Ingram RH, et al: Effects of atropine on potentiation of exercise-induced bronchospasm by cold air. J Appl Physiol 45:238, 1978.

873. Griffin MP, Fung KF, Ingram RH Jr, et al: Dose-response effects of atropine on thermal stimulus-response relationships in asthma. J Appl Physiol 53:1576, 1982.

874. O'Byrne PM, Thomson NC, Morris M, et al: The protective effect of inhaled chlorpheniramine and atropine on bronchoconstriction stimulated by airway cooling. Am Rev Respir Dis 128:611, 1983.

875. Chen WY, Brenner AM, Weiser PC, et al: Atropine and exercise-induced bronchoconstriction. Chest 79:651, 1981.

876. Sheppard D, Epstein J, Holtzman MJ, et al: Effect of route of atropine delivery on bronchospasm from cold air and methacholine. J Appl Physiol 54:130, 1983.

877. Wilson NM, Barnes PJ, Vickers H, et al: Hyperventilation-induced asthma: Evidence for two mechanisms. Thorax 37:657, 1982.

878. Kerrebijn KF (ed): Pulmonary infection and antibiotic treatment in patients with cystic fibrosis. Chest (Suppl) 94:97S, 1988.

879. Souhrada M, Souhrada JF: The direct effect of temperature on airway smooth muscle. Respir Physiol 44:311, 1981.

880. Black JL, Armour CL, Shaw J: The effect of alteration in temperature on contractile responses in human airways in vitro. Respir Physiol 57:269, 1984.

881. McFadden ER, Lenner KAM, Strohl KP: Post-exertion at airway rewarming and thermally induced asthma: New insights into pathophysiology and possible pathogenesis. J Clin Invest 78:18, 1986.

882. Miller WS: The Lung. Springfield, Ill, Charles C Thomas, 1947, p 69.

883. Larsson K, Hjemdahl P, Martinsson A: Sympathoadrenal reactivity in exercise-induced asthma. Chest 82:561, 1982.

884. Hartley JPR, Davies CJ, Charles TJ, et al: Plasma cyclic nucleotide levels in exercise-induced asthma. Thorax 36:823, 1981.

885. Chryssanthopoulos C, Barboriak JJ, Fink JN, et al: Adrenergic responses of asthmatic and normal subjects to submaximal and maximal work levels. J Allergy Clin Immunol 61:17, 1978.

886. Schwartz S, Davies S, Juers JA: Life-threatening cold and exercise-induced asthma potentiated by administration of propranolol. Chest 78:100, 1980.

887. Edmunds AT, Tooley W, Godfrey S: The refractory period after exercise-induced asthma. Its duration and relation to the severity of exercise. Am Rev Respir Dis 117:247, 1978.

888. Haas F, Levin N, Pasierski S, et al: Reduced hyperpnea-induced bronchospasm following repeated cold air challenge. J Appl Physiol 61:210, 1986.

889. Weiler-Ravell D, Godfrey S: Do exercise-induced and antigen-induced asthma utilize the same pathways—antigen provocation in patients rendered refractory to exercise-induced asthma. J Allergy Clin Immunol 67:391, 1981.

890. Rosenthal RR, Laube B, Jaeger JJ: Methacholine sensitivity is unchanged during the refractory period following an exercise or isocapnic challenge. Am Rev Respir Dis 129:A250, 1984.

891. Hahn AG, Nograday SG, Tumulty D, et al: Histamine reactivity during the refractory period after exercise induced asthma. Thorax 39:919, 1984.

892. Lee TH, Belcher NG, Dalton N, et al: Serum neutrophil chemotactic activity (NCA) and plasma catecholamine concentrations in the refractory period after exercise-induced asthma. J Allergy Clin Immunol 77:164A, 1986.

893. Anderson SD, Schoeffel RE: Respiratory heat and water loss during exercise in patients with asthma—effect of repeated exercise challenge. Eur J Respir Dis 63:472, 1982.

894. Ben-Dov I, Gur I, Bar-Yishay E, et al: Refractory period following induced asthma: Contributions of exercise and isocapnic hyperventilation. Thorax 38:849, 1983.

895. Satake T, Kato M, Takagi K, et al: Role of prostaglandins in exercise-induced asthma. Adv Physiol Sci 10:369, 1981.

896. O'Byrne PM, Jones GL: The effect of indomethacin on exercise-induced bronchoconstriction and refractoriness after exercise. Am Rev Respir Dis 134:69, 1986.

897. Ben-Dov I, Bar-Yishay E, Godfrey S: Refractory period after exercise-induced asthma is unexplained by respiratory heat loss. Am Rev Respir Dis 125:530, 1982.

898. Bar-Yishay E, Godfrey S: Mechanisms of exercise-induced asthma. Lung 162:195, 1984.

899. Hahn A, Nograday S, Burton G, et al: Absence of refractoriness in asthmatic subjects after exercise with warm, humid inspirate. Thorax 40:418, 1985.

900. Tam E, Geffroy B, Myers D, et al: Effect of eucapnic hypoxia on bronchomotor tone and on the bronchomotor response to dry air in asthmatic subjects. Am Rev Respir Dis 132:690, 1985.

901. Schiffman PL, Ryan A, Whipp BJ, et al: Hyperoxic attenuation of exercise-induced bronchospasm in asthmatics. J Clin Invest 63:30, 1979.

902. Resnick AD, Deal EC, Ingram RH, et al: A critical assessment of the mechanism by which hyperoxia attenuates exercise-induced asthma. J Clin Invest 64:541, 1979.

903. Vecchiet L, Flacco L, Marini I, et al: Effects of cold stimulus of the chest wall on bronchial resistance. Respiration 47:253, 1985.

904. Horton DJ, Chen WY: Effects of breathing warm humidified air on bronchoconstriction induced by body cooling and by inhalation of methacholine. Chest 75:24, 1979.

905. Wilson NM, Dixon C, Silverman M: Increased bronchial responsiveness caused by ingestion of ice. Eur J Respir Dis 66:25, 1985.

906. Schnall RP, Landau LI: Protective effects of repeated short sprints in exercise-induced asthma. Thorax 35:828, 1980.

907. Bierman CW: A comparison of late reactions to antigen and exercise. J Allergy Clin Immunol 73(Suppl):654, 1984.

908. Bierman C, Spiro S, Petheram I: Characterization of the late response in exercise-induced asthma. J Allergy Clin Immunol 74:701, 1984.

909. Feldman CH, Fox J, Kraut E, et al: Exercise-induced asthma (EIA): Treatment for early and late responses. Am Rev Respir Dis (Suppl) 125:195A, 1982.

910. Iikura Y, Inui H, Nagakura T, et al: Factors predisposing to exercise-induced late asthmatic responses. J Allergy Clin Immunol 75:285, 1985.

911. Boulet LP, Legris C, Turcotte H: Prevalence and characteristics of late asthmatic responses to exercise in an adult population. J Allergy Clin Immunol 77:163A, 1986.

912. Tuncotte H, Legris C, Boulet LP: Non-specific bronchial responsiveness to histamine after repeated exercise. J Allergy Clin Immunol 77:164A, 1986.

913. Rubinstein I, Levison H, Slutsky AS, et al: Immediate and delayed bronchoconstriction after exercise in patients with asthma. N Engl J Med 317:482, 1987.

914. Neijens HJ, Wesselius T, Kerrebijn KF: Exercise-induced bronchoconstriction as an expression of bronchial hyperreactivity—a study of its mechanisms in children. Thorax 36:517, 1981.

915. Weiss JW, Rossing TH, McFadden ER, et al: Relationship between bronchial responsiveness to hyperventilation with cold and methacholine in asthma. J Allergy Clin Immunol 72:140, 1983.

916. Hodgson WC, Cotton DJ, Warner GD, et al: Relationship between bronchial response to respiratory heat exchange and nonspecific airways reactivity in asthmatic patients. Chest 85:465, 1984.

917. O'Byrne PM, Ryan G, Morris M, et al: Asthma induced by cold air and its relation to nonspecific bronchial responsiveness to methacholine. Am Rev Respir Dis 125:281, 1982.

918. Mellis CM, Kattan M, Keens TG, et al: Comparative study of histamine and exercise challenges in asthmatic children. Am Rev Respir Dis 117:911, 1978.

919. Chatham M, Bleecker ER, Smith PL, et al: A comparison of histamine, methacholine, and exercise on airway reactivity in normal and asthmatic subjects. Am Rev Respir Dis 126:235, 1982.

920. Banner AS, Green J, O'Connor M: Relation of respiratory water loss to coughing after exercise. N Engl J Med 311:883, 1984.

921. Banner AS, Chausow A, Green J: The tussive effect of hyperpnea with cold air. Am Rev Respir Dis 131:362, 1985.

922. Hall WJ, Hall CB: Alterations in pulmonary function following respiratory viral infection. Chest 76:458, 1979.

923. Similä S, Linna O, Lanning P, et al: Chronic lung damage caused by adenovirus type 7; a 10 year follow-up study. Chest 80:127, 1981.

924. Hall WJ, Hall CB, Speers DM: Respiratory syncytial virus infection in adults. Clinical, virologic, and serial pulmonary function studies. Ann Intern Med 88:203, 1978.

925. O'Connor SA, Jones DP, Collinsa JV, et al: Changes in pulmonary function after naturally acquired respiratory infection in normal persons. Am Rev Respir Dis 120:1087, 1979.

926. Little JW, Hall WJ, Douglas RG Jr, et al: Airway hyperreactivity and peripheral airway dysfunction in influenza A infection. Am Rev Respir Dis 118:295, 1978.

927. Aquilina AT, Hall WJ, Douglas RG Jr, et al: Airway reactivity in subjects with viral upper respiratory tract infections: The effects of exercise and cold air. Am Rev Respir Dis 122:3, 1980.

928. Hafermann DR, Cissik JH, Byrd RB, et al: Effects of influenza vaccination on the peripheral airways of healthy human volunteers. Chest 75:468, 1979.

929. Banks J, Bevan C, Fennerty A, et al: Association between rise in antibodies and increase in airway sensitivity after intramuscular injection of killed influenza virus in asthmatic patients. Eur J Respir Dis 66:268, 1985.

930. DeJongste JC, Degenhart HJ, Neijens HJ, et al: Bronchial respon-

siveness and leucocyte reactivity after influenza vaccine in asthmatic patients. Eur J Respir Dis 65:196, 1984.

931. Jenkins CR, Breslin ABX: Upper respiratory tract infections and airway reactivity in normal and asthmatic subjects. Am Rev Respir Dis 130:879, 1984.

932. Hudgel DW, Langston L, Selner JC, et al: Viral and bacterial infections in adults with chronic asthma. Am Rev Respir Dis 120:393, 1979.

933. Lambert HP, Stern H: Infective factors in exacerbations of bronchitis and asthma. Br Med J 3:323, 1972.

934. Minor TE, Dick EC, DeMeo AN, et al: Viruses as precipitants of asthma attacks in children. JAMA 227:292, 1974.

935. Clarke CW: Relationship of bacterial and viral infections to exacerbations of asthma. Thorax 34:344, 1979.

936. Seggev JS, Lis I, Siman-Tov R, et al: Mycoplasma pneumoniae is a frequent cause of exacerbation of bronchial asthma in adults. Ann Allergy 57:263, 1986.

937. Kava T: Effect of respiratory infections on exacerbation of asthma in adult patients. A six-month follow-up. Allergy 41:556, 1986.

938. Davies RJ, Holford-Strevens VC, Wells ID, et al: Bacterial precipitins and their immunoglobulin class in atopic asthma, non-atopic asthma, and chronic bronchitis. Thorax 31:419, 1976.

939. Stevenson DD, Mathison DA, Tan EM, et al: Provoking factors in bronchial asthma. Arch Intern Med 135:777, 1975.

940. Giraldo B, Blumenthal MN, Spink WW: Aspirin intolerance in asthma, a clinical and immunological study. Ann Intern Med 71:479, 1969.

941. Settipane GA, Chafee FH, Klein DK: Aspirin intolerance. 2. A prospective study of an atopic and normal population. J Allergy Clin Immunol 53:200, 1974.

942. Slepian IK, Mathews KP, McLean JA: Aspirin-sensitive asthma. Chest 87:386, 1985.

943. Ogino S, Harada T, Okawachi I, et al: Aspirin-induced asthma and nasal polyps. Acta Otolaryngol [Suppl] (Stockh) 430:21, 1986.

944. Weltman JK, Szaro RP, Settipane GA: An analysis of the role of IgE in intolerance to aspirin and tartrazine. Allergy 33:273, 1978.

945. Pleskow WW, Stevenson DD, Mathison DA, et al: Aspirin-sensitive rhinosinusitis/asthma—spectrum of adverse reactions to aspirin. J Allergy Clin Immunol 71:574, 1983.

946. Pleskow WW, Stevenson DD, Mathison DA, et al: Aspirin desensitization in aspirin-sensitive asthmatic patients—clinical manifestations and characterizations of the refractory period. J Allergy Clin Immunol 69:11, 1982.

947. Chiu JT: Improvement in aspirin-sensitive asthmatic subjects after rapid aspirin desensitization and aspirin maintenance (ADAM) treatment. J Allergy Clin Immunol 71:560, 1983.

948. Szmidt M, Grzelewska-Rzymowska I, Kowalski ML, et al: Tolerance to acetylsalicylic acid (ASA) induced in ASA-sensitive asthmatics does not depend on initial adverse reaction. Allergy 42:102, 1987.

949. Hollingsworth HM, Center DM: Neutrophil chemotactic factor (NCF) in aspirin-induced bronchospasm. Chest 87:167S, 1985.

950. Hollingsworth HM, Downing ET, et al: Identification and characterization of neutrophil chemotactic activity in aspirin-induced asthma. Am Rev Respir Dis 130:373, 1984.

951. Martelli NA, Usandivaras G: Inhibition of aspirin-induced bronchoconstriction by sodium cromoglycate inhalation. Thorax 32:684, 1977.

952. Martelli NA: Bronchial and intravenous provocation tests with indomethacin in aspirin-sensitive asthmatics. Am Rev Respir Dis 120:1073, 1979.

953. Grzelewska-Rzymowska I, Bogucki A, Szmidt M, et al: Migraine in aspirin-sensitive asthmatics. Allergol Immunopathol (Madr) 13:13, 1985.

954. Ameisen JC, Capron A, Joseph M, et al: Aspirin-sensitive asthma: abnormal platelet response to drugs inducing asthmatic attacks. Diagnostic and physiopathological implications. Int Arch Allergy Appl Immunol 78:438, 1985.

955. Dajani BM, Sliman NA, Shubair KS, et al: Bronchospasm caused by intravenous hydrocortisone sodium succinate (Solu-Cortef) in aspirin-sensitive patients. J Allergy Clin Immunol 68:201, 1981.

956. Szczeklik A, Nizankowska E, Czerniawska-Mysik G, et al: Hydrocortisone and airflow impairment in aspirin-induced asthma. J Allergy Clin Immunol 76:530, 1985.

957. Szczeklik A, Nizankowska E, Czerniawska-Mysik G, et al: Hydrocortisone and airflow impairment in aspirin-induced asthma. J Allergy Clin Immunol 76:530, 1985.

958. Allen CJ, Newhouse MT: Gastroesophageal reflux and chronic respiratory disease. Am Rev Respir Dis 129:645, 1984.

959. Boyle JT, Tuchman DN, Altschuler SM, et al: Mechanisms for the association of gastroesophageal reflux and bronchospasm. Am Rev Respir Dis 131:S16, 1985.

960. Ducolone A, Vandevenne A, Jouin H, et al: Gastroesophageal reflux in patients with asthma and chronic bronchitis. Am Rev Respir Dis 135:327, 1987.

961. Spaulding HS, Mansfield LE, Stein MR, et al: Further investigation of the association between gastroesophageal reflux and bronchoconstriction. J Allergy Clin Immunol 69:516, 1982.

962. Perpiña M, Ponce J, Marco V, et al: The prevalence of asymptomatic gastroesophageal reflux in bronchial asthma and in non-asthmatic individuals. Eur J Respir Dis 64:582, 1983.

963. Davis RS, Larsen GL, Grunstein MM: Respiratory response to intraesophageal acid infusion in asthmatic children during sleep. J Allergy Clin Immunol 72:393, 1983.

964. Andersen LI, Schmidt A, Bundgaard A: Pulmonary function and acid application in the esophagus. Chest 90:358, 1986.

965. Perpiña M, Pellicer C, Marco V, et al: The significance of the reflex bronchoconstriction provoked by gastroesophageal reflux in bronchial asthma. Eur J Respir Dis 66:91, 1985.

966. Herve P, Denjean A, Jian R, et al: Intraesophageal perfusion of acid increases the bronchomotor response to methacholine and to isocapnic hyperventilation in asthmatic subjects. Am Rev Respir Dis 134:986, 1986.

967. Goodall RJR, Earis JE, Cooper DN, et al: Relationship between asthma and gastro-oesophageal reflux. Thorax 36:116, 1981.

968. Sontag S, O'Connell S, Greenlee H, et al: Is gastroesophageal reflux a factor in some asthmatics? Am J Gastroenterol 82:119, 1987.

969. Nelson HS: Gastroesophageal reflux and pulmonary disease. J Allergy Clin Immunol 73:547, 1984.

970. Spector S, Luparello TJ, Kopetzky MT, et al: Response of asthmatics to methacholine and suggestion. Am Rev Respir Dis 113:43, 1976.

971. Wright GLT: Asthma and the emotions: Aetiology and treatment. Med J Aust 1:961, 1965.

972. Horton DJ, Suda WL, Kinsman RA, et al: Bronchoconstrictive suggestion in asthma: A role for airways hyperreactivity and emotions. Am Rev Respir Dis 117:1029, 1978.

973. Lewis RA, Lewis MN, Tattersfield AE: Asthma induced by suggestion—Is it due to airway cooling? Am Rev Respir Dis 129:691, 1984.

974. Baraff AA, Cunningham AP: Asthmatic and normal children. JAMA 192:13, 1965.

975. Demeter SL, Cordasco EM: Hyperventilation syndrome and asthma. Am J Med 81:989, 1986.

976. Ussetti P, Roca J, Agusti AGN, et al: Another asthma outbreak in Barcelona. Role of oxides of nitrogen. Lancet 1:156, 1984.

977. Avol E, Linn W, Shamoo D, et al: Respiratory effects of photochemical oxidant air pollution in exercising adolescents. Am Rev Respir Dis 132:619, 1985.

978. Hazucha MJ, Ginsberg JF, McDonnell WF, et al: Effects of 0.1 ppm nitrogen dioxide on airways of normal and asthmatic subjects. J Appl Physiol 54:730, 1983.

979. Koenig JQ, Pierson WE, Horike M, et al: Bronchoconstrictor responses to sulfur dioxide or sulfur dioxide plus sodium chloride droplets in allergic, nonasthmatic adolescents. J Allergy Clin Immunol 69:339, 1982.

980. Jaeger MJ, Tribble D, Wittig HJ: Effect of 0.5 ppm sulfur dioxide on the respiratory function of normal and asthmatic subjects. Lung 156:119, 1979.

981. Folinsbee LJ, Bedi JF, Horvath SM: Pulmonary response to threshold levels of sulfur dioxide (1.0 ppm) and ozone (0.3 ppm). J Appl Physiol 58:1783, 1985.

982. Snashall PD, Baldwin C: Mechanisms of sulphur dioxide induced bronchoconstriction in normal and asthmatic man. Thorax 37:118, 1982.

983. Sheppard D, Saisho AK, Nadel JA, et al: Exercise increases sulfur dioxide-induced bronchoconstriction in asthmatic subjects. Am Rev Respir Dis 123:486, 1981.

984. Bethel RA, Epstein J, Sheppard D, et al: Sulfur dioxide-induced bronchoconstriction in freely breathing, exercising, asthmatic subjects. Am Rev Respir Dis 128:987, 1983.

985. Sheppard D, Wong WS, Uehara CF, et al: Lower threshold and greater bronchomotor responsiveness of asthmatic subjects to sulfur dioxide. Am Rev Respir Dis 122:873, 1980.

986. Roger LJ, Kehrl HR, Hazucha M, et al: Bronchoconstriction in asthmatics exposed to sulfur dioxide during repeated exercise. J Appl Physiol 59:784, 1985.

987. Linn WS, Venet TG, Shamoo DA, et al: Respiratory effects of sulfur dioxide in heavily exercising asthmatics—a dose-response study. Am Rev Respir Dis 127:278, 1983.

988. Kehrl HR, Roger LJ, Hazucha MJ, et al: Differing response of asthmatics to sulfur dioxide exposure with continuous and intermittent exercise. Am Rev Respir Dis 135:350, 1987.

989. Sheppard D, Nadel JA, Boushey HA: Effect of the oronasal breathing route on sulfur dioxide-induced bronchoconstriction in exercising asthmatic subjects. Am Rev Respir Dis 125:627, 1982.

990. Bethel RA, Erle DJ, Epstein J, et al: Effect of exercise rate and route of inhalation on sulfur dioxide-induced bronchoconstriction in asthmatic subjects. Am Rev Respir Dis 128:592, 1983.

11

991. Sheppard D, Eschenbacher WL, Boushey HA, et al: Magnitude of the interaction between the bronchomotor effects of sulfur dioxide and those of dry (cold) air. Am Rev Respir Dis 130:52, 1984.

992. Bethel RA, Sheppard D, Epstein J, et al: Interaction of sulphur dioxide and dry cold air causing bronchoconstriction in asthmatic subjects. J Appl Physiol 57:419, 1984.

993. Linn WS, Shamoo DA, Anderson KR, et al: Effects of heat and humidity on the responses of exercising asthmatics to sulfur dioxide exposure. Am Rev Respir Dis 131:221, 1985.

994. Kulle TJ, Sauder LR, Hebel JR, et al: Ozone response relationships in healthy nonsmokers. Am Rev Respir Dis 132:36, 1985.

995. Linn WS, Buckley RD, Spier CE, et al: Health effects of ozone exposure in asthmatics. Am Rev Respir Dis 117:835, 1978.

996. Lauritzen SK, Adams WC: Ozone inhalation effects consequent to continuous exercise in females: Comparison to males. J Appl Physiol 59:1601, 1985.

997. McDonnell W, Chapman R, Leigh M, et al: Respiratory responses of vigorously exercising children to 0.12 ppm ozone exposure. Am Rev Respir Dis 132:875, 1985.

998. Hackney JD, Linn WS, Mohler JG, et al: Experimental studies on human health effects of air pollutants. II. Four-hour exposure to ozone alone and in combinations with other pollutant gases. Arch Environ Health 30:379, 1975.

999. Bates DV, Ball GM, Burnham CD, et al: Short-term effects of ozone on the lung. J Appl Physiol 32:176, 1972.

1000. Hazucha M, Silverman F, Parent C, et al: Pulmonary function in a man after short-term exposure to ozone. Arch Environ Health 27:183, 1973.

1001. Hackney JD, Linn WS, Law DC, et al: Experimental studies on human health effects of air pollutants. III. Two-hour exposure to ozone and in combination with other pollutant gases. Arch Environ Health 30:385, 1975.

1002. Hackney JD, Linn WS, Buckley RD, et al: Scientific communications. Experimental studies on human health effects of air pollutants. I. Design considerations. Arch Environ Health 30:373, 1975.

1003. Kerr HD, Kulle TJ, McIlhany ML, et al: Effects of ozone on pulmonary function in normal subjects. An environmental-chamber study. Am Rev Respir Dis 111:763, 1975.

1004. Kagawa J, Toyama T: Effects of ozone and brief exercise on specific airway conductance in man. Arch Environ Health 30:36, 1975.

1005. Golden JA, Nadel JA, Boushey HA: Bronchial hyperirritability in healthy subjects after exposure to ozone. Am Rev Respir Dis 118:287, 1978.

1006. Holtzman MJ, Cunningham JH, Sheller JR, et al: Effect of ozone on bronchial reactivity in atopic and nonatopic subjects. Am Rev Respir Dis 120:1059, 1979.

1007. Holtzman MJ, Fabbri LM, O'Byrne PM, et al: Importance of airway inflammation for hyperresponsiveness induced by ozone. Am Rev Respir Dis 127:686, 1983.

1008. O'Byrne PM, Walters EH, Gold BD, et al: Neutrophil depletion inhibits airway hyperresponsiveness induced by ozone exposure. Am Rev Respir Dis 130:214, 1984.

1009. O'Byrne PM, Walters EH, Alzawa H, et al: Indomethacin inhibits the airway hyperresponsiveness but not the neutrophil influx induced by ozone in dogs. Am Rev Respir Dis 130:220, 1984.

1010. Fabbri LM, Aizawa H, Alpert SE, et al: Airway hyperresponsiveness and changes in cell counts in bronchoalveolar lavage after ozone exposure in dogs. Am Rev Respir Dis 129:288, 1984.

1011. Bauer MA, Utell MJ, Morrow PE, et al: Inhalation of 0.30 ppm nitrogen dioxide potentiates exercise-induced bronchospasm in asthmatics. Am Rev Respir Dis 134:1203, 1986.

1012. Bylin G, Lindvall T, Rehn T, et al: Effects of short-term exposure to ambient nitrogen dioxide concentrations on human bronchial reactivity and lung function. Eur J Respir Dis 66:205, 1985.

1013. Lewis R, Gilkeson M, McCaldin RO: Air pollution and New Orleans asthma. Public Health Rep 77:947, 1962.

1014. Weill H, Ziskind MM, Derbes V, et al: Further observations on New Orleans asthma. Arch Environ Health 8:184, 1964.

1015. Weill H, Ziskind MM, Dickerson RC, et al: Epidemic asthma in New Orleans. JAMA 190:811, 1964.

1016. Smith RBW, Kolb EJ, Phelps HW, et al: Tokyo-Yokohawa asthma. An area specific air pollution disease. Arch Environ Health 8:805, 1964.

1017. Phelps HW, Koike S: Tokyo-Yokohama asthma. The rapid development of respiratory distress presumably due to air pollution. Am Rev Respir Dis 86:55, 1962.

1018. Oshima Y, Ishizaki T, Miyamoto T, et al: Air pollution and respiratory diseases in the Tokyo-Yokohama area. Am Rev Respir Dis 90:572, 1964.

1019. Schoettlin CE, Landau E: Air pollution and asthmatic attacks in the Los Angeles area. Public Health Rep 76:545, 1961.

1020. Parham WM, Shepard RH, Norman PS, et al: Analysis of time course and magnitude of lung inflation effects on airway tone—relation to airway reactivity. Am Rev Respir Dis 128:240, 1983.

1021. Orehek J, Charpin D, Velardocchio JM, et al: Bronchomotor effect of bronchoconstriction-induced deep inspirations in asthmatics. Am Rev Respir Dis 121:297, 1980.

1022. Fish JE, Kehoe TJ, Cugell DW: Effect of deep inspiration on maximum expiratory flow rates in asthmatic subjects. Respiration 36:57, 1978.

1023. Zamel N, Hughes D, Levison H, et al: Partial and complete maximum expiratory flow-volume curves in asthmatic patients with spontaneous bronchospasm. Chest 83:35, 1983.

1024. Beaupré A, Badier M, Delpierre S, et al: Airways response of asthmatics to carbachol and to deep inspiration. Eur J Respir Dis 64:108, 1983.

1025. Brusasco V, Rocchi D: Effects of volume history and time dependence of flow-volume curves on assessment of bronchial response to inhaled methacholine in normals. Respiration 41:106, 1981.

1026. Beaupré A, Orehek J: Factors influencing the bronchodilator effect of a deep inspiration in asthmatic patients with provoked bronchoconstriction. Thorax 37:124, 1982.

1027. Hida W, Arai M, Shindoh C, et al: Effect of inspiratory flow rate on bronchomotor tone in normal and asthmatic subjects. Thorax 39:86, 1984.

1028. Day A, Zamel N: Failure of cholinergic blockade to prevent bronchodilatation following deep inspiration. J Appl Physiol 58:1449, 1985.

1029. Burns CB, Taylor WR, Ingram RH Jr: Effects of deep inhalation in asthma: Relative airway and parenchymal hysteresis. J Appl Physiol 59:1590, 1985.

1030. Ayres JG, Clark TJH: Alcoholic drinks and asthma—a survey. Br J Dis Chest 77:370, 1983.

1031. Gong H, Tashkin DP, Calvarese BM: Alcohol-induced bronchospasm in an asthmatic patient—pharmacologic evaluation of the mechanism. Chest 80:167, 1981.

1032. Geppert EF, Boushey HA: An investigation of the mechanism of ethanol-induced bronchoconstriction. Am Rev Respir Dis 118:135, 1978.

1033. Genton C, Frei PC, Pécoud A: Value of oral provocation tests to aspirin and food additives in the routine investigation of asthma and chronic urticaria. J Allergy Clin Immunol 76:40, 1985.

1034. Bush RK, Taylor SL, Holden K, et al: Prevalence of sensitivity to sulfiting agents in asthmatic patients. Am J Med 81:816, 1986.

1035. Stevenson DD, Simon RA: Sensitivity to ingested metabisulfites in asthmatic subjects. J Allergy Clin Immunol 68:26, 1981.

1036. Dahl R, Henriksen JM, Harving H: Red wine asthma: A controlled challenge study. J Allergy Clin Immunol 78:1126, 1986.

1037. Koepke JW, Christopher KL, Chai H, et al: Dose-dependant bronchospasm from sulfites in isoetharine. JAMA 251:2982, 1984.

1038. Shim C, Williams MH Jr: Effect of odors in asthma. Am J Med 80:18, 1986.

1039. Dahms TE, Bolin JF, Slavin RG: Passive smoking—Effects on bronchial asthma. Chest 80:530, 1981.

1040. Higenbottam TW, Feyeraband C, Clark TJH: Cigarette smoking in asthma. Br J Dis Chest 74:279, 1980.

1041. Hillerdahl G, Rylander R: Asthma and cessation of smoking. Clin Allergy 14:45, 1984.

1042. Murray AB, Harrison BJ: The effect of cigarette smoke from the mother on bronchial responsiveness and severity of symptoms in children with asthma. J Allergy Clin Immunol 77:575, 1986.

1043. Gibbs C, Coutts II, Lock R, et al: Premenstrual exacerbation of asthma. Thorax 39:833, 1984.

1044. Hanley SP: Asthma variation with menstruation. Br J Dis Chest 75:306, 1981.

1045. Eliasson O, Scherzer HH, DeGraff AC Jr: Morbidity in asthma in relation to the menstrual cycle. J Allergy Clin Immunol 77:87, 1986.

1046. Louie S, Krzanowski JJ Jr, Bukantz SC, et al: Effects of ergometrine on airway smooth muscle contractile responses. Clin Allergy 15:173, 1985.

1047. Packe GE, Ayres JG: Asthma outbreak during a thunderstorm. Lancet 2(8448):199, 1985.

1048. Chan-Yeung N: Occupational assessment of asthma. Chest 82:24S, 1982.

1049. Belin L: Hyperreactivity in clinical practice—induction by occupational factors. Eur J Respir Dis (Suppl 131) 64:285, 1983.

1050. Manireda J, Holford-Strevens V, Cheang M, et al: Acute symptoms following exposure to grain dust in farming. Environ Health Perspect 66:73, 1986.

1051. Hendrick DJ: Editorial: Contaminated humidifiers and the lung. Thorax 40:244, 1985.

1052. Burge PS, Finnegan M, Horsfield N, et al: Occupational asthma in a factory with a contaminated humidifier. Thorax 40:248, 1985.

1053. Bryant DH: Asthma due to insecticide sensitivity. Aust NZ J Med 15:66, 1985.

1054. Petry RW, Voss MJ, Kroutil LA, et al: Monkey dander asthma. J Allergy Clin Immunol 75:268, 1985.

1055. Lutsky I, Teichtahl H, Bar-Sela S: Occupational asthma due to poultry mites. J Allergy Clin Immunol 73:56, 1984.

1056. Burge SB, Hendy M, Hodgson ES: Occupational asthma, rhinitis, and dermatitis due to tetrazene in a detonator manufacturer. Thorax 39:470, 1984.

1057. Van Hage-Hamsten HI, Johansson SS, Höglund S, et al: Storage site allergy is common in a farming population. Clin Allergy 15:555, 1985.

1058. Spieksma FT, Vooren PH, Kramps JA, et al: Respiratory allergy to laboratory fruit flies (Drosophila melanogaster). J Allergy Clin Immunol 77:108, 1986.

1059. Kino T, Oshima S: Allergy to insects in Japan. 1. Reaginic sensitivity to moth and butterfly in patients with bronchial asthma. J Allergy Clin Immunol 61:10, 1978.

1060. Kaufman GL, Baldo BA, Tovey ER, et al: Inhalant allergy following occupational exposure to blowflies. Clin Allergy 16:65, 1986.

1061. Gold B, Mathews K, Burge H: Occupational asthma caused by sewer flies. Am Rev Respir Dis 131:949, 1985.

1062. Ostrom NK, Swanson MC, Agarwal MK, et al: Occupational allergy to honeybee-body dust in a honey-processing plant. J Allergy Clin Immunol 77:736, 1986.

1063. Prichard M, Turner KJ: Acute hypersensitivity to ingested processed pollen. Aust NZ J Med 15:346, 1985.

1064. Cartier A, Malo JL, Forest F, et al: Occupational asthma in snow crab-processing workers. J Allergy Clin Immunol 74:261, 1984.

1065. Prichard MG, Ryan G, Walsh BJ, et al: Skin test and RAST responses to wheat and common allergens and respiratory disease in bakers. Clin Allergy 15:203, 1985.

1066. Osterman K, Johansson SGO, Zetterström O: Diagnostic tests in allergy to green coffee. Allergy 40:336, 1985.

1067. Karr RM, Lehrer SB, Butcher BT, et al: Coffee workers asthma—A clinical appraisal using radioallergosorbent test. J Allergy Clin Immunol 62:143, 1978.

1068. Topping MD, Henderson RTS, Luczynska CM, et al: Castor bean allergy among workers in the felt industry. Allergy 37:603, 1982.

1069. Davison AG, Britton MG, Forrester JA, et al: Asthma in merchant seamen and laboratory workers caused by allergy to castor beans: Analysis of allergens. Clin Allergy 13:553, 1983.

1070. Twiggs JT, Yunginger JW, Agarwal MK, et al: Occupational asthma in a florist caused by the dried plant, baby's breath. J Allergy Clin Immunol 69:474, 1982.

1071. Falleroni AE, Zeiss CR, Levitz D: Occupational asthma secondary to inhalation of garlic dust. J Allergy Clin Immunol 68:156, 1981.

1072. Lybarger JA, Gallagher JS, Pulver SW: Occupational asthma induced by inhalation and ingestion of garlic. J Allergy Clin Immunol 69:448, 1982.

1073. van Toorenenbergen AW, Dieges PH: Immunoglobulin E antibodies against coriander and other spices. J Allergy Clin Immunol 76:477, 1985.

1074. Wiessman KJ, Baur X: Occupational lung disease following long-term inhalation of pancreatic extracts. Eur J Respir Dis 66:13, 1985.

1075. Cartier A, Malo JL, Pineau L, et al: Occupational asthma due to pepsin. J Allergy Clin Immunol 73:574, 1984.

1076. Losada E, Hinojosa M, Moneo I, et al: Occupational asthma caused by cellulase. J Allergy Clin Immunol 77:635, 1986.

1077. Harries MG, Sherwood Burge P, Samson M, et al: Isocyanate asthma: Respiratory symptoms due to 1,5-naphthylene di-isocyanate. Thorax 34:762, 1979.

1078. Tse KS, Johnson A, Chan H, et al: A study of serum antibody activity in workers with occupational exposure to diphenylmethane diisocyanate. Allergy 40:314, 1985.

1079. Butcher BT, Karr RM, O'Neill CE, et al: Inhalation challenge and pharmacologic studies of toluene diisocyanate (TDI)-sensitive work. J Allergy Clin Immunol 64:146, 1979.

1080. Zammit-Tabona M, Sherkin M, Kijek K, et al: Asthma caused by diphenylmethane diisocyanate in foundry workers—clinical, bronchial provocation, and immunologic studies. Am Rev Respir Dis 128:226, 1983.

1081. Venables KM, Dally MB, Burge PS, et al: Occupational asthma in a steel coating plant. Br J Indern Med 42:517, 1985.

1082. Alexandersson R, Gustafsson P, Hedenstierna G, et al: Exposure to naphthalene-diisocyanate in a rubber plant: Symptoms and lung function. Arch Environ Health 41:85, 1986.

1083. Moller DR, Gallagher JS, Bernstein DI, et al: Detection of IgE-mediated respiratory sensitization in workers exposed to hexahydrophthalic anhydride. J Allergy Clin Immunol 75:663, 1985.

1084. Meadway J: Asthma and atopy in workers with an epoxy adhesive. Br J Dis Chest 74:149, 1980.

1085. Howe W, Venables KM, Topping MD, et al: Tetrachlorophthalic anhydride asthma—Evidence for specific IgE antibody. J Allergy Clin Immunol 71:5, 1983.

1086. Bush RK, Yunginger JW, Reed CE: Asthma due to African zebrawood (Microberlinia) dust. Am Rev Respir Dis 117:601, 1978.

1087. Cartier A, Chan N, Malo JL, et al: Occupational asthma caused by eastern white cedar (Thuja occidentalis) with demonstration that alicatic acid is present in this wood dust and is the causal agent. J Allergy Clin Immunol 77:639, 1984.

1088. Lung disease in dental laboratory technicians. Lancet 1:1200, 1985.

1089. Simonsson BG, Sjoberg A, Rolf C, et al: Acute and long-term airway hyperreactivity in alumin-salt exposed workers with nocturnal asthma. Eur J Respir Dis 66:105, 1985.

1090. Field GB: Pulmonary function in aluminium smelters. Thorax 39:743, 1984.

1091. Sorić M, Godnić-Cyar J, Gomzi M, et al: The role of atopy in potroom workers' asthma. Am J Indern Med 9:239, 1986.

1092. Gheysens B, Auwerx J, Van den Eeckhout A, et al: Cobalt-induced bronchial asthma in diamond polishers. Chest 88:740, 1985.

1093. Blainey AD, Ollier S, Cundell D, et al: Occupational asthma in a hairdressing salon. Thorax 41:42, 1986.

1094. Malo JL, Pineau L, Cartier A: Occupational asthma due to azobisformamide. Clin Allergy 15:261, 1985.

1095. Graham VAL, Coe MJS, Davies RJ: Occupational asthma after exposure to a diazonium salt. Thorax 36:950, 1981.

1096. Corrado OJ, Osman J, Davies RJ: Asthma and rhinitis after exposure to glutaraldehyde in endoscopy units. Hum Toxicol 5:325, 1986.

1097. Cockcroft DW, Cartier A, Jones G, et al: Asthma caused by occupational exposure to a furan-based binder system. J Allergy Clin Immunol 66:458, 1980.

1098. Lozewicz S, Davison AG, Hopkirk A, et al: Occupational asthma due to methyl methacrylate and cyanoacrylates. Thorax 40:836, 1985.

1099. Krumpe PE, Finley TN, Martinez NN: The search for expiratory obstruction in meat wrappers studied on the job. Am Rev Respir Dis 119:611, 1979.

1100. Baser ME, Tockman MS, Kennedy TP: Pulmonary function and respiratory symptoms in polyvinylchloride fabrication workers. Am Rev Respir Dis 131:203, 1985.

1101. Gandevia B: Occupational asthma. Med J Aust 2:332, 1970.

1102. Brooks SM, Weiss MA, Bernstein IL: Reactive airways dysfunction syndrome (RADS): Persistent asthma syndrome after high level irritant exposures. Chest 88:376, 1985.

1103. Mustchin CP, Pickering CAC: "Coughing water": bronchial hyperreactivity induced by swimming in a chlorinated pool. Thorax 34:682, 1979.

1104. Cinkotai FF, Sharpe TC, Gibbs ACC: Circadian rhythms in peak expiratory flow rate in workers exposed to cotton dust. Thorax 39:759, 1984.

1105. Tockman MS, Baser M: Is cotton dust exposure associated with chronic effects? Am Rev Respir Dis 130:1, 1984.

1106. Schachter EN, Maunder LR, Beck GJ: The pattern of lung function abnormalities in cotton textile workers. Am Rev Respir Dis 129:523, 1984.

1107. Beck GJ, Schacter EN, Maunder LR: The relationship of respiratory symptoms and lung function loss in cotton textile workers. Am Rev Respir Dis 130:6, 1984.

1108. Schachter EN, Brown S, Zuskin E, et al: Airway reactivity in cotton bract-induced bronchospasm. Am Res Respir Dis 123:273, 1981.

1109. Schachter EN, Zuskin E, Buck MG, et al: Airway reactivity and cotton bract-induced bronchial obstruction. Chest 87:51, 1986.

1110. Edwards JH, Alzubaidy TS, Altikriti R, et al: Byssinosis; inhalation challenge with polyphenol. Chest 85:215, 1984.

1111. Rylander R, Haglind P, Lundholm M: Endotoxin in cotton dust and respiratory function decrement among cotton workers in an experimental cardroom. Am Rev Respir Dis 131:209, 1985.

1112. Castellan RM, Olenchock SA, Hankinson JL, et al: Acute bronchoconstriction induced by cotton dust: Dose-related response to endotoxin and other dust factors. Ann Intern Med 101:159, 1984.

1113. Wilson MR, Sehul A, Ory R, et al: Activation of the alternative complement pathway by extracts of cotton dust. Clin Allergy 10:303, 1980.

1114. Pernis B, Vigliani EC, Cavagna C, et al: The role of bacterial endotoxins on occupational diseases caused by inhaling vegetable dusts. Br J Ind Med 18:120, 1961.

1115. Dopico GA, Flaherty D, Bhansali P, et al: Grain fever syndrome induced by inhalation of airborne grain dust. J Allergy Clin Immunol 69:435, 1982.

1116. Cockcroft AE, McDermott M, Edwards JH, et al: Grain exposure symptoms and lung function. Eur J Respir Dis 64:189, 1983.

1117. doPico GA, Reddan W, Anderson S, et al: Acute effects of grain dust exposure during a work shift. Am Rev Respir Dis 128:399, 1983.

1118. Chan-Yeung M, Giclas PC, Henson PM: Activation of complement by plicatic acid, the chemical compound responsible for asthma due to western red cedar (Thujaplicata). J Allergy Clin Immunol 65:333, 1980.

11

1119. Banaszak EF, Thiede WH, Fink JW: Hypersensitivity pneumonia due to contamination of an air conditioner. N Engl J Med 283:271, 1970.

1120. Asai S, Krzanowski JJ, Anderson WH, et al: Effects of the toxin of red tide, Ptychodiscus brevis, on canine tracheal smooth muscle—a possible new asthma-triggering mechanism. J Allergy Clin Immunol 69:418, 1982.

1121. Bernstein IL: Isocyanate-induced pulmonary diseases: a current perspective. J Allergy Clin Immunol 70:24, 1982.

1122. Chester EH, Martinez-Catinchi FL, Schwartz HJ, et al: Patterns of airway reactivity to asthma produced by exposure to toluene diisocyanate. Chest 75:229, 1979.

1123. McKay RT, Brooks SM: Effects of toluene diisocyanate on beta-adrenergic receptor function—biochemical and physiologic studies. Am Rev Respir Dis 128:50, 1983.

1124. Agrup G, Belin L, Sjöstedt L, et al: Allergy to laboratory animals in laboratory technicians and animal keepers. Br J Ind Med 43:192, 1986.

1125. Dosman JA, Graham BL, Cotton DJ: Chronic bronchitis and exposure to cereal grain dust (editorial). Am Rev Respir Dis 120:477, 1979.

1126. Broder I, Mintz S, Hutcheon M: Comparison of respiratory variables in grain elevator workers and civic outside workers of Thunder Bay, Canada. Am Rev Respir Dis 119:193, 1979.

1127. Mink JT, Gerrard JW, Cockcroft DW, et al: Increased bronchial reactivity to inhaled histamine in nonsmoking grain workers with normal lung function. Chest 77:28, 1980.

1128. Cookson WO, Ryan G, MacDonald S, et al: Atopy, non-allergic bronchial reactivity, and past history as determinants of work related symptoms in seasonal grain handlers. Br J Ind Med 43:396, 1986.

1129. Chan-Yeung M, Wong R, Maclean L: Respiratory abnormalities among grain elevator workers. Chest 75:461, 1979.

1130. Cotton DJ, Graham BL, Li KYR, et al: Effects of smoking and occupational exposure on peripheral airway function in young cereal grain workers. Am Rev Respir Dis 126:660, 1982.

1131. Tabona M, Chan-Yeung M, Enarson D, et al: Host factors affecting longitudinal decline in lung spirometry among grain elevator workers. Chest 85:782, 1984.

1132. Yach D, Myers J, Bradshaw D, et al: A respiratory epidemiologic survey of grain mill workers in Cape-Town, South Africa. Am Rev Respir Dis 131:505, 1985.

1133. Enarson DA, Vedal S, Chan-Yeung M: Rapid decline in FEV₁ in grain handlers—relation to level of dust exposure. Am Rev Respir Dis 132:814, 1985.

1134. Enarson DA, Chan-Yeung M, Tabona M, et al: Predictors of bronchial hyperexcitability in grain handlers. Chest 87:452, 1985.

1135. Thiel H, Ulmer WNT: Baker's asthma: Development and possibility of treatment. Chest 78:S400, 1980.

1136. Mitchell CA, Gandevia B: Respiratory symptoms and skin test sensitivity in works exposed to proteolytic enzyme in detergent industry. Am Rev Respir Dis 104:1, 1971.

1137. Franz T, McMurran KD, Brooks S, et al: Clinical immunologic and physiologic observations in factory workers exposed to B. subtilis enzyme dust. J Allergy 42:170, 1971.

1138. Milne J, Gandevia B: Occupational asthma and rhinitis due to western red cedar (Thuja plicata). Med J Aust 2:741, 1967.

1139. Lam S, Tan F, Chan H, et al: Relationship between types of asthmatic reaction, nonspecific bronchial reactivity, and specific IgE antibodies in patients with red cedar asthma. J Allergy Clin Immunol 72:134, 1983.

1140. Chan-Yeung M: Immunologic and nonimmunologic mechanisms in asthma due to western red cedar (Thuja plicata). J Allergy Clin Immunol 70:32, 1982.

1141. Chan-Yeung M: Fate of occupational asthma: A follow-up study of patients with occupational asthma due to western red cedar (Thuja plicata). Am Rev Respir Dis 116:1023, 1977.

1142. Chan-Yeung M, Vedal S, Kus J, et al: Symptoms, pulmonary function and bronchial hyperreactivity in western red cedar workers compared to those in office workers. Am Rev Respir Dis 130:1038, 1984.

1143. Vedal S, Chan-Yeung M, Enarson DA, et al: Plicatic acid-specific IgE and nonspecific bronchial hyperresponsiveness in western red-cedar workers. Allergy Clin Immunol 78:1103, 1986.

1144. Paggiaro PL, Chan-Yeung M: Pattern of specific airway response in asthma due to western red cedar (Thuja plicata): Relationship with length of exposure and lung function measurements. Clin Allergy 17:333, 1987.

1145. Cockcroft DW, Cotton DJ, Mink JT: Nonspecific bronchial hyper-reactivity after exposure to western red cedar. Am Rev Respir Dis 119:505, 1979.

1146. Vedal S, Chan-Yeung M, Enarson D, et al: Symptoms and pulmonary function in western red cedar workers related to duration of employment and dust exposure. Arch Environ Health 41:179, 1986.

1147. Chan-Yeung M, Grzybowski S: Prognosis in occupational asthma (editorial). Thorax 40:241, 1985.

1148. Venables KM, Topping MD, Nunn AJ, et al: Immunologic and functional consequences of chemical (tetrachlorophthalic anhydride)-induced asthma after four years of avoidance of exposure. J Allergy Clin Immunol 80:212, 1987.

1149. Hudson P, Cartier A, Pineau L, et al: Follow-up of occupational asthma caused by crab and various agents. J Allergy Clin Immunol 76:682, 1985.

1150. Chan-Yeung M, MacLean L, Paggiaro PL: Follow-up study of 232 patients with occupational asthma caused by western red cedar (Thuja plicata). J Allergy Clin Immunol 79:792, 1987.

1151. Bardana EJ Jr, Andrasch RH: Occupational asthma secondary to low molecular weight agents used in the plastic and resin industries. Eur J Respir Dis 64:241, 1983.

1152. Zeiss CR, Wolkonsky P, Pruzansky JJ, et al: Clinical and immunologic evaluation of trimellitic anhydride workers in multiple industrial settings. J Allergy Clin Immunol 70:15, 1982.

1153. Bernstein DI, Zeiss CR, Wolkonsky P, et al: The relationship of total serum IgE and blocking antibody in trimellitic anhydride induced occupational asthma. J Allergy Clin Immunol 72:714, 1983.

1154. Moller DR, Gallagher JS, Bernstein DI, et al: Detection of IgE-mediated respiratory sensitization in workers exposed to hexahydrophthalic anhydride. J Allergy Clin Immunol 75:663, 1985.

1155. Bernstein DI, Roach DE, McGrath KG, et al: The relationship of airborne trimellitic anhydride concentrations to trimellitic anhydride-induced symptoms and immune responses. J Allergy Clin Immunol 72:709, 1983.

1156. Moller DR, McKay RT, Bernstein IL, et al: Persistent airways disease caused by toluene diisocyanate. Am Rev Respir Dis 134:175, 1986.

1157. Moller DR, Brooks SM, McKay RT, et al: Chronic asthma due to toluene diisocyanate. Chest 90:494, 1986.

1158. Zeiss CR, Kanellakes TM, Bellone JD, et al: Immunoglobulin E-mediated asthma and hypersensitivity pneumonitis with precipitating anti-hapten antibodies due to diphenylmethane disocyanate (Mdi) exposure. J Allergy Clin Immunol 65:346, 1980.

1159. Fink JN, Schlueter DP: Bathtub refinisher's lung: An unusual response to toluene diisocyanate. Am Rev Respir Dis 118:955, 1978.

1160. Mapp CE, Dal Vecchio L, Boschetto P, et al: Toluene diisocyanate-induced asthma without airway hyperresponsiveness. Eur J Respir Dis 68:89, 1986.

1161. Chester EH, Martinez-Catinchi FL, Schwartz HJ, et al: Patterns of airway reactivity to asthma produced by exposure to toluene diisocyanate. Chest 75:229, 1979.

1162. Paggiaro PL, Innocenti A, Bacci E, et al: Specific bronchial reactivity to toluene diisocyanate: Relationship with baseline clinical findings. Thorax 41:279, 1986.

1163. Fabbri LM, Chiesura-Corona P, Delvecchio L, et al: Prednisone inhibits late asthmatic reactions and the associated increase in airway responsiveness induced by toluene-diisocyanate in sensitized subjects. Am Rev Respir Dis 132:1010, 1985.

1164. McKay RT, Brooks SM: Hyperreactive airway smooth muscle responsiveness after inhalation of toluene diisocyanate vapors. Am Rev Respir Dis 129:296, 1984.

1165. Burge PS, Harries MG, Lam WK, et al: Occupational asthma due to formaldehyde. Thorax 40:255, 1985.

1166. Frigas E, Filley W, Reed C: Bronchial challenge with formaldehyde gas: Lack of bronchoconstriction in 13 patients suspected of having formaldehyde-induced asthma. Mayo Clin Proc 59:295, 1984.

1167. Frigas E, Filley WV, Reed CE: Asthma induced by dust from urea-formaldehyde foam insulating material. Chest 79:706, 1981.

1168. Cockcroft DW, Hoeppner VH, Colovich J: Occupational asthma caused by cedar urea formaldehyde particle board. Chest 82:49, 1982.

1169. Eisen EA, Hegman DH, Smith TJ: Across-shift changes in the pulmonary function of meat-wrappers and other workers in the retail food industry. Scand J Work Environ Health 11:21, 1985.

1170. Perks WH, Burge PS, Pepys J, et al: Respiratory disease in an electronics factory. Br J Dis Chest 72:257, 1978.

1171. Burge PS, Perks W, O'Brien IM, et al: Occupational asthma in an electronics factory. Thorax 34:13, 1979.

1172. Ozhiganoua VN, Ivanoua IS, Dueva LA: Bronchial asthma in radio equipment assemblers. Sov Med 4:139, 1977.

1173. Perks WH, Burge PS, Rehahn M, et al: Work-related respiratory disease in employees leaving an electronics factory. Thorax 34:19, 1979.

1174. Pepys J, Pickering CAC, Hughes EG: Asthma due to inhaled chemical agents: Complex salts of platinum. Clin Allergy 2:391, 1972.

1175. Malo JL, Cartier A, Doepner M, et al: Occupational asthma caused by nickel sulfate. J Allergy Clin Immunol 69:55, 1982.

1176. Metals and the lung. Lancet 2:903, 1984.
1177. Sprince NL, Chamberlin RI, Hales CA, et al: Respiratory disease in tungsten carbide production workers. Chest 86:549, 1984.
1178. Gheysens B, Auwerx J, Van den Eeckhout A, et al: Cobalt-induced bronchial asthma in diamond polishers. Chest 88:740, 1985.
1179. Burge SP, Perks WH, O'Brien IM, et al: Occupational asthma in an electronics factory: A case control study to evaluate aetiological factors. Thorax 34:300, 1979.
1180. Burge SP, O'Brien IM, Harries MG: Peak flow rate records in the diagnosis of occupational asthma due to colophony. Thorax 34:308, 1979.
1181. Burge SP, O'Brien IM, Harries MG: Peak flow rate records in the diagnosis of occupational asthma due to isocyanates. Thorax 34:317, 1979.
1182. Lam S, Tan F, Chan H, et al: Relationship between types of asthmatic reaction, non-specific bronchial reactivity and specific IgE antibodies in patients with red cedar asthma. J Allergy Clin Immunol 72:134, 1983.
1183. Cockcroft DW, Hoeppner VH, Werner GD: Recurrent nocturnal asthma after bronchoprovocation with western red cedar sawdust: Association with acute increase in non-allergic bronchial responsiveness. Clin Allergy 14:61, 1984.
1184. Hodson ME, Simon G, Batten JC: Radiology of uncomplicated asthma. Thorax 29:296, 1974.
1185. Rebuck AS: Radiological aspects of severe asthma. Australas Radiol 14:264, 1970.
1186. Simon G, Connolly N, Littlejohns DW, et al: Radiological abnormalities in children with asthma and their relation to the clinical findings and some respiratory function tests. Thorax 28:115, 1973.
1187. Hodson CJ, Trickey SE: Bronchial wall thickening in asthma. Clin Radiol 11:183, 1960.
1188. Gillies JD, Reed MH, Simons FE: Radiologic findings in acute childhood asthma. J Can Assoc Radiol 29:28, 1978.
1189. Petheram IS, Kerr IH, Collins JV: Value of chest radiographs in severe acute asthma. Clin Radiol 32:281, 1981.
1190. Zieverink SF, Harper AP, Holden RW, et al. Emergency room radiography of asthma: An efficacy study. Radiology 145:27, 1982.
1191. Scannel JG: An anatomic approach to segmental resection. J Thorac Surg 18:64, 1949.
1192. Simonsson BG: Chronic cough and expectoration in patients with asthma and in patients with alpha₁-antitrypsin deficiency. Eur J Respir Dis 118:123, 1982.
1193. Fitch KD, Godfrey S: Asthma and athletic performance. JAMA 236:152, 1976.
1194. Lee HY, Stretton TB: Asthma in the elderly. Br Med J 4:93, 1972.
1195. McFadden ER Jr: Exertional dyspnea and cough as prelude to acute attacks of bronchial asthma. N Engl J Med 292:555, 1975.
1196. Baumann UA, Haerdi E, Keller R: Relations between clinical signs and lung function in bronchial asthma: how is acute bronchial obstruction reflected in dyspnoea and wheezing? Respiration 50:294, 1986.
1197. McFadden ER Jr, Kiser R, de Groot WJ: Acute bronchial asthma: Relations between clinical and physiologic manifestations. N Engl J Med 288:221, 1973.
1198. Editorial. Spirometry in asthma. N Engl J Med 288:262, 1973.
1199. Pratter MR, Hingston DM, Irwin RS: Diagnosis of bronchial asthma by clinical evaluation: An unreliable method. Chest 84:42, 1983.
1200. Pardee NE, Winterbauer RH, Morgan EH, et al: Combinations of 4 physical signs as indicators of ventilatory abnormality in obstructive pulmonary syndromes. Chest 77:354, 1980.
1201. Knowles GK, Clark TJH: Pulsus paradoxus as a valuable sign indicating severity of asthma. Lancet 2:1356, 1973.
1202. Rebuck AS, Reed J: Assessment and management of severe asthma. Am J Med 51:788, 1971.
1203. Rebuck AS, Pengally LD: Development of pulsus paradoxus in the presence of airways obstruction. N Engl J Med 288:66, 1973.
1204. Galant SP, Groncy CE, Shaw KC: The value of pulsus paradoxus in assessing the child with status asthmaticus. Pediatrics 61:46, 1978.
1205. Bellamy D, Collins JV: "Acute" asthma in adults. Thorax 34:36, 1979.
1206. Arnold AG, Lane DJ, Zapata E: The speed of onset and severity of acute severe asthma. Br J Dis Chest 76:157, 1982.
1207. Stellman JL, Spicer JE, Clayton RM: Morbidity from chronic asthma. Thorax 37:218, 1982.
1208. Banner AS, Shah RS, Addington WW: Rapid prediction of need for hospitalization in acute asthma. JAMA 235:1337, 1976.
1209. Senior RM, Lefrak RS, Korenblat PE: Status asthmaticus. JAMA 231:1277, 1972.
1210. Leading article: Treatment of status asthmaticus. Br Med J 4:563, 1972.
1211. Alston WC, Patel KR, Kerr JW: Response of leukocyte adenyl cyclase to isoprenaline and effect of alpha-blocking drugs in extrinsic bronchial asthma. Br Med J 1:90, 1974.

1212. Heilpern S, Rebuck AS: Effect of disodium cromoglycate (Intal) on sputum protein composition. Thorax 27:726, 1972.
1213. Brogan TD, Ryley HC, Neale L, et al: Soluble proteins of bronchopulmonary secretions from patients with cystic fibrosis, asthma, and bronchitis. Thorax 30:72, 1975.
1214. Laurenzi GA, Yin S: Studies of mucus flow in the mammalian respiratory tract. I. The beneficial effects of acetyl ouabain on respiratory tract mucus flow. Am Rev Respir Dis 103:800, 1971.
1215. Sackner MA, Epstein S, Wanner A: Effect of beta-adrenergic agonists aerosolized by freon propellant on tracheal mucous velocity and cardiac output. Chest 69(Suppl):593, 1976.
1216. Grieco MH: Catecholamines and the lung. Chest 69:579, 1976.
1217. Todisco T, Grassi V, Sorbini C: Circadian rhythms of respiratory functions in asthmatics. Respiration 40:128, 1980.
1218. Connolly CK: Diurnal rhythms in airway obstruction. Br J Dis Chest 73:357, 1979.
1219. Bahous J, Cartier A, Malo JL: Monitoring of peak expiratory flow rates in subjects with mild airway hyperexcitability. Bull Eur Physiol Respir 21:25, 1985.
1220. Turner-Warwick M: On observing patterns of airflow obstruction in chronic asthma. Br J Dis Chest 71:73, 1977.
1221. Sakula A: Sir John Floyer's "A Tratise of the Asthma" (1698). Thorax 39:248, 1984.
1222. Johansson SG, Wuthrich B, Zortea-Caflish C: Nightly asthma caused by allergens in silk-filled bed quilts: Clinical and immunologic studies. J Allergy Clin Immunol 75:452, 1985.
1223. Jönsson E, Mossberg B: Impairment of ventilatory function by supine posture in asthma. Eur J Respir Dis 65:496, 1984.
1224. Barnes P, Fitzgerald G, Brown M, et al: Nocturnal asthma and changes in circulating epinephrine, histamine and cortisol. N Engl J Med 303:263, 1980.
1225. Al-Damluji S, Thompson PJ, Citron KM, et al: Effect of naloxone on circadian rhythm in lung function. Thorax 38:914, 1983.
1226. Hetzel MR, Clark TJH: Does sleep cause nocturnal asthma? Thorax 34:749, 1979.
1227. Catterall JR, Rhind GB, Stewart IC, et al: Effect of sleep deprivation on overnight bronchoconstriction in nocturnal asthma. Thorax 41:676, 1986.
1228. Montplaisir J, Walsh J, Malo JL: Nocturnal asthma—features of attacks, sleep and breathing patterns. Am Rev Respir Dis 125:18, 1982.
1229. Shapiro CM, Catterall JR, Montgomery I, et al: Do asthmatics suffer bronchoconstriction during rapid eye movement sleep? Br Med J 292:1161, 1986.
1230. Soutar CA, Costello J, Ijaduola O, et al: Nocturnal and morning asthma: Relationship to plasma corticosteroids and response to cortical infusion. Thorax 30:436, 1975.
1231. Carpentiere G, Marino S, Castello F: Effects of inhaled fenoterol on the circadian rhythm of expiratory flow in allergic bronchial asthma. Chest 83:211, 1983.
1232. Soutar CA, Carruthers M, Pickering CAC: Nocturnal asthma and urinary adrenaline and noradrenaline excretion. Thorax 32:677, 1977.
1233. Bellia V, Cibella F, Migliara G, et al: Characteristics and prognostic value of morning dipping of peak expiratory flow rate in stable asthmatic subjects. Chest 88:89, 1985.
1234. Kelsen SG, Fleegler B, Altose MD: The respiratory neuromuscular response to hypoxia, hypercapnia and obstruction to airflow in asthma. Am Rev Respir Dis 120:517, 1979.
1235. Zackon H, Despas PJ, Anthonisen NR: Occlusion pressure responses in asthma and chronic obstructive lung disease. Am Rev Respir Dis 114:917, 1976.
1236. Pack AI, Hertz BC, Ledlie JF, et al: Reflex effects of aerosolized histamine on phrenic nerve activity. J Clin Invest 70:424, 1982.
1237. Kassabian J, Miller KD, Lavietes MH: Respiratory center output and ventilatory timing in patients with acute airway (asthma) and alveolar (pneumonia) disease. Chest 81:536, 1982.
1238. Chapman KR, Rebuck AS: Inspiratory and expiratory resistive loading as a model of dyspnea in asthma. Respiration 44:425, 1983.
1239. Burki NK, Mitchell K, Chaudhary BA, et al: The ability of asthmatics to detect added resistive loads. Am Rev Respir Dis 117:71, 1978.
1240. Gottfried SB, Altose MD, Kelsen SG, et al: Perception of changes in airflow resistance in obstructive pulmonary disorders. Am Rev Respir Dis 124:566, 1981.
1241. Issa FG, Sullivan CE: Respiratory muscle activity and thoracoabdominal motion during acute episodes of asthma during sleep. Am Rev Respir Dis 132:999, 1985.
1242. Tabachnick E, Müller NL, Levison H, et al: Chest wall mechanics and pattern of breathing during sleep in asthmatic adolescents. Am Rev Respir Dis 124:269, 1981.
1243. Hutchison AA, Olinski A: Hypoxic and hypercapnic response in asthmatic subjects with previous respiratory failure. Thorax 36:759, 1981.

11

1244. Corrao WM, Braman SS, Irwin RS: Chronic cough as the sole presenting manifestation of bronchial asthma. N Engl J Med 300:633, 1979.

1245. Poe RH, Israel RH, Utell MJ, et al: Chronic cough—bronchoscopy or pulmonary function testing? Am Rev Respir Dis 126:160, 1982.

1246. Cohen RM, Grant W, Lieberman P, et al: The use of methacholine inhalation, methacholine skin testing, distilled water inhalation challenge and eosinophil counts in the evaluation of patients presenting with cough and/or nonwheezing dyspnea. Ann Allergy 56:308, 1986.

1247. Puolijoki H, Lahdensuo A: Chronic cough as a risk indicator of broncho-pulmonary disease. Eur J Respir Dis 71:77, 1987.

1248. Eschenbacher WL, Boushey HA, Sheppard D: Alteration in osmolarity of inhaled aerosols causes bronchoconstriction and cough, but absence of a permeant anion causes cough alone. Am Rev Respir Dis 129:211, 1984.

1249. Higenbottam T: Essay. Cough induced by changes of ionic composition of airway surface liquid. Bull Eur Physiol Respir 20:553, 1985.

1250. Pounsford J, Birch M, Saunders K: Effect of bronchodilators on the cough response to inhaled citric acid in normal and asthmatic subjects. Thorax 40:662, 1985.

1251. Sheppard D, Rizk NW, Boushey HA, et al: Mechanism of cough and bronchoconstriction induced by distilled water aerosol. Am Rev Respir Dis 127:691, 1983.

1252. Arnup NE, Fleetham JA: Cough threshold: Variation within a normal population and relationship to bronchial reactivity. Am Rev Respir Dis 123:A129, 1981.

1253. Pounsford J, Saunders K: Diurnal variation and adaptation of the cough response to citric acid in normal subjects. Thorax 40:657, 1985.

1254. Irwin RS, Pratter MR, Holland PS, et al: Postnasal drip causes cough and is associated with reversible upper airway obstruction. Chest 85:346, 1984.

1255. O'Connell JM, Baird LI, Campbell AH: Sputum eosinophilia in chornic bronchitis and asthma. Respiration 35:65, 1978.

1256. Strang LB: Eosinophilia in children with asthma and bronchiectasis. Br Med J 1:167, 1960.

1257. Lowell FC: The total eosinophil count in obstructive pulmonary disease. N Engl J Med 292:1182, 1975.

1258. Horn BR, Robin ED, Theordore J, et al: Total eosinophil counts in the management of bronchial asthma. N Engl J Med 292:1152, 1975.

1259. Karetzky MS: Blood studies in untreated patients with acute asthma. Am Rev Respir Dis 112:607, 1975.

1260. Usher DJ, Shepherd RJ, Deegan T: Serum lactate dehydrogenase isoenzyme activities in patients with asthma. Thorax 29:685, 1976.

1261. Szczeklik A, Turowska B, Czerniawska-Mysik G, et al: Serum alpha$_1$-antitrypsin in bronchial asthma. Am Rev Respir Dis 109:487, 1974.

1262. Singleton R, Moel DI, Cohn RA: Preliminary observation of impaired water excretion in treated status asthmaticus. Am J Dis Child 140:59, 1986.

1263. Baker JW, Yerger S, Segar WE: Elevated plasma antidiuretic hormone levels in status asthmaticus. Mayo Clin Proc 51:31, 1976.

1264. Benfield GFA, Odoherty K, Davies BH: Status asthmaticus and the syndrome of inappropriate secretion of antidiuretic hormone. Thorax 37:147, 1982.

1265. Beers Ray F Jr: Skin tests. In Samter M, Alexander HL (eds): Immunologic Disorders. Boston, Little, Brown & Co, 1965, p 539.

1266. Greaves MW, Yamamoto S, Fairley VM: New in-vitro test for IgE-mediated hypersensitivity in man. Br Med J 2:623, 1972.

1267. Pepys J: Current concepts: Inhalation challenge tests in asthma. N Engl J Med 293:758, 1975.

1268. Gunstone RF: Right heart pressures in bronchial asthma. Thorax 26:39, 1971.

1269. Ahonen A: Analysis of the changes in ECG during status asthmaticus. Respiration 37:85, 1979.

1270. Gelb AF, Lyons HA, Fairshter RD, et al: P-Pulmonale in status asthmaticus. J Allergy Clin Immunol 64:18, 1979.

1271. Woolcock AJ, Vincent NJ, Macklem PT: Frequency dependence of compliance as a test for obstruction in the small airways. J Clin Invest 48:1097, 1969.

1272. Orzalesi MM, Cook CD, Hart MC: Pulmonary function in symptom-free asthmatic patients. Acta Paediatr Scand 53:401, 1964.

1273. Burrows D, Penman RWB: Prognosis of the eczema-asthma syndrome. Br Med J 2:825, 1960.

1274. Rubinfeld AR, Pain MCF: Perception of asthma. Lancet 1:882, 1976.

1275. Jones RHT, Jones RS: Ventilatory capacity in young adults with a history of asthma in childhood. Br Med J 2:976, 1966.

1276. Hill DJ, Landau LI, Phelan PD: Small airway disease in asymptomatic asthmatic adolescents. Am Rev Respir Dis 106:873, 1972.

1277. McCarthy D, Milic-Emili J: Closing volume in asymptomatic asthma. Am Rev Respir Dis 107:559, 1973.

1278. Morgan EJ, Hall DR: Abnormalities of lung function in hay fever. Thorax 31:80, 1976.

1279. Levine G, Housley E, MacLeod P, et al: Gas exchange abnormalities in mild bronchitis and asymptomatic asthma. N Engl J Med 282:1277, 1970.

1280. Palmer KNV, Kelman GR: Pulmonary function in asthmatic patients in remission. Br Med J 1:485, 1975.

1281. Wolf B, Gaultier C, Lopez C, et al: Hypoxemia in attack free asthmatic children: Relationship with lung volumes and lung mechanics. Bull Eur Physiopathol Respir 19:471, 1983.

1282. Wagner PD, Dantzker DB, Iacovoni VE, et al: Ventilation-perfusion inequality in asymptomatic asthma. Am Rev Respir Dis 118:511, 1978.

1283. Graff-Lonnevig V, Bevegard S, Eriksson BO: Ventilation and pulmonary gas exchange at rest and during exercise in boys with bronchial asthma. Eur J Respir Dis 61:357, 1980.

1284. Corte P, Young IH: Ventilation-perfusion relationships in symptomatic asthma; response to oxygen and clemastine. Chest 88:167, 1985.

1285. Loke J, Ganeshananthan M, Palm CR, et al: Site of airway obstruction in asymptomatic asthmatic children. Lung 159:35, 1981.

1286. Fairshter RD, Wilson AF: Relationship between the site of airflow limitation and localization of the bronchodilator response in asthma. Am Rev Respir Dis 122:27, 1980.

1287. Despas PJ, Leroux M, Macklem PT: Site of airway obstruction in asthma as determined by measuring maximal expiratory flow breathing air and a helium-oxygen mixture. J Clin Invest 51:3235, 1972.

1288. Chan-Yeung M, Abboud R, Tsao MS, et al: Effect of helium on maximal expiratory flow in patients with asthma before and during induced bronchoconstriction. Am Rev Respir Dis 113:433, 1976.

1289. Benatar SR, Clark TJR, Cochrane GM: Clinical relevance of the flow rate response to low density gas breathing in asthmatics. Am Rev Respir Dis 111:126, 1975.

1290. Partridge MR, Saunders KB: The site of airflow limitation in asthma—the effect of time, acute exacerbations of disease and clinical features. Br J Dis Chest 75:263, 1981.

1291. Antic R, Macklem PT: Influence of clinical factors on the site of airways obstruction in asthma. Am Rev Respir Dis 114:851, 1976.

1292. Metzger WJ, Nugent K, Richerson HB: Site of airflow obstruction during early and late phase asthmatic responses to allergen bronchoprovocation. Chest 88:369, 1985.

1293. Meisner P, Hugh-Jones P: Pulmonary function in bronchial asthma. Br Med J 1:470, 1968.

1294. Olive JT Jr, Hyatt RE: Maximal expiratory flow and total respiratory resistance during induced bronchoconstriction in asthmatic subjects. Am Rev Respir Dis 106:366, 1972.

1295. Clark TJH, Godfrey S, Pride NB: Physiology. In Clark TJH, Godfrey S (eds): Asthma. London, Chapman and Hall, 1983, p 12.

1296. Wang T-R, Levison H: Pulmonary function in children with asthma at acute attack and symptom-free status. Am Rev Respir Dis 99:719, 1969.

1297. Blackhall MI, Jones RS: Lung volume and its subdivisions in normal and asthmatic males. Thorax 28:89, 1973.

1298. Palmer KNV, Kelman GR: A comparison of pulmonary function in extrinsic and intrinsic bronchial asthma. Am Rev Respir Dis 107:940, 1973.

1299. Mayfield JD, Paez PN, Nicholson DP: Static and dynamic lung volumes and ventilation-perfusion abnormality in adult asthma. Thorax 26:591, 1971.

1300. Pedersen OF, Thiessen B, Naeraa N, et al: Factors determining residual volume in normal and asthmatic subjects. Eur J Respir Dis 65:99, 1984.

1301. Woolcock AJ, Read J: Lung volumes in exacerbations of asthma. Am J Med 41:259, 1966.

1302. Martin J, Powell E, Shore S, et al: The role of respiratory muscles in the hyperinflation of bronchial asthma. Am Rev Respir Dis 121:441, 1980.

1303. Müller N, Bryan AC, Zamel N: Tonic inspiratory muscle activity as a cause of hyperinflation in asthma. J Appl Physiol 50:279, 1981.

1304. Macklem PT: Hyperinflation (editorial). Am Rev Respir Dis 129:1, 1984.

1305. Ringel ER, Loring SH, McFadden ER, et al: Chest wall configurational changes before and during acute obstructive episodes in asthma. Am Rev Respir Dis 128:607, 1983.

1306. Lennox S, Mengeot PM, Martin JG: The contributions of rib cage and abdominal displacements to the hyperinflation of acute bronchospasm. Am Rev Respir Dis 132:679, 1985.

1307. Woolcock AJ, Read J: Improvement in bronchial asthma not reflected in forced expiratory volume. Lancet 2:1323, 1965.

1308. Martin JG, Shore SA, Engel LA: Mechanical load and inspiratory muscle action during induced asthma. Am Rev Respir Dis 128:455, 1983.

1309. Woolcock AJ, Rebuck AS, Cade JF, et al: Lung volume changes in asthma measured concurrently by two methods. Am Rev Respir Dis 104:703, 1971.

1310. Shore S, Miolic-Emili J, Martin JG: Reassessment of body plethysmographic technique for the measurement of thoracic gas volume in asthmatics. Am Rev Respir Dis 126:515, 1982.

1311. Stanescu DC, Rodenstein D, Cauberghs M, et al: Failure of body plethysmography in bronchial asthma. J Appl Physiol 52:939, 1982.

1312. Rodenstein D, Stanescu DC: Elastic properties of the lung in acute induced asthma. J Appl Physiol 54:152, 1983.

1313. Kirby JG, Juniper EF, Hargreave FE, et al: Total lung capacity does not change during methacholine-stimulated airway narrowing. J Appl Physiol 61:2144, 1986.

1314. Brown R, Ingram RH, McFadden ER: Problems in the plethysmographic assessment of changes in total lung capacity in asthma. Am Rev Respir Dis 118:685, 1978.

1315. Woolcock AJ, Read J: The static elastic properties of the lungs in asthma. Am Rev Respir Dis 98:788, 1968.

1316. Holmes PW, Campbell AH, Barter CE: Acute changes of lung volumes and lung mechanics in asthma and in normal subjects. Thorax 33:394, 1978.

1317. Hillman DR, Finucane KE: The effect of hyperinflation on lung elasticity in healthy subjects. Respir Physiol 54:295, 1983.

1318. Greaves IA, Colebatch HJ: Large lungs after childhood asthma: A consequence of enlarged air spaces. Aust NZ J Med 15:427, 1985.

1319. Ohman JL Jr, Schmidt-Nowara W, Lawrence M, et al: The diffusing capacity in asthma. Effect of airflow obstruction. Am Rev Respir Dis 107:932, 1973.

1320. Lawther PJ, Brooks AG, Waller RE: Respiratory function measurements in a cohort of medical students. Thorax 25:172, 1970.

1321. Ogilvie CM: Pulmonary function in asthma. Br Med J 1:768, 1968.

1322. Keens TG, Mansell A, Krastins IRB, et al: Evaluation of the single-breath diffusing capacity in asthma and cystic fibrosis. Chest 76:41, 1979.

1323. Graham BL, Mink JT, Cotton DJ, et al: Overestimation of the single-breath carbon monoxide diffusing capacity in patients with air-flow obstruction. Am Rev Respir Dis 129:403, 1984.

1324. Palmer KNV, Diament ML: Dynamic and static lung volumes and blood-gas tensions in bronchial asthma. Lancet 1:591, 1969.

1325. McFadden ER Jr, Lyons HA: Arterial-blood gas tension in asthma. N Engl J Med 278:1027, 1968.

1326. Tai E, Read J: Blood-gas tensions in bronchial asthma. Lancet 1:644, 1967.

1327. Simpson H, Forfar JO, Grubb DJ: Arterial blood gas tensions and pH in acute asthma in childhood. Br Med J 3:460, 1968.

1328. Wagner PD, Hedenstierna G, Bylin G: Ventilation-perfusion inequality in chronic asthma. Am Rev Respir Dis 136:605, 1987.

1329. Roncoroni AJ, Adrogué HJA, De Obrutsky CW, et al: Metabolic acidosis in status asthmaticus. Respiration 33:85–94, 1976.

1330. Alberts WM, Williams JH, Ramsdell JW: Metabolic acidosis as a presenting feature in acute asthma. Ann Allergy 57:107, 1986.

1331. Rees HA, Millar JS, Donald KW: A study of the clinical course and arterial blood gas tensions of patients in status asthmaticus. Q Med J 37:541, 1968.

1332. Palmer KNV, Diament ML: Relative contributions of obstructive and restrictive ventilatory impairment in the production of hypoxaemia and hypercapnia in chronic bronchitis. Lancet 1:1233, 1968.

1333. Stanescu DC, Teculescu DB: Pulmonary function in status asthmaticus: Effect of therapy. Thorax 25:581, 1970.

1334. Young IH, Corte P, Schoeffel RE: Pattern and time course of ventilation-perfusion inequality in exercise-induced asthma. Am Rev Respir Dis 125:304, 1982.

1335. Olgiati R, Birch S, Rao A, et al: Differential effects of methacholine and antigen challenge on gas exchange in allergic subjects. J Allergy Clin Immunol 67:325, 1981.

1336. Rubinfield AR, Wagner PD, West JB: Gas exchange during acute experimental canine asthma. Am Rev Respir Dis 118:525, 1978.

1337. Freyschuss U, Hedlin G, Hedenstierna G: Ventilation-perfusion relationships during exercise-induced asthma in children. Am Rev Respir Dis 130:888, 1984.

1338. Wilson AF, Suprenant EL, Beall GN, et al: The significance of regional pulmonary function changes in bronchial asthma. Am J Med 48:416, 1970.

1339. Rebuck AS, Read J: Patterns of ventilatory response to carbon dioxide during recovery from severe asthma. Clin Sci 41:13, 1971.

1340. Hudgel DW, Weil JV: Depression of hypoxic and hypercapnic ventilatory drives in severe asthma. Chest 68:493, 1975.

1341. Hudgel DW, Weil JV: Asthma associated with decreased hypoxia. Ann Intern Med 80:622, 1974.

1342. Eggleston PA, Ward BH, Pierson WE, et al: Radiographic abnormalities in acute asthma in children. Pediatrics 54:442, 1974.

1343. Gershel JC, Goldman HS, Stein EK, et al: The usefulness of chest radiographs in first asthma attacks. N Engl J Med 309:336, 1983.

1344. Findley LF, Sahn SA: The value of chest roentgenograms in acute asthma in adults. Chest 80:535, 1981.

1345. Bendkowski B: Asian influenza (1957) in allergic patients. Br Med J 2:1314, 1958.

1346. Luhr J: Atelectasis in bronchial asthma during childhood. Nord Med 60:1198, 1958.

1347. Dees SC, Spock A: Right middle lobe syndrome in children. JAMA 197:8, 1966.

1348. Bierman CW: Pneumomediastinum and pneumothorax complicating asthma in children. Am J Dis Child 114:42, 1967.

1349. Ozonoff MB: Pneumomediastinum associated with asthma and pneumonia in children. Am J Roentgenol 95:112, 1965.

1350. D'Assumpcao C, Smith WG: Spontaneous mediastinal and subcutaneous emphysema complicating bronchial asthma. Med J Aust 1:328, 1967.

1351. Dattwyler RJ, Goldman MA, Bloch KJ: Pneumomediastinum as a complication of asthma in teenage and young adult patients. J Allergy Clin Immunol 63:412, 1979.

1352. Macklin CC: Pneumothorax with massive collapse from experimental local overinflation of the lung substance. Can Med Assoc J 36:414, 1937.

1353. Macklin MT, Macklin CC: Malignant interstitial emphysema of the lungs and mediastinum as an important occult complication in many respirator diseases and other conditions: An interpretation of the clinical literature in the light of laboratory experiment. Medicine 23:281, 1944.

1354. Lewis M, Kallenbach J, Zaltzman M, et al: Acute respiratory failure in a young asthmatic patient. Chest 84:733, 1983.

1355. Toledo TM, Moore WL, Nash DA, et al: Spontaneous pneumopericardium in acute asthma. Case report and review of the literature. Chest 62:118, 1972.

1356. Segal AJ, Wasserman M: Arterial air embolism: A cause of sudden death in status asthmaticus. Radiology 99:271, 1971.

1357. Knudson RJ, Constantine HP: An effect of isoproterenol on ventilation-perfusion in asthmatic versus normal subjects. J Appl Physiol 22:402, 1967.

1358. Daly JJ, Howard P: Effect of intravenous aminophylline on the arterial oxygen saturation in chronic bronchitis. Thorax 20:324, 1965.

1359. Palmer KNV, Diament ML: Effect of aerosol isoprenaline on blood-gas tensions in severe bronchial asthma. Lancet 2:1232, 1967.

1360. Rees HA, Millar JS, Donald KW: Adrenaline in bronchial asthma. Lancet 2:1164, 1967.

1361. Rees HA, Borthwick RC, Millar JS, et al: Aminophylline in bronchial asthma. Lancet 2:1167, 1967.

1362. Palmer KNV, Diament ML: Effect of salbutamol on spirometry and blood gas tensions in bronchial asthma. Br Med J 1:31, 1969.

1363. Watanabe S, Renzetti A Jr, Bigler A: Bronchodilator and corticosteroid effects on regional and total airway resistance in patients with asthma, chronic bronchitis and chronic pulmonary emphysema. Am Rev Respir Dis 106:392, 1972.

1364. Gazioglu K, Condemi JJ, Hyde RW, et al: Effect of isoproterenol on gas exchange during air and oxygen breathing in patients with asthma. Am J Med 50:185, 1971.

1365. Halmagyi DF, Cotes JE: Reduction in systemic blood oxygen as a result of procedures affecting the pulmonary circulation in patients with chronic pulmonary disease. Clin Sci 18:475, 1959.

1366. Ingram RH Jr, Krumpe PE, Duffell GM, et al: Ventilation-perfusion changes after aerosolized isoproterenol in asthma. Am Rev Respir Dis 101:364, 1970.

1367. Chick TW, Nicholson DP, Johnson RL Jr: Effects of isoproterenol on distribution of ventilation and perfusion in asthma. Am Rev Respir Dis 107:869, 1973.

1368. Gazioglu K, Kaltreider NL, Hyde RW: Effect of isoproterenol on gas exchange during air and oxygen breathing in patients with chronic pulmonary diseases. Am Rev Respir Dis 104:188, 1971.

1369. Stolley PD: Asthma mortality. Why the United States was spared an epidemic of deaths due to asthma. Am Rev Respir Dis 105:883, 1972.

1370. Paterson JW, Sudlow MF, Walker SR: Blood-levels of fluorinated hydrocarbons in asthmatic patients after inhalation of pressurized aerosols. Lancet 2:565, 1971.

1371. Milledge JS, Benjamin S: Arterial desaturation after sodium bicarbonate therapy in bronchial asthma. Am Rev Respir Dis 105:126, 1972.

1372. Selikoff IJ, Churg J, Hammond EC: Asbestos exposure, smoking, and neoplasia. JAMA 204:106, 1968.

1373. Steinberg I, Finby N: Lipoid (mineral oil) pneumonia and cor pulmonale due to cardiospasm. Report of a case. Am J Roentgenol 76:108, 1956.

1374. Casey JF: Chronic cor pulmonale associated with lipoid pneumonia. JAMA 177:896, 1961.

1375. Higenbottam TW, Heard BE: Opportunistic pulmonary strongyloidiasis complicating asthma treated with steroids. Thorax 31:226, 1976.

1376. El-Shaboury AH, Hayes TM: Hyperlipidaemia in asthmatic patients receiving long-term steroid therapy. Br Med J 2:85, 1973.

11

1377. Smith AP: Patterns of recovery from acute severe asthma. Br J Dis Chest 75:132, 1981.

1378. Jenkins PF, Benfield GFA, Smith AP: Predicting recovery from acute severe asthma. Thorax 36:835, 1981.

1379. Centor RM, Yarbrough B, Wood JP: Inability to predict relapse in acute asthma. N Engl J Med 310:577, 1984.

1380. Fischl MA, Pitchenik A, Gardner LB: An index predicting relapse and need for hospitalization in patients with acute bronchial asthma. N Engl J Med 305:783, 1981.

1381. Benfield GFA, Smith AP: Predicting rapid and slow response to treatment in acute severe asthma. Br J Dis Chest 77:249, 1983.

1382. Ogilvie AG: Asthma: A study in prognosis of 1,000 patients. Thorax 17:183, 1962.

1383. Blackhall MI: Effect of age on fixed and labile components of airway resistance in asthma. Thorax 26:325, 1971.

1384. Lloyd TC Jr, Wright GW: Evaluation of methods used in detecting changes of airway resistance in man. Am Rev Respir Dis 87:529, 1963.

1385. Rackemann FN, Edwards MC: Asthma in children. A follow-up study of 688 patients after an interval of twenty years. N Engl J Med 246:815, 1952.

1386. Rackemann FN, Edwards MC: Asthma in children. A follow-up study of 688 patients after an interval of twenty years (concluded). N Engl J Med 246:858, 1952.

1387. Cserhati E, Mezei G, Kelemen J: Late prognosis of bronchial asthma in children. Respiration 46:160, 1984.

1388. Brown PJ, Greville HW, Finucane KE: Asthma and irreversible airflow obstruction. Thorax 39:131, 1984.

1389. Peat JK, Woolcock AJ, Cullen K: Rate of decline of lung function in subjects with asthma. Eur J Respir Dis 70:171, 1986.

1390. Alexander HL: A historical account of death from asthma. J Allergy 34:305, 1963.

1391. Speizer FE, Doll R: A century of asthma deaths in young people. Br Med J 3:245, 1968.

1392. Speizer FE, Doll R, Heaf P: Observtions on recent increase in mortality from asthma. Br Med J 1:335, 1968.

1393. Speizer FE, Doll R, Heaf P, et al: Investigation into use of drugs preceding death from asthma. Br Med J 1:339, 1968.

1394. Leading article: Asthma deaths: A question answered. Br Med J 4:443, 1972.

1395. Stableforth DE: Death from asthma. Thorax 38:801, 1983.

1396. Stewart CJ, Nunn AJ: Are asthma mortality rates changing. Br J Dis Chest 79:229, 1985.

1397. Bateman JRM, Clarke SW: Sudden death in asthma. Thorax 34:40, 1979.

1398. Sears MR, Rea HH, Beaglehole R, et al: Asthma mortality in New Zealand: a two year national study. NZ Med J 98:271, 1985.

1399. Sutherland DC, Beaglehole R, Fenwick J, et al: Death from asthma in Auckland: Circumstances and validation of causes. NZ Med J 97:845, 1984.

1400. Sears MR: Why are deaths from asthma increasing? Eur J Respir Dis 147(Suppl):175, 1986.

1401. Paulozzi LJ, Coleman JJ, Buist AS: A recent increase in asthma mortality in the northwestern United States. Ann Allergy 56:392, 1986.

1402. Evans R, Mullally DI, Wilson RW, et al: National trends in the morbidity and mortality of asthma in the U.S. Prevalence, hospitalization and death from asthma over two decades: 1965–1984. Chest 91(6 Suppl):65S, 1987.

1403. Burney PG: Asthma mortality in England and Wales: Evidence for a further increase, 1974–84. Lancet 2:323, 1986.

1404. Picado C, Montserrat JM, Roca J, et al: Mechanical ventilation in severe exacerbation of asthma. Study of 26 cases with six deaths. Eur J Respir Dis 64:102, 1983.

1405. Sears MR, Rea HH, Fenwick J: Deaths from asthma in New Zealand. Arch Dis Child 61:6, 1986.

1406. Strunk RC, Mrazek DA, Fuhrmann GS, et al: Physiologic and psychological characteristics associated with deaths due to asthma in childhood. A case-controlled study. JAMA 254:1193, 1985.

1407. Eason J, Markowe HL: Controlled investigation of deaths from asthma in hospitals in the North East Thames region. Br Med J 294:1255, 1987.

1408. Crompton GK, Grant IWB: Edinburgh emergency asthma admission service. Br Med J 4:680, 1975.

1409. Crompton GK, Grant IW, Chapman BJ, et al: Edinburgh Emergency Asthma Admission Service: Report on 15 years' experience. Eur J Respir Dis 70:266, 1987.

1410. Turner KJ, Baldo BA, Hilton JMN: IgE antibodies and Dermatophagoides pteronyssinus (house dust mite), Aspergillus fumigatus, and β-lactoglobulin in sudden infant death syndrome. Br Med J 1:357, 1975.

1411. Burrows B: Foreword, symposium on chronic respiratory disease. Med Clin North Am 57:545, 1973.

1412. Friedman D, Dales LG, Ury HK, et al: Mortality in middle-aged smokers and non-smokers. N Engl J Med 300:213, 1979.

1413. Ferris B Jr: Chronic bronchitis and emphysema: Classification and epidemiology. Med Clin North Am 57:637, 1973.

1414. Peto R, Speizer FE, Cochrane AL, et al: The relevance in adults of air-flow obstruction, but not of mucus hypersecretion, to mortality from chronic lung disease—results from 20 years of prospective observation. Am Rev Respir Dis 128:491, 1983.

1415. Burrows B, Knudson RJ, Camilli AE, et al: The "horse-racing effect" and predicting decline in forced expiratory volume in one second from screening spirometry. Am Rev Respir Dis 135:788, 1987.

1416. Laennec RTH: A Treatise on the Diseases of the Chest and on Mediate Auscultation, 4th ed, John Forbes, Translator. New York, Wood, 1835.

1417. Turner-Warwick M: Some clinical problems in patients with airways obstruction. Chest 82:3S, 1982.

1418. Fletcher CM, Pride NB: Editorial: Definitions of emphysema, chronic bronchitis, asthma, and airflow obstruction: 25 years on from the CIBA symposium. Thorax 39:81, 1984.

1419. Becklake MR: Chronic airflow limitation: Its relationship to work in dusty occupations. Chest 88:608, 1985.

1420. Macklem PT, Thurlbeck WM, Fraser RG, et al: Chronic obstructive disease of small airways. Ann Intern Med 74:167, 1971.

1421. American Thoracic Society (Statement by Committee on Diagnostic Standards for Nontuberculous Respiratory Diseases): Definitions and classification of chronic bronchitis, asthma, and pulmonary emphysema. Am Rev Respir Dis 85:762, 1962.

1422. Lebowitz MD, Burrows B: Comparison of questionnaires: The BMRC and NHLI respiratory questionnaires and a new self-completion questionnaire. Am Rev Respir Dis 113:627, 1976.

1423. Report of the conclusions of a Ciba Guest Symposium: Terminology, definitions and classification of chronic pulmonary emphysema and related conditions. Thorax 14:286, 1959.

1424. Snider GL, Kleinerman JL, Thurlbeck WM, et al: The definition of emphysema—report of a national heart-lung-and-blood institute, Division of Lung Diseases Workshop. Am Rev Respir Dis 132:182, 1985.

1425. Oswald NC: Chronic bronchitis and emphysema: A symposium II. Clinical aspects of chronic bronchitis. Br J Radiol 32:289, 1959.

1426. Fletcher CM: Chronic bronchitis. Its prevalence, nature, and pathogenesis. Am Rev Respir Dis 80:483, 1959.

1427. Reid DD, Anderson DO, Ferris BG, et al: An Anglo-American comparison of the prevalence of bronchitis. Br Med J 2:1487, 1964.

1428. Dodge R, Cline MG, Burrows B: Comparisons of asthma, emphysema, and chronic bronchitis diagnoses in a general population sample. Am Rev Respir Dis 133:981, 1986.

1429. Keith TA III, Schreiner AW: Hemophilus influenzae in adult bronchopulmonary infection. Ann Intern Med 56:27, 1962.

1430. College of General Practitioners: Chronic bronchitis in Great Britain. A national survey carried out by the Respiratory Diseases Study Group of the College of General Practitioners. Br Med J 2:973, 1961.

1431. Tager I, Speizer FE: Role of infection in chronic bronchitis. N Engl J Med 292:563, 1975.

1432. Zuskin E, Valie F: Effect of short term cigarette smoking on simple tests of ventilatory capacity in medical students. Am Rev Respir Dis 110:198, 1974.

1433. Grimes CA, Hanes B: Influence of cigarette smoking on the spirometric evaluation of employees of a large insurance company. Am Rev Respir Dis 108:273, 1973.

1434. Higgins MW, Keller JB, Becker M, et al: An index of risk for obstructive airway disease. Am Rev Respir Dis 125:144, 1982.

1435. Higgins MW, Keller JB, Landis JR, et al: Risk of chronic obstructive pulmonary disease—collaborative assessment of the validity of the Tecumseh Index of Risk. Am Rev Respir Dis 130:380, 1984.

1436. Rimington J: Chronic bronchitis: Method of cigarette smoking. Br Med J 1:776, 1973.

1437. Rimington J: Cigarette smoker's bronchitis: The effect of relighting. Br Med J 2:591, 1974.

1438. Webster JR Jr, Kettel LJ, Moran F, et al: Chronic obstructive pulmonary disease. A comparison between men and women. Am Rev Respir Dis 98:1021, 1968.

1439. Oswald NC, Medvei VC, Waller RE: Chronic bronchitis: A 10-year follow-up. Thorax 22:279, 1967.

1440. Fletcher CM, Elmes PC, Fairbairn AS, et al: The significance of respiratory symptoms and the diagnosis of chronic bronchitis in a working population. Br Med J 2:257, 1959.

1441. Seltzer CC, Siegelaub AB, Friedman GD, et al: Differences in pulmonary function related to smoking habits and race. Am Rev Respir Dis 110:598, 1974.

1442. Miller GJ: Cigarette smoking and irreversible airways obstruction in the West Indies. Thorax 29:495, 1974.

1443. Emirgil C, Sobol BJ, Heymann B, et al: Pulmonary function in alcoholics. Am J Med 57:69, 1974.

1444. Sobol BJ, Herbert WH, Emirgil C: The high incidence of pulmonary functional abnormalities in patients with coronary artery disease. Chest 65:148, 1974.

1445. Burrows B, Niden AH, Barclay WR, et al: Chronic obstructive lung disease. 1. Clinical and physiologic findings in 175 patients and their relationship to age and sex. Am Rev Respir Dis 91:521, 1965.

1446. Clément J, Van de Woestijne KP. Rapidly decreasing forced expiratory volume in one second or vital capacity and development of chronic airflow obstruction. Am Rev Respir Dis 125:553, 1982.

1447. Beaty TH, Menkes HA, Cohen BH, et al: Risk factors associated with longitudinal change in pulmonary function. Am Rev Respir Dis 129:660, 1984.

1448. Pride NB: Which smokers develop progressive airflow obstruction. Eur J Respir Dis 64(Suppl 126):79, 1983.

1449. Cullen KJ, Stenhouse NS, Welborn TA, et al: Chronic respiratory disese in a rural community. Lancet 2:657, 1968.

1450. Dysinger PW, Lemon FR, Crenshaw GL, et al: Pulmonary emphysema in a non-smoking population. Dis Chest 43:17, 1963.

1451. Payne M, Kjelsberg M: Respiratory symptoms, lung function, and smoking habits in an adult population. Am J Public Health 54:261, 1964.

1452. Thurlbeck WM: Chronic Airflow Obstruction in Lung Disease: Major Problems in Pathology, Vol 5. Philadelphia, WB Saunders Co, 1976.

1453. Boucot KR, Cooper DA, Weiss W: Smoking and the health of older men. 1. Smoking and chronic cough. Arch Environ Health 4:59, 1962.

1454. Wynder EL, Lemon FR, Mantel N: Epidemiology of persistent cough. Am Rev Respir Dis 91:679, 1965.

1455. Peters GA, Miller RD: Effect of smoking on asthma and emphysema. Mayo Clin Proc 35:353, 1960.

1456. Anderson DO, Ferris BG Jr: Role of tobacco smoking in the causation of chronic respiratory disease. N Engl J Med 267:787, 1962.

1457. Mueller RE, Keble DL, Plummer J, et al: The prevalence of chronic bronchitis, chronic airway obstruction, and respiratory symptoms in a Colorado city. Am Rev Respir Dis 103:209, 1971.

1458. Brinkman GL, Coates EO Jr: The effect of bronchitis, smoking, and occupation on ventilation. Am Rev Respir Dis 87:684, 1963.

1459. Barker GS: Lung function in elderly male heavy smokers and nonsmokers. Am Rev Respir Dis 91:409, 1965.

1460. Wilson RH, Meador RS, Jay BE, et al: The pulmonary pathologic physiology of persons who smoke cigarettes. N Engl J Med 262:956, 1960.

1461. Sharp JT, Paul O, Lepper MH, et al: Prevalence of chronic bronchitis in an American male urban industrial population. Am Rev Respir Dis 91:510, 1965.

1462. Bower G: Respiratory symptoms and ventilatory function in 172 adults employed in a bank. Am Rev Respir Dis 83:684, 1961.

1463. Weiss W, Boucot KR, Cooper DA, et al: Smoking and the health of older men. II. Smoking and ventilatory function. Arch Environ Health 7:538, 1963.

1464. Larson RK: The chronic effect of cigarette smoking on pulmonary ventilation. Am Rev Respir Dis 88:630, 1963.

1465. Franklin W, Lowell FC: Unrecognized airway obstruction associated with smoking: A probable forerunner of obstructive pulmonary emphysema. Ann Intern Med 54:379, 1961.

1466. Beck GJ, Doyle CA, Schachter EN, et al: Smoking and lung function. Am Rev Respir Dis 123:149, 1981.

1467. Tager IB, Muñoz A, Rosner B, et al: Effect of cigarette smoking on the pulmonary function of children and adolescents. Am Rev Respir Dis 131:752, 1985.

1468. Paoletti P, Camilli AE, Holberg CJ, et al: Respiratory effects in relation to estimated tar exposure from current and cumulative cigarette consumption. Chest 88:849, 1985.

1469. Tobin MJ, Sackner MA: Monitoring smoking patterns of low and high tar cigarettes with inductive plethysmography. Am Rev Respir Dis 126:258, 1982.

1470. Medici TC, Unger S, Rüegger M, et al: Smoking pattern of smokers with and without tobacco smoke-related lung diseases. Am Rev Respir Dis 131:385, 1985.

1471. Taylor DR, Reid WD, Pare PD, et al: Cigarette smoke inhalation patterns and bronchial reactivity. Thorax 43:65–70, 1988.

1472. Smaldone GC, Messina MS: Enhancement of particle deposition by flow-limiting segments in humans. J Appl Physiol 49:509, 1985.

1473. Rodenstein D, Stănescu D: Pattern of inhalation of tobacco smoke in pipe, cigarette, and never smokers. Am Rev Respir Dis 132:628, 1985.

1474. Sparrow D, Stefos T, Bossé R, et al: The relationship of tar content to decline in pulmonary function in cigarette smokers. Am Rev Respir Dis 127:56, 1983.

1475. Lehrer SB, Barbandi F, Taylor JP, et al: Tobacco smoke sensitivity—is there an immunologic basis? J Allergy Clin Immunol 240:73, 1984.

1476. Lehrer SB, Wilson MR, Salvaggio JE, et al: Immunogenic properties of tobacco smoke. J Allergy Clin Immunol 62:368, 1978.

1477. Guyatt AR, Berry G, Alpers JH, et al: Relationship of airway conductance and its immediate change on smoking to smoking habits and symptoms of chronic bronchitis. Am Rev Respir Dis 101:44, 1970.

1478. Nadel JA, Comroe JH Jr: Acute effects of inhalation of cigarette smoke on airway conductance. J Appl Physiol 16:713, 1961.

1479. Sterling GM: Mechanism of bronchoconstriction caused by cigarette smoking. Br Med J 3:275, 1967.

1480. Costello JF, Sudlow MF, Douglas NJ, et al: Acute effects of smoking tobacco and a tobacco substitute on lung function in man. Lancet 2:678, 1975.

1481. McCarthy DS, Craig DB, Cherniack RM: The effect of acute, intensive cigarette smoking on maximal expiratory flows and the single-breath nitrogen washout trace. Am Rev Respir Dis 113:301, 1976.

1482. Chiang ST, Wang BC: Acute effects of cigarette smoking on pulmonary function. Am Rev Respir Dis 101:860, 1970.

1483. Higenbottam T, Hamilton D, Feyerband C, et al: Acute effects of smoking a single cigarette on the airway resistance and the maximal and partial forced expiratory flow volume curves. Br J Dis Chest 74:37, 1980.

1484. Taveira DA, Silva AM, Hamosh P: Airways response to inhaled tobacco smoke: Time course, dose dependence and effect of volume history. Respiration 41:96, 1981.

1485. McIntyre EL, Ruffin RE, Alpers JH, et al: Lack of short-term effects of cigarette smoking on bronchial sensitivity to histamine and methacholine. Eur J Respir Dis 63:535, 1982.

1486. Malo JL, Filiatrault S, Martin RR, et al: Bronchial responsiveness to inhaled methacholine in young asymptomatic smokers. J Appl Physiol 52:1464, 1982.

1487. Taylor RG, Clarke SW: Bronchial reactivity to histamine in young male smokers. Eur J Respir Dis 66:390, 1985.

1488. Kabiraj MU, Simonsson BG, Groth S, et al: Bronchial reactivity, smoking, and alpha₁-antitrypsin: a population-based study of middle-aged men. Am Rev Respir Dis 126:864, 1982.

1489. Buczko GB, Zamel N: Combined effect of cigarette smoking and allergic rhinitis on airway responsiveness to inhaled methacholine. Am Rev Respir Dis 129:15, 1984.

1490. Weiss ST, Tager IB, Schenker M, et al: The health effects of involuntary smoking. Am Rev Respir Dis 128:933, 1983.

1491. Bake B: Effects in humans. Does environmental tobacco smoke affect lung function? In Rylander R, Peterson Y, Snella M-C (eds): Environmental Tobacco Smoke: Report from a workshop on effects and exposure levels held on March 15–17, 1983, Geneva, Switzerland. Eur J Respir Dis 65(Suppl 133):85, 1984.

1492. Hiller FC, McCusker KT, Mazumder MK, et al: Deposition of sidestream cigarette smoke in the human respiratory tract. Am Rev Respir Dis 125:405, 1982.

1493. Jarvis MJ, Russell MAH, Feyerabend C, et al: Absorption of nicotine and carbon monoxide from passive smoking under natural conditions of exposure. Thorax 31:829, 1983.

1494. Tashkin DP, Clark VA, Simmons M, et al: The UCLA population studies of chronic obstructive respiratory disease: Relationship between parental smoking and children's lung function. Am Rev Respir Dis 129:891, 1984.

1495. Weiss ST, Taher IB, Speizer FE, et al: Passive smoking; its relationship to respiratory symptoms, pulmonary function and non-specific bronchial responsiveness. Chest 84:651, 1983.

1496. Burchfiel CM, Higgins MW, Keller JB, et al: Passive smoking in childhood. Respiratory conditions and pulmonary function in Tecumseh, Michigan. Am Rev Respir Dis 133:966, 1986.

1497. Tsimoyianis GV, Jacobson MS, Feldman JG: Reduction in pulmonary function and increased frequency of cough associated with passive smoking in teenage athletes. Pediatrics 80:32, 1987.

1498. Tager B, Weiss T, Muñoz A, et al: Longitudinal study of the effects of maternal smoking on pulmonary function in children. N Engl J Med 309:699, 1983.

1499. Comstock GW, Meyer MB, Helsing KJ, et al: Respiratory effects of household exposures to tobacco smoke and gas cooking. Am Rev Respir Dis 124:143, 1981.

1500. White RW, Froeb F: Small airways dysfunction in nonsmokers chronically exposed to tobacco smoke. N Engl J Med 302:720, 1980.

1501. Colley JRT, Holland WW, Corkhill RT: Influence of passive smoking and parental phlegm on pneumonia and bronchitis in early childhood. Lancet 2:1031, 1974.

1502. Tashkin DP, Shapiro BJ, Lee YE, et al: Subacute effects of heavy marihuana smoking on pulmonary function in healthy men. N Engl J Med 294:125, 1976.

1503. Tashkin DP, Coulson AH, Clark VA, et al: Respiratory symptoms and lung function in habitual heavy smokers of marijuana alone, smokers of marijuana and tobacco, smokers of tobacco alone, and nonsmokers. Am Rev Respir Dis 135:209, 1987.

1504. DaCosta JL, Tock EPC, Boey HK: Lung disease with chronic obstruction in opium smokers in Singapore. Thorax 26:555, 1971.

11

1505. Morgan WKC: On dust, disability and death (editorial). Am Rev Respir Dis *134*:639, 1986.

1506. Nadel JA, Comroe JH Jr: Acute effects of inhalation of cigarette smoke on airway conductance. J Appl Physiol *16*:713, 1961.

1507. Megahed GE, Senna GA, Eissa MH, et al: Smoking versus infection as the aetiology of bronchial mucous gland hypertrophy in chronic bronchitis. Thorax *22*:271, 1967.

1508. Mitchell RS, Ryan SF, Petty TL, et al: The significance of morphologic chronic hyperplastic bronchitis. Am Rev Respir Dis *93*:720, 1966.

1509. Sanderud K: Squamous metaplasia of the respiratory tract epithelium. An autopsy study of 214 cases. 2. Relation to tobacco smoking, occupation and residence. Acta Pathol Microbiol Scand *43*:47, 1958.

1510. Bates DV: Air pollutants and the human lung. The James Waring memorial lecture. Am Rev Respir Dis *105*:1, 1972.

1511. Lebowitz MD, Bendheim P, Cristea G, et al: The effect of air pollution and weather on lung function in exercising children and adolescents. Am Rev Respir Dis *109*:262, 1974.

1512. Lawther PJ, Waller RE, Henderson M: Air pollution and exacerbations of bronchitis. Thorax *25*:525, 1970.

1513. Bates DV, Sizto R: A study of hospital admissions and air pollutants in Southern Ontario. *In* Lee SD, Schneider T, Grant LD, et al (eds): Aerosols. Chelsea, Mich, Lewis Publishers, Inc., 1986.

1514. Cohen CA, Hudson AR, Clausen JL, et al: Respiratory symptoms, spirometry, and oxidant air pollution in nonsmoking adults. Am Rev Respir Dis *105*:251, 1972.

1515. Zepletal A, Jech J, Paul T, et al: Pulmonary function studies in children living in an air-polluted area. Am Rev Respir Dis *107*:400, 1973.

1516. Lambert PM, Reid DD: Smoking, air pollution, and bronchitis in Britain. Lancet *1*:853, 1970.

1517. Van der Lende R, Rijcken B: Longitudinal versus cross-sectional studies in measuring effect of smoking, air pollution and hyperreactivity on VC and FEV_1. Bull Eur Physiopathol Respir *19*:85, 1983.

1518. Solic J, Hazucha J, Bromberg A, et al: The acute effects of 0.2 ppm ozone in patients with chronic obstructive pulmonary disease. Am Rev Respir Dis *125*:664, 1982.

1519. Linn S, Fischer D, Medway A, et al: Short-term respiratory effects of 0.12 ppm ozone exposure in volunteers with chronic obstructive pulmonary disease. Am Rev Respir Dis *125*:658, 1982.

1520. Kehrl HR, Hazucha MJ, Solic JJ, et al: Responses of subjects with chronic obstructive pulmonary disease after exposures to 0.3 ppm ozone. Am Rev Respir Dis *131*:719, 1985.

1521. Clini V, Pozzi G, Ferrara A, et al: Bronchial hyperreactivity and arterial carboxyhemoglobin as detectors of air pollution in Milan: A study on normal subjects. Respiration *47*:1, 1985.

1522. Dohan FC, Taylor EW: Air pollution and respiratory disease. A preliminary report. Am J Med Sci *240*:337, 1960.

1523. Holland WW, Reid DD: The urban factor in chronic bronchitis. Lancet *1*:445, 1965.

1524. Ferris BG Jr, Higgins ITT, Higgins MW, et al: Chronic nonspecific respiratory disease in Berlin, New Hampshire, 1961 to 1967. A follow-up study. Am Rev Respir Dis *107*:110, 1973.

1525. Ferris BG Jr, Higgins ITT, Higgins MW, et al: Chronic non specific respiratory disease, Berlin, New Hampshire, 1961–1967: A cross-sectional study. Am Rev Respir Dis *104*:232, 1971.

1526. Storms WW, DoPico GA, Reed CE: Aerosol Sch 1000. An anticholinergic bronchodilator. Am Rev Respir Dis *111*:419, 1975.

1527. Douglas JWB, Waller RE: Air pollution and respiratory infection in children. Br J Prev Soc Med *20*:1, 1966.

1528. Lunn JE, Knowelden J, Handyside AJ: Patterns of respiratory illness in Sheffield infant schoolchildren. Br J Prev Soc Med *21*:7, 1967.

1529. Ware JH, Dockery DW, Spiro A, et al: Passive smoking, gas cooking and respiratory health of children living in 6 cities. Am Rev Respir Dis *129*:366, 1984.

1530. Ekwo EE, Weinberger MM, Lachenbruch PA, et al: Relationship of parental smoking and gas cooking to respiratory disease in children. Chest *662*:84, 1983.

1531. Pandey MR: Prevalence of chronic bronchitis in a rural community of the hill region of Nepal. Thorax *39*:331, 1984.

1532. Pandey MR: Domestic smoke pollution and chronic bronchitis in a rural community of the hill region of Nepal. Thorax *39*:337, 1984.

1533. Woolcock AJ, Blackburn CRB, Freeman MH, et al: Studies of chronic (nontuberculous) lung disease in New Guinea populations. The nature of the disease. Am Rev Respir Dis *102*:575, 1970.

1534. Jones HL Jr: COPD in women in developing countries. Chest *65*:704, 1974.

1535. Cullen KJ, Elder J, Adams AR, et al: Additional factors in chronic bronchitis. Br Med J *1*:394, 1970.

1536. Medical Research Council: Chronic bronchitis and occupation. M.R.C. report. Br Med J *1*:101, 1966.

1537. Lane RE: Chronic bronchitis and occupation. Br J Tuberc *52*:11, 1958.

1538. McDonald JC: Epidemiology. *In* Weill H, Turner-Warwick M (eds): Occupational Lung Diseases: Research Approaches and Methods. New York, M Dekker, 1981, p 373.

1539. Korn RJ, Dockery DW, Speizer FE, et al: Occupational exposures and chronic respiratory symptoms. A population-based study. Am Rev Respir Dis *136*:298, 1987.

1540. Diem JE, Jones RN, Hendrick DJ, et al: Five year longitudinal study of workers employed in a new toluene diisocyanate manufacturing plant. Am Rev Respir Dis *126*:420, 1982.

1541. Attfield MD: Longitudinal decline in FEV_1 in United States coalminers. Thorax *40*:132, 1985.

1542. Soutar CA, Hurley JF: Relation between dust exposure and lung function in miners and ex-miners. Br J Ind Med *43*:307, 1986.

1543. Morgan WKC: Industrial bronchitis. Br J Ind Med *35*:285, 1978.

1544. Cohen BM, Adasczik A, Cohen EM, et al: Small airways changes in workers exposed to asbestos. Respiration *45*:296, 1984.

1545. Sue D, Oren A, Hansen J, et al: Lung function and exercise performance in smoking and non-smoking asbestos-exposed workers. Am Rev Respir Dis *132*:612, 1985.

1546. Bégin R, Boileau R, Péloquin S: Asbestos exposure, cigarette smoking, and airflow limitation in long-term Canadian chrysotile miners and millers. Am J Industr Med *11*:55, 1987.

1547. Sparrow D, Bossé R, Rosner B, et al: The effect of occupational exposure on pulmonary function. Am Rev Respir Dis *125*:319, 1982.

1548. Ruckley VA, Gauld SJ, Chapman JS, et al: Emphysema and dust exposure in a group of coal workers. Am Rev Respir Dis *129*:528, 1984.

1549. Becklake MR, Irwig L, Kielkowski D, et al: The predictors of emphysema in South African gold miners. Am Rev Respir Dis *135*:1234, 1987.

1550. Chan-Yeung M, Wong R, MacLean L, et al: Respiratory survey of workers in a pulp and paper mill in Powell River, British Columbia. Am Rev Respir Dis *122*:249, 1980.

1551. Colley JRT, Reid DD: Urban and social origins of childhood bronchitis in England and Wales. Br Med J *2*:213, 1970.

1552. Colley JRT, Douglas JWB, Reid DD: Respiratory disease in young adults: Influence of early childhood lower respiratory tract illness, social class, air pollution, and smoking. Br Med J *3*:195, 1973.

1553. Cederlöf R, Edfors ML, Friberg L, et al: Hereditary factors, "spontaneous cough" and "smoker's cough." A study of 7,800 twin-pairs with the aid of mailed questionnaires. Arch Environ Health *14*:401, 1967.

1554. Britten N, Davies JM, Colley JR: Early respiratory experience and subsequent cough and peak expiratory flow rate in 36 year old men and women. Br Med J *294*:1317, 1987.

1555. Boule M, Gaultier C, Tournier G, et al: Lung function in children with recurrent bronchitis. Respiration *38*:127, 1979.

1556. Woolcock AJ, Leeder SR, Peat JK, et al: The influence of lower respiratory illness in infancy and childhood and subsequent cigarette smoking on lung function in Sydney school children. Am Rev Respir Dis *120*:5, 1979.

1557. Woolcock A, Peat J, Leeder S, et al: The development of lung function in Sydney children: Effects of respiratory illness and smoking. A ten year study. Eur J Respir Dis *65*:1, 1985.

1558. Moreno R, McCormack GS, Mullen JBM, et al: The effect of intravenous papain on the tracheal pressure volume curves in rabbits. J Appl Physiol *60*:247, 1986.

1559. Holland WW: Beginnings of bronchitis. Thorax *37*:401, 1982.

1560. Hallett WY: Infection: The real culprit in chronic bronchitis and emphysema? Med Clin North Am *57*:735, 1973.

1561. Gurwitz D, Corey M, Levison H, et al: Pulmonary function and bronchial reactivity in children after croup. Am Rev Respir Dis *122*:95, 1980.

1562. Barker DJ, Osmond C: Childhood respiratory infection and adult chronic bronchitis in England and Wales. Br Med J *293*:1271, 1986.

1563. Medici TC, Buergi H: The role of immunoglobulin A in endogenous bronchial defense mechanisms in chronic bronchitis. Am Rev Respir Dis *103*:784, 1971.

1564. Lewis DM, Lapp N, Burrell R: Quantitation of secretory immunoglobulin A in chronic pulmonary disease. Am Rev Respir Dis *101*:55, 1970.

1565. Siegler DIM, Citron KM: Serum and parotid salivary IgA in chronic bronchitis and asthma. Thorax *29*:313, 1974.

1566. Falk GA, Okinaka AJ, Siskind GW: Immunoglobulins in the bronchial washings of patients with chronic obstructive pulmonary disease. Am Rev Respir Dis *105*:14, 1972.

1567. Orfanakis MG, Smith CB, Klauber MR, et al: Factors related to serum and secretory immunoglobulin concentrations in patients with chronic obstructive pulmonary disease. Am Rev Respir Dis *107*:728, 1974.

1568. Gump DW, Christmas WA, Forsyth BR, et al: Serum and secretory antibodies in patients with chronic bronchitis. Arch Intern Med *132*:847, 1973.

1569. Medici TC, Chodosh S: Sputum cell dynamics in bacterial exacerbations of chronic bronchial disease. Arch Intern Med 129:597, 1972.

1570. Ritts RE, Miller RD, LeDuc PV, et al: Phagocytosis and cutaneous delayed hypersensitivity in patients with chronic obstructive pulmonary disease. Chest 69:474, 1976.

1571. Massala C, Amendolea MA, Bonini S: Mucus antibodies in pulmonary tuberculosis and chronic obstructive lung disease. Lancet 2:821, 1976.

1572. Picken JJ, Niewoehner DE, Chester EH: Prolonged effects of viral infections of the upper respiratory tract upon small airways. Am J Med 52:738, 1972.

1573. Fridy WW Jr, Ingram RH Jr, Hierholzer JC, et al: Airway function during mild viral respiratory illness. Ann Intern Med 80:150, 1974.

1574. Blair HT, Greenberg SB, Stevens PM, et al: Effects of rhinovirus infection on pulmonary function of healthy human volunteers. Am Rev Respir Dis 114:95, 1976.

1575. McFarlane JT, Morris MJ: Abnormalities in lung function following clinical recovery from Mycoplasma pneumoniae pneumonia. Eur J Respir Dis 63:337, 1982.

1576. Macklem PT: Obstruction in small airways. Am J Med 52:721, 1972.

1577. May JR, Peto R, Tinker CM, et al: A study of Hemophilus influenzae precipitins in the serum of working men in relation to smoking habits, bronchial infection, and airway obstruction. Am Rev Respir Dis 108:460, 1973.

1578. Bates DV: The fate of the chronic bronchitic: A report of the ten-year follow-up in the Canadian Department of Veteran's Affairs coordinated study of chronic bronchitis. Am Rev Respir Dis 108:1043, 1973.

1579. Kass EH: Changing ecology of bacterial infections. Arch Environ Health 6:19, 1963.

1580. Laurenzi GA, Potter RT, Kass EH: Bacteriologic flora of the lower respiratory tract. N Engl J Med 265:1273, 1961.

1581. Pecora DV, Yegian D: Bacteriology of the lower respiratory tract in health and chronic diseases. N Engl J Med 258:71, 1958.

1582. Edwards G: Acute bronchitis—aetiology, diagnosis, and management. Br Med J 1:963, 1966.

1583. Fisher M, Akhtar AJ, Calder MA, et al: Pilot study of factors associated with exacerbations in chronic bronchitis. Br Med J 4:187, 1969.

1584. Burns MW, May JR: Haemophilus influenzae precipitins in the serum of patients with chronic bronchial disorders. Lancet 1:354, 1967.

1585. May JR, Delves DM: The survival of Haemophilus influenzae and pneumococci in specimens of sputum sent to the laboratory by post. J Clin Pathol 17:254, 1964.

1586. May JR, May DS: Bacteriology of sputum in chronic bronchitis. Tubercle 44:162, 1963.

1587. Jenne JW, MacDonald FM, Lapinski EM, et al: The course of chronic Hemophilus bronchitis treated with massive doses of penicillin combined with streptomycin. Am Rev Respir Dis 101:907, 1970.

1588. Reichek N, Lewin EB, Rhoden DL, et al: Antibody responses to bacterial antigens during exacerbations of chronic bronchitis. Am Rev Respir Dis 101:238, 1970.

1589. Smith CB, Golden CA, Kanner RE, et al: Haemophilus influenzae and Haemophilus parainfluenzae in chronic obstructive pulmonary disease. Lancet 1:1253, 1976.

1590. Cooper AW, Williamson GM, Zinnemann K, et al: Chronic bronchitis. Changes in the bacterial flora of the sputum associated with exacerbations and long-term antibacterial treatment. Br J Dis Chest 55:23, 1961.

1591. Hennessy AV: An attempt to demonstrate a viral etiology for chronic bronchitis. Am Rev Respir Dis 86:350, 1962.

1592. Jack I, Gandevia B: Virus studies in chronic bronchitis. Am Rev Respir Dis 82:482, 1960.

1593. McNamara MJ, Phillips IA, Williams OB: Viral and Mycoplasma pneumoniae infections in exacerbations of chronic lung disease. Am Rev Respir Dis 100:19, 1969.

1594. Sommerville RG: Respiratory syncytial virus in acute exacerbations of chronic bronchitis. Lancet 2:1247, 1963.

1595. Stark JE, Heath RB, Curwen MP: Infection with influenza and parainfluenza viruses in chronic bronchitis. Thorax 20:124, 1965.

1596. Ross CAC, McMichael S, Eadie MB, et al: Infective agents and chronic bronchitis. Thorax 21:461, 1966.

1597. Eadie MB, Stott EJ, Grist NR: Virological studies in chronic bronchitis. Br Med J 2:671, 1966.

1598. Stenhouse AC: Viral antibody levels and clinical status in acute exacerbations of chronic bronchitis: A controlled prospective study. Br Med J 3:287, 1968.

1599. Grist NR: Group discussion: Virus infections in chronic bronchitis. 1. In acute exacerbations. In Tyrrell DAJ (ed): College of Pathologists, Acute Respiratory Diseases. Symposium organized by the College of Pathologists, London, February 1968. J Clin Pathol 21(Suppl 2):98, 1968.

1600. Stern H: Group discussion: Virus infections in chronic bronchitis. A family study. In Tyrrell DAJ (ed): College of Pathologists, Acute Respiratory Diseases. Symposium organized by the College of Pathologists, London, February 1968. J Clin Pathol 21(Suppl 2):99, 1968.

1601. Lamy ME, Pouthier-Simon F, Debacker-Willame E: Respiratory viral infections in hospital patients with chronic bronchitis. Chest 63:336, 1973.

1602. Gump DW, Phillips CA, Forsyth BR, et al: Role of infection in chronic bronchitis. Am Rev Respir Dis 113:465, 1976.

1603. Carilli AD, Gohd RS, Gordon W: A virologic study of chronic bronchitis. N Engl J Med 270:123, 1964.

1604. Snider GL, Doctor L, Demas TA, et al: Obstructive airway disease in patients with treated pulmonary tuberculosis. Am Rev Respir Dis 103:625, 1971.

1605. Govindaraj M: The effect of dehydration on the ventilatory capacity in normal subjects. Am Rev Respir Dis 105:842, 1972.

1606. Andersen IB, Lundqvist GR, Proctor DF: Human nasal mucosal function under four controlled humidities. Am Rev Respir Dis 106:438, 1972.

1607. Greenburg L, Field F, Reed JI, et al: Asthma and temperature change. An epidemiological study of emergency clinic visits for asthma in three large New York hospitals. Arch Environ Health 8:642, 1964.

1608. Cornwall CJ, Raffle PAB: Bronchitis—sickness absence in London transport. Br J Industr Med 18:24, 1961.

1609. Burrows B, Lebowitz MD: Characteristics of chronic bronchitis in a warm, dry region. Am Rev Respir Dis 112:365, 1975.

1610. Wells RE Jr, Walker JEC, Hickler RB: Effects of cold air on respiratory airflow resistance in patients with respiratory-tract disease. N Engl J Med 263:268, 1960.

1611. Hsieh Y-C, Frayser R, Ross JC: The effect of cold-air inhalation on ventilation in normal subjects and in patients with chronic obstructive pulmonary disease. Am Rev Respir Dis 98:613, 1968.

1612. Arnup ME, Mendella LA, Anthonisen NR, et al: Effects of cold air hyperpnea in patients with chronic obstructive lung disease. Am Rev Respir Dis 128:236, 1983.

1613. Ramsdale E, Roberts R, Morris M, et al: Differences in responsiveness to hyperventilation and methacholine in asthma and chronic bronchitis. Thorax 40:422, 1985.

1614. Tockman MS, Khoury MJ, Cohen BH: The epidemiology of COPD. In Petty TL (ed): Chronic Obstructive Disease: Lefant C (ed): Lung Biology in Health and Disease. New York, M Dekker, 1985, p 43.

1615. Eriksson S: Pulmonary emphysema and alpha₁-antitrypsin deficiency. Acta Med Scand 175:197, 1964.

1616. Lilienfeld AM, Lilienfeld D: Foundations of Epidemiology, 2nd ed. New York, Oxford University Press, 1980, pp 346–347.

1617. Morse JO: Alpha₁-antitrypsin deficiency. N Engl J Med 299:1045, 1978.

1618. Welch MH, Reinecke ME, Hammarsten JF, et al: Antitrypsin deficiency in pulmonary disease: The significance of intermediate levels. Ann Intern Med 71:533, 1969.

1619. Cooper DM, Hoeppner V, Cox D: Lung function in alpha₁-antitrypsin heterozygotes (Pi type MZ). Am Rev Respir Dis 110:708, 1974.

1620. Macklem PT, Hogg WE, Brunton J: Peripheral airways obstruction and particulate deposition in the lung. Arch Intern Med 131:93, 1973.

1621. Cox DW, Hoeppner VH, Levison H: Protease inhibitors in patients with chronic obstructive pulmonary disease: The alpha₁-antitrypsin heterozygote controversy. Am Rev Respir Dis 113:601, 1976.

1622. Mittman C, Lieberman J, Miranda A, et al: Pulmonary disease and intermediate alpha₁-antitrypsin deficiency. In Mittman C (ed): Pulmonary Emphysema and Proteolysis. New York, Academic Press, 1972, p 33.

1623. Barnett TB, Gottovi D, Johnson AM: Protease inhibitors in chronic obstructive pulmonary disease. Am Rev Respir Dis 111:587, 1975.

1624. Mittman C, Lieberman J, Rumsfeld J: Prevalence of abnormal protease inhibitor phenotypes in patients with chronic obstructive lung disease. Am Rev Respir Dis 109:295, 1974.

1625. Madison R, Mittan C, Afifi AA, et al: Risk factors for obstructive lung disease. Am Rev Respir Dis 149:124, 1981.

1626. Bartmann K, Fooke-Achterrath M, Koch G, et al: Heterozygosity in the Pi-system as a pathogenetic cofactor in chronic obstructive pulmonary disease (COPD). Eur J Respir Dis 66:184, 1985.

1627. Lieberman J, Winter B, Sastre A: Alpha₁-antitrypsin Pi-types in 963 COPD patients. Chest 89:370, 1986.

1628. Fagerhol MK: The incidence of alpha₁-antitrypsin variants in chronic obstructive pulmonary disease. In Mittman C (ed): Pulmonary Emphysema and Proteolysis. New York, Academic Press, 1972, p 51.

1629. Gelb AF, Klein E, Lieberman J: Pulmonary function in nonsmoking subjects with alpha₁-antitrypsin deficiency (MZ phenotype). Am J Med 62:93, 1977.

11

1630. Hepper NG, Westbrook PR, Miller RD, et al: The prevalence of alpha₁-antitrypsin deficiency in selected groups of patients with chronic obstructive lung disease. *In* Mittman C (ed): Pulmonary Emphysema and Proteolysis. New York, Academic Press, 1972, p 55.

1631. Kueppers F, Donhardt A: Obstructive lung disease in heterozygotes for alpha₁-antitrypsin deficiency. Ann Intern Med *80*:209, 1974.

1632. Shigeoka JW, Hall WJ, Hyde RW, et al: The prevalence of alpha₁-antitrypsin heterozygotes (Pi MZ) in patients with obstructive pulmonary disease. Am Rev Respir Dis *114*:1077, 1976.

1633. McDonagh DJ, Nathan SP, Knudson RJ, et al: Assessment of Alpha₁-antitrypsin deficiency heterozygosity as a risk factor in the etiology of emphysema—physiological comparison of adult normal and heterozygous protease inhibitor phenotype subjects from a random population. J Clin Invest *63*:299, 1979.

1634. Buist S, Sexton G, Azzam AH, et al: Pulmonary function in heterozygotes for alpha₁-antitrypsin deficiency: A case-control study. Am Rev Respir Dis *120*:759, 1979.

1635. Bruce RM, Cohen BH, Diamond EL, et al: Collaborative study to assess risk of lung disease in Pi MZ phenotype subjects. Am Rev Respir Dis *130*:386, 1984.

1636. Tattersall SF, Pereira RP, Hunter D, et al: Lung distensibility and airway function in intermediate alpha₁-antitrypsin deficiency (pi MZ). Thorax *34*:637, 1979.

1637. Mittman C: Editorial: The Pi MZ phenotype: Is it a significant risk factor for the development of chronic obstructive lung disease? Am Rev Respir Dis *118*:649, 1978.

1638. Kalsheker NA, Hodgson IJ, Watkins GL, et al: Deoxyribonucleic acid (DNA) polymorphism of the alpha₁-antitrypsin gene in chronic lung disease. Br Med J *294*:1511, 1987.

1639. Naseem SM, Tishler PV, Tager IB, et al: The relationship of host factors to the pathogenesis of chronic bronchitis and obstructive airway disease: Lymphoblast aryl hydrocarbon hydroxylase. Am Rev Respir Dis *117*:647, 1978.

1640. Khoury MJ, Beaty TH, Newill CA, et al: Genetic-environmental interactions in chronic airways obstruction. Int J Epidemiol *15*:65, 1986.

1641. Krzyzanowski M, Jedrychowski W, Wysocki M: Factors associated with the change in ventilatory function and the development of chronic obstructive pulmonary disease in a 13-year follow-up of the Cracow Study. Risk of chronic obstructive pulmonary disease. Am Rev Respir Dis *134*:1011, 1986.

1642. Kauffman F, Kleisbauer JP, De Mouzon C, et al: Genetic markers in chronic air-flow limitation: a genetic epidemiologic study. Am Rev Respir Dis *127*:263, 1983.

1643. Meine F, Grossman H, Forman W, et al: The radiographic findings in congenital cutis laxa. Radiology *113*:687, 1974.

1644. Lally JF, Gohel VK, Dalinka MK, et al: The roentgenographic manifestations of cutis laxa (generalized elastolysis). Radiology *113*:605, 1974.

1645. Rasmussen FV: Associations between housing conditions, smoking habits and ventilatory lung function in men with clean jobs. Br J Dis Chest *72*:261, 1978.

1646. Rasmussen FV, Borchsenius L, Winslow JB, et al: Associations between housing conditions, smoking habits and ventilatory lung function in men with clean jobs. Scand J Respir Dis *59*:264, 1978.

1647. Cohen BH, Celentano DD, Chase GA, et al: Alcohol consumption and airways obstruction. Am Rev Respir Dis *121*:205, 1980.

1648. Pratt PC, Vollmer RT: The beneficial effect of alcohol consumption on the prevalence and extent of centrilobular emphysema. Chest *85*:372, 1984.

1649. Girard F, Puchelle E, Aug F, et al: Protein evolution in bronchial secretions during an episode of superinfection in chronic bronchitis. Bull Eur Physiopathol Respir *15*:513, 1979.

1650. Puchelle E, Zahm J-M, Aug F: Viscoelasticity, protein content and ciliary transport rate of sputum in patient with recurrent and chronic bronchitis. Biorheology *18*:659, 1981.

1651. Puchelle E, Zahm JM, Girard F, et al: Mucociliary transport in vivo and in vitro. Relations to sputum properties in chronic bronchitis. Eur J Respir Dis *61*:254, 1980.

1652. Weiss T, Dorow P, Felix R: Regional mucociliary removal of inhaled particles in smokers with small airways disease. Respiration *44*:338, 1983.

1653. Foster WM, Langenback E, Bergofsky E, et al: Disassociation in the mucociliary function of central and peripheral airways of asymptomatic smokers. Am Rev Respir Dis *132*:633, 1985.

1654. Goodman RM, Yergin BM, Landa JF, et al: Relationship of smoking history and pulmonary function tests to tracheal mucous velocity in non-smokers, young smokers, ex-smokers and patients with chronic bronchitis. Am Rev Respir Dis *117*:205, 1978.

1655. Matthys H, Vastag E, Kohler D, et al: Mucociliary clearance in patients with chronic bronchitis and bronchial carcinoma. Respiration *44*:329, 1983.

1656. Agnew JE, Little F, Pavia D, et al: Mucus clearance from the airways in chronic bronchitis: Smokers and ex-smokers. Bull Eur Physiopathol Respir *18*:473, 1982.

1657. Lauque D, Aug F, Puchelle E, et al: Efficiency of mucociliary clearance and cough in bronchitis. Bull Eur Physiopathol Respir *20*:145, 1985.

1658. Yeates DB: The role of mucociliary transport in the pathogenesis of chronic obstructive pulmonary disease. *In* Chantler EEN, Elder JB, Elstein M (eds): Mucus in Health and Disease, No. 2, Advances in Experimental Medicine and Biology. New York, Plenum Press, 1982, pp 411–415.

1659. Oldenburg FA Jr, Dolovich MD, Montgomery JM, et al: Effects of postural drainage, exercise and cough on mucus clearance in chronic bronchitis. Am Rev Respir Dis *120*:739, 1979.

1660. Lungarella G, Fonzi L, Ermini G, et al: Abnormalities of bronchial cilia in patients with chronic bronchitis. Lung *161*:147, 1983.

1661. Welsh JM: Cigarette smoke inhibition of ion transport in canine tracheal epithelium. J Clin Invest *71*:1615, 1983.

1662. Mossberg B, Camner P: Impaired mucociliary transport as a pathogenetic factor in obstructive pulmonary diseases. Chest *77*:265, 1980.

1663. Pavia D, Thomson ML, Clarke SW: Enhanced clearance of secretions from the human lung after the administration of hypertonic saline aerosol. Am Rev Respir Dis *117*:199, 1978.

1664. Mossberg B, Strandbert K, Camner P: Stimulatory effect of beta-adrenergic drugs on mucociliary transport. Scand J Respir Dis *101*(Suppl):71, 1977.

1665. Weiss ST, Speizer FE: Increased levels of airways responsiveness as a risk factor for development of chronic obstructive lung disease: what are the issues? Chest *86*:3, 1984.

1666. Barter CE, Campbell AH: Relationship of constitutional factors and cigarette smoking to decrease in one second forced expiratory volume. Am Rev Respir Dis *113*:305, 1976.

1667. Taylor RG, Joyce H, Gross E, et al: Bronchial reactivity to inhaled histamine and annual rate of decline in FEV₁ in male smokers and ex-smokers. Thorax *40*:9, 1985.

1668. Kanner RE: The relationship between airways responsiveness and chronic airflow limitation. Chest *86*:54, 1984.

1669. Postma DS, de Vries K, Köeter GH, et al: Independent influence of reversibility of air-flow obstruction and nonspecific hyperreactivity on the long-term course of lung function in chronic air-flow obstruction. Am Rev Respir Dis *134*:276, 1986.

1670. Pare PD, Armour C, Taylor S, et al: Airway hyperreactivity in COPD; Cause or effect, an *in vivo, in vitro* comparison. Chest *91*:405, 1987.

1671. Anthonisen NR, Wright EC, Hodgkin JE: Prognosis in chronic obstructive pulmonary disease. Am Rev Respir Dis *133*:14, 1986.

1672. Rijcken B, Schouten JP, Weiss ST, et al: The relationship of nonspecific bronchial responsiveness to respiratory symptoms in a random population sample. Am Rev Respir Dis *136*:62, 1987.

1673. Taylor RG, Gross E, Joyce H, et al: Smoking, allergy, and the differential white blood cell count. Thorax *40*:17, 1985.

1674. Burrows B, Lebowitz MD, Barbee RA, et al: Interactions of smoking and immunologic factors in relation to airways obstruction. Chest *84*:657, 1983.

1675. Burrows B, Hasan FM, Barbee RA, et al: Epidemiologic observations on eosinophilia and its relation to respiratory disorders. Am Rev Respir Dis *122*:709, 1980.

1676. Casterline CL: Interaction of immunoglobulin E and cigarette smoke: Predisposition to symptomatic lung disease? Chest *84*:652, 1983.

1677. Pauwels R, Van Der Straeten M: Total serum IgE levels in normals and patients with chronic non-specific lung diseases. Allergy *33*:254, 1978.

1678. Burrows B, Halonen M, Barbee RA, et al: The relationship of serum immunoglobulin-E to cigarette smoking. Am Rev Respir Dis *124*:523, 1981.

1679. Bloom JW, Halonen M, Dunn AM, et al: Pneumococcus-specific immunoglobulin E in cigarette smokers. Clin Allergy *16*:25, 1986.

1680. Habib MP, Klink ME, Knudson DE, et al: Physiologic characteristics of subjects exhibiting accelerated deterioration of ventilatory function. Am Rev Respir Dis *136*:638, 1987.

1681. Janoff A: Elastase in tissue injury. Annu Rev Med *36*:207, 1985.

1682. Janoff A: Elastases and emphysema—current assessment of the protese-antiprotease hypothesis. Am Rev Respir Dis *132*:417, 1985.

1683. Snider GL: The pathogenesis of emphysema—20 years of progress. Am Rev Respir Dis *124*:321, 1981.

1684. Anderson LL, Oikarinen AI, Ryhänen L, et al: Characterization and partial purification of a neutral protease from the serum of a patient with autosomal recessive pulmonary emphysema and cutis laxa. J Lab Clin Med *105*:537, 1985.

1685. Gadek JE, Fells GA, Zimmerman RL, et al: Antielastases of the human alveolar structures—implications for the protease-antiprotease theory of emphysema. J Clin Invest *68*:889, 1981.

1686. Hoidal JR, Niewoehner DE: Pathogenesis of emphysema. Chest *83*:679, 1983.

1687. Kuhn C, Senior RM: The role of elastases in the development of emphysema. Lung 155:185, 1978.

1688. Sparrow D, Glynn RJ, Cohen M, et al: The relationship of the peripheral leukocyte count and cigarette smoking to pulmonary function among adult men. Chest 86:383, 1984.

1689. Chan Yeung M, Dy Buncio A: Leukocyte count, smoking and lung function. Am J Med 76:31, 1984.

1690. Ludwig P, Schwartz B, Hoidal J, et al: Cigarette smoking causes accumulation of polymorphonuclear leukocytes in alveolar septum. Am Rev Respir Dis 131:828, 1985.

1691. Martin T, Raghu G, Maunder R, et al: The effects of chronic bronchitis and chronic airflow obstruction on lung cell populations recovered by bronchoalveolar lavage. Am Rev Respir Dis 132:254, 1985.

1692. Bridges RB, Wyatt RJ, Rehm SR: Effects of smoking on inflammatory mediators and their relationship to pulmonary dysfunction. Eur J Respir Dis 146(Suppl):145, 1986.

1693. Hunninghake GW, Crystal RG: Cigarette smoking and lung destruction—accumulation of neutrophils in the lungs of cigarette smokers. Am Rev Respir Dis 128:833, 1983.

1694. Hobson JE, Wright JL, Wiggs BR, et al: Comparison of the cell content of lung lavage fluid with the presence of emphysema and peripheral airways inflammation in resected lungs. Respiration 50:1, 1986.

1695. Hogg JC: Neutrophil kinetics and lung injury. Physiol Rev 67:1249, 1987.

1696. Muir AL, Cruz M, Martin BA, et al: Leukocyte kinetics in the human lung. Role of exercise and catecholamines. J Appl Physiol 57:711, 1984.

1697. Hogg JC, Martin BA, Lee S, et al: Regional differences in erythrocyte transit in normal. J Appl Physiol 59:1266, 1985.

1698. MacNee W, Martin BA, Tanco S, et al: Cigarette smoking delays polymorphonuclear leukocyte (PMN) transit through the pulmonary circulation. Am Rev Respir Dis 135:A146, 1987.

1699. Kew RR, Ghebrehiwet B, and Janoff A, et al: Cigarette smoke can activate the alternative pathway of complement in vitro by modifying the third component of complement. J Clin Invest 75:1000, 1985.

1700. Lam S, Chan-Yeung M, Abboud R, et al: Interrelationships between serum chemotactic factor inactivator, alpha₁-antitrypsin deficiency and chronic obstructive lung disease. Am Rev Respir Dis 121:507, 1980.

1701. Blue M-L, Janoff A: Possible mechanisms of emphysema in cigarette smokers. Release of elastase from human polymorphonuclear leukocytes by cigarette smoke condensate in vitro. Am Rev Respir Dis 117:317, 1978.

1702. Rodriguez JR, Seals JE, Radin A, et al: Neutrophil lysosomal elastase activity in normal subjects and in patients with chronic obstructive pulmonary disease. Am Rev Respir Dis 119:409, 1979.

1703. Abboud RT, Rushton J-M, Grzybowski S, et al: Interrelationships between neutrophil elastase, serum alpha₁-antitrypsin, lung function, and chest radiography in patients with chronic airflow obstruction. Am Rev Respir Dis 120:31, 1979.

1704. Kramps JA, Bakker W, Dijkman JH, et al: A matched-pair study of the leukocyte elastase-like activity in normal persons and in emphysematous patients with and without alpha₁-antitrypsin deficiency. Am Rev Respir Dis 121:253, 1980.

1705. Bridges RB, Wyatt RJ, Rehm SR: Effect of smoking on peripheral blood leukocytes and serum antiproteases. Eur J Respir Dis 139(Suppl):24, 1985.

1706. Finley TN, Swenson EW, Curran WS, et al: Bronchopulmonary lavage in normal subjects and patients with obstructive lung disease. Ann Intern Med 66:651, 1967.

1707. Harris JO, Olsen GN, Castle JR, et al: Comparison of proteolytic enzyme activity in pulmonary alveolar macrophages and blood leukocytes in smokers and nonsmokers. Am Rev Respir Dis 111:579, 1975.

1708. Harris JO, Swenson EW, Johnson JE III: Human alveolar macrophages: Comparison of phagocytic ability, glucose utilization, and ultrastructure in smokers and nonsmokers. J Clin Invest 49:2086, 1970.

1709. The Fourth International Pneumoconiosis Conference: Working party on the definition of pneumoconiosis report. Geneva, 1971.

1710. Cohen AB: The effects in vivo and in vitro of oxidative damage to purified alpha₁-antitrypsin and to the enzyme-inhibiting activity of plasma. Am Rev Respir Dis 119:953, 1979.

1711. Carp H, Janoff A: Possible mechanisms of emphysema in smokers: In vitro suppression of serum elastase-inhibitory capacity by fresh cigarette smoke and its prevention by antioxidants. Am Rev Respir Dis 118:617, 1978.

1712. Janoff A, Dearing R: Alpha₁-proteinase inhibitor is more sensitive to inactivation by cigarette smoke than is leukocyte elastase. Am Rev Respir Dis 126:691, 1982.

1713. Taylor JC, Madison R, Kosinska D: Is antioxidant deficiency related to chronic obstructive pulmonary disease? Am Rev Respir Dis 134:285, 1986.

1714. Lellouch J, Claude JR, Martin JP, et al: Smoking does not reduce the functional activity of serum alpha₁ proteinase inhibitor—an epidemiologic study of 719 healthy men. Am Rev Respir Dis 132:818, 1985.

1715. Chowdhury P, Bone RC, Louria DB, et al: Effect of cigarette smoke on human serum trypsin inhibitory capacity and antitrypsin concentrations. Am Rev Respir Dis 126:177, 1982.

1716. Martin WJ II, Taylor JC: Abnormal interaction of alpha₁-antitrypsin and leukocyte elastolytic activity in patients with chronic obstructive pulmonary disease. Am Rev Respir Dis 120:411, 1979.

1717. Binder R, Stone RJ, Calore JD, et al: Serum antielastase and neutrophil elastase levels in PiM phenotype cigarette smokers with airflow obstruction. Respiration 47:267, 1985.

1718. Fera T, Abboud RT, Johal SS, et al: Effect of smoking on functional activity of plasma alpha₁-protease inhibitor. Chest 91:346, 1987.

1719. Abboud RT, Fera T, Johal S, et al: Effects of smoking on plasma neutrophil elastase levels. J Lab Clin Med 108:294, 1986.

1720. Damiano VV, Tsang A, Kucich U, et al: Immunolocalization of elastase in human emphysematous lungs. J Clin Invest 78:482, 1986.

1721. Stockley RA, Burnett D: Alpha₁-antitrypsin and leukocyte elastase in infected and noninfected sputum. Am Rev Respir Dis 120:1081, 1979.

1722. Abboud RT, Fera T, Richter A, et al: Acute effect of smoking on the functional activity of alpha₁-protease inhibitor in bronchoalveolar lavage fluid. Am Rev Respir Dis 131:79, 1985.

1723. Galdston M, Levytska V, Schwartz MS, et al: Ceruloplasmin: Serum concentration and impaired antioxidant activity in cigarette smokers, and ability to prevent suppression of elastase inhibitory capacity of alpha₁-protease inhibitor. Am Rev Respir Dis 129:258, 1984.

1724. Rasche B, Hochstrasser K, Albrecht GJ, et al: An elastase-specific inhibitor from human bronchial mucus. Respiration 44:397, 1983.

1725. Pelham F, Wewers M, Crystal R, et al: Urinary excretion of desmosine (elastin cross-links) in subjects with PiZZ alpha-1-antitrypsin deficiency, a phenotype associated with hereditary predisposition to pulmonary emphysema. Am Rev Respir Dis 132:821, 1985.

1726. Gross P, Pfitzer EA, Tolker E, et al: Experimental emphysema: Its production with papain in normal and silicotic rats. Arch Environ Health 11:50, 1965.

1727. Martin RR: Altered morphology and increased acid hydrolase content of pulmonary macrophages from cigarette smokers. Am Rev Respir Dis 107:596, 1973.

1728. Marco V, Meranze DR, Bentivoglio LG, et al: Papain-induced experimental emphysema in the dog. Fed Proc 28:526, 1969.

1729. Pushpakom R, Hogg JC, Woolcock AJ, et al: Experimental papain-induced emphysema in dogs. Am Rev Respir Dis 102:778, 1970.

1730. Kilburn KH, Dowell AR, Pratt PC: Morphological and biochemical assessment of papain-induced emphysema. Arch Intern Med 127:884, 1971.

1731. Goldring IP, Park SS, Greenberg L, et al: Sequential anatomic changes in lungs exposed to papain and other proteolytic enzymes. In Mittman C (ed): Pulmonary Emphysema and Proteolysis. New York, Academic Press, 1972, p 389.

1732. Kleinerman J, Rynbrandt DJ: Papain-induced emphysema in hamsters: The effect of agents that increase serum alpha₁-antitrypsin. In Mittman C (ed): Pulmonary Emphysema and Proteolysis. New York, Academic Press, 1972, p 421.

1733. Harley RA: Pulmonary vascular changes in experimental papain emphysema. In Mittman C (ed): Pulmonary Emphysema and Proteolysis. New York, Academic Press, 1972, p 449.

1734. Caldwell EJ: The physiologic and anatomic effects of papain on the rabbit lung. In Mittman C (ed): Pulmonary Emphysema and Proteolysis. New York, Academic Press, 1972, p 487.

1735. Johanson WG Jr, Reynolds RC, Scott TC, et al: Connective tissue damage in emphysema. An electron microscopic study of papain-induced emphysema in rats. Am Rev Respir Dis 107:589, 1973.

1736. Weinbaum G, Marco V, Ikeda T, et al: Enzymatic production of experimental emphysema in the dog. Route of exposure. Am Rev Respir Dis 109:351, 1974.

1737. Snider GL, Hayes JA, Franzblau C, et al: Relationship between elastolytic activity and experimental emphysema-inducing properties of papain preparations. Am Rev Respir Dis 110:254, 1974.

1738. Martorana PA, Share NN: Effect of human alpha₁-antitrypsin on papain-induced emphysema in the hamster. Am Rev Respir Dis 113:607, 1976.

1739. Karlinsky JB, Catanese A, Honeychurch C, et al: In vitro effects of elastase and collagenase on mechanical properties of hamster lungs. Chest 69:275, 1976.

1740. Karlinsky JB, Snider GL, Franzblau C, et al: In vitro effects of elastase and collagenase on mechanical properties of hamster lungs. Am Rev Respir Dis 113:769, 1976.

11

1741. Marco V, Mass B, Meranze DR, et al: Induction of experimental emphysema in dogs using leukocyte homogenates. Am Rev Respir Dis 104:595, 1971.

1742. Kimbel P, Mass B, Ikeda T, et al: Emphysema in dogs induced by leukocyte contents. In Mittman C (ed): Pulmonary Emphysema and Proteolysis. New York, Academic Press, 1972, p 411.

1743. Mass B, Ikeda T, Meranze DR, et al: Induction of experimental emphysema. Cellular and species specificity. Am Rev Respir Dis 106:384, 1974.

1744. Karlinsky JB, Snider GL: State of the art: Animal models of emphysema. Am Rev Respir Dis 117:1109, 1978.

1745. Senior RM, Tegner H, Kuhn C, et al: The induction of pulmonary emphysema with human leukocyte elastase. Am Rev Respir Dis 116:469, 1977.

1746. Hyman AL, Spannhake EW, Kadowitz RJ, et al: Physiologic and morphologic observations of the effects of intravenous elastase on the lung. Am Rev Respir Dis 117:97, 1978.

1747. Martorana AP, Schaper J, Van Even P, et al: The effect of physical exercise on elastase-induced emphysema in hamsters. Am Rev Respir Dis 120:1209, 1979.

1748. Polzin JK, Napier JS, Taylor JC, et al: Effect of elastase and ventilation on elastic recoil of excised dog lungs. Am Rev Respir Dis 119:377, 1979.

1749. Blackwood RA, Correta JM, Manol I, et al: Alpha₁-antitrypsin deficiency and increased susceptibility to elastase-induced experimental emphysema in a rat model. Am Rev Respir Dis 120:1375, 1979.

1750. Martorana PA, Richard JW, McKeel NW, et al: Inhibition of papain-induced emphysema in the hamster by human alpha₁-antitrypsin. Can J Physiol Pharmacol 52:758, 1974.

1751. Kaplan PD, Kuhn C, Pierce JA: The induction of emphysema with elastase. I. The evolution of the lesion and the influence of serum. J Lab Clin Med 82:349, 1973.

1752. Tarján E, Petö L, Appel J, et al: Prevention of elastase-induced emphysema by aerosol administration of a specific synthetic elastase inhibitor. Eur J Respir Dis 64:442, 1983.

1753. Gudapaty SR, Liener IE, Hoidal JR, et al: The prevention of elastase-induced emphysema in hamsters by the intratracheal administration of a synthetic elastase inhibitor bound to albumin microspheres. Am Rev Respir Dis 159:132, 1985.

1754. Kucich U, Christner P, Weinbaum G, et al: Immunologic identification of elastin-derived peptides in the serums of dogs with experimental emphysema. Am Rev Respir Dis 122:461, 1980.

1755. Guenter CA, Coalson JJ, Jacques J, et al: Emphysema associated with intravascular leukocyte sequestration: Comparison with papain induced emphysema. Am Rev Respir Dis 123:79, 1981.

1756. Wittels EH, Coalson JJ, Welch MH, et al: Pulmonary intravascular leukocyte sequestration. A potential mechanism of lung injury. Am Rev Respir Dis 109:502, 1974.

1757. McKusick VA: Heritable Disorders of Connective Tissue, 4th ed. St. Louis, CV Mosby Co, 1972, p 187.

1758. Kida K, Thurlbeck WM: Lack of recovery of lung structure and function after the administration of beta aminoproprionitrile in the postnatal period. Am Rev Respir Dis 122:467, 1980.

1759. O'Dell BL, Kilburn KH, McKenzie WN, et al: The lung of the copper-deficient rat. Am J Pathol 91:413, 1978.

1760. Soskel NT, Watanabe S, Hammond E, et al: A copper-deficient, zinc-supplemented diet produces emphysema in pigs. Am Rev Respir Dis 126:316, 1982.

1761. Sparrow D, Silkert JE, Weiss ST, et al: The relationship of pulmonary function to copper concentrations in drinking water. Am Rev Respir Dis 126:312, 1982.

1762. Fisk DE, Kuhn C: Emphysema-like changes in the lungs of the blotchy mouse. Am Rev Respir Dis 113:787, 1976.

1763. Snider GL, Hayes JA, Korthy AL, et al: Centrilobular emphysema experimentally induced by cadmium chloride aerosol. Am Rev Respir Dis 108:40, 1973.

1764. Thurlbeck WM, Foley FD: Experimental pulmonary emphysema: The effect of intratracheal injection of cadmium chloride solution in the guinea pig. Am J Pathol 42:431, 1963.

1765. Lewis GP, Lyle H, Miller S: Association between elevated hepatic water-soluble protein-bound cadmium levels and chronic bronchitis and/or emphysema. Lancet 2:1330, 1969.

1766. Freeman G, Haydon GB: Emphysema after low-level exposure to NO₂. Arch Environ Health 8:125, 1964.

1767. Freeman G, Crane SC, Stephens RJ, et al: Pathogenesis of the nitrogen dioxide-induced lesion in the rat lung: A review and presentation of new observations. Am Rev Respir Dis 98:429, 1968.

1768. Freeman G, Crane SC, Furiosi NJ, et al: Covert reduction in ventilatory surface in rats during prolonged exposure to subacute nitrogen dioxide. Am Rev Respir Dis 106:563, 1972.

1769. Reid L: Measurement of the bronchial mucous gland layer: A diagnostic yardstick in chronic bronchitis. Thorax 15:132, 1960.

1770. Thurlbeck WM, Angus GE: A distribution curve for chronic bronchitis. Thorax 19:436, 1964.

1771. Hayes JA: Distribution of bronchial gland measurements in a Jamaican population. Thorax 24:619, 1969.

1772. Scott KWM: An autopsy study of bronchial mucous gland hypertrophy in Glasgow. Am Rev Respir Dis 107:239, 1973.

1773. Jamal K, Cooney TP, Fleetham JA, et al: Chronic bronchitis—correlation of morphologic findings to sputum production and flow rates. Am Rev Respir Dis 129:719, 1984.

1774. Jamal K, Cooney TP, Fleetham JA, et al: Chronic bronchitis. Correlation of morphologic findings to sputum production and flow rates. Am Rev Respir Dis 129:719, 1984.

1775. Oberholzer M, Dalquen P, Wyss M, et al: The applicability of the gland/wall ratio (Reid-Index) to clinicopathological correlation studies. Thorax 33:779, 1978.

1776. Hayes JA: Distribution of bronchial gland measurements in a Jamaican population. Thorax 24:619, 1969.

1777. Mitchell RS, Ryan SF, Petty TL, et al: The significance of morphologic chronic hyperplastic bronchitis. Am Rev Respir Dis 93:720, 1966.

1778. Thurlbeck WM, Angus GE: A distribution curve for chronic bronchitis. Thorax 19:436, 1964.

1779. Takizawa T, Thurlbeck WM: A comparative study of four methods of assessing the morphologic changes in chronic bronchitis. Am Rev Respir Dis 103:774, 1971.

1780. Martin CJ, Katsura S, Cochran TH: The relationship of chronic bronchitis to the diffuse obstructive pulmonary syndrome. Am Rev Respir Dis 102:362, 1970.

1781. Wang NS, Ying WL: Morphogenesis of human bronchial diverticulum. A scanning electron microscopic study. Chest 69:201, 1976.

1782. Nagai A, West W, Paul J, et al: The National Institutes of Health Intermittent Positive-Pressure Breathing Trial—Pathology studies. 1. Interrelationship between morphologic lesions. Am Rev Respir Dis 132:937, 1985.

1783. Tandon MK, Campbell AH: Bronchial cartilage in chronic bronchitis. Thorax 24:607, 1969.

1784. Thurlbeck WM, Pun R, Toth J, et al: Bronchial cartilage in chronic obstructive lung disease. Am Rev Respir Dis 109:73, 1974.

1785. Maisel JC, Silvers GW, Mitchell RS, et al: Bronchial atrophy and dynamic expiratory collapse. Am Rev Respir Dis 98:988, 1968.

1786. Maisel JC, Silvers GW, George MS, et al: The significance of bronchial atrophy. Am J Pathol 67:371, 1972.

1787. Macklem PT, Fraser RG, Brown WG: Bronchial pressure measurements in emphysema and bronchitis. J Clin Invest 44:897, 1965.

1788. Macklem PT, Wilson NJ: Measurement of intrabronchial pressure in man. J Appl Physiol 20:653, 1965.

1789. Restrepo GL, Heard BE: Air trapping in chronic bronchitis and emphysema. Measurements of the bronchial cartilage. Am Rev Respir Dis 90:395, 1964.

1790. Linhartova A, Anderson AE, Foraker AG: Site predilection of airway inflammation by emphysema type. Arch Pathol Lab Med 108:662, 1984.

1791. Baier H, Zarzecki S, Wanner A, et al: Influence of lung inflation on the cross-sectional area of central airways in normals and in patients with lung disease. Respiration 41:145, 1981.

1792. McCormack G, Moreno R, Hogg JC, et al: Lung mechanics in papain treated rabbits. J Appl Physiol 60:242, 1986.

1793. Bowen JH, Woodard BH, Pratt PC: Bronchial collapse in obstructive lung disease. Chest 80:510, 1981.

1794. Hossain S, Heard BE: Hyperplasia of bronchial muscle in chronic bronchitis. J Pathol 101:171, 1970.

1795. Carlile A, Edwards C: Structural variation in the named bronchi of the left lung. A morphometric study. Br J Dis Chest 77:344, 1983.

1796. Mullen JBM, Wright JL, Wiggs BR, et al: Reassessment of inflammation of airways in chronic bronchitis. Br Med J 291:1235, 1985.

1797. Ellefsen P, Tos M: Goblet cells in the human trachea. Quantitative studies of a pathological biopsy material. Arch Otolaryngol 95:547, 1972.

1798. Reid L: Bronchial mucus production in health and disease. In Liebow AA, Smith DE (eds): International Academy of Pathology, Monographs in Pathology, Vol. 8, 1968: The Lung. Baltimore, Williams & Wilkins, 1968, pp 87–108.

1799. Hogg JC, Macklem PT, Thurlbeck WM: Site and nature of airway obstruction in chronic obstructive lung disease. N Engl J Med 278:1355, 1968.

1800. Cosio MG, Ghezzo H, Hogg JC, et al: The relations between structural changes in small airways and pulmonary function tests. N Engl J Med 298:1277, 1977.

1801. Wright JL, Cosio M, Wiggs BJ, et al: A morphologic grading scheme for membranous and respiratory bronchioles. Arch Pathol Lab Med 109:163, 1985.

1802. Wright JL, Paré PD, Nelems JM, et al: The nature of peripheral airway inflammations in emphysema. Fed Proc 39:332A, 1980.

1803. Wright JL, Hobson J, Wiggs BR, et al: Effect of cigarette smoke on structure of the small airways. Lung 165:91, 1987.

1804. Berend N, Woolcock AJ, Marlin GK: The relationship between bronchial and arterial diameters in normal human lungs. Thorax 34:354, 1979.
1805. Matsuba K, Thurlbeck WM: Disease of the small airways in chronic bronchitis. Am Rev Respir Dis 107:552, 1973.
1806. Berend N, Wright JL, Thurlbeck WM, et al: Small airways disease—reproducibility of measurements and correlation with lung function. Chest 79:263, 1981.
1807. Petty TL, Silvers GW, Stanford RE, et al: Small airway disease is associated with elastic recoil changes in excised human lungs. Am Rev Respir Dis 130:42, 1984.
1808. Scott KWM, Steiner GM: Postmortem assessment of chronic airways obstruction by tantalum bronchography. Thorax 30:405, 1975.
1809. Petty TL, Silvers GW, Stanford RE, et al: Radial traction and small airway disease in excised human lungs. Am Rev Respir Dis 133:132, 1986.
1810. Cosio MG, Shiner RJ, Saetta M, et al: Alveolar fenestrae in smokers: Relationship with light microscopic and functional abnormalities. Am Rev Respir Dis 133:126, 1986.
1811. Cosio MG, Hale KA, Niewoehner DE, et al: Morphologic and morphometric effects of prolonged cigarette smoking on the small airways. Am Rev Respir Dis 122:265, 1980.
1812. Niewoehner DE, Knoke JD, Kleinerman J, et al: Peripheral airways as a determinant of ventilatory function in the human lung. J Clin Invest 60:139, 1970.
1813. Niewoehner DE, Kleinerman J: Morphologic basis of pulmonary resistance in the human lung and effects of aging. J Appl Physiol 36:412, 1974.
1814. Salmon RB, Saidel GM, Inkley SR, et al: Relationship of ventilation inhomogeneity to morphologic variables in excised human lungs. Am Rev Respir Dis 126:686, 1982.
1815. Berend N, Thurlbeck WM: Correlations of maximum expiratory flow with small airway dimensions and pathology. J Appl Physiol 52:346, 1982.
1816. Petty TL, Silvers G, Stanford RE, et al: Small airway pathology is related to increased closing capacity and abnormal slope of phase III in excised lungs. Am Rev Respir Dis 121:449, 1980.
1817. Berend N, Woolcock AJ, Marlin GE, et al: Correlation between the function and structure of the lung in smokers. Am Rev Respir Dis 119:695, 1979.
1818. Wright JL, Lawson LM, Paré PD, et al: The detection of small airways disease. Am Rev Respir Dis 129:989, 1984.
1819. Petty TL, Silvers GW, Stanford RE, et al: Small airway dimension and size distribution in human lungs with an increased closing capacity. Am Rev Respir Dis 125:535, 1982.
1820. Berend N, Skoog C, Thurlbeck WM, et al: Single-breath nitrogen test in excised human lungs. J Appl Physiol 51:1568, 1981.
1821. Colebatch HJH, Greaves IA: Chronic airflow obstruction. Evolution of disordered function in cigarette smokers. Med J Aust 142:607, 1985.
1822. Nagai A, West W, Thurlbeck WM, et al: The National Institutes of Health Intermittent Positive-Pressure Breathing Trial—Pathology Studies. 2. Correlation between morphologic findings, clinical findings, and evidence of expiratory air-flow obstruction. Am Rev Respir Dis 132:946, 1985.
1823. Paré PD, Brooks LA, Coppin CA, et al: Density-dependence of maximal expiratory flow and its correlation with small airway disease in smokers. Am Rev Respir Dis 131:521, 1985.
1824. Linhartová A, Anderson AE: Small airways in severe panlobular emphysema—mural thickening and premature closure. Am Rev Respir Dis 127:42, 1983.
1825. Hale KA, Ewing SL, Gosnell BA, et al: Lung disease in long-term cigarette smokers with and without chronic air-flow obstruction. Am Rev Respir Dis 130:716, 1984.
1826. Berend N: Lobar distribution of bronchiolar inflammation in emphysema. Am Rev Respir Dis 124:218, 1981.
1827. Wright JL, Wiggs BJ, Hogg JC, et al: Airway disease in upper and lower lobes in lungs of patients with and without emphysema. Thorax 282:39, 1984.
1828. Thurlbeck WM: The pathology of small airways in chronic airflow limitation. Eur J Respir Dis 63:9, 1982.
1829. Thurlbeck WM: Chronic airflow obstruction in lung disease, Vol V in the Series. Major Problems in Pathology. Philadelphia, WB Saunders Co, 1976.
1830. Pump KK: The pattern of development of emphysema in the human lung. Am Rev Respir Dis 108:610, 1973.
1831. Saetta M, Ghezzo H, Kim W, et al: Loss of alveolar attachments in smokers—a morphometric correlate of lung function impairment. Am Rev Respir Dis 132:894, 1985.
1832. Linhartová A: Lesions in resected lung parenchyma with regard to possible initial phase of pulmonary emphysema. An ultrastructural study. Pathol Res Pract 181:71, 1986.
1833. McLean KH: The histology of generalized pulmonary emphysema. I. The genesis of the early centrolobular lesion: Focal emphysema. Australas Ann Med 6:124, 1957.
1834. Thurlbeck WM: Chronic obstructive lung disease. Pathol Annu 3:367, 1968.
1835. Leopold JG, Gough J: The centrilobular form of hypertrophic emphysema and its relation to chronic bronchitis. Thorax 12:219, 1957.
1836. Anderson AE Jr, Foraker AG: Centrilobular emphysema and panlobular emphysema: Two different diseases. Thorax 28:547, 1973.
1837. Sweet HC, Wyatt JP, Fritsch AJ, et al: Panlobular and centrilobular emphysema. Correlation of clinical findings with pathologic patterns. Ann Intern Med 55:565, 1961.
1838. Snider GL, Brody JS, Doctor L: Subclinical pulmonary emphysema. Incidence and anatomic features. Am Rev Respir Dis 85:666, 1962.
1839. Cockcroft DW, Horne SL: Localization of emphysema within the lung. Chest 82:483, 1982.
1840. Silvers GW, Petty TL, Stanford RE, et al: The elastic properties of lobes of excised human lungs. Am Rev Respir Dis 120:207, 1979.
1841. Berend N, Skoog C, Thurlbeck WM, et al: Exponential analysis of lobar pressure-volume characteristics. Thorax 36:452, 1981.
1842. Boren HG: Alveolar fenestrae. Relationship to the pathology and pathogenesis of pulmonary emphysema. Am Rev Respir Dis 85:328, 1962.
1843. Thurlbeck WM: Pulmonary emphysema. Am J Med Sci 246:332, 1963.
1844. Horsfield K, Cumming G, Hicken P. A morphologic study of airway disease using bronchial casts. Am Rev Respir Dis 93:900, 1966.
1845. Thurlbeck WM: The incidence of pulmonary emphysema with observations on the relative incidence and spatial distribution of various types of emphysema. Am Rev Respir Dis 87:206, 1963.
1846. Anderson AE Jr, Furlaneto JA, Foraker AG: Bronchopulmonary derangements in nonsmokers. Am Rev Respir Dis 101:518, 1970.
1847. Sutinen S, Vaajalahti P, Pääkkö P, et al: Prevalence, severity and types of pulmonary emphysema in a population of deaths in a Finnish city. Correlation with age, sex and smoking. Scand J Respir Dis 59:101, 1978.
1848. Snider GL, Kleinerman JL, Thurlbeck WM, et al: The definition of emphysema. Report of a national heart, lung, and blood institute, division of lung diseases workshop. Am Rev Respir Dis 132:182, 1985.
1849. Osborne S, Hogg JC, Wright JL, et al: Exponential analysis of the pressure-volume curve: Correlation with mean linear intercept and emphysema in human lungs. Am Rev Respir Dis 137:1083, 1988.
1850. Thurlbeck WM: Post-mortem lung volumes. Thorax 34:735, 1979.
1851. Thurlbeck WM: Smoking, airflow limitation and the pulmonary circulation. Am Rev Respir Dis 122:183, 1980.
1852. Thurlbeck WM: Aspects of chronic airflow obstruction. Chest 72:341, 1977.
1853. Berend N, Thurlbeck WM: Exponential analysis of pressure-volume relationship in excised human lungs. J Appl Physiol 52:838, 1982.
1854. Petty TL, Silvers GW, Stanford RE, et al: Functional correlations with mild and moderate emphysema in excised human lungs. Am Rev Respir Dis 124:700, 1981.
1855. Silvers GW, Petty TL, Stanford RE, et al: Elastic recoil changes in early emphysema. Thorax 35:490, 1980.
1856. Haber PS, Colebatch HJH, Ng CKY, et al: Alveolar size as a determinant of pulmonary distensibility in mammalian lungs. J Appl Physiol 54:837, 1983.
1857. Greaves IA, Colebatch HJH: Elastic behaviour and structure of normal and emphysematous lungs post-mortem. Am Rev Respir Dis 121:127, 1980.
1858. Hogg JC, Nepszy SJ, Macklem PT, et al: Elastic properties of the centrilobular emphysematous space. J Clin Invest 48:1306, 1969.
1859. Alpert JS: Pulmonary hypertension and cardiac function in chronic obstructive pulmonary disease. Chest 75:651, 1979.
1860. Wright JL, Lawson L, Paré PD, et al: The structure and function of the pulmonary vasculature in mild chronic obstructive pulmonary disease—the effect of oxygen and exercise. Am Rev Respir Dis 128:702, 1983.
1861. Hale KA, Niewoehner DE, Cosio MG, et al: Morphologic changes in the muscular pulmonary arteries: Relationship to cigarette smoking, airway disease and emphysema. Am Rev Resp Dis 122:273, 1980.
1862. Scott KWM: Quantitation of thick-walled peripheral lung vessels in chronic airway obstruction. Thorax 31:315, 1976.
1863. Reid JA, Heard BE: The capillary network of normal and emphysematous human lungs studied by injections of Indian ink. Thorax 18:201, 1963.
1864. Cudkowicz L, Armstrong JB: The bronchial arteries in pulmonary emphysema. Thorax 8:46, 1953.
1865. Jacobson G, Turner AF, Balchum O, et al: Pulmonary arteriovenous shunts in emphysema demonstrated by wedge arteriography. Am J Roentgenol 93:868, 1965.

11

1866. Simon G, Galbraith HJB: Radiology of chronic bronchitis. Lancet 265:850, 1953.

1867. Bates DV, Gordon CA, Paul GI, et al: Chronic bronchitis: Report on the third and fourth stages of the co-ordinated study of chronic bronchitis in the Department of Veterans Affairs, Canada. Med Serv J Can 22:5, 1966.

1868. Simon G: Chronic bronchitis and emphysema: A symposium. III. Pathological findings and radiological changes in chronic bronchitis and emphysema. (b) Radiological changes in chronic bronchitis. Br J Radiol 32:292, 1959.

1869. Simon G: Principles of Chest X-Ray Diagnosis. 3rd ed. London, Butterworth, 1971.

1870. Fraser RG, Fraser RS, Renner JW, et al: The roentgenologic diagnosis of chronic bronchitis: A reassessment with emphasis on parahilar bronchi seen end-on. Radiology 120:1, 1976.

1871. Feigin DS, Abraham JL: "Increased pulmonary markings"—A radiologic-pathologic correlation study (abstr). Invest Radiol 15:425, 1980.

1872. Christoforidis AJ, Nelson SW, Tomashefski JF: Effects of bronchography on pulmonary function. Am Rev Respir Dis 85:127, 1962.

1873. Suprenant E, Wilson A, Bennett L, et al: Changes in regional pulmonary function following bronchography. Radiology 91:736, 1968.

1874. Simon G: Radiology and emphysema. Clin Radiol 15:293, 1964.

1875. Thurlbeck WM, Henderson JA, Fraser RG, et al: Chronic obstructive lung disease. A comparison between clinical, roentgenologic, functional and morphological criteria in chronic bronchitis, emphysema, asthma and bronchiectasis. Medicine 49:81, 1970.

1876. Fraser RG, Bates DV: Body section roentgenography in the evaluation and differentiation of chronic hypertrophic emphysema and asthma. Am J Roentgenol 82:39, 1959.

1877. Dunnill MS: Quantitative methods in study of pulmonary pathology. Thorax 17:320, 1962.

1878. Thurlbeck WM: Internal surface area and other measurements in emphysema. Thorax 22:483, 1967.

1879. Nicklaus TM, Stowell DW, Christiansen WR, et al: The accuracy of the roentgenologic diagnosis of chronic pulmonary emphysema. Am Rev Respir Dis 93:889, 1966.

1880. Simon G, Pride NB, Jones NL, et al: Relation between abnormalities in the chest radiograph and changes in pulmonary function in chronic bronchitis and emphysema. Thorax 28:15, 1973.

1881. Thomson KR, Eyssen GE, Fraser RG: Discrimination of normal and overinflated lungs and prediction of total lung capacity based on chest film measurements. Radiology 119:721, 1976.

1882. Burki NK: Conventional chest films can identify air flow obstruction. Chest 93:675, 1988.

1883. Pratt PC: Chest radiographs cannot identify airflow obstruction. Letter to the Editor. Chest 93:1120, 1988.

1884. Reich SB, Weinshelbaum A, Yee J: Correlation of radiographic measurements and pulmonary function tests in chronic obstructive pulmonary disease. AJR 144:695, 1985.

1885. Barnhard HJ, Pierce JA, Joyce JW, et al: Roentgenographic determination of total lung capacity. A new method evaluated in health, emphysema and congestive heart failure. Am J Med 28:51, 1960.

1886. Loyd HM, String ST, DuBois AB: Radiographic and plethysmographic determination of total lung capacity. Radiology 86:7, 1966.

1887. Glenn WB Jr, Greene R: Rapid computer-aided radiographic calculation of total lung capacity (TLC). Radiology 117:269, 1975.

1888. Mori PA, Anderson AE Jr, Eckert P: The radiological spectrum of aging and emphysematous lungs. Radiology 83:48, 1964.

1889. Järvinen KAJ, Thomander K: The diagnosis of obstructive pulmonary emphysema in mass radiography. Ann Med Int Fenn 48:151, 1959.

1890. Simon G: The appearance of the chest radiograph in old persons. Radiol Clin North Am 3:293, 1965.

1891. Horn C, Robertson M: Assessment of obstructive airways disease by whole lung tomograms. Australas Radiol 12:32, 1968.

1892. Milne ENC, Bass H: Roentgenologic and functional analysis of combined chronic obstructive pulmonary disease and congestive cardiac failure. Invest Radiol 4:129, 1969.

1893. Laws JW, Heard BE: Emphysema and the chest film: A retrospective radiological and pathological study. Br J Radiol 35:750, 1962.

1894. Abbott OA, Hopkins WA, Van Fleit WE, et al: A new approach to pulmonary emphysema. Thorax 8:116, 1953.

1895. Schoenmackers J, Vieten H: Das verhalten der Lungengefässe bei verändertem Luftgehalt der Lunge. (Alteration of lung vasculature with various air contents of the lungs.) Fortschr Roentgenstr 76:24, 1952.

1896. Barden RP: The interpretation of some radiologic signs of abnormal pulmonary function. Radiology 59:481, 1952.

1897. Dulfano MJ, DiRienzo A: Laminagraphic observations of the lung vasculature in chronic pulmonary emphysema. Am J Roentgenol 88:1043, 1962.

1898. Scarrow GD: The pulmonary angiogram in chronic bronchitis and emphysema. Clin Radiol 17:54, 1966.

1899. Jacobson G, Turner AF, Balchum OJ, et al: Vascular changes in pulmonary emphysema: The radiologic evaluation by selective and peripheral pulmonary wedge angiography. Am J Roentgenol 100:374, 1967.

1900. Scarrow GD: The pulmonary angiogram in chronic bronchitis and emphysema. Proc R Soc Med 58:684, 1965.

1901. Simon G: Complexities of emphysema. In Simon M, Potchen EJ, LeMay M (eds): Frontiers of Pulmonary Radiology. New York, Grune & Stratton, Inc., 1969, pp 142–153.

1902. Musk AW: Relation of pulmonary vessel size to transfer factor in subjects with airflow obstruction. Am J Roentgenol 141:915, 1983.

1903. Barden RP: Glimpses through the pulmonary window. Interpretation of the radiologic evidence in disorders of the lungs. Hickey Lecture, 1966. Am J Roentgenol 98:269, 1966.

1904. Bell RS: The radiographic manifestations of alpha-1 antitrypsin deficiency. An important recognizable pattern of chronic obstructive pulmonary disease (COPD). Radiology 95:19, 1970.

1905. Rosen RA, Dalinka MK, Gralino BJ Jr, et al: The roentgenographic findings in alpha-1 antitrypsin deficiency (AAD). Radiology 95:25, 1970.

1906. Jones MC, Thomas GO: Alpha$_1$-antitrypsin deficiency and pulmonary emphysema. Thorax 26:652, 1971.

1907. Martelli NA, Hutchison DCS, Barter CE: Radiological distribution of pulmonary emphysema. Thorax 29:81, 1974.

1908. Bentivoglio LG, Beerel F, Stewart PB, et al: Studies of regional ventilation and perfusion in pulmonary emphysema using xenon[133]. Am Rev Respir Dis 88:315, 1963.

1909. Nairn JR, Prime FJ, Simon G: Association between radiological findings and total and regional function in emphysema. Thorax 24:218, 1969.

1910. Medina JR, Lillehei JP, Loken MK, et al: Use of the scintillation angle camera and xenon-133 in the study of chronic obstructive lung disease. JAMA 208:985, 1969.

1911. Ramanna L, Tashkin DP, Taplin GV, et al: Radioaerosol lung imaging in chronic obstructive pulmonary disease—comparison with pulmonary function tests and roentgenography. Chest 68:634, 1975.

1912. Muir VY: Diagnosing emphysema from the lung scan. Thorax 26:712, 1971.

1913. Morgan TE, Finley TN, Huber GL, et al: Alterations to pulmonary surface active lipids during exposure to increased oxygen tension. J Clin Invest 44:1737, 1965.

1914. Levant MN, Bass H, Anthonisen N, et al: Microvascular circulation of the lungs in emphysema: Correlation of results obtained with roentgenologic and radioactive-isotope techniques. J Can Assoc Radiol 19:130, 1968.

1915. Goddard PR, Nicholson EM, Laszlo G, et al: Computed tomography in pulmonary emphysema. Clin Radiol 33:379, 1982.

1916. Murata K, Itoh H, Todo G, et al: Centrilobular lesions of the lung: Demonstration by high-resolution CT and pathologic correlation. Radiology 161:641, 1986.

1917. Meziane MA, Hruban RH, Zerhouni EA, et al: High resolution CT of the lung parenchyma with pathologic correlation. Radiographics 8:27, 1988.

1918. Foster WL Jr, Pratt PC, Roggli VL, et al: Centrilobular emphysema: CT-pathologic correlation. Radiology 159:27, 1986.

1919. Wigh RE: On defining microcardia: Application in pulmonary emphysema. South Med J 71:150, 1978.

1920. Dornhorst AD: Respiratory insufficiency. Lancet 1:1185, 1955.

1921. Fraser RG, Paré JAPP: Diagnosis of Diseases of the Chest: An Integrated Study Based on the Abnormal Roentgenogram. Philadelphia, WB Saunders Co, 1970.

1922. Lieberman J: Alpha$_1$-antitrypsin deficiency. Med Clin North Am 57:691, 1973.

1923. Burrows B, Fletcher CM, Heard BE, et al: Emphysematous and bronchial types of chronic airways obstruction: Clinicopathological study of patients in London and Chicago. Lancet 1:830, 1966.

1924. Milne ENC, Bass H: Roentgenologic diagnosis of early chronic obstructive pulmonary disease. J Can Assoc Radiol 30:3, 1969.

1925. Reid L: The Pathology of Emphysema. London, Lloyd-Luke (Medical Books) Ltd, 1967.

1926. Reid L: Chronic bronchitis and emphysema: A symposium. III. Pathological findings and radiological changes in chronic bronchitis and emphysema. (a) Pathological findings in chronic bronchitis. Br J Radiol 32:291, 1959.

1927. Heitzman ER: The Lung. Radiologic-Pathologic Correlations. St. Louis, CV Mosby Co, 1973, p 350.

1928. Heitzman ER, Markarian B, Soloman J: Chronic obstructive pulmonary disease: Review, emphasizing roentgen pathologic correlations. Radiol Clin North Am 11:49, 1973.

1929. Thurlbeck WM: Chronic Airflow Obstruction in Lung Disease. Philadelphia, WB Saunders Co, 1976, p 220.

1930. Sutinen S, Christoforidis AJ, Klugh GA, et al: Roentgenologic criteria for the recognition of nonsymptomatic pulmonary emphysema. Correlation between roentgenologic findings and pulmonary pathology. Am Rev Respir Dis 91:69, 1965.

1931. Reid LM, Millard FJC: Correlation between radiological diagnosis and structural lung changes in emphysema. Clin Radiol 15:307, 1964.

1932. Thurlbeck WM: Clinico-pathological study of emphysema in American hospitals. Thorax 18:59, 1963.

1933. Thurlbeck WM, Simon G: Radiographic appearance of the chest in emphysema. Am J Roentgenol 130:429, 1978.

1934. Pratt PC: Role of conventional chest radiography in diagnosis and exclusion of emphysema. Am J Med 82:998, 1987.

1935. Pratt PC: Radiographic appearance of the chest in emphysema. Invest Radiol 22:927, 1987.

1936. Fletcher CM, Jones NL, Burrows B, et al: American emphysema and British bronchitis. A standardized comparative study. Am Rev Respir Dis 90:1, 1964.

1937. Burrows B, Petty TL: Long-term effects of treatment in patients with chronic airway obstruction. Chest 60:25, 1971 (Suppl to August 1971 issue).

1938. Fraser RG: The radiologist and obstructive airway disease: Caldwell lecture, 1973. Am J Roentgenol 120:737, 1974.

1939. Reid LM: Role of chronic bronchitis in production of "chronic obstructive pulmonary emphysema." J Am Women's Assoc 20:633, 1965.

1940. Reid LM: Emphysema: Classification and clinical significance. Br J Dis Chest 60:57, 1966.

1941. Reid LM: The Pathology of Emphysema. London, Lloyd-Luke (Medical Books), Ltd, 1967.

1942. Dayman H: Mechanics of airflow in health and in emphysema. J Clin Invest 30:1175, 1951.

1943. Fry DL, Hyatt RE: Pulmonary mechanics. A unified analysis of the relationship between pressure, volume and gas flow in the lungs of normal and diseased human subjects. Am J Med 29:672, 1960.

1944. Campbell EJM, Martin HB, Riley RL: Mechanics of airway obstruction. Bull Johns Hopkins Hosp 101:329, 1957.

1945. Dayman H: Expiratory spirogram. Am Rev Respir Dis 83:842, 1961.

1946. Dekker E, Defarges JG, Heemstra H: Direct measurement of intrabronchial pressure; its application to location of check-valve mechanism. J Appl Physiol 13:35, 1958.

1947. Einthoven W: Über die Wirkung der Bronchialmuskeln nach einer neuen Methode untesucht, und über Asthma nervosum. Pfluegers Arch 51:367, 1892.

1948. Fry DL, Ebert RV, Stead WW, et al: Mechanics of pulmonary ventilation in normal subjects and in patients with emphysema. Am J Med 16:80, 1954.

1949. Koblet H, Wyss F: Das klinische und funktionelle bild des genuinen Bronchialkollapses mit Lungenemphysem. (The clinical and functional picture of genuine bronchial collapse in emphysema of the lungs.) Hel Med Acta 23:553, 1956.

1950. Mead J, Turner JM, Macklem PT, et al: Significance of relationship between lung recoil and maximum expiratory flow. J Appl Physiol 22:95, 1967.

1951. Fraser RG: Measurements of the caliber of human bronchi in three phases of respiration by cinebronchography. J Can Assoc Radiol 12:102, 1961.

1952. Fraser RG, Macklen PT, Brown WG: Airway dynamics in bronchiectasis: A combined cinefluorographic-manometric study. Am J Roentgenol 93:821, 1965.

1953. Fraser RG, Macklen PT: Bronchial dynamics in health and obstructive airway disease: Physiology and roentgenology. In Simon M, Potchen EJ, LeMay M (eds): Frontiers of Chest Radiology. New York, Grune & Stratton, Inc, 1969, pp 76–101.

1954. Wright RR: Bronchial atrophy and collapse in chronic obstructive pulmonary emphysema. Am J Pathol 37:63, 1960.

1955. DiRienzo S: Functional bronchial stenosis. Surgery 27:853, 1950.

1956. Greening RR, Atkins JP: Radiologic and bronchoscopic observations in diffuse narrowing of lumen of tracheobronchial tree. Ann Otol 62:828, 1963.

1957. Herzog H: Exspiratorische stenose der Trachea und der grossen Bronchien durch die erschlaffte Pars membranacea. Operative Korrektur durch Spanskplastik. (Expiratory stenosis of the trachea and great bronchi by loosening of the membraneous portion; plastic chip repair.) Thoraxchirurgie 5:281, 1958.

1958. Macklem PT, Proctor DF, Hogg JC: Stability of peripheral airways. Respir Physiol 8:191, 1970.

1959. Green GM: Lung defense mechanisms. Med Clin North Am 57:547, 1973.

1960. Burrows B, Niden AH, Barclay WR, et al: Chronic obstructive lung disease. II. Relationship of clinical and physiologic findings to the severity of airways obstruction. Am Rev Respir Dis 92:665, 1965.

1961. Kass I, O'Brien LE, Zamel N, et al: Lack of correlation between clinical background and pulmonary function tests in patients with chronic obstructive pulmonary diseases. A retrospective study of 140 cases. Am Rev Respir Dis 107:64, 1973.

1962. Miller RD, Hepper NGG, Kueppers F, et al: Host factors in chronic obstructive pulmonary disease in an upper mid-west rural community: Design, case selection and clinical characteristics in a matched pair study. Mayo Clin Proc 51:709, 1976.

1963. Sharp JT, Drutz WS, Moisan T, et al: Postural relief of dyspnea in severe chronic obstructive pulmonary disease. Am Rev Respir Dis 122:201, 1980.

1964. Seward JB, Hayes DL, Smith HC, et al: Platypnea-orthodeoxia: Clinical profile, diagnostic workup, management, and report of seven cases. Mayo Clin Proc 59:221, 1984.

1965. Minh VD, Chun D, Fairshter RD, et al: Supine change in arterial oxygenation in patients with chronic obstructive pulmonary disease. Am Rev Respir Dis 133:820, 1986.

1966. Shim C, Chun KJ, Williams MH Jr, et al: Positional effects on distribution of ventilation in chronic obstructive pulmonary disease. Ann Intern Med 105:346, 1986.

1967. Burrows B, Fletcher CM, Heard BE, et al: The emphysematous and bronchial types of chronic airways obstruction. Lancet 1:830, 1966.

1968. Bates DV: The J. Burns Amberson lecture—The fate of the chronic bronchitic: A report of the ten-year follow-up in the Canadian Department of Veterans' Affairs coordinated study of chronic bronchitis. Am Rev Respir Dis 108:1043, 1973.

1969. Burrows B, Earle RH: Course and prognosis of chronic obstructive lung disease. A prospective study of 200 patients. N Engl J Med 280:397, 1969.

1970. Mitchell RS: Outlook in emphysema and chronic bronchitis. N Engl J Med 280:445, 1969.

1971. Jones NL, Burrows B, Fletcher CM: Serial studies of 100 patients with chronic airway obstruction in London and Chicago. Thorax 22:327, 1967.

1972. Vandenbergh E, Clement J, de Woestijne KP: Course and prognosis of patients with advanced chronic obstructive pulmonary disease. Evaluation by means of functional indices. Am J Med 55:736, 1973.

1973. Burk RH, George RB: Acute respiratory failure in chronic obstructive pulmonary disease. Arch Intern Med 132:865, 1973.

1974. Moser KM, Shibel EM, Beamon AJ: Acute respiratory failure in obstructive lung disease. JAMA 225:705, 1973.

1975. Ude AC, Howard P: Controlled oxygen therapy and pulmonary heart failure. Thorax 26:572, 1971.

1976. Moore LG, Rohr AL, Maisenback JK, et al: Emphysema mortality is increased in Colorado residents at high altitude. Am Rev Respir Dis 126:225, 1982.

1977. Nocturnal Oxygen Therapy Trial Group: Continuous or nocturnal oxygen therapy in hypoxemic chronic obstructive lung disease. Ann Intern Med 93:391, 1980.

1978. Medical Research Council Working Party: Long term domiciliary oxygen therapy in chronic hypoxic cor pulmonale complicating chronic bronchitis and emphysema. Lancet 1:681, 1981.

1979. Timms RM, Khaja FU, Williams GW: The nocturnal oxygen therapy trial group. Hemodynamic response to oxygen therapy in chronic obstructive pulmonary disease. Ann Intern Med 102:29, 1985.

1980. Flick MR, Block AJ: Nocturnal vs diurnal cardiac arrhythmias in patients with chronic obstructive pulmonary disease. Chest 75:8, 1979.

1981. Sassoon CSH, Hassell KT, Mahutte CK, et al: Hyperoxic-induced hypercapnia in stable chronic obstructive pulmonary disease. Am Rev Respir Dis 135:907, 1987.

1982. Aubier M, Murciano D, Milic-Emili J, et al: Effects of the administration of O_2 on ventilation and blood gases in patients with chronic obstructive pulmonary disease during acute respiratory failure. Am Rev Respir Dis 122:747, 1980.

1983. Arnold WH Jr, Grant JL: Oxygen-induced hypoventilation. Am Rev Respir Dis 95:255, 1967.

1984. McNicol MW, Campbell EJM: Severity of respiratory failure. Arterial blood-gases in untreated patients. Lancet 1:336, 1965.

1985. Filley GF: Acid regulation and CO_2 retention. Chest 58:417, 1970.

1986. Vanier T, Dulfano MJ, Wu C, et al: Emphysema, hypoxia and the polycythemic response. N Engl J Med 269:169, 1963.

1987. Lertzman M, Israels LG, Cherniack RM: Erythropoiesis and ferrokinetics in chronic respiratory disease. Ann Intern Med 56:821, 1962.

1988. Gallo RC, Fraimow W, Cathcart RT, et al: Erythropoietic response in chronic pulmonary disease. Arch Intern Med 113:559, 1964.

1989. Calverley MA, Leggett RJ, McElderry L, et al: Cigarette smoking and secondary polycythemia in hypoxic cor pulmonale. Am Rev Respir Dis 125:507, 1982.

1990. Fielding J, Zorab PA: Polycythaemia and iron deficiency in pulmonary "emphysema." Lancet 2:284, 1964.

11

1991. Wedzicha JA, Cotes PM, Empey DW, et al: Serum immunoreactive erythropoietin in hypoxic lung disease with and without polycythaemia. Clin Sci 69:413, 1985.

1992. Chamberlain DA, Millard FJC: The treatment of polycythaemia secondary to hypoxic lung disease by continuous oxygen administration. Q J Med 32:341, 1963.

1993. Patakas DA, Christaki PI, Louridas GE, et al: Control of breathing in patients with chronic obstructive lung diseases and secondary polycythemia after venesection. Respiration 49:257, 1986.

1994. Palmer KNV, Gardiner AJS: Effect of partial gastrectomy on pulmonary physiology. Br Med J 1:347, 1964.

1995. Dines DE, Clagett OT, Payne WS: Spontaneous pneumothorax in emphysema. Mayo Clin Proc 45:481, 1970.

1996. Schwartz JS, Bencowitz HZ, Moser KM, et al: Air travel hypoxemia with chronic obstructive pulmonary disease. Ann Intern Med 100:473, 1984.

1997. Fanta CH, Wright TC, McFadden ER, et al: Differentiation of recurrent pulmonary emboli from chronic obstructive lung disease as a cause of cor pulmonale. Chest 79:92, 1981.

1998. Lippmann M, Fein A: Pulmonary embolism in the patient with chronic obstructive pulmonary disease—a diagnostic dilemma. Chest 79:39, 1981.

1999. Openbrier DR, Irwin MM, Rogers RM, et al: Nutritional status and lung function in patients with emphysema and chronic bronchitis. Chest 83:17, 1983.

2000. Braun SR, Keim NL, Dixon RM, et al: The prevalence and determinants of nutritional changes in chronic obstructive pulmonary disease. Chest 86:558, 1984.

2001. Goldstein SA, Thomashow B, Askanazi J: Functional changes during nutritional repletion in patients with lung disease. Clin Chest Med 7:141, 1986.

2002. Goldstein S, Askanazi J, Weissman C, et al: Energy expenditure in patients with chronic obstructive pulmonary disease. Chest 91:222, 1987.

2003. Wilson DO, Rogers RM, Sanders MH, et al: Nutritional intervention in malnourished patients with emphysema. Am Rev Respir Dis 134:672, 1986.

2004. Massaro DJ, Katz S, Luchsinger PC: The use of a carbon buffer (trishydroxymethylaminomethane) in the treatment of respiratory acidosis. Am Rev Respir Dis 86:353, 1962.

2005. Swanson AG: Potential harmful effects of treating pulmonary encephalopathy with a carbon dioxide buffering agent. Am J Med Sci 240:433, 1960.

2006. Hamilton JD, Gross NJ: Unusual neurological and cardiovascular complications of respiratory failure. Br Med J 2:1092, 1963.

2007. Kilburn KH: Neurologic manifestations of respiratory failure. Arch Intern Med 116:409, 1965.

2008. Block AJ, Ball WC Jr: Acute respiratory failure. Observations on the use of the Mörch Piston Respirator. Ann Intern Med 65:957, 1966.

2009. Addington WW, Kettle LJ, Cugell DW: Alkalosis due to mechanical hyperventilation in patients with chronic hypercapnia. Am Rev Respir Dis 93:736, 1966.

2010. White RJ, Woodings DF: Impaired water handling in chronic airways disease. Br Med J 2:561, 1971.

2011. Telfer N, Weiner JM, Merrill Q: Distribution of sodium and potassium in chronic obstructive pulmonary disease. Am Rev Respir Dis 111:166, 1975.

2012. Kilburn KH, Dowell AR: Renal function in respiratory failure. Arch Intern Med 127:754, 1971.

2013. Editorial: Renal function in respiratory failure. JAMA 216:131, 1971.

2014. Schloerb PR, King CR, Kerby G, Ruth WE: Potassium depletion in patients with chronic respiratory failure. Am Rev Respir Dis 102:53, 1970.

2015. Turino GM, Goldring RM, Heinemann HO: Renal response to mechanical ventilation in patients with chronic hypercapnia. Am J Med 56:151, 1974.

2016. Marks A: Chronic bronchitis and emphysema: Clinical diagnosis and evaluation. Med Clin North Am 57:707, 1973.

2017. Marini JJ, Pierson DJ, Hudson LD, et al: The significance of wheezing in chronic airflow obstruction. Am Rev Respir Dis 120:1069, 1979.

2018. Campbell EJM: Physical signs of diffuse airways obstruction and lung distention. Thorax 24:1, 1969.

2019. Christie RV: Emphysema of the lungs. Br Med J 1:105, 1944.

2020. Hoover CF: Definitive percussion and inspection in estimating size and contour of heart. JAMA 75:1626, 1920.

2021. Ashutosh K, Gilbert R, Auchincloss JH Jr, et al: Asynchronous breathing movements in patients with chronic obstructive pulmonary disease. Chest 67:553, 1975.

2022. Sharp JT, Goldberg NB, Druz WS, et al: Thoracoabdominal motion in chronic obstructive pulmonary disease. Am Rev Respir Dis 115:47, 1977.

2023. Godfrey S, Edwards RHT, Campbell EJM, et al: Clinical and physiological associations of some physical signs observed in patients with chronic airways obstruction. Thorax 25:285, 1970.

2024. Boushy SF, Adhikari PK, Sakamoto A, et al: Factors affecting prognosis in emphysema. Dis Chest 45:402, 1964.

2025. Thurlbeck WM: Diaphragm and body weight in emphysema. Thorax 33:483, 1978.

2026. Sánchez J, Medrano G, Debesse B, et al: Muscle fibre types in costal and crural diaphragm in normal men and in patients with moderate chronic respiratory disease. Clin Respir Physiol 21:351, 1985.

2027. Campbell JA, Hughes RL, Saghal V, et al: Alterations in intercostal muscle morphology and biochemistry in patients with obstructive lung disease. Am Rev Respir Dis 122:679, 1980.

2028. Sánchez J, Bastien C, Medrano G, et al: Metabolic enzymatic activities in the diaphragm of normal men and patients with moderate chronic obstructive pulmonary disease. Bull Eur Physiopathol Respir 20:535, 1985.

2029. Kelsen SG, Wolanski T, Supinski GS, et al: The effect of elastase-induced emphysema on diaphragmatic muscle structure in hamsters. Am Rev Respir Dis 127:330, 1983.

2030. Supinski GS, Kelsen SG: Effect of elastase-induced emphysema on the force-generating ability of the diaphragm. J Clin Invest 70:978, 1982.

2031. Gaultier C, Boulé M, Tourmier G, et al: Inspiratory force reserve of the respiratory muscles in children with chronic obstructive pulmonary disease. Am Rev Respir Dis 132:811, 1985.

2032. Rochester DF, Braun NMT: Determinants of maximal inspiratory pressure in chronic obstructive pulmonary disease. Am Rev Respir Dis 132:42, 1985.

2033. Grassino A, Macklem PT: Respiratory muscle fatigue and ventilatory failure. Annu Rev Med 35:625, 1984.

2034. Bellemare F, Grassino A: Force reserve of the diaphragm in patients with chronic obstructive pulmonary disease. J Appl Physiol 55:8, 1983.

2035. Aubier M, Murciano D, Lecocguic Y, et al: Bilateral phrenic stimulation: A simple technique to assess diaphragmatic fatigue in humans. J Appl Physiol 58:58, 1985.

2036. Bye P, Esau S, Levy R, et al: Ventilatory muscle function during exercise in air and oxygen in patients with chronic air-flow limitation. Am Rev Respir Dis 236:132, 1985.

2037. Wilson SH, Cooke NT, Moxham J, et al: Sternomastoid muscle function and fatigue in normal subjects and in patients with chronic obstructive pulmonary disease. Am Rev Respir Dis 129:460, 1984.

2038. Aldrich TK: The application of muscle endurance training techniques to the respiratory muscles in COPD. Lung 163:15, 1985.

2039. Belman MJ, Mittman C (with the technical assistance of Robert Weir): Ventilatory muscle training improves exercise capacity in chronic obstructive pulmonary disease. Am Rev Respir Dis 121:273, 1980.

2040. Pardy RL, Rivington RN, Despas PJ, et al: The effects of inspiratory muscle training on exercise performance in chronic airflow limitation. Am Rev Respir Dis 123:426, 1981.

2041. Pardy RL, Rivington RN, Despas PJ, et al: Inspiratory muscle training compared with physiotherapy in chronic airflow limitation. Am Rev Respir Dis 123:421, 1981.

2042. Schrijen F, Urtiaga B: Pulmonary blood volume in chronic lung disease—changes with legs raised and during exercise. Chest 81:544, 1982.

2043. Albert RK, Muramoto A, Caldwell J, et al: Increases in intrathoracic pressure do not explain the rise in left ventricular end-diastolic pressure that occurs during exercise in patients with chronic obstructive pulmonary disease. Am Rev Respir Dis 132:623, 1985.

2044. Light RW, Mintz HM, Linden GS, et al: Hemodynamics of patients with severe chronic obstructive pulmonary disease during progressive upright exercise. Am Rev Respir Dis 130:391, 1984.

2045. Weitzenblum E, Hirth C, Parini JP, et al: Clinical, functional and pulmonary hemodynamic course of patients with chronic obstructive pulmonary disease followed-up over 3 years. Respiration 36:1, 1978.

2046. Weitzenblum E, Jezek V: Evolution of pulmonary hypertension in chronic respiratory disease. Bull Eur Physiopathol Respir 20:73, 1985.

2047. Degaute JP, Domenighetti G, Naeije R, et al: Oxygen delivery in acute exacerbation of chronic obstructive pulmonary disease—effects of controlled oxygen therapy. Am Rev Respir Dis 124:26, 1981.

2048. Block AJ, Boysen PG, Wynne JW, et al: The origins of cor pulmonale—a hypothesis. Chest 75:109, 1979.

2049. Midgren B, White T, Petersson K, et al: Nocturnal hypoxaemia and cor pulmonale in severe chronic lung disease. Bull Eur Physiopathol Respir 21:527, 1985.

2050. Sturani C, Bassein L, Schiavina M, et al: Oral nifedipine in chronic cor pulmonale secondary to severe chronic obstructive pulmonary disease (COPD). Chest 84:135, 1983.

2051. Naeije R, Mélot C, Mols P, et al: Reduction in pulmonary hypertension by prostaglandin-E₁ in decompensated chronic obstructive pulmonary disease. Am Rev Respir Dis 125:1, 1982.

2052. Mélot C, Naaije R, Rothschild T, et al: Improvement in ventilation-perfusion matching by almitrine in COPD. Chest 83:528, 1983.

2053. Weitzenblum E, Ehrhart M, Schneider JC, et al: Effects of intravenous almitrine on pulmonary haemodynamics in chronic bronchitics with respiratory insufficiency. Bull Eur Physiopathol Respir 18:765, 1982.

2054. Weitzenblum E, Loiseau A, Hirth C, et al: Course of pulmonary hemodynamics in patients with chronic obstructive pulmonary disease. Chest 75:656, 1979.

2055. Schrijen F, Uffholtz H, Polu JM, et al: Pulmonary and systemic hemodynamic evolution in chronic bronchitis. Am Rev Respir Dis 117:25, 1978.

2056. Gluskowski J, Jedrzejewska-Makowska M, Hawrylkiewicz I, et al: Effects of prolonged oxygen therapy on pulmonary hypertension and blood viscosity in patients with advanced cor pulmonale. Respiration 44:177, 1983.

2057. Weitzenblum E, Sautegeau A, Ehrhart M, et al: Long-term oxygen therapy can reverse the progression of pulmonary hypertension in patients with chronic obstructive pulmonary disease. Am Rev Respir Dis 131:493, 1985.

2058. Fletcher EC, Levin DC: Cardiopulmonary hemodynamics during sleep in subjects with chronic obstructive pulmonary disease. Chest 85:6, 1984.

2059. Ashutosh K, Dunsky M: Noninvasive tests for responsiveness of pulmonary hypertension to oxygen. Prediction of survival in patients with chronic obstructive lung disease and cor pulmonale. Chest 92:393, 1987.

2060. Lindsay DA, Read J: Pulmonary vascular responsiveness in the prognosis of chronic obstructive lung disease. Am Rev Respir Dis 105:242, 1972.

2061. Rebuck AS, Vandenberg RA: The relationship between pulmonary arterial pressure and physiologic dead space in patients with obstructive lung disease. Am Rev Respir Dis 107:423, 1973.

2062. Soroldoni M, Ferrarini F, Biffi E, et al: M-mode subxiphoid echocardiography in assessing pulmonary hypertension. Its usefulness in chronic obstructive pulmonary disease. Respiration 47:164, 1985.

2063. Williams IP, Boyd MJ, Humberstone AM, et al: Pulmonary arterial hypertension and emphysema. Br J Dis Chest 78:211, 1984.

2064. Taha RA, Boushy SF, Thompson HK Jr, et al: The electrocardiogram in chronic obstructive pulmonary disease. Am Rev Respir Dis 107:1067, 1973.

2065. Tandon MK: Correlations of electrocardiographic features with airway obstruction in chronic bronchitis. Chest 63:146, 1973.

2066. Murphy ML, Hutcheson F: The electrocardiographic diagnosis of right ventricular hypertrophy in chronic obstructive pulmonary disease. Chest 65:622, 1974.

2067. Olvey SK, Reduto LA, Stevens PM, et al: First pass radionuclide assessment of right and left ventricular ejection fraction in chronic pulmonary disease effect of oxygen upon exercise response. Chest 78:4, 1980.

2068. MacNee W, Morgan A, Wathen C, et al: Right ventricular performance during exercise in chronic obstructive pulmonary disease: The effects of oxygen. Respiration 48:206, 1985.

2069. Macnee W, Xue QF, Hannan WJ, et al: Assessment by radionucleide angiography of right and left ventricular function in chronic bronchitis and emphysema. Thorax 38:494, 1983.

2070. Burghuber O, Bergmann H, Silberbauer K, et al: Right ventricular performance in chronic air flow obstruction. Respiration 45:124, 1984.

2071. Mahler D, Brent B, Loke J, et al: Right ventricular performance and central circulatory hemodynamics during upright exercise in patients with chronic obstructive pulmonary disease. Am Rev Respir Dis 130:722, 1984.

2072. Bertoli L, Rizzato G, Sala G, et al: Echocardiographic and hemodynamic assessment of right heart impairment in chronic obstructive lung disease. Respiration 44:282, 1983.

2073. Yamaoka S, Yonekura Y, Koide H, et al: Noninvasive method to assess cor pulmonale in patients with chronic obstructive pulmonary disease. Chest 92:10, 1987.

2074. Seibold H, Roth U, Lippert R, et al: Left heart function in chronic obstructive lung disease. Klin Wochenschr 64:433, 1986.

2075. Jardin F, Gueret P, Prost JF, et al: 2-dimensional echocardiographic assessment of left ventricular function in chronic obstructive pulmonary disease. Am Rev Respir Dis 129:135, 1984.

2076. Roux JJ, Deveze JL, Escojido H, et al: Left ventricular function in chronic obstructive pulmonary disease after decompensation. Respiration 38:43, 1979.

2077. Edwards CW: Left ventricular hypertrophy in emphysema. Thorax 29:75, 1974.

2078. Murphy ML, Adamson J, Hutcheson F: Left ventricular hypertrophy in patients with chronic bronchitis and emphysema. Ann Intern Med 81:307, 1974.

2079. Hudson LD, Kurt TL, Petty TL, et al: Arrhythmias associated with acute respiratory failure in patients with chronic airway obstruction. Chest 63:661, 1973.

2080. Corazzo LJ, Pastor BH: Cardiac arrhythmias in chronic cor pulmonale. N Engl J Med 259:862, 1958.

2081. Holford FD, Mithoefer JC: Cardiac arrhythmias in hospitalized patients with chronic obstructive pulmonary disease. Am Rev Respir Dis 108:879, 1973.

2082. Bishop JM, Cross KW: Physiological variables and mortality in patients with various categories of chronic respiratory disease. Bull Eur Physiopathol Respir 20:495, 1985.

2083. Burrows B, Kettel LJ, Niden AH, et al: Patterns of cardiovascular dysfunction in chronic obstructive lung disease. N Engl J Med 286:912, 1972.

2084. Weitzenblum E, Hirth C, Ducolone A, et al: Prognostic value of pulmonary artery pressure in chronic obstructive pulmonary disease. Thorax 36:752, 1981.

2085. Traver GA, Cline MG, Burrows B, et al: Predictors of mortality in chronic obstructive pulmonary disease. A 15-year follow-up study. Am Rev Respir Dis 119:895, 1979.

2086. Finlay M, Middleton HC, Peake MD, et al: Cardiac output, pulmonary hypertension, hypoxemia and survival in patients with chronic obstructive airways disease. Eur J Respir Dis 64:252, 1983.

2087. Kawakami Y, Terai T, Yamamoto H, et al: Exercise and oxygen inhalation in relation to prognosis of chronic obstructive pulmonary disease. Chest 81:182, 1982.

2088. Kok-Jensen A, Ebbehoj K: Prognosis of chronic obstructive lung disease in relation to radiology and electrocardiogram. Scand J Respir Dis 58:304, 1977.

2089. Postma DS, Burema J, Gimeno F, et al: Prognosis in severe chronic obstructive pulmonary disease. Am Rev Respir Dis 119:356, 1979.

2090. Camilli AE, Burrows B, Knudson RJ, et al: Longitudinal changes in forced expiratory volume in one second in adults: Effect of smoking and smoking cessation. Am Rev Respir Dis 135:794, 1987.

2091. Buist AS, Ghezzo H, Anthonisen NR, et al: Relationship between the single-breath N₂ test and age, sex and smoking habit in three North American cities. Am Rev Respir Dis 120:305, 1979.

2092. Becklake MR, Leclerc M, Strobach H, et al: The N₂ closing volume test in population studies: Sources of variation and reproducibility. Am Rev Respir Dis 111:141, 1975.

2093. Becklake MR, Permutt S: Evaluation of tests of lung function for "screening" for early detection of chronic obstructive lung disease. In Macklem PT, Permutt S (eds): The Lung in the Transition Between Health and Disease. New York, Marcel Dekker, 1979, p 345.

2094. Martin PR, Lindsay D, Despas P, et al: The early detection of airway obstruction. Am Rev Respir Dis 111:119, 1975.

2095. Murtagh PS, Proctor DF, Permutt S, et al: Bronchial closure with mechoyl in excised dog lobes. J Appl Physiol 31:409, 1971.

2096. Wright JL, Lawson LM, Paré PD, et al: The detection of small airways disease. Am Rev Respir Dis 129:989, 1984.

2097. Demedts M, Cosemans J, De Roo M, et al: Emphysema with minor airway obstruction and abnormal tests of small airway disease. Respiration 35:148, 1978.

2098. Van de Woestijne KP: Are the small airways really quiet? Eur J Respir Dis 63:19, 1982.

2099. Detels R, Tashkin DP, Simmons MS, et al: The UCLA population studies of chronic obstructive respiratory disease. 5. Agreement and disagreement of tests in identifying abnormal lung function. Chest 82:630, 1982.

2100. Dosman JA, Cotton DJ, Graham BL, et al: Sensitivity and specificity of early diagnostic tests of lung function in smokers. Chest 79:6, 1981.

2101. Nemery B, Moavero NE, Brasseur L, et al: Significance of small airway tests in middle-aged smokers. Am Rev Respir Dis 124:232, 1981.

2102. Walter S, Nancy NR, Collier CR, et al: Changes in the forced expiratory spirogram in young male smokers. Am Rev Respir Dis 119:717, 1979.

2103. Solomon DA: Clinical significance of pulmonary function tests: Are small airways tests helpful in the detection of early airflow obstruction? Chest 74:567, 1978.

2104. Olofsson J, Bake B, Svardsudd K, et al: The single breath N₂-test predicts the rate of decline in FEV₁. Eur J Respir Dis 69:46, 1986.

2105. Buist AS, Vollmer WM, Johnson LR, et al: Does the single-breath test identify the susceptible individual? Chest 85:105, 1984.

2106. Bake B: Is maximum mid-expiratory flow rate sensitive to small airways obstruction? Eur J Respir Dis 62:150, 1981.

2107. Marrero O, Beck GJ, Schachter EN: Discriminating power of measurements from maximum expiratory flow-volume curves. Respiration 49:263, 1986.

2108. Herzog H, Keller R, Perruchoud A, et al: The combined flow-volume pressure-resistance diagram for classification of airways obstruction. *In* DeKock MA, Nadel JA, Lewis CM (eds): Mechanisms of Airways Obstruction in Human Respiratory Disease. Cape Town, South Africa, A. A. Balkema, 1979, p 333.

2109. Colebatch HJH, Greaves IA: Chronic airflow obstruction. Evolution of disordered function in cigarette smokers. Med J Aust *142*:607, 1985.

2110. Hyatt RE, Rodarte JR: Changes in lung mechanics. *In* Macklem PT, Permutt S (eds): The Lung in the Transition Between Health and Disease. New York, Marcel Dekker, 1979, p 73.

2111. Paré PD, Coppin CA, Brooks LA, et al: Upstream resistance in COPD patients with emphysema and small airway inflammation. Am Rev Respir Dis *127*:256A, 1983.

2112. Rossoff LJ, Csima A, Zamel N, et al: Reproducibility of maximum expiratory flow in severe chronic obstructive pulmonary disease. Bull Eur Physiopathol Respir *15*:1129, 1979.

2113. Jadue C, Greville H, Coalson JJ, et al: Forced expiration and HeO$_2$ response in canine peripheral airway obstruction. J Appl Physiol *58*:1788, 1985.

2114. Mink SN: Expiratory flow limitation and the response to breathing a helium-oxygen gas mixture in a canine model of pulmonary emphysema. J Clin Invest *73*:1321, 1984.

2115. Anthonisen NR, Wright EC: Bronchodilator response in chronic obstructive pulmonary disease. Am Rev Respir Dis *133*:814, 1986.

2116. Wardman AG, Binns V, Clayden AD, et al: The diagnosis and treatment of adults with obstructive airways disease in general practice. Br J Dis Chest *80*:19, 1986.

2117. Dawkins KD, Muers MF: Diurnal variation in airflow obstruction in chronic bronchitis. Thorax *36*:618, 1981.

2118. Ramsdale EH, Morris MM, Hargreave FE: Interpretation of the variability of peak flow rates in chronic bronchitis. Thorax *41*:771, 1986.

2119. Chester EJ, Schwartz HJ, Fleming GM, et al: Adverse effect of propranolol on airway function in nonasthmatic chronic obstructive lung disease. Chest *79*:540, 1981.

2120. Postma DS, Keyzer JJ, Koëter GH, et al: Influence of the parasympathetic and sympathetic nervous system on nocturnal bronchial obstruction. Clin Sci *69*:251, 1985.

2121. Emmett PC, Love RG, Hannan WJ, et al: The relationship between the pulmonary distribution of inhaled fine aerosols and tests of small airway function. Bull Eur Physiopathol Respir *20*:325, 1984.

2122. Barter SJ, Cunningham DA, Lavender JP, et al: Abnormal ventilation scans in middle-aged smokers—comparison with tests of overall lung function. Am Rev Respir Dis *132*:148, 1985.

2123. Fairshter RD: Airway hysteresis in normal subjects and individuals with chronic airflow obstruction. J Appl Physiol *48*:1505, 1985.

2124. Guillemi S, Coppin C, Osborne S, et al: Density dependence of maximum expiratory flow and pulmonary resistance—correlation with small airway pathology in smokers. Am Rev Respir Dis *133*:A31, 1986.

2125. Clément J, Làndsér FJ, Van de Woestijne KP, et al: Total resistance and reactance in patients with respiratory complaints with and without airways obstruction. Chest *83*:215, 1983.

2126. Higenbottom T, Payne J: Glottis narrowing in lung disease. Am Rev Respir Dis *125*:746, 1982.

2127. Hogg JC, Wright JL, Paré PD, et al: Airway disease: Evolution, pathology, and recognition. Med J Aust *142*:605, 1985.

2128. York EL, Jones RL: Effects of smoking on regional residual volume in young adults. Chest *79*:12, 1981.

2129. Hughes JA, Hutchison DCS: Errors in the estimation of vital capacity from expiratory flow-volume curves in pulmonary emphysema. Br J Dis Chest *76*:279, 1982.

2130. Fleury B, Murciano D, Talamo C, et al: Worth of breathing in patients with chronic obstructive pulmonary disease in acute respiratory failure. Am Rev Respir Dis *131*:822, 1985.

2131. Fleury B, Murciano D, Talamo C, et al: Work of breathing in patients with chronic obstructive pulmonary disease in acute respiratory failure. Am Rev Respir Dis *131*:822, 1985.

2132. Brancatisano TP, Dodd DS, Collett PW, et al: Effect of expiratory loading on glottic dimensions in humans. J Appl Physiol *58*:605, 1985.

2133. Marini JJ, Tyler ML, Hudson LD, et al: Influence of head-dependent positions on lung volume and oxygen saturation in chronic air-flow obstruction. Am Rev Respir Dis *129*:101, 1984.

2134. Farkas GA, Roussos CH: Adaptability of the hamster diaphragm to exercise and/or emphysema. J Appl Physiol *53*:1263, 1982.

2135. Paré PD, Coppin CA: Errors in the measurement of total lung capacity in patients with chronic obstructive pulmonary disease. Thorax *38*:468, 1983.

2136. Burns CB, Scheinhorn DJ: Evaluation of single-breath helium dilution total lung capacity in obstructive lung disease. Am Rev Respir Dis *130*:580, 1985.

2137. Rodenstein DO, Stănescu DC: Reassessment of lung volume measurement by helium dilution and by body plethysmography in chronic air-flow obstruction. Am Rev Respir Dis *126*:1040, 1982.

2138. Piquet J, Harf A, Lorino H, et al: Lung volume measurements by plethysmography in chronic obstructive pulmonary disease. Influence of the panting pattern. Bull Eur Physiopathol Respir *20*:31, 1985.

2139. Bégin P, Peslin R: Influence of panting frequency on thoracic gas volume measurements in chronic obstructive pulmonary disease. Am Rev Respir Dis *130*:121, 1984.

2140. Rodenstein DO, Stănescu DC: Frequency dependence of plethysmographic volume in healthy and asthmatic subjects. J Appl Physiol *54*:159, 1983.

2141. Colebatch HJH, Greaves IA, Ng CKY, et al: Exponential analysis of elastic recoil and aging in healthy males and females. J Appl Physiol *47*:683, 1979.

2142. Gibson GJ, Pride NB, Davis J, et al: Exponential description of the static pressure-volume curve of normal and diseased lungs. Am Rev Respir Dis *120*:799, 1979.

2143. Knudson RJ, Kaltenborn WT: Evaluation of lung elastic recoil by exponential curve analysis. Respir Physiol *46*:29, 1981.

2144. Colebatch HJH, Greaves IA, Ng CKY, et al: Pulmonary distensibility and ventilatory function in smokers. Bull Eur Physiopathol Respir *21*:439, 1985.

2145. Corbin RP, Loveland M, Martin RR, et al: A four-year follow-up study of lung mechanics in smokers. Am Rev Respir Dis *120*:293, 1979.

2146. Paré PD, Brooks LA, Bates J, et al: Exponential analysis of the lung pressure-volume curve as a predictor of pulmonary emphysema. Am Rev Respir Dis *126*:54, 1982.

2147. Knudson RJ, Bloom JW, Knudson DE, et al: Subclinical effects of smoking. Chest *86*:20, 1984.

2148. Berend N, Glanville AR, Grunstein MM, et al: Determinants of the slope of phase III of the single breath nitrogen test. Bull Eur Physiopathol Respir *20*:521, 1985.

2149. De Troyer A, Yernault JC, Rodenstein D, et al: Influence of beta2-agonist aerosols on pressure-volume characteristics of the lungs. Am Rev Respir Dis *118*:987, 1978.

2150. Zamel N, Webster PM: Improved expiratory air flow dynamics with smoking cessation. Bull Eur Physiopathol Respir *20*:19, 1985.

2151. Wagner PD, Dantzker DR, Dueck R, et al: Ventilation-perfusion inequality in chronic obstructive pulmonary disease. J Clin Invest *59*:203, 1977.

2152. Marthan R, Castaing Y, Manier G, et al: Gas exchange alterations in patients with chronic obstructive lung disease. Chest *87*:470, 1985.

2153. Comroe JH Jr, Fowler WS: Lung function studies. VI. Detection of uneven alveolar ventilation during a single breath of oxygen. Am J Med *10*:408, 1951.

2154. Darling RC, Cournand A, Mansfield JS, et al: Studies on the intrapulmonary mixture of gases. I. Nitrogen elimination from blood and body tissues during high oxygen breathing. J Clin Invest *19*:591, 1940.

2155. Meneely GR, Kaltreider NL: The volume of the lung determined by helium dilution. Description of the method and comparison with other procedures. J Clin Invest *28*:129, 1949.

2156. Bates DV, Christie RV: Intrapulmonary mixing of helium in health and in emphysema. Clin Sci *9*:17, 1950.

2157. Anthonisen NR, Bass H, Heckscher T, et al: Recent observation on the measurement of regional V̇/Q̇ ratios in chronic lung disease. J Nucl Biol Med *11*:73, 1967.

2158. Bentivoglio LG, Beerel F, Stewart PB, et al: Studies of regional ventilation and perfusion in pulmonary emphysema using xenon[133]. Am Rev Respir Dis *88*:315, 1963.

2159. Dore EK, Poe ND, Ellestad MH, et al: Lung perfusion and inhalation scanning in pulmonary emphysema. Am J Roentgenol *104*:770, 1968.

2160. Pontoppidan H, Hedley-Whyte J, Bendixen HH, et al: Ventilation and oxygen requirements during prolonged artificial ventilation in patients with respiratory failure. N Engl J Med *273*:401, 1965.

2161. Kamat SR, Dulfano MJ, Segal MS: The effects of intermittent positive pressure breathing (IPPB/I) with compressed air in patients with severe chronic nonspecific obstructive pulmonary disease. Am Rev Respir Dis *86*:360, 1962.

2162. Torres G, Lyons HA, Emerson P: The effects of intermittent positive pressure breathing on the intrapulmonary distribution of inspired air. Am J Med *29*:946, 1960.

2163. Aubier M, Murciano D, Fournier M, et al: Central respiratory drive in acute respiratory failure of patients with chronic obstructive pulmonary disease. Am Rev Respir Dis *122*:191, 1980.

2164. Guenard H, Verhas M, Todd-Prokopek A, et al: Effects of oxygen breathing on regional distribution of ventilation and perfusion in hypoxemic patients with chronic lung disease. Am Rev Respir Dis *125*:12, 1982.

2165. Lee J, Read J: Effect of oxygen breathing on distribution of pulmonary blood flow in chronic obstructive lung disease. Am Rev Respir Dis *96*:1173, 1967.

2166. Mithoefer JC, Ramirez C, Cook W, et al: The effect of mixed venous oxygenation on arterial blood chronic obstructive pulmonary disease. The basis for a classification. Am Rev Respir Dis 117:259, 1978.

2167. Paré PD, Brooks LA, Baile EM, et al: The effect of systemic venous hypertension on pulmonary function and lung water. J Appl Physiol 51:592, 1981.

2168. Parot S, Saunier C, Schrijen F, et al: Concomitant changes in function tests, breathing pattern and $PacO_2$ in patients with chronic obstructive pulmonary disease. Bull Eur Physiopathol Respir 18:145, 1982.

2169. Parot S, Miara B, Milic-Emili J, et al: Hypoxemia, hypercapnia and breathing pattern in patients with chronic obstructive pulmonary disease. Am Rev Respir Dis 126:822, 1982.

2170. Mountain R, Zwillich C, Weil J, et al: Hypoventilation in obstructive lung disease: The role of familial factors. N Engl J Med 298:521, 1978.

2171. Kawakami Y, Irie T, Kishi F, et al: Familial aggregation of abnormal ventilatory control and pulmonary function in chronic obstructive pulmonary disease. Eur J Respir Dis 62:56, 1981.

2172. Kawakami Y, Irie T, Shida A, et al: Familial factors affecting arterial blood gas values and respiratory chemosensitivity in chronic obstructive pulmonary disease. Am Rev Respir Dis 125:420, 1982.

2173. Milic-Emili J: Recent advances in clinical assessment of control of breathing. Lung 160:1, 1982.

2174. Fahey PJ, Hyde RW: "Won't breathe" vs "Can't breathe": Detection of depressed ventilatory drive in patients with obstructive pulmonary disease. Chest 81:19, 1983.

2175. Bradley CA, Fleetham JA, Anthonisen NR, et al: Ventilatory control in patients with hypoxemia due to obstructive lung disease. Am Rev Respir Dis 120:21, 1979.

2176. Hedemark LL, Kronenberg RS: Chemical regulation of respiration. Chest 82:488, 1982.

2177. Santiago TV, Remolina C, Scoles V III, et al: Endorphins and the control of breathing. Ability of naloxone to restore flow-resistive load compensation in chronic obstructive pulmonary disease. N Engl J Med 304:1190, 1981.

2178. Tobin MJ, Jenouri G, Sackner MA, et al: Effect of naloxone on breathing pattern in patients with chronic obstructive pulmonary disease with and without hypercapnia. Respiration 44:419, 1983.

2179. Montserrat JM, Ballester E, Sopeña JJ, et al: Effect of naloxone on arterial gases in chronically obstructed patients with acute respiratory failure. Eur J Respir Dis 66:77, 1985.

2180. Flenley DC, Franklin DH, Millar JS, et al: The hypoxic drive to breathing in chronic bronchitis and emphysema. Clin Sci 38:503, 1970.

2181. Oliven A, Kelsen SG, Deal EC Jr, et al: Respiratory pressure sensation. Relationship to changes in breathing pattern and PCO_2 during acute increase in airway resistance in patients with chronic obstructive pulmonary disease. Am Rev Respir Dis 132:1214, 1985.

2182. Loveridge B, West P, Anthonisen N, et al: Breathing patterns in patients with chronic obstructive pulmonary disease. Am Rev Respir Dis 130:730, 1984.

2183. Pardy RL, Rivington RN, Milic-Emili J, et al: Control of breathing in chronic obstructive pulmonary disease—the effect of histamine inhalation. Am Rev Respir Dis 125:6, 1982.

2184. Oliven A, Cherniack NS, Deal EC, et al: The effects of acute bronchoconstriction on respiratory activity in patients with chronic obstructive pulmonary disease. Am Rev Respir Dis 131:236, 1985.

2185. Fennerty AG, Banks J, Bevan C, et al: Role of airway receptors in the breathing pattern of patients with chronic obstructive lung disease. Thorax 40:268, 1985.

2186. Muriciano D, Aubier M, Viau F, et al: Effects of airway anesthesia on pattern of breathing and blood gases in patients with chronic obstructive pulmonary disease during acute respiratory failure. Am Rev Respir Dis 126:113, 1982.

2187. Gottfried SB, Redline S, Altose MD, et al: Respiratory sensation in chronic obstructive pulmonary disease. Am Rev Respir Dis 132:954, 1985.

2188. Fleetham JA, Bradley CA, Kryger MH, et al: The effect of low flow oxygen therapy on the chemical control of ventilation in patients with hypoxemic COPD. Am Rev Respir Dis 122:833, 1980.

2189. Burki NK: Breathlessness and mouth occlusion pressure in patients with chronic obstruction of the airways. Chest 76:527, 1979.

2190. Koo KW, Sax DS, Snider GL: Arterial blood gases and pH during sleep in chronic obstructive pulmonary disease. Am J Med 58:663, 1975.

2191. Flick MR, Block AJ: Continuous in-vivo monitoring of arterial oxygenation in chronic obstructive lung disease. Ann Intern Med 86:725, 1977.

2192. Fleetham J, West P, Mezon B, et al: Sleep, arousals, and oxygen desaturation in chronic obstructive pulmonary disease—the effect of oxygen therapy. Am Rev Respir Dis 126:429, 1982.

2193. Calverley PMA, Brezinova V, Douglas NJ, et al: The effect of oxygenation on sleep quality in chronic bronchitis and emphysema. Am Rev Respir Dis 126:206, 1982.

2194. Guilleminault C, Cummiskey J, Motta J, et al: Chronic obstructive airflow disease and sleep studies. Am Rev Respir Dis 122:397, 1980.

2195. Douglas NJ, Calverley PMA, Leggett RJE, et al: Transient hypoxemia during sleep in chronic bronchitis and emphysema. Lancet 1:1(8106), 1979.

2196. George CF, West P, Kryger MH: Oxygenation and breathing pattern during phasic and tonic REM in patients with chronic obstructive pulmonary disease. Sleep 10:234, 1987.

2197. DeMarco FJ, Wynne JW, Block AJ, et al: Oxygen desaturation during sleep as a determinant of the "blue and bloated" syndrome. Chest 79:621, 1981.

2198. Perez-Padilla R, Conway W, Roth T, et al: Hypercapnia and sleep O_2 desaturation in chronic obstructive pulmonary disease. Sleep 10:216, 1987.

2199. Goldstein RS, Ramcharan V, Bowes G, et al: Effect of supplemental nocturnal oxygen on gas exchange in patients with severe obstructive lung disease. N Engl J Med 310:425, 1984.

2200. Arand DL, McGinty DJ, Littner MR, et al: Respiratory patterns associated with hemoglobin desaturation during sleep in chronic obstructive pulmonary disease. Chest 80:183, 1981.

2201. Littner MR, McGinty DJ, Arand DL, et al: Determinants of oxygen desaturation in the course of ventilation during sleep in chronic obstructive pulmonary disease. Am Rev Respir Dis 122:849, 1980.

2202. Tatsumi K, Kimura H, Kunitomo F, et al: Sleep arterial oxygen desaturation and chemical control of breathing during wakefulness in COPD. Chest 90:68, 1986.

2203. Dolly FR, Block AJ: Medroxyprogesterone acetate and COPD; effect on breathing and oxygenation in sleeping and awake patients. Chest 84:394, 1983.

2204. Boysen PG, Block AJ, Wynne JW, et al: Nocturnal pulmonary hypertension in patients with chronic obstructive pulmonary disease. Chest 76:536, 1979.

2205. Stone DJ, Zaldivar C, Keltz H: The effects of very low doses of nebulized isoproterenol, nebulized saline, and intravenous isoproterenol on blood gases in patients with chronic bronchitis. Am Rev Respir Dis 101:511, 1970.

2206. Pflug AE, Cheney FW Jr, Butler J: The effects of an ultrasonic aerosol on pulmonary mechanics and arterial blood gases in patients with chronic bronchitis. Am Rev Respir Dis 101:710, 1970.

2207. Rao S, Wilson DB, Brooks RC, et al: Acute effects of nebulization of N-acetylcysteine on pulmonary mechanics and gas exchange. Am Rev Respir Dis 102:17, 1970.

2208. Stone DJ, Keltz H, Samortin T, et al: The effect of β-adrenergic inhibition on respiratory gas exchange and lung function. Am Rev Respir Dis 103:503, 1971.

2209. Minh VD, Lee HM, Dolan GF, et al: Hypoxemia during exercise in patients with chronic obstructive pulmonary disease. Am Rev Respir Dis 120:787, 1979.

2210. Raffestin B, Escourrou P, Legrand A, et al: Circulatory transport of oxygen in patients with chronic airflow obstruction exercising maximally. Am Rev Respir Dis 125:426, 1982.

2211. Stewart RI, Lewis CM: Arterial oxygenation and oxygen transport during exercise in patients with chronic obstructive pulmonary disease. Respiration 49:161, 1986.

2212. Owens G, Rogers R, Pennock B, et al: The diffusing capacity as a predictor of arterial oxygen desaturation during exercise in patients with chronic obstructive pulmonary disease. N Engl J Med 310:1218, 1984.

2213. Van Meerhaeghe A, Sergysels R: Control of breathing during exercise in patients with chronic airflow limitation with or without hypercapnia. Chest 84:565, 1983.

2214. Giminez M, Servera E, Candina R, et al: Hypercapnia during maximal exercise in patients with chronic airflow obstruction. Bull Eur Physiopathol Respir 20:113, 1985.

2215. Scano G, van Meerhaeghe A, Willeput R, et al: Effect of oxygen on breathing during exercise in patients with chronic obstructive lung disease. Eur J Respir Dis 63:23, 1982.

2216. Bradley BL, Garner AE, Billiu D, et al: Oxygen-assisted exercise in chronic obstructive lung disease. The effect on exercise capacity and arterial blood gas tensions. Am Rev Respir Dis 118:239, 1978.

2217. Stein DA, Bradley BL, Miller WC, et al: Mechanism of oxygen effects on exercise in patients with chronic obstructive pulmonary disease. Chest 81:6, 1982.

2218. Brown SE, Wiener S, Brown RA, et al: Exercise performance following a carbohydrate load in chronic airflow obstruction. J Appl Physiol 58:1340, 1985.

2219. Brown SE, Nagendran RC, McHugh JW, et al: Effects of a large carbohydrate load on walking performance in chronic air-flow obstruction. Am Rev Respir Dis 132:960, 1985.

2220. Lockhart A: Exercise limiting factors in chronic obstructive lung diseases. Bull Eur Physiopathol Respir 15:305, 1979.

11

2221. Brown HV, Wasserman K: Exercise performance in chronic obstructive pulmonary disease. Med Clin N Am 65:525, 1981.

2222. Dillard T, Piantadosi S, Rajagopal K, et al: Prediction of ventilation at maximal exercise in chronic airflow obstruction. Am Rev Respir Dis 143:230, 1985.

2223. Killian KJ, Jones NL: The use of exercise testing and other methods in the investigation of dyspnea. Clin Chest Med 5:99, 1984.

2224. Delgado HR, Braun SR, Skatrud JB, et al: Chest wall and abdominal motion during exercise in patients with chronic obstructive pulmonary disease. Am Rev Respir Dis 126:200, 1982.

2225. Dodd DS, Brancatisano T, Engel LA, et al: Chest wall mechanics during exercise in patients with severe chronic air-flow obstruction. Am Rev Respir Dis 129:33, 1984.

2226. Ingram RH Jr, Miller RB, Tate LA: Acid-base response to acute carbon dioxide changes in chronic obstructive pulmonary disease. Am Rev Respir Dis 108:225, 1973.

2227. Eldridge F: Blood lactate and pyruvate in pulmonary insufficiency. N Engl J Med 274:878, 1966.

2228. Merwath CR, Sieker HO, Manfredi F: Acid-base relations between blood and cerebrospinal fluid in normal subjects and patients with respiratory insufficiency. N Engl J Med 265:310, 1961.

2229. Dunkin RS, Bondurant S: The determinants of cerebrospinal fluid P_{O_2}. The effects of oxygen and carbon dioxide breathing in patients with chronic lung disease. Ann Intern Med 64:71, 1966.

2230. Miller A, Thornton JC, Warshaw R, et al: Single breath diffusing capacity in a representative sample of the population of Michigan, a large industrial state—predicted values, lower limits of normal, and frequencies of abnormality by smoking history. Am Rev Respir Dis 127:270, 1983.

2231. Gonzalez E, Weill H, Ziskind MM, et al: The value of the single breath diffusing capacity in separating chronic bronchitis from pulmonary emphysema. Dis Chest 53:229, 1968.

2232. Georg J, Lassen NA, Millemgaard K, et al: Diffusion in the gas phase of the lungs in normal and emphysematous subjects. Clin Sci 29:525, 1965.

2233. Williams MH Jr, Park SS: Diffusion of gases within the lungs of patients with chronic obstructive pulmonary disease. Am Rev Respir Dis 98:210, 1968.

2234. Michaels R, Sigurdson M, Thurlbeck S, et al: Elastic recoil of the lung in cigarette smokers: The effect of nebulized bronchodilator and cessation of smoking. Am Rev Respir Dis 119:707, 1979.

2235. Zamel N, Leroux M, Ramcharan V, et al: Decrease in lung recoil pressure after cessation of smoking. Am Rev Respir Dis 119:205, 1979.

2236. Buist AS, Nagy JM, Sexton GJ, et al: The effect of smoking cessation on pulmonary function. A 30-month follow-up of two smoking cessation clinics. Am Rev Respir Dis 120:953, 1979.

2237. Bossé R, Sparrow D, Rose CL, et al: Longitudinal effect of age and smoking cessation on pulmonary function. Am Rev Respir Dis 123:378, 1981.

2238. Tashkin D, Clark V, Coulson A, et al: The UCLA population studies of chronic obstructive respiratory disease. VIII. Effects of smoking cessation on lung function—a prospective study of a free-living population. Am Rev Respir Dis 130:707, 1984.

2239. Simonsson BG, Rolf C: Bronchial reactivity to methacholine in ten non-obstructive heavy smokers before and up to one year after cessation of smoking. Eur J Respir Dis 63:526, 1982.

2240. Ad Hoc Committee to Review Antitrypsin Methods: Statement on methods for detecting alpha₁-antitrypsin abnormalities. In Mittman C (ed): Pulmonary Emphysema and Proteolysis. Academic Press, 1972, p 141.

2241. Heimburger N: Introductory remarks. Proteinase inhibition in human serum. Identification, concentration, chemical properties, enzymatic specificity. In Mittman C (ed): Pulmonary Emphysema and Proteolysis. New York, Academic Press, 1972, p 307.

2242. Geratz JD: Specific low-molecular-weight inhibitors of trypsin. Their structure, activity relationships, and possible clinical uses. In Mittman C (ed): Pulmonary Emphysema and Proteolysis. New York, Academic Press, 1972, p 325.

2243. Ihrig J, Kleinerman J, Rynbrandt DJ: Serum antitrypsins in animals: Studies of species variations, components, and the influence of certain irritants. Am Rev Respir Dis 103:377, 1971.

2244. Tan BH, Gans H: The isolation and purification of bovine alpha₁ antitrypsin. In Mittman C (ed): Pulmonary Emphysema and Proteolysis. New York, Academic Press, 1972, p 361.

2245. Kueppers F: The major proteinase inhibitor in rabbit serum. In Mittman C (ed): Pulmonary Emphysema and Proteolysis. New York, Academic Press, 1972, p 355.

2246. Rosenberg M, Roegner V, Becker FF: Isolation and characterization of two alpha₁-protease inhibitors in rat serum. Am Rev Respir Dis 113:779, 1976.

2247. Talamo RC, Langley CE, Hyslop NE Jr: A comparison of functional and immunochemical measurements of serum alpha₁-antitrypsin. In Mittman C (ed): Pulmonary Emphysema and Proteolysis. New York, Academic Press, 1972, p 167.

2248. Laurell CB: Antigen-antibody crossed electrophoresis. Anal Biochem 10:358, 1965.

2249. Laurell CB: Variation of the alpha₁-antitrypsin level of plasma. In Mittman C (ed): Pulmonary Emphysema and Proteolysis. New York, Academic Press, 1972, p 161.

2250. Moskowitz RW, Heinrich G: Bacterial inactivation of human serum alpha₁-antitrypsin: A possible factor in the pathogenesis of pulmonary disease related to antitrypsin deficiency states. In Mittman C (ed): Pulmonary Emphysema and Proteolysis. New York, Academic Press, 1972, p 261.

2251. Talamo RC, Langley CE, Levine BW, et al: Genetic vs. quantitative analysis of serum alpha₁-antitrypsin. N Engl J Med 287:1067, 1972.

2252. Pierce JA: More on antitrypsin (Editorial). N Engl J Med 287:1095, 1972.

2253. Ashley MJ, Corey P, Chan-Yeung M, et al: Smoking, dust exposure and serum alpha₁-antitrypsin. Am Rev Respir Dis 121:783, 1980.

2254. Fagerhol MK: Genetics of a Pi system. In Mittman C (ed): Pulmonary Emphysema and Proteolysis. New York, Academic Press, 1972, p 123.

2255. Lieberman J, Gaidulis L, Garoutte B, et al: Identification and characteristics of the common alpha₁-antitrypsin phenotypes. Chest 62:557, 1972.

2256. Lieberman J: Elastase, collagenase, emphysema, and alpha₁-antitrypsin deficiency. Chest 70:62, 1976.

2257. Fagerhol MK: Serum Pi types in Norwegians. Acta Pathol Microbiol Scand 70:421, 1967.

2258. Pierce JA, Eradio B, Dew TA: Antitrypsin phenotypes in St. Louis. JAMA 231:609, 1975.

2259. Webb DR, Hyde RW, Schwartz RH, et al: Serum alpha₁-antitrypsin variants, prevalence and clinical spirometry. Am Rev Respir Dis 108:918, 1973.

2260. Cole RB, Nevin NC, Blundell G, et al: Relation of alpha₁-antitrypsin phenotype to the performance of pulmonary function tests and to the prevalence of respiratory illness in a working population. Thorax 31:149, 1976.

2261. Talamo RC, Thurlbeck WM: Alpha₁-antitrypsin Pi types in post-mortem blood. Am Rev Respir Dis 112:201, 1975.

2262. Falk GA, Briscoe WA: Alpha₁-antitrypsin deficiency in chronic obstructive pulmonary disease. Ann Intern Med 72:430, 1970.

2263. Alper CA: Deficiency of alpha₁-antitrypsin. Ann Intern Med 78:298, 1973.

2264. Leading article: Enzyme deficiency and emphysema. Br Med J 3:655, 1971.

2265. Buist AS, Adams BE, Azzam AH, et al: Pulmonary function in young children with alpha₁-antitrypsin deficiency: Comparison with matched control subjects. Am Rev Respir Dis 122:817, 1980.

2266. Falk GA, Briscoe WA: Alpha₁-antitrypsin deficiency in chronic obstructive pulmonary disease. Ann Intern Med 72:430, 1970.

2267. Hutchison DCS, Cook PJL, Barter CE, et al: Pulmonary emphysema and alpha₁-antitrypsin deficiency. Br Med J 1:689, 1971.

2268. Leading article: Alpha₁-antitrypsin deficiency and liver disease in childhood. Br Med J 1:758, 1973.

2269. Kueppers F, Black LF: Alpha₁-antitrypsin and its deficiency. Am Rev Respir Dis 110:176, 1974.

2270. Tobin MJ, Cook PJL, Hutchison DCS, et al: Alpha₁-antitrypsin deficiency—the clinical and physiological features of pulmonary emphysema in subjects homozygous for Pi-type-Z—a survey by the British Thoracic Association. Br J Dis Chest 77:14, 1983.

2271. Black LF, Kueppers F: Alpha₁-antitrypsin deficiency in nonsmokers. Am Rev Respir Dis 117:421, 1978.

2272. Janus ED, Phillips NT, Carrell RW, et al: Smoking, lung function and alpha₁-antitrypsin deficiency. Lancet 1:152, 1985.

2273. Mittman C, Lieberman J, Marasso F, et al: Smoking and chronic obstructive lung disease in alpha₁-antitrypsin deficiency. Chest 60:214, 1971.

2274. Glasgow JFT, Lynch MJ, Hercz A, et al: Alpha₁-antitrypsin deficiency in association with both cirrhosis and chronic obstructive lung disease in two sibs. Am J Med 54:181, 1973.

2275. Orell SR, Mazodier P: Pathological findings in alpha₁-antitrypsin deficiency. In Mittman C (ed): Pulmonary Emphysema and Proteolysis. New York, Academic Press, 1972, p 69.

2276. Mittman C: Summary of symposium on pulmonary emphysema and proteolysis. Am Rev Respir Dis 105:430, 1972.

2277. Lieberman J, Gaidulis L, Roberts L: Racial distribution of alpha₁-antitrypsin variants among junior high school students. Am Rev Respir Dis 114:1194, 1976.

2278. Jeppsson JO, Larsson C, Eriksson S: Characterization of alpha₁-antitrypsin in the inclusion bodies from the liver in alpha₁-antitrypsin deficiency. N Engl J Med 293:576, 1975.

2279. Lieberman J: Heat lability of alpha₁-antitrypsin variants. Chest 64:579, 1973.

2280. Lieberman J, Mittman C, Gordon HW: Alpha₁-antitrypsin in the livers of patients with emphysema. Science 175:63, 1972.

2281. Pääkö P, Ryhänen L, Rantala H, et al: Pulmonary emphysema in a nonsmoking patient with Salla disease. Am Rev Respir Dis *135*: 979, 1987.

2282. Eriksson S, Larsson C: Purification and partial characterization of PAS-positive inclusion bodies from the liver in alpha₁-antitrypsin deficiency. N Engl J Med *292*:176, 1975.

2283. Sharp H, Freier E, Bridges R: Alpha₁-globulin deficiency in familial infantile liver disease. Pediatr Res *2*:298, 1968.

2284. Kueppers F, Dickson ER, Summerskill WHJ: Alpha₁-antitrypsin phenotypes in chronic active liver disease and primary biliary cirrhosis. Mayo Clin Proc *51*:286, 1976.

2285. Porter CA, Mowat AP, Cook PJL, et al: Alpha₁-antitrypsin deficiency and neonatal hepatitis. Br Med J *3*:435, 1972.

2286. Sveger T: Liver disease in alpha₁-antitrypsin deficiency detected by screening of 200,000 infants. N Engl J Med *294*:1316, 1976.

2287. Sharp H, Freier MS: Familial cirrhosis. *In* Mittman C (ed): Pulmonary Emphysema and Proteolysis. New York, Academic Press, 1972, p 101.

2288. Wagener JS, Sobonya RE, Taussig LM, et al: Unusual abnormalities in adolescent siblings with alpha₁-antitrypsin deficiency. Chest *83*:464, 1983.

2289. Berg NO, Eriksson S: Liver disease in adults with alpha₁-antitrypsin deficiency. N Engl J Med *287*:1264, 1972.

2290. Cohen KL, Rubin PE, Echevarria RA, et al: Alpha₁-antitrypsin deficiency, emphysema, and cirrhosis in an adult. Ann Intern Med *78*:227, 1973.

2291. Kumar P, Lancaster-Smith M, Cook P, et al: Antitrypsin deficiency in chronic liver disease and a report of cirrhosis and emphysema in adult members of a family. Br Med J *1*:366, 1974.

2292. Powell LW, Galdabini JJ: Cholestasis and cholangitis in a man with alpha₁-antitrypsin deficiency. N Engl J Med *289*:1301, 1973.

2293. Donlan CJ Jr, Ross DG, Golembieski M, et al: Pulmonary emphysema and liver disease. JAMA *232*:1147, 1975.

2294. Triger DR, Millward-Sadler GH, Czaykowski AA, et al: Alpha₁ antitrypsin deficiency and liver disease in adults. Q J Med *45*:351, 1976.

2295. Lieberman J: Emphysema, cirrhosis, and hepatoma with alpha₁-antitrypsin deficiency. Ann Intern Med *81*:850, 1974.

2296. Schleissner JA, Cohen AH: Alpha₁-antitrypsin deficiency and hepatic carcinoma. Am Rev Respir Dis *111*:863, 1975.

2297. Rawlings W Jr, Moss J, Cooper HS, et al: Hepatocellular carcinoma and partial deficiency of alpha₁-antitrypsin (MZ). Ann Intern Med *81*:771, 1974.

2298. Campra JL, Craig JR, Peters RL, et al: Cirrhosis associated with partial deficiency of alpha₁-antitrypsin in an adult. Ann Intern Med *78*:233, 1973.

2299. Morin T, Martin JP, Feldman G, et al: Heterozygous alpha₁-antitrypsin deficiency and cirrhosis in adults. A fortuitous association. Lancet *1*:250, 1975.

2300. Greenwald AJ, Johnson DS, Oskvig RM, et al: Antitrypsin deficiency, emphysema, cirrhosis and intestinal mucosal atrophy. JAMA *231*:273, 1975.

2301. Freeman HJ, Weinstein WM, Shnitka TK, et al: Alpha₁-antitrypsin deficiency and pancreatic fibrosis. Ann Intern Med *85*:73, 1976.

2302. Rubenstein HM, Jaffer AM, Kudrna JC, et al: Alpha₁-antitrypsin deficiency with severe panniculitis. Ann Intern Med *86*:742, 1977.

2303. Kidd VJ, Golbus MS, Wallace RB, et al: Prenatal diagnosis of α₁-antitrypsin deficiency by direct analysis of the mutation site in the gene. N Engl J Med *310*:639, 1984.

2304. Lieberman J, Gaidulus L, Klotz SD: A new deficient variant of alpha₁-antitrypsin (M_duarte). Inability to detect the heterozygous state by antitrypsin phenotyping. Am Rev Respir Dis *113*:31, 1976.

2305. Hutchison DC, Tobin MJ, Cook PJL, et al: Alpha₁-antitrypsin deficiency—clinical and physiological features in heterozygotes of Pi type SZ. A survey by the British Thoracic Association. Br J Dis Chest *77*:28, 1983.

2306. Lieberman J, Gaidulis L, Schleissner PJA: Intermediate alpha₁-antitrypsin deficiency from a null gene (M. phenotypes). Chest *70*:532, 1976.

2307. Bencze K, Sabatke L, Fruhmann G, et al: Alpha₁-antitrypsin—the PIMM subtypes—do they play a role in development of chronic obstructive pulmonary diseases. Chest *77*:761, 1980.

2308. Carrico RJ, Lieberman J, Yeager F: The source of a minor alpha₁-antitrypsin in variant serum. Am Rev Respir Dis *114*:53, 1976.

2309. Lieberman J: A new "double ring" screening test for alpha₁-antitrypsin variants. Am Rev Respir Dis *108*:248, 1973.

2310. Stevens PM, Hnilica VS, Johnson PC, et al: Pathophysiology of hereditary emphysema. Ann Intern Med *74*:672, 1971.

2311. Levine BW, Talamo RC, Shannon DC, et al: Alteration in distribution of pulmonary blood flow. Ann Intern Med *73*:397, 1970.

2312. Eriksson S, Hedenstierna G, Soderholm B: Lung function in homozygous alpha₁-antitrypsin deficiency: Mechanics and regional function in an asymptomatic male. *In* Mittman C (ed): Pulmonary Emphysema and Proteolysis. New York, Academic Press, 1972, p 25.

2313. Eriksson S, Berven H: Lung function and homozygous alpha₁-antitrypsin deficiency: Studies in patients with severe disease. *In* Mittman C (ed): Pulmonary Emphysema and Proteolysis. New York, Academic Press, 1972, p 7.

2314. Simonsson BG: Chronic cough and expectoration in patients with asthma and in patients with alpha₁-antitrypsin deficiency. Eur J Respir Dis *118*:123, 1982.

2315. Quigley MJ, Fraser RS: Pulmonary Pneumatocele: Pathology and pathogenesis. AJR *150*:1275, 1988.

2316. Laurenzi GA, Turino GM, Fishman AP: Bullous disease of the lung. Am J Med *32*:361, 1962.

2317. Boushy SF, Kohen R, Billig DM, et al: Bullous emphysema: Clinical, roentgenologic and physiologic study of 49 patients. Dis Chest *54*:327, 1968.

2318. Viola AR, Zuffardi EA: Physiologic and clinical aspects of pulmonary bullous disease. Am Rev Respir Dis *94*:574, 1966.

2319. Stone DJ, Schwartz A, Feltman JA: Bullous emphysema. A long-term study of the natural history and the effects of therapy. Am Rev Respir Dis *82*:493, 1960.

2320. Richards DW: Pulmonary emphysema: Etiologic factors and clinical forms. Ann Intern Med *53*:1105, 1960.

2321. Ohata M, Suzuki H: Pathogenesis of spontaneous pneumothorax with special reference to the ultrastructure of emphysematous bullae. Chest *77*:771, 1980.

2322. Dermksian G, Lamb LE: Spontaneous pneumothorax in apparently healthy flying personnel. Ann Intern Med *51*:39, 1959.

2323. Morgan MD, Denison DM, Strickland B, et al: Value of computed tomography for selecting patients with bullous lung disease for surgery. Thorax *41*:855, 1986.

2324. Jensen KM, Miscall L, Steinberg I: Angiocardiography in bullous emphysema: Its role in selection of the case suitable for surgery. Am J Roentgenol *85*:229, 1961.

2325. Pue RH, Wellman HN, Berke RA, et al: Perfusion-ventilation scintiphotography in bullous disease of the lung. Am Rev Respir Dis *107*:946, 1973.

2326. Lopez-Majano V, Kieffer RF Jr, Marine DN, et al: Pulmonary resection in bullous disease. Am Rev Respir Dis *99*:554, 1969.

2327. Pride NB, Barter CE, Hugh-Jones P: The ventilation of bullae and the effect of their removal on thoracic gas volumes and tests of overall pulmonary function. Am Rev Respir Dis *107*:83, 1973.

2328. Douglas AC, Grant IWB: Spontaneous closure of large pulmonary bullae. A report of three cases. Br J Tuberc *51*:335, 1957.

2329. Rubin EH, Buchberg AS: Capricious behavior of pulmonary bullae developing fluid. Dis Chest *54*:546, 1968.

2330. Jay SJ, Johanson WG Jr: Massive intrapulmonary hemorrhage: An uncommon complication of bullous emphysema. Am Rev Respir Dis *110*:497, 1974.

2331. Berry BE, Ochsner A Jr: Massive hemoptysis associated with localized pulmonary bullae requiring emergency surgery. A case report. J Thorac Cardiovasc Surg *63*:94, 1972.

2332. Grimes OF, Farber SM: Air cysts of the lung. Surg Gynecol Obstet *113*:720, 1961.

2333. Bersack SR: Fluid collection in emphysematous bullae. Am J Roentgenol *83*:283, 1960.

2334. Lenk R: Die Röntgendiagnose der 'Pseudoabszesse' der Lunge. (Roentgen diagnosis of pseudo-abscesses of the lung.) Acta Radiol *28*:405, 1947.

2335. Gibson GJ: Familial pneumothoraces and bullae. Thorax *32*:88, 1977.

2336. Stark P, Gadziala N, Green R: Fluid accumulation in preexisting pulmonary air spaces. Am J Roentgenol *134*:701, 1980.

2337. Angstodt JD, Cohn HE, Steiner RM, et al: Unilateral hyperlucent lung due to bullous disease. Chest *90*:437, 1986.

2338. Gaensler EA, Cugell DW, Knudson RJ, et al: Surgical management of emphysema. Clin Chest Med *4*:443, 1983.

2339. Bourgouin P, Cousineau G, Lemire P, et al: Computed tomography used to exclude pneumothorax in bullous lung disease. J Can Assoc Radiol *36*:341, 1985.

2340. Wimpfheimer F, Schneider L: Familial emphysema. Am Rev Respir Dis *83*:697, 1961.

2341. Wood JR, Bellamy D, Child AH, et al: Pulmonary disease in patients with Marfan Syndrome. Thorax *39*:780, 1984.

2342. Ayers JG, Pope FM, Reudy JF, et al: Abnormalities of the lungs and thoracic cage in the Ehlers-Danlos syndrome. Thorax *40*:300, 1985.

2343. Boushy SF, Billig DM, Kohen R: Changes in pulmonary function after bullectomy. Am J Med *47*:916, 1969.

2344. Gelb AF, Gold WM, Nadel JA: Mechanisms limiting airflow in bullous lung disease. Am Rev Respir Dis *107*:571, 1973.

2345. Pride NB, Hugh-Jones P, O'Brien EN, et al: Changes in lung function following the surgical treatment of bullous emphysema. Q J Med *39*:49, 1970.

2346. Foreman S, Weill H, Duke R, et al: Bullous disease of the lung. Physiologic improvement after surgery. Ann Intern Med *69*:757, 1968.

2347. Hirschfeld JH: Bronchography in localized (lobar) bullous emphysema. A report of two cases and discussion of certain bronchographic findings. Am Rev Respir Dis 85:92, 1962.

2348. Pierce JA, Growdon JH: Physical properties of the lungs in giant cysts: Report of a case treated surgically. N Engl J Med 267:169, 1962.

2349. Neidhart P, Suter PM: Pulmonary bullae and sudden death in a young aeroplane passenger. Intensive Care Med 11:45, 1985.

2350. Thomas MP, Storer J, Grierson AC: Bilateral giant pulmonary air cysts. Chest 52:291, 1967.

2351. Swyer PR, James GCW: A case of unilateral pulmonary emphysema. Thorax 8:133, 1953.

2352. MacLeod WM: Abnormal transradiancy of one lung. Thorax 9:147, 1954.

2353. Warrell DA, Hughes JMB, Rosenzweig DY: Cardiopulmonary performance at rest and during exercise in seven patients with increased transradiancy of one lung (Macleod's syndrome). Thorax 25:587, 1970.

2354. Reid L, Simon G: Unilateral lung transradiancy. Thorax 17:230, 1962.

2355. Reid L, Simon G: The role of alveolar hypoplasia in some types of emphysema. Br J Dis Chest 58:158, 1964.

2356. Rakower J, Morgan E: Unilateral hyperlucent lung (Swyer-James syndrome). Am J Med 33:864, 1962.

2357. Fouché RF, Spears JR, Ogilvie C: Unilateral emphysema. Br Med J 1:1312, 1960.

2358. Houk VN, Kent DC, Fosburg RG: Unilateral hyperlucent lung: A study in pathophysiology and etiology. Am J Med Sci 253:406, 1967.

2359. Leahy DJ: Increased transradiancy of one lung. Br J Dis Chest 55:72, 1961.

2360. Peters ME, Dickie HA, Crummy AB, et al: Swyer-James-Macleod syndrome: A case with a baseline normal chest radiograph. Pediatr Radiol 12:211, 1982.

2361. Gold RE, Wilt JC, Adhikari TK, et al: Adenoviral pneumonia and its complications in infancy and childhood. J Can Assoc Radiol 20:218, 1969.

2362. Culiner MM: The hyperlucent lung, a problem in differential diagnosis. Dis Chest 49:578, 1966.

2363. Margolin HN, Rosenberg LS, Felson B, et al: Idiopathic unilateral hyperlucent lung: A roentgenographic syndrome. Am J Roentgenol 82:63, 1959.

2364. McKenzie SA, Allison DJ, Singh MP, et al: Unilateral hyperlucent lung: The case for investigation. Thorax 35:745, 1980.

2365. O'Dell CW Jr, Taylor A, Higgins CB, et al: Ventilation-perfusion lung images in the Swyer-James syndrome. Radiology 121:423, 1976.

2366. Daniel TL, Woodring JH, Vandiviere HM, et al: Swyer-James syndrome—unilateral hyperlucent lung syndrome. A case report and review. Clin Geriatr 23:393, 1984.

2367. Gottlieb LS, Turner AF: Swyer-James (MacLeod's) syndrome—variations in pulmonary-bronchial arterial blood flow. Chest 69:62, 1976.

2368. Hekali P, Halttunen P, Korhola O, et al: Chronic unilateral hyperlucent lung. A consecutive series of 40 patients. Fortschr Rontgenstr 136:41, 1982.

2369. Prowse OM, Fuchs JE, Kaufman SA, et al: Chronic obstructive pseudoemphysema. A rare cause of unilateral hyperlucent lung. N Engl J Med 271:127, 1964.

2370. Nairn JR, Prime FJ: A physiological study of Macleod's syndrome. Thorax 22:148, 1967.

2371. Dornhorst AC, Heaf PJ, Semple SJG: Unilateral "emphysema." Lancet 2:873, 1957.

2372. Bates DV, Macklem PT, Christie RV: Respiratory Function in Disease: An Introduction to the Integrated Study of the Lung, 2nd ed. Philadelphia, WB Saunders Co, 1971.

2373. Llamas R, Schwartz A, Gupta SK, et al: Unilateral hyperlucent lung with polycythemia and cor pulmonale. Chest 59:690, 1971.

2374. Mont JL, Botey A, Subias R, et al: Unilateral pulmonary hemorrhage in a patient with Goodpasture's and Swyer-James' syndrome. Eur J Respir Dis 67:145, 1985.

2375. Glauser EM, Cook CD, Harris GBC: Bronchiectasis: A review of 187 cases in children with follow-up pulmonary function studies in 58. Acta Paediatr Scand 165(Suppl):1, 1966.

2376. Sanderson JM, Kennedy MCS, Johnson MF, et al: Bronchiectasis: Results of surgical and conservative management (a review of 393 cases). Thorax 29:407, 1974.

2377. Barker AF, Bardana EJ: Bronchiectasis: Update of an orphan disease. Am Rev Respir Dis 137:969, 1988.

2378. Croxatto OC, Lanari A: Pathogenesis of bronchiectasis. Experimental study and anatomic findings. J Thorac Surg 27:51, 1954.

2379. Cole PJ: Inflammation: A two-edged sword—the model of bronchiectasis. Eur J Respir Dis 69(Suppl 147):6, 1986.

2380. Hoeffler HB, Schweppe HI, Greenberg SD: Bronchiectasis following pulmonary ammonia burn. Arch Pathol Lab Med 106:686, 1982.

2381. Landau LI, Phelan PD, Williams HE: Ventilatory mechanics in patients with bronchiectasis starting in childhood. Thorax 29:304, 1974.

2382. Banner AS, Muthuswamy P, Shah RS, et al: Bronchiectasis following heroin-induced pulmonary edema—rapid clearing of pulmonary infiltrates. Chest 69:552, 1976.

2383. Steinberg I, Lyons HA: Ipsilateral hypoplasia of a pulmonary artery in advanced bronchiectasis. Am J Roentgenol 101:939, 1967.

2384. Reid L: Reduction in bronchial subdivision in bronchiectasis. Thorax 5:233, 1950.

2385. Whitwell F: A study of the pathology and pathogenesis of bronchiectasis. Thorax 7:213, 1952.

2386. Cudkowicz L: Bronchiectasis and Bronchial Artery Circulation. In Moser KM (ed): Pulmonary Vascular Diseases. (Lung Biology in Health and Disease Series, Vol 14.) New York, Marcel Dekker, 1979, p 165.

2387. Clark NS: Bronchiectasis in childhood. Br Med J 1:80, 1963.

2388. Hessén I: Bronchiectasis of the apical segment of the lower lobe. Acta Radiol 48:7, 1957.

2389. Gudbjerg CE: Bronchiectasis; radiological diagnosis and prognosis after operative treatment. Acta Radiol (Suppl):143, 1957.

2390. Gudbjerg CE: Roentgenologic diagnosis of bronchiectasis. An analysis of 112 cases. Acta Radiol 43:209, 1955.

2391. Bateson EM, Woo-Ming M: Destroyed lung. A report of cases in West Indians and Australian aborigines. Clin Radiol 27:223, 1976.

2392. Müller NL, Bergin CJ, Ostrow DN, et al: Role of computed tomography in the recognition of bronchiectasis. AJR 143:971, 1984.

2393. Grenier P, Maurice F, Musset D, et al: Bronchiectasis: Assessment by thin-section CT. Radiology 161:95, 1986.

2394. Joharjy IA, Bashi SA, Adbullah AK: Value of medium-thickness CT in the diagnosis of bronchiectasis. AJR 149:1133, 1987.

2395. Pontius JR, Jacobs LG: The reversal of advanced bronchiectasis. Radiology 68:204, 1957.

2396. Nelson SW, Christoforidis A: Reversible bronchiectasis. Radiology 71:375, 1958.

2397. Brogan TD, Davies BH, Ryley HC, et al: Composition of bronchopulmonary secretions from patients with bronchiectasis. Thorax 35:624, 1980.

2398. Caughey JE, Wilson RF, Borrie J: Peripheral neuropathy (peripheral neuritis) with bronchiectasis. Thorax 13:59, 1958.

2399. Hilton AM, Hasleton PS, Bradlow A, et al: Cutaneous vasculitis and immune complexes in severe bronchiectasis. Thorax 39:185, 1984.

2400. Moore JR, Kobernick SD, Wiglesworth FW: Bronchiectasis: A study of the segmental distribution of the pathologic lesions. Surg Gynecol Obstet 89:145, 1949.

2401. Cherniack N, Vosti KL, Saxton GA, et al: Pulmonary function tests in fifty patients with bronchiectasis. J Lab Clin Med 53:693, 1959.

2402. Bahous J, Cartier A, Pineau L, et al: Pulmonary function tests and airway responsiveness to methacholine in chronic bronchiectasis of the adult. Bull Eur Physiopathol Respir 20:375, 1984.

2403. Currie DC, Pavia D, Agnew JE, et al: Impaired tracheobronchial clearance in bronchiectasis. Thorax 42:126, 1987.

2404. Lourenço RV, Loddenkemper R, Carton RW: Patterns of distribution and clearance of aerosols in patients with bronchiectasis. Am Rev Respir Dis 106:857, 1972.

2405. Helm WH, Thompson VC: The long-term results of resection for bronchiectasis. Q J Med 27:353, 1958.

2406. Chesterman JT: Recurrence after resection for bronchiectasis. Br J Surg 45:155, 1957.

2407. Avery ME, Riley MC, Weiss A: The course of bronchiectasis in childhood. Bull Hopkins Hosp 109:20, 1961.

2408. Perry KMA, King DS: Bronchiectasis—a study of prognosis based on a follow-up of 400 patients. Am Rev Tuberc 41:531, 1940.

2409. Konietzko NFJ, Carton RW, Leroy EP: Causes of death in patients with bronchiectasis. Am Rev Respir Dis 100:852, 1969.

2410. Sanderson JM, Kennedy MCS, Johnson MF, et al: Bronchiectasis: Results of surgical and conservative management; a review of 393 cases. Thorax 29:407, 1974.

2411. Ellis DA, Thornley PE, Wightman AJ, et al: Present outlook in bronchiectasis: Clinical and social study and review of factors influencing prognosis. Thorax 31:659, 1981.

2412. Kartagener M: Zur Pathogenese der bronchiektasien; bronchiektasien bei situs viscerum inversus. Beitr Klin Tuberk 83:489, 1933.

2413. Solomon MH, Winn KJ, White RD, et al: Kartagener's syndrome with corrected transposition—conducting system studies and coronary arterial occlusion complicating valvular replacement. Chest 69:677, 1976.

2414. Holmes LB, Blennerhassett JB, Austen KF: A reappraisal of Kartagener's syndrome. Am J Med Sci 255:13, 1968.

2415. Todd NW Jr, Yodaiken RE: A patient with Kartagener and Paterson-Brown-Kelly syndromes. JAMA 234:1248, 1975.

2416. Overholt EL, Bauman DF: Variants of Kartagener's syndrome in the same family. Ann Intern Med 48:574, 1958.

2417. Camner P, Mossberg B, Afzelius BA: Evidence for congenitally nonfunctioning cilia in the tracheobronchial tract in two subjects. Am Rev Respir Dis 112:807, 1975.

2418. Afzelius BA: Immotile-cilia syndrome and ciliary abnormalities induced by infection and injury. Am Rev Respir Dis 124:107, 1981.

2419. Pedersen M, Mygind N: Ciliary motility in the "immotile cilia syndrome". First results of microphoto-oscillographic studies. Br J Dis Chest 74:239, 1980.

2420. Rossman CM, Forrest JB, Lee RMKW: The dyskinetic cilia syndrome—abnormal ciliary motility in association with abnormal ciliary ultrastructure. Chest 80:860, 1981.

2421. Pedersen M: Specific types of abnormal ciliary motility in Kartagener's syndrome and analogous respiratory disorders. A quantified microphoto-oscillographic investigation of 27 patients. Eur J Respir Dis 127:78, 1983.

2422. van der Baan S, Veerman AJ, Wulffraat N, et al: Primary ciliary dyskinesia: Ciliary activity. Acta Otolaryngol 102:274, 1986.

2423. Katsuhara K, Kawamoto S, Wakabayashi T, et al: Situs inversus totalis and Kartagener's syndrome in a Japanese population. Chest 61:56, 1972.

2424. Waite D, Wakefield SJ, Steele R, et al: Cilia and sperm tail abnormalities in Polynesian bronchiectatics. Lancet 2:132, 1978.

2425. Wakefield SJ, Waite D: Abnormal cilia in Polynesians with bronchiectasis. Am Rev Respir Dis 121:1003, 1980.

2426. Waite DA, Wakefield SJ, Mackay JB, et al: Mucociliary transport and ultrastructural abnormalities in Polynesian bronchiectasis. Chest 80:896, 1981.

2427. Fox B, Bull T: Abnormal cilia in Polynesians with bronchiectasis. (Letter to Editor) Am Rev Respir Dis 123:142, 1981.

2428. Clarke SW, Lopez-Vidriero MT, Pavia D, et al: Abnormal cilia in Polynesians with bronchiectasis (Letter to Editor) Am Rev Respir Dis 123:141, 1981.

2429. Waite DA, Wakefield SJ, Moriarty KM, et al: Polynesian bronchiectasis. Eur J Respir Dis 127:31, 1983.

2430. Moreno A, Murphy EA: Inheritance of Kartagener syndrome. Am J Hum Genet 8:305, 1981

2431. Rott HD: Genetics of Kartagener's syndrome. Eur J Respir Dis 127:1, 1983.

2432. Chao J, Turner JA, Sturgess JM, et al: Genetic heterogeneity of dynein-deficiency in cilia from patients with respiratory disease. Am Rev Respir Dis 126:302, 1982.

2433. Jonsson MS, McCormick JR, Gillies CG, et al: Kartagener's syndrome with motile spermatozoa. N Engl J Med 307:1131, 1982.

2434. Matwijiw I, Thliveris JA, Faiman C: Aplasia of nasal cilia with situs inversus, azoospermia and normal sperm flagella: A unique variant of the immotile cilia syndrome. J Urol 137:522, 1987.

2435. Moryan A, Guay AT, Kurtz S, et al: Familial ciliary dyskinesis: A cause of infertility without respiratory disease. Fertil Steril 44:539, 1985.

2436. Ras GJ, Van Wyk CJ: Primary ciliary dyskinesia in association with Marfan's syndrome. A case report. S Afr Med J 61:212, 1983.

2437. Sturgess JM, Chao J, Wong J, et al: Cilia with defective radial spokes. A cause of human respiratory disease. N Engl J Med 300:53, 1979.

2438. Wilton LJ, Teichtahl H, Temple-Smith PD, et al: Kartagener's syndrome with motile cilia and immotile spermatozoa: Axonemal ultrastructure and function. Am Rev Respir Dis 134:1233, 1986.

2439. Sturgess JM, Chao J, Turner JAP, et al: Transposition of ciliary microtubules. Another cause of impaired ciliary motility. N Engl J Med 303:318, 1980.

2440. Moreau MF, Chretien MF, Dubin J, et al: Transposed ciliary microtubules in Kartagener's syndrome. A case report with electron microscopy of bronchial and nasal brushings. Acta Cytol 29:248, 1985.

2441. Antonelli M, Modesti A, Quattrucci S, et al: Supernumerary microtubules in the cilia of two siblings causing "immotile cilia syndrome." Eur J Respir Dis 64:607, 1983.

2442. Lungarella G, De Santi MM, Palatresi R, et al: Ultrastructural observations on basal apparatus of respiratory cilia in immotile cilia syndrome. Eur J Respir Dis 66:165, 1985.

2443. Afzelius BA, Gargani G, Romano C: Abnormal length of cilia as a possible cause of defective mucociliary clearance. Eur J Respir Dis 66:173, 1985.

2444. Herzon FS, Murphy S: Normal ciliary ultrastructure in children with Kartagener's syndrome. Ann Otol 89:81, 1980.

2445. Greenstone MA, Dewar A, Cole PJ: Ciliary dyskinesia with normal ultrastructure. Thorax 38:875, 1983.

2446. Escudier E, Escalier D, Homasson JP, et al: Unexpectedly normal cilia and spermatozoa in an infertile man with Kartagener's syndrome. Eur J Respir Dis 70:180, 1987.

2447. Gonzalez S, von Bassewitz DB, Grundmann E, et al: Atypical cilia in hyperplastic, metaplastic, and dysplastic human bronchial mucosa. Ultrastr Pathol 8:345, 1985.

2448. Fox B, Bull TB, Makey AR, et al: The significance of ultrastructural abnormalities of the human cilia. Chest 80:796, 1981.

2449. Lee RMKW, Rossman CM, O'Brodovich H, et al: Ciliary defects associated with the development of bronchopulmonary dysplasia—ciliary motility and ultrastructure. Am Rev Respir Dis 129:190, 1984.

2450. Rossman CM, Lee RMKW, Forrest JB, et al: Nasal ciliary ultrastructure and function in patients with primary ciliary dyskinesia compared with that in normal subjects and in subjects with various respiratory diseases. Am Rev Respir Dis 129:161, 1984.

2451. Englander LL, Malech HL: Abnormal movement of polymorphonuclear neutrophils in the immotile cilia syndrome. Cinemicrographic analysis. Exp Cell Res 135:468, 1981.

2452. Valerius NH, Knudsen BB, Pedersen M, et al: Defective neutrophil motility in patients with primary ciliary dyskinesia. Eur J Clin Invest 13:489, 1983.

2453. Afzelius BA, Ewetz L, Palmblad J, et al: Structure and function of neutrophil leukocytes from patients with the immotile-cilia syndrome. Acta Med Scand 208:145, 1980.

2454. Nadel HR, Stringer DA, Levison H, et al: The immotile cilia syndrome: Radiological manifestations. Radiology 154:651, 1985.

2455. Turner JAP, Corkey CW, Lee JY, et al: Clinical expressions of immotile cilia syndrome. Pediatrics 67:805, 1981.

2456. Kollberg H, Mossberg B, Afzelius BA, et al: Cystic fibrosis compared with the immotile-cilia syndrome. A study of mucociliary clearance, ciliary ultrastructure, clinical picture and ventilatory function. Scand J Respir Dis 59:297, 1978.

2457. Camner P, Mossberg B, Afzelius BA, et al: Measurements of tracheobronchial clearance in patients with immotile-cilia syndrome and its value in differential diagnosis. Eur J Respir Dis 127:57, 1983.

2458. Evander E, Arborelius M Jr, Johnson B, et al: Lung function and bronchial reactivity in six patients with immotile cilia syndrome. Eur J Respir Dis 127:137, 1983.

2459. Corkey CW, Levison H, Turner JA, et al: The immotile cilia syndrome. A longitudinal study. Am Rev Respir Dis 124:544, 1981.

2460. Handelsman DJ, Conway AJ, Boylan LM, et al: Young's syndrome. Obstructive azoospermia and chronic sinopulmonary infections. N Engl J Med 310:3, 1984.

2461. Schanker HM, Rajfer J, Saxon A: Recurrent respiratory disease, azoospermia, and nasal polyposis. A syndrome that mimics cystic fibrosis and immotile cilia syndrome. Arch Intern Med 145:2201, 1985.

2462. Hughes TM, Skolnick JL, Belker AM: Young's syndrome: An often unrecognized correctable cause of obstructive azoospermia. J Urol 137:1238, 1987.

2463. Pavia D, Agnew JE, Bateman JRM, et al: Lung mucociliary clearance in patients with Young's syndrome. Chest 80:892, 1981.

2464. Jequier AM: Obstructive azoospermia: A study of 102 patients. Clin Reprod Fertil 3:21, 1985.

2465. Davis PB, Hubbard VS, Garvin AJ: Bronchiectasis and oligospermia: Two families. Thorax 40:376, 1985.

2466. Samman PD, White WF: The "yellow nail" syndrome. Br J Dermatol 76:153, 1964.

2467. Emerson PA: Yellow nails, lymphedema, and pleural effusion. Thorax 21:247, 1966.

2468. Nordkild P, Kormann-Andersen H, Struve-Christensen E: Yellow nail syndrome: the triad of yellow nails, lymphedema and pleural effusions. Acta Med Scand 219:221, 1986.

2469. Yellow nails (editorial). Lancet 1:1492, 1973.

2470. Leading article: Yellow nails and oedema. Br Med J 4:130, 1972.

2471. Bowers D: Unequal breasts, yellow nails, bronchiectasis and lymphedema. Can Med Assoc J 100:437, 1969.

2472. Hassard AD, Martin J, Ross J: Yellow nail syndrome and chronic sinusitus. J Otolaryngol 13:318, 1984.

2473. Solal-Celigny P, Cormier Y, Fournier M: The yellow nail syndrome—light and electron microscopic aspects of the pleura. Arch Pathol Lab Med 107:183, 1983.

2474. Hiller E, Rosenow EC III, Olsen AM: Pulmonary manifestations of the yellow nail syndrome. Chest 61:452, 1972.

2475. Battaglia A, Di Ricco G, Mariani G, et al: Pleural effusion and recurrent broncho-pneumonia with lymphedema, yellow nails and protein-losing enteropathy. Eur J Respir Dis 66:65, 1985.

2476. Knuckles MLF, Hodge SJ, Roy TM, et al: Yellow nail syndrome in association with sleep apnea. Int. J Dermatol 25:588, 1986.

2477. Dilley JJ, Kierland RR, Randall RV, et al: Primary lymphedema associated with yellow nails and pleural effusions. JAMA 204:670, 1968.

2478. McNicholas WT, Quigley C, Fitzgerald MX: Upper lobe bronchiectasis in the yellow nail syndrome: Report of a case. Ir J Med Sci 153:394, 1984.

2479. di Sant'Agnese PA, Darling RC, Perera GA, et al: Abnormal electrolyte composition of sweat in cystic fibrosis of the pancreas. Clinical significance and relationship to the disease. Pediatrics 12:549, 1953.

11

2480. Wood RE, Boat TF, Doershuk CF: Cystic fibrosis. Am Rev Respir Dis 113:833, 1976.

2481. Addington WW, Cugell DW, Zelkowitz PS, et al: Cystic fibrosis of the pancreas—a comparison of the pulmonary manifestations in children and young adults. Chest 59:306, 1971.

2482. Danes BS, Bearn AG: A genetic cell marker in cystic fibrosis of the pancreas. Lancet 1:1061, 1968.

2483. di Sant'Agnese PA, Talamo RC: Pathogenesis and physiopathology of cystic fibrosis of the pancreas (concluded). N Engl J Med 277:1399, 1967.

2484. di Sant'Agnese PA, Talamo RC: Pathogenesis and physiopathology of cystic fibrosis of the pancreas (continued.) N Engl J Med 277:1344, 1967.

2485. di Sant'Agnese PA, Talamo RC: Pathogenesis and physiopathology of cystic fibrosis of the pancreas. Fibrocystic disease of the pancreas (mucoviscidosis). N Engl J Med 277:1287, 1967.

2486. Rosenstein BJ, Langbaum TS, Metz SJ, et al: Cystic fibrosis: Diagnostic considerations. Johns Hopkins Med J 150:113, 1982.

2487. Nice CM Jr: Exocrine gland dysfunction (mucoviscidosis) in adults. Radiology 81:828, 1963.

2488. Coates EO Jr: Characteristics of cystic fibrosis in adults. A report of seven patients. Dis Chest 49:195, 1966.

2489. Ball RE Jr, Ellis CA Jr, Jones HL Jr: Mucoviscidosis in young adults. Report of a case in a twenty-year-old female. N Engl J Med 265:31, 1961.

2490. Cece JD, Henry JP, Toigo A: Pancreatic cystic fibrosis in an adult. JAMA 181:31, 1962.

2491. Hunt B, Geddes DM: Newly diagnosed cystic fibrosis in middle and later life. Thorax 40:23, 1985.

2492. Fitzpatrick SB, Rosenstein BJ, Langbaum TS, et al: Diagnosis of cystic fibrosis during adolescence. J Adolesc Health Care 7:38, 1986.

2493. di Sant'Agnese PA, Davis PB: Research in cystic fibrosis (first of three parts). N Engl J Med 295:481, 1976.

2494. Danks DM, Allan J, Phelan PD, et al: Mutations at more than one locus may be involved in cystic fibrosis—evidence based on first-cousin and direct counting of cases. Am J Hum Genet 35:838, 1983.

2495. Bowman BH, Mangos JA: Current concepts in genetics: Cystic fibrosis. N Engl J Med 294:937, 1976.

2496. Polymenidis Z, Ludwig H, Gotz M: Cystic fibrosis and HL-A antigens. Lancet 2:1452, 1973.

2497. Hodson ME: Genetic heterogeneity in cystic fibrosis. Br J Dis Chest 72:260, 1978.

2498. Rosenstein BJ, Levine J, Langbaum TS, et al: Cystic fibrosis in adults: Delayed diagnosis in three siblings. South Med J 79:319, 1986.

2499. Qureshi AR, Punnett HH: Carrier detection in cystic fibrosis. J Pediatr 106:913, 1985.

2500. Ceder O, Hosli P, Vogt E, et al: Diagnosis of cystic fibrosis homozygotes and heterozygotes from plasma and fibroblast cultures. A three-generation family study. Clin Genet 23:298, 1983.

2501. Theile H, Gressmann HW, Winiecki P, et al: Detection of cystic fibrosis heterozygotes using a modified loading with bromide. Hum Genet 69:277, 1985.

2502. Brock D, Bedgood D, Barron L, et al: Prospective prenatal diagnosis of cystic fibrosis. Lancet 1(8439):1175, 1985.

2503. Nadler HL, Mesirow K, Rembelski P, et al: Prenatal detection of cystic fibrosis. Prog Clin Biol Res 103:533, 1982.

2504. di Sant'Agnese PA, Davis PB: Research in cystic fibrosis (third of three parts). N Engl J Med 295:597, 1976.

2505. Kuzemko JA: Evolution of lung disease in cystic fibrosis. Lancet 1:448, 1983.

2506. Sahu S, Lynn WS: Lipid composition of airway secretions from patients with asthma and patients with cystic fibrosis. Am Rev Respir Dis 115:233, 1977.

2507. Wood RE, Wanner A, Hirsch J, et al: Tracheal mucociliary transport in patients with cystic fibrosis and its stimulation by terbutaline. Am Rev Respir Dis 111:733, 1975.

2508. Yeates DB, Sturgess JM, Kahn SR, et al: Mucociliary transport in trachea of patients with cystic fibrosis. Arch Dis Child 51:28, 1976.

2509. King M: Is cystic fibrosis mucus abnormal? Pediatr Res 15:120, 1981.

2510. Puchelle E, Jacquot J, Beck G, et al: Rheological and transport properties of airway secretions in cystic fibrosis—relationships with the degree of infection and severity of the disease. Eur J Clin Invest 15:389, 1985.

2511. Speck A, Heick HM, Cress H, et al: Abnormal serum factor in patients with cystic fibrosis of the pancreas. Pediatr Res 1:173, 1967.

2512. Rutland J, Penketh A, Griffin WM, et al: Cystic fibrosis serum does not inhibit human ciliary beat frequency. Am Rev Respir Dis 128:1030, 1983.

2513. Wanner A: Clinical aspects of mucociliary transport. Am Rev Respir Dis 116:73, 1977.

2514. Conover JH, Conod EJ, Hirschhorn K: Complement components in cystic fibrosis. Lancet 2:1501, 1973.

2515. Lieberman J: Carboxypeptidase B-like activity and C3 in cystic fibrosis. Am Rev Respir Dis 111:100, 1975.

2516. Wilson GB, Fudenberg HH, Parise MT, et al: Cystic fibrosis ciliary dyskinesia substances and pulmonary disease. Effects of ciliary dyskinesia substances on neutrophil movement in vitro. J Clin Invest 68:171, 1981.

2517. Danes BS: Association of cystic-fibrosis factor to metachromasia of the cultured cystic fibrosis fibroblast. Lancet 2:765, 1973.

2518. Wilson GB, Monsher MT, Fudenberg HH: Studies on cystic fibrosis using isoelectric focusing. III. Correlation between cystic fibrosis protein and ciliary dyskinesia activity in serum shown by a modified rabbit tracheal bioassay. Pediatr Res 11:143, 1977.

2519. Nagy E, Khan S, Sturgess JM: Serum factor in cystic fibrosis: Correlation with clinical parameters. Pediatr Res 13:729, 1979.

2520. Smallman LA, Hill SL, Stockley RA: Reduction of ciliary beat frequency in vitro by sputum from patients with bronchiectasis: A serine proteinase effect. Thorax 39:663, 1984.

2521. Stockley RA, Hill SL, Morrison HM, et al: Elastolytic activity of sputum and its relation to purulence and lung function in patients with bronchiectasis. Thorax 39:408, 1984.

2522. Rutland J, Cole PJ: Nasal mucociliary clearance and ciliary beat frequency in cystic fibrosis compared with sinusitis and bronchiectasis. Thorax 36:654, 1981.

2523. Katz SM, Holsclaw DS Jr: Ultrastructural features of respiratory cilia in cystic fibrosis. Am J Clin Pathol 73:682, 1980.

2524. Katz SM, Holsclaw DS Jr: Ultrastructural features of respiratory cilia in cystic fibrosis. Am J Clin Pathol 73:682, 1980.

2525. Cromwell O, Walport MJ, Morris HR, et al: Identification of leukotrienes D and B in sputum from cystic fibrosis patients. Lancet 2:164, 1981.

2526. Davis PB, Shelhamer JR, Kaliner M: Abnormal adrenergic and cholinergic sensitivity in cystic fibrosis. N Engl J Med 302:1453, 1980.

2527. Davis PB: Physiologic implications of the autonomic aberrations in cystic fibrosis. Horm Metab Res 18:217, 1986.

2528. Davis PB, Dieckman L, Boat TF, et al: Beta adrenergic receptors in lymphocytes and granulocytes from patients with cystic fibrosis. J Clin Invest 71:1787, 1983.

2529. Sato K, Sato F: Defective beta adrenergic response of cystic fibrosis sweat glands in vivo and in vitro. J Clin Invest 73:1763, 1984.

2530. McPherson MA, Dormer RL, Dodge JA, et al: Adrenergic secretory response of submandibular tissues from control subjects and cystic fibrosis patients. Clin Chim Acta 148:229, 1985.

2531. McPherson MA, Dormer RL, Bradbury NA, et al: Defective beta-adrenergic secretory responses in submandibular acinar cells from cystic fibrosis patients. Lancet 2:1007, 1986.

2532. Wiesmann UN, Boat TF, di Sant'Agnese PA: Flow-rates and electrolytes in minor-salivary-gland saliva in normal subjects and patients with cystic fibrosis. Lancet 2:510, 1972.

2533. Warton KL, Blomfield J: Hydroxyapatite in the pathogenesis of cystic fibrosis. Br Med J 3:570, 1971.

2534. Mangos JA, McSherry NR, Benke PJ: A sodium transport inhibitory factor in the saliva of patients with cystic fibrosis of the pancreas. Pediatr Res 1:436, 1967.

2535. Mangos JA, McSherry NR: Sodium transport: Inhibitory factor in sweat of patients with cystic fibrosis. Science 158:135, 1967.

2536. Knowles M, Gatzy J, Boucher R, et al: Increased bioelectric potential difference across respiratory epithelia in cystic fibrosis. N Engl J Med 305:1489, 1981.

2537. Hay JB, Geddes DM: Transepithelial potential difference in cystic fibrosis. Thorax 40:493, 1985.

2538. Yankaskas JR, Cotton CU, Knowles MR, et al: Culture of human nasal epithelial cells on collagen matrix supports. A comparison of bioelectric properties of normal and cystic fibrosis epithelia. Am Rev Respir Dis 132:1281, 1985.

2539. Boucher RC, Stutts MJ, Knowles MR, et al: Na+ transport in cystic fibrosis respiratory epithelia. Abnormal basal rate and response to adenylate cyclase activation. J Clin Invest 78:1245, 1986.

2540. Anderson CM: Hypothesis revisited: Cystic fibrosis: a disturbance of water and electrolyte movement in exocrine secretory tissue associated with altered prostaglandin (PGE2) metabolism? J Pediatr Gastroenterol 3:15, 1984.

2541. Thomassen MJ, Demko CA, Klinger JD, et al: Pseudomonas cepacia colonization among patients with cystic fibrosis. A new opportunist. Am Rev Respir Dis 131:791, 1985.

2542. Klinger JD, Thomassen MJ: Occurrence and antimicrobial susceptibility of gram-negative nonfermentative bacilli in cystic fibrosis patients. Diagn Microbiol Infect Dis 3:149, 1985.

2543. Bruns WT, Brown BA: L forms in patients with cystic fibrosis. Am Rev Respir Dis 101:935, 1970.

2544. Matthews WJ Jr, Williams M, Oliphint B, et al: Hypogammaglobulinemia in patients with cystic fibrosis. N Engl J Med 302:245, 1980.

2545. Mearns M, Longbottom J, Batten J: Precipitating antibodies to *Aspergillus fumigatus* in cystic fibrosis. Lancet *1*:538, 1967.

2546. Wilson GB, Fudenberg HH: Does a primary host defence abnormality involving monocytes-macrophages underlie the pathogenesis of lung disease in cystic fibrosis? Med Hypotheses *8*:527, 1982.

2547. Ravia Y, Avivi L, Goldman B, et al: Differences between cystic fibrosis and normal cells in the degree of satellite association. Hum Genet *71*:294, 1985.

2548. Shryock TR, Mollé JS, Klinger JD, et al: Association with phagocytic inhibition G antibody subclass levels in serum from patients with cystic fibrosis. J Clin Microbiol *23*:513, 1986.

2549. Fick RB Jr, Olchowski J, Squier SU, et al: Immunoglobulin-G subclasses in cystic fibrosis. IgG2 response to *Pseudomonas aeruginosa* lipopolysaccaride. Am Rev Respir Dis *133*:418, 1986.

2550. Moss RB, Hsu YP, Sullivan MM, et al: Altered antibody isotype in cystic fibrosis: Possible role in opsonic deficiency. Pediatr Res *20*:453, 1986.

2551. May JR, Roberts DE: Bronchial infection in cystic fibrosis. Lancet *1*:602, 1969.

2552. Hodson ME, Beldon I, Batten JC, et al: Circulating immune complexes in patients with cystic fibrosis in relation to clinical features. Clin Allergy *15*:363, 1985.

2553. Disis ML, McDonald TL, Colombo JL, et al: Circulating immune complexes in cystic fibrosis and their correlation to clinical parameters. Pediatr Res *20*:385, 1986.

2554. Wisnieski JJ, Todd EW, Fuller RK, et al: Immune complexes and complement abnormalities in patients with cystic fibrosis. Increased mortality associated with circulating immune complexes and decreased function of the alternative complement pathway. Am Rev Respir Dis *132*:770, 1985.

2555. Moss RB, Hsu YP, Lewiston NJ, et al: Association of systemic immune complexes, complement activation, and antibodies to *Pseudomonas aeruginosa* lipopolysaccharide and exotoxin A with mortality in cystic fibrosis. Am Rev Respir Dis *133*:648, 1986.

2556. Rush PJ, Shore A, Coblentz C, et al: The musculoskeletal manifestations of cystic fibrosis. Semin Arthritis Rheum *15*:213, 1986.

2557. Wönne R, Hoffmann D, Posselt HG, et al: Bronchial allergy in cystic fibrosis. Clin Allergy *15*:455, 1985.

2558. Tobin MJ, Maguire O, Reen D, et al: Atopy and bronchial reactivity in older patients with cystic fibrosis. Thorax *35*:807, 1980.

2559. Laufer P, Fink JN, Bruns WT, et al: Allergic bronchopulmonary aspergillosis in cystic fibrosis. J Allerg Clin Immunol *73*:44, 1984.

2560. McFarlane H, Holzel A, Brenchley P, et al: Immune complexes in cystic fibrosis. Br Med J *1*:423, 1975.

2561. Wilmott RW, Tyson SL, Matthew DJ, et al: Cystic fibrosis survival rates. The influences of allergy and *Pseudomonas aeruginosa*. Am J Dis Child *139*:669, 1985.

2562. Pitcher-Wilmott RW, Levinsky RJ, Gordon I, et al: *Pseudomonas* infection, allergy, and cystic fibrosis. Arch Dis Child *57*:582, 1982.

2563. Galant SP, Rucker RW, Groncy CE, et al: Incidence of serum antibodies to several *Aspergillus* species and to *Candida albicans* in cystic fibrosis. Am Rev Respir Dis *114*:325, 1976.

2564. Murphy MB, Reen DJ, Fitzgerald MX: Atopy, immunological changes and respiratory function in bronchiectasis. Thorax *39*:179, 1984.

2565. Brock DJ, Hayward C, Super M: Controlled trial of serum isoelectric focusing in the detection of the cystic fibrosis gene. Hum Genet *60*:30, 1982.

2566. Heeley AF, Watson D: Cystic fibrosis—its biochemical detection. Clin Chem *29*:2011, 1983.

2567. Dorin JRM, Novak RE, Hill DJH, et al: A clue to the basic defect in cystic fibrosis from cloning the CF antigen gene. Nature *326*:614, 1987.

2568. Kraemer R: Onset of pulmonary involvement in cystic fibrosis. Eur J Pediatr *139*:239, 1982.

2569. Chow CW, Landau LI, Taussig LM, et al: Bronchial mucous glands in the newborn with cystic fibrosis. Eur J Paediatr *139*:240, 1982.

2570. Bhagavan BS, Rao DRG, Weinberg T: Histoplasmosis producing broncholithiasis. Arch Pathol *91*:577, 1971.

2571. Guidotti TL, Line BR, Leutzeler J, et al: Cystic fibrosis related lung disease in young adults with minimal impairment. Respiration *44*:351, 1983.

2572. Vawter GF, Shwachman H: Cystic fibrosis in adults. An autopsy study. *In* Sommers SC, Rosen PP (eds): Pathology Annual, Part 2, Vol 14. New York, Appleton-Century-Crofts, 1979, p 357.

2573. Tomashefski JF Jr, Bruce M, Stern RC, et al: Pulmonary air cysts in cystic fibrosis: Relation of pathologic features to radiologic findings and history of pneumothorax. Hum Pathol *16*:253, 1985.

2574. Wentworth P, Gough J, Wentworth JE: Pulmonary changes and cor pulmonale in mucoviscidosis. Thorax *23*:582, 1968.

2575. Esterly JR, Oppenheimer EH: Cystic fibrosis of the pancreas: Structural changes in peripheral airways. Thorax *23*:670, 1968.

2576. Polgar G, Denton R: Cystic fibrosis in adults. Studies of pulmonary function and some physical properties of bronchial mucus. Am Rev Respir Dis *85*:319, 1962.

2577. Tomashefski JF, Bruce M, Goldberg HI, et al: Regional distribution of macroscopic lung disease in cystic fibrosis. Am Rev Respir Dis *133*:535, 1986.

2578. Sobonya RE, Taussig LM: Quantitative aspects of lung pathology in cystic fibrosis. Am Rev Respir Dis *134*:290, 1986.

2579. Rezek PR, Talbert WM Jr: Kongenitale (familiäre) zystiche Fibrose der Lunge. Beziehungen zur Metaplasie und dem Carcinoma in situ. (Congenital cystic fibrosis of the lung. Relationship to metaplasia and carcinoma in situ.) Wien Klin Wochenschr *74*:869, 1962.

2580. Ryland D, Reid L: The pulmonary circulation in cystic fibrosis. Thorax *30*:285, 1975.

2581. Iacocca VF, Sibinga MS, Barbero GJ: Bacteriological studies in cystic fibrosis of the pancreas. Am J Dis Child *102*:543, 1961.

2582. Huang NN, Van Loon EL, Sheng KT: The flora of the respiratory tract of patients with cystic fibrosis of the pancreas. J Pediatr *59*:512, 1961.

2583. Iacocca VF, Sibinga MS, Barbero GJ: Respiratory tract bacteriology in cystic fibrosis. Am J Dis Child *106*:315, 324, 1963.

2584. Bryan GT, Owen GM, Knight V: Effects of antimicrobial therapy on the bacterial flora of the respiratory tract in cystic fibrosis of the pancreas. Am J Dis Child *102*:539, 1961.

2585. Katznelsen D, Vawter GF, Foley GE, et al: Botryomycosis, a complication of computed tomography and plain chest radiographs. Report of 7 cases. J Pediatr *65*:525, 1964.

2586. Stur O: Lungenveränderungen bei Mucoviscidose. (Pulmonary changes in mucoviscidosis.) Fortschr Roentgenstr *99*:625, 1963.

2587. Reinig JW, Sanchez FW, Thomason DM, et al: The distinctly visible right upper lobe bronchus on the lateral chest: A clue to adolescent cystic fibrosis. Pediatr Radiol *15*:222, 1985.

2588. Hodson CJ, France NE: Pulmonary changes in cystic fibrosis of the pancreas. A radio-pathological study. Clin Radiol *13*:54, 1962.

2589. White H: Fibrocystic disease of the pancreas: Roentgen manifestations. Radiology *71*:816, 1958.

2590. Griscom NT, Vawter GF, Stigol LC: Radiologic and pathologic abnormalities of the trachea in older patients with cystic fibrosis. AJR *148*:691, 1987.

2591. Waring WW, Brunt CH, Hilman BC: Mucoid impaction of the bronchi in cystic fibrosis. Pediatrics *39*:166, 1967.

2592. di Sant'Agnese PA: The pulmonary manifestations of fibrocystic disease of the pancreas. Dis Chest *27*:654, 1955.

2593. Hinshaw HC, Garland LH: Diseases of the Chest, 3rd ed. Philadelphia, WB Saunders Co, 1969.

2594. Schwartz EE, Holsclaw DS: Pulmonary involvement in adults with cystic fibrosis. Am J Roentgenol *122*:708, 1974.

2595. Mearns MB, Simon G: Patterns of lung and heart growth as determined from serial radiographs of 76 children with cystic fibrosis. Thorax *28*:537, 1973.

2596. Fiel SB, Friedman AC, Caroline DF, et al: Magnetic resonance imaging in young adults with cystic fibrosis. Chest *91*:181, 1987.

2597. Jacobsen LE, Houston CS, Habbick BF, et al: Cystic fibrosis: A comparison of computed tomography and plain chest radiographs. J Can Assoc Rad *37*:17, 1986.

2598. Hernanz-Schulman M, Kirkpatrick J Jr, Shwachman H, et al: Pneumatosis intestinalis in cystic fibrosis. Radiology *160*:497, 1986.

2599. Hodson ME, Mearns MB, Batten JC: Meconium ileus equivalent in adults with cystic fibrosis of pancreas: A report of six cases. Br Med J *2*:790, 1976.

2600. Schwachman H: Meconium ileus: Ten patients over 28 years of age. J Pediatr Surg *18*:570, 1983.

2601. Lober CW, Seigler HF, Spock A: Cystic fibrosis in a black woman. JAMA *235*:1140, 1976.

2602. Lees AW, Roberts GBS: Fibrocystic disease of the pancreas presenting as bronchiectasis in an adolescent. Br J Dis Chest *53*:365, 1959.

2603. Gilljam H, Malmborg AS, Strandvik B: Conformity of bacterial growth in sputum and contamination free endobronchial samples in patients with cystic fibrosis. Thorax *41*:641, 1986.

2604. Holsclaw DS, Grand RJ, Shwachman H: Massive hemoptysis in cystic fibrosis. J Pediatr *76*:829, 1970.

2605. Leading Article: Haemoptysis in cystic fibrosis. Br Med J *4*:702, 1970.

2606. Matthay MA, Matthay RA, Mills DM, et al: Hypertrophic osteoarthropathy in adults with cystic fibrosis. Thorax *31*:572, 1976.

2607. Cohen AM, Yulish BS, Wasser KB, et al: Evaluation of pulmonary hypertrophic osteoarthropathy in cystic fibrosis. A comprehensive study. Am J Dis Child *140*:74, 1986.

2608. Lemen RJ, Gates AJ, Mathe AA, et al: Relationships among digital clubbing, disease severity, and serum prostaglandins F2alpha and E concentrations in cystic fibrosis patients. Am Rev Respir Dis *117*:639, 1978.

2609. Boat TF, di Sant'Agnese PA, Warwick WJ, et al: Pneumothorax in cystic fibrosis. JAMA *209*:1498, 1969.

2610. McLaughlin FJ, Matthews WJ, Strieder DJ, et al: Pneumothorax in cystic fibrosis: Management and outcome. J Pediatr *100*:863, 1982.

11

2611. Mitchell-Heggs PF, Batten JC: Pleurectomy for spontaneous pneumothorax in cystic fibrosis. Thorax 25:165, 1970.

2612. Stowe SM, Boat TF, Mendelsohn H, et al: Open thoracotomy for pneumothorax in cystic fibrosis. Am Rev Respir Dis 111:611, 1975.

2613. Geggel RL, Dozor AJ, Fyler DC, et al: Effect of vasodilators at rest and during exercise in young adults with cystic fibrosis and chronic cor pulmonale. Am Rev Respir Dis 131:531, 1985.

2614. Goldring RM, Fishman AP, Turino GM, et al: Pulmonary hypertension and cor pulmonale in cystic fibrosis of the pancreas. J Pediatr 65:501, 1964.

2615. Kaplan E, Shwachman H, Perlmutter AD, et al: Reproductive failure in males with cystic fibrosis. N Engl J Med 279:65, 1968.

2616. Taussig LM, Lobeck CC, di Sant'Agnese PA, et al: Fertility in males with cystic fibrosis. N Engl J Med 287:586, 1972.

2617. Kredentser JV, Pokrant C, McCoshen JA, et al: Intrauterine insemination for infertility due to cystic fibrosis. Fertil Steril 45:425, 1986.

2618. Palmer J, Dillon-Baker C, Tecklin JS, et al: Pregnancy in patients with cystic fibrosis. Ann Intern Med 99:596, 1983.

2619. Seale TW, Flux M, Rennert OM, et al: Reproductive defects in patients of both sexes with cystic fibrosis: A review. Ann Clin Lab Sci 15:152, 1985.

2620. Shepherd RW, Holt TL, Thomas BJ, et al: Nutritional rehabilitation in cystic fibrosis: Controlled studies of effects on nutritional growth retardation, body protein turnover, and course of pulmonary disease. J Pediatr 109:788, 1986.

2621. Holt TL, Ward LC, Francis PJ, et al: Whole body protein turnover in malnourished cystic fibrosis patients and its relationship to pulmonary disease. Am J Clin Nutr 41:1061, 1985.

2622. Masaryk TJ, Achkar E: Pancreatitis as initial presentation of cystic fibrosis in young adults. A report of two cases. Dig Dis Sci 28:874, 1983.

2623. Abdul-Karim FW, Dahms BB, Velasco ME, et al: Islets of Langerhans in adolescents and adults with cystic fibrosis. A quantitative study. Arch Pathol Lab Med 110:602, 1986.

2624. Kulczycki LL, Shwachman H: Studies in cystic fibrosis of the pancreas. Occurrence of rectal prolapse. N Engl J Med 259:409, 1958.

2625. Gross K, Desanto A, Grosfeld JL, et al: J Pediatr Surg 20:431, 1985.

2626. McGlennen RC, Burke BA, Dehner LP: Systemic amyloidosis complicating cystic fibrosis. Arch Pathol Lab Med 110:879, 1986.

2627. Travis WD, Castile R, Vawter G, et al: Secondary (AA) amyloidosis in cystic fibrosis. A report of three cases. Am J Clin Pathol 85:419, 1986.

2628. Castile R, Schwachman H, Travis W, et al: Amyloidosis as a complication of cystic fibrosis. Am J Dis Child 139:728, 1985.

2629. Shwachman H, Gahm N: Studies in cystic fibrosis of the pancreas. A simple test for the detection of excessive chloride on the skin. N Engl J Med 255:999, 1956.

2630. Gibson LE, Cooke RE: A test for concentration of electrolytes in sweat in cystic fibrosis of the pancreas utilizing pilocarpine by iontophoresis. Pediatrics 23:545, 1959.

2631. Jones JD, Steige H, Logan GB: Variations of sweat sodium values in children and adults with cystic fibrosis and other diseases. Mayo Clin Proc 45:768, 1970.

2632. Warwick WJ, Huang NN, Waring WW, et al: Evaluation of a cystic fibrosis screening system incorporating a miniature sweat stimulator and disposable chloride sensor. Clin Chem 32:850, 1986.

2633. Corkey CW, Corey M, Gaskin K, et al: Prognostic value of sweat-chloride levels in cystic fibrosis: A negative report. Eur J Respir Dis 64:434, 1983.

2634. Franck J, Shmerling DH: The use of sweat osmolarity in the diagnosis of cystic fibrosis. Helv Pediatr Acta 39:347, 1984.

2635. Chapman AL, Fegley B, Cho CT, et al: X-ray microanalysis of chloride in nails from cystic fibrosis and control patients. Eur J Respir Dis 66:218, 1985.

2636. Anderson CM, Freeman M, Allan J, et al: Observations on (i) sweat sodium levels in relation to chronic respiratory disease in adults and (ii) the incidence of respiratory and other disease in parents and siblings of patients with fibrocystic disease of the pancreas. Med J Aust 1:965, 1962.

2637. Hallett WY, Knudson AG Jr, Massey FJ Jr: Absence of detrimental effect of the carrier state for the cystic fibrosis gene. Am Rev Respir Dis 92:714, 1965.

2638. Orzalesi MM, Kohner D, Cook CD, et al: Anamnesis, sweat electrolyte and pulmonary function studies in parents of patients with cystic fibrosis of the pancreas. Acta Paediatr 52:267, 1963.

2639. Batten J, Muir D, Simon G, et al: The prevalence of respiratory disease in heterozygotes for the gene for fibrocystic disease of the pancreas. Lancet 1:1348, 1963.

2640. Karlish AJ, Tárnoky AL: Mucoviscidosis and chronic lung disease in adults. Am Rev Respir Dis 88:810, 1963.

2641. Coates EO Jr, Brinkman GL: Sweat chloride in patients with chronic bronchial disease and its relation to mucoviscidosis (cystic fibrosis). Am Rev Respir Dis 87:673, 1963.

2642. Bernard E, Israel L, Debris MM: Chronic bronchitis and mucoviscidosis. Am Rev Respir Dis 85:22, 1962.

2643. Wood JA, Fishman AP, Reemtsma K, et al: A comparison of sweat chlorides and intestinal fat absorption in chronic obstructive pulmonary emphysema and fibrocystic disease of the pancreas. N Engl J Med 260:951, 1959.

2644. Muir D, Batten J, Simon G: Mucoviscidosis and adult chronic bronchitis. Their possible relationship. Lancet 1:181, 1962.

2645. Sekelj P, Belmonte M, Rasmussen K: Survey of electrolytes of unstimulated sweat from the hand in normal and diseased adults. Am Rev Respir Dis 108:603, 1973.

2646. Stephan U, Busch EW, Kollberg H, et al: Cystic fibrosis detection by means of a test-strip. Pediatrics 55:35, 1975.

2647. Weber AM, Roy CC, Morin CL, et al: Malabsorption of bile acids in children with cystic fibrosis. N Engl J Med 289:1001, 1973.

2648. Durie PR, Forstner GG, Gaskin KJ, et al: Age-related alterations of immunoreactive pancreatic cationic trypsinogen in sera from cystic fibrosis patients with and without pancreatic insufficiency. Pediatr Res 20:209, 1986.

2649. Cleghorn G, Benjamin L, Corey M, et al: Serum immunoreactive pancreatic lipase and cationic trypsinogen for the assessment of exocrine pancreatic function in older patients with cystic fibrosis. Pediatrics 77:301, 1986.

2650. Bollbach R, Becker M, Rotthauwe HW, et al: Serum immunoreactive trypsin and pancreatic lipase in cystic fibrosis. Eur J Pediatr 144:167, 1985.

2651. Swobodnik W, Wolf A, Wechsler JG, et al: Ultrasound characteristics of the pancreas in children with cystic fibrosis. JCU 13:469, 1985.

2652. Graham N, Manhire AR, Stead RJ, et al: Cystic fibrosis: ultrasonographic findings in the pancreas and hepatobiliary system correlated with clinical data and pathology. Clin Radiol 36:199, 1985.

2653. Deren JJ, Arora B, Toskes PP, et al: Malabsorption of crystalline vitamin B_{12} in cystic fibrosis. N Engl J Med 288:949, 1973.

2654. Lee PA, Roloff DW, Howatt WF: Hypoproteinemia and anemia in infants with cystic fibrosis—a presenting complex often misdiagnosed. JAMA 228:585, 1974.

2655. Featherby EA, Weng T-R, Crozier DN, et al: Dynamic and static lung volumes, blood gas tensions, and diffusing capacity in patients with cystic fibrosis. Am Rev Respir Dis 102:737, 1970.

2656. Neuburger N, Levison H, Kruger B: Transit time analysis of the forced expiratory vital capacity in cystic fibrosis. Am Rev Respir Dis 114:753, 1976.

2657. Landau LI, Phelan PD: The spectrum of cystic fibrosis. A study of pulmonary mechanics in 46 patients. Am Rev Respir Dis 108:593, 1973.

2658. Harrison GM, Vallbona C, Murray J: Quantitative studies of intrapulmonary gas mixing and distribution in children with cystic fibrosis. Am J Dis Child 100:530, 1960.

2659. DeMuth GR, Howatt W, Talner N: Intrapulmonary gas distribution in cystic fibrosis. Am J Dis Child 100:582, 1960.

2660. DeMuth GR, Howatt WF, Talner NS: Intrapulmonary gas distribution in cystic fibrosis. Am J Dis Child 103:129, 1962.

2661. Beier FR, Renzetti AD Jr, Mitchell M, et al: Pulmonary pathophysiology in cystic fibrosis. Am Rev Respir Dis 94:430, 1966.

2662. Tomashefski JF, Christoforidis AJ, Abdullah AK: Cystic fibrosis in young adults—An overlooked diagnosis with emphasis on pulmonary function and radiological patterns. Chest 57:28, 1970.

2663. Lebecque P, Lapierre JG, Lamarre A, et al: Diffusion capacity and oxygen desaturation effects on exercise in patients with cystic fibrosis. Chest 91:693, 1987.

2664. Chang N, Levison H: The effect of a nebulized bronchodilator administered with or without intermittent positive pressure breathing on ventilatory function in children with cystic fibrosis and asthma. Am Rev Respir Dis 106:867, 1972.

2665. Zach MS, Oberwaldner B, Forche G, et al: Bronchodilators increase airway instability in cystic fibrosis. Am Rev Respir Dis 131:537, 1985.

2666. Larsen GL, Barron RJ, Cotton EK, et al: A comparative study of inhaled atropine sulfate and isoproterenol hydrochloride in cystic fibrosis. Am Rev Respir Dis 119:399, 1979.

2667. Mansell A, Dubrawsky C, Levison H, et al: Lung elastic recoil in cystic fibrosis. Am Rev Respir Dis 109:190, 1974.

2668. Landau LI, Taussig LM, Macklem PT, et al: Contribution of inhomogeneity of lung units to the maximal expiratory flow-volume curve in children with asthma and cystic fibrosis. Am Rev Resp Dis 111:725, 1975.

2669. Dantzker DR, Patten GA, Bower JS: Gas exchange at rest and during exercise in adults with cystic fibrosis. Am Rev Respir Dis 125:400, 1982.

2670. Coates AL, Desmond KJ, Milic-Emili J, et al: Ventilation, respiratory center output, and contribution of the rib cage and abdominal components to ventilation during CO_2 rebreathing in children with cystic fibrosis. Am Rev Respir Dis 124:526, 1981.

2671. Dantzker DR, Patten GA, Bower JS, et al: Gas exchange at rest and during exercise in adults with cystic fibrosis. Am Rev Respir Dis 125:400, 1982.

2672. Muller NL, Francis PW, Gurwitz D, et al: Mechanism of hemoglobin desaturation during rapid-eye-movement sleep in normal subjects and patients with cystic fibrosis. Am Rev Respir Dis 121:463, 1980.

2673. Tepper RS, Skatrud JB, Dempsey JA, et al: Ventilation and oxygenation changes during sleep in cystic fibrosis. Chest 84:388, 1983.

2674. Stokes DC, Wohl ME, Khaw KT, et al: Postural hypoxemia in cystic fibrosis. Chest 87:785, 1985.

2675. Lwin N, Giammona ST: Ventilatory responses to inspired CO_2 in patients with cystic fibrosis. Chest 61:206, 1972.

2676. Szeinberg A, England S, Mindorff C, et al: Maximal inspiratory and expiratory pressures are reduced in hyperinflated, malnourished, young adult male patients with cystic fibrosis. Am Rev Respir Dis 132:766, 1985.

2677. Marks J, Pasterkamp H, Tal A, et al: Relationship between respiratory muscle strength, nutritional status, and lung volume in cystic fibrosis and asthma. Am Rev Respir Dis 133:414, 1986.

2678. O'Neill S, Leahy F, Pasterkamp H, et al: The effects of chronic hyperinflation, nutritional status, and posture on respiratory muscle strength in cystic fibrosis. Am Rev Respir Dis 128:1051, 1983.

2679. Corey M, Levison H, Crozier D: Five-to-seven years course of pulmonary function in cystic fibrosis. Am Rev Respir Dis 114:1085, 1976.

2680. Reilly BJ, Featherby EA, Weng T-R, et al: The correlation of radiological changes with pulmonary function in cystic fibrosis. Radiology 98:281, 1971.

2681. Alderson PO, Secker-Walker RH, Strominger DB, et al: Quantitative assessment of regional ventilation and perfusion in children with cystic fibrosis. Radiology 111:151, 1974.

2682. Wilmott RW, Tyson SL, Dinwiddie R, et al: Survival rates in cystic fibrosis. Arch Dis Child 58:835, 1983.

2683. Berkin KE, Alcock SR, Stack BH, et al: Cystic fibrosis: A review of 26 adolescent and adult patients. Eur J Respir Dis 67:103, 1985.

2684. Brusilow SW: Cystic fibrosis in adults. Annu Rev Med 21:99, 1970.

2685. Shwachman H, Kulczycki LL, Khaw K-T: Studies in cystic fibrosis. A report on sixty-five patients over 17 years of age. Pediatrics 36:689, 1965.

2686. Phelan P, Hey E: Cystic fibrosis mortality in England and Wales and in Victoria, Australia 1976–1980. Arch Dis Child 59:71, 1984.

2687. Wesley AW, Stewart AW: Cystic fibrosis in New Zealand: Incidence and mortality. NZ Med J 98:321, 1985.

2688. Wilcken B, Chalmers G: Reduced morbidity in patients with cystic fibrosis detected by neonatal screening. Lancet 2(8468):1319, 1985.

2689. Doershuk CF, Matthews LW, Tucker AS, et al: Evaluation of a prophylactic and therapeutic program for patients with cystic fibrosis. Pediatrics 36:675, 1965.

2690. Huang NN, Schidlow DV, Szatrowski TH, et al: Clinical features, survival rate, and prognostic factors in young adults with cystic fibrosis. Am J Med 82:871, 1987.

2691. Schwachman H, Kulczycki LL: Long term study of one hundred and five patients with cystic fibrosis. Am J Dis Child 96:6, 1958.

2692. Riley CM, Day RL, Greeley D, et al: Central autonomic dysfunction with defective lacrimation. I. Report of five cases. Pediatrics 3:468, 1949.

2693. Brunt PW, McKusick VA: Familial dysautonomia: A report of genetic and clinical studies, with a review of the literature. Medicine 49:343, 1970.

2694. Weinshilboum RM, Axelrod J: Reduced plasma dopamine-β-hydroxylase activity in familial dysautonomia. N Engl J Med 285:938, 1971.

2695. Siggers DC, Rogers JG, Boyer SH, et al: Increased nerve-growth-factor β-chain cross reacting material in familial dysautonomia. N Engl J Med 295:629, 1976.

2696. Levi-Montalcini R: Nerve-growth factor in familial dysautonomia. N Engl J Med 295:671, 1976.

2697. Kirkpatrick RH, Riley CM: Roentgenographic findings in familial dysautonomia. Radiology 68:654, 1957.

2698. Moloshok RE, Moseley JE: Familial dysautonomia: Pulmonary manifestations. Pediatrics 17:327, 1956.

2699. Bartels J, Mazzia VDB: Familial dysautonomia. JAMA 212:318, 1970.

2700. Eisele JH, Cross CE, Rausch DC, et al: Abnormal respiratory control in acquired dysautonomia. N Engl J Med 285:366, 1971.

2701. Riley CM, Moore RH: Familial dysautonomia differentiated from related disorders. Case reports and discussions of current concepts. Pediatrics 37:435, 1966.

2702. Moersch HJ, Schmidt HW: Broncholithiasis. Ann Otol 68:548, 1959.

2703. Gordonson J, Sargent EN: Nephrobroncholithiasis: Report of a case secondary to renal lithiasis with a nephrobronchial fistula. Am J Roentgenol 110:701, 1970.

2704. Hotchi M, Schwarz J: Etiology of pigmented scars in the bronchial mucosa. Am J Clin Pathol 58:654, 1972.

2705. Unfug HV: Vocal-cord paralysis from calcified hilar lymph node cured by spontaneous broncholithoptysis. N Engl J Med 272:527, 1965.

2706. Gosink BB, Friedman PJ, Liebow AA: Bronchiolitis obliterans: Roentgenologic-pathologic correlation. Am J Roentgenol 117:816, 1973.

2707. Guerry-Force ML, Müller NL, Wright JL, et al: A comparison of bronchiolitis obliterans with organizing pneumonia, usual interstitial pneumonia, and small airway disease. Am Rev Respir Dis 135:705, 1987.

2708. Chandler PW, Shin MS, Friedman SE, et al: Radiographic manifestations of bronchiolitis obliterans with organizing pneumonia vs usual interstitial pneumonia. AJR 147:899, 1986.

2709. Epler GR, Colby TV: The spectrum of bronchiolitis obliterans. Chest 83:161, 1983.

2710. Seggev JS, Mason UG, Worthen S, et al: Bronchiolitis obliterans: Report of three cases with detailed physiologic studies. Chest 83:169, 1983.

2711. Kirkpatrick B, Bass JB: Severe obstructive lung disease after smoke inhalation. Chest 76:108, 1979.

2712. Ramirez FJ: The first death from nitrogen dioxide fumes. The story of a man and his dog. JAMA 229:1181, 1974.

2713. Ramirez RJ, Dowell AR: Silo-filler's disease: Nitrogen dioxide–induced lung injury. Long term follow-up and review of the literature. Ann Intern Med 74:569, 1971.

2714. Tse RL, Bockman AA: Nitrogen dioxide toxicity. Report of four cases in firemen. JAMA 212:1341, 1970.

2715. Jones GR, Proudfoot AT, Hall JI: Pulmonary effects of acute exposure to nitrous fumes. Thorax 28:61, 1973.

2716. Wohl M, Chernick V: State of the art: Bronchiolitis. Am Rev Respir Dis 118:759, 1978.

2717. Beem M, Egerer R, Fasan D, et al: Investigation of the etiology of acute bronchiolitis of infants. Am J Dis Child 102:461, 1961.

2718. Beem M, Wright FH, Fasan DM: Observations on the etiology of acute bronchiolitis in infants. J Pediatr 61:864, 1962.

2719. Sandiford BR, Spencer B: Respiratory syncytial virus in epidemic bronchiolitis of infants. Br Med J 2:881, 1962.

2720. Simpson H, Matthew DJ, Inglis JM, et al: Virological findings and blood gas tensions in acute lower respiratory tract infections in children. Br Med J 2:629, 1974.

2721. Heycock JB, Noble TC: 1,230 cases of acute bronchiolitis in infancy. Br Med J 2:879, 1962.

2722. Buckley CE III, Tucker DH, Thorne NA, et al: Bronchiolectasis. The clinical syndrome and its relationship to chronic lung disease. Am J Med 38:190, 198, 1965.

2723. Sturtevant HN, Knudson HW: Bronchiolar ectasia: A report of twelve cases. Am J Roentgenol 83:279, 1960.

2724. Wisoff CP: Bronchiolectasis in bronchitis. Radiology 70:848, 1958.

2725. Koch DA: Roentgenologic considerations of capillary bronchiolitis. Am J Roentgenol 82:433, 1959.

2726. Engel S: Bronchiolitis. Br J Dis Chest 53:125, 1959.

2727. Sawazaki H, Watabe S, Onoki S, et al: Two cases of bronchiolitis obliterans. Jap J Chest Dis 21:635, 1962.

2728. Felson B, Felson H: Acute diffuse pneumonia of asthmatics. Am J Roentgenol 74:235, 1955.

2729. Ham JC: Acute infectious obstructing bronchiolitis. A potentially fatal disease in the adult. Ann Intern Med 60:47, 1964.

2730. Hogg JC, Williams J, Richardson JB, et al: Age as a factor in the distribution of lower-airway conductance and in the pathologic anatomy of obstructive lung disease. N Engl J Med 282:1283, 1970.

2731. Geddes DM, Corrin B, Brewerton DA, et al: Progressive airway obliteration in adults and its association with rheumatoid disease. Q J Med 46:427, 1977.

2732. Epler GR, Snider GL, Gaensler EA, et al: Bronchiolitis and bronchitis in connective tissue disease, a possible relationship to the use of penicillamine. JAMA 242:528, 1979.

2733. Chebat J, Seigneur F, Lechien J, et al: Severe bronchiolitis in three cases of rheumatoid polyarthritis treated with D-penicillamine. Rev Fr Mal Respir 9:147, 1981.

2734. Herzog CA, Miller RR, Hoidal JR, et al: Bronchiolitis and rheumatoid arthritis. Am Rev Respir Dis 124:636, 1981.

2735. Murphy KC, Atkins CJ, Offer RC, et al: Obliterative bronchitis in two rheumatoid arthritis patients treated with penicillamine. Arthritis Rheum 24:557, 1981.

2736. Jacobs P, Bonnyns M, Depierreux M, et al: Rapidly fatal bronchiolitis obliterans with circulating antinuclear and rheumatoid factors. Eur J Respir Dis 65:384, 1984.

2737. Gibson JM, O'Hara MD, Beare JM, et al: Bronchial obstruction in a patient with Behcet's disease. Eur J Respir Dis 63:356, 1982.

2738. Turton CW, Williams G, Green M, et al: Cryptogenic obliterative bronchiolitis in adults. Thorax 36:805, 1981.

11

2739. Green M, Turton CW: Bronchiolitis and its manifestations. Eur J Respir Dis 63:36, 1982.

2740. Roca J, Graneña A, Rodriguez-Roisin R, et al: Fatal airway disease in an adult with chronic graft-versus-host disease. Thorax 37:77, 1982.

2741. Ralph DD, Springmeyer SC, Sullivan KM, et al: Rapidly progressive air-flow obstruction in marrow transplant recipients: Possible association between obliterative bronchiolitis and chronic graft-versus-host disease. Am Rev Respir Dis 129:641, 1984.

2742. Johnson FL, Stokes DC, Ruggiero M, et al: Chronic obstructive airways disease after bone marrow transplantation. J Pediatr 105:370, 1984.

2743. Epler GR, Colby TV, McCloud TC, et al: Bronchiolitis obliterans organizing pneumonia. N Engl J Med 312:152, 1985.

2744. Macklem PT, Thurlbeck WM, Fraser RG: Chronic obstructive disease of small airways. Ann Intern Med 74:167, 1971.

2745. Homma H, Yamanaka A, Tanimoto S, et al: Diffuse panbronchiolitis. A disease of the transitional zone of the lung. Chest 83:63, 1983.

2746. Maeda M, Saiki S, Yamanaka A: Serial section analysis of the lesions in diffuse panbronchiolitis. Acta Pathol Jpn 37:693, 1987.

2747. Akira M, Kitatani F, Yong-Sik L, et al: Diffuse panbronchiolitis: Evaluation with high-resolution CT[1]. Radiology 168:433, 1988.

2748. Vincken WG, Gauthier SG, Dollfuss RE, et al: Involvement of upper airway muscles in extrapyramidal disorders: A cause of airflow limitation. N Engl J Med 311:438, 1984.

2749. Alexander HL, Paddock R: Bronchial asthma: Response to pilocarpin and epinephrine. Arch Intern Med 27:184, 1921.

2750. Michoud MC, Jeanneret-Grosjean A, Cohen A, Amyot R: Reflex decrease of histamine-induced bronchoconstriction after laryngeal stimulation in asthmatic patients. Am Rev Respir Dis 138:1548, 1988.

2751. Baile EM, Dahlby R, Wiggs BR, et al: Effect of warm and dry air hyperventilation on canine airway blood flow. J Appl Physiol 62:526, 1987.

2752. Schoeffel RE, Anderson SD, Altounyan REC: Bronchial hyperreactivity in response to inhalation of ultrasonically nebulized solutions of distilled water and saline. Br J Med 23:1285, 1981.

2753. Elwood RK, Hogg JC, Paré PD: Airway responses to osmolar challenge in asthma. Am Rev Respir Dis 125:61A, 1982.

2754. Finney MJB, Anderson SD, Black JL: The effect of non-isotonic solutions on human isolated airway smooth muscle. Respir Physiol 69:277, 1987.

2755. McGregor M: Current concepts: Pulsus paradoxus. N Engl J Med 301:480, 1979.

2756. Dodd DF, Kelly S, Collett PW, et al: Pressure-time product, work rate, and endurance during resistive breathing in humans. J Appl Physiol 64:1397, 1988.

2757. Collett PW, Perry C, Engel L: Pressure-time product, flow, and O_2 cost of resistive breathing in humans. J Appl Physiol 58:1263, 1965.

2758. Paré PD, Brooks LA, Coppin CA, et al: Density dependence of maximum expiratory flow and its correlation with small airway pathology in smokers. Am Rev Respir Dis 131:521, 1985.

2759. Sanders C, Nath PH, Bailey WC: Detection of emphysema with computed tomography. Correlation with pulmonary function tests and chest radiography. Invest Radiol 23:262, 1988.

2760. Genereux GP: Radiology and pulmonary immunopathologic lung disease. In Steiner, RE (ed): Recent Advances in Radiology and Medical Imaging. New York, Churchill Livingstone, 1983, pp 213–240.

2761. Blair DN, Coppage L, Shaw C: Medical imaging in asthma. J Thorac Imag 1:23, 1986.

2762. Sostman HD, Gottschalk AG: The stripe sign: A new sign for diagnosis of nonembolic defects on pulmonary perfusion scintigraphy. Radiology 142:737, 1982.

2763. Thurlbeck WM: The morphology of chronic bronchitis, asthma, and bronciectasis. In Chronic Airflow Obstruction in Lung Disease. Philadelphia, WB Saunders Co, 1976, p 31.

2764. Felson B, Felson H: Acute diffuse pneumonia in asthmatics. Am J Roentgenol 74:235, 1955.

2765. Douglas AN: Quantitative study of bronchial mucous gland enlargement. Thorax 35:198, 1980.

2766. McDowell EM, Barrett LA, Harris CC, et al: Abdominal cilia in human bronchial epithelium. Arch Pathol Lab Med 100:429, 1976.

2767. Ailsby RL, Ghadially FN: Atypical cilia in human bronchial mucosa. J Pathol 109:75, 1973.

2768. Smallman LA, Gregory J: Ultrastructural abnormalities of cilia in the human respiratory tract. Hum Pathol 17:848, 1986.

2769. Lungarella G, Fonzi L, Ermini G: Abnormalities of bronchial cilia in patients with chronic bronchitis. An ultrastructural and quantitative analysis. Lung 161:147, 1983.

2770. Wisseman CL, Simel DL, Spock A, et al: The prevalence of abnormal cilia in normal pediatric lungs. Arch Pathol Lab Med 105:552, 1981.

2771. Fox B, Bull TB, Makey AR, et al: The significance of ultrastructural abnormalities of human cilia. Chest 80:796, 1981.

2772. Woodring JH, Barrett PA, Rehm SR, et al: Acquired tracheomegaly in adults as a complication of diffuse pulmonary fibrosis. AJR 152:743, 1989.

2773. Partinen M, Jamieson A, Guilleminault C: Long-term outcome for obstructive sleep apnea syndrome patients. Mortality. Chest 94:1200, 1988.

2774. Larsson SG, Gislason T, Lindholm CE: Computed tomography of the oropharynx in obstructive sleep apnea. Acta Radiol 29:401, 1988.

2775. Agosta JM, Sprenger JD, Lum LG, et al: Transfer of allergen-specific IgE-mediated hypersensitivity with allogeneic bone marrow transplantation. N Engl J Med 319:1623, 1988.

2776. Turner KJ, Stewart GA, Woolcock AJ, et al: Relationship between mite densities and the prevalence of asthma: Comparative studies in two populations in the Eastern Highlands of Papua, New Guinea. Clin Allergy 18:331, 1988.

2777. James AL, Paré PD, Hogg JC: The mechanics of airway narrowing in asthma. Am Rev Respir Dis 132:242, 1989.

2778. Whicker SD, Armour CL, Black JL: Responsiveness of bronchial smooth muscle from asthmatic patients to relaxant and contractile agonists. Pulmonary Pharmacol 1:25, 1988.

2779. Durham SR, Craddock CF, Cookson WD, et al: Increases in airway responsiveness to histamine precede allergen-induced late asthmatic responses. J Allergy Clin Immunol 82:764, 1988.

2780. Reiff, DB, Choudry NB, Pride NB, et al: The effect of prolonged submaximal warm-up exercise on exercise-induced asthma. Am Rev Respir Dis 139:479, 1989.

2781. Ekström T, Tibbling L: Gastro-oesophageal reflux and triggering of bronchial asthma: A negative report. Eur J Respir Dis 71:177, 1987.

2782. Allen DH, Delohery J, Baker G: Monosodium L-glutamate–induced asthma. J Allergy Clin Immunol 80:530, 1987.

2783. Roca J, Ramis L, Rodriguez-Roison R, et al: Serial relationships between ventilation-perfusion inequality and spirometry in acute severe asthma requiring hospitalization. Am Rev Respir Dis 137:1055, 1988.

2784. Rodriguez-Roison R, Ballester E, Roca J, et al: Mechanisms of hypoxemia in patients with status asthmaticus requiring mechanical ventilation. Am Rev Respir Dis 139:732, 1989.

2785. Okrent DG, Tessler S, Twersky RA, et al: Metabolic acidosis not due to lactic acidosis in patients with severe acute asthma. Crit Care Med 15:1098, 1987.

2786. Mountain RD, Sahn SA: Clinical features and outcome in patients with acute asthma presenting with hypercapnia. Am Rev Respir Dis 138:535, 1988.

2787. Lecks HI, Whitney T, Wood D, et al: Newer concepts in occurrence of segmental atelectasis in acute bronchial asthma and status asthmaticus in children. J Asthma Res 4:65, 1966.

2788. Jenkins MA, Hurley SF, Jolley DJ, et al: Trends in Australian mortality of asthma, 1979–1985. Med J Aust 149:620, 1988.

2789. Sly RM: Mortality from asthma, 1979–1984. J Allergy Clin Immunol 82:705, 1988.

2790. Sears MR, Rea HH, Fenwick J, et al: 75 deaths in asthmatics prescribed home nebulizers. Br Med J 294:477, 1987.

2791. Richards GA, Theron AJ, Van Der Merwe CA, et al: Spirometric abnormalities in young smokers correlate with increased chemiluminescence responses of activated blood phagocytes. Am Rev Respir Dis 139:181, 1989.

2792. Paré JP, Cote G, Fraser RS: Long term follow-up of drug abusers with intravenous talcosis. Am Rev Respir Dis 139:233, 1989.

2793. Fernie JM, McLean A, Lamb D: Significant intimal abnormalities in muscular pulmonary arteries of patients with early obstructive lung disease. J Clin Pathol 41:730, 1988.

2794. Magee F, Wright JL, Wiggs BR, et al: Pulmonary vascular structure and function in chronic obstructive pulmonary disease. Thorax 43:183, 1988.

2795. Miller RR, Müller NL, Vedal S, et al: Limitations of computed tomography in the assessment of emphysema. Am Rev Respir Dis 139:980, 1989.

2796. Bates DV, Macklem PT, Christie RV: Respiratory Function in Disease: An Introduction to the Integral Study of Lung, 2nd ed. Philadelphia, WB Saunders Co, 1971.

2797. Brantly ML, Paul LD, Miller BH, et al: Clinical features and history of the destructive lung disease associated with alpha₁-antitrypsin deficiency of adults with pulmonary symptoms. Am Rev Respir Dis 138:327, 1988.

2798. Cox DW, Levison H: Emphysema of early onset associated with a complete deficiency of alpha₁-antitrypsin (null homozygotes). Am Rev Respir Dis 137:371, 1988.

2799. Bohadana AB, Peslin R, Uffholtz H, et al: Pulmonary function and clinical pattern in homozygous (PiZ) alpha₁-antitrypsin deficiency. Respiration 37:167, 1979.

2800. Tarver RD, Conces DJ Jr, Godwin JD: Motion artifacts on CT simulate bronchiectasis. AJR 151:1117, 1988.

2801. Zeaske R, Bruns WT, Fink JN, et al: Immune responses to Aspergillus in cystic fibrosis. J Allergy Clin Immunol 82:73, 1988.

2802. Myers JL, Katzenstein ALA: Ultrastructural evidence of alveolar epithelial injury in idiopathic bronchiolitis obliterans—organizing pneumonia. Am J Pathol 132:102, 1988.

2803. Burke CM, Glanville AR, Theodore J, et al: Lung immunogenicity, rejection, and obliterative bronchiolitis. Chest 92:547, 1987.

2804. Malo J-L, Cartier A, Ghezzo H, et al: Patterns of improvement in spirometry, bronchial hyperresponsiveness, and specific IgE antibody levels after cessation of exposure in occupational asthma caused by snow-crab processing. Am Rev Respir Dis 138:807, 1988.

2805. Robertson AS, Weir DC, Burge PS: Occupational asthma due to oil mists. Thorax 43:200, 1988.

2806. Choudat D, Neukirch F, Brochard P, et al: Allergy and occupational exposure to hydroquinone and to methionine. Br J Ind Med 45:376, 1988.

2807. Musk AW, Peach S, Ryan G: Occupational asthma in a mineral analysis laboratory. Br J Ind Med 45:381, 1988.

11

12

Pleuropulmonary Disease Caused by Inhalation of Inorganic Dust (Pneumoconiosis)

The Fourth International Pneumoconiosis Conference[1] held in Bucharest in 1971 defined *pneumoconiosis* as "the accumulation of dust in the lungs and the tissue reactions to its presence." Dust itself can be regarded as an aerosol composed of solid particles that can be inorganic or organic in nature. The *inorganic* dust pneumoconioses are caused by inhalation of minerals or other inorganic particles and their retention in the lung parenchyma. The accumulation of these substances over time generally results in one or both of two pathologic reactions:

1. *Fibrosis*, which can be focal and nodular (as in silicosis) or diffuse (as in asbestosis). It is probably related to a toxic effect of the inhaled substance on pulmonary epithelial or inflammatory cells; the fibrosis often results in roentgenographic abnormalities and, if extensive enough, in significant functional impairment.

2. *Aggregates of particle-laden macrophages* with minimal or no accompanying fibrosis; this reaction is typically seen with inert dusts such as iron, tin, and barium. Although sometimes associated with chronic roentgenographic abnormalities, this reaction usually causes few if any functional or clinical manifestations.

In contrast to disease caused by inorganic particles, the *organic dust* pneumoconioses, such as byssinosis and the hypersensitivity pneumonitides, are characteristically unassociated with the accumulation of particles within the lungs; for this reason and because of the strong evidence for an immunopathogenesis, these conditions are discussed in the chapter on immunologic lung disease (*see* page 1266). Although features similar to those of the organic dust pneumoconioses are found with inhalation of some inorganic particles (such as beryllium), these substances have traditionally been included among the inorganic pneumoconioses and are discussed in this chapter.

The establishment of a causal relationship between an inhaled dust and an adverse biologic effect requires careful study of exposed populations and demands evidence of pulmonary involvement by the demonstration of abnormalities in pulmonary function, the chest roentgenogram, or lung structure. Analysis of the concentration and particle size of the dust in the workers' "breathing zone" is important, and the results are taken into consideration whenever available. In addition, a detailed occupational history is of the utmost importance

because certain jobs not usually regarded as harmful can become so if carried out in proximity to other, potentially hazardous occupations such as welding and sandblasting.[2] Even when all investigations have shown convincing evidence for the presence of a pneumoconiosis, the precise etiology may not be evident, even with a detailed pathologic examination. This statement is lent emphasis by the fact that individuals in many occupations are exposed to more than one type of dust particle; an analysis of lung tissue can reflect this multiplicity, and it is sometimes difficult to attribute pathologic changes to one specific substance. For example, shale miners sometimes develop progressive massive fibrosis (PMF) similar to that seen in coal miners and kaolin workers and their lungs have been shown to contain dust composed of a combination of kaolinite, mica, and silica,[3] each of which can itself cause pulmonary disease. Individuals in numerous other occupations, such as locomotive drivers and stokers,[4] dental technicians,[5–7] foundry workers,[8, 9] oxyacetylene torch workers,[10] and miners and millers of many minerals,[11] are also at risk for the development of pneumoconiosis caused by inhalation of more than one dust (thus the term "mixed dust pneumoconiosis").[12]

The identification of foreign substances in lung tissue requires one or more of a number of techniques: (1) routine light and electron microscopy, (2) dark field microscopy, (3) polarization microscopy, (4) histochemical staining, (5) microincineration and bulk chemical analysis, and (6) analytical electron microscopy.[13, 14] The last-named is carried out with a standard electron microscope fitted with analytical equipment; both transmission and scanning electron microscopy can be employed, permitting nondestructive structural and elemental analysis of lung and other tissues *in situ*. Its various facets have been described by McMahon.[13] Selected-area electron diffraction is an electron microscopic imaging technique that permits sequential morphologic and crystallographic analysis of mineral particles found in thin tissue sections or lung digestates. Energy-dispersive x-ray analysis is an *in situ* nondestructive analytical technique for recording the presence of elements ranging from fluoride (atomic number [Z] = 9) to uranium (Z = 92) within a biopsy or surgical specimen. Lung particulate load can be quantified either by *in situ* analytical electron microscopy or by counting with light or electron microscopy the mineral residues found after low-temperature ashing or sodium hypochlorite (bleach) digestion; the former procedure is perhaps more useful because it equates the local burden with regional differences in tissue response.

The inorganic dust pneumoconioses are in large measure occupational diseases. In recent years, however, it has become increasingly apparent that they can develop in individuals who live in the vicinity of industrial plants (particularly those handling asbestos or beryllium) but who do not work there. Such "para-occupational" disease occurs particularly in spouses and children of workers who transport hazardous material on clothing from the worksite into the home.[15] It is important, therefore, that in any individual in whom the presence of pneumoconiosis is suspected, an occupational history should be obtained not only from the patient but also from his or her spouse; in addition, the site of the patient's residence in relation to industrial plants should be considered.

The entire subject of inorganic dust pneumoconiosis has been discussed in detail in the excellent monographs by Parkes[16] and by Morgan and Seaton.[17]

GENERAL PATHOGENETIC FEATURES

The reaction of the lung to inhaled inorganic dust depends on several factors, each of which is important by itself but all of which must be considered in combination, because they are to a certain extent interdependent. Eight factors are predominant: (1) the chemical nature of the dust, (2) the size and shape of dust particles, (3) the rate and pattern of breathing, (4) the distribution of inhaled dust particles, (5) the concentration of dust particles, (6) the duration of exposure, (7) individual susceptibility, and (8) the clearance of inhaled dust particles.

THE CHEMICAL NATURE OF THE DUST

The majority of inorganic dusts, if inhaled in sufficient quantity over a long enough time, cause pulmonary fibrosis. Even though a few dusts are "inert" and are not fibrogenic (for example, tin, iron, and barium), they can produce some degree of functional impairment if inhaled in sufficient quantity over a sufficient period. To expect the lung to act as a "physiologic dust trap" without its function being impaired to some extent is unreasonable. It is important to appreciate that chronic inhalation of certain dusts—for example, barium—can produce an awesome-looking chest roentgenogram in a patient who is relatively asymptomatic, simply because of the physical presence of much nonreactive radiopaque material within the lungs. At the other end of the scale are those dusts—for example, asbestos—that can cause incapacitating clinical symptoms and severe functional impairment, even though the chest roentgenogram is almost normal.

THE SIZE AND SHAPE OF DUST PARTICLES

Four main physical processes determine particle deposition in the lungs:

1. *Inertial impaction* occurs when the momentum of a particle being carried in an air current causes it to impinge on an airway wall when the latter changes direction. This is the principal mechanism by which large particles (ranging in diameter from 2 to 100 μm) are deposited in the respiratory tract.[18] Because of its anatomic complexity, the nose is the most important site for such a mechanism and, in fact, the majority of particles larger than 10 μm in diameter are deposited here.[18] The bend in the nasopharynx and the increased velocity of airflow at this site serve to trap most larger particles that have avoided impaction in the nasal passages.[19, 20] Inertial impaction also occurs at the bifurcation of bronchi and, to a lesser extent, bronchioles.

2. *Sedimentation* is the mechanism by which particles are deposited on airway walls as a result of the influence of gravity. Such deposition depends on the density and diameter of the particle; the larger and denser the particle, the more rapid the settling. This is an important mechanism of deposition of particles ranging from 0.5 to 2 μm in diameter and occurs mostly in the bronchi and membranous bronchioles.

3. *Diffusion or brownian movement* causes small particles to move randomly as a result of energy transfer from adjacent gas molecules and to impinge by chance on an airway or alveolar wall. This mechanism plays a role in the deposition of particles up to 2 μm in diameter; it is the major mechanism of deposition of those 0.5 μm or less and the only mechanism for particles less than 0.2 μm in diameter. Diffusion is most important in particle deposition within the alveolar airspaces, although some particles can also settle out in the larger conducting airways by this means.

4. *Interception.* The first three mechanisms of dust deposition relate predominantly to particles that are approximately spherical. As the length-diameter ratio of particles increases, they are termed *fibers*, and a fourth mechanism comes into play (a fiber being defined as a particle whose length-diameter ratio is approximately 3:1). Such fibrous particulates, especially those with a large real or effective cross-sectional diameter (the latter consisting of fibers such as chrysotile asbestos, which are curled or irregular in shape) are likely to come into contact with the airway wall. By contrast, fibers with a straight configuration and a relatively small diameter can penetrate into the lung periphery.[21]

In summary, most particles 5 μm or greater are deposited on the walls of the nose, nasopharynx, trachea, and bronchial bifurcations as a result of inertial impaction and, to a lesser extent, sedimentation. Many particles smaller than 2 μm in diameter are deposited in the respiratory bronchioles and alveoli, chiefly by diffusion but partly by sedimentation. Particles less than 0.5 μm in diameter tend to be exhaled, and the majority are not retained within the lung, at least during quiet breathing.

In addition to influencing the site within the respiratory tract at which a fiber or particle is deposited, size and shape can have a role in determining the host reaction. This is particularly true of asbestos; for example, there is abundant evidence that asbestos fibers with a high length-diameter ratio are important in the pathogenesis of mesothelioma.[22–25]

THE RATE AND PATTERN OF BREATHING

Because the majority of large particles are trapped within the nasal mucosa, a greater concentration of particles tends to reach the lower respiratory tree in habitual mouth-breathers or individuals engaged in heavy labor, in which there is excessive mouth-breathing. In addition, the increased pulmonary ventilation that accompanies heavy labor can be expected to result in a greater number of particles reaching the lung in a given period.

THE DISTRIBUTION OF INHALED DUST PARTICLES

Little experimental work has been performed to determine the distribution of inhaled inorganic particles in normal lungs, but because ventilation in the erect position is relatively greater in lower than in upper lung regions, it might be expected that the lower regions would be slightly more susceptible to lung damage. However, it is clear that other factors must be implicated, as indicated by the predominant involvement of upper lung zones in patients with silicosis and coal worker's pneumoconiosis; whether this anatomic predilection is caused by the initial distribution of particles, perhaps influenced by variations in bronchial anatomy,[26] or by other regional differences in lung function, such as alveolar clearance,[27] is unknown. The size of an individual's central airways relative to lung volume can influence particle deposition; the smaller the airways, the greater the proximal deposition.[28] As might be expected, intrinsic lung disease such as emphysema can have an appreciable effect on particle deposition.[29] In addition, particulate deposits on both large and small airways can induce bronchospasm, which can influence regional distribution,[30, 31] even in normal lungs. This effect is considerably enhanced in the presence of established lung disease because of diversion of inspired gas to unobstructed airways.[32, 33]

THE CONCENTRATION OF DUST PARTICLES

Davies[34] showed that the ability of the healthy lung to cope with the introduction of dust particles into the alveoli appears to relate roughly to the concentration of airborne dust inhaled. A concentration of less than ten particles of 5 μm or less per ml can be completely eliminated, whereas only about 90 per cent of a concentration of approximately 1,000 such particles/ml will be eliminated, and the retained 10 per cent can produce a slowly developing pneumoconiosis. With concentrations as high as 1,000,000 particles/ml, a very large proportion is retained and lung disease can develop rapidly.

THE DURATION OF EXPOSURE

The great majority of cases of pneumoconiosis develop only after many years of dust exposure. Occasionally, however, severe progressive lung disease develops after only relatively brief exposure—a few months, for example. In these instances, it is probable that two factors are chiefly responsible: a very high concentration of dust and an individual susceptibility.

INDIVIDUAL SUSCEPTIBILITY

Individual susceptibility is a difficult factor to assess, but there is no doubt that different individuals with identical dust exposure may have different reactions; for example, one may be free of disease while another may show advanced progressive massive fibrosis. The precise reasons for such individual variation are not clear but may relate to differences in airway geometry, immunologic status, variation in the efficiency of dust clearance,[35] and the presence of other disease such as tuberculosis.

CLEARANCE OF INHALED DUST PARTICLES

Clearance of inhaled inorganic particles is accomplished by one or both of two mechanisms— transport up the mucociliary escalator and lymphatic drainage. In normal subjects, nasal mucous flow rates vary considerably, ranging from zero to more than 20 mm/minute,[19] and a similar variation exists for the efficiency of tracheobronchial mucous transport. Thus, although particles deposited on the tracheobronchial tree are usually transported rapidly to the pharynx, where they are either expectorated or swallowed along with mucus, transport can be prolonged in some individuals. In addition to inherent individual variation in mucous flow rates, environmental factors such as cigarette smoke may also influence the efficiency of mucociliary clearance and predispose to greater dust retention.[766]

As discussed previously, small particles that reach the transitional airways and alveoli are thought to be deposited on the epithelial surface predominantly by diffusion or sedimentation. Once deposited, the majority are probably phagocytosed by alveolar macrophages. These dust-containing macrophages then make their way along the alveolar ducts and respiratory bronchioles to the mucociliary escalator, on which they are transported to the pharynx, where they are expectorated or swallowed in the same manner as free dust particles. In addition to this mechanism, dust particles, either free or within macrophages, can enter the peribronchial or peribronchiolar interstitial tissue. Although some particles remain at this site for an indefinite period, others are transported either centripetally to central lymphatics or centrifugally to perilobular lymphatics. Histologic studies have shown that clearance time of particles via lymphatics in peribronchovascular bundles ranges from 1 to 14 days, whereas particles that reach a subpleural location in paraseptal or perivascular lymphatics can remain in the lungs for months.[36] Regional differences in lymphatic flow[27] or mucociliary clearance may explain some of the variations in anatomic localization of disease in different pneumoconioses; individual differences in these clearance mechanisms may also partly explain individual susceptibility to disease. In the presence of active inflammation and exudation or overwhelming particle deposition, some dust particles can enter the bloodstream and be carried to various organs of the body, particularly the spleen and liver.[36]

INTERNATIONAL CLASSIFICATION OF RADIOGRAPHS OF THE PNEUMOCONIOSES, AND RECOMMENDED TERMINOLOGY

The chest roentgenogram is an important epidemiologic tool that is useful not only in detecting the effects of dust particle deposition in the lungs but also in measuring progression.[37] In order for the roentgenogram to be useful in epidemiologic studies, however, it is essential that an international classification of extent of involvement be followed and an acceptable nomenclature be employed. A multitude of such classifications have been developed over the years, all of which have evolved from the first International Labour Office (ILO) classification contained in the "Report of the International Conference on Silicosis," Johannesburg, 1930.[38] This codification scheme was employed for almost 30 years, but was extensively modified in 1958 in the publication of the ILO "International Classification of Persistent Radiological Opacities in the Lung Fields Provoked by the Inhalation of Mineral Dusts."[39]

In response to a growing need for an internationally acceptable system for coding the changes seen on chest roentgenograms of individuals exposed to asbestos, a committee of l'Union Internationale Contre le Cancer (the International Union Against Cancer, UICC), together with other groups, met in Cincinnati in 1967 for the purpose of developing a new classification. This was subsequently adopted and became known as the UICC/Cincinnati (U/C) classification.[40] Shortly thereafter, the ILO 1958 classification was revised (based in part on the U/C 1968 classification) and became known as the ILO 1968 classification. Following a period of experience with these two classifications, a meeting was convened in 1971 at the Medical Research Council Pneumoconiosis Unit in Penarth, Wales, and it was recommended that the ILO 1968 and U/C classifications, including standard reference roentgenograms, be combined. The obvious benefits to be derived from such a combination were the establishment of uniform international standards and the ability to compare results around the world. These recommendations were approved in 1971 and subsequently modified once again in 1980, thus giving official recognition to the classification now widely used throughout the world, the ILO 1980 International Classification of Radiographs of the Pneumoconioses.

The object of the classification is to codify the roentgenographic changes of the pneumoconioses in a simple, reproducible manner. It does not define pathologic entities but possesses the considerable advantage of providing a uniform method of reporting the type and extent of pneumoconiosis, thus leading to international comparability of pneumoconiosis statistics. The classification provides a means of systematically recording the roentgenographic changes in the chest caused by the inhalation of all types of mineral dusts, including coal, silica, carbon, asbestos, and beryllium. Because the classification employs roentgenologic descriptors that are somewhat different from those generally used throughout this book, a short glossary of terms is reproduced here. A more extensive description of the classification may be obtained from *Medical Radiography and Photography*,[41] from which publication much of the material in this section has been gleaned.

The complete classification is intended primarily for a comprehensive and semiquantitative description of the roentgenographic changes of all the principal features, including those of the pleura; it is likely to be particularly useful for epidemiologic studies. Standard reference roentgenograms have been selected to illustrate the ILO 1980 classification and have been superbly reproduced in the publication *Medical Radiography and Photography*[41] for ready reference.*

GLOSSARY OF TERMS USED TO DESCRIBE ROENTGENOGRAPHIC CHANGES IN THE PNEUMOCONIOSES

Terms requiring explanation are discussed here. All other terms used in the classification are self-explanatory and identical in context to the same terms used elsewhere in this book.

---

*In North America, a set of the ILO 1980 Standard Reference Radiographs can be purchased from the regional center of the International Labour Office, 1750 New York Avenue NW, Washington, DC 20006. In other parts of the world, it can be purchased from the International Labour Office, Geneva, Switzerland.

SMALL ROUNDED OPACITIES

These are well-circumscribed opacities or nodules ranging in diameter from barely visible up to 10 mm. The qualifiers p, q, and r subdivide the predominant opacities into three diameter ranges—up to 1.5 mm, 1.5 to 3 mm, and 3 mm to 10 mm, respectively.

SMALL IRREGULAR OPACITIES

This term is employed to describe a pattern that, elsewhere in this book, has been designated "linear," "reticular," or "reticulonodular"—in other words, a netlike pattern. Although the nature of these opacities is such that the establishment of quantitative dimensions is considerably more difficult than with rounded opacities, the ILO has seen fit to establish three categories—s (width up to about 1.5 mm), t (width exceeding 1.5 mm and up to about 3 mm), and u (width exceeding 3 mm and up to about 10 mm).

To record shape and size, two letters must be used. Thus, if the reader considers that all or virtually all opacities are one shape and size, this should be noted by recording the symbol twice, separated by an oblique stroke (for example, q/q). If, however, another shape or size is seen, this should be recorded as the second letter (for example, q/t). The designation q/t would mean that the predominant small opacity is round and of size q, but that there are, in addition, significant numbers of small irregular opacities of size t. In this way, any combination of small opacities may be recorded.

PROFUSION

This term denotes the number of small rounded or small irregular opacities per unit area or zone of lung. There are four basic categories:

Category 0: small opacities absent or less profuse than in category 1.

Category 1: small opacities definitely present but few in number. The normal markings are usually visible.

Category 2: numerous small opacities. The normal lung markings are usually partly obscured.

Category 3: very numerous small opacities. The normal lung markings are usually totally obscured.

These categories can be further subdivided by employing the 12-point scale designed by Liddell,[42, 43] by which the classification recognizes the existence of a continuum of changes from complete normality to the most advanced category or grade. The 12-point scale is listed as follows:

0/−	0/0	0/1
1/0	1/1	1/2
2/1	2/2	2/3
3/2	3/3	3/+

Employing this scale, profusion of opacities is categorized as follows: the roentgenogram is classified in the usual way into one of the four categories, 0, 1, 2, or 3. If during the process the category above or below is considered as a serious alternative, this is recorded, e.g., a roentgenogram in which profusion is considered to be Category 2 but for which Category 1 was seriously considered as an alternative would be graded Category 2/1. If no alternative was considered—i.e., the profusion was definitely Category 2—it would be classified 2/2.

A subdivision is also possible within Categories 0 and 3. Category 0/1 is profusion of Category 0 with Category 1 seriously considered as an alternative. Category 0/0 is a radiograph in which there are no small opacities or one in which a few opacities are thought to be present but are not sufficiently definite or numerous for Category 1 to be considered. If the absence of small opacities is particularly obvious, profusion should be recorded as 0/−. A radiograph that shows profusion markedly higher than that classifiable as 3/3 would be recorded as 3/+.

LARGE OPACITIES

This term is used for opacities that are larger than the maximum permitted for small rounded opacities, i.e., greater than 10 mm. Three categories are recognized:

Category A: an opacity having a greatest diameter exceeding 1 cm and up to and including 5 cm, or several opacities each greater than 1 cm, the sum of whose greatest diameters does not exceed 5 cm.

Category B: one or more opacities larger or more numerous than in category A whose combined area does not exceed the equivalent of the right upper zone.

Category C: one or more opacities whose combined area exceeds the equivalent of the right upper zone.

EXTENT

Each lung is divided into three zones—upper, middle, and lower—by horizontal lines drawn at one-third and two-thirds of the vertical distance between the apex of the lung and the dome of the diaphragm.

ROENTGENOLOGIC INTERPRETATION

Since enactment in 1969 by the Congress of the United States of the Federal Coal Miners' Health and Safety Act, which provided certain benefits to coal miners with pneumoconiosis, much attention has been directed toward decision-making processes and observer error in the roentgenologic diagnosis of pneumoconiosis.[44–46] Common to all these reports has been an exceptionally high degree of inter-reader variability and observer error, which has been attributed to a combination of lack of experience with the classification systems employed, lack of familiarity with the roentgenologic manifestations of pneumoconiosis, and poor film quality. As a result of these deficiencies, the National Institute of Occupational Safety and Health (NIOSH) has established an examination that is administered to physicians who wish to be certified as interpreters of chest roentgenograms in pneumoconiosis programs; the examination is preceded by a weekend course administered by the American College of Radiology. Completion of the course establishes the physician as an "A reader;" successful completion of the examination results in the designation "B reader."

Turner and colleagues[47] have reported on a study of the value of automated computer screening of chest roentgenograms for the presence of pneumoconiosis (specifically, coal worker's pneumoconiosis). They found that two complementary computer approaches yielded classification results comparable to those obtained by experienced radiologists.

In a report of the workshop set up to study the value of the chest roentgenogram as an epidemiologic tool,[48] one of the conclusions was as follows: "It is anticipated that in the foreseeable future automated image transformation and recognition, and nonphysician describers or classifiers, may be used in epidemiologic investigations of occupational dust diseases. However, there are still technical problems to be overcome." The workshop recommended, "Further study should be addressed to developing information about sensory perception in pattern recognition of pneumoconioses."

In assessing roentgenologic progression of simple pneumoconiosis in individual miners, Liddell,[49] in common with others,[37, 46] recommends the viewing of all films together in known temporal order, recording into the most detailed classification available. Side-by-side reading has been shown to lead to substantially lower observer error and variability than independent reading.

THE INORGANIC DUSTS

SILICA

Silica is an ubiquitous and abundant mineral composed of regularly arranged molecules of silicon dioxide (SiO_2). It exists in three forms: (1) *crystalline*, which, depending on the temperature of formation, occurs primarily as quartz, tridymite, or cristobalite; (2) *microcrystalline*, consisting of minute crystals of quartz bonded together by amorphous silica and exemplified by flint and chert; and (3) *amorphous*, which is noncrystalline and consists of kieselguhr (composed of the skeletal remains of diatoms) or vitreous (derived by heating and rapid cooling of the crystalline types) forms. Occupational exposure to and the fibrogenic potential of these different forms vary, a fact that is important in understanding the development of disease in different individuals.

Pure "free" silica (composed predominantly of silicon dioxide) must be distinguished from other substances in which SiO_2 is combined with an appreciable proportion of various cations ("combined" silica); such silicates include asbestos, talc, and mica, and are associated with different clinicopathologic forms of disease (*see* later).

Epidemiology

Exposure to a concentration of silica high enough to result in roentgenologic and pathologic manifestations of silicosis can occur in many occupations; only a brief overview is given here, and the reader is referred to more comprehensive sources for further details.[16, 17, 50, 51] The most important occupations at risk are the following:

1. *Mining, tunneling, and quarrying.* Because of the ubiquity of silica in the earth's crust, such work almost inevitably leads to some exposure unless it involves pure limestone or marble.[52] Thus, the mining of gold, tin, iron, copper, nickel, silver, tungsten, barium[53, 54] and uranium[17] has been associated with the development of silicosis. The mining of other minerals recognized as causes of pneumoconiosis, such as coal, can also be accompanied by silica exposure, and there is no doubt that the lung disease in some affected individuals results from the silica, at least in part.

2. *Foundry work* involving the production of molds, knocking out of castings, and cleaning and polishing (fettling) of the final product.[55]

3. The *ceramic industry*, in which workers are exposed to potter's clay and powdered flint.[56]

4. Workers exposed to *diatomaceous earth*[57–63] in the manufacture of paints, varnishes, and insecticides, and in filtration and other processes. Although generally considered to be relatively inert in its amorphous form, diatomaceous earth is converted into cristobalite and tridymite when heated,[17] and exposure to these substances has been associated with a rare but apparently virulent form of disease.

5. In *a variety of other occupations*, including sandblasting; boiler scaling; the manufacture of artificial grinding wheels,[64] glass and silica bricks, and crucibles; in slate pencil manufacturing in India;[65, 66] in the use of ochre,[67] granite,[68, 767] bentonite,[69] and enamel;[70] and in the manufacture and use of silica flour.[71] The last-named is a finely ground silica reportedly composed of 99 per cent silicon dioxide and used as an abrasive, paint extender, and filler for cosmetics and other manufactured items. Its use as an abrasive scouring powder was among the earliest recognized causes of the acute variety of silicosis (*see* later);[72, 73] more recently, its use as a polisher or buffer has been reported to be responsible for cases of silicosis in gemstone[74] and jade[75] workers in Hong Kong and in furniture workers in Japan.[76]

Although the nature of the occupations involved in exposure to silica dust limits the disease mainly to men, roughly half the 20,000 employees at risk in the pottery industry in England are women, many of whom have exhibited typical features of pneumoconiosis.[77] In fact, one form of environmental lung disease characterized by increased silica deposition is apparently unique to women—that associated with the inhalation of fine sand particles by Bedouin females in the Negev desert of Israel.[78] Histopathologic examination of the lungs of a number of these women has revealed only increased silica deposition without the usual silicotic reaction, leading to the designation simple siliceous pneumoconiosis (rather than silicosis). This disease is both environmental and occupational, because it results from the work habits of these women, which involve increased dust inhalation in the tents, particularly during the making of cloth from sheep's wool. It is analogous to the Transkei silicosis that is restricted to Bantu females, who grind their food with sandstone, thus freeing large amounts of silica particles into the air.[79] An extraordinarily high incidence of silicosis has been reported among workers in sandstone quarries in northern Nigeria.[80] Of 126 stone cutters, 49 had roentgenographic evidence of silicosis. It is expected that in future years the true incidence of pneumoconiosis in the developing countries will become evident as a result of dissemination of knowledge and thorough epidemiologic studies.

The U.S. Public Health Service statements of *concentration* of dust particles in the atmosphere describe primary and secondary thresholds. *The primary threshold* consists of 5×10^6 particles less than 10 μm in size per cubic foot; exposure to concentrations below this level does not result in silicosis. *The secondary threshold* consists of 100×10^6 particles of the same size per cubic foot; all persons exposed at or above this level will acquire silicosis.

Pathogenesis

In addition to clinical and pathologic observations, numerous investigations of experimental animals and cell cultures have resulted in the recognition of a variety of factors that may be important in the pathogenesis of silica-induced pulmonary disease. Such factors must attempt to explain the two fundamental histologic reactions to inhaled silica: (1) the *silicotic nodule*, which is characterized by dense, often concentric lamellae of collagen and which, when conglomerated, is termed progressive massive fibrosis (PMF); and (2) *silicoproteinosis*, which typically occurs in individuals or animals exposed to very high concentrations of silica and which is characterized by alveolar filling by lipoproteinaceous material similar to that seen in idiopathic alveolar proteinosis. The majority of experimental investigations have focused on the first of these reactions because it is by far the more common; these investigations are only briefly summarized here, more detailed information being available in other, more extensive texts and monographs.[16, 51, 81]

Two of the early hypotheses dealing with fibrogenesis and silica have now been largely abandoned. The suggestion that small electric currents generated on the surface of quartz crystals could damage cells (the so-called piezoelectric effect)[82] has been found to be inconsistent with the electrical properties of various forms of silica and other minerals.[16] Similarly, the idea that tissue damage and fibrosis are caused by silicic acid derived from the gradual solubilization of crystalline silica has not been confirmed. It has been shown that the solubility of different forms of silica correlates poorly with their ability to cause fibrosis[16] and, more importantly, that silica contained within a capsule whose membrane is permeable to simple silicic acid and that is placed subcutaneously in an experimental animal does not result in a significant fibrotic reaction.[83]

The latter observation led to the conclusion that direct contact between cells or tissue and silica particles is necessary for the production of a pathologic effect. The logical candidate for such contact is the alveolar macrophage, and there is now abundant evidence that this cell is intimately involved in the pathogenesis of silica-induced fibrosis. When silica is added to a macrophage cell culture, it is rapidly ingested and incorporated within phagosomes.[84–86] Lysosomes subsequently fuse with and release their enzymes into the phagosomes, but instead of being destroyed the silica remains intact and by mechanisms as yet unclear, the lysosomal membrane ruptures. Silica and numerous toxic enzymes are thus released into the cell cytoplasm and, upon cell death, back into the culture medium. Among the substances released from the dead macrophages is an agent that causes fibroblasts to produce collagen.[87, 88] These experimental observations have led to the concept that silica induces lung fibrosis by causing lysosomal rupture, macrophage death, and the release of fibrogenic substances; ingestion of the released silica by new generations of macrophages and their subsequent death would then be responsible for increasing tissue injury. Injection of quartz into Sprague-Dawley rats has provided evidence that the process of fibrosis alternates with periods of collagen lysis;[89] extending such a finding to the human might explain the long interval between exposure and roentgenographic evidence of disease.

Although this hypothetical mechanism explains many of the features of both experimental and clinical silicosis, it has become clear that the theory is an oversimplification. First, not all investigators have been able to demonstrate the release of fibrogenic substances from dying macrophages.[81, 90] Second, more detailed studies of the interaction between macrophages and fibroblasts have shown that macrophage-derived chemical mediators can both stimulate and inhibit the production of collagen;[90] in addition, as previously noted, experimental studies have shown that when quartz is injected into Sprague-Dawley rats, the process of fibrosis alternates with periods of lysis of collagen;[89] both of these observations imply that additional factors may be important in affecting whether or not and to what degree fibrosis will occur. Third, there is evidence that a process other than lysosomal rupture is responsible for silica-associated macrophage death. Kane and associates[85] have shown that such death depends on the presence of calcium ions; in their absence, intracellular lysosomal rupture occurs without cell destruction. These authors suggested that macrophage death may be mediated instead by toxic damage to the plasma membrane's function as a permeability barrier. Finally, there is evidence that the time course of silica-induced macrophage injury is much more prolonged *in vivo* than in tissue culture;[81, 91] for this and other reasons, it has been suggested that silica affects macrophages by altering their function while they are still alive rather than by causing their death and dissolution.[81, 92] This in turn suggests that other cells or cell products might be important in the pathogenesis of disease. Lymphocytes, particulary T-helper cells,[768] are increased in number in bronchoalveolar lavage (BAL) fluid in both experimental and clinical silicosis, leading Davis[81] to hypothesize that macrophage-lymphocyte interactions and the production of inflammatory mediators such as interleukin-1 may be important in pathogenesis. There is also evidence that polymorphonuclear leukocytes can modulate the tissue reaction to silica.[81, 93]

In many individuals with silicosis, the finding of an increased number of lymphocytes in both BAL fluid and tissue sections, and the presence of a variety of serologic abnormalities—including rheumatoid factor (RF), antinuclear antibodies (ANA), immune complexes,[94, 95] and a polyclonal increase in gamma-globulin,[95, 96]—and in some cases clinical evidence of immune disturbance,[97, 98] particularly with reference to kidney disease,[97, 98, 99] have suggested the possibility of immune-related tissue damage in the pathogenesis of the disease. Protein adsorbed onto the silicon dioxide can theoretically act as an antigen, and it has been speculated[96] that the silicotic nodule contains antigen-antibody precipitates as well as collagen. Because (1) plasma cells can be prominent in relation to some silicotic nodules[81] and (2) some nodules are reported to contain immunoglobulins,[16] it is possible that a local immunoglobulin reaction might be important. There is also some evidence, both *in vivo*[100] and *in vitro*,[101] that cell-mediated immunity may play a role. Other factors that have been proposed as increasing the risk for the development of silicosis include infective[102] and genetic[103] influences, the latter because of an increased prevalence of HLA-Aw19.

The reasons behind the development of PMF by some individuals and not by others are unclear. Using immunohistochemical techniques, one group of investigators[104] identified fibronectin in PMF lesions of silicosis and other pneumoconioses; however, the significance of this observation is uncertain. In general, a high content of quartz is correlated with the development of conglomerate silicotic masses.[105]

In contrast to the fibrosis associated with chronic, relatively low dose exposure to silica, it is perhaps surprising that acute exposure to large amounts in both animals[106] and humans[107, 108] results in little collagen deposition. Instead, abundant intra-alveolar proteinaceous debris, virtually identical histologically and ultrastructurally to that seen in alveolar proteinosis, is typically produced.[108] The precise pathogenesis of this reaction is unclear. Experimentally, instillation of silica into the lungs has been associated with type 1 alveolar cell injury and concomitant reparative type 2 cell hyperplasia,[93] suggesting that this might be a factor. It is also possible that the silica stimulates type 2 cells to produce excessive alveolar lining material or disturbs the ability of macrophages to handle normally produced material,[109] or a combination of both factors. Vallyathan and colleagues have shown that freshly fractured silica possesses a greater biologic reactivity than the aged form;[769] since acute silicoproteinosis is associated with occupations in which fractured silica is likely to be generated, these authors speculated that this fracture may be important in the pathogenesis of the disease. The reason for the lack of fibrosis in acute silicoproteinosis is also unclear, although it has been shown that coating silica particles with alveolar lining material results in significantly less cytotoxicity for the ingesting macrophages and does not disturb phagocytosis.[110]

Altered macrophage function probably underlies the greater susceptibility to tuberculosis of patients with both fibrotic silicosis and acute silicoproteinosis; *Mycobacterium tuberculosis* grows much more rapidly in cultures of macrophages exposed to sublethal doses of quartz than in those without such exposure.[111]

Pathologic Characteristics

The pathologic features of silicosis have recently been reviewed in detail in a report by the Silicosis and Silicate Disease Committee of the National Institute for Occupational Safety and Health, United States.[770] Grossly, silicotic nodules range from 1 to 10 mm in diameter (although some authorities accept 2 cm as the cutoff between a single nodule and PMF[770]) and typically are more numerous in the upper lobes and parahilar regions than elsewhere (Fig. 12–1). Cut sections show the nodules to be more or less well-defined, spherical or irregularly shaped, and firm to hard in texture; calcification or ossification is occasionally present. Depending on the admixture of other dusts, the nodules and lungs themselves can show varying degrees of pigmentation ranging from slate gray to dense black. Coalescence of nodules results in larger masses that can occupy virtually an entire lobe (PMF) (Fig. 12–2). Such masses are usually associated with adjacent emphysema and may be cavitated

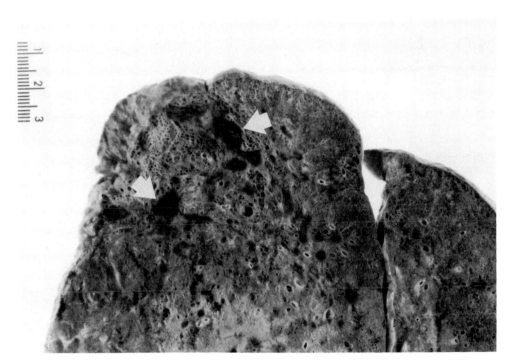

Figure 12–1. Silicosis: Silicotic Nodules. A slice of an upper lobe and superior segment of the lower lobe shows multiple well-defined, somewhat irregularly shaped nodules within the lung parenchyma *(arrows)*. The nodules are black as a result of the presence of abundant anthracotic pigment.

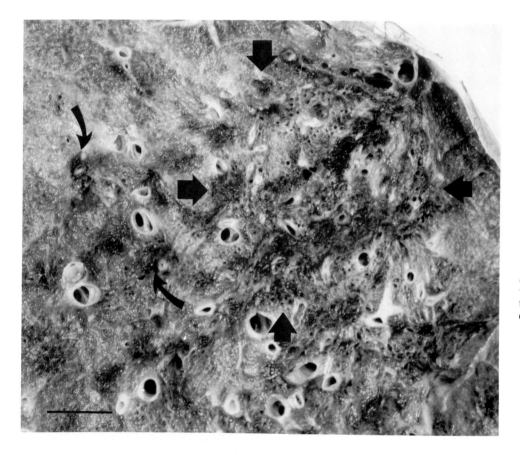

Figure 12–2. Silicosis: Progressive Massive Fibrosis. A magnified view of the posterior segment of the right upper lobe shows several small discrete silicotic nodules *(curved arrows).* In addition, confluence of nodules has resulted in an irregularly shaped area of fibrosis approximately 3 × 4 cm in extent *(indicated by large arrows).* A small focus of emphysema is present in the uppermost region. (Bar = 1 cm).

as a result of ischemia, tuberculosis, or anaerobic infection. Bronchopulmonary and hilar lymph nodes are often somewhat enlarged and rubbery in consistency; extension of fibrous tissue outside the capsule may obscure the limits of the node and is not infrequently associated with distortion of the underlying bronchial anatomy (Fig. 12–3).

Microscopically, the earliest lesions are located characteristically in the peribronchiolar, paraseptal, and subpleural interstitial tissues. Initially, they consist predominantly of macrophages with scattered reticulin fibers. As the lesions enlarge, the central portions become relatively acellular and composed of mature collagen, often in relatively well-defined, more or less concentric lamellae; a peripheral zone of macrophages and lesser numbers of plasma cells and lymphocytes surrounds this central portion (Fig. 12–4). Occasionally, the inflammation may be granulomatous in nature, similar to that seen in Caplan's lesions of coalworker's pneumoconiosis (CWP) (see farther on). Type 2 cells adjacent to the fibrotic region may be hyperplastic and presumably are the source from which these cells have been identified in BAL specimens.[266] In the cellular areas, a variable number of needle-shaped birefringent silicate crystals 1 to 3 μm in length can usually be identified; these can also be seen by metachromatic staining with toluidine blue.[112] Occasionally, the crystals are not apparent with standard microscopy, and more sophisticated examination such as scanning electron microscopy is required to reveal their presence.[113]

The larger conglomerate lesions are also composed of hyalinized collagen, although the concentric lamellar appearance of the smaller nodules is frequently not as evident. Focal necrosis is common in the central portions (Fig. 12–5) and is occasionally associated with granulomatous inflammation, implying tuberculous infection. In one report, anaerobic organisms were cultured from material obtained by transtracheal and transthoracic needle aspiration.[114] The diagnosis of silicosis has been made by needle biopsy; in one study, the core of tissue was considered to be compatible with such a diagnosis in 63 per cent of patients in whom the final diagnosis of silicosis was confirmed.[115]

The pathologic findings in *acute heavy silica exposure* differ dramatically from those described previously. Although there may be mild interstitial fibrosis and focal small nodular lesions, the well-defined collagenous nodule is typically absent. Instead, airspaces are more or less diffusely filled by PAS-positive, finely granular proteinaceous material. Macrophages are present in increased numbers, and adjacent alveolar type 2 cells show a varying degree of hyperplasia. Ultrastructurally, the intra-alveolar material contains macrophages and desquamated type 2 cells as well as numerous aggregates of membranous material resembling that seen in the normal alveolar lining layer.[108]

Macrophage aggregates and fibrotic nodules identical to those found in the lungs can also be identified elsewhere in the body. As might be expected, they are most common in the hilar and mediastinal lymph nodes; in these sites they are sometimes identified in individuals with no history of significant occupational dust exposure.[116] These nodules are also occasionally found in the liver,

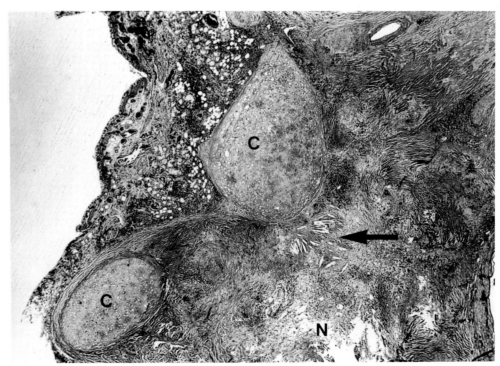

Figure 12–3. Silicosis: Bronchial Wall Fibrosis. A focus of fibrosis caused by silicosis has extended outside a peribronchial lymph node into the adjacent bronchial wall (the node itself is not visible in the illustration). The fibrous tissue and pigment-laden macrophages extend into the submucosa; the bronchial cartilage plates (C) are somewhat distorted. Note the cholesterol clefts *(arrow)* and focal necrosis (N) indicating the histologic changes of progressive massive fibrosis. (× 15.)

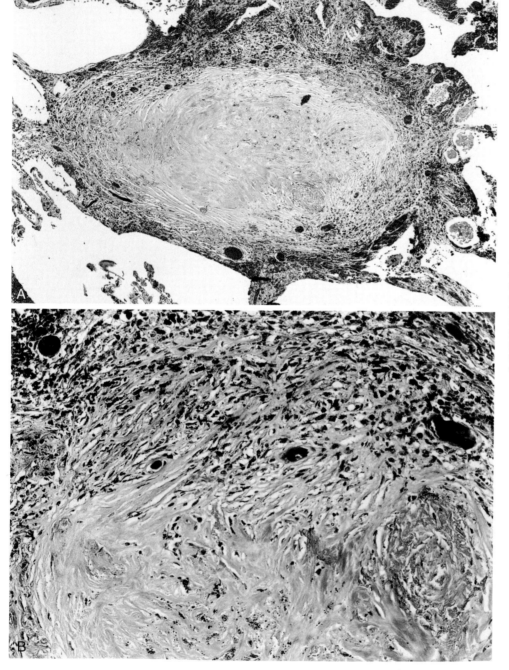

Figure 12–4. Silicotic Nodule. A histologic section *(A)* shows a typical silicotic nodule consisting of a central zone of dense collagen and a peripheral rim of macrophages in which abundant foreign particulate material is situated. A section at higher magnification *(B)* shows these characteristics to better advantage. (*A*, × 40; *B*, × 150.)

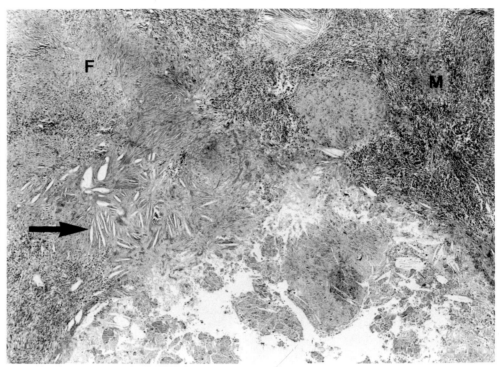

Figure 12–5. Silicosis: Progressive Massive Fibrosis. A histologic section from the central portion of the confluent nodular mass illustrated in Figure 12–2 reveals fibrosis (F), aggregates of pigment-laden macrophages (M), and multiple cholesterol clefts *(arrow)*. The tissue in the lower half of the illustration is necrotic and has undergone liquefaction. (× 25.)

spleen, intra-abdominal lymph nodes, and bone marrow.[99, 117]

Roentgenographic Manifestations

Ten to 20 years' exposure usually is necessary before the appearance of roentgenographic abnormality,[118] although the onset of silicosis sometimes is acute, particularly in patients exposed to high concentrations of dust in a relatively confined area (Figs. 12–6 and 12–7).[119]

The classic roentgenographic pattern of silicosis consists of multiple nodular opacities ranging from 1 to 10 mm in diameter (Fig. 12–8). The nodules tend to be fairly well circumscribed and of uniform density. Profusion can be fairly even throughout both lungs but commonly shows considerable upper zonal predominance. Calcification occurs more frequently than is realized. In one series of 724 miners who showed roentgenographic evidence of pneumoconiosis, calcification of nodules was present in 20 per cent.[120] J. A. Louw and G. K. Sluis-Cremer of the South African Department of Health and Welfare have recently informed us in personal communication that although calcification of silicotic nodules was fairly common in the decades following 1920, the incidence has fallen off dramatically in recent years, possibly as a result of a marked reduction in dust levels in the mines. There is a tendency for calcified nodules to be subpleural in location. We have encountered such calcification only rarely, but its presence creates an awesome appearance on the chest roentgenogram (Fig. 12–9).

The nodular pattern may be preceded by or associated with a reticular pattern—the small irregular opacities of the ILO 1980 classification—which sometimes is the earliest roentgenographic abnormality (Figure 12–10). With nodulation—or even with reticulation only—hilar lymph node enlargement can occur (Figs. 12–6, 12–7, and 12–10), but seldom during either stage is there evidence of pleural abnormality. Although nodularity is usually stressed as the typical roentgenographic pattern in uncomplicated silicosis, correlative studies of roentgenologic and pathologic material suggest that the linear or reticular pattern (including Kerley A and B lines) may be present without visible nodules and may be associated with severe clinical disability.[121] In fact, lack of correlation of roentgenographic appearances and pathologic changes may be considerable. A necropsy study of 100 white gold miners[122] revealed silicotic nodules not apparent on premortem chest roentgenograms in many cases.

Silicosis secondary to diatomaceous earth exposure appears to present a somewhat different roentgenographic pattern from that of quartz silicosis;[57, 58] nodularity either is absent or is so minute that appreciation is extremely difficult. More characteristically, however, a linear or reticular pattern is seen, particularly in the early stages of the disease and predominantly in the upper lung zones. Progressive massive fibrosis and emphysema are common.

The roentgenographic pattern of small round or irregular opacities is commonly referred to as "simple" silicosis, in contrast to "complicated" silicosis, which is characterized by large opacities or conglomerate shadows (Fig. 12–11). Large opacities represent homogeneous areas of consolidation of nonsegmental distribution usually affecting the

Text continued on page 2300

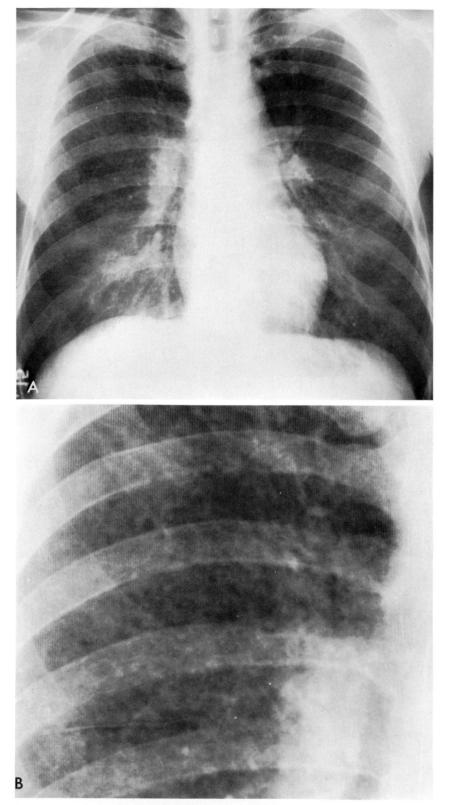

Figure 12–6. *See legend on opposite page.*

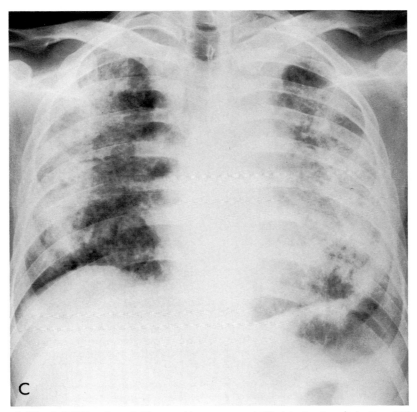

Figure 12–6. *Continued.* **"Acute" Silicosis.** A 29-year-old man was admitted to the hospital with a history of increasing dyspnea for 6 months and cough productive of thick yellow sputum for 1 week. During the previous 3 years, he had been employed full time as a sandblaster inside huge, nonventilated metal tanks. He was provided with a loosely-fitting face mask with a continuous flow of supposedly sand-free air (although the air flow was not filtered). He frequently worked without the air hose connected. On admission, a posteroanterior roentgenogram *(A)* and a magnified view of the right upper lung *(B)* revealed multiple fairly well-circumscribed nodules scattered diffusely throughout both lungs but more numerous in the upper and mid zones. The nodules ranged in size from bare visibility to 3 mm in diameter. Bilateral hilar lymph node enlargement was present. Poorly defined shadows of increased density in both apical zones suggested early conglomeration. Pulmonary function studies showed lung volumes, mixing efficiency, and flow rates to be normal; the diffusing capacity at rest was low and did not rise with exercise. Blood gases and mechanical properties of the lung were within the normal range. Lung biopsy revealed gross disorganization of much of the pulmonary parenchyma suggestive of silicosis. Ashing of the lung biopsy specimen showed a residuum of 20 per cent silicon dioxide. The patient's subsequent course was progressively and rapidly downhill, leading to severe respiratory failure. A roentgenogram 2 years after the initial study *(C)* reveals marked loss of lung volume, much of the lung parenchyma showing a very coarse reticular pattern, which in many areas is confluent as a result of conglomeration.

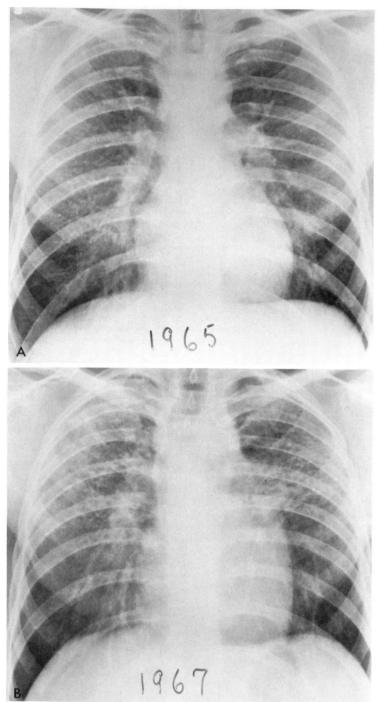

Figure 12–7. Silicosis Showing Rapid Progression. Roentgenograms of a 27-year-old man, brother to the patient illustrated in Figure 12–6 and involved in the same occupation, showed similar but somewhat less "acute" manifestations of his disease. In 1965, a postero-anterior roentgenogram *(A)* revealed diffuse, predominantly irregular opacities more prominent in the upper lung zones; hilar lymph nodes were enlarged. By 1967 *(B)*, lung volume had reduced somewhat, particularly in the upper lung zones (note the upward displacement of both hila). The opacities in the upper lungs were showing early coalescence.

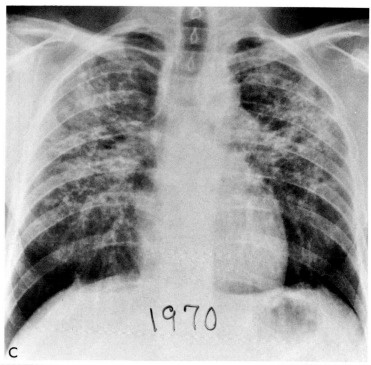

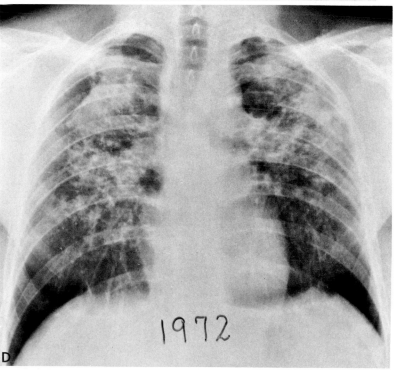

Figure 12–7. *Continued*. Three years later *(C)*, large opacities had developed in the upper lung zones, and by 1972 *(D)*, 7 years after he was originally seen, the large opacities had become much larger. Note the sharply defined lateral margin of the large opacity on the right.

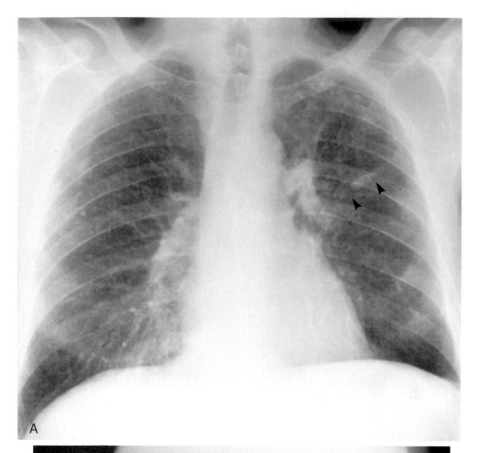

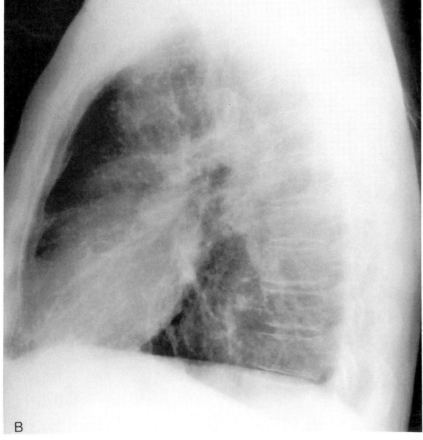

Figure 12–8. Silicosis. Posteroanterior *(A)* and lateral *(B)* chest roentgenograms of a 48-year-old sandblaster reveal an admixture of fine reticular and nodular shadows predominating in the mid and upper lung zones bilaterally. A larger opacity *(arrowheads)* is located in the left upper zone; the left hilum is elevated, and there is faint stippled calcification in the ipsilateral lymph nodes.

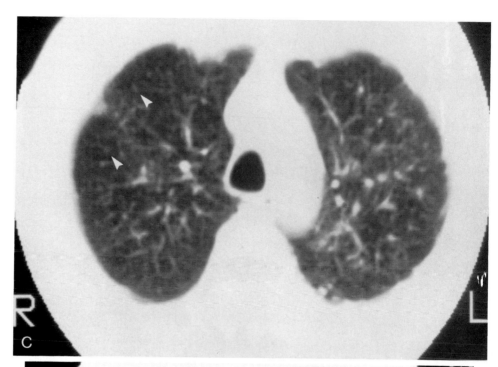

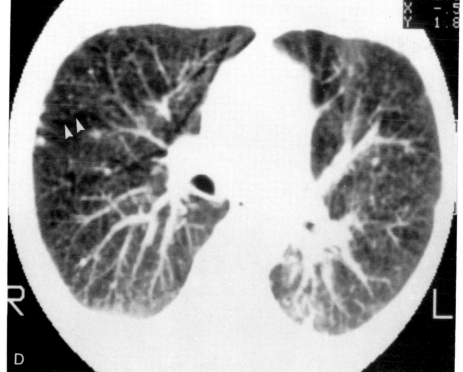

Figure 12–8. *Continued.* CT scans through the upper *(C)* and lower *(D)* thorax confirm the presence of multiple nodules measuring 2 to 5 mm *(arrowheads)*. The larger opacity in *A* proved to be calcified and was assumed to be a healed tuberculous scar.

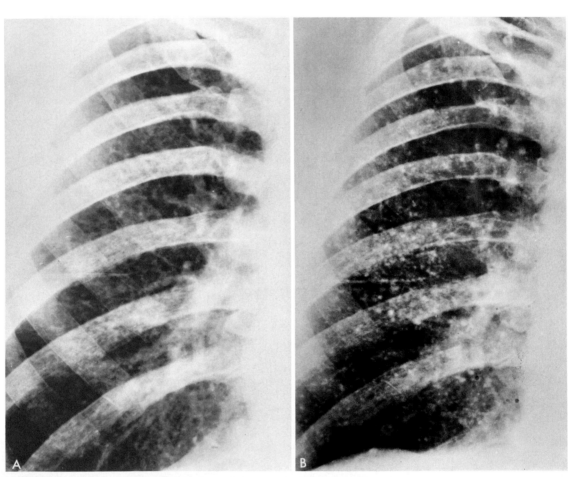

Figure 12–9. Calcification of Silicotic Nodules. *A*, A view of the right hemithorax from a posteroanterior roentgenogram of a 32-year-old South African black man revealed involvement of all lung zones by small irregular opacities of unit density. *B*, Eighteen years later, multiple punctate calcifications had developed throughout the right lung, representing calcification of silicotic nodules. The patient had a history of 26 years in South African gold mines. (Courtesy of Dr. Raymond Glynn-Thomas, Medical Bureau for Occupational Diseases, Johannesburg, South Africa.)

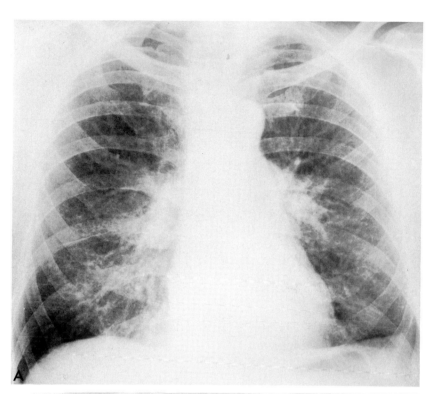

Figure 12–10. Silicosis with Predominant Irregular Opacities. A posteroanterior roentgenogram *(A)* and a magnified view of the upper portion of the right lung *(B)* reveal a rather coarse reticular pattern evenly distributed throughout both lungs. Hilar lymph nodes are enlarged bilaterally. This patient, a 57-year-old man, had worked underground in a gold mine for many years.

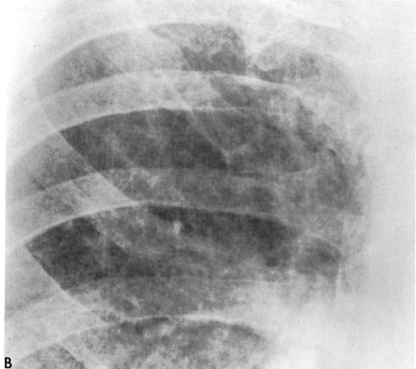

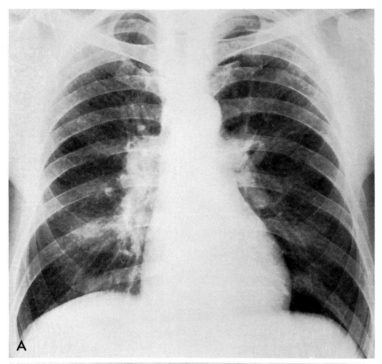

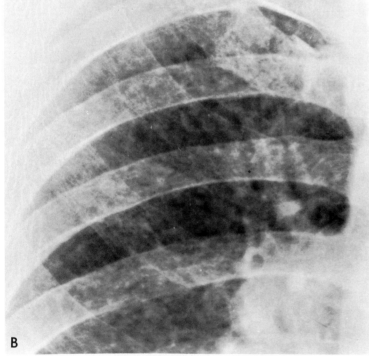

Figure 12–11. Silicosis Progressing from Simple to Conglomerate. A 54-year-old foundry worker was asymptomatic at the time of the roentgenogram reproduced in *A.* The opacities throughout both lungs are predominantly small and rounded, although possessing a reticular component, and are more evident in the upper and mid zones than in the bases. The nodules are relatively discrete, as revealed in a magnified view of the right upper lung *(B).* An exceptional degree of hilar lymph node enlargement is present bilaterally.

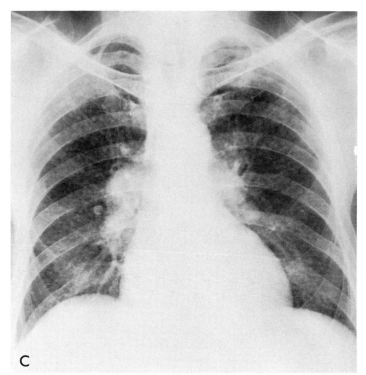

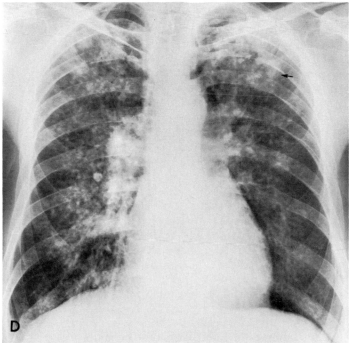

Figure 12–11. *Continued.* Four years later *(C)*, the nodules are more numerous and in the subapical zones bilaterally have become confluent so as to form shadows of homogeneous density (conglomeration). A roentgenogram *(D)* taken 7 years after *C* reveals marked progression of the disease; not only are the nodules more numerous, but their density is considerably greater than had been observed earlier. By this time, confluence of shadows in the subapical zones had progressed considerably, and one of the confluent shadows on the left had undergone cavitation *(arrow)*.

upper lobes and measuring more than 1 cm in diameter; they may become very large (Fig. 12–12), some even exceeding the volume of an upper lobe. The shadow margins sometimes are irregular and somewhat ill-defined, with multiple "pseudopodia" extending outward from their edges;[123] perhaps more commonly, however, the lateral margin can be very smooth, creating an interface that parallels the lateral chest wall. These shadows represent confluence of individual silicotic nodules, sometimes associated with superimposed tuberculous infection. They commonly develop in the midzone or periphery of the lung and tend to migrate later toward the hilum, leaving overinflated emphysematous lung tissue between the consolidation and the pleural surface (Figure 12–13).[124] The more extensive the progressive massive fibrosis, the less the apparent nodularity in the remainder of the lungs.[124] This unique characteristic presumably is caused by gradual incorporation of nodular lesions into the massive consolidation in the upper lungs. The conglomerate lesions may cavitate (Figure 12–11). In an arteriographic study of six patients with silicosis, four with large and two with small opacities, Tada and associates[125] selectively opacified the bronchial arteries and in all four cases with large opacities found enlargement of the bronchial arterial trunk, considerable neovascularization, and peripheral bronchopulmonary arterial shunts. The findings were compatible with any chronic inflammatory process in the lungs. The two patients with small opacities showed normal bronchial arteries.

Hilar lymph node enlargement is a common roentgenographic finding and may occur at any stage of silicosis.[124] So-called egg-shell calcification is caused by the deposition of calcium salts in the periphery of enlarged lymph nodes and is almost pathognomonic of silicosis (Fig. 12–14), although it is seen occasionally in sarcoidosis.[126] Of 1,905 cases of silicosis reported by Bellini, it was identified in 4.7 per cent,[127] and its occurrence in coal and metal miners was attributed by him to exposure to silicon dioxide.[128] Egg-shell calcification involves not only the hilar lymph nodes[127] but also (rarely) lymph nodes in the anterior and posterior mediastinum, the thoracic wall,[127] and the intraperitoneal and retroperitoneal areas.[126] Enlarged lymph nodes with peripheral calcification and without pulmonary parenchymal lesions have been described in miners but must be a rare presenting picture in silicosis.[128] Enlarged silicotic nodes may encroach upon the phrenic nerve, resulting in unilateral diaphragmatic paralysis.[129]

Two other variants of the classic roentgenographic changes of the disease are the acute silicosis of sandblasters (see Figs. 12–6 and 12–7) and the nodular lesions of Caplan's syndrome.[130] Acute silicoproteinosis is associated with a pattern of diffuse airspace disease, similar if not identical to that of alveolar proteinosis.[131] Caplan's syndrome consists of the presence of large necrobiotic nodules super-

imposed on a background of simple silicosis (Fig. 12–15). It is a manifestation of rheumatoid lung disease and is seen more commonly in CWP than in silicosis. In a controlled study of patients who had silicosis with and without rheumatoid arthritis,[132] the rate of progression of the silicosis was found to be greater in the former, as was the probability that the silicosis was manifested by larger nodules (type r) at the time of presentation.[132]

Roentgenographic progression of silicosis after removal from exposure is a well-accepted phenomenon. In a study of 1,902 workers who had no roentgenographic evidence of PMF a maximum of 4 years before leaving the occupation, 172 subsequently developed PMF on follow-up examination.[133] Despite the development of conglomerate lesions after leaving employment, this cohort of workers showed no overall progression or regression of the grades of simple pneumoconiosis.

Two groups of workers have reported the results of studies designed to test the value of computed tomography (CT) in the assessment of silicosis. In a study of 58 workers with long-term exposure to silica in the granite and foundry industries of Quebec, Bégin and associates[135, 771] found that CT and conventional chest roentgenograms yielded similar average scores for the detection (profusion) of small nodules but that CT identified significantly more coalescence and large opacities in patients with simple silicosis. Similar results were obtained by Bergin and colleagues[134] in their study of 17 patients, particularly with respect to the evaluation of profusion of small opacities; however, this group also found that emphysema associated with silicosis was easily detected on CT but not on conventional roentgenograms.

Clinical Manifestations

SYMPTOMS AND SIGNS

The diagnosis of silicosis usually is based on the identification of a diffuse nodular or reticulonodular pattern on the chest roentgenogram of a patient with an occupational history compatible with exposure to dust containing high concentrations of silicon dioxide. Although most hazardous occupations have been recognized for many years and the majority have been rendered less risky through preventive measures, new sources of significant silica exposure are still being identified, such as that of bentonite workers in Wyoming.[69] Many patients are totally asymptomatic when first seen. Some may complain of shortness of breath, first noted on exertion only but becoming progressively more severe as the roentgenographic changes worsen. With progressive destruction of functioning pulmonary tissue, pulmonary hypertension develops, resulting in cor pulmonale and, eventually, right-sided heart failure.

Dyspnea was found to be more common in a group of patients with roentgenographic evidence

Text continued on page 2306

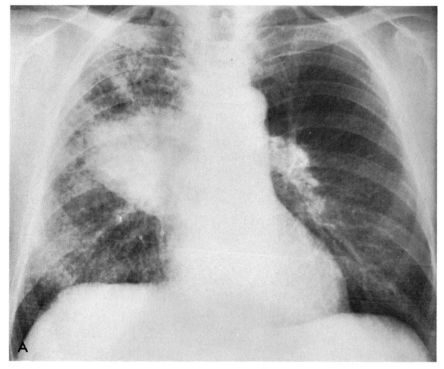

Figure 12–12. Silicosis with Conglomeration (PMF). A posteroanterior roentgenogram *(A)* of a 58-year-old miner reveals combined rounded and irregular opacities throughout both lungs, much more marked on the right than on the left. Large nodular shadows measuring up to 8 mm in diameter are present throughout the apical and subapical zones of the right lung, and a large mass of homogeneous density is situated in the parahilar area. A tomographic section of the right lung *(B)* shows the homogeneity of the large parahilar mass to be disturbed by a well-defined air bronchogram; the mass is remarkably well circumscribed. At thoracotomy, the mass was found to be extremely hard in consistency; biopsy revealed typical conglomerate silicosis. Although such an appearance could be produced by bronchogenic carcinoma associated with silicosis, the presence of the air bronchogram should favor the diagnosis of PMF.

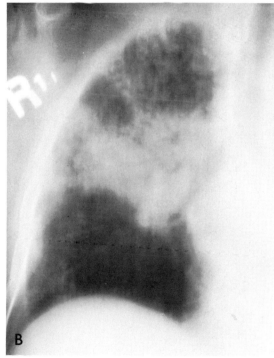

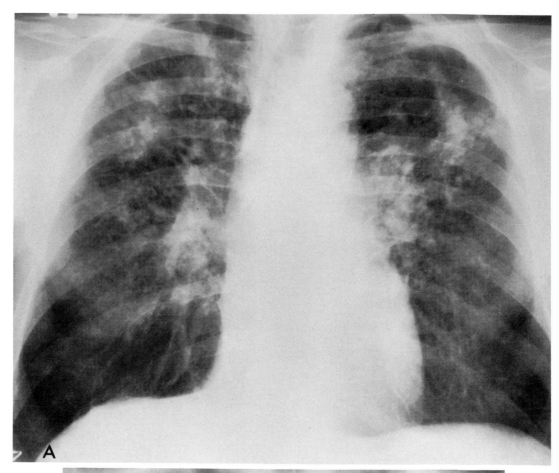

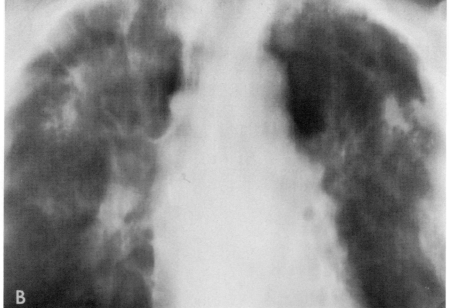

Figure 12–13. Silicosis with Conglomeration (PMF).   A posteroanterior roentgenogram *(A)* and an anteroposterior tomogram *(B)* of a 54-year-old foundry worker reveal extensive irregular opacities involving predominantly the upper and mid lung zones. In the subapical regions bilaterally, poorly defined shadows of homogeneous density represent large opacities (category B).

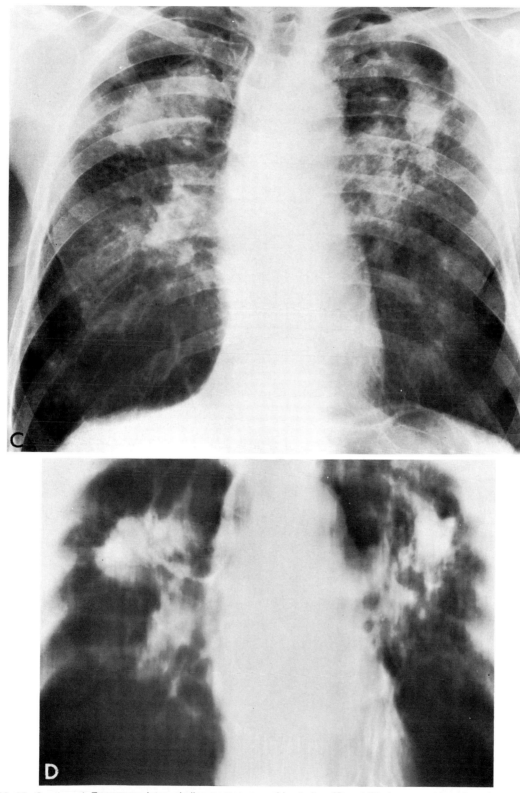

Figure 12–13. *Continued.* Four years later, similar roentgenographic studies *(C* and *D)* show considerable enlargement of the large opacities, which are now category C. Most of the enlargement appears to have occurred hilarward, suggesting medial "migration" of the lesions. The lung peripheral to the zones of PMF has shown a loss of markings, suggesting the development of emphysema; the lower lung zones also have shown signs of progressive emphysema.

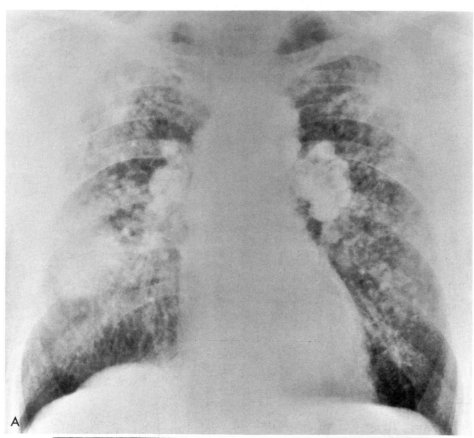

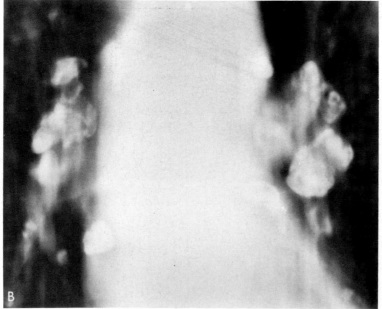

Figure 12–14. Eggshell Calcification of Lymph Nodes in Silicosis. A 62-year-old man had worked in a foundry for 30 years. A posteroanterior roentgenogram *(A)* reveals general involvement of both lungs by small rounded opacities with conglomeration in the upper lobes bilaterally and in the right lower zone. Extensive calcification of hilar lymph nodes is readily apparent. An anteroposterior tomogram of the hilar region *(B)* reveals dense calcification of the nodes bilaterally, the distribution being largely peripheral. (Courtesy of Dr. J. F. Meakins, Royal Victoria Hospital, Montreal.)

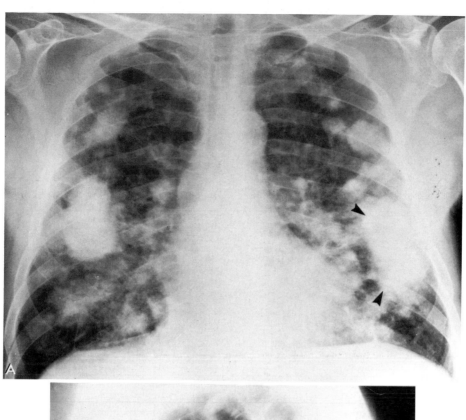

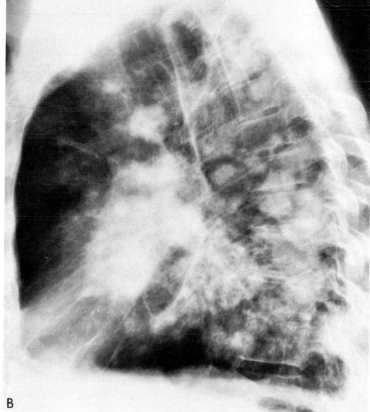

Figure 12–15. Caplan's Syndrome.   Posteroanterior *(A)* and lateral *(B)* roentgenograms reveal a multitude of fairly well-circumscribed nodules ranging in diameter from 1 to 5 cm, scattered randomly throughout both lungs with no notable anatomic predilection. No cavitation is apparent, nor is there evidence of calcification. This patient, a 56-year-old man, had been a coal miner for many years and in recent years had developed arthralgia, which proved to be due to rheumatoid arthritis. As a means of establishing the nature of the pulmonary nodules, a percutaneous needle aspiration was carried out on the large mass situated in the lower portion of the left lung *(arrowheads in A)*: several milliliters of inky black fluid were aspirated. The necrotic nature of this mass was thus established, as was the presence of large quantities of coal dust within it.

Illustration continued on following page

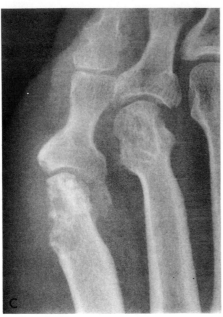

Figure 12–15 *Continued* A view of the fourth and fifth metatarsophalangeal joints of the right foot *(C)* shows changes typical of moderately advanced rheumatoid arthritis. (Courtesy of Dr. Michael O'Donavan, Montreal General Hospital.)

of silicosis than among a control group matched for silica exposure, age, and gender whose chest roentgenograms were normal.[136] In a series of hospitalized patients with silicosis, rales and wheezes were found to be present in the majority;[137] however, in our experience, asymptomatic ambulatory patients with silicosis usually have no adventitial signs on auscultation; this is in contrast to asbestos-exposed individuals, who often have bilateral rales despite an absence of roentgenographic abnormality in the chest. As with many other chronic pulmonary diseases, silicosis is accompanied by a rise in angiotensin converting enzyme, although usually when the reaction is more granulomatous in nature;[138–140] high levels of this enzyme in the serum have been found to correlate with active progression of the disease.[140]

Unlike many other inhalation diseases caused by inorganic and organic dusts, the fibrosis and associated disability in silicosis frequently are progressive, even after removal of the patient from the dusty environment.[132, 141] Thus, it is not uncommon for these patients to present with symptoms many years after leaving the occupation responsible for the dust exposure. This is an important point to remember, because only a complete occupational history, ranging over a patient's entire working life, may provide the clue to the diagnosis.

In contrast to classic chronic silicosis, in which the great majority of patients are asymptomatic and an exposure of 10 to 20 years is required before the disease becomes roentgenographically manifest, an acute, rapidly progressive form has been recognized since the turn of the century, when more than 10 per cent of 1,000 men who milled quartzite ore in Nevada died of silicosis after less than 5 years of dust exposure.[142] In 1929, the development of acute and accelerated silicosis was reported in the scouring powder industry.[72, 73] More recently, silicoproteinosis has been described in tunnelers[145] and sandblasters.[107, 144, 772] These workers often remove their masks after sandblasting and then proceed to paint in the dusty atmosphere; they usually die in respiratory failure, not uncommonly with a complicating pneumothorax.[144]

Although the combination of a positive history and typical roentgenographic changes usually suffices to permit confident diagnosis in most cases, confirmation may be required for such purposes as medical compensation. Pathologic examination by simple microscopy of material obtained by needle biopsy[115, 145] or direct lung biopsy may confirm the diagnosis. In some cases, more specialized procedures may be used, such as the chemical determination of ash content, scanning electron microscopy, and x-ray energy spectrometry.[51, 146] Regardless of the validity of such methods, often it is necessary to prove *clinical disability*, and for this purpose pulmonary function tests are essential.

PULMONARY FUNCTION TESTS

Function may be normal in the early stages of disease.[147, 148] When dyspnea is present, impairment of function may be obstructive or restrictive, or a combination of both.[149] Diffusing capacity may be decreased,[147, 149] and the combination of this finding with hyperinflation and decrease in flow rates constitutes a pattern of functional impairment identical to that of uncomplicated pulmonary emphysema. In fact, because miners are usually cigarette smokers, difficulty may be encountered in assessing the specific factor responsible for pulmonary dysfunction. Further compounding the situation is the distinct possibility that symptoms of cough and dyspnea may be caused by chronic bronchitis secondary to a nonspecific effect from the dust itself. In a study of 1,973 white gold miners in South Africa,[150] symptoms of chronic bronchitis were equally common in patients with and without silicosis. However, although mean forced vital capacity (FVC) was the same in the two groups, forced expiratory volume in 1 second (FEV_1) and midexpiratory flow were significantly lower in the silicotic group, two findings almost entirely attributable to their higher exposure to dust in the mines. Although arterial oxygen saturation may be normal at rest, exercise often gives rise to hypoxemia, at least in patients with progressive massive fibrosis.[149, 771] In the late stages of the disease, carbon dioxide retention may develop.[151]

Relationship to Pulmonary Tuberculosis

There appears to be little question that silicosis predisposes to tuberculosis. It is customary to suspect this complication with the development of PMF, although sputum cultures of acid-fast bacilli are positive in as many patients with nodular opacities alone as in those with conglomerate shadows.[152] Even PMF does not necessarily indicate the presence of tuberculous infection, because such shadows may develop in patients in whom the response to repeated Mantoux testing is negative.[153] It may be extremely difficult to isolate tubercle bacilli during life in patients with progressive massive fibrosis, despite subsequent postmortem demonstration of active tuberculous infection.[152] A study carried out in Sweden found that the incidence of tuberculosis was significantly higher in silicotic subjects than in control subjects; in addition, individuals who developed silicosis in the mining, quarrying, and tunneling occupations showed a higher risk of lung cancer.[154]

COAL AND CARBON

The inhalation and retention in the lung of dust composed predominantly of carbon (often termed "anthracosis") is seen in many individuals,[155] particularly those who smoke or live in a city or industrial environment. Microscopically, such material is easily recognized as dense black particles, mostly 1 to 2 μm in size, within macrophages adjacent to terminal or proximal respiratory bronchioles and in the pleura. The material is also commonly present in bronchopulmonary, hilar, and mediastinal lymph nodes. Although predominantly composed of carbon, the particles also contain traces of other substances, such as silica and iron. Nevertheless, associated fibrosis or emphysema is invariably minimal or absent (except when associated with cigarette smoking), and it is generally believed that the presence of such particles is of no pathologic or functional significance.

Such innocuous environmental anthracosis is caused by the inhalation of relatively small amounts of dust; it is clear, however, that inhalation of large amounts of carbonaceous material, either in the form of coal dust or as substances derived from coal or petroleum products, can be associated with significant pulmonary disease. Because quantity is important in this effect, disease occurs almost exclusively in the workplace, where the concentration of these materials is much greater than that in nonoccupational settings. The most important occupation in terms of the number of individuals affected is coal mining, the resulting disease being called appropriately *coalworker's pneumoconiosis*. Workers involved in the production or use of graphite,[156–160] carbon black,[161] and carbon electrodes[162] are affected less often. The possibility that pulmonary disease can occasionally be caused by inhalation of fly-ash has also been suggested.[163]

Epidemiology

Coal is a sedimentary rock formed by the action of pressure, temperature, and chemical reactions on vegetable material. The percentage of pure carbon varies with different types, brown coal and lignite containing the least and anthracite the most.[164] The degree of exposure to carbon dust thus depends to some extent on the type of coal being mined, a feature that at least in part may explain the variability in incidence of CWP from colliery to colliery. Perhaps more important in this regard are local geologic variations;[165] some coal seams are very thick (up to 100 feet),[164] whereas others are much thinner and are separated by seams of siliceous rock. Mining in the latter situation can result in a significant concomitant exposure to silica and other substances, a feature that probably explains the occurrence of classic silicosis in a small percentage of coal miners.[165–168] Certain occupations within the coal mine can also influence the probability of developing disease and the form that it may take; for example, because the majority of dust is produced at the coal face, workers of cutting and loading machines are exposed to the highest concentration of coal dust,[164] whereas surface coal miners drilling through quartz[167] and workers involved in the maintenance or construction of underground roadways or the transportation of coal to the surface by railway (during which time sand may be put on the rails to increase traction) are more likely to come in contact with silica.[164]

Although the great majority of reports on CWP have originated in the United Kingdom and continental Europe, the disease is also recognized in the United States.[170–180] Epidemiologic studies carried out in the early 1970s in the Appalachian region showed approximately 10 per cent of coal miners to have pneumoconiosis and about a third of these to have progressive massive fibrosis (PMF).[169, 181] A more recent assessment of 1,438 surface coal miners in the United States revealed 59 (4 per cent) to have roentgenographic evidence of pneumoconiosis; only seven of these patients were interpreted as having opacities in category 2 or higher.[182] Most of the affected miners had worked in underground coal mines for prolonged periods. Similarly, in Great Britain[179] there has been a significant decline in the incidence of coal worker's pneumoconiosis of category 2 or more, attributed to both a decrease in the number of coal miners and a drop in the levels of dust concentration. Three decades ago, the incidence of PMF was particularly high in South Wales, a fact Cochrane[183] attributed to the very young age at which boys began work at the coal face in that area.

Fly-ash is the solid residue that remains after the combustion of coal; the particles so formed are composed of a variety of elements, including silicon, aluminum, and iron.[163] Workers in occupations associated with a high concentration of fly-ash are theoretically at risk for developing pneumoconiosis; in fact, a high content of such particles has been demonstrated in the lungs of some individuals with pulmonary fibrosis.[163] Nevertheless, the majority of clinical and experimental evidence suggests that this material is not fibrogenic.[184]

Graphite (crystalline carbon) occurs both naturally as a mineral and as an artificial substance derived from heated coal or coke. It is used in the manufacture of steel, lubricants, lead pencils, nuclear reactors, and electrodes,[52] and in electrotyping.[160] Pulmonary disease identical to CWP has been described in individuals engaged in these occupations.[156–160] In the lungs, crystals of graphite are coated with deposits of iron-enriched protein[185] and can be recognized in tissue sections and by digestion techniques.[186]

Carbon black is produced from the flames of natural gas and various petroleum products. It is used as a filler in rubber,[161] plastics, records, and inks, and in the manufacture of carbon paper and carbon electrodes. Rare examples of pneumoconiosis attributed to heavy exposure during the manufacture of such products have been reported.[161, 162, 187] In a report of the results of a survey of process workers and their environment in a factory producing *continuous filament carbon fiber*, the manufacture of which was begun some 20 years ago, no evidence of ill effects on the lungs was found by roentgenographic, spirometric, or clinical assessments.[188]

Pathologic, roentgenographic, and clinical findings in workers exposed to large amounts of carbon in whatever form are similar; however, because the vast majority of such individuals are involved in coal mining, the literature reflects this fact and much of the following description relates to CWP.

Pathogenesis and Pathologic Characteristics

The two morphologic findings characteristic of CWP are the *coal macule* and PMF.[164, 189, 190] The former is characterized by deposits of anthracotic pigment unassociated with fibrosis, a finding sometimes referred to as "simple" pneumoconiosis. PMF is defined as a focus of irregular fibrosis and pigment deposition larger than 1 cm in diameter and is sometimes designated "complicated" pneumoconiosis. In addition, small foci of fibrous tissue and pigmented macrophages, comprising so-called nodular lesions,[164, 190] can be found in many cases, unassociated with features of PMF.

Grossly, coal macules are stellate or round, nonpalpable black foci that range in size from 1 to 5 mm (Fig. 12–16); they are scattered fairly uniformly throughout the lung parenchyma, although they tend to be more numerous at the apex than at the base. In uncomplicated disease, lung tissue between the macules is typically relatively normal in

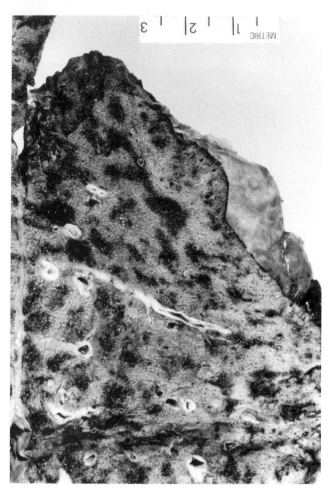

Figure 12–16. Coalworker's Pneumoconiosis: The Coal Macule. A magnified view of the superior segment of a lower lobe shows multiple foci of dense black pigmentation that are of irregular shape but are fairly evenly spaced. Emphysema is present but is difficult to appreciate in this thick formalin-fixed section. Note also the dense zone of subpleural pigment deposition.

structure and color, although interlobular septa and peribronchial connective tissue and lymph nodes are usually also heavily pigmented. Microscopically, the macule relates to respiratory bronchioles and consists of numerous pigment-laden macrophages in the interstitium (Fig. 12–17); fine reticulin fibers can be identified between the macrophages, but mature collagen is minimal or absent. Aggregates of pigment-laden macrophages can also be seen in adjacent alveolar airspaces, especially in lung tissue derived from active miners. Depending on the type of coal or form of carbon dust that has been inhaled,[164] the particulate material within the macrophages differs somewhat in shape, size, color, and translucency. Ferruginous bodies composed of coal can be identified occasionally (Fig. 12–18); they are similar to those that occur with asbestos exposure, except for having relatively large, black cores. Although the coal macule is the characteristic feature of CWP, it should be emphasized that identical lesions can be found in individuals in other envi-

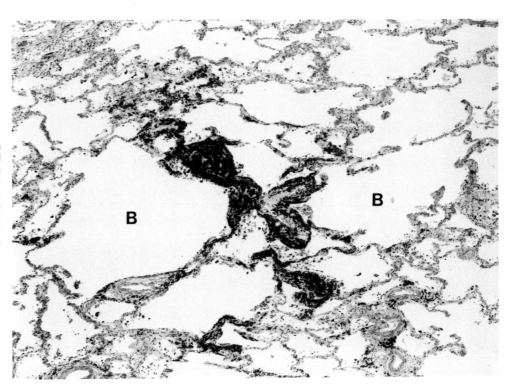

Figure 12–17. Coalworker's Pneumoconiosis: The Coal Macule. A histologic section shows numerous alveolar macrophages containing abundant anthracotic pigment situated in the interstitial tissue adjacent to respiratory bronchioles (B). No fibrosis is evident. The bronchioles are moderately dilated. (× 40.)

ronments,[155] and the simple presence of a "macule" does not necessarily constitute evidence of occupational dust exposure. Microscopic foci of macrophage aggregates similar to those in the coal macule can also be identified in regional lymph nodes and occasionally outside the thorax in tissues such as bone marrow.[194]

Bronchioles adjacent to the macrophage aggregates in the macules are frequently distended (Fig. 12–17), a finding often designated "focal emphysema."[170, 181] The pathogenesis of this abnormality has been debated. It was suggested by Gough and Heppleston[195] that involvement of the parenchyma around the respiratory bronchioles prevents expansion of this tissue, so that the tension normally expended on surrounding alveoli during inspiration is instead transmitted to the respiratory bronchioles. This process, together with atrophy of bronchiolar smooth muscle, was hypothesized to be the major cause of dilatation of respiratory bronchioles. On the basis of a necropsy study of fixed inflated lungs, Duguid and Lambert[196] proposed instead that as dust is deposited on alveolar lining cells to form anthracotic foci, consolidation, organization, fibrosis, and shrinkage occur, with focal emphysema developing as a compensatory process. Other investigators have questioned both these views and have suggested that focal emphysema is basically similar to the more common centrilobular emphysema associated with cigarette smoking.[155, 197]

Palpable gray or black nodules smaller than 1 cm in diameter can also be found in the lungs of many coal workers. Although these are described separately, it is important to realize that at the light microscopic level they blend imperceptibly with the macule on the one hand and with PMF on the other,[198] and it is likely that the nodules represent steps in a spectrum of changes rather than pathogenetically distinct lesions. The nodules can be stellate or round and are fairly well delimited from adjacent lung. They have a variable histologic composition, some consisting of a haphazard mixture of pigment-laden macrophages, free dust, and reticulin and collagen fibers (Fig. 12–19), and others possessing a relatively discrete central zone of pigment-free collagen surrounded by pigment-laden macrophages resembling small silicotic nodules. Degenerative changes identical to those seen in PMF are present occasionally.[164] Other palpable nodules, such as rheumatoid nodules of Caplan's syndrome (see page 1216) and infectious granulomas, are present less frequently.

Nodular lesions or masses larger than 1 cm (or, according to some definitions, 2 or even 3 cm)[190] are arbitrarily termed *progressive massive fibrosis*. Despite this designation, it should be understood that some lesions do not appear to be progressive, and according to the size definition, many are clearly not massive. Nevertheless, the term is firmly entrenched in the literature and will continue to be used in this text. The lesions of PMF are easily palpable and are firm or somewhat rubbery and either round or stellate. They may be unilateral or bilateral, and develop most often in the posterior segment of an upper lobe or superior segment of a lower lobe,[162, 195, 200] a localization that is thought by some to be related to poor lymphatic drainage.[27] The lesion can extend across a fissure into an

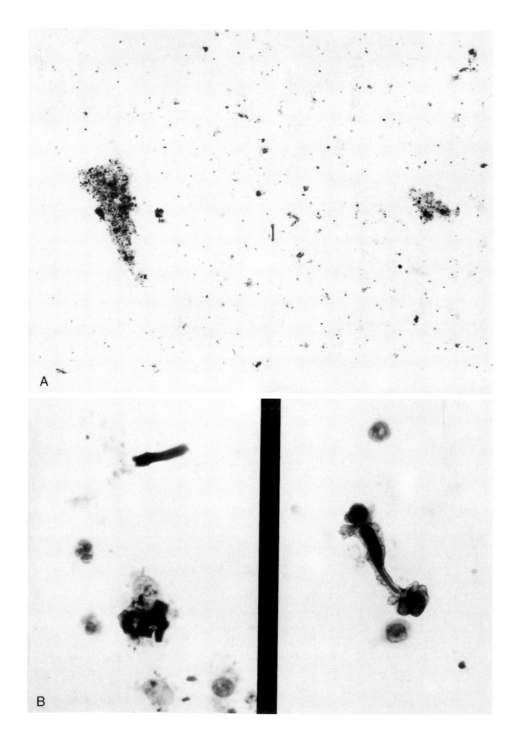

Figure 12–18. Coalworker's Pneumoconiosis: Transthoracic Needle Aspirate. A filter preparation from a transthoracic needle aspirate *(A)* shows single and clustered cells, many of which appear to contain foreign material. Magnified views of two foci *(B)* show this material to be black, irregular in shape, and localized both within macrophages (on the left) and free (on the right). The latter particle is a ferruginous body, consisting of a central black core (representing the coal particle) and a transparent somewhat nodular iron-protein coat. This material was aspirated from a patient with an upper lobe mass that looked like a carcinoma. *(A,* × 100; *B,* × 800; Papanicolaou stain.)

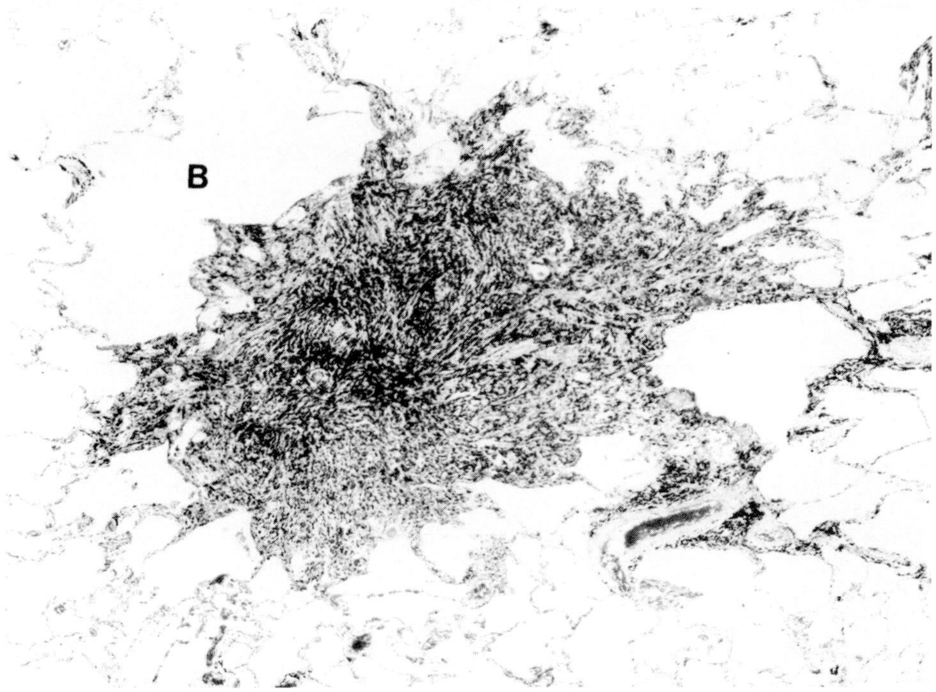

Figure 12–19. Coalworker's Pneumoconiosis: Nodular Lesion. A histologic section shows a stellate focus of pigmented macrophages adjacent to two respiratory bronchioles, one of which is mildly dilated (B). Connective tissue stains showed abundant reticulin fibers but only mild collagen deposition. In contrast to the typical coal macule, this lesion was grossly palpable. ($\times$ 40.)

adjacent lobe. Adjacent emphysema is not uncommon. Cut section often reveals a center of necrotic dark black fluid that can be washed away, leaving a cavity. In most cases, the pathogenesis of the necrosis is ischemia;[201, 202] as discussed later, vascular obliteration both within and adjacent to the region of PMF is a common histologic feature, and, in fact, avascular zones can be demonstrated by lung perfusion scanning.[178] Occasionally, cavitation is caused by tuberculous infection.

The microscopic features of PMF are similar to those of the smaller palpable nodules already described. Bundles of haphazardly arranged, sometimes hyalinized bands of collagen are interspersed with numerous pigment-laden macrophages and abundant free pigment; the latter tends to be more evident in the central regions (Fig. 12–20). Foci of degenerated and frankly necrotic tissue, cholesterol clefts, and chronic inflammatory cells are often present. Although the hyalinized tissue is usually assumed to be collagen, biochemical analysis has shown a high proportion of a noncollagenous, insoluble protein,[203] at least some of which is probably fibronectin.[204] Airways and blood vessels can be incorporated within and destroyed by the expanding fibrotic process (Fig. 12–20), and vessels at the periphery of the lesion frequently show endarteritis obliterans.

The etiology and pathogenesis of PMF are unclear, and several agents or processes, either alone or in combination, may be responsible. The lesion is more likely to occur in coal workers with heavy dust exposure and with large amounts of dust

in the lungs at autopsy, suggesting that the quantity of coal dust itself may be important.[180, 205, 206–209] Seal and colleagues[210] found a high degree of correlation between the presence of PMF and the degree and type of associated pathologic change in perihilar lymph nodes; in this preliminary study, they hypothesized that increasing dust concentration in these nodes results in obliteration of nodal architecture and eventually in the spread of dust outside the capsule and into the wall of adjacent pulmonary arteries and bronchi; rupture through the bronchial wall can then send dust-laden cells back into the lungs to produce PMF.

Because classic silicosis is associated with lesions that are similar both pathologically and radiologically to those of coalworker's PMF, it has been suggested that contamination of coal dust by silica may be responsible for these lesions.[198] However, at least three observations militate against the involvement of silica in the pathogenesis of PMF in most workers exposed to coal dust: (1) there is a wide variation in the amount of silica in the lungs of coalworkers with PMF;[164] (2) in at least some studies, the severity of CWP is more closely related to total dust content of the lung than to the concentration of quartz;[179] and (3) workers involved with carbon black or carbon electrodes who are exposed almost exclusively to carbon sometimes develop lesions similar to those that occur in underground coalworkers.[157, 160–162, 187] Despite the foregoing observations, it is possible that silica is responsible for the development of PMF in some cases; in their study of the lungs of 490 British coal miners, Davis and

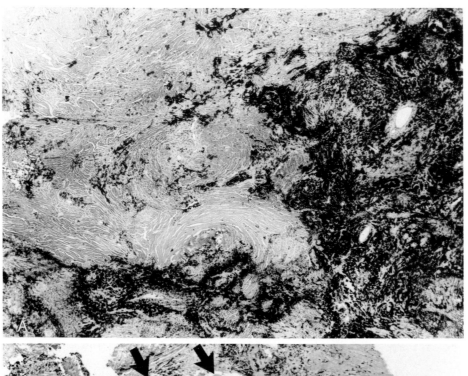

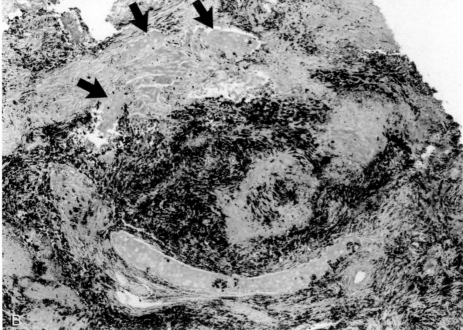

Figure 12–20. Coalworker's Pneumoconiosis: Progressive Massive Fibrosis. A histologic section *(A)* from a 4-cm mass in the upper lobe of a retired coalworker shows abundant anthracotic pigment as well as extensive collagen deposition. No necrosis is evident. At slightly higher magnification, another focus *(B)* shows the lumen of a subsegmental bronchus completely obliterated by similar tissue (*arrows* denote residual, partly destroyed cartilage plates). (*A*, × 25; *B*, × 35.)

colleagues[198] found evidence for two distinct histologic varieties of PMF, one apparently formed by conglomeration of several nodular lesions and the other by enlargement of a single lesion. The two patterns were associated with lung dust content and with colliery rank, the former being associated with low colliery rank and the latter with high colliery rank; the authors suggested that the effect of silica (perhaps itself affected by the presence of other inhaled substances such as kaolinite and mica) might be important in pathogenesis.

In the past, an increased mortality rate from tuberculosis in coal miners and the frequent isolation of mycobacteria from the lesions of PMF[164, 211] suggested that tuberculosis might be responsible in part for the development of these lesions. More recent studies have suggested, however, that these relationships are rather weak,[164] and it now seems likely that tuberculosis is a complicating rather than a pathogenetic feature of PMF.

The presence in coal miners of hypergammaglobulinemia,[212] rheumatoid factor, and antinuclear or anti-lung antibodies has raised the possibility of an immunologic mechanism in the pathogenesis of CWP. Although titers of rheumatoid factor and antibodies have been found to be higher than in control subjects before the development of roentgenographic abnormality,[213] in most series levels have been shown to rise with increasing severity of roentgenographically determined category of disease.[213-218] In one study, the incidence of humoral anti-lung antibodies and lymphocyte-mediated cellular cytotoxicity was found to be higher in smoking than in nonsmoking miners.[219]

Caplan[220] originally reported the association between rheumatoid arthritis and CWP (see page 1216). In addition, he and his coworkers[216] described an increased incidence of rheumatoid factor in miners with the r type of small rounded opacities and in those with irregular, large opacities unassociated with overt rheumatoid arthritis. Other studies have confirmed and extended these observations. For example, in one investigation of 109 coalworkers with pneumoconiosis, circulating antinuclear antibody and rheumatoid factor were found in 13 per cent of miners with simple pneumoconiosis and in 45 per cent of those with category C PMF.[214] Other studies have shown positive test results for rheumatoid factor in 30 to 40 per cent[215] and for antinuclear antibodies in 74 per cent[217] of patients with PMF. In addition, lung-reactive antibodies have been identified in the serum of miners[221] and in rats and mice exposed to coal dust.[222] Although positive titers of these serum antibodies are not in the same range as those found in connective tissue diseases, in most cases their level has been recorded as at least 1/10, a finding observed in only 2 to 3 per cent of the normal male population.[214] Tissue-bound rheumatoid factor and antinuclear antibodies have been demonstrated in some cases.[215] Despite this abundant evidence suggesting a role for immunologic factors in the development of PMF, precise details of possible pathogenetic mechanisms are not understood. Three studies have failed to reveal an association between either simple or complicated CWP and any specific histocompatibility antigens.[223-225]

Pathologic evidence of cor pulmonale is frequently found at necropsy in patients with complicated CWP, and occasionally in those with the simple form of the disease.[226-228] In most patients in the latter group, this evidence can be explained on the basis of associated chronic bronchitis and emphysema or silicosis, but in some the sole explanation appears to be simple pneumoconiosis itself, characterized roentgenographically by the smaller type of pinpoint (p) opacities.[226, 229, 230] Of possible significance is a study in which inhalation of a monodispersed aerosol (mean diameter 0.55 μm)[231] showed that coal miners with type p opacities have small conducting airways that are narrower and peripheral airspaces that are larger than miners with type q opacities or without pneumoconiosis; in such cases, focal emphysema may play a role in the development of cor pulmonale.

In several investigations emphysema has been shown to be present more often and to be more severe in patients with CWP than in those without it;[232, 233] emphysema also correlates with the degree of exposure to coal dust.[234] In one study, this correlation was demonstrated to be independent of age and cigarette smoking and to be positively related to the dust content of macules.[233] Coalworkers are also susceptible to COPD.[235-238]

Roentgenographic Manifestations

The roentgenographic pattern of "simple" pneumoconiosis is typically one of small, round opacities (nodular)[239-241] but may be composed predominantly of small, irregular opacities (a reticular pattern), particularly in the early stages (Fig. 12–21). The nodules range from 1 to 5 mm in diameter, tend to be somewhat less well defined than those of silicosis, and are of a "granular" density unlike the homogeneous density of silicotic nodules. Roentgenologic-pathologic correlative studies suggest that the opacity of individual nodules cannot be entirely attributed to the coal dust, whose density is only slightly greater than unity.[242] Despite the foregoing, it is generally agreed that the roentgenographic changes of coalworker's pneumoconiosis cannot be distinguished from those of silicosis with any degree of confidence.

Although it has been stated that pulmonary nodules rarely calcify,[243] calcification occurs in at least a few of the nodules in up to 10 per cent of older coal miners, particularly anthracite workers.[175] The calcification begins as a central dot, thus helping to differentiate these nodules from those of silicosis, in which the calcification tends to be diffuse. Eggshell calcification of lymph nodes is un-

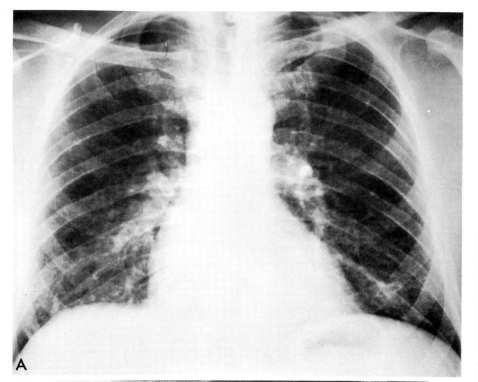

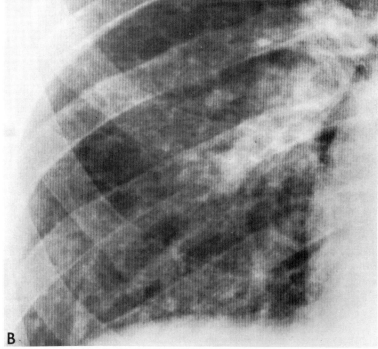

Figure 12–21. Coalworker's Pneumoconiosis. This posteroanterior roentgenogram *(A)* and magnified view of the lower half of the right lung *(B)* reveal a coarse reticulonodular pattern throughout both lungs, affecting the upper lung zones least. Both hila are enlarged and possess a contour suggestive of lymph node enlargement. The patient, a 45-year-old miner, was admitted to the hospital complaining of increasing shortness of breath. Approximately 15 years previously he had worked underground in a Belgian coal mine for 7 years and had been exposed to heavy concentrations of dust but had never worn a mask. At the time of admission, he stated that he was short of breath after walking 100 yards on level ground or climbing seven to ten steps. Pulmonary function studies were within normal limits except for a slight reduction in functional residual capacity; studies of lung mechanics revealed normal compliance and airway resistance.

common in coalworker's pneumoconiosis, occurring in only 1.3 per cent of 1,063 coal miners[175] whose chest roentgenograms showed evidence of pneumoconiosis. All had worked 20 or more years in the mines.

The appearance of large opacities (larger than 1 cm in diameter) indicates the development of "complicated" pneumoconiosis—PMF. These lesions range from a minimum of 1 cm in diameter to the volume of a whole lobe and are almost always restricted to the upper half of the lungs. They usually develop on a background of simple pneumoconiosis but have been observed in miners whose initial chest roentgenograms 4 to 5 years earlier were considered to be within normal limits.[245] PMF is said to develop in about 30 per cent of patients with diffuse bilateral opacities.[169, 244] It typically starts near the periphery of the lung and manifests as a mass with a smooth, well-defined lateral border that parallels the rib cage and projects 1 to 3 cm from it.[175] The medial margin of the mass is often ill-defined in contrast to its sharp lateral border. This configuration was observed in 22 of 50 cases of PMF in coal miners studied by Williams and Moller.[175] These authors have drawn attention to the unusual shape of the masses of PMF, which they regard as highly suggestive of the diagnosis. They point out that such masses tend to be thicker in one dimension than the other; for example, they tend to produce a broad face on a posteroanterior roentgenogram and a thin shape on a lateral roentgenogram, frequently paralleling the major fissure. As might be expected, this spindle-shaped configuration creates a roentgenographic opacity that is considerably less dense in one projection than in the other.

Both the smooth, sharply defined lateral border and the somewhat flattened configuration characteristic of these lesions can be employed to considerable advantage in differentiation from pulmonary carcinoma, whose borders tend to be less well-defined and whose configuration is typically spherical. PMF is usually homogeneous in density unless cavitation, which occurs only occasionally, has developed. As with the conglomerate shadows of silicosis, PMF usually originates in the lung periphery and gradually migrates toward the hilum, leaving a zone of overinflated emphysematous lung between it and the chest wall. The presence of a large homogeneous mass in the parahilar area of one lung may closely simulate pulmonary carcinoma (see Fig. 12–12). Such an error in diagnosis may lead to useless thoracotomy unless a background of pneumoconiosis is present and is recognized in the rest of the lungs. However, PMF is occasionally unassociated with roentgenographic evidence of nodularity,[175] and in such cases the correct diagnosis would not be suspected in the absence of an appropriate occupational history; even with such a history, the possibility of carcinoma would be difficult to exclude short of performing thoracotomy, although TTNA

may provide confirmatory evidence of the nature of the lesion in some cases (see Fig. 12–18). Occasionally, masses caused by PMF contain small calcifications, an obvious aid in differentiating the lesion from pulmonary carcinoma. Linear calcifications occur at times along the border of PMF, always along the lateral margin.[175] Coalworker's PMF may develop after exposure to coal dust has ceased and, unlike simple pneumoconiosis, may progress in the absence of further exposure.[169, 240, 246]

The pulmonary nodules described by Caplan[220] in coalworkers with rheumatoid disease are more regular in contour and more peripherally located than the masses of PMF. They range in size from 0.5 to 5 cm in diameter and are seen most often in workers who manifest subcutaneous rheumatoid nodules clinically and whose chest roentgenograms are classified as category 0 or 1 simple pneumoconiosis.[170]

The roentgenographic changes correlate well with pathology in coalworker's pneumoconiosis,[242, 247] unlike similar comparisons in silicosis. A number of articles have appeared in which the effects of film quality and other factors on the roentgenographic categorization of coalworker's pneumoconiosis have been analyzed.[176, 177, 248]

Clinical Manifestations

SYMPTOMS AND SIGNS

Unlike patients with silicosis, coalworkers with simple pneumoconiosis suffer little clinical disability and seldom show progress of their disease if removed from their dust-ridden environment.[249, 250] Symptoms, which usually develop only when the disease becomes complicated with PMF, include cough, mucoid expectoration, dyspnea on exertion, hemoptysis, frequent attacks of acute purulent bronchitis, and the expectoration of jet-black fluid.[251] Copious amounts of black sputum are produced when an ischemic lesion of PMF liquefies and ruptures into a bronchus, in which circumstance a cavity should be visible roentgenographically.[251, 252] With progression of the disease, dyspnea usually worsens; cor pulmonale and right-sided heart failure may ensue.

The degree of breathlessness appears to be directly related to the stage of the disease. In simple pneumoconiosis, there is usually no breathlessness on exertion, despite increasing roentgenographic abnormality. By contrast, in complicated pneumoconiosis, breathlessness is nearly always severe and increases with progression of roentgenographic changes.[253] The incidence of chronic bronchitis among coal miners is high, and several observers believe that coal dust may represent an etiologic factor in addition to the more significant factor of cigarette smoking.[169, 181, 254, 255, 773] For example, in one study of 8,000 working American coal miners, the incidence of symptoms increased with greater dust exposure even among nonsmokers, implicating dust in pathogenesis.[256] Although it is difficult to attribute specific causes to symptoms in coalworkers, especially those who smoke, some investigators[244, 257] are of the opinion that simple nodular pneumoconiosis may lead to significant disability, an attitude that is supported by the results of pulmonary function testing. Physical examination may reveal decreased breath sounds and a few rales. A patient has been described who developed vocal cord paralysis as a result of involvement of the recurrent laryngeal nerve by PMF.[258]

Mortality studies in coal miners[259] and coke oven workers[260] have shown no increase in the standardized mortality rate despite an increase in the incidence of death from respiratory disease; in both these studies, this apparent paradox was explained on the basis of a significant decrease in the incidence of death from heart disease.

PULMONARY FUNCTION TESTS

The results of pulmonary function testing in coal workers are at variance, largely because of differences in population groups studied. Nonworking miners show more impairment than those who are working, an apparent paradox that presumably results from the fact that the former have left the job because of disability. Other variables that influence results include cigarette smoking and particle size of coal dust inhaled. An often cited study of pulmonary function of patients with simple pneumoconiosis compared with a control group of the same age, published in 1955, showed no significant differences apart from minor disturbances in gas distribution.[261] More recently, however,[207] in a long-term follow-up of a group of coal miners who did not have PMF but were selected because of a suspicion that they may have suffered greater than average effects from dust exposure, it was found that the relationship between exposure and FEV_1 suggested that in some miners, even moderate exposure to dust can cause severe impairment of lung function. Others have reported longitudinal studies in which a deterioration in FEV_1 was shown to be related to cumulative dust exposure in coalworkers whose chest roentgenograms were normal.[206, 773] Most observers have found that a decrease in ventilatory capacity (as measured by FEV_1 and FVC) in patients with simple CWP can be explained largely on the basis of either smoking or heavy dust exposure (or both), but that patients with PMF show defects that are larger than those of appropriate normal controls.[170, 262] In an investigation of 95 coalworkers with pneumoconiosis aged 65 years or older who had had an average experience underground of 43 years, Hildick-Smith[263] found that 72 (76 per cent) had normal spirometry results for age; in the remainder, there was no clear-cut relationship between impaired function and the severity of pneumoconiosis, whether simple or complicated.

Diffusing capacity can be reduced in miners who smoke but is usually normal in nonsmoking miners with simple pneumoconiosis.[264, 265] On the other hand, focal impairment of $\dot{V}/\dot{Q}$ ratios resulting in impaired gas exchange has been described in nonsmoking coal miners despite normal spirometric findings.[774]

In contrast to simple CWP, PMF is frequently associated with physiologic evidence of airway obstruction, reduced diffusing capacity, abnormal blood gases, and increased pulmonary arterial pressures.[267, 268] In a study in which pathology and function were correlated, Lyons and Campbell[269] attributed these changes in function not only to PMF and the extent of emphysema but also to small airway disease and interstitial fibrosis. One assessment of lung mechanics in the early stages of simple CWP has shown a loss of elastic recoil,[270] suggesting the presence of focal emphysema.

Reduced diffusion, impaired gas exchange, and pulmonary hypertension have been described in coalworkers who manifest the micronodular roentgenologic pattern (category p).[169, 257, 271, 272] In a correlative roentgenologic, physiologic, pathologic, and clinical study of 247 coal miners, Ryder and associates[232] found that extensive emphysema was commoner in patients with this micronodular pattern than in those with larger nodules, whether the pneumoconiosis was simple or complicated. Others have related the development of physiologic obstruction and emphysema to the late appearance of small irregular opacities (type s or t).[240, 241, 273]

A comparative study of pulmonary function in coalworkers with Caplan's syndrome and with nonrheumatoid PMF[274] has shown significantly less obstruction in the patients with Caplan's syndrome but no significant difference in DL_{CO}; the authors interpret these findings as reflecting different pathologic features of the two entities.

ASBESTOS

Asbestos is the general term given to a group of minerals that are fibrous in nature and are resistant to high temperatures and various chemical insults. These minerals represent combinations of silicic acid with magnesium, calcium, sodium, and iron. They are divided mineralogically into two major groups, the *serpentines*, of which the only member of commercial importance is chrysotile, and the *amphiboles*, which include amosite (brown asbestos), crocidolite (blue asbestos), anthophyllite, tremolite, and actinolite. Chrysotile, amosite, and crocidolite are responsible for the vast majority of pleuropulmonary disease. Chrysotile fibers are curved or curly, whereas the amphiboles are straight and rectilinear (Fig. 12–22). These physical properties, as well as chemical differences, are responsible for the varying uses of asbestos; for example, chrysotile fibers are particularly suitable for textile manufac-

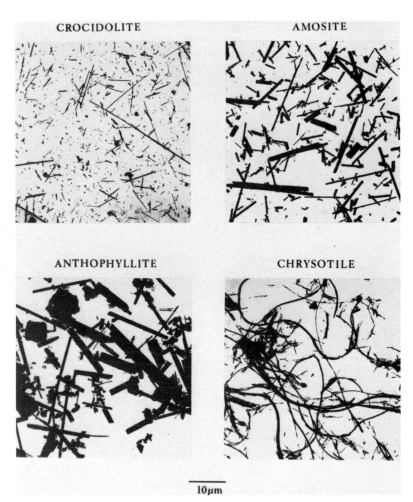

Figure 12–22. Types of Asbestos Fiber. Electron microscopic views of four different types of asbestos fiber. (Reproduced from Timbrell B: Physical factors as etiologic mechanisms. I.A.R.C. Scientific Publication No. 8, Lyons, 1973, p. 295.)

ture because they are long and pliable, whereas crocidolite and amosite are of greater value for marine insulation because they are more acid-resistant. The different types of asbestos fiber show some variation in disease-producing potential, related at least partly to fiber size.

The spectrum of asbestos-related pleuropulmonary disease is discussed in greater detail in the monograph by Preger[298] and the more recent articles by Craighead and Mossman[21] and Becklake.[299] The medical, legal, and engineering aspects of asbestos disease have been covered thoroughly in a sourcebook by Peters and Peters.[300]

Epidemiology

The use of asbestos in industry increased enormously during the first three quarters of this century; for example, world production jumped from 500 tons in 1900 to three million tons in 1968[275] and an estimated six million tons in 1981.[276] Although recognition of the harmful effects of asbestos exposure has resulted in better control of dust levels and, undoubtedly, an overall decrease in total exposure, the potential for the development of serious disease still exists.[277, 278] It has been esti-

mated, for example, that in the United States, eight[279] to nine[280] million people have been occupationally exposed to asbestos.

The three major sources of exposure to asbestos dust are (1) the primary occupations of asbestos mining and its processing in a mill, (2) numerous secondary occupations involving its use in a variety of industrial and commercial products, and (3) nonoccupational exposure to contaminated air. In some individuals, such as those living adjacent to asbestos mines, nonoccupational exposure can be substantial, but in the majority it is minimal and is evidenced only by the presence of asbestos bodies in concentrated digests of lung tissue.

The major producers of asbestos are the Soviet Union, Canada, and South Africa. Amosite is produced largely in the Transvaal, crocidolite in Capetown, and chrysotile in the Soviet Union and Quebec; anthophyllite is mined exclusively in Finland. Chrysotile is the most important form commercially, accounting for about 90 per cent of the total asbestos marketed in the United States and elsewhere.[21] In mining and milling, exposure occurs predominantly to only one type of fiber, although small amounts of other types may be present, even in commercially "pure" preparations.[21] By contrast, mixtures of fibers are commonly employed in construction and in the manufacture of textiles.

The secondary uses of asbestos are numerous (Table 12–1). The most important are in the construction industry, in which asbestos is extensively incorporated in cement piping, tiles, moldings, and panelings; shipbuilding and ship repair;[281, 282] railroad occupations (particularly during the era of the steam engine);[283] the manufacture of textiles and plastics;[284] the manufacture and repair of gaskets, brake linings, and gas masks[285] in dentistry, by dentists and dental technicians;[775] and in the jewelry industry.[776] Although the risk of exposure applies during the manufacturing process, it is even greater during repair and demolition. Although the fiber is generally assumed to be well bound and harmless once it is incorporated into manufactured products,[777] a report of significant levels of airborne asbestos in a 10-year-old office building whose ceilings had been sprayed with a crocidolite-containing material and whose floors were covered with vinyl-chrysotile tiles[286] leaves even this assumption in doubt.

Environmental exposure to asbestos dust also occurs in individuals not directly involved in asbestos-related occupations.[287] The prevalence of this mineral throughout the world is indicated by the frequency with which asbestos bodies are found in routine necropsies, the incidence ranging from 1 per cent in rural Italy[288] to 60 per cent in New York City.[289] In urban areas such as Miami,[290] Glasgow,[289] London,[291] Pittsburgh,[292] Melbourne,[293] and Montreal,[294] the prevalence rate has ranged from 25 to 50 per cent. Although the finding of asbestos bodies in the lungs in routine necropsies indicates that such exposure is almost universal, there is no evi-

Table 12–1. Occupations at Risk for Asbestos Exposure:
Mining, Milling, Manufacturing, and Secondary Uses

PROCESS	PRODUCTS MADE OR USED	JOBS POTENTIALLY AT RISK
Production		
Mining		Rock mining, loading, trucking
Milling		Crushing, milling
Handling		Transport workers, dockers, loaders, those who unpack jute sacks (recently replaced with sacks that do not permit fibers to escape)
Primary uses		
Spray insulation	Spray of fiber mixed with oil	Spray insulators (construction, shipbuilding)
Filler and grouting		
Manufacturing of		
Textiles	Cloth, curtains, lagging, protective clothing, mailbags, padding, conveyor belts	Blending, carding, spinning, twisting, winding, braiding, weaving, slurry mixing, laminating, molding, drying
Cement products	Sheets, pipes, roofing shingles, gutters, ventilation shafts, flower pots	Blending, slurry preparation, rolling, pressing, pipe cutting
"Paper" products	Millboard, roofing felt, fine-quality electrical papers, flooring felt, fillers	
Friction materials	Automotive products: gaskets, clutch plates, brake linings	
Insulation products	Pipe and boiler insulation, bulkhead linings for ships	
Applications		
Construction		
New construction	Boards and tiles; putties, caulk, paints, joint fillers; cement products (tiles, pipes, siding, shingles)	Direct: carpenters, laggers, painters, tile layers, insulation workers, sheet metal and heating equipment workers, masons Indirectly: all other workers on construction sites, such as plumbers, welders, electricians
Repair, demolition		Demolition workers for all of these
Shipbuilding		
Construction	Insulation materials (boards, mattresses, cloth) for engines, hull, decks, lagging of ventilation and water pipes, cables	Laggers, refitters, strippers, steam fitters, sailmakers, joiners, shipwrights, engine fitters, masons, painters, welders, caulkers
Repair, refits	Insulation materials, as described for "Construction"	Directly: all above jobs on refits, dry dock, and other repair operations Indirectly: maintenance fitters and repairers, electricians, plumbers, welders, carpenters
Automotive industry		
Manufacture	Gaskets, brake linings, undercoating	Installation of brake linings, gaskets, and so on
Repair	Gaskets, brake linings, undercoating	Service people, brake repairers, body repairers, auto mechanics

Modified from Becklake MR: Am Rev Respir Dis *114*:187, 1976.

dence to date that in most individuals[295] this finding represents a significant risk for the development of pleuropulmonary disease. On the other hand, there is irrefutable evidence that individuals who live in the vicinity of a mine, mill, or factory associated with heavy asbestos dust pollution have a greater incidence of pleural plaques and mesothelioma.[296, 301–304] In fact, these abnormalities can develop in persons whose only exposure is the repeated handling of the clothes of asbestos workers.[305–308] In a roentgenographic study of 93 women over 40 years of age, all of whom were wives of insulation workers exposed to asbestos, Sider and associates[309] found 18 (19 per cent) to have pleural changes consistent with asbestos exposure; these included chest wall plaques in 16 patients, diaphragmatic plaques in five, pleural calcification in three, and diffuse pleural thickening in one. Of 17 husbands of the 18 women, 14 demonstrated more severe roentgenographic abnormalities than their wives. A history of such environmental asbestos exposure may not be readily apparent from a cursory inquiry, because the exposure may have occurred many years prior to the recognition of disease and may have been of short duration. An example of how remote nonoccupational exposure may be is illustrated by the story of two brothers aged 27 and 33 years who presented with chest wall and diaphragmatic pleural calcification and whose only exposure was playing in childhood in the cellar of their home, which was also used by their father in a muffler repair business.[308]

Although disease caused by asbestos exposure, particularly mesothelioma, has been described in workers who manufacture friction materials, such as brake and clutch linings,[310] the fear that there may be excessive release of asbestos dust from automobile brakes has been eliminated by studies showing that the high heat of friction on application of brakes converts asbestos to an inert nonfibrous silicate known as fosterite.[52, 311] A high incidence of nonoccupational asbestos-related disease has been reported from the Metsovo area of northwest Greece[312, 313] and from isolated villages in Turkey,[314–316] where the soil, which contains tremolite, has been used as a whitewash for buildings; manifestations have been largely pleural, most of the inhabitants having pleural plaques, and many, mesothelioma.

The discovery that asbestos fibers can be found in drinking water,[317–319, 320] wine,[320] and even intravenous medications[803] has led to some concern regarding the potential hazard associated with ingestion or administration of these liquids.[321] A study from the San Francisco Bay area found an increased incidence of gastrointestinal malignancy in a population exposed to high concentrations of asbestos fibers in drinking water.[322] However, in an experimental study in which rats were administered water contaminated by asbestos fibers in the concentration reported to occur in drinking water failed to show

a significantly higher incidence of malignant tumors than that in controls.[323]

Pathogenesis and Pathologic Characteristics

Pathologic abnormalities in the chest caused by asbestos inhalation can occur in the pleura, lung parenchyma, airways, and lymph nodes. Pleural disease is the most common, and it most often takes the form of parietal pleural plaques; localized visceral pleural fibrosis, more or less diffuse pleural fibrosis, and mesothelioma (each of which can be associated with pleural effusion) also occur. It has been estimated that there may be as many as 1.3 million people in the United States with roentgenographically detectable occupational pleural thickening.[279] Pulmonary manifestations include diffuse interstitial fibrosis (asbestosis), round atelectasis, and pulmonary carcinoma. Fibrosis has also been described in relation to membranous and respiratory bronchioles and alveolar ducts,[324] but at the time of writing, it has not been established whether this finding represents an early form of asbestosis or a pathogenetically separate lesion.

In addition to these pathologic abnormalities, evidence of asbestos exposure can also be seen in tissue sections by the identification of iron-coated asbestos fibers. These asbestos bodies are most often found in lung parenchyma, but also occur in airway walls and intrathoracic lymph nodes. It should be emphasized that the discovery of one or more such bodies in tissue sections by itself does not signify the presence of pleuropulmonary disease, but indicates only that the patient has been exposed to the mineral.

PLEURAL MANIFESTATIONS

Pleural Plaques. As indicated, pleural plaques are almost certainly the most common form of asbestos-related pleuropulmonary disease and are not infrequently present without any other pathologic abnormality.[325–328] Grossly, they consist of well-defined, pearly-white foci of firm fibrous tissue, usually 2 to 5 mm thick and up to 10 cm in diameter;[329] they may have a smooth surface or show a fine or coarse nodularity and can be round, elliptical, or irregularly shaped (Fig. 12–23).[330] Foci of calcification are not uncommon and are occasionally extensive. Characteristically, plaques are located on the parietal pleura overlying the ribs and on the domes of the diaphragm. They are generally absent from the apices, costophrenic angles, and anterior chest wall, and are almost always bilateral.

Histologically, plaques consist of rather dense, virtually acellular bands of collagen often arranged in a "basket weave" configuration (Fig. 12–23).[327, 329, 330] Asbestos bodies are invariably absent, although uncoated fibers may be demonstrated when

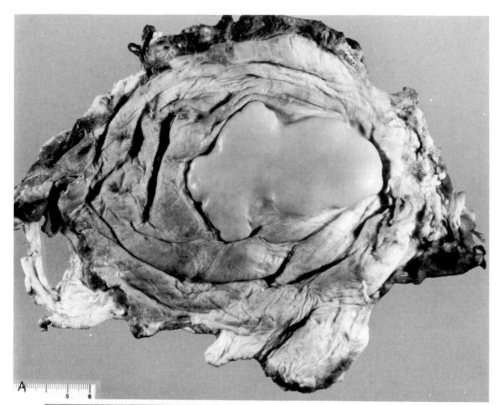

Figure 12–23. Pleural Plaque Secondary to Asbestos Exposure. A gross specimen of a hemidiaphragm *(A)* reveals a smooth, pearly-white, well-circumscribed focus of fibrosis on the tendinous portion. A histologic section *(B)* shows dense, almost acellular collagen with a "basket-weave" appearance. (× 40.) This was an incidental finding in a construction worker whose lung contained occasional asbestos bodies.

tissue is dissolved or ashed and examined under polarized light or by electron microscopy.[305, 325, 331, 332]

Parietal pleural plaques are common, the incidence in consecutive routine autopsies ranging from 4 to 12 per cent.[327, 329] In most cases, there is evidence of prior asbestos exposure, as indicated by either an appropriate occupational history or the presence of a substantial number of coated or uncoated asbestos fibers within the lungs.[325–329] In several series of individuals in whom pleural plaques have been discovered at autopsy,[333–335] a history of asbestos exposure has been obtained in approximately 60 per cent. In some patients, however, asbestos bodies or fibers are not demonstrable,[325, 326, 778] in which case the plaques cannot be regarded as *absolute* evidence of an asbestos etiology although they are certainly highly suggestive. To what extent these plaques are caused by trauma, infection, or inhalation of nonasbestos fibers often cannot be established. The pathogenesis of pleural plaques is unclear, and numerous mechanical, chemical, and immunologic mechanisms have been invoked to explain their formation.[314]

Focal Visceral Pleural Fibrosis. Relatively discrete foci of pleural fibrosis morphologically distinct from pleural plaques are not uncommon in association with asbestos exposure, and occur on the visceral rather than the parietal pleura. They consist of round or elliptical areas of gray or white fibrous tissue that often appear to radiate from a central focus (Fig. 12–24). The underlying lung may show partial or complete collapse (round atelectasis; *see* farther on). Histologically, the lesion consists of mature fibrous tissue and a variable number of chronic inflammatory cells. The areas of fibrosis usually measure only 1 to 2 mm thick and, unless associated with round atelectasis or located in a fissure, are unlikely to be detected on conventional chest roentgenograms.

Diffuse Pleural Fibrosis. In contrast to the morphologically distinctive, relatively discrete foci of visceral and parietal pleural fibrosis described previously, some patients show more diffuse pleural thickening that can be progressive and can be associated with clinical and functional abnormalities (*see* farther on).[280] Although the fibrosis can be restricted to either the parietal[280] or visceral[336] pleura, it usually involves both and is accompanied by interpleural adhesions (*see* Fig. 12–25). The fibrosis can extend to adjacent interlobar fissures and interlobular septa[280] and even into the mediastinum.[337] Histologically, the lesions are composed of mature collagen, in some cases possessing a "basket weave" pattern resembling discrete pleural plaques;[336] a variable number of chronic inflammatory cells are usually present. An acute fibrinous pleuritis is sometimes associated.[280] In seven cases studied by Stephens and associates,[336] interstitial fibrosis was present in and limited to the adjacent pulmonary parenchyma (*see* Fig. 12–25).

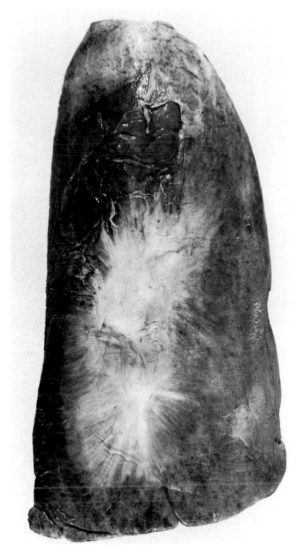

Figure 12–24. Localized Visceral Pleural Fibrosis Secondary to Asbestos Exposure. The lateral surface of this lower lobe shows a rather poorly demarcated area of fibrosis that appears to radiate out from two central foci. The fibrosis is limited to the visceral pleura, although multiple plaques were identified on the parietal pleura of the chest wall and hemidiaphragms. The underlying lung was unremarkable. The patient was a former construction worker with known asbestos exposure.

It is not clear whether this form of diffuse fibrosis represents an extension of one or both of the other two forms of fibrosis or is a pathogenetically separate process. In their study of seven patients with diffuse pleural fibrosis, Miller and colleagues[280] identified one or more episodes of pleural effusion and suggested that organization of the effusion might have been responsible for the chronic changes. In some cases, the presence of numerous inflammatory cells within the fibrous tissue has raised the possibility of an immunologic pathogenesis.[337]

Pleural Effusion. In patients with benign asbestos effusion, histologic examination of the pleura

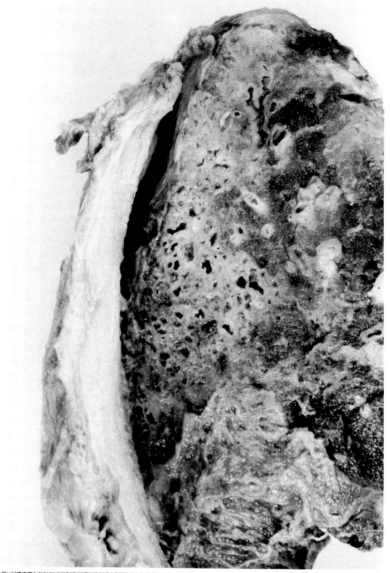

A

Figure 12–25. Diffuse Pleural Fibrosis and Asbestosis. A gross section of a lower lobe *(A)* shows severe pleural thickening and underlying parenchymal interstitial fibrosis. The pleural lesion consists of fibrous tissue, focally calcified, which extends over most of the costal surface; although focally it appears to be related predominantly to the parietal pleura, interpleural adhesions are present in many areas. A histologic section of subpleural lung parenchyma *(B)* shows severe disorganization of normal lung architecture; in its place are broad bands of fibrous tissue and cystic spaces focally lined by metaplastic bronchiolar epithelium ("honeycomb lung"). (× 30.)

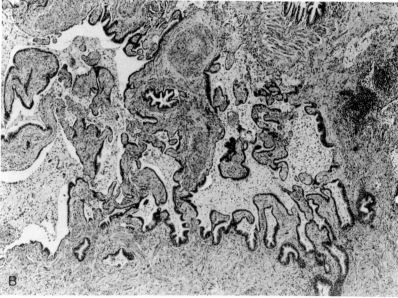

B

has shown only fibrosis and nonspecific chronic inflammation.[338, 339] In many cases the fibrosis is a microscopic finding only, although in some it has also been associated with grossly identifiable diffuse pleural fibrosis.[280] Mesothelial hyperplasia may be present and must be differentiated from mesothelioma. As with other forms of asbestos-related pleural disease, the pathogenesis of non-neoplastic effusion is unclear. It has been suggested by Shore and colleagues,[340] on the basis of experimental studies in rabbits, that interaction between asbestos fibers and pleural tissue results in the release of non–complement-related chemotactic factors that cause the effusion; this hypothesis has been supported by a study by Antony and colleagues[779] which showed that tissue cultures of rabbit mesothelial cells stimulated by asbestos fibers are capable of releasing a substance that possesses chemotactic activity for neutrophils.

Mesothelioma. There is now no doubt of the association between asbestos exposure and the development of mesothelioma. The pathologic features and pathogenesis of these tumors are discussed in greater detail later (*see* page 2347).

PULMONARY MANIFESTATIONS

Asbestosis. Asbestosis can be defined as a pneumoconiosis characterized by more or less diffuse parenchymal interstitial fibrosis secondary to the inhalation of asbestos fibers. Digestion techniques characteristically reveal a large number of asbestos bodies and fibers in lung tissue,[341] and the condition is usually associated with high exposure levels. As-

bestos bodies are also often visible in tissue sections and may be present in great numbers.

Grossly,[330, 344] the fibrosis is most prominent in the subpleural regions of the lower lobes and varies from a moderately coarse appearance of the parenchyma to obvious "honeycomb" change (Fig. 12–25). Fibrosis of adjacent visceral pleura is common and is often accompanied by parietal adhesions. As might be expected from the gross description, the microscopic appearance varies from a slight increase in interstitial collagen to complete obliteration of normal lung architecture and the formation of thick fibrous bands and cystic spaces (Fig. 12–25). The spaces may be lined by metaplastic bronchiolar cells or by hyperplastic type II cells; the latter sometimes contain within their cytoplasm well-demarcated eosinophilic inclusions that are identical histochemically and ultrastructurally to alcoholic (Mallory's) hyaline (Fig. 12–26).[342, 343] Although when first described[342] these inclusions were thought to be related to injury by asbestos, it is now apparent that they can be caused by a variety of pulmonary insults.[343] A grading system to assess the severity of interstitial fibrosis on a systematic basis has been proposed.[330]

The earliest histologic change in asbestosis is considered by some authorities to consist of fibrosis in the walls of respiratory bronchioles.[21, 330, 780] According to this view, the process begins in the most proximal of such airways and extends in time to involve terminal and more distal respiratory bronchioles and adjacent alveolar interstitium; as the disease progresses, greater portions of lung parenchyma are affected in a centrifugal fashion. Al-

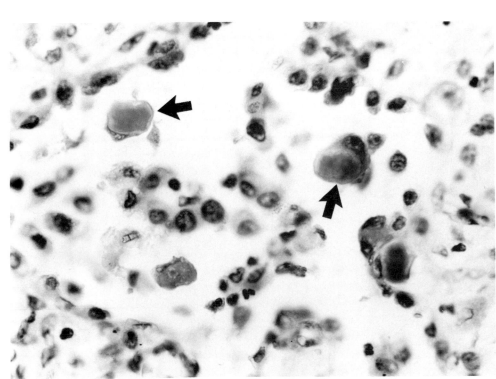

Figure 12–26. Asbestosis: Type II Cell Inclusions. A magnified photomicrograph of lung parenchyma with asbestosis shows macrophages and hyperplastic type II cells, some of which contain smudged, densely eosinophilic cytoplasmic inclusions *(arrows)*; they are similar to those seen in hepatocytes secondary to alcohol toxicity (Mallory's hyaline). (× 600.)

though there is no doubt that peribronchiolar fibrosis exists in association with asbestos exposure (Fig. 12–27), some workers have suggested that it may represent a distinct process pathogenetically separate from pulmonary parenchymal fibrosis (i.e., asbestosis).[35, 324, 345] In a study of patients with known asbestos exposure, Wright and Churg[324] found fibrosis, pigment deposition, and chronic inflammation in the walls of membranous and respiratory bronchioles and alveolar ducts; although such changes were also present in the membranous bronchioles of individuals without asbestos exposure who were matched for age, sex, and smoking history, these findings were substantially less severe and less common in the more peripheral airways. The authors thus suggested that fibrosis at these sites is highly suggestive of asbestos inhalation. However, the results of subsequent studies by the same authors have suggested that this may not be the case;[324, 346] for example, Churg and Wright[345] identified similar airway abnormalities in patients with a history of exposure to mineral dust other than asbestos, implying that these pathologic changes may be a nonspecific reaction to dust inhalation rather than a specific manifestation of asbestos toxicity. Experimental studies in sheep have also demonstrated evidence for two distinct pulmonary reactions, one related to small airways and the other to the parenchymal interstitium.[35] Whatever its relationship to interstitial fibrosis, the peribronchiolar and alveolar duct fibrosis seems likely to be related to the airflow obstruction that is observed in both patients[347–351] and experimental animals.[35, 352, 353]

The pathogenesis of asbestosis is incompletely understood. In experimental animals, inhaled asbestos fibers small enough to reach the lung parenchyma appear to be deposited preferentially at alveolar duct bifurcations.[354, 355] Such deposition is rapidly followed by the accumulation of alveolar macrophages,[355, 356] possibly as a result of direct activation by asbestos of a complement-dependent chemo-attractant.[357, 358] Further, there is evidence that macrophages that come in contact with asbestos fibers can release substances that stimulate growth of fibroblasts with resulting collagen production.[359, 360] Experiments in which human alveolar macrophages have been cultured in varying concentrations of amosite asbestos have shown no decrease in cell viability within 24 hours at concentrations less than 100 µg/ml; however, at 48 hours at these concentrations and at 24 hours at concentrations up to 300 µg/ml, significant cytotoxicity has been evident.[361] These observations suggest direct physical or chemical damage, possibly resulting in cell death; however, it is also conceivable that less severe damage results simply in abnormalities in macrophage function similar to those proposed for silicosis (see page 2283).

Although the majority of inhaled asbestos is transported out of the lung via the mucociliary escalator,[362] a variable proportion enters the interstitium, the amount depending on the efficiency of fiber clearance and the asbestos dose itself. Passage from the airspace lumen to the interstitium may be accomplished by one or more of at least three mechanisms: (1) within macrophages, (2) directly within or between epithelial cells,[363] or (3) by incorporation into the interstitium through organization of intraluminal exudate secondary to epithelial necrosis.[360]

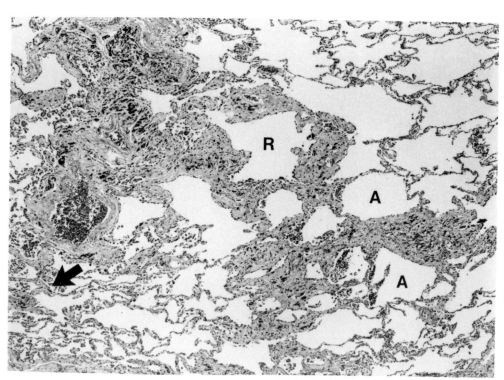

Figure 12–27. Peribronchiolar Fibrosis Associated with Asbestos Exposure. In this histologic section the wall of a respiratory bronchiole (R) and its distal divisions (A) (identified as alveolar ducts on serial sections) are substantially thickened by fibrous tissue, pigmented macrophages, and a mild lymphocytic infiltrate. The adjacent parenchyma is mostly normal, although focal interstitial fibrosis is present *(arrow)*. The patient was a 55-year-old man employed as an insulator; asbestos bodies were easily identified in lung parenchyma. (× 40.)

As indicated previously, the development of asbestosis depends in part on both the degree and length of exposure, clinical manifestations usually not becoming manifest until 20 to 40 years after the initial contact with the mineral. However, not all individuals with heavy exposure show harmful effects,[28] the dose-response relationship being weaker in asbestosis than in other pneumoconioses such as CWP. Both of these observations have raised the possibility that other extrinsic agents or intrinsic host factors may be important in the pathogenesis of the disease. The most extensively studied *extrinsic agent* is cigarette smoke. Although there is some disagreement,[364, 781] most investigators[365-371] have demonstrated an apparent synergistic effect of cigarette smoking on the development of roentgenographically detectable asbestosis. The pathogenetic basis for the cigarette smoke–asbestosis association is unclear. However, experimental studies in guinea pigs[372] have shown that cigarette smoke appears to increase the penetration of asbestos fibers into the walls of respiratory bronchioles, suggesting that the resulting larger interstitial fiber burden may be related to more severe fibrosis. The incidence of pleural plaques in asbestos workers has been found by some[369, 370] but not by others[371, 373] to be higher in cigarette smokers than in nonsmokers.

Intrinsic host factors that might be important in determining individual susceptibility to the harmful effects of asbestos include the efficiency of alveolar and tracheobronchial clearance, underlying lung structure,[28] and immunologic status. The last-named has been the most thoroughly studied. Evidence for an autoimmune factor in the pathogenesis of asbestosis lies chiefly in the presence in asbestos workers of circulating rheumatoid and antinuclear factors; Turner-Warwick and Parkes[374] identified the former in 28 per cent and the latter in 27 per cent of asbestos workers with positive chest roentgenograms. In this study, the autoantibodies were of the IgM type and were present in titers considerably lower than those usually identified in connective tissue diseases. In workers exposed to asbestos, other investigators have found hypergammaglobulinemia, a variety of additional autoantibodies, and even immune complexes.[375-377] Although such B-cell hyperactivity appears to correlate with roentgenographic progression of asbestosis,[377] there is as yet no clear-cut evidence that it is directly involved in the pathogenesis of the disease.[375, 376] Cell-mediated immunity, as measured by delayed skin hypersensitivity tests and *in vitro* methods, is reduced in patients with more advanced asbestosis but not in those with mesothelioma;[378-380] the results of one study suggest that this defect may antedate the roentgenographic appearance of fibrosis.[380]

Although the studies just cited have suggested an immunologic factor in the pathogenesis of asbestosis, not all investigations have confirmed this suggestion. For example, studies of anthophyllite asbestos workers in Finland have shown the incidence of rheumatoid factor to be similar to that found in healthy control groups.[381] In addition, in a study of 72 long-term workers of the mines and mills of Quebec (40 of whom had asbestosis) and a reference population of 150 residents, Bégin and colleagues[382] documented 53 phenotypes of the human leukocyte antigen (HLA)-A,B,C, and DR but were unable to find any significant difference in the frequency of these phenotypes in the two groups.

In patients with asbestosis and in asbestos-exposed individuals, light microscopic examination of fluid obtained by BAL has been employed as a means of both identifying asbestos fibers and determining the type and degree of cellular activity. Using this technique, exposure to asbestos can be readily documented; by contrast, in nonoccupationally exposed controls or those with other pulmonary disease, significant exposure can be excluded by either the complete absence of asbestos bodies[383, 384] or the presence of a small number.[385] In one study, quantitative analysis did not serve to distinguish asbestos workers with disease from those without;[384] however, in another study, the highest levels of asbestos body counts were found in patients with clinical evidence of asbestosis.[385] In individuals who are occupationally exposed but who lack asbestos bodies by light microscopy, electron microscopy readily reveals fibers in the BAL fluid.[133] Asbestos body counts have been found to be higher in patients with interstitial lung disease than in those with mesothelioma; in one study, BAL was positive for asbestos bodies in only nine of 13 patients with the neoplasm.[386]

The cellular content of BAL fluid provides evidence for a neutrophil-eosinophil alveolitis in asbestos-exposed workers;[384, 387, 388] this in turn correlates with the presence of crackles on auscultation[384, 388] and with PaO_2 and A–a (PO_2) but not with other physiologic changes or with roentgenographic abnormality.[388] Analysis of BAL supernatant reveals high levels of neutrophil chemotactic factors in asbestos-exposed individuals.[782] The ratio of T-helper to T-suppressor lymphocytes has been reported to be both increased[389] and decreased[390] in BAL fluid of workers exposed to asbestos. Other findings in BAL fluid that point to a cell-mediated pathogenetic mechanism include a reduction in natural killer cell activity[783] and an increased production of gamma interferon.[784] Using BAL, Gellert and coworkers[391, 392] demonstrated greater pulmonary epithelial permeability in patients with asbestosis.

Gallium-67 lung scans have been shown to be positive in patients with asbestosis and in sheep exposed to asbestos, attributable according to Bégin and coworkers[393] to the enhanced serum protein leakage binding with gallium-67 and macrophage uptake of the isotope in the alveoli. These same authors have shown that fibronectin and procollagen 3 levels are elevated in BAL fluid both in sheep exposed to chrysotile asbestos and in patients with asbestos-associated alveolitis and asbestosis; Bégin and coworkers[393] consider levels of these substances to correlate with fibrogenic activity.

The Asbestos Body. The asbestos body, seen commonly in tissue sections in association with asbestos pleuropulmonary disease, consists of a core composed of a transparent asbestos fiber surrounded by a variably thick coat of iron and protein (Fig. 12–28). Most bodies measure between 2 and 5 μm in width and 20 to 50 μm in length; the asbestos cores themselves range from 0.1 to 1.5 μm in diameter.[395] The shape is quite variable depending on the length of the asbestos core, the amount and pattern of deposition of the protein-iron coat, and whether the body is whole or fragmented. The coat is often segmented over the length of the fiber and sometimes forms bulbous projections at both ends, resulting in a drumstick appearance (Fig. 12–28). The majority are straight, although curved and angulated forms are seen occasionally. The core of most asbestos bodies consists of amphiboles, especially amosite and crocidolite.[395, 396] The relative paucity of chrysotile cores probably results from the tendency of this substance to fragment into forms that are too short to form bodies or from the fact that they have dissolved in lung fluids.[398]

In tissue sections, asbestos bodies are usually found within either interstitial fibrous tissue or airspaces; they are rarely present in pleural plaques. They can also be present in hilar and mediastinal lymph nodes and even in extrathoracic visceral organs,[395, 399, 400] where they can cause a fibrotic reaction.[397] Their presence in the sputum of individuals with occupational exposure has been well documented,[401, 402, 476] and they are sometimes identifiable in specimens obtained by TTNA.[403] Staining for iron can be helpful for identification, especially when few bodies are present.

It is believed that the body is formed within the alveolar macrophage by deposition around a phagocytosed asbestos fiber of a glycoprotein matrix and iron.[395, 404] The source of the iron is unclear; it has been suggested that it is derived either from hemorrhage related to the inhalation of asbestos or from circulating iron stores.[395] The encasement of foreign material by an iron-glycoprotein coat is not unique to asbestos; it can occur in experimental animals around fiber glass or synthetic aluminum silicate particles[405] and in humans around a variety of particles, including talc, mica, carbon (see Fig. 12–18), diatomaceous earth, rutile, fly ash,[406, 407] zeolite,[408] and even iron itself.[409] With the exception of zeolite, such nonasbestos ferruginous bodies can usually be distinguished from true asbestos bodies by the appearance of the asbestos fiber core, which is thin and translucent.[406, 407]

Although for practical reasons, asbestos bodies are most often identified in tissue sections, their true number is best estimated by examining concentrates of digested lung tissue;[410] for example, it has

been estimated that microscopic examination of 30 to 40 fields at a magnification of 400 would be necessary to find a single asbestos body in a tissue section from lung that contains 5,000 bodies per gram.[411] In fact, the digestion technique permits identification of asbestos bodies in virtually 100 per cent of the general population,[341, 412] whereas tissue sections reveal them only rarely in the absence of occupational exposure.

Attempts have been made to correlate the number of asbestos bodies on tissue sections with the number identified in tissue digests. In a study of six individuals with asbestosis or asbestos-related neoplasia, Roggli and Pratt[413] found that an average of two asbestos bodies on 2 × 2 cm iron-stained tissue sections 5 μm thick was equivalent to approximately 200 asbestos bodies per gram of wet-fixed lung tissue. Subsequently, Vollmer and Roggli[411] devised a mathematical model that they claim is even more accurate for predicting total lung asbestos body concentration from the number of asbestos bodies in tissue sections. Warrock and Wolery[785] have shown, however, that in the presence of fibrosis and a high asbestos fiber burden, asbestos bodies are scarce or absent in tissue sections from some subjects.

Although the presence of asbestos bodies in tissue sections or digested lung samples examined by ordinary light or phase contrast microscopy is a reliable indicator of asbestos exposure, it is clear that the absolute number of asbestos bodies identified by these means is a gross underestimation of the total number of uncoated asbestos fibers as determined by electron microscopic examination.[341, 395, 414] Thus, the ratio of uncoated to coated fibers in lung digests ranges from approximately 7:1 to 5000:1 in different series.[341] In individuals without occupational exposure, most of these uncoated fibers are short (less than 5 μm in length) and consist of chrysotile or noncommercial amphiboles such as tremolite and anthophyllite.[415] As with asbestos bodies, a great variety of nonasbestos fibers can be found in human lung digests.[344]

The number of asbestos bodies and fibers per gram of digested lung tissue is roughly proportional to both the presence and severity of disease and the degree of occupational exposure.[341, 344, 395, 412] Thus, individuals with well-documented high exposure generally have a 20- to 100-fold increase in the total number of fibers within the lung compared with controls;[341] individuals with asbestosis or mesothelioma usually have a 100- to 1,000-fold relative increase.[341] Similarly, an asbestos worker might have 10^5 to 10^7 asbestos bodies per gram of wet lung, whereas members of the general population have between 0 and 50.[395] Individuals with environmental (nonoccupational) asbestos exposure have levels between these two extremes; for example, Case and Sebastien[416] found that persons living close to a large open-pit chrysotile asbestos mine demonstrated asbestos body counts intermediate between

Figure 12–28. Asbestos Bodies. A histologic section *(A)* reveals a typical asbestos body consisting of a slightly curved, elongated structure with a finely beaded iron-protein coat. The asbestos fiber itself can be identified as a thin line in the center of the coat near one end of the body *(arrow)*. In another section *(B)*, other asbestos bodies show a more prominent iron-protein coat obscuring the enclosed asbestos fiber; some bodies are fragmented *(curved arrows)*. A characteristic drumstick form is taken by one *(straight arrow)*. (*A* and *B*, × 400.)

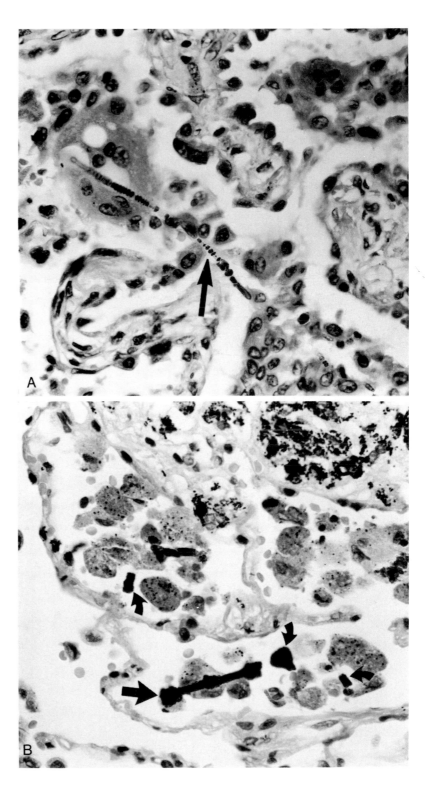

those of nonexposed controls and those of miners and millers.

Round Atelectasis. Round atelectasis, a condition originally described by Blesovsky,[417] consists of a localized zone of collapsed parenchyma in the periphery of the lung, partly surrounded by thickened, invaginated pleura. Its nature has been repeatedly confirmed pathologically following pulmonary resection for suspected pulmonary carcinoma.[418–421] The majority of cases are associated with asbestos-related pleural fibrosis.[422–424, 786] Grossly, the atelectatic lung is poorly defined and appears to blend imperceptibly with adjacent normal lung parenchyma (Fig. 12–29).[418] The overlying pleura is invariably fibrotic and shows one or more invaginations 1 mm to 3 cm in length into the adjacent lung. Pleural wrinkling and folding and a variable degree of alveolar collapse and fibrosis are seen microscopically (Fig. 12–29). The pathogenesis of round atelectasis has been discussed in Chapter 4 (*see* page 489) and in greater detail by Menzies and Fraser.[418]

Pulmonary Carcinoma. As with mesothelioma, there is now no doubt about the very significant relationship between asbestos exposure and pulmonary carcinoma, particularly in cigarette smokers. This subject is considered in detail farther on (*see* page 2347).

Roentgenographic Manifestations

The roentgenographic changes in the chest in asbestos-related disease can be both pleural and parenchymal, but in most reported series the former are far more striking than the latter.[425–427] Of 56 patients with asbestos-related disease described by Freundlich and Greening,[426] 48 per cent showed pleural thickening alone, 41 per cent combined pleural and parenchymal manifestations, and only 11 per cent parenchymal changes alone. A similar predominance of pleural over parenchymal changes was reported by Anton:[428] of 40 patients with asbestos exposure, only five had parenchymal changes in the lung bases, pleural plaques being the sole manifestation of disease in the other 35. In a study of 133 Finnish patients with roentgenographic evidence of asbestosis, Zitting and coworkers[429] found 88 (66 per cent) to have pleural changes; in 78 patients, pleural calcification was present.

PLEURAL MANIFESTATIONS

Four types of roentgenographic changes occur in the pleura—plaque formation, diffuse pleural thickening, calcification, and pleural effusion—each of which may occur alone or in combination with the others. It has been estimated that there may be as many as 1.3 million people in the United States with roentgenographically detectable asbestos-related pleural thickening.[279]

Pleural Plaques. Pleural plaques usually are more prominent in the lower half of the thorax and tend to follow the rib contours.[305, 430–432] They may be smooth or nodular in contour and can measure up to 1 cm in thickness, although they are usually thinner (Fig. 12–30). They occur most commonly on the domes of the diaphragm, on the posterolateral chest wall between the seventh and tenth ribs, and on the lateral chest wall between the sixth and ninth ribs (Fig. 12–31).[296, 427, 433–435] The earliest appearance of a pleural plaque is as a thin line of unit density visible under a rib in the axillary region, usually the seventh or eighth rib on one side or both sides. Although they are usually multiple, occasionally only a single plaque is identifiable (Fig. 12–32). They may be very difficult to identify particularly when viewed en face, and tangential roentgenograms may be necessary. In fact, the frequency with which plaques occur along the posterolateral or anterolateral portion of the thorax suggested to Fletcher and Edge[427] that oblique projections of the thorax should be standard in the roentgenographic investigation of patients suspected of having asbestos-related disease. The value of 45-degree oblique projections has also been stressed by MacKenzie,[436] who regards the space between the inner border of the ribs and the lung margin, where a localized expansion occurs in the presence of hyaline plaques, as being an important diagnostic area. In a study of 127 long-term asbestos workers, Bégin and associates[437] evaluated the diagnostic content of three types of examination—a single posteroanterior (PA) roentgenogram, roentgenograms in four projections (PA, lateral, and both 45-degree oblique views), and CT. They found that the four-view roentgenograms revealed more sites of pleural plaques and the CT scans more calcified pleural plaques than could be identified on the single PA roentgenograms. More recent studies indicate that high-resolution CT is even more useful than conventional CT in detecting both pleural and parenchymal asbestos-related disease.[438, 439] It is important to realize that depending on the criteria for diagnosis, the frequency with which plaques are recognized roentgenographically ranges from only 8.3 to 40.3 per cent of cases in which they are demonstrated at autopsy.[327]

Although it is generally thought that pleural plaques or thickening is usually bilateral and fairly symmetric, this has not been found in all studies; for example, in a review of the roentgenograms of 200 individuals with known or suspected asbestos exposure, Fisher[441] found that plaques or thickening (with or without calcification) occurred solely or predominantly on the left side in 90, on the right side in 32, and equally on the two sides in 44. Thus, in this series at least, asymmetry was common, leading the author to conclude that apparently unilateral changes should prompt a search for more subtle changes elsewhere.

Text continued on page 2335

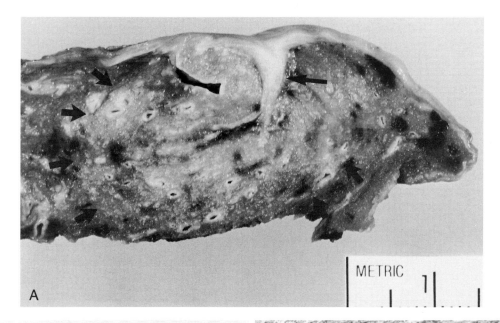

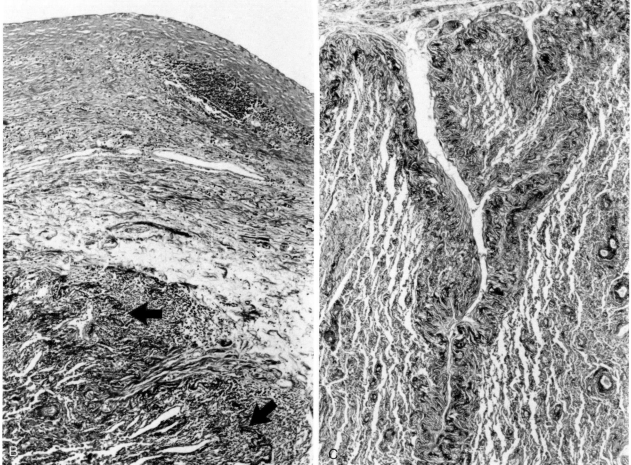

Figure 12–29. Round Atelectasis: Pathologic Characteristics. A slice of an uninflated lower lobe *(A)* from a patient with roentgenographic evidence of typical round atelectasis shows a poorly defined, somewhat rounded focus of atelectasis *(short arrows)* that blends almost imperceptibly with normal lung. The overlying visceral pleura is fibrotic and focally invaginates into the underlying parenchyma *(long arrow)*. A histologic section *(B)* shows pleural fibrosis and wrinkling of the pleural elastic lamina *(arrows)*. A section through one of the deep pleural invaginations *(C)* reveals more extensive wrinkling. The adjacent lung is atelectatic and shows mild fibrosis. *(B,* × 60; *C,* × 40; both Verhoeff–van Gieson). (From Menzies R, Fraser R: Am J Surg Pathol *11*:674, 1987.)

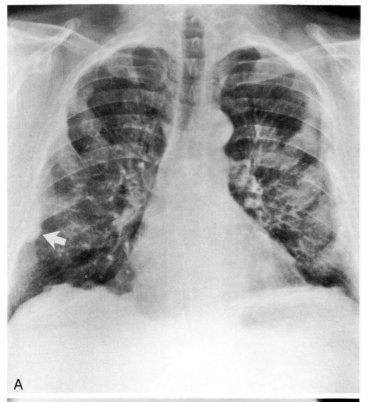

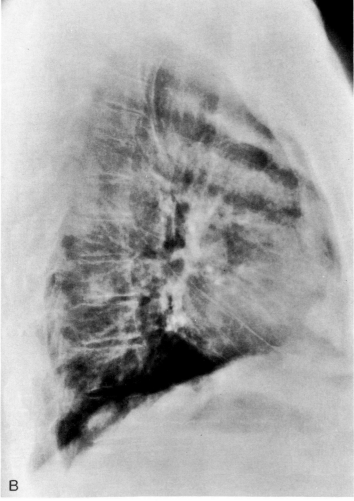

Figure 12–30. Pleural Plaques. Posteroanterior *(A)* and lateral *(B)* roentgenograms of the chest reveal multiple pleura-based opacities situated on all aspects of the chest wall and diaphragm. Several are viewed tangentially, the largest measuring 15 mm in width *(arrow)*, but perhaps the majority are ill defined and rather hazy, indicating their origin from the posterolateral and anterolateral chest wall. The diaphragmatic plaques have created an irregular configuration of both hemidiaphragms. Even the anterior and posterior chest walls are severely affected, as revealed in *B*. The patient is a 54-year-old man with a long history of occupational asbestos exposure; he had no symptoms referable to his thorax.

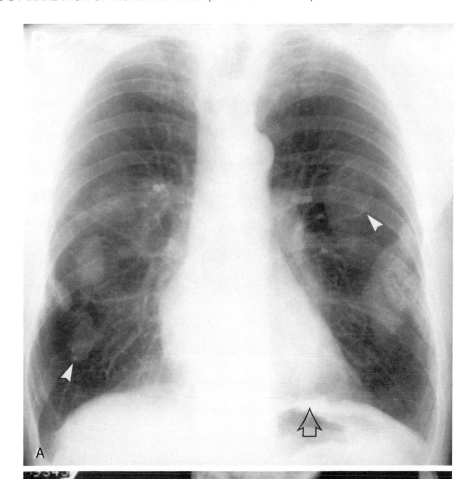

Figure 12–31. Calcification of Pleural Plaques. A posteroanterior chest roentgenogram *(A)* reveals multiple round and elliptical opacities located peripherally between the sixth and tenth ribs posteriorly. Faint curvilinear and nodular calcification *(arrowheads)* can be identified in several of the lesions. There is slight irregularity on the superomedial portion of the left hemidiaphragm *(open arrow)* consistent with plaque formation. Two 10-mm-thick CT scans *(B)* through the lower lobes reveals bilateral posteromedial nodular *(arrow)* and hemispheric *(arrowheads)* opacities.

Illustration continued on following page

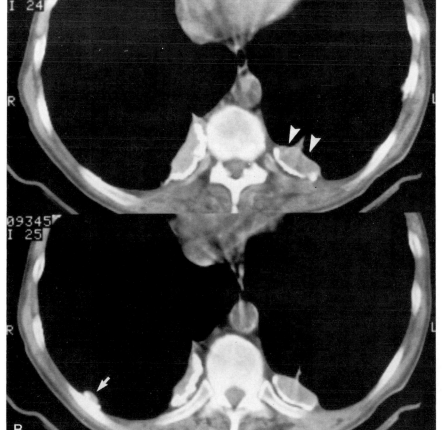

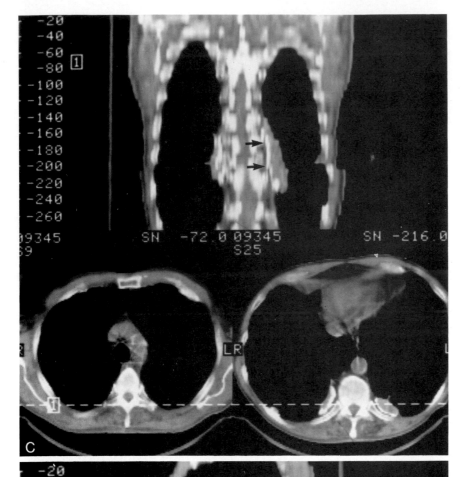

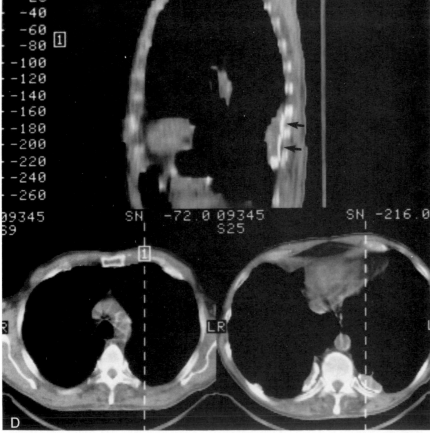

Figure 12–31. *Continued.* Coronal *(C)* and sagittal *(D)* CT re-formations (with appropriate transverse images) through the lower lobes and medial part of the left lung, respectively, show the full extent of the nearly symmetrical posteromedial fibrocalcific plaques. Note that the calcification *(small arrows)* within the plaques is peripheral, involving the parietal pleura. The patient is a middle-aged man.

Figure 12–32. Unilateral Pleural Plaque Formation. A posteroanterior chest roentgenogram *(A)* discloses a vague semilunar opacity *(curved arrow)* in the axillary portion of the right hemithorax. Its configuration suggests that it is closely related to the pleural surface. A thin curvilinear opacity *(arrowheads)* extends obliquely through the right lower hemithorax.

Illustration continued on following page

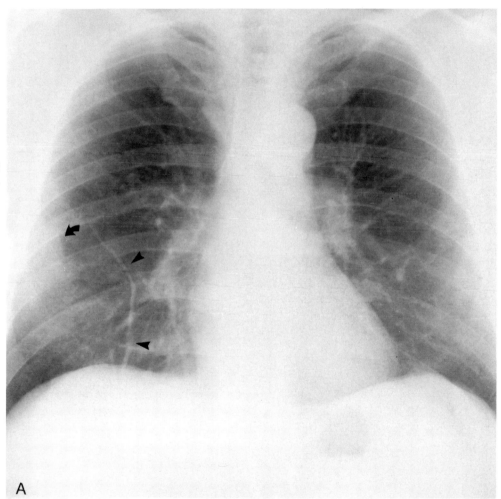

A

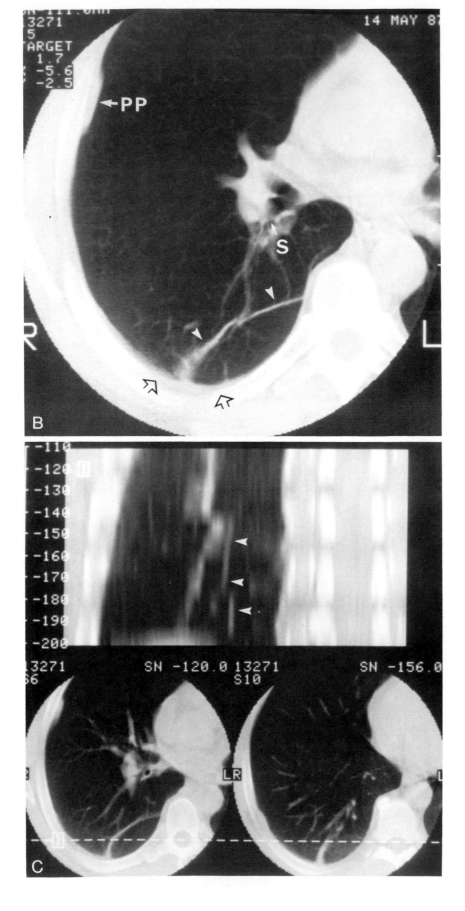

Figure 12–32. *Continued.* A transverse CT scan *(B)* and a coronal CT re-formation of the right lower lobe (with appropriate transverse images) *(C)* show that the semilunar opacity in *A* represents a solitary pleural plaque (PP). The vertically oriented curvilinear shadow *(arrowheads)* in the posteromedial part of the lower lobe subtends a small focal area of pleural thickening *(open arrows)*. Bronchovascular bundles that originate in the superior (S) segment are retracted toward and incorporated within the line. The precise nature of the line is uncertain, although it may be an unusual manifestation of plate-like atelectasis or an early presentation of round atelectasis. The patient is a middle-aged man with a history of asbestos exposure.

The greatest problem in the roentgenologic diagnosis of diffuse pleural thickening and early plaque formation lies in distinguishing them from normal companion shadows of the chest wall—not those that are associated with the first three ribs, because this area is rarely involved in asbestos-related pleural disease—but those muscle and fat shadows that may be identified in as many as 75 per cent of normal posteroanterior roentgenograms along the inferior convexity of the thorax. In fact, sometimes it is impossible to differentiate pleural plaques from companion shadows with conviction. Sargent and colleagues[442] have pointed out the frequency with which subpleural collections of fat can mimic noncalcified pleural plaques and diffuse pleural thickening. In a study of 30 patients involved in compensation and medicolegal problems resulting from exposure to asbestos dust, conventional and oblique roentgenograms revealed pleural shadows of uncertain origin in all. In order to clarify their nature, CT examination was performed, and it proved that in 14 patients (47 per cent), the pleural opacities were the result of subpleural fat accumulation (of the remaining 16 patients, ten had definite pleural plaques, four had no evidence of either plaques or fat, and two demonstrated shadows that could not be attributed with certainty to either plaques or fat). Despite these difficulties, it is clear that when noncalcified plaques can be positively identified, they can be regarded as strongly suggestive evidence of asbestos exposure. In fact, Anton[428] believes that the roentgenographic appearance of multiple pleural plaques is so specific that exposure to asbestos definitely can be concluded, provided that there has been no occupational history of exposure to the related minerals talc or mica.

Diffuse Pleural Thickening. In contrast to a pleural plaque, which is a local circumscribed thickening of the pleura, diffuse thickening is a generalized, more or less uniform increase in pleural width. Although the term is not precisely defined in the 1980 ILO classification, an acceptable definition has been provided by McLoud and colleagues: "a smooth, non-interrupted pleural density extending over a least one-fourth of the chest wall, with or without costophrenic angle obliteration."[443] (In their definition, Sargent and coworkers[444] specified "without nodularity of contour," a wise addition, we think.) In a study designed to determine the prevalence and causes of diffuse pleural thickening in an asbestos-exposed population, McLoud and colleagues[443] evaluated the chest roentgenograms of 1,373 exposed individuals and 717 control subjects, interpretations being made by two B readers according to the 1980 ILO scheme. Among the exposed group, plaques and diffuse thickening occurred with almost equal frequency, 16.5 and 13.5 per cent, respectively. Of the 185 cases with diffuse thickening, the changes were most often considered to be either the residuum of benign asbestos pleural effusion (31.3 per cent) or a confluence of pleural plaques (25.4 per cent). Of considerable interest was the observation that only 10.2 per cent of the 185 patients had coexistent asbestosis, indicating that extension of fibrosis from pulmonary parenchyma into pleura is an untenable theory of pathogenesis.

Two studies have documented the advantages of high-resolution CT in the evaluation of asbestos-related pleural and parenchymal disease, in comparison with both conventional roentgenograms and conventional CT. In a study of 60 men with a history of occupational asbestosis exposure, Friedman and colleagues[445] compared findings on conventional roentgenograms and high-resolution CT and found the predictive value (the likelihood that a positive interpretation is correct) for pleural disease to be 79 per cent for roentgenograms and 100 per cent for CT; comparable figures for parenchymal disease (asbestosis) were 83 and 100 per cent, respectively. These authors also stressed the value of CT in eliminating false-positive diagnoses of asbestos-related pleural disease caused by subpleural fat. In another study of 29 patients with occupational asbestos exposure and 34 age-similar control subjects, Aberle and coworkers[446] found that high-resolution CT was more sensitive than conventional CT in the detection of both pleural and parenchymal abnormalities. For example, in patients with clinical asbestosis, high-resolution CT demonstrated parenchymal abnormality in 96 per cent, compared with 83 per cent for CT. These authors also advocate scanning with the patient in the prone position, a maneuver that effectively permits distinction of structural abnormalities from gravity-related physiologic phenomena.

In a roentgenographic study of an asbestos-exposed population and a control group, Rockoff and his coworkers[440] evaluated the interlobar fissures for evidence of visceral pleural thickening. They found an incidence of fissural thickening in asbestos workers of 54.5 per cent, compared with 16.0 per cent in the unexposed control group; there was a strong positive statistical effect of asbestos exposure beyond that attributable to age. Fissural thickening was present in 85 per cent of workers with parietal pleural plaques and in 36 per cent of those without plaques; it was very common (85 per cent) in patients with pulmonary fibrosis but was identified in only 45 per cent of those without evidence of asbestosis.

Calcification. Although noncalcified pleural plaque formation is probably the commonest roentgenographic manifestations of asbestos-related disease, the most striking abnormality is calcification of pleural plaques. The frequency of pleural calcification is variable. Anton[428] reported finding calcified and noncalcified plaques in roughly equal numbers of his 40 cases, whereas Freundlich and Greening[426] observed calcification in only 21 per cent of their 56 cases. In an American survey of 261 workers exposed to asbestos in industry, pleural calcification was found in none,[454] whereas in Finland it is common,[296] a difference in incidence that probably relates to the variety of asbestos concerned. Calcified plaques vary from small linear or circular shadows, commonly situated over the diaphragmatic domes, to complete encirclement of the lower portion of the lungs.[455] When calcification is minimal, a roentgenogram overexposed at maximal inspiration facilitates visibility.[456] No portion of the pleura is immune to calcification, although the most common site is the diaphragm (Fig. 12–33).[457] There appears to be a dose-response relationship with regard to the development of pleural plaques and calcification. Pleural calcification generally does not develop until at least 20 years after the first exposure to asbestos,[427, 457] although the occupational exposure can be relatively short. Two patients have been described in whom isolated calcific diaphragmatic pleural plaques developed approximately 20 years after occupational exposure of only 8 and 11 months.[458]

Pleural Effusion. The third pleural manifestation of asbestos-related disease, which often is not appreciated, is pleural effusion (Fig. 12–34).[459–461] The most comprehensive report of the prevalence and incidence of pleural effusion in an asbestos-exposed population was by Epler and colleagues,[461] who studied 1,135 exposed workers and 717 control subjects. Benign asbestos effusion was defined by (1) history of exposure to asbestos, (2) confirmation by roentgenograms or thoracentesis or both, (3) no other disease related to pleural effusion, and (4) no malignant tumor within 3 years. These authors found 34 benign effusions among the exposed workers (3 per cent), compared with no otherwise unexplained effusions among the control subjects. Prevalence was dose-related. The latency period was shorter than for other asbestos-related disorders, benign effusion being the most common abnormality during the first 20 years after exposure. Most effusions were small, 28 per cent recurred, and 66 per cent were asymptomatic.

The major differential diagnoses must include tuberculosis and mesothelioma. Of the 12 patients in the Gaensler and Kaplan series,[459] the presence of mesothelioma was recognized in one patient 9 years after the first documented effusion. Of four patients in one other series,[462] two eventually developed mesothelioma. Differentiation from a tuberculous pleural effusion can be made with confidence only if the effusion is persistently negative for *Mycobacterium tuberculosis* on culture.

Mesothelioma. The relationship between mesothelioma and asbestos exposure is now well recognized and is discussed in some detail farther on (see page 2347). Similarly, the pathologic and roentgenographic features of this neoplasm are discussed in Chapter 18, and it will suffice here to describe briefly certain roentgenographic features that relate to other forms of asbestos-related disease.

In a comparative study of mesothelioma and asbestosis using CT and conventional chest roentgenography, Rabinowitz and colleagues[447] found that the major pathologic features of both asbestosis and mesothelioma were well demonstrated by both modalities, although CT demonstrated the findings more frequently and in greater detail; Katz and Kreel[448] also found CT to be significantly more sensitive in the detection of both pleural and parenchymal disease except for thickened fissures. Of interest in the Rabinowitz[447] study was the observation that no features distinguishing between pleural plaques and mesothelioma could be established on the basis of configuration and size of the lesion; many pleural plaques associated with advanced asbestosis were large and irregular and resembled those associated with mesothelioma. Features that predominated in mesothelioma included nodular involvement of the pleural fissures, pleural effusion, and ipsilateral volume loss with a fixed mediastinum. Others have described identical roentgenographic features of mesothelioma.[449, 450] This neoplasm is frequently associated with pleural calcification, as in seven of 14 patients in one series;[450] however, the calcification is almost invariably within pleural plaques, and only rarely is it found pathologically to be within the tumor itself.[451, 452]

PULMONARY MANIFESTATIONS

The roentgenographic changes of asbestosis occur in two forms, small and large opacities.

Small Opacities. These opacities may be round (a nodular pattern) or irregular (a reticular pattern) or a combination of the two. Changes caused by small opacities may be divided into three stages:[463]

1. A fine reticulation occupying predominantly the lower lung zones and associated with a "ground-glass" appearance that is probably the result of combined pleural thickening[428] and early interstitial pneumonitis or fibrosis.

2. A stage in which irregular small opacities become more marked, creating a prominent interstitial reticulation (Fig. 12–35). A combination of parenchymal and pleural changes leads to partial obscuration of the heart border—the so-called shaggy heart sign—and of the diaphragm.

3. A late stage in which reticulation becomes visible in the mid and upper lung zones and the cardiac and diaphragmatic contours become more obscured.[124, 463] Hilar lymph node enlargement is seldom if ever notable.[456]

The small irregular opacities of asbestosis are best detected on a conventional PA roentgenogram, other views contributing little to their identification. Computed tomography,[464] particularly with high resolution,[438, 439] has been proposed as a sensitive and reliable method of detecting parenchymal opacities. In one study, workers exposed to asbestos cement showed greater attenuation of lung paren-

Text continued on page 2345

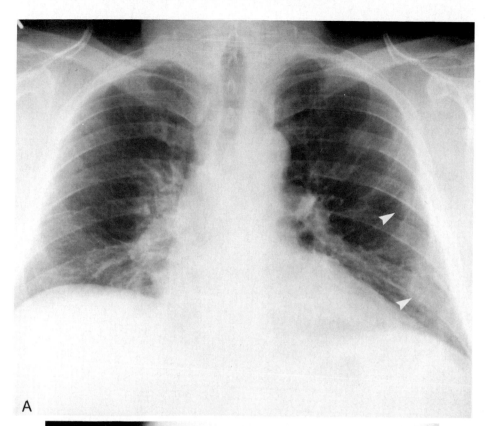

A

Figure 12–33. Asbestos-Induced Pleuropulmonary Disease. Posteroanterior *(A)* and lateral *(B)* chest roentgenograms show multiple ill-defined peripheral opacities *(arrowheads)*, predominantly on the left. The right hemidiaphragm is elevated, and the posterior costophrenic sulcus *(small arrows)* is blunted. Note the curvilinear calcification *(open arrows)* on the posterior aspect of the right hemidiaphragm.

Illustration continued on following page

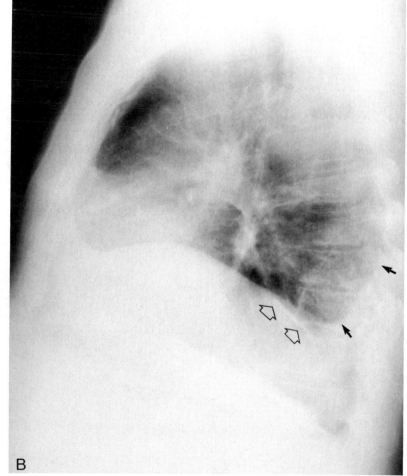

B

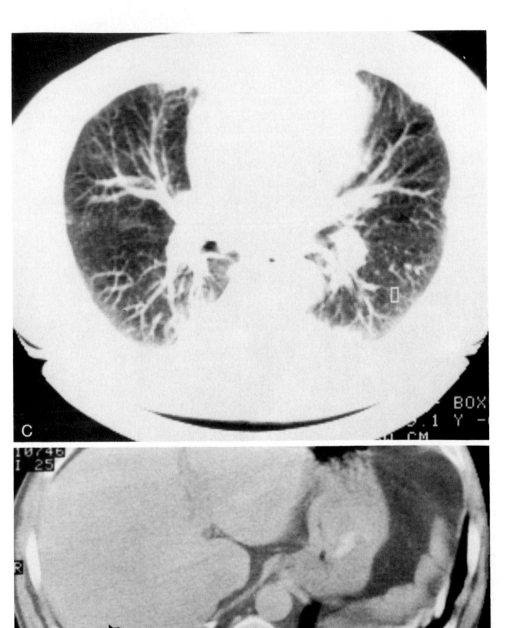

Figure 12–33. *Continued.* A CT scan though the lower lungs *(C)* reveals evidence of a reticular pattern consistent with mild interstitial fibrosis; attenuation values (−767 Hounsfield units) within the left lower lobe are abnormally high. A CT scan through the lower thorax *(D)* reveals bilateral, predominantly right-sided posteromedial diaphragmatic pleural thickening and calcification *(arrowheads)*. Scans at a higher level showed the opacities in *A* to be typical pleural plaques.

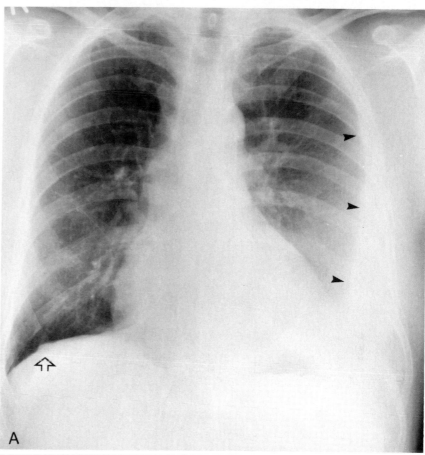

Figure 12–34. Asbestos-Induced Pleural Effusion, Plaque Formation, and Round Atelectasis. A posteroanterior chest roentgenogram *(A)* shows a left pleural effusion of moderate size *(arrowheads)*. A small plaque *(open arrow)* is present on the right hemidiaphragm. A vague opacity is visible behind the right atrial shadow. A posteroanterior roentgenogram taken six months later *(B)* reveals regression of the pleural effusion, although there is residual pleural fibrosis.

Illustration continued on following page

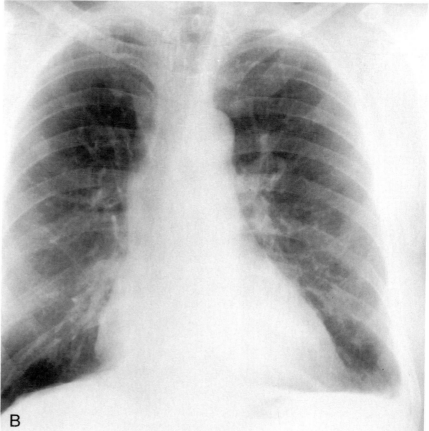

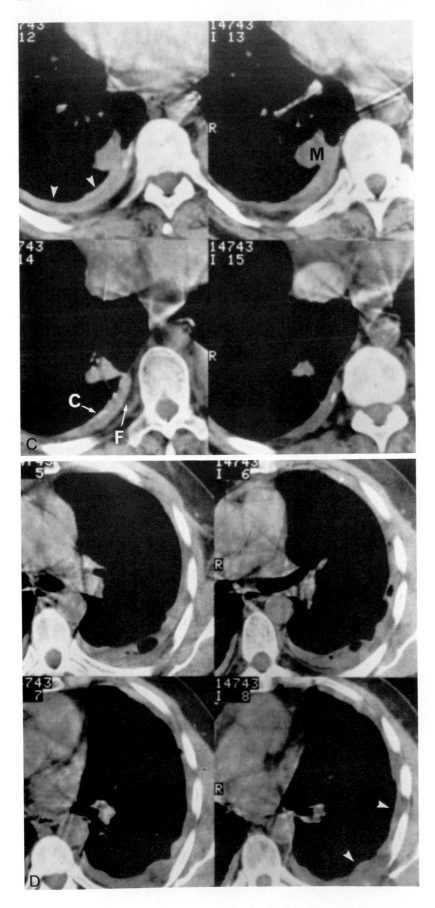

Figure 12–34. *Continued.* Contiguous 10-mm-thick CT scans (obtained on the same day as the roentgenogram in *B*) through the right *(C)* and left *(D)* lower lobes demonstrate extensive bilateral posteromedial pleural thickening *(arrowheads)*. Note the linear calcifications (C) and increased fat (F) in relation to the thickened pleura on the right. A mass (M) is present adjacent to the thickened pleura.

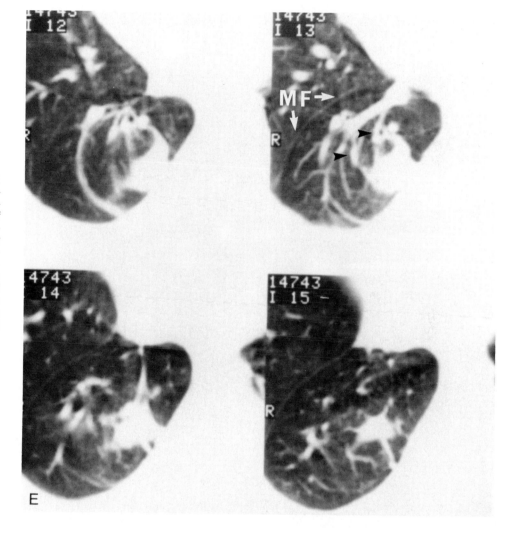

Figure 12–34. *Continued.* CT scans with lung window technique *(E)* through the mass demonstrate the typical features of round atelectasis: Note the curvilinear displacement of the nearby bronchovascular bundles ("comet-tail" sign) *(arrowheads)*. The major fissure (MF) is displaced posteromedially, indicating loss of volume of the right lower lobe. The patient is a 55-year-old man with a history of occupational asbestos exposure.

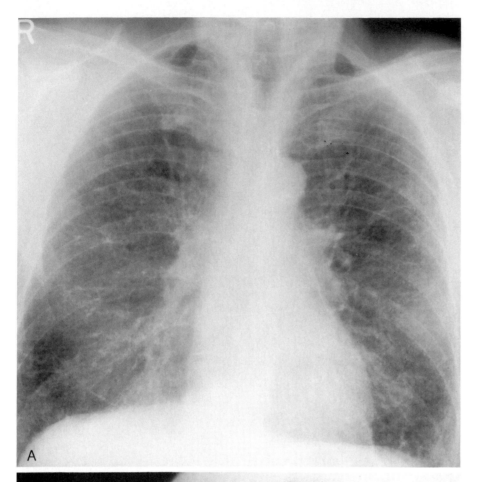

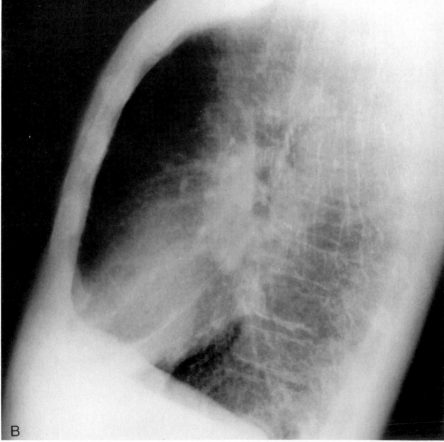

Figure 12–35. Asbestosis. Posteroanterior *(A)* and lateral *(B)* chest roentgenograms disclose a diffuse medium reticular or reticulonodular pattern throughout both lungs with some middle and lower zone predominance. No pleural abnormalities can be identified.

Figure 12–35. *Continued.* CT scans through the middle *(C)* and lower *(D)* lung zones confirm the presence of widespread interstitial disease: at the middle level, cystic spaces measuring 2 to 3 cm can be identified, surrounded by thick walls *(C)*. The lower lobe disease shows rather marked posterior predominance and in many areas is actually confluent *(arrowheads)*. Open lung biopsy in the patient, a 48-year-old man, revealed numerous asbestos bodies and severe interstitial fibrosis consistent with asbestosis.

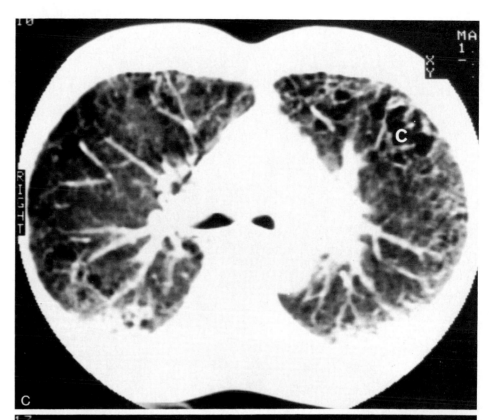

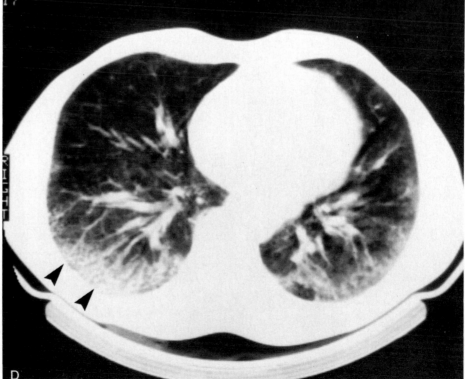

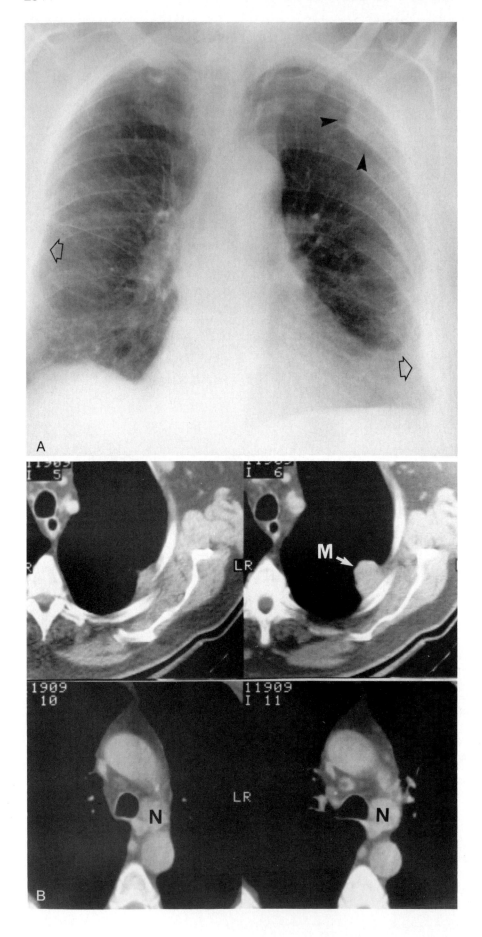

Figure 12–36. Subpleural Curvilinear Shadow Associated with Asbestosis. A posteroanterior chest roentgenogram *(A)* shows a medium reticular pattern throughout both lungs indicating diffuse interstitial disease. A vaguely defined opacity *(arrowheads)* is present in the left upper lobe, and bilateral pleural thickening *(open arrows)* is suggestive of plaque formation. CT scans *(B)* through the left upper lobe opacity (M) *(top)* and subaortic arch *(bottom)* reveal enlarged lymph notes (N) in the aortopulmonary window; the mass was subsequently shown by TTNA to be an adenocarcinoma.

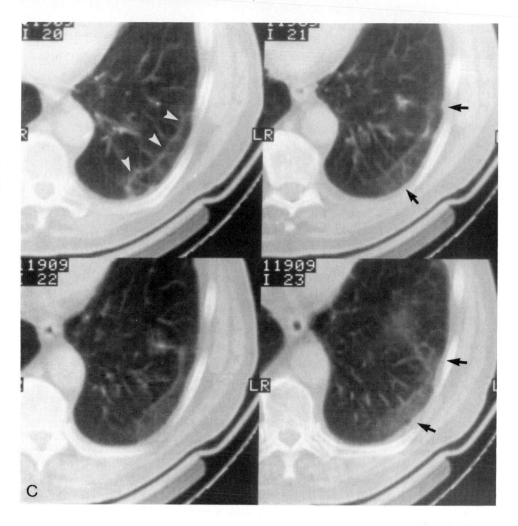

Figure 12–36. *Continued. A series of contiguous 10-mm-thick CT scans through the left lower lobe (C) demonstrate a thin curvilinear opacity (arrowheads) in the posterolateral part of the lung. Similar but less pronounced findings were present in the right lower lobe (not illustrated). Note that the 5-mm to 7-mm zone peripheral to the linear opacity is distinctly abnormal (high CT attenuation and fine reticulation) as a result of interstitial lung disease. Pleural plaques are clearly visible (arrows). The patient is a 52-year-old man.*

chyma on CT than did normal controls, even in the presence of a normal chest roentgenogram; pulmonary function tests revealed reduced static lung volumes and lung compliance.[465]

An unusual manifestation of asbestosis has been described by Toshimura and associates[466] on high-resolution CT scans. Of 19 patients with established disease, 15 showed a subpleural curvilinear opacity that paralleled the inner chest wall (Fig. 12–36). The majority ranged in length from 5 to 10 cm and (judging from the published illustrations) from 2 to 5 mm in width; they showed marked lower lobe predominance. In most patients, the pulmonary fibrosis was relatively mild, suggesting to the authors that the process may represent the initial manifestation of fibrosing bronchioloalveolitis (sic).

Although asbestosis characteristically exhibits considerable mid and lower zonal predominance, a group of cases has been reported in which slowly progressive pleural and parenchymal fibrosis occurred in the lung apices.[467] Of 1,251 patients with asbestos-related pleural or parenchymal abnormalities observed roentgenographically, 16 manifested slowly progressive loss of volume of the upper lobes associated with homogeneous opacities occupying the apical lung zones; these changes were observed most frequently in patients with bilaterally rounded costophrenic sulci and diffuse pleural thickening. Tuberculosis and other possible causes for the apical opacities were excluded, and the author hypothesized that the changes were caused by asbestos exposure. In view of the extensive pleural fibrosis present in these patients, we wonder whether some of the opacities may have represented round atelectasis.

Large Opacities. These opacities measure 1 cm or more in diameter and are an uncommon manifestation of asbestosis. These conglomerate shadows are invariably associated with widespread interstitial fibrosis[468] and usually with calcified or uncalcified pleural plaques. According to Solomon and colleagues,[468] these lesions consist pathologically of diffuse hyaline fibrosis with or without foci of concentric fibrosis, necrosis, and calcification. The hyaline and concentric fibrosis observed by these authors was of the silicotic type, suggesting that quartz may have been responsible for the lesions. South African asbestos rock has a quartz content of approximately 16 per cent, although the amount of quartz in air-borne dust probably does not exceed

1 per cent.[468] Although an association between tuberculosis and large opacities, as in the massive fibrosis of silicotics, cannot be positively denied, no acid-fast bacilli could be identified pathologically in the four cases studied at necropsy by Solomon and colleagues.[468] Roentgenographically, the large opacities may be well- or ill-defined, are nonsegmental in distribution, may be multiple, and may become very large. Although they may occur in both upper and lower lung zones, they tend to show a lower zonal predominance, in contrast to the upper lobe predominance of the large opacities of silicosis.[468] Unlike the large opacities of silicosis or CWP, the massive fibrosis of asbestosis does not appear to "migrate" toward the center of the lung. Further, the opacities have not been known to undergo roentgenographically demonstrable cavitation.

Until recent years, the accuracy with which the commonly accepted roentgenographic signs of asbestosis may be recognized has been rather poor. In their 1960 study of observer error, Williams and Hugh-Jones[507] showed wide disparity in the opinions registered by 11 experienced observers in assessing the roentgenograms of patients with established asbestosis. In recent years, possibly as a result of the general acceptance of the ILO 1980 International Classification, observer variability appears to have diminished somewhat. For example, in an epidemiologic study of 13,021 mine and mill workers in the chrysotile asbestos industry of Quebec, Rossiter and colleagues[508] obtained results that were thought to be well within acceptable limits in comparison with previous observer variation in pneumoconiosis studies. The most repeatable indices were pleural calcification and costophrenic angle obliteration, with irregular small opacities being the least repeatable.

Clinical Manifestations

SYMPTOMS AND SIGNS

The great majority of patients with pleuropulmonary asbestos-related disease probably have no symptoms.[296, 463] Occasionally an acute pleural effusion is associated with pleural pain.[339, 469–471] Such effusions can occur in the absence of symptoms[472] and are recurrent in 15[472] to 30 per cent[471] of cases. They are usually smaller than 500 ml, are often serosanguineous,[339, 471, 472] and persist from 2 weeks to 6 months.[471, 472] Although effusions can occur in the absence of pleural plaques, more often plaques are present at the time of effusion.[472] In one study of 22 patients with benign pleural effusion attributed to asbestos exposure, the mean duration of exposure was 5.5 years (in one case it was said to occur after only 2 weeks!), and the mean interval between exposure and presentation was 16.3 years.[471]

In asbestos-related pleuropulmonary disease, breathlessness is almost invariably associated with interstitial fibrosis, although it can occasionally be caused partly (in rare cases largely) by thickened pleura.[280, 473–475, 787] Dyspnea is usually progressive despite discontinuation of asbestos exposure. In patients with asbestosis, shortness of breath seldom develops sooner than 20 to 30 years after initial exposure.[476, 477]

Prolonged asbestos exposure can cause cough that can be dry or productive of mucopurulent sputum; this symptom can be present with or without dyspnea on exertion and in the absence of roentgenographic or physiologic evidence of asbestosis.[788] In a study of respiratory symptoms in an age-stratified random sample of 1,015 male employees in Quebec chrysotile asbestos mines and mills, the prevalence of cough, sputum production, and wheezing increased with age and was much higher in smokers than in nonsmokers or ex-smokers. There was little or no evidence of any association between these symptoms and dust exposure, except perhaps in men over 50 years. In contrast, breathlessness appeared more closely related to dust exposure than to smoking, although it also occurred more frequently with rising age.

Physical examination may reveal evidence of deformity of the thoracic cage caused by underlying pleural disease, even in symptom-free patients. Pleural effusion may be suggested by unilateral or bilateral dullness on percussion and decreased breath sounds. Crepitations (fine rales or crackles) are common at the lung bases in workers with prolonged exposure to asbestos;[478] in two separate studies, the incidence of crepitations was virtually identical, being identified in 32 per cent of workers compared with only 5 per cent in control populations.[479, 480] Because the presence of rales correlates with derangement of pulmonary function,[481] most observers would compensate the worker for asbestosis on the basis of this physical sign, even in the absence of roentgenographic abnormality and providing that the history suggested sufficiently heavy exposure and that pulmonary function tests showed decreased compliance.[482, 483] Basal rales are even more common in patients in whom the diagnosis of asbestosis has been made on the basis of their chest roentgenograms[481]—in 58 per cent in one series[484] and in 64 per cent in another.[485]

Finger clubbing is also a frequent sign in asbestosis,[477] having been observed in 32 per cent of patients in one series[484] and in 42 per cent in another.[485] In 167 cases of asbestosis certified by the London Pneumoconiosis Medical Panel from 1958 to 1975, the prognostic significance of finger clubbing was evaluated.[486] Clubbing was found to develop early in the clinical course of the disease and to be associated with a lower diffusing capacity, a higher mortality rate, and a greater likelihood of progression of pulmonary fibrosis than was observed among patients without finger clubbing. Thus, its presence is an indication of a more severe form of disease; however, finger clubbing was not associated with heavier asbestos exposure. If the patient lives long enough and survives complicating mesothelioma or pulmonary carcinoma, signs of cor pulmonale may develop. Rarely, patients with asbestosis have developed chronic constrictive pericarditis.[789]

It is well known that the incidence of radiation-induced lung damage is higher in patients receiving chemotherapy and in those with pulmonary consolidation and atelectasis; it has now been suggested that asbestosis may also increase the risk.[453]

PULMONARY FUNCTION TESTS

Patients with interstitial fibrosis caused by asbestos inhalation usually show a restrictive pattern of pulmonary function, with decreased vital capacity, residual volume, and diffusion capacity, and preservation of relatively good ventilatory function. However, because (1) most are cigarette smokers and (2) there is good evidence that the inhalation of asbestos fibers can cause some degree of airway obstruction (see farther on), the measurement of total lung capacity (TLC) alone is thought to be an insensitive means of assessing functional impairment in asbestosis.[487] Hypoxemia may be observed on exercise but the P_{CO_2} is normal or low. Pulmonary compliance characteristically is greatly reduced.[149, 477, 478, 488–490] Employing a combination of electron microscopy and stereologic principles, Divertie and colleagues[491] concluded that measurable diffusion abnormalities were caused chiefly by ventilation-perfusion imbalance rather than increased thickness of the alveolar membrane. Cookson and coworkers[492] compared the roentgenographic and functional characteristics of patients with asbestosis and with cryptogenic fibrosing alveolitis; they found that although there were functional, pathologic, and roentgenographic similarities, pulmonary function was better in patients with asbestosis than in those with cryptogenic fibrosing alveolitis who had the same degree of roentgenographic parenchymal abnormality.

The extensive pleural thickening that can occur as a result of asbestos exposure can seriously restrict lung expansion; in such circumstances, correction of the diffusing capacity for alveolar volume will give a higher coefficient of diffusion that does not accurately reflect the severity of the parenchymal fibrosis.[493, 494] In a study of pulmonary function profiles of over 1,000 Quebec chrysotile asbestos workers, Fournier-Massey and Becklake[495] found an obstructive pulmonary function pattern in smokers that could not be explained solely on the basis of cigarette consumption. This finding may be analogous to the greater prevalence of pulmonary fibrosis in asbestos workers who smoke[365] and to the additive or synergistic carcinogenic effect of cigarette smoking and asbestos exposure reported by Selikoff and colleagues.[497] In a group of 120 asbestos-exposed workers who were seeking compensation, Agostoni and associates[496] carried out an evaluation by clinical exercise testing; they found a surprising number to be limited by cardiac function and concluded that the complaint of dyspnea was usually caused by cardiac rather than ventilatory dysfunction.

Although lung function tests are not generally considered to be more useful than the chest roentgenogram in the early detection of asbestosis,[295] in one epidemiologic study of exposed individuals who manifested no clinical or roentgenographic evidence of disease and whose routine lung function tests were normal, changes in the mechanical properties of the lung (specifically a decrease in compliance and an increase in calculated upstream resistance) were detectable in subjects with heavier dust exposure.[498]

Diagnosis

In the presence of characteristic roentgenographic findings, the diagnosis of asbestos-related disease should be based primarily on a complete occupational history;[499] inquiry should also be directed towards the possibility of a nonoccupational environmental exposure. This approach applies to women as well as to men, not only because of the potential for significant asbestos dust exposure from the cleaning of clothes of occupationally exposed male members of the family, but also because women may have been occupationally exposed as well, however remotely.[307, 308, 500] The combination of a history of exposure, positive roentgenographic findings, bibasilar fine rales, and impaired pulmonary function (including significant reductions in vital capacity, diffusing capacity, and compliance) is virtually diagnostic.[281] Because the number of asbestos bodies found in BAL fluid has been found to correlate with the number in lung tissue sections,[501, 790] BAL can be useful in establishing a diagnosis; the same cannot be said for sputum whose content does not correlate with bronchial washings.[791] Direct lung biopsy can confirm a suspected diagnosis but is seldom indicated; in fact, in the presence of advanced disease, it can be a hazardous procedure.[502] A poorly defined opacity in the periphery of a lung of a patient with asbestos-related pleural disease often represents round atelectasis whose roentgenographic appearance is characteristic, particularly on CT; however, transthoracic needle aspiration may occasionally be required to rule out the possibility of pulmonary carcinoma.[420, 421, 503, 504]

In contrast to the acknowledged risk of tuberculosis in patients with silicosis, those with asbestosis do not appear to be at greater risk than the general population;[505] however, one large study of causes of death among miners and millers of crocidolite in Western Australia showed an excess mortality from tuberculosis, the standardized mortality ratio being 4.87.[506]

Relationship to Neoplasia

Of all non-neoplastic pulmonary diseases, those related to asbestos have the highest incidence of associated neoplasia, especially pulmonary carcinoma (Fig. 12–37) and pleural mesothelioma (Fig. 12–38).[509] Since it was first investigated scientifically in 1955,[510] the relationship has been documented in many pathologic and epidemiologic studies.[510, 511] A latent period of at least 20 years from the time of first exposure to the development of malignancy is characteristic.[512]

The degree of exposure, as indicated by occupational history and the number of asbestos bodies or fibers in lung tissue, is usually high,[284, 513–519] although in some cases of mesothelioma it may be deceptively low (see farther on). Most[499, 520] but not all[513] studies indicate that the relationship between malignancy and asbestos exposure is linear. According to Becklake[499] the relationship has no threshold below which there is no risk.

As pointed out by Selikoff and Hammond,[521] the burden of risk for asbestos-associated pulmonary cancer is borne predominantly by workers who smoke. These investigators reported on a 10-year follow-up study of 8,220 asbestos insulation workers who had volunteered their histories of smoking at the outset of the study in 1967; 6,841 had a history of cigarette smoking, 1,379 did not. For comparison, a group of 73,763 men in the American Cancer Society's prospective cancer prevention study was analyzed as controls; these men had the same distribution of smoking habits and were alike in most other respects except that they had not been exposed to asbestos. Death rates for lung cancer (per 100,000 man-years, standardized for age) were as follows: 11.3 for men who neither worked with asbestos nor smoked cigarettes; 58.4 for men who worked with asbestos but did not smoke; 122.6 for cigarette smokers who had not worked with asbestos; and 601.6 for men who had been exposed to both cigarettes and asbestos. The bottom line is ominous indeed: among asbestos workers who smoke, one in every five deaths is caused by lung cancer. Equally ominous is the mortality rate for pulmonary carcinoma and mesothelioma in asbestos workers in whom the presence of asbestosis had been established: in one study, almost 50 per cent died from these malignancies.[522]

Pathologically, asbestosis is frequently[524] but not invariably[499, 523] present when pulmonary carcinoma develops in association with asbestos exposure (Fig. 12–39); however, even when identified histologically, the fibrosis may not be detectable roentgenographically or by pulmonary function studies.[511] The cell type most commonly reported in asbestos-associated lung cancer is adenocarcinoma,[511] although a predominance of squamous cell carcinoma[527] has been reported in some series. It has been stated that asbestos-related carcinoma occurs more commonly in lower than in upper lobes,[511] although some studies have found no such association.[527]

The incidence of associated neoplasia relates in part to the type of asbestos involved.[792] This is particularly true for mesothelioma, in which the most commonly implicated dust is crocidolite, a relationship first described from both occupational and environmental exposure in the mining area of Northwest Cape, South Africa.[302] In contrast to the experience in the Northwest Cape, despite the fact that 20 per cent of the crocidolite produced in South Africa comes from the Transvaal, mesotheliomas only rarely occur in this region and then only in association with amosite asbestos mining.[311] Wagner[528] explains this apparent contradiction by the much larger diameter of the crocidolite fiber in the Transvaal than in Northwest Cape, the larger fiber theoretically being unable to penetrate to the visceral pleura. However, Webster[529] has offered an alternative explanation by invoking the high concentration of manganese—a known inhibitor of benzpyrene—in Transvaal ore. It is generally agreed that the risk of developing mesothelioma is somewhat less for amosite and considerably less for chrysotile than for crocidolite.[295, 301, 530]

The risk of developing both pulmonary carcinoma[531] and mesothelioma with crocidolite and chrysotile exposure appears to be higher in manufacturing industries than in mining and milling. Several studies have demonstrated a possible relationship between the development of mesothelioma and the manufacturing and secondary uses of asbestos, including chrysotile.[523, 524] In recent years, tremolite[312–314, 526, 535, 536] and crocidolite[525, 537–539] have also been implicated as a cause of mesothelioma; these amphiboles are present in small quantities in chrysotile deposits in both mining and milling and as contaminants in industrial use. Despite a thorough search, mesothelioma has not been found to be associated with anthophyllite asbestos production in Finland.[540]

Most investigations directed towards an assessment of the association of asbestos and mesothelioma find it to be strong, the incidence ranging from 70 per cent[541] to 80 per cent,[311, 542] occasionally even higher.[543–545] As with other neoplasms, a genetic susceptibility has been considered, in this instance based on the occurrence of mesothelioma in siblings with relatively mild exposure to asbestos.[546] Some studies, particularly one from the Massachusetts General Hospital in Boston,[547] throw some doubt on the acceptance of asbestos as the almost invariable cause of mesothelioma: in a retrospective study of 36 patients with mesothelioma who had no history of exposure to asbestos, 19 showed no evidence of asbestos bodies at autopsy. This lack of association between mesothelioma and asbestos may be the result of an inadequate occupational history or the possibility that mesothelioma is related to more than one etiologic factor. The facts that women survive longer than men[393, 793] and that patients with mesothelioma but without a history of exposure to asbestos have longer survival times[519] support the latter possibility. An example of other possible etiologic factors has been reported by Antman and

Text continued on page 2354

Figure 12–37. Asbestosis and Pulmonary Carcinoma. A posteroanterior chest roentgenogram *(A)* reveals a coarse reticular pattern throughout both lungs with marked basal predominance. The right hilum is enlarged and lobulated in contour, suggesting lymph node enlargement. Similarly, the lateral interface of the aortopulmonary window *(arrowhead)* is convex, indicating the probability of enlarged nodes. A posteroanterior roentgenogram taken 7 months later *(B)* reveals a marked increase in the size of both hila, greater prominence of the aortopulmonary window nodes, and widening of the upper mediastinum. A poorly defined opacity *(arrowhead)* can be identified in the right lower lobe. At autopsy, performed several months after *B* was obtained, the lungs were found to be the site of severe interstitial fibrosis; hilar and mediastinal lymph nodes were markedly enlarged by metastatic small cell carcinoma, although the primary site was not identified. Many asbestos bodies were present throughout the lung parenchyma. The patient was an elderly man with a long history of asbestos exposure and cigarette smoking.

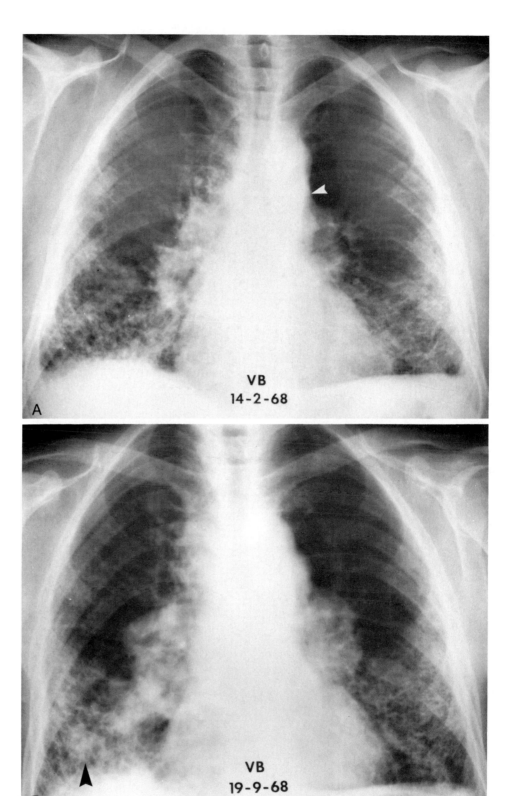

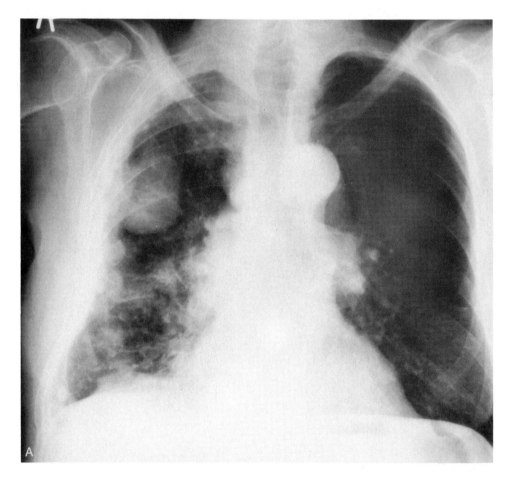

Figure 12–38. Diffuse Mesothelioma. An overpenetrated posteroanterior chest roentgenogram *(A)* shows a reduction in volume of the right hemithorax. There is marked thickening of the pleura over the whole of the right lung, including its mediastinal surface. The thickening is very irregular and nodular and is associated with a large mass in the upper axillary region.

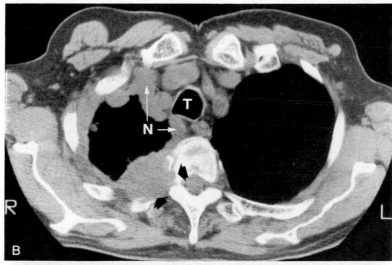

Figure 12–38. *Continued.* High-resolution CT scans through the upper *(B)*, middle *(C)*, and lower *(D)* thorax confirm the extensive right pleural thickening *(arrowheads)* and demonstrate extrapleural extension of the neoplasm in and around the ribs and vertebra *(closed arrows)* and within some of the mediastinal lymph nodes (N). The diagnosis of mesothelioma was confirmed at autopsy several months later.

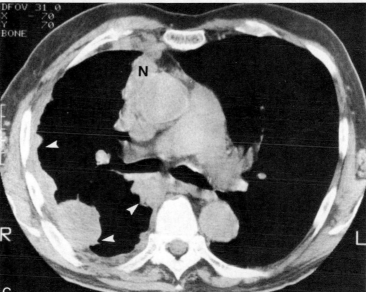

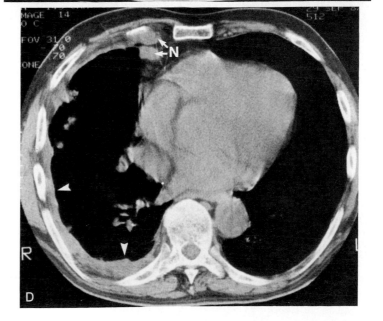

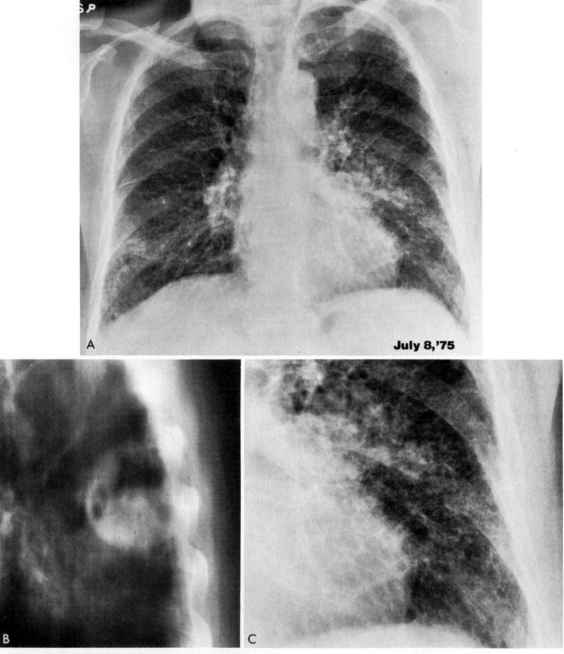

Figure 12–39. Double Primary Pulmonary Carcinoma in a Patient with Asbestosis. A 64-year-old woman had a long history of asbestos exposure. In July 1975, shortly after an episode of hemoptysis, there was roentgenographic evidence *(A)* of a poorly defined mass projected in the plane of the left hilum. A lateral tomogram obtained at that time *(B)* showed a sharply circumscribed mass in the superior segment of the left lower lobe with central cavitation. At the time of these examinations, the poorly defined opacity situated in the plane of the lower portion of the right hilum was not commented upon. Note the rather coarse reticular pattern throughout both lungs, consistent with asbestosis and seen to advantage in a magnified view of the lower half of the left lung *(C)*. The left lower lobe was resected, the specimen revealing squamous cell carcinoma on a background of asbestosis.

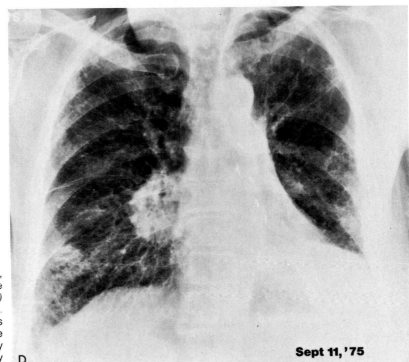

Sept 11, '75

D

Figure 12-39. *Continued.* Two months later, the patient returned for a routine postoperative check-up, and a posteroanterior roentgenogram *(D)* revealed a large mass projected over the right hilum. A tomogram in anteroposterior projection *(E)* shows a 5-cm mass in the right lower lobe; its margins are spiculated in a manner characteristic of primary carcinoma. In view of the patient's limited respiratory reserve, further surgical intervention was considered contraindicated. However, because sputum cytology was positive at this time, the diagnosis of a second primary carcinoma may be regarded as reasonably certain.

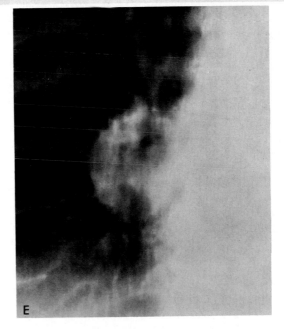

E

associates,[548] who described four patients and discovered five others in the literature in whom mesothelioma originated at the site of therapeutic radiation administered many years earlier. The occurrence of mesothelioma in patients previously treated for Wilms' tumor in childhood[549, 550] may reflect a similar pathogenesis. The bulk of evidence indicates that smoking plays no role in the pathogenesis of mesothelioma.[499, 551]

In contrast to other manifestations of asbestos-related pleuropulmonary disease, the relationship between dose and the development of mesothelioma is considerably weaker; for example, cases have been described in which the duration of exposure was one year or less.[542, 552] However, the latent period between exposure and the development of clinical signs usually exceeds 20 years[553] and more often is in the vicinity of 40 years.[554] In one case, the development of a mesothelioma 7.5 years after occupational exposure suggested to the authors that the patient must have had an unrecognized exposure at an earlier date.[555]

A variety of extrathoracic neoplasms have also been noted with increased frequency following asbestos exposure, the one with the closest association probably being peritoneal mesothelioma;[556, 557] Enticknap and Smithers[557] described 11 patients with this rare malignancy, all of whom had worked in the same asbestos factory. A number of studies have shown evidence for an increased incidence of gastrointestinal,[295, 558] renal,[521] oropharyngeal,[521] and laryngeal[559–561] carcinoma as well as leukemia[794] and lymphoma[562] in workers exposed to asbestos.

OTHER SILICATES

Talc

Talc is a hydrated magnesium silicate that usually occurs in the form of sheet-like crystals that are easily cleaved into thin plates.[563] It is used in the manufacture of such diverse products as leather, rubber, paper, textiles, ceramic tiles, and roofing material. It is also employed as an additive in paint, food, many pharmaceuticals, insecticides, and herbicides. Individuals in any of these occupational settings may be exposed to potentially harmful levels of dust. Others at risk include workers involved in talc mining and milling,[564–566] individuals who work with soapstone,[567, 568] and people exposed to commercial talcum powder, either as an occupational hazard[569–573] or environmentally, the latter usually as an obsession (Fig. 12–40).[571] Although pulmonary disease related to talc most often results from chronic dust inhalation in one of the previously mentioned settings, it can also be seen in three other situations.

1. Acute fatal respiratory insufficiency has been reported in small children caused by accidental inhalation of talcum powder and resultant tracheobronchial obstruction.[574, 575]

2. Chronic pulmonary disease can occur secondary to the intravenous injection of oral medications containing talc as a filler, a form of microembolization discussed in detail in Chapter 9 (*see* page 1794).

3. One case has been described in which bilateral interstitial disease and pleural effusion developed following talc pleurodesis.[576]

Because other elements such as iron and nickel are usually incorporated within the talc crystal and because the substance is often found in association with other minerals such as quartz and various types of asbestos, the composition of commercially available talc is quite variable from region to region and from industry to industry.[563, 566, 577] As a result, the pattern of pulmonary disease associated with its inhalation is highly variable, leading to the use of such terms as "talco-asbestosis," "talco-silicosis," and "pure talcosis."[578] Although there is no doubt that talc can induce a foreign body giant cell reaction, its ability in *pure form* to induce fibrosis has been questioned in both epidemiologic and animal studies;[563] in fact, it has even been suggested that the majority if not all of the functionally and roentgenologically significant pulmonary abnormalities are caused by substances other than talc. It seems likely, however, that true inhalational talcosis does occur, as evidenced by reported cases in which significant pulmonary disease has been caused by exposure to dust apparently uncontaminated by asbestos or silica.[568, 578, 579]

Pathologic findings are variable[568, 578] and as previously indicated may be caused in some cases by asbestos or silica rather than talc alone. Abnormalities include pleural fibrosis (sometimes with calcification and plaque formation similar to that seen in asbestos-related pleural disease), focal nodular parenchymal fibrosis, more or less diffuse interstitial fibrosis, non-necrotizing granulomatous inflammation,[580] and peribronchiolar and perivascular macrophage infiltrates. Multinucleated giant cells containing irregularly shaped birefringent plates or needle-like crystals, representing macrophage-ingested talc, are common. Occasionally, the amount of talc is minimal, its presence being evidenced only with the use of scanning electron microscopy.[580] In suspected cases, optical and electron microscopy may reveal talc particles in BAL fluid.[576, 577]

Roentgenographically, the hallmark in the diagnosis of talc-related disease is pleural plaque formation. These are often diaphragmatic, and may be massive, often bizzare in shape, extending over much of the surface of both lungs;[565, 566, 581–583] they sometimes involve the pericardium. The incidence of pleural abnormality in talcosis is similar to that in asbestosis. In a study of 221 workers exposed to tremolite talc, Smith[454] found pleural plaques in 14 (6.3 per cent). Parenchymal involvement is said to be similar to that in asbestosis,[582, 584, 585] the roentgenographic pattern being one of general haziness, nodulation, and reticulation, with sparing of the apices and costophrenic sinuses.[565, 585] Some cases

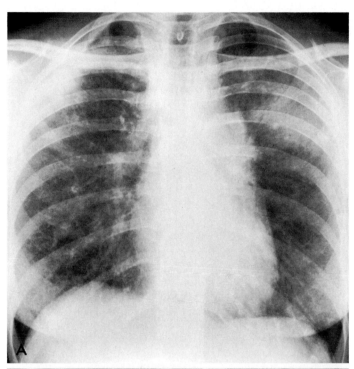

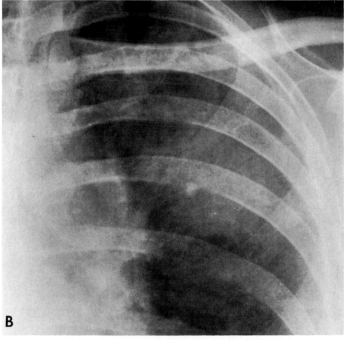

Figure 12–40. Pulmonary Talcosis. A 31-year-old woman had noted the onset of dyspnea on exertion several months previously and at the time of this roentgenographic examination could climb only ten stairs without stopping. She had to use two pillows to sleep, and on occasion she awoke during the night gasping for breath. There was no cough or recent hemoptysis. A posteroanterior roentgenogram *(A)* reveals extensive involvement of both lungs by a rather coarse reticular pattern. In the upper axillary zone on the right and in the left midlung *(B)* are two areas of homogeneous consolidation possessing poorly defined margins. Paratracheal lymph node enlargement is present bilaterally, more marked on the left. At thoracotomy, biopsy specimens obtained from lung and lymph node revealed multiple foci of dense fibrosis lying in close proximity to blood vessels and containing extremely numerous, doubly refractile crystals. In view of these findings, the patient was questioned further and finally admitted to an extraordinary history of excessive inhalation of lavender-scented talcum powder during a 3-month-period when she was pregnant 2 years previously. She was in the habit of spreading the talcum powder liberally over her pillow and blankets at night and actually inhaled it in large amounts from her cupped hands. Subsequent assay of the doubly refractile particles observed histologically proved them to be talc.

may show confluence of lesions, creating large opacities (Fig. 12–40).[586]

Symptoms are similar to those of any other disabling pneumoconiosis and include dyspnea and productive cough. Decreased breath sounds (presumably due to pleural thickening), rales at the lung bases, limited chest expansion, and finger clubbing are found on physical examination.[582, 587] Levels of serum angiotensin converting enzyme are increased in some patients.[588] In a study of 110 men employed in the mining and processing of soapstone in Sweden, Ahlmark and associates[567] found five persons with at least 20 years' exposure who showed minimal roentgenographic evidence of pneumoconiosis and no restriction of work capacity. Others have commented on an association between the degree of exposure and the development of pleuropulmonary disease.[566] An investigation into the cause of death among talc miners and millers in New York State indicated an increased incidence of pulmonary and pleural neoplasms.[589]

Decreases in vital capacity (VC), TLC, and carbon monoxide diffusing capacity have been reported to occur in many exposed workers.[590, 591] Diffusing capacity is said to correlate with the extent of parenchymal involvement seen roentgenographically. We studied one case, proven by biopsy, in which both VC and residual volume (RV) were moderately decreased and repeated measurement of the steady state DL_{CO} was less than 50 per cent of predicted normal. Restrictive pulmonary function impairment has been described in patients with pleural disease only.[566, 583]

Mica

Micas are complex aluminum silicates of which three forms are commercially available: (1) *muscovite*, a potassium compound that, because of its transparency and resistance to heat and electricity, is used in the manufacture of windows for stoves and furnaces, (2) *phlogopite*, a magnesium compound that is used in the electrical industry, and (3) *vermiculite*, another magnesium compound whose uses relate primarily to its fire resistance and its insulation and ion-exchange properties. The last-named substance is also used as a soil additive, an animal feed bulking agent, and a carrier for various chemicals, including herbicides, insecticides, fungicides, and fertilizers.[592]

Like talc, micas are often associated with other minerals, particularly tremolite,[592] and the possibility that micas can cause disease by themselves has been questioned.[593] For example, workers exposed to vermiculite contaminated with fibrous tremolite have been found to have a high incidence of benign pleural effusion, plaques, and pleural thickening,[592] abnormalities well known to be caused by asbestos alone. In addition, although there have been many reports of possible pneumoconiosis caused by micas,[592, 594–596] the documentation of the relationship

between occupational exposure and pathologic findings has not always excluded other etiologic agents. Thus, a literature review in 1985 found 66 cases reported as mica pneumoconiosis, but the evidence that it was caused by mica exposure alone was reasonably convincing in only 26.[597]

Animal experiments have demonstrated little or no fibrogenic activity caused by mica,[16] although the validity of these studies has been questioned.[597] Despite these uncertainties, occasional cases have been reported in which apparently pure mica exposure has been associated with pulmonary fibrosis,[593] and it seems reasonable to conclude that the risk of developing pulmonary disease from mica inhalation is present but slight.

When present, roentgenographic and clinical manifestations of significant exposure to mica are virtually indistinguishable from those of exposure to asbestos or talc.[454, 575]

Fuller's Earth

Fuller's earth is an aluminum silicate containing iron and magnesium, formerly used in the process of fulling (removing grease from wool) and now employed in the refining of oils, as a filtering agent, as a filler in cosmetics and other products, and in the bonding of molding sands in foundry work. Prolonged exposure to this dust can produce simple pneumoconiosis and, occasionally, massive fibrosis.[52] The pathologic changes, which occur mainly in the upper lobes, consist of an increase in reticulin surrounding dust particles, with little actual collagen formation or cellular reaction.[598, 599] Roentgenographic changes are said to consist of a prominence of bronchovascular markings[599, 600] and, occasionally, PMF.[600]

Kaolin (China Clay)

The term kaolin (china clay) derives from the chinese "Kauling" or high ridge, the name given a hill near Jauchau Fu, China, where the clay was first mined.[601] It actually designates a group of clays of which *kaolinite*, a hydrated aluminum silicate, is the most important member. This substance is used industrially as a filler in plastics, rubber, paints, and adhesives, as a coating for paper, as an absorbent,[602] and in the making of firebricks.[603]

Although water is usually employed in quarrying or strip mining to minimize the risk of dust exposure, subsequent drying, bagging, and transporting of kaolin can result in high concentrations of aerosolized dust and the potential for pulmonary disease. For example, in a study of 65 workers in a Georgia kaolin mine,[604] pneumoconiosis occurred only in workers exposed in the processing area, where the mean respirable dust level was over 12 times that in the mine itself. Although it seems likely that kaolinite alone can cause pulmonary disease,[602, 605] it is probable that some cases are complicated by the inhalation of other particulates,[606] partly because the purity of raw clay varies considerably. For example, although in some regions, such as Georgia, the kaolin is relatively silica free,[602] in others there can be substantial amounts of admixed quartz and other minerals. Exposure to kaolinite can also occur in workers involved in the mining, crushing, or grinding of china stone,[606] in which quartz is likely to be an important contaminant. The lungs of Scottish shale miners have been shown to contain high concentrations of kaolinite.[3]

The incidence of significant chest disease varies in reported series. In one study of 5,130 workers in the kaolin industry,[607] it was concluded that their general state of health varied little from that of the regional general population of corresponding age and race. By contrast, in a study of 553 Cornish china clay workers exposed to kaolin dust for periods exceeding 5 years, 48 (9 per cent) showed clinical and roentgenographic evidence of disease. Abnormalities were present in 23 per cent of those exposed for more than 15 years.[608] In a more recent roentgenographic study of 1676 china clay workers from the same area by three observers using the ILO 1980 International Classification, 77.4 per cent were judged to be in category 0, 17.9 per cent in category 1, and 4.7 per cent in categories 2 and 3; 19 workers (1.1 per cent) were considered to have large opacities of progressive massive fibrosis.[501] The prevalence of pneumoconiosis in Georgia kaolin workers has been estimated to be about 10 per cent.[609]

Despite these figures, most patients have no disability and show only slight increase in lung markings roentgenographically, even after many years' exposure. Disabling pneumoconiosis is believed to develop in only a small proportion of these workers.[610] However, in workers who processed kaolin in a Georgia mine, a significant degree of restrictive pulmonary dysfunction was found that correlated with the number of years of exposure.[604]

Pathologic features have been described in workers from Georgia[602] and Cornwall.[606] In the former study,[602] the features were similar to those of CWP, consisting of peribronchiolar macules (composed of numerous pigment-laden macrophages and interspersed reticulin fibers) and of larger masses measuring up to 12 cm in diameter. The latter were composed almost entirely of macrophages with only small amounts of interspersed collagen; coagulation necrosis and obliterative vascular changes similar to those seen in CWP were also present. In their description of the pathologic changes in Cornish workers, Wagner and colleagues[606] described variable degrees of both interstitial and nodular fibrosis, the latter correlating with the pulmonary quartz content.

The roentgenographic pattern varies widely. There may be no more than a general increase in lung markings; with prolonged and severe exposure, a diffuse nodular and miliary mottling is present, and a late manifestation is bilateral progressive massive fibrosis identical to that seen in silicosis, talcosis, and coalworker's pneumoconiosis.[611, 612]

Of an entirely different nature is the pulmonary reaction that occurs following the use of a liquid kaolin suspension for pleural poudrage in the treatment of recurrent spontaneous pneumothorax; in the case reported by Herman and colleagues,[613] multiple nodular opacities measuring up to 2 cm in diameter developed that proved pathologically to be granulomas containing numerous birefringent crystals that were assumed to be kaolin; the nodules were apparently situated in lung parenchyma. This reaction appears to be identical to the previously mentioned parenchymal talcosis that developed in patients treated with talc pleurodesis.

Nepheline Rock Dust

Nepheline is a mineral composed of sodium, potassium, and aluminum silicates that occurs in crystalline form in many igneous rocks; SiO_2 is not free but is bound in a complex crystal lattice. The rock is milled to a fine powder and is used in the production of pottery glazes. At least three cases have been reported in which pneumoconiosis occurred as a result of exposure to this dust.[614, 615] In the two cases reported by Olscamp and associates,[615] the roentgenographic changes consisted of diffuse interstitial lung disease, bilateral lymph node enlargement, and focal areas of atelectasis that were presumably the result of airway compression by enlarged nodes.

Zeolites (Erionite)

Zeolites are a group of over 30 naturally occurring minerals composed of hydrated aluminum silicates that are found in deposits of volcanic ash.[616] They are widely used as absorbents and for filtration. Most do not have a fibrous form and are not considered toxic; *erionite*, however, is fibrous and has been associated with a variety of pulmonary abnormalities. The richest deposits of this material are in Turkey and the western United States, particularly Nevada and Utah. The initial indication that the substance might be harmful came from Turkey, where epidemiologic studies revealed a high incidence of pleural plaques, mesothelioma, and pulmonary carcinoma,[617–620] apparently unassociated with asbestos exposure. Subsequent reports have also documented the presence of interstitial fibrosis.[315, 616, 617, 620]

INERT RADIOPAQUE DUSTS

Iron

Workers in many occupations are exposed to dust containing a high content of iron, usually in the form of iron oxide (Fe_2O_3). When this substance is inhaled in sufficient quantity, it causes *siderosis*, a condition generally believed to be unassociated with fibrosis or functional impairment. When the iron is admixed with a substantial quantity of silica, however, the result is *silicosiderosis*, a condition that can be associated with appreciable pulmonary fibrosis and disability. The majority of affected individuals are electric arc or oxyacetylene torch workers, who are exposed to iron oxide in fumes derived from melted and boiled iron emitted during the welding process.[10] Other cases of silicosiderosis are found among individuals involved in the mining and processing of iron ore and metallic pigments such as ocher, workers in iron and steel rolling mills, foundry workers (particularly those involved with cleaning steel castings),[8, 9] boiler scalers, silver polishers (*see* farther on), and workers exposed to magnetite (FeO_4).[622]

As indicated previously, iron oxide inhaled in relatively pure form is believed to cause no significant inflammatory reaction or pulmonary fibrosis.[623] This belief is supported by experimental studies in animals in which various iron compounds inhaled or injected intratracheally have not caused a fibrotic reaction.[624, 625] In addition, persons exposed for many years to iron oxide in high concentration are usually not disabled and show little evidence of fibrosis at necropsy,[9, 623, 626, 627] even when the iron content of their lungs is very high. Despite the relative benignity of pure siderosis, it is important to realize that occupations associated with iron dust or fume production frequently generate other noxious materials; for example, the mineral content of fumes derived from the welding process may be quite variable, depending on the composition of the

metal being welded or of the welding electrode itself, or both. Among the additional materials that may be present are carbon, manganese, titanium, aluminum, various silicates (including asbestos), and free silica.[10, 628, 629] As the proportion of these substances in the fumes or dusts increases, the propensity for the development of pulmonary fibrosis also increases, resulting in the clinical, roentgenographic, and pathologic features characteristic of mixed dust pneumoconiosis (silicosiderosis), particularly if welding or other work is carried out in inadequately ventilated areas.[628, 630, 631] Although free silica is probably the most important admixed agent responsible for the development of pulmonary disease in these circumstances, microanalysis of elements in tissue and BAL fluid by energy-dispersive x-ray microprobe and scanning electron microscopy has suggested that there may be a fibrogenic reaction in some cases of welder's pneumoconiosis in the absence of significant silica content.[632–634] In another process not directly related to metal inhalation, the lungs of welders can also be damaged as a result of the direct effect on the tracheobronchial tree of ozone or nitrogen oxides created during welding.

Pathologically, pure siderosis is characterized by the presence of large granular or amorphous deposits of iron oxide situated predominantly in macrophages in the peribronchovascular interstitium.[10, 629, 630] Iron-containing macrophages can also be present within alveolar airspaces, particularly in individuals who were active welders at the time of death or biopsy (Fig. 12–41); these macrophages can frequently be detected in sputum specimens.[635] Fibrosis is usually absent or minimal in cases of

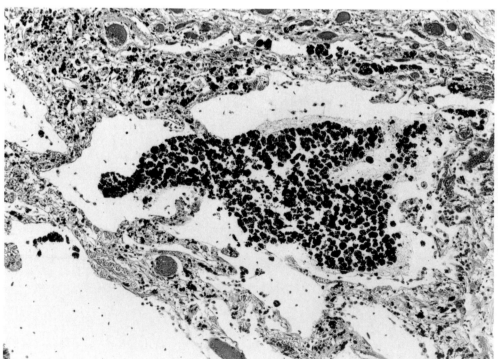

Figure 12–41. Siderosis. A histologic section shows a large cluster of iron-containing macrophages within pulmonary airspaces. A smaller amount of iron is also present in the adjacent bronchial wall. Although there is some fibrosis in both airway wall and lung parenchyma, it is mild and present only focally. The patient was an electric arc welder who died accidentally. ($\times$ 100.)

pure Fe_2O_3 inhalation but is present to a variable degree if fibrogenic substances are also present;[630] in this situation, the appearance is similar to that of silicosis and is characterized by solitary or conglomerate nodules, the latter occasionally being large enough to be designated PMF (Fig. 12–42). Unlike pure silicosis, however, the nodules are usually rather poorly defined and stellate. Aggregates of iron oxide, either free or within macrophages, can often be found admixed within the fibrous tissue.

The *roentgenographic pattern* in pure siderosis is reticulonodular and widely disseminated (Fig. 12–43). In a roentgenographic evaluation of 661 British electric arc welders,[621] 7 per cent showed small rounded opacities of 0/1 category or higher, there being a clear association between prevalence and years of exposure; only ten workers showed changes higher than 2/2. Opacities have been shown experimentally to correlate with localized aggregates of Fe_2O_3-laden macrophages[625] and are caused by the density of the iron oxide itself.[636] Individual shadows appear to be of lesser density than the nodules of silicosis. In contrast to the majority of cases of pneumoconiosis, the roentgenographic abnormalities can disappear partly or completely when patients are removed from dust exposure.[4, 637] In siderosilicosis, the pattern depends somewhat on the concentration of free silica in the inhaled dust; when it is relatively low (less than 10 per cent), the appearance is similar to that of pure siderosis or CWP,[8] but when the concentration is high, the pattern is identical to that of silicosis.[626]

Clinically, patients with siderosis have no symptoms of chest disease, and pulmonary function studies of welders have shown values considered to be within normal limits.[10, 627, 629] Some patients with siderosilicosis complain of cough and dyspnea. Even in the absence of roentgenographic abnormality, arc welders[638] and foundry workers[639] have been found to have a higher incidence of bronchitis than control subjects; symptoms tended to be worse after the Monday work-shift, suggesting the possibility that they were occasioned by fumes and vapors derived from the molding process.

The incidence of pulmonary carcinoma is significantly higher in patients with siderosis or silicosiderosis than in the general population.[8, 9, 640–642] In addition, squamous metaplasia, in many cases with atypical features, has been reported in a substantial number of iron foundry workers.[635] In one epidemiologic and environmental study in Scotland,[643] higher standardized mortality rates for lung cancer were grouped in residential areas most exposed to pollution from the foundries. Despite these findings, there is no direct evidence linking iron oxide *per se* with the development of carcinoma.

Iron and Silver

Argyrosiderosis results from the use of jeweler's rouge, which is composed in part of iron oxide, as a polishing agent in the finishing of silver products. When it is applied with a buffer, small particles of Fe_2O_3 and silver are generated that may be inhaled. The roentgenographic manifestation in these patients is rather characteristic, consisting of a fine stippled pattern in contrast to the reticulonodular pattern of siderosis. Pathologic examination shows the presence of iron within macrophages in a similar distribution to that of pure siderosis; in addition, the inhaled silver is found localized to the alveolar walls and to the elastic tissue of smaller arteries and veins, particularly the internal elastic laminae.[644] Patients are typically asymptomatic.

Tin

Pneumoconiosis caused by inhalation of tin *(stannosis)* is uncommon; the hazard exists predominantly for individuals employed in the handling of the ore after it has been mined, especially in industries in which tin oxide fumes are created. Although the condition is of no functional significance, the high density of tin (atomic number 50) results in a dramatic roentgenographic appearance (*see* farther on). In one study of 215 individuals exposed to tin oxide fumes,[645] 95 per cent of whom had worked in the environment for at least 3 years, 121 (56 per cent) showed an abnormality on the chest roentgenogram; none of the 121 subjects had symptoms or signs referable to the chest.

Pathologically, the findings simulate the macule of coalworker's pneumoconiosis, pigment-laden macrophages being found in alveoli, interlobular septa, and most prominently in aggregates around terminal bronchioles and proximal respiratory bronchioles; fibrosis is minimal or absent.[646] Unlike CWP, focal emphysema is not a prominent feature.[646]

The *roentgenographic pattern* consists of multiple tiny shadows of high density, about 1 mm in diameter, distributed evenly throughout the lungs.[645] Linear opacities may be present in the paramediastinal zone, in the vicinity of the diaphragm, and in the costophrenic angles. Lymph node enlargement has not been observed. A second type of pattern, described by Robertson,[647] consists of larger, somewhat less numerous nodules; this pattern is seen chiefly in furnace workers in the tin ore industry.

Barium

Barium and its salts, particularly barium sulfate, have a wide variety of industrial uses, including as coloring or weighting agents, as fillers in numerous products, and in the manufacture of glass. Involvement in many of these occupations, as well as in mining of the ore, can theoretically cause pulmonary disease *(barytosis)*. Originally described in Italian workers,[626, 648] this disease has been reported in the German,[649] French,[650] American,[651]

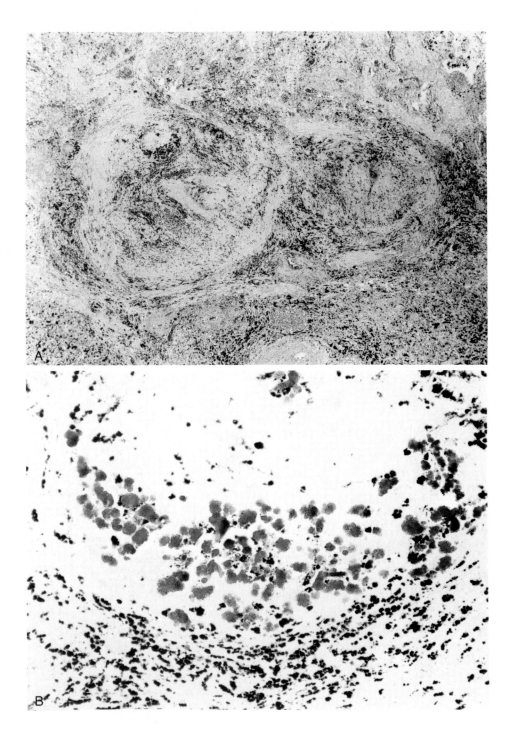

Figure 12–42. Silicosiderosis. A histologic section *(A)* from a 3-cm irregular mass in the upper lobe of a retired oxyacetylene torch welder shows extensive fibrosis with abundant interspersed pigment. Note the two rounded areas in the central portion that suggest that the mass was formed by confluence of multiple nodules. A magnified view of the pigmented material *(B)* shows it to consist of small black particles (anthracotic and other pigments) and larger, rather amorphous granules representing iron dioxide. *(A,* × 25; *B,* × 250.)

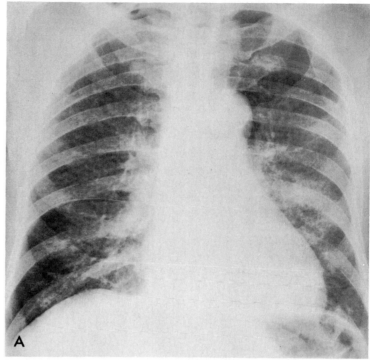

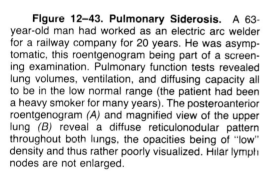

Figure 12–43. Pulmonary Siderosis. A 63-year-old man had worked as an electric arc welder for a railway company for 20 years. He was asymptomatic, this roentgenogram being part of a screening examination. Pulmonary function tests revealed lung volumes, ventilation, and diffusing capacity all to be in the low normal range (the patient had been a heavy smoker for many years). The posteroanterior roentgenogram *(A)* and magnified view of the upper lung *(B)* reveal a diffuse reticulonodular pattern throughout both lungs, the opacities being of "low" density and thus rather poorly visualized. Hilar lymph nodes are not enlarged.

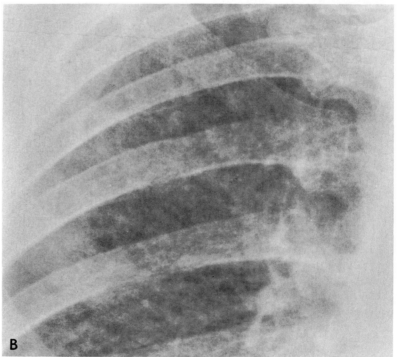

and British[652] literature also. Approximately 50 per cent of 118 Algerian workers exposed to dust containing a high percentage of barium sulfate had abnormal chest roentgenograms.[650]

Pendergrass and Greening[651] reported pathologic changes observed in one case at necropsy. The patient had worked in a coal mine also, and there was morphologic evidence of both dusts. Particles of barium were found in the interstitial tissues and were unassociated with fibrosis.

Owing to the high radiopacity of barium (atomic number 56), the discrete shadows in the chest roentgenogram are extremely dense, creating an awesome appearance. The apices and bases usually are spared, and massive shadows do not occur.[652] Roentgenographic abnormalities may develop after only relatively brief exposure. Of the nine affected patients described by Doig,[652] two were exposed for periods of only 18 and 21 months. The lesions characteristically regress roentgenographically after the patient is removed from the dust-filled environment.[626, 649, 652]

Some of the Algerian workers already referred to complained of chronic cough, expectoration, and asthma-like attacks; however, the degree of pulmonary function impairment was similar in those with and those without roentgenographic abnormality.[650]

Antimony

Antimony is procured mainly from the mineral stibnite and is handled either as unrefined ore or as a fine white powder.[653] The main exposures are to antimony trioxide and, to a lesser extent, antimony pentoxide.[654] It is used in cosmetics, in the manufacture of batteries, pewter, printing type, and electrodes, in the compounding of rubber, in textiles, paints, and plastics as a flame retardant, and in ceramics as an opacifier.[653]

There has been little pathologic description of the effects of antimony on the lungs; in one brief report, McCallum[653] documented the presence of dust-laden macrophages in alveolar septa and perivascular tissue unaccompanied by fibrosis. There is also experimental evidence confirming the lack of fibrogenic potential.[655] The chest roentgenogram reveals minute dense opacites scattered widely throughout both lungs.[655] In one report of 51 workers exposed for at least a decade to dust containing a high concentration of antimony,[654] the roentgenographic pattern was described as showing numerous p and occasional q opacities; PMF was not seen. Respiratory symptoms and pulmonary function tests were judged to be similar to those found in other pneumoconioses. Approximately 50 per cent of workers had pustular skin lesions. There is no evidence that the dust causes disturbances in lung function.

Rare Earths

The rare earth elements include cerium—quantitatively the most important—scandium, yttrium, lanthanum, and 14 other minerals. Their atomic numbers range from 51 to 71, explaining the great density of the roentgenographic shadows. The elements are used in reactor control rods, in manufacturing and polishing of colored glass, in the manufacture of flints, and as part of the alloy in cast iron, light metals, and heating conductors. Industrial exposure occurs chiefly in workers in the graphic arts and in factories producing cored carbon for arc lamps.

There are few pathologic descriptions of the effects of rare earths on the lung. In animal experiments, Hoschek[656] found that these elements were practically inert, inducing only small collections of macrophages around the dust deposits. However, Caine and colleagues[657] described granulomatous inflammation and parenchymal fibrosis in some cases; the extent and progression of disease depended to some extent on the thorium content of the dust. In one patient who was exposed for many years to rare earth fumes and dusts emitted from carbon arc lamps, the chest roentgenogram was described as showing severe pulmonary fibrosis; high concentrations of these rare earth elements (mostly cerium, neodymium, lanthanum, and samarium) were found in the tissues, particularly the lungs and lymph nodes.[658] The typical roentgenographic pattern consists of widely disseminated punctate opacities of great density, in one patient categorized as q opacities of 2/3 severity;[659] like others described in the literature,[660] this patient was asymptomatic despite the spirometric demonstration of a restrictive impairment.

MISCELLANEOUS INORGANIC DUSTS

Beryllium

EPIDEMIOLOGY

The major commercial source of beryllium is beryl, a beryllium aluminum silicate. Its industrial use is related to three commodities—beryllium alloys, beryllium oxides, and metallic beryllium. The interested reader may refer to detailed lists of the uses of this metal in industry compiled by Hardy[661] and by an American College of Chest Physicians committee on occupational diseases of the chest.[662] During and immediately before the 1940s, when the toxicity of this substance was first appreciated, the majority of cases resulted from exposure to beryllium in refineries, to beryllium alloys in metal working, and to fluorescent phosphor production (the ore of beryl apparently does not cause disease). In 1949, in an attempt to eradicate this disease, industrial plants instituted controls designed to keep the beryllium content of the air at less than 2 micrograms per cubic meter (averaged over an 8-hour work day). Presumably as a result of the establishment of these precautionary measures, the disease appeared to be almost totally eradicated, as illustrated by the fact that not a single new case was recorded at the Beryllium Diseases Registry at the Massachusetts General Hospital from 1949 to 1962.[663] However, almost 100 new cases have been reported since 1966,[664-667] in half of which the patients were exposed to beryllium after 1949. In a 1973 survey of workers in a beryllium extraction and processing plant that had been in operation for 14 years, 31 of 214 workers had roentgenographic changes compatible with interstitial disease, and it was determined that they had been exposed to dust concentrations well above the recommended level.[668] Cases that have been reported most recently have been associated with the processing and handling of beryllium compounds in the aerospace industry, in the manufacture of gyroscopes and nuclear reactors,[664, 666] and with exposure in a precious metal refinery.[667]

Berylliosis may occur in an acute or chronic form, the latter being much more common.[669] A 1972 progress report from the United States Beryllium Case Registry described 832 cases of beryllium disease, 211 of which were acute, 577 chronic, and 44 both acute and chronic.[665]

ACUTE BERYLLIOSIS

The majority of patients are exposed to the dust while working in beryllium refineries. Depending on the intensity of exposure, the clinical presentation may be either fulminating or insidious. In both presentations, the pathologic changes are relatively nonspecific, being identical to those seen in other forms of acute chemical pneumonitis. They consist of bronchitis, bronchiolitis, and various stages of diffuse alveolar damage (interstitial and airspace edema, hyaline membranes, and fibrosis).[670, 671] Granulomatous inflammation does not occur.

The fulminating variety develops rapidly following an overwhelming exposure. Its clinical and roentgenographic manifestations are those of acute pulmonary edema, which may be rapidly fatal.[672]

The insidious variety produces symptoms weeks or even months after the initial exposure.[673] The onset is heralded by a dry cough, substernal pain, shortness of breath on exertion, anorexia, weakness, and weight loss. Auscultatory findings include rales and, in some cases, rhonchi, suggesting asthma.[662] Various nonpulmonary manifestations, including rhinitis, pharyngitis, tracheobronchitis, conjunctivitis, and various dermatitides, may occur with or without clinical and roentgenologic evidence of involvement of the lungs.[662]

The chest roentgenogram usually does not become abnormal until 1 to 4 weeks after the onset of symptoms. Diffuse, symmetric, bilateral "haziness" is seen in the earliest stage of the disease, with subsequent development of irregular patchy opacities scattered rather widely throughout the lungs. Subsequently, discrete or confluent mottling may be observed.[662, 672] Complete roentgenographic clearing may take 2 to 3 months.[662, 674]

Pulmonary function studies in the insidious form of acute disease have shown hyperventilation, reduction in VC, normal RV, and normal MBC.[673] In some cases arterial oxygen saturation is greatly decreased during exercise and even at rest, with an increase in the alveolar-arterial gradient for oxygen. Removal from exposure to the dust results in gradual return to normal function.

CHRONIC BERYLLIOSIS

The chronic variety of berylliosis, described in the United States in 1946 by Hardy and Tabershaw,[675] is much more common and more serious than the acute disease. It is a widespread systemic disease, producing lesions in the lungs, lymph nodes, liver, spleen, kidneys, myocardium, skin, skeletal muscle, and pleura. In the majority of patients in the earlier reports, the disease resulted from exposure in the fluorescent phosphor industry or from working with beryllium alloys.[662] In some patients, however, the only known source of exposure was contaminated work clothes at home or atmospheric contamination from neighboring beryllium plants.[671]

Pathogenesis. The frequent delay in onset of disease from the time of exposure, the decrease in beryllium content of the lungs of affected individuals with time (*see* farther on), the common presence of granulomatous inflammation, and the poor correlation between the degree of exposure and the development of disease all suggest that the pathogenesis of chronic berylliosis is immunologic, most likely mediated by a type IV hypersensitivity reaction. Several clinical and experimental immunologic findings support this conclusion. Cutaneous granulomatous inflammation develops in approximately 70 per cent of patients on skin testing, and blast transformation and the production of macrophage inhibition factor occur in an equal number when their lymphocytes are cultured in the presence of beryllium.[676-680] The total number of cells obtained by bronchoalveolar lavage is increased, principally owing to larger numbers of lymphocytes;[679] most are T cells, and there is an increased helper-to-suppressor ratio. A proliferative response of bronchoalveolar lymphocytes to beryllium has been proposed as a useful diagnostic test.[667, 681, 682] In their study of a small number of patients with chronic berylliosis, one group of workers found this test to show 100 per cent sensitivity and specificity.[682]

Although the precise pathogenesis of chronic berylliosis is not understood, it has been proposed that the metal binds to a tissue or blood protein and acts as a hapten; this complex can then be recognized by the immune system as foreign, inducing a cellular immune response.[679]

Pathologic Characteristics. The characteristic pulmonary abnormality in chronic berylliosis is interstitial pneumonitis,[671] which may appear on pathologic examination as: (1) a more or less diffuse mononuclear cell infiltrate unassociated with granulomatous inflammation (Fig. 12–44), (2) a similar infiltrate containing loose epithelial cell aggregates and scattered multinucleated giant cells, frequently containing calcified intracellular inclusions, or (3) well-formed, discrete, non-necrotizing granulomas indistinguishable from those of sarcoidosis (Fig. 12–44). Interstitial fibrosis is also common, occurring either diffusely within the parenchymal interstitium or in the form of well-defined nodules, often with central hyalinization or necrosis, or both.

In contrast to most other dusts that cause pneumoconiosis, beryllium is largely removed from the lungs with time and excreted in the urine (although it may be stored in bone and liver for many years); as a result, quantitative studies show significantly less tissue content of beryllium in chronic than in acute disease.[671] Despite this, the substance can be detected within affected tissues by laser probe and emission spectroscopy[683] and by laser ion mass analysis.[684] Although there is overlap, in most affected individuals the beryllium content of the lung and mediastinal lymph nodes is greater than that of normal individuals and of patients with sarcoidosis.[685]

Roentgenographic Manifestations. The roentgenographic pattern is neither specific nor diagnostic.[686] When the degree of involvement is relatively minor, the pattern is described as a diffuse, finely granular "haziness" with a tendency to sparing of the apices and bases.[687] With more severe involvement, ill-defined nodules of moderate size are scattered diffusely throughout the lungs, sometimes with associated lymph node enlargement. Calcification of nodules occurs and, when present, permits differentiation from sarcoidosis.[688] In a group of 17 patients in whom the presence of chronic berylliosis was established by means of a positive lymphocyte proliferation test on BAL fluid, Aronchick and colleagues[689] found that the most common roentgenographic abnormality consisted of diffuse, small, round and irregular opacities. Hilar node enlargement, linear scars, lung distortion, bullae, and pleural thickening were found less commonly. These changes did not correlate with pulmonary function abnormalities.

In advanced cases, the pattern may be chiefly reticular and may be associated with great decrease in volume and with some conglomeration of nodular shadows. Areas of emphysema may be identified, usually in the upper lobes. Spontaneous pneumothorax occurs in slightly more than 10 per cent of cases.[688] A complicating mycetoma has been reported that proved to be fatal.[795]

Clinical Manifestations. The majority of reported cases of chronic berylliosis have had a history of dust exposure of more than 2 years' duration. Because there is strong evidence that berylliosis represents an immunologic reaction, it would be expected that the severity of exposure, including both dust and fume concentration, would not be a major factor in pathogenesis; two reports of the development of disease with an air concentration of beryllium below the permissible exposure limit of 2 micrograms per cubic meter[667, 690] appear to bear out this hypothesis.

Rarely, patients with proven disease may be asymptomatic. Usually, however, symptoms develop insidiously after a latent period that may be as long as 15 years following the last exposure to dust.[661, 662, 691] Early symptoms include minimal cough, fatigue, weight loss, increasing dyspnea on exertion, and, sometimes, migratory arthralgia. Occasionally, adventitious sounds may be heard on auscultation, and the liver and spleen may be palpable; up to 10 per cent of patients develop renal calculi. With progression of the disease, cyanosis may become obvious, and in approximately 30 per cent of patients, clubbing of the fingers and toes develops; cor pulmonale is frequent. Hypergammaglobulinemia, hypercalciuria, and polycythemia are not uncommon findings.[661, 662, 691] In one study, 25 of 48 patients were reported to show hypergammaglobulinemia.[692] In two other studies, immunoelectrophoresis showed this to be caused chiefly by elevated levels of serum IgG[693] and IgA.[676] Hyperuricemia, which has been reported to occur in somewhat less than 50 per cent of patients with sarcoidosis,[694] was noted in six of 15 patients with chronic beryllium poisoning.[695]

Cotes and coworkers[690] believe that the disease can be precipitated by certain trigger factors, including pregnancy, withdrawal from exposure, and the performance of a beryllium patch test. A reduction in the air concentration of beryllium can result in a significant improvement in lung function; for example, of 20 men who had hypoxemia at the time air pollution was reduced in 1971, 13 showed improvement in arterial blood gases and lower alveolar-arterial gradients in a follow-up study 3 years later; some of these showed an improvement in the severity of roentgenographic abnormalities.[696]

Results of pulmonary function studies may be normal or may indicate some degree of restrictive insufficiency.[149, 697] In many cases the arterial oxygen tension is decreased, even at rest. Diffusing capacity may be reduced, and the alveolar-arterial oxygen difference increased, suggesting that the diffusion abnormality is caused primarily by $\dot{V}/\dot{Q}$ inequality. A few patients have functional impairment suggestive of emphysema, and others have impairment almost identical to that of sarcoidosis.[697] Andrews and associates[698] performed pulmonary function tests on 41 patients with chronic berylliosis and found impairment in 39. Sixteen manifested an

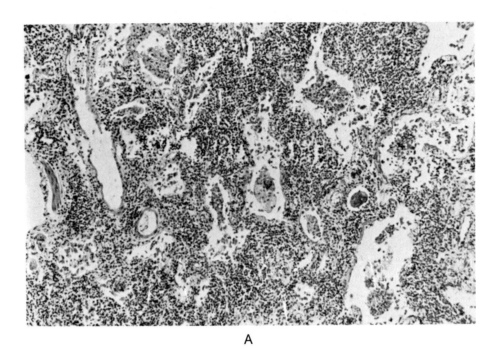

A

Figure 12–44. Chronic Berylliosis. A histologic section *(A)* shows severe interstitial infiltration by mononuclear inflammatory cells unassociated with granuloma formation. A different histologic pattern is shown in *B*, consisting of patchy, non-necrotizing granulomatous inflammation within the pulmonary interstitium, indistinguishable from sarcoidosis. (From Freiman DG, Hardy HL. Hum Pathol *1*:30, 1970.)

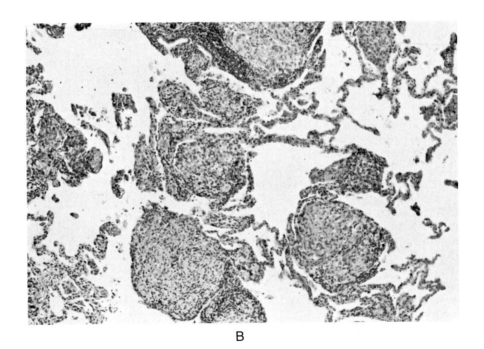

B

obstructive pattern, and eight a restrictive one, and 15 had diminished diffusing capacity without evidence of either obstruction or restriction. Patients with obstructive lung disease were not necessarily smokers. The prognosis in this group was poor.

The diagnosis of chronic beryllium disease may be suspected from a history of exposure to the dust and a chest roentgenogram showing diffuse nodular disease. Confirmation may be obtained by a patch test showing hypersensitivity to beryllium[699, 700] or by blastogenic transformation of blood[676-680] or alveolar[662, 681, 682] lymphocytes. Diagnostically, this disease may be confused with sarcoidosis, a disease that is much more frequently asymptomatic and carries a better prognosis. At least two recent reports indicate that chronic berylliosis is sometimes misdiagnosed as sarcoidosis.[666, 667] Helpful points in differentiation include absence of involvement of the uveal tract, tonsils, parotid glands, and bones in berylliosis (although conjunctivitis is seen in both sarcoidosis and the acute form of berylliosis). There is no change in tuberculin reactivity unless the patient is receiving corticosteroid therapy. In such circumstances, even hypersensitivity to beryllium on patch testing may be abolished.

Aluminum

Individuals can be exposed to the potential toxic effects of aluminum in four situations:

1. During the manufacture of the abrasive corundum from bauxite (so-called Shaver's disease).[701] Although bauxite itself is generally believed to be innocuous, one report has suggested that it may also be associated with pulmonary fibrosis.[702]

2. During the preparation or use of aluminum powder derived from either stamping of cold metal (flake type) or directly from molten metal (granular type).[703-707]

3. During aluminum arc-welding.[708-710]

4. During the grinding or polishing of aluminum products.[191, 711]

Although each of these situations can be associated with pulmonary disease, it is not certain that aluminum is the pathogenetic agent in every case, because often there is concomitant exposure to other substances of potential toxicity. This pathogenetic uncertainty is underlined by several experimental and clinical studies. For example, following the observation by Denny and colleagues[712] that silicosis did not develop in rabbits that inhaled dust containing one part of aluminum to 100 parts of freshly fractured quartz, aluminum was added prophylactically to dust inhaled by miners exposed to silica; such addition apparently has had no untoward effects.[713] In addition, several animal experiments have shown either minimal or no pulmonary reaction to inhaled aluminum;[192, 193, 796] however, some investigators have shown a significant fibrotic reaction, implying that, at least in some cases, true toxicity is present.[199] Although it is possible that

differences in the form of aluminum employed in the experimental studies may underlie these discrepant findings, it has been hypothesized that host factors, perhaps mediated by immunologic mechanisms, may also be responsible.[707, 710]

Pathologic findings in the lungs of individuals exposed to aluminum are variable and, as indicated previously, may be caused in some cases by substances other than aluminum itself. In their study of the lungs of patients who had been exposed to bauxite fumes, Wyatt and Riddell[714] found diffuse parenchymal fibrosis, often accompanied by emphysema; well-defined nodules suggestive of silicosis were not identified. Gilks and Churg[715] studied the lungs of a 50-year-old man who had worked in the aluminum smelting industry for 19 years and had died of respiratory insufficiency; using electron optical techniques, they found numerous fibrous and nonfibrous aluminum particles in the diffusely fibrotic lungs, and raised the possibility that fibers may have played a role in the pathogenesis of the disease. Other histologic reactions that have been reported include desquamative interstitial pneumonitis,[708] alveolar proteinosis,[711] and diffuse granulomatous inflammation.[707, 710]

Roentgenographic abnormalities may become apparent after a few months or several years of exposure.[149, 705] Fully developed changes consist of a fine to coarse reticular pattern widely distributed throughout the lungs (Fig. 12–45), sometimes with a nodular component.[705] Lung volume may be greatly decreased, and the pleura may become thickened; spontaneous pneumothorax is a frequent complication (Fig. 12–45).

Breathlessness is the chief symptom and may be severely disabling. Death may occur from pulmonary insufficiency.[704, 705] The few pulmonary function studies that have been reported have shown both restrictive and obstructive disease with reduction in diffusing capacity.[149] Two epidemiologic studies carried out in aluminum smelting plants indicate that exposure to aluminum particles can cause chronic bronchitis; respiratory symptoms and a reduction in flow rates were found to correlate with the degree of exposure.[716, 717]

Cobalt and Tungsten Carbide

The term *hard metal* is usually used to refer to an alloy of tungsten, carbon, and cobalt, occasionally with the addition of small amounts of other metals such as titanium, tantalum, nickel, and chromium.[718, 719] The resulting product is extremely hard and resistant to heat and is used extensively in the drilling and polishing of other metals. Exposure to dust can occur during either the manufacture or use of the metal and is well recognized as a cause of interstitial pneumonitis and fibrosis.

The precise pathogenesis of disease is unclear. Experimental studies in animals suggest that cobalt is the etiologic agent,[719, 720] a hypothesis supported

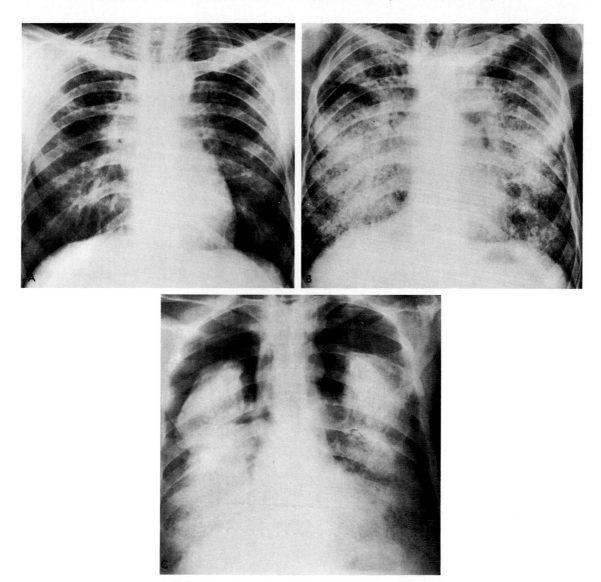

Figure 12–45. Bauxite Pneumoconiosis (Shaver's Disease). A 29-year-old man had been exposed for a number of years to bauxite in the manufacture of corundum. The first posteroanterior roentgenogram *(A)* revealed a coarse reticulonodular pattern throughout both lungs and involving predominantly the upper and middle lung zones. Slightly more than 1 year later *(B)*, the disease had extended to a remarkable degree, the reticulonodular shadows being confluent in many areas. Shortly after this second roentgenogram was obtained, the patient suffered bilateral pneumothorax *(C)* associated with marked collapse of both lungs. This was one of several similar episodes of pneumothorax, some of which were unilateral and others bilateral. The prompt application of therapy resulted in the patient's survival of this and all other episodes of pneumothorax. (Courtesy of Montreal Chest Hospital Center.)

by the finding of disease in diamond polishers,[721] who are exposed to high concentrations of cobalt alone; their pulmonary disease is virtually identical to that seen in hard metal workers. However, there is evidence that the effects of cobalt are enhanced by the presence of tungsten carbide,[719] and in some autopsy studies of patients with interstitial fibrosis and a history of exposure to hard metals, cobalt has not been found in the lung tissue.[722, 723] It has been suggested that the disease may result from a hypersensitivity reaction analogous to that seen in berylliosis.[720] In addition to the well-documented cases of irreversible fibrosis, some cases of asthma have been associated with cobalt exposure;[724, 725] there is

some evidence that this is also caused by an immunologically mediated hypersensitivity reaction.[797]

Pathologic findings are predominantly those of interstitial pneumonitis with a variable degree of fibrosis.[718, 720] Characteristically, numerous macrophages are present in alveolar airspaces, creating a pattern simulating desquamative interstitial pneumonitis. In some cases, multinucleated giant cells are prominent, both in the airspaces and lining alveolar walls, resembling giant cell interstitial pneumonitis;[718, 726] these cells can be seen in cytology specimens obtained by bronchial washing.[727] Bronchiolitis obliterans has been noted occasionally.[718, 726]

The chest roentgenogram is said to show a

diffuse micronodular and reticular pattern, sometimes with lymph node enlargement; the reticulation may be very coarse[728] and in advanced disease may be accompanied by small cystic shadows.[720, 729]

Symptoms include a dry cough and dyspnea on exertion; severe respiratory insufficiency sometimes develops and can prove fatal.[728, 730] Pulmonary function tests reveal both restrictive and obstructive patterns,[731] and diffusion may be reduced.[720, 729]

Silicon Carbide

Silicon carbide (carborundum) is produced by fusion at high temperature of high-grade sand, finely ground carbon (coke), salt, and wood dust.[732] The resulting product is extremely hard and is used as an abrasive. Although the findings in experimental studies in animals have suggested that the substance is inert,[732, 798] occasional individuals with apparently pure or predominant silicon carbide exposure have shown pathologic evidence of interstitial fibrosis and macrophage accumulation accompanied by roentgenographic and pulmonary function abnormalities.[732, 798, 799] There is evidence that these changes may be caused by silica derived from the sand or by silicon carbide fibers produced during the manufacturing process or perhaps by both.[798]

Polyvinyl Chloride

In its pure form, polyvinyl chloride is a white powder that is produced by polymerization under pressure of the gas vinyl chloride;[733] it is used in the manufacture of plastics, synthetic fibers, and numerous other commercial products. There is some evidence that its inhalation, during either its production or its use in the manufacture of other materials, may be associated with chronic pulmonary disease. In one study of 1,215 workers employed in a polyvinyl chloride production plant, 20 were considered to have roentgenographic abnormalities consistent with pneumoconiosis.[734] Occasional case reports have documented a possible association between exposure and the presence of interstitial pneumonitis and fibrosis or the accumulation of interstitial and intra-alveolar macrophages.[733, 735, 736] Experimental studies in animals have also provided evidence for the development of pulmonary fibrosis.[737] This subject is discussed at greater length in Chapter 14.

Titanium Dioxide

Titanium dioxide is derived from the ore ilmenite and is used chiefly as a pigment in paints, paper, and other products, as a mordant in dyeing, and as an alloy in some hard metals. Pathologic examination of affected lungs has shown alveolar and interstitial accumulation of macrophages but no[738] or minimal[739, 740] fibrosis. The apparent inertness of the material has been corroborated by experimental studies in animals.[739] Non-necrotizing granulomatous inflammation has been documented in a biopsy specimen from one patient;[741] because of a positive lymphocyte transformation test on exposure to titanium, the authors considered the possibility of an hypersensitivity reaction similar to that proposed for berylliosis. In macrophages, titanium dioxide appears as small black granules virtually identical to anthracotic pigment; in contrast to the latter, however, they are strongly birefringent.[739, 740]

Roentgenographic changes considered consistent with pneumoconiosis have been reported in some workers involved in pigment production.[738-740] A cross-sectional survey of 209 titanium metal production workers showed a reduction in ventilatory capacity and roentgenographic evidence of pleural plaques and thickening not clearly attributable to asbestos exposure.[742]

Volcanic Dust

Volcanic eruption occurs when magma (liquid rock) is extruded from the depths of the earth to its surface. Although the magma may simply flow over the rim of the volcano onto the adjacent earth (where it is known as lava), violent eruption into the atmosphere can also occur and can produce large amounts of ash (tephra). Depending on the severity and nature of the eruption—e.g., whether it is vertical or at an angle to the earth's surface—and on the composition of the magma itself, significant quantities of potentially harmful ash may be generated into the atmosphere.

The best-studied volcanic eruption from the point of view of human health was at Mount Saint Helen's in 1980.[743] As of 1981, 35 individuals were known to have died directly as a result of the eruption;[744] among the 25 who underwent autopsy, the majority were considered to have asphyxiated as a result of major airway plugging by mucus and inhaled volcanic ash.[745] In individuals outside the areas of most severe damage, there was a mild increase in the number of acute respiratory complaints such as cough, wheezing, and dyspnea,[743] probably secondary to airway irritation. A considerable increase in emergency room attendance by asthmatics and bronchitics was recorded at local hospitals.[746] The long-term consequences, if any, of volcanic ash inhalation are unclear; Craighead and colleagues[743] estimated that free crystalline silicates formed about 3 to 7 per cent of the ash of the Mount Saint Helen's eruption, and it is conceivable that persons who suffered heavy exposure might develop chronic pulmonary disease, called appropriately pneumonoultramicroscopicsilicovolcanoconiosis.[800] Whether individuals exposed to ash derived from other volcanic sites have a greater risk for the development of disease is also unclear.

Synthetic Mineral Fibers

Synthetic mineral fibers are amorphous silicates derived from slag, rock, or glass. Their diameter and length vary considerably, depending on the specific use to which they are put;[747] for example, those fibers used in textiles and as reinforcement in plastics and other materials are mostly between 9 and 25 μm in diameter, whereas those employed in insulation are generally smaller (3 to 6 μm). Unlike natural silicates such as asbestos, synthetic fibers break transversely rather than longitudinally when traumatized, resulting in small fragments whose diameter is the same as that of their parents.[747] Because the potential for causing disease is related to a high length-diameter ratio, at least in part,[747, 748] this effect may be important in explaining the relative lack of toxicity of these substances.

The bulk of evidence suggests that inhaled synthetic mineral fibers have little, if any, harmful effects on the lungs.[747] An autopsy study by Gross and colleagues[749] found no gross or microscopic abnormality in the lungs of workers exposed to fiber glass; in addition, the total number of fibers per gram of dry lung was similar to that of a control group, implying adequate clearance of inhaled particles. Inhalation of synthetic mineral fibers by rats, hamsters, and monkeys has failed to cause significant fibrosis or neoplasia;[747, 750] no alteration of pulmonary structure or inflammatory reaction has been observed except for the presence of alveolar macrophages during the early stages and the development of proteinosis after 90 days of inhalation.[751]

In addition to these experimental pathologic studies, most epidemiologic investigations, roentgenographic surveys, tests of pulmonary function, and mortality rates of workers involved with synthetic mineral fibers have shown no differences from those of appropriate controls.[747, 750, 752, 753] Although these results imply a lack of pathogenicity, it has been suggested that they may simply reflect the very low doses to which these workers had been exposed.[753, 754] In fact, some studies have raised the possibility that synthetic mineral fibers can cause significant tissue damage. For example, in their study of 1,448 fiberglass workers, Bayliss and colleagues[755] found no overall increase in the mortality rate, but there was a statistically significant increase in the number of deaths caused by respiratory disease other than cancer and pneumonia. In another comparative epidemiologic analysis of men exposed to either asbestos or synthetic mineral fibers, Goldsmith[756] concluded that on the basis of fiber or particle counts, synthetic fibers appear to be the more potent of the two as a cause of chronic pulmonary disease. In one study of pulmonary function tests, lung elastic recoil was found to be slightly higher in a group of sheet metal workers exposed to fiber glass.[757]

In contrast to the apparent benignity of inhaled synthetic mineral fibers, instillation of these substances directly into either the pleural or peritoneal cavities of experimental animals has been shown to be associated with the development of mesothelioma.[748] This property is considered to be a function of the dimension and durability of the fibers rather than their physicochemical characteristics.[748]

Pneumoconiosis associated with exposure to glass and abrasive particles is perhaps properly included in this section: a patient with a history of decorating glass fixtures by means of abrasive etching showed roentgenologic abnormality and functional impairment;[758] mineralogic analysis of specimens obtained by lung biopsy showed particles whose composition was consistent with the glasses etched and abrasives used.

Wollastonite

Wollastonite is a naturally occurring acicular or fibrous metasilicate used in ceramics and as a substitute for asbestos in some applications; it is similar in form, length, and diameter to amphiboles.[759] There is fairly convincing roentgenographic and functional evidence that this substance can cause interstitial fibrosis,[759–761] although we are unaware of any pathologic studies confirming it.

Taconite

Taconite is a low-grade ore consisting of iron, quartz, and numerous silicates, including cummingtonite-grunerite, a relative of amosite asbestos. It is unlikely that this substance is either fibrinogenic or carcinogenic despite some evidence to the contrary.[762, 763]

Dental Technician's Powder

This form of pneumoconiosis has been attributed to silicon dioxide, although it is probable that other agents can be implicated as well; for example, air concentration exposure studies and mineralogic analyses of BAL fluid and lung tissue have disclosed chromium-cobalt-molybdenum[7] and cobalt-beryllium[6] constituents, acrylic resin,[801] and alginate powder.[802]

Cement Dust

In a survey of 195 cement workers, Sander[764] found that many years' exposure to a high concentration of raw and mixed cement dust can result in roentgenographic evidence of accentuation of linear markings and ill-defined micronodulation; however, other epidemiologic studies have found little or no evidence of roentgenographic abnormality.[16, 764] Although McDowell[765] found an increased incidence of cancer of the stomach among cement workers, he observed no increase in the mortality from respiratory disease. It is possible that any changes that have been observed have been caused by the quartz that is present in varying amounts in some cement.

REFERENCES

1. The Fourth International Pneumoconiosis Conference: Working Party on the Definition of Pneumoconiosis Report. Geneva, 1971.
2. Weill H: Epidemiologic methods in the investigation of occupational lung disease. Am Rev Respir Dis 112:1, 1975.
3. Seaton A, Lamb D, Brown WR, et al: Pneumoconiosis of shale miners. Thorax 36:412, 1981.
4. Harris DK: Some hazards in the manufacture and use of plastics. Br J Ind Med 16:221, 1959.
5. Morgenroth K, Kronenberger H, Michalke G, et al: Morphology and pathogenesis of pneumoconiosis in dental technicians. Pathol Respir Pract 179:528, 1985.
6. Rom WN, Lockey JE, Lee JS, et al: Pneumoconiosis and exposures of dental laboratory technicians. Am J Public Health 74:1252, 1984.
7. De Vuyst P, Vande Weyer R, De Coster A, et al: Dental technician's pneumoconiosis: A report of two cases. Am Rev Respir Dis 133:316, 1986.
8. McLaughlin AIG: Pneumoconiosis in foundry workers. Br J Tuberc 51:297, 1957.
9. McLaughlin AIG, Harding HE: Pneumoconiosis and other causes of death in iron and steel foundry workers. AMA Arch Ind Health 14:350, 1956.
10. Morgan WKC, Kerr HD: Pathologic and physiologic studies of welders' siderosis. Ann Intern Med 58:293, 1963.
11. Edstrom HW, Rice DMD: "Labrador lung": An unusual mixed dust pneumoconiosis. CMA J 126:27, 1982.
12. Mark GJ, Monroe CB, Kazemi H: Mixed pneumoconiosis: Silicosis, asbestosis, talcosis, and berylliosis. Chest 75:726, 1979.
13. McMahon JT: Analytical electron microscopy in pneumoconiosis. Cleve Clin Q 52:503, 1985.
14. Brady AR, Vallyathan NV, Craighead JE: Use of scanning electron microscopy and x-ray energy spectrometry to determine the elemental content of inclusions in human tissue lesions. In Becker RP, Johari O (eds): Scanning Electron Microscopy/1978/II. AMF O'Hare, Ill, Scanning Electron Microscopy, Inc, 1978, pp 615–621.
15. Knishkowy B, Baker EL: Transmission of occupational disease to family contacts. Am J Ind Med 9:543, 1986.
16. Parkes WR: Occupational Lung Disorders, 2nd ed. London, Butterworths, 1982.
17. Morgan WKC, Seaton A: Occupational Lung Diseases. Philadelphia, WB Saunders Co, 1984.
18. Stuart BO: Deposition of inhaled aerosols. Arch Intern Med 131:60, 1973.
19. Proctor DF, Andersen I, Lundqvist G: Clearance of inhaled particles from the human nose. Arch Intern Med 131:132, 1973.
20. Gross P, Detreville RTP: The lung as an embattled domain against inanimate pollutants. A precis of mechanisms. Am Rev Respir Dis 106:684, 1972.
21. Craighead JE, Mossman BT: The pathogenesis of asbestos-associated diseases. N Engl J Med 306:1446, 1982.
22. Hillerdal G: Malignant mesothelioma 1982: Review of 4,710 published cases. Br J Dis Chest 77:321, 1983.
23. Churg A, Wiggs B: Fiber size and number in amphibole asbestos-induced mesothelioma. Am J Pathol 115:437, 1984.
24. Amosite asbestos and mesothelioma (editorial). Lancet 2:1397, 1981.
25. Elmes PC: Mesotheliomas, minerals, and man-made mineral fibres. Thorax 35:561, 1980.
26. Pinkerton KE, Plopper CG, Mercer RR, et al: Airway branching patterns influence asbestos fiber location and the extent of tissue injury in the pulmonary parenchyma. Lab Invest 55:688, 1986.
27. Goodwin RA, Des Prez RM: Apical localization of pulmonary tuberculosis, chronic pulmonary histoplasmosis, and progressive massive fibrosis of the lung. Chest 83:801, 1983.
28. Becklake MR, Toyota B, Stewart M, et al: Lung structure as a risk factor in adverse pulmonary responses to asbestos exposure. A case-referent study in Quebec chrysotile miners and millers. Am Rev Respir Dis 128:385, 1983.
29. Sweeney TD, Brain JD, Leavitt SA, et al: Emphysema alters the deposition pattern of inhaled particles in hamsters. Am J Pathol 128:19, 1987.
30. Nadel JA: Aerosol effects on smooth muscle and airway visualization technique. Arch Intern Med 131:83, 1973.
31. Swartenaren M, Philipson K, Linnman L, et al: Regional deposition of particles in human lung after induced bronchoconstriction. Exp Lung Res 10:223, 1986.
32. Macklem PT, Hogg WE, Brunton J: Peripheral airways obstruction and particulate deposition in the lung. Arch Intern Med 131:93, 1973.
33. Goldberg IS, Lourenço RV: Deposition of aerosols in pulmonary disease. Arch Intern Med 131:88, 1973.
34. Davies CN: The handling of particles by the human lungs. Br Med Bull 19:49, 1963.
35. Bégin R, Massé S, Sébastien P, et al: Asbestos exposure and retention as determinants of airway disease and asbestos alveolitis. Am Rev Respir Dis 134:1176, 1986.
36. Green GM: Alveolobronchiolar transport mechanisms. Arch Intern Med 131:109, 1973.
37. Amandus HE, Reger RB, Pendergrass EP, et al: The pneumoconioses: Methods of measuring progression. Chest 63:736, 1973.
38. International Labor Office (League of Nations): Silicosis. Records of the international conference held at Johannesburg 13–27 August 1930. International Labour Office, Studies and Reports, Series F (Industrial Hygiene), No. 13. Geneva, International Labor Office, 1930, pp 86–93.
39. International Classification of Persistent Radiological Opacities in the Lung Fields Provoked by the Inhalation of Mineral Dusts. Safety Health 9:63, 1959.
40. UICC–Cincinnati classification of the radiographic appearances of pneumoconioses. A cooperative study by the UICC committee. Chest 58:57, 1970.
41. Russell AR (ed): Classification of radiographs of the pneumoconioses. Med Radiogr Photogr 57:2, 1981.
42. Liddell FDK: An experiment in film reading. Br J Ind Med 20:300, 1963.
43. Liddell FDK, Lindars DC: An elaboration of the I.L.O. classification of simple pneumoconiosis. Br J Ind Med 26:89, 1969.
44. Felson B, Morgan WKC, Bristol LJ, et al: Observations on the results of multiple readings of chest films on coal miners' pneumoconiosis. Radiology 109:19, 1973.
45. Morgan RH, Donner MW, Gayler BW, et al: Decision processes and observer error in the diagnosis of pneumoconiosis by chest roentgenography. Am J Roentgenol 117:757, 1973.
46. Amandus HE, Pendergrass EP, Dennis JM, et al: Pneumoconiosis: Inter-reader variability in the classification of the type of small opacities in the chest roentgenogram. Am J Roentgenol 122:740, 1974.
47. Turner AF, Kruger RP, Thompson WB: Automated computer screening of chest radiographs of pneumoconiosis. Invest Radiol 11:258, 1976.
48. Weill H, Jones R (eds): The chest roentgenogram as an epidemiologic tool. Report of a workshop. Arch Environ Health 30:435, 1975.
49. Liddell FDK: Assessment of radiological progression of simple pneumoconiosis in individual miners. Br J Ind Med 31:185, 1974.
50. Lapp NL: Lung disease secondary to inhalation of nonfibrous minerals. Clin Chest Med 2:219, 1981.
51. Ziskind M, Jones RN, Weill H: Silicosis. Am Rev Respir Dis 113:643, 1976.
52. Morgan WKC, Seaton A: Occupational Lung Disease. Philadelphia, WB Saunders Co, 1975, p 241.
53. Seaton A, Ruckley VA, Addison J, et al: Silicosis in barium miners. Thorax 41:591, 1986.
54. Trapp E, Renzetti AD Jr, Kobayashi T, et al: Cardiopulmonary function in uranium miners. Am Rev Respir Dis 101:27, 1970.
55. Landrigan PJ, Cherniack MG, Lewis FA, et al: Silicosis in a grey iron foundry: The persistence of an ancient disease. Scand J Work Environ Health 12:32, 1986.
56. Gerhardsson L, Ahlmark A: Silicosis in women: Experience from the Swedish Pneumoconiosis Register. J Occup Med 27:347, 1985.
57. Oechsli WR, Jacobson G, Brodeur AE: Diatomite pneumoconiosis: Roentgen characteristics and classification. Am J Roentgentol 85:263, 1961.
58. Caldwell DM: The coalescent lesion of diatomaceous earth pneumoconiosis. Am Rev Tuberc 77:644, 1958.
59. Ahlmark A, Bruce T, Nyström Å: Pneumoconiosis in diatomaceous earth workers. Nord Med 59:289, 1958.
60. Dutra FR: Diatomaceous earth pneumoconiosis. Arch Environ Health 11:613, 1965.
61. Smart RH, Anderson WM: Pneumoconiosis due to diatomaceous earth. Clinical and x-ray aspects. Ind Med Surg 21:509, 1952.
62. Beskow R: Silicosis in diatomaceous earth factory workers in Sweden. Scand J Respir Dis 59:216, 1978.

63. Cooper WC, Sargent EN: A 26-year radiographic follow-up of workers in a diatomite mine and mill. J Occup Med 26:456, 1984.

64. Posner E: Pneumoconiosis in makers of artificial grinding wheels, including a case of Caplan's syndrome. Br J Ind Med 17:109, 1960.

65. Saiyed HN, Parikh DJ, Ghodasara NB, et al: Silicosis in slate pencil workers: I. An environmental and medical study. Am J Ind Med 8:127, 1985.

66. Saiyed HN, Chatterjee BB: Rapid progression of silicosis in slate pencil workers: II. A follow-up study. Am J Ind Med 8:135, 1985.

67. Roche AD, Picard D, Vernhes A: Silicosis of ocher workers. A clinical and anatomopathologic study. Am Rev Tuberc 77:839, 1958.

68. Hale LW, Sheers G: Silicosis in West Country granite workers. Br J Ind Med 20:218, 1963.

69. Phibbs BP, Sundin RE, Mitchell RS: Silicosis in Wyoming bentonite workers. Am Rev Respir Dis 103:1, 1971.

70. Erdélyi J, Ökrös A: Über die durch emaileinatmung bewirkten erkrankungen. (Enamel pneumoconiosis.) Fortschr Röntgenstr 92:235, 1960.

71. Banks DE, Morring KL, Boehlecke BA, et al: Silicosis in silica flour workers. Am Rev Respir Dis 124:445, 1981.

72. Middleton EL: The present position of silicosis in industry in Britain. Br Med J 2:485, 1929.

73. Gong H Jr, Tashkin DP: Silicosis due to intentional inhalation of abrasive scouring powder: Case report with long-term survival and vasculitic sequelae. Am J Med 67:358, 1979.

74. Ng TP, Tsin TW, O'Kelly FJ, et al: A survey of the respiratory health of silica-exposed gemstone workers in Hong Kong. Am Rev Respir Dis 135:1249, 1987.

75. Ng TP, Allan WG, Tsin TW, et al: Silicosis in jade workers. Br J Ind Med 42:761, 1985.

76. Kawakami M, Sato S, Takishima T: Silicosis in workers dealing with tonoko: Case reports and analyses of tonoko. Chest 72:635, 1977.

77. Cunningham CDB, Hugh AE: Pneumoconiosis in women. Clin Radiol 24:491, 1973.

78. Hirsch M, Bar-Ziv J, Lehmann E, et al: Simple siliceous pneumoconiosis of Bedouin females in the Negev desert. Clin Radiol 25:507, 1974.

79. Palmer PES, Daynes G: Transkei silicosis. S Afr Med J 41:1182, 1967.

80. Warrell DA, Harrison BDW, Fawcett TN, et al: Silicosis among grindstone cutters in the north of Nigeria. Thorax 30:389, 1975.

81. Davis GS: Pathogenesis of silicosis: Current concepts and hypotheses. Lung 164:139, 1986.

82. Evans SM, Zeit W: Tissue responses to physical forces. J Lab Clin Med 34:592, 1949.

83. Curran RC, Rowsell EV: The application of the diffusion-chamber technique to the study of silicosis. J Pathol Bacteriol 76:561, 1958.

84. Allison AC, Harington JS, Birbeck M: An examination of the cytotoxic effects of silica on macrophages. J Exp Med 124:141, 1966.

85. Kane AB, Stanton RP, Raymond EG, et al: Dissociation of intracellular lysosomal rupture from the cell death caused by silica. J Cell Biol 87:643, 1980.

86. Gee JBL: Cellular mechanisms in occupational lung disease. Chest 78 (Suppl):384, 1980.

87. Heppleston AG: The fibrinogenic action of silica. Br Med Bull 25:282, 1969.

88. Heppleston AG, Styles JA: Activity of a macrophage factor in collagen formation by silica. Nature 214:521, 1967.

89. Chvapil M, Eskelson CD, Stiffel V, et al: Early changes in the chemical composition of the rat lung after silica administration. Arch Environ Health 34:402, 1979.

90. Gritter HL, Adamson IYR, King GM: Modulation of fibroblast activity by normal and silica-exposed alveolar macrophages. J Pathol 148:263, 1986.

91. Lowrie DB: What goes wrong with the macrophage in silicosis? Eur J Respir Dis 63:180, 1982.

92. What goes wrong with the macrophage in silicosis (editorial)? Eur J Respir Dis 63:180, 1982.

93. Bowden DH, Adamson IYR: The role of cell injury and the continuing inflammatory response in the generation of silicotic pulmonary fibrosis. J Pathol 144:149, 1984.

94. Jones RN, Turner-Warwick M, Ziskind M, et al: High prevalance of anti-nuclear antibodies in sandblasters' silicosis. Am Rev Respir Dis 113:393, 1976.

95. Doll NJ, Stankus RP, Hughes J, et al: Immune complexes and autoantibodies in silicosis. J Allergy Clin Immunol 68:281, 1981.

96. Vigliani EC, Pernis B: Immunological factors in the pathogenesis of the hyaline tissue of silicosis. Br J Ind Med 15:8, 1958.

97. Giles RD, Sturgill BC, Suratt PM, et al: Massive proteinuria and acute renal failure in a patient with acute silicoproteinosis. Am J Med 64:336, 1978.

98. Banks DE, Milutinovic J, Desnick RJ, et al: Silicon nephropathy mimicking Fabry's disease. Am J Nephrol 3:279, 1983.

99. Slavin RE, Swedo JL, Brandes D, et al: Extrapulmonary silicosis: A clinical, morphologic, and ultrastructural study. Hum Pathol 16:393, 1985.

100. Schuyler M, Ziskind M, Salvaggio J: Cell-mediated immunity in silicosis. Am Rev Respir Dis 116:147, 1977.

101. Schuyler MR, Ziskind MM, Salvaggio J: Function of lymphocytes and monocytes in silicosis. Chest 75:340, 1979.

102. Chiappino G, Vigliani EC: Role of infective, immunological and chronic irritative factors in the development of silicosis. Br J Ind Med 39:253, 1982.

103. Koskinen H, Tiilikainen A, Nordman H: Increased prevalence of HLA-Aw19 and of phenogroup Aw19,B18 in advanced silicosis. Chest 83:848, 1983.

104. Wagner JC, Burns J, Munday DE, et al: Presence of fibronectin in pneumoconiotic lesions. Thorax 37:54, 1982.

105. Leibowitz MC, Goldstein B: Some investigations into the nature and cause of massive fibrosis (MF) in the lungs of South African gold, coal, and asbestos mine workers. Am J Ind Med 12:129, 1987.

106. Heppleston AG, Wright MA, Stewart JA: Experimental alveolar lipo-proteinosis following the inhalation of silica. J Pathol 101:293, 1970.

107. Buechner HA, Ansari A: Acute silicoproteinosis. A new pathologic variant of acute silicosis in sandblasters, characterized by histologic features resembling alveolar proteinosis. Dis Chest 55:274, 1969.

108. Hoffman EO, Lamberty J, Pizzolato P, et al: The ultrastructure of acute silicosis. Arch Pathol 96:104, 1973.

109. Miller BE, Hook GER: Isolation and characterization of hypertrophic Type II cells from the lungs of silica-treated rats. Lab Invest 58:565, 1988.

110. Emerson RJ, Davis GS: Effect of alveolar lining material-coated silica on rat alveolar macrophages. Environ Health Perspect 51:81, 1983.

111. Allison AC, Hart PD: Potentiation by silica of the growth of Mycobacterium tuberculosis in macrophage cultures. Br J Exp Pathol 49:465, 1968.

112. Curran RC: Observations on the formation of collagen in quartz lesions. J Pathol Bacteriol 66:271, 1953.

113. Craighead JE, Vallyathan MV: Cryptic pulmonary lesions in workers occupationally exposed to dust containing silica. JAMA 244:1939, 1980.

114. del Campo JM, Hitado J, Gea G, et al: Anaerobes: A new aetiology in cavitary pneumoconiosis. Br J Ind Med 39:392, 1982.

115. Tukiainen P, Taskinen E, Korhola O, et al: TruCutR needle biopsy in asbestosis and silicosis: Correlation of histological changes with radiographic changes and pulmonary function in 41 patients. Br J Ind Med 35:292, 1978.

116. Tosi P, Franzinelli A, Miracco C, et al: Silicotic lymph node lesions in non-occupationally exposed lung carcinoma patients. Eur J Respir Dis 68:362, 1986.

117. Eide J, Gylseth B, Skaug V: Silicotic lesions of the bone marrow: Histopathology and microanalysis. Histopathology 8:693, 1984.

118. Paterson JF: Silicosis in hardrock miners in Ontario: The problem and its prevention. Can Med Assoc J 84:594, 1961.

119. Michel RD, Morris JF: Acute silicosis. Arch Intern Med 113:850, 1964.

120. Felson B: Chest Roentgenology. Philadelphia, WB Saunders Co, 1973.

121. Oosthuizen SF, Theron CP: Correlation between the radiographic and pathological findings in silicosis. Med Proc 10:337, 1964.

122. Theron CP, Walters LG, Webster I: The international classification of radiographs of the pneumoconioses. Based on the findings in 100 deceased white South African gold miners. An evaluation. Med Proc (Johannesburg) 10:352, 1964.

123. Greening RR, Heslep JH: The roentgenology of silicosis. Semin Roentgenol 2:265, 1967.

124. Pendergrass EP: Caldwell Lecture 1957—Silicosis and a few of the other pneumoconioses: Observations on certain aspects of the problem, with emphasis on the role of the radiologist. Am J Roentgenol 80:1, 1958.

125. Tada S, Yasukochi H, Shida H, et al: Bronchial arteriography in silicosis. Am J Roentgenol 120:810, 1974.

126. Jacobs LG, Gerstl B, Hollander AG, et al: Intra-abdominal egg-shell calcifications due to silicosis. Radiology 67:527, 1956.

127. Bellini F, Ghislandi E: "Egg-shell" calcifications at extrahilar sites in a silicotuberculotic patient. Med Lav 51:600, 1960.

128. Jacobson G, Felson B, Pendergrass EP, et al: Eggshell calcifications in coal and metal workers. Semin Roentgenol 2:276, 1967.

129. Nicod J-L, Gardiol D: Silicose et paralysie du diaphragme. (Silicosis and paralysis of the diaphragm.) Schweiz Med Wochenschr 94:1461, 1964.

130. Nice CM Jr, Ostrolenk DG: Asbestos and nodular lesions of the lung: A radiologic study. Dis Chest 54:226, 1968.

131. Buechner HA, Ansari A: Acute silicoproteinosis. A new pathologic variant of acute silicosis in sandblasters, characterized by histologic features resembling alveolar proteinosis. Dis Chest 55:274, 1969.

132. Sluis-Cremer GK, Hessel PA, Hnizdo E, et al: Relationship between silicosis and rheumatoid arthritis. Thorax 41:596, 1986.

12

133. MacLaren WM, Soutar CA: Progressive massive fibrosis and simple pneumoconiosis in ex-miners. Br J Ind Med 42:734, 1985.
134. Bergin CJ, Müller NL, Vedall S, et al: CT in silicosis: Correlation with plain films and pulmonary function tests. AJR 146:477, 1986.
135. Bégin R, Bergeron D, Samson R, et al: CT assessment of silicosis in exposed workers. AJR 148:509, 1987.
136. Koskinen H: Symptoms and clinical findings in patients with silicosis. Scand J Work Environ Health 11:101, 1985.
137. Munakata M, Homma Y, Matsuzaki M, et al: Rales in silicosis. A correlative study with physiological and radiological abnormalities. Respiration 48:140, 1985.
138. Gronhagen-Riska C, Kurppa K, Fyhrquist F, et al: Angiotensin-converting enzyme and lysozyme in silicosis and asbestosis. Scand J Respir Dis 59:228, 1978.
139. Bucca C, Veglio F, Rolla G, et al: Serum angiotensin converting enzyme (ACE) in silicosis. Eur J Respir Dis 65:477, 1984.
140. Nordman H, Koskinen H, Froseth B: Increased activity of angiotensin-converting enzyme in progressive silicosis. Chest 86:203, 1984.
141. Nozaki S, Sawada Y: Progress of simple pulmonary silicosis in retired miners. Jpn J Clin Tuberc 18:154, 1959.
142. Betts WW: Chalicosis pulmonum or chronic interstitial pneumonia induced by stone dust. JAMA 34:70, 1900.
143. Gardner LU: Pathology of the so-called acute silicosis. Am J Public Health 23:1240, 1933.
144. Bailey WC, Brown M, Buechner HA, et al: Silico-mycobacterial disease in sandblasters. Am Rev Respir Dis 110:115, 1974.
145. Mann B, Sinha CN: Jack needle lung biopsy in pneumoconiosis. Dis Chest 50:504, 1966.
146. Funahashi A, Schlueter DP, Pintar K, et al: Value of in situ elemental microanalysis in the histologic diagnosis of silicosis. Chest 85:506, 1984.
147. Teculescu DR, Stănescu DC: Carbon monoxide transfer factor for the lung in silicosis. Scand J Respir Dis 51:150, 1970.
148. Renzetti AD Jr, Kobayshi T, Bigler A, et al: Regional ventilation and perfusion in silicosis and in the alveolar-capillary block syndrome. Am J Med 49:5, 1970.
149. Becklake MR: Pneumoconioses. In Fenn WO, Rahn H (eds): Handbook of Physiology, Section III, Vol 2. Baltimore, Waverly Press, 1965, pp 1601–1614.
150. Irwiq LM, Rocks P: Lung function and respiratory symptoms in silicotic and nonsilicotic gold miners. Am Rev Respir Dis 117:429, 1978.
151. Bates DV, Macklem PT, Christie RV: Respiratory function in Disease; An Introduction to the Integrated Study of the Lung, 2nd ed, Philadelphia, WB Saunders Co, 1971.
152. Brink GC, Grzybowski S, Lane GB: Silicotuberculosis. Can Med Assoc J 82:959, 1960.
153. Gilson JC: Industrial pulmonary disease. In Schilling RSF (ed): Modern Trends in Occupational Health. London, Butterworth, 1960, p 50.
154. Westerholm P, Ahlmark A, Maasing R, et al: Silicosis and risk of lung cancer or lung tuberculosis: A cohort study. Environ Res 41:339, 1986.
155. Fisher ER, Watkins G, Lam NV, et al: Objective pathological diagnosis of coal workers' pneumoconiosis. JAMA 245:1829, 1981.
156. Lister WB: Carbon pneumoconiosis in a synthetic graphite worker. Br J Ind Med 18:114, 1961.
157. Miller AA, Ramsden F: Carbon pneumoconiosis. Br J Ind Med 18:103, 1961.
158. Pendergrass EP, Vorwald AJ, Mishkin MM, et al: Observations on workers in the graphite industry. Part I. Med Radiogr Photogr 43:70, 1967.
159. Pendergrass EP, Vorwald AJ, Mishkin MM, et al: Observations on workers in the graphite industry. Part II. Med Radiogr Photogr 44:2, 1968.
160. Gaensler EA, Cadigan JB, Sasahara AA, et al: Graphite pneumoconiosis of electrotypers. Am J Med 41:864, 1966.
161. Miller AA, Ramsden F: Carbon pneumoconiosis. Br J Ind Med 18:103, 1961.
162. Watson AJ, Black J, Doig AT, et al: Pneumoconiosis in carbon electrode makers. Br J Ind Med 16:274, 1959.
163. Golden EB, Varnock ML, Hulett LD Jr, et al: Fly ash lung: A new pneumoconiosis? Am Rev Respir Dis 125:108, 1982.
164. Green FHY, Laqueur WA: Coal workers' pneumoconiosis. Pathol Ann 15:333, 1980.
165. Naeye RL, Mahon JK, Dellinger WS: Rank of coal and coal workers' pneumoconiosis. Am Rev Respir Dis 103:350, 1971.
166. Seaton A, Dodgson J, Dick JA, et al: Quartz and pneumoconiosis in coalminers. Lancet 2:1272, 1981.
167. Seaton A, Dick JA, Dodgson J, et al: Quartz and pneumoconiosis in coalminers. Lancet 2:1272, 1981.
168. Banks DE, Bauer MA, Castellan RM, et al: Silicosis in surface coalmine drillers. Thorax 38:275, 1983.
169. Morgan WKC: Respiratory disease in coal miners. JAMA 231:1347, 1975.
170. Morgan WKC, Lapp NL: Respiratory disease in coal miners. Am Rev Respir Dis 113:531, 1976.
171. Martin JE Jr: Breathless coal workers as seen at the Golden Clinic. AMA Arch Ind Health 15:494, 1957.
172. Reed ES, Wells PO, Wicker EH: Coal miners' pneumoconiosis. Radiology 71:661, 1958.
173. Wyatt JP: Morphogenesis of pneumoconiosis occurring in southern Illinois bituminous workers. AMA Arch Ind Health 21:445, 1960.
174. Hyatt RE, Kistin AD, Mahan TK: Respiratory disease in southern West Virginia coal miners. Am Rev Respir Dis 89:387, 1964.
175. Williams JL, Moller GA: Solitary mass in the lungs of coal miners. Am J Roentgenol 117:765, 1973.
176. Pendergrass EP: An evaluation of some of the radiologic patterns of small opacities in coal workers' pneumoconiosis. Am J Roentgenol 115:457, 1972.
177. Reger RB, Smith CA, Kibelstis JA, et al: The effect of film quality and other factors on the roentgenographic categorization of coal workers' pneumoconiosis. Am J Roentgenol 115:462, 1972.
178. Seaton A, Lapp NL, Chang CEJ: Lung perfusion scanning in coal workers' pneumoconiosis. Am Rev Respir Dis 103:338, 1971.
179. Seaton A: Coalworkers pneumoconiosis in Britain today and tomorrow. Br Med J 284:1507, 1982.
180. Douglas AN, Robertson A, Chapman JS, et al: Dust exposure, dust recovered from the lung, and associated pathology in a group of British coalminers. Br J Ind Med 43:795, 1986.
181. Penman RW: Conference on pneumoconiosis: A summary of the conclusions from an international conference on coal workers' pneumoconiosis. Am Rev Respir Dis 102:243, 1970.
182. Pairman RP, O'Brien RJ, Swecker S, et al: Respiratory status of surface coal miners in the United States. Arch Environ Health 32:211, 1977.
183. Cochrane AL: Epidemiology of coal workers' pneumoconiosis. In King EJ, Fletcher CM (eds): Industrial Pulmonary Diseases: A Symposium held at the Postgraduate Medical School of London, 18–20 September 1957 and 25–27 March 1958. London, J & A Churchill, 1960, pp 221–231.
184. Bonnell JA, Schilling CJ, Massey PMO: Clinical and experimental studies of the effects of pulverized fuel ash. A review. Ann Occup Hyg 23:159, 1980.
185. Town JD: Pseudoasbestos bodies and asteroid giant cells in a patient with graphite pneumoconiosis. Can Med Assoc J 98:100, 1968.
186. Johnson FB: Identification of graphite in tissue sections. Arch Pathol Lab Med 104:491, 1980.
187. Crosbie WA: The respiratory health of carbon black workers. Arch Environ Health 41:346, 1986.
188. Jones HD, Jones TR, Lyle WH: Carbon fibre: Results of a survey of process workers and their environment in a factory producing continuous filament. Ann Occup Hyg 26:861, 1982.
189. Heppleston AG: The essential lesion of pneumokoniosis in Welsh coal workers. J Pathol Bacteriol 59:453, 1947.
190. Kleinerman J, Green F, Harley RA, et al: Pathology standards for coal workers' pneumoconiosis. Arch Pathol Lab Med 103:375, 1979.
191. DeVuyst P, Dumortier P, Rickaert F, et al: Occupational lung fibrosis in an aluminium polisher. Eur J Respir Dis 68:131, 1986.
192. Pigott GH, Gaskell BA, Ishmael J: Effects of long term inhalation of alumina fibres in rats. Br J Exp Pathol 62:323, 1981.
193. Gross P, Harley RA Jr, deTreville RTP: Pulmonary reaction to metallic aluminum powders. Arch Environ Health 26:227, 1973.
194. Pelstring RJ, Kim CK, Lower EE, et al: Marrow granulomas in coal workers' pneumoconiosis. A histological study with elemental analysis. Am J Clin Pathol 89:553, 1988.
195. Gough J, Heppleston AG: The pathology of the pneumoconioses. In King EJ, Fletcher CM (eds): Industrial Pulmonary Diseases: A Symposium held at the Postgraduate Medical School of London, 18–20 September 1957 and 25–27 March 1958. London, J & A Churchill, 1960, pp 23–26.
196. Duguid JB, Lambert MW: The pathogenesis of coal miner's pneumoconiosis. J Pathol Bacteriol 88:389, 1964.
197. Reid L: The Pathology of Emphysema. Chicago, Year Book Medical Publishers, 1967.
198. Davis JMG, Chapman J, Collings P, et al: Variations in the histological patterns of the lesions of coal workers' pneumoconiosis in Britain and their relationship to lung dust content. Am Rev Respir Dis 128:118, 1983.
199. King EJ, Harrison CV, Mohanty GP: The effect of various forms of alumina on the lungs of rats. J Pathol Bacteriol 69:81, 1955.
200. Lyons JP, Campbell H: Relation between progressive massive fibrosis, emphysema, and pulmonary dysfunction in coalworkers' pneumoconiosis. Br J Ind Med 38:125, 1981.
201. Prignot J, Van de Velde R: La cavitation aseptique des pseudotumeurs dans l'anthraco-silicose. Etude clinique et radiologique. (Aseptic cavitation of pseudotumors in anthracosilicosis: Clinical and radiological study.) J Fr Med Chir Thorac 12:623, 1958.
202. Theodos PA, Cathcart RT, Fraimow W: Ischemic necrosis in anthracosilicosis. Arch Environ Health 2:609, 1961.

203. Wagner JC, Wusteman FS, Edwards JH, et al: The composition of massive lesions in coal miners. Thorax 30:382, 1975.

204. Wagner JC, Burns J, De Munday JM: Presence of fibronectin in pneumoconiotic lesions. Thorax 37:54, 1982.

205. King EJ, Maguire BA, Nagelschmidt G: Further studies of the dust in lungs of coal-miners. Br J Ind Med 13:9, 1956.

206. Love RG, Miller BG: Longitudinal study of lung function in coal-miners. Thorax 37:193, 1982.

207. Hurley JF, Soutar CA: Can exposure to coalmine dust cause a severe impairment of lung function? Br J Ind Med 43:150, 1986.

208. Hurley JF, Alexander WP, Hazledine DJ, et al: Exposure to respirable coalmine dust and incidence of progressive massive fibrosis. Br J Ind Med 444:661, 1987.

209. Soutar CA, Collins HP: Classification of progressive massive fibrosis of coalminers by type of radiographic appearance. Br J Ind Med 41:334, 1984.

210. Seal RME, Cockcroft A, Kung I, et al: Central lymph node changes and progressive massive fibrosis in coalworkers. Thorax 41:531, 1986.

211. James WRL: The relationship of tuberculosis to the development of massive pneumokoniosis in coal workers. Br J Tuberc 48:89, 1954.

212. Robertson MD, Boyd JE, Collins HP, et al: Serum immunoglobulin levels and humoral immune competence in coalworkers. Am J Ind Med 6:387, 1984.

213. Rom WN, Turner WG, Kanner RE, et al: Antinuclear antibodies in Utah coal miners. Chest 83:515, 1983.

214. Soutar CA, Turner-Warwick M, Parkes WR: Circulating antinuclear antibody and rheumatoid factor in coal pneumoconiosis. Br Med J 3:145, 1974.

215. Wagner JC, McCormick JN: Immunological investigations of coal workers' disease. J R Coll Physicians Lond 2:49, 1967.

216. Caplan A, Payne RB, Withey JL: A broader concept of Caplan's syndrome related to rheumatoid factors. Thorax 17:205, 1962.

217. Lippman M, Eckert IIL, Hahon N, et al: Circulating antinuclear and rheumatoid factors in coal miners. A prevalence study in Pennsylvania and West Virginia. Ann Intern Med 79:807, 1973.

218. Pearson DJ, Mentnech MS, Elliot JA, et al: Serologic changes in pneumoconiosis and progressive massive fibrosis of coal workers. Am Rev Respir Dis 124:696, 1981.

219. Robertson MD, Boyd JE, Fernie JM, et al: Some immunological studies on coalworkers with and without pneumoconiosis. Am J Ind Med 4:467, 1983.

220. Caplan A: Certain unusual radiological appearances in the chest of coal-miners suffering from rheumatoid arthritis. Thorax 8:29, 1953.

221. Burrell R: Immunological aspects of coal workers' pneumoconiosis. Ann NY Acad Sci 200:94, 1972.

222. Burrell R, Flaherty DK, Schreiber JK: Immunological studies of experimental coal workers' pneumoconiosis. Presented at the Fourth International Conference on Inhaled Particles, Edinburgh, September 1975.

223. Heise ER, Mentnech MS, Olenchock SA, et al: HLA-A1 and coal-workers' pneumoconiosis. Am Rev Respir Dis 119:903, 1979.

224. Rasche B, Reisner MTR, Islam MS, et al: Individual factors in the development of coal miners pneumoconiosis. Ann Occup Hyg 26:713, 1982.

225. Soutar CA, Coutts I, Parkes WR, et al: Histocompatibility antigens in coal miners with pneumoconiosis. Br J Ind Med 40:34, 1983.

226. Lapp NL, Seaton A, Kaplan KC, et al: Pulmonary hemodynamics in symptomatic coal miners. Am Rev Respir Dis 104:418, 1971.

227. Naeye RL, Laqueur WA: Chronic cor pulmonale. Its pathogenesis in Appalachian bituminous coal workers. Arch Pathol 90:487, 1970.

228. Fernie JM, Douglas AN, Lamb D, et al: Right ventricular hypertrophy in a group of coalworkers. Thorax 38:436, 1983.

229. James WRL, Thomas AJ: Cardiac hypertrophy in coal miners' pneumoconiosis. Br J Ind Med 13:24, 1956.

230. Wells NA, Laquer WA: Right ventricular hypertrophy in West Virginia coal miners. Report of communication to International Academy of Pathology, US Department of Health, Education, and Welfare Public Health Service, 1966.

231. Hankinson JL, Palmes ED, Lapp NL: Pulmonary air space size in coal miners. Am Rev Respir Dis 119:391, 1979.

232. Ryder R, Lyons JP, Campbell H, et al: Emphysema in coal workers' pneumoconiosis. Br Med J 3:481, 1970.

233. Cockcroft A, Seal RME, Wagner JC, et al: Postmortem study of emphysema in coalworkers and noncoalworkers. Lancet 2:600, 1982.

234. Leigh J, Outhred KG, McKenzie HI, et al: Quantified pathology of emphysema, pneumoconiosis, and chronic bronchitis in coal workers. Br J Ind Med 40:258, 1983.

235. Rom WN, Kanner RE, Renzetti AD Jr, et al: Respiratory disease in Utah coal miners. Am Rev Respir Dis 123:372, 1981.

236. Douglas AN, Lamb D, Ruckley VA: Bronchial gland dimensions in coalminers: Influence of smoking and dust exposure. Thorax 37:760, 1982.

237. Leigh J, Wiles AN, Glick M: Total population study of factors affecting chronic bronchitis prevalence in the coal mining industry of New South Wales, Australia. Br J Ind Med 43:263, 1986.

238. Marine WM, Gurr D, Jacobsen M: Clinically important respiratory effects of dust exposure and smoking in British coal miners. Am Rev Respir Dis 137:106, 1988.

239. Cockcroft AE, Wagner JC, Seal EM, et al: Irregular opacities in coalworkers' pneumoconiosis: Correlation with pulmonary function and pathology. Ann Occup Hyg 26:767, 1982.

240. Musk AW, Cotes JE, Bevan C, et al: Relationship between type of simple coalworkers pneumoconiosis and lung function: A 9-year follow-up study of subjects with small rounded opacities. Br J Ind Med 38:313, 1981.

241. Cockcroft A, Lyons JP, Andersson N, et al: Prevalence and relation to underground exposure of radiological irregular opacities in South Wales coal workers with pneumoconiosis. Br J Ind Med 40:169, 1983.

242. Gough J, James WRL, Wentworth JE: A comparison of the radiological and pathological changes in coalworkers' pneumoconiosis. J Fac Radiol 1:28, 1949.

243. Lyons JP, Watson AJ: The significance of radiographic "calcification" in the lungs of coalworkers. Tubercle 42:457, 1961.

244. Davies D: Disability and coal workers' pneumoconiosis. Br Med J 2:652, 1974.

245. Shennan DH, Washington JS, Thomas DJ, et al: Factors predisposing to the development of progressive massive fibrosis in coal miners. Br J Ind Med 38:321, 1981.

246. Seaton A, Soutar CA, Melville AWT: Radiological changes in coal-miners on leaving the industry. Br J Dis Chest 74:310, 1980.

247. Caplan A: Correlation of radiological category with lung pathology in coal workers' pneumoconiosis. Br J Ind Med 19:171, 1962.

248. Reger RB, Amandus HE, Morgan WKC: On the diagnosis of coal workers' pneumoconiosis. Anglo-American disharmony. Am Rev Respir Dis 108:1186, 1973.

249. Cochrane AL, Moore F: A 20-year follow-up of men aged 55–64 including coal-miners and foundry workers in Staveley, Derbyshire. Br J Ind Med 37:226, 1980.

250. Morgan WKC, Lapp NL, Seaton D: Respiratory disability in coal miners. JAMA 243:2401, 1980.

251. Ball J: The natural history and management of coal workers' pneumoconiosis. In King EJ, Fletcher CM (eds): Industrial Pulmonary Diseases: A Symposium held at the Postgraduate Medical School of London, 18–20 September 1957 and 25–27 March 1958. London, J & A Churchill, 1960, pp 241–254.

252. Cathcart RT, Theodos PA, Fraimow W: Anthracosilicosis. Selected aspects related to the evaluation of disability, cavitation, and the unusual x-ray. Arch Intern Med 106:368, 1960.

253. Pendergrass EP: The Pneumoconiosis Problem, with Emphasis on the Role of the Radiologist. Springfield Ill, Charles C Thomas, 1958, pp 16–17.

254. Ashford JR, Morgan DC, Rae S, et al: Respiratory symptoms in British coal miners. Am Rev Respir Dis 102:370, 1970.

255. Gilson JC: The disability of coal worker in Wales. AMA Arch Ind Health 15:487, 1957.

256. Kibelstis JA, Morgan EJ, Reger R, et al: Prevalence of bronchitis and airway obstruction in American bituminous coal miners. Am Rev Respir Dis 108:886, 1973.

257. Rasmussen DL, Laquer WA, Futterman P, et al: Pulmonary impairment in Southern West Virginia coal miners. Am Rev Respir Dis 98:658, 1968.

258. Sherani TM, Angelini GD, Passani SP, et al: Vocal cord paralysis associated with coalworkers' pneumoconiosis and progressive massive fibrosis. Thorax 39:683, 1984.

259. Cochrane AL, Moore F, Moncrieff CB: Are coalminers, with low "risk factors" for ischaemic heart disease at greater risk of developing progressive massive fibrosis? Br J Ind Med 39:265, 1982.

260. Davies GM: A mortality study of coke oven workers in two South Wales integrated steelworks. Br J Ind Med 34:291, 1977.

261. Gilson J, Hugh-Jones P: Lung function in coal workers' pneumoconiosis. Medical Research Council, Special Report 290, HMSO London, 1955.

262. Zhicheng S: A study of lung function in coalworkers' pneumoconiosis. Br J Ind Med 43:644, 1986.

263. Hildick-Smith M: Natural history of coal-workers pneumoconiosis in men over 65. J R Coll Physicians Lond 17:111, 1983.

264. Kibelstis JA: Diffusing capacity in bituminous coal miners. Chest 63:501, 1973.

265. Seaton A, Lapp NL, Morgan WKC: The relationship of pulmonary impairment in simple coal workers' pneumoconiosis to type of radiologic capacity. Br J Ind Med 29:50, 1972.

266. Schuyler MR, Gaumer HR, Stankus RP, et al: Bronchoalveolar lavage in silicosis: Evidence of type II cell hyperplasia. Lung 157:95, 1980.

267. Morgan WKC, Lapp NL: Respiratory disease in coal miners. Am Rev Respir Dis 113:531, 1976.

268. Musk AW, Cotes JE, Bevan C, et al: Relationship between type of simple coal workers' pneumoconiosis and lung function. A nine-year follow-up study of subjects with small rounded opacities. Br J Ind Med 38:313, 1981.

269. Lyons JP, Campbell H: Relation between progressive massive fibrosis, emphysema, and pulmonary dysfunction in coal workers' pneumoconiosis. Br J Ind Med 38:125, 1981.

270. Legg SJ, Cotes JE, Bevan C: Lung mechanics in relation to radiographic category of coalworkers' simple pneumoconiosis. Br J Ind Med 40:28, 1983.

271. Lyons JP, Clarke WG, Hall AM, et al: Transfer factor (diffusing capacity) for the lung in simple pneumoconiosis of coal workers. Br Med J 4:772, 1967.

272. Rasmussen DL, Nelson CW: Respiratory function in Southern Appalachian coal miners. Am Rev Respir Dis 103:240, 1971.

273. Cockcroft A, Berry G, Cotes JE, et al: Shape of small opacities and lung function in coalworkers. Thorax 37:765, 1982.

274. Constantinidis K, Musk AW, Jenkins JP, et al: Pulmonary function in coal workers with Caplan's syndrome and non-rheumatoid complicated pneumoconiosis. Thorax 33:764, 1978.

275. Leading article: Asbestosis. Br Med J 3:62, 1967.

276. Selikoff IJ: Household risks with inorganic fibers. Bull NY Acad Med 57:947, 1981.

277. Elmes PC, Simpson MJ: Insulation workers in Belfast: A further study of mortality due to asbestos exposure. Br J Ind Med 34:174, 1977.

278. Peto J, Doll R, Howard SV, et al: A mortality study among workers in an English asbestos factory. Br J Ind Med 34:169, 1977.

279. Rogan WJ, Gladen BC, Ragan ND, et al: U.S. prevalence of occupational pleural thickening: A look at chest x-rays from the first National Health and Nutrition Examination Survey. Am J Epidemiol 126:893, 1987.

280. Miller A, Teirstein AS, Selikoff IJ: Ventilatory failure due to asbestos pleurisy. Am J Med 75:911, 1983.

281. Murphy RLH Jr, Gaensler EA, Ferris BG, et al: Diagnosis of "asbestosis": Observations from a longitudinal survey of shipyard pipe coverers. Am J Med 65:488, 1978.

282. Kilburn KH, Warshaw R, Thornton JC: Asbestosis, pulmonary symptoms and functional impairment in shipyard workers. Chest 88:254, 1985.

283. Oliver LC, Eisen EA, Greene RE, et al: Asbestos-related disease in railroad workers: A cross-sectional study. Am Rev Respir Dis 131:499, 1985.

284. McDonald AD, Fry JS, Woolley AJ, et al: Dust exposure and mortality in an American factory using chrysotile, amosite, and crocidolite in mainly textile manufacture. Br J Ind Med 40:368, 1983.

285. Acheson ED, Gardner MJ, Pippard EC, et al: Mortality of two groups of women who manufactured gas masks from chrysotile and crocidolite asbestos: A 40-year follow-up. Br J Ind Med 39:344, 1982.

286. Sebastien P, Bignon J, Martin M: Indoor airborne asbestos pollution: From the ceiling and the floor. Science 216:1410, 1982.

287. Young I, West S, Jackson J, et al: Prevalence of asbestos related lung disease among employees in non-asbestos industries. Med J Aust 1:464, 1981.

288. Peacock PR, Biancifiori C, Bucciarelli E: Examination of lung smears for asbestos bodies in 109 consecutive necropsies in Perugia. Eur J Cancer 5:155, 1969.

289. Roberts GH: Asbestos bodies in lungs at necropsy. J Clin Pathol 20:570, 1967.

290. Thomson JG, Graves WM Jr: Asbestos as an urban air contaminant. Arch Pathol 81:458, 1966.

291. Donisch I, Swettenham KV, Hathorn MKS: Prevalence of asbestos bodies in a necropsy series in East London: Association with disease, occupation, and domiciliary address. Br J Ind Med 32:16, 1975.

292. Cauna D, Totten RS, Gross P: Asbestos bodies in human lungs at autopsy. JAMA 192:371, 1965.

293. Xipell JM, Bhathal PS: Asbestos bodies in lungs: An Australian report. Pathology 1:327, 1969.

294. Anjilvel L, Thurlbeck WM: The incidence of asbestos bodies in the lungs in random necropsies in Montreal. Can Med Assoc J 95:1179, 1966.

295. Becklake MR: Asbestos-related diseases of the lung and other organs: Their epidemiology and implications for clinical practice. Am Rev Respir Dis 114:187, 1976.

296. Kiviluoto R: Pleural calcification as a roentgenologic sign of non-occupational endemic anthophyllite-asbestosis. Acta Radiol (Suppl): 194, 1960.

297. Van De Water JM, Kagey KS, Miller IT, et al: Oxygen response of the lung to six to 12 hours of 100 per cent inhalation in normal man. N Engl J Med 283:621, 1970.

298. Preger L: Asbestos-Related Disease. New York, Grune & Stratton, 1978.

299. Becklake MR: Exposure to asbestos and human disease. N Engl J Med 306:1480, 1982.

300. Peters A, Peters J: Source-book on Asbestos Diseases: Medical, Legal, and Engineering Aspects. New York, Garland STPM Press, 1980.

301. Webster I: Asbestosis. S Afr Med J 38:870, 1964.

302. Wagner JC, Sleggs CA, Marchand P: Diffuse pleural mesothelioma and asbestos exposure in the north western Cape Province. Br J Ind Med 7:260, 1960.

303. Parkes WR: Asbestos-related disorders. Br J Dis Chest 67:261, 1973.

304. Newhouse ML: A study of the mortality of workers in an asbestos factory. Br J Ind Med 26:294, 1969.

305. Hourihane DO, Lessof L, Richardson PC: Hyaline and calcified pleural plaques as an index of exposure to asbestos. A study of radiological and pathological features of 100 cases with a consideration of epidemiology. Br Med J 1:1069, 1966.

306. Champion P: Two cases of malignant mesothelioma after exposure to asbestos. Am Rev Respir Dis 103:821, 1971.

307. Vianna NJ, Polan AK: Non-occupational exposure to asbestos and malignant mesothelioma in females. Lancet 1:1061, 1978.

308. Epler GR, Fitzgerald MX, Gaensler EA, et al: Asbestos-related disease from household exposure. Respiration 39:229, 1980.

309. Sider L, Holland EA, Davis TM Jr, et al: Changes on radiographs of wives of workers exposed to asbestos. Radiology 164:723, 1987.

310. Berry G, Newhouse ML: Mortality of workers manufacturing friction materials using asbestos. Br J Ind Med 40:1, 1983.

311. Wright GW: Asbestos and health in 1969. Am Rev Respir Dis 100:467, 1969.

312. Constantopoulos SH, Goudevenos JA, Saratzis N, et al: Metsovo lung: Pleural calcification and restrictive lung function in northwestern Greece: Environmental exposure to mineral fiber as etiology. Environ Res 38:319, 1985.

313. Constantopoulos SH, Saratzis NA, Kontogiannis D, et al: Tremolite whitewashing and pleural calcifications. Chest 92:709, 1987.

314. Yazicioglu S, Ilcayto R, Balci K, et al: Pleural calcification, pleural mesotheliomas, and bronchial cancers caused by tremolite dust. Thorax 35:564, 1980.

315. Baris YI, Sahin AA, Erkan ML: Clinical and radiological study in sepiolite workers. Arch Environ Health 35:343, 1980.

316. De Vuyst P, Mairesse M, Gaudichet A, et al: Mineralogical analysis of bronchoalveolar lavage fluid as an aid to diagnosis of "imported" pleural asbestosis. Thorax 38:628, 1983.

317. Round the World, United States: Asbestos in water. Lancet 2:1256, 1973.

318. Masson TJ, McKay FW, Miller RW: Asbestos-like fibers in Duluth water supply: Relation to cancer mortality. JAMA 228:1019, 1974.

319. Leading article: Asbestos hazards. Br Med J 4:312, 1973.

320. Cunningham HM, Pontefract R: Asbestos fibres in beverages and drinking water. Nature 232:332, 1971.

321. Asbestos in water (editorial). Lancet 2:132, 1981.

322. Conforti PM, Kanarek MS, Jackson LA, et al: Asbestos in drinking water and cancer in the San Francisco bay area: 1969–1974 incidence. J Chronic Dis 34:211, 1981.

323. Hilding AC, Hilding DA, Larson DM, et al: Biological effects of ingested amosite asbestos, taconite tailings, diatomaceous earth and Lake Superior water in rats. Arch Environ Health 36:298, 1981.

324. Wright JL, Churg A: Morphology of small-airway lesions in patients with asbestos exposure. Hum Pathol 15:68, 1984.

325. Warnock ML, Prescott BT, Kuvahara TJ: Numbers and types of asbestos fibers in subjects with pleural plaques. Am J Pathol 109:37, 1982.

326. Churg A: Asbestos fibers and pleural plaques in a general autopsy population. Am J Pathol 109:88, 1982.

327. Wain SL, Roggli VL, Foster WL Jr: Parietal pleural plaques, asbestos bodies, and neoplasia. Chest 86:707, 1984.

328. Churg A, Golden J: Current problems in the pathology of asbestos-related disease. Pathol Ann 17(pt. 2):33, 1982.

329. Roberts GH: The pathology of parietal pleural plaques. J Clin Pathol 24:348, 1971.

330. Craighead JE, Abraham JL, Churg A, et al: The pathology of asbestos-associated diseases of the lungs and pleural cavities: Diagnostic criteria and proposed grading schema. Arch Pathol Lab Med 106:544, 1982.

331. Meurman L: Asbestos bodies and pleural plaques in a Finnish series of autopsy cases: Introduction. Acta Pathol Microbiol Scand 181(Supple):7, 1966.

332. Meurman L: Asbestos bodies and pleural plaques in a Finnish series of autopsy cases. Acta Pathol Microbiol Scand (Suppl)181:97, 1966.

333. Francis D, Jussuf A, Mortensen T, et al: Hyaline pleural plaques and asbestos bodies in 198 randomized autopsies. Scand J Respir Dis 58:193, 1977.

334. Hillerdal G: Pleural plaques in a health survey material: Frequency, development and exposure to asbestos. Scand J Respir Dis 59:257, 1978.

335. Albelda SM, Epstein DM, Gefter WB, et al: Pleural thickening: Its

significance and relationship to asbestos dust exposure. Am Rev Respir Dis 126:621, 1982.

336. Stephens M, Gibbs AR, Pooley FD, et al: Asbestos induced diffuse pleural fibrosis: Pathology and mineralogy. Thorax 42:583, 1987.

337. O'Brien CJ, Franks AJ: Paraplegia due to massive asbestos-related pleural and mediastinal fibrosis. Histopathology 11:541, 1987.

338. Sluis-Cremer GK, Webster I: Acute pleurisy in asbestosis exposed persons. Environ Res 5:380, 1972.

339. Gaensler EA, Kaplan AI: Asbestos pleural effusion. Ann Intern Med 74:178, 1971.

340. Shore BL, Daughaday CC, Spilberg I: Benign asbestos pleurisy in the rabbit. Am Rev Respir Dis 128:481, 1983.

341. Churg A: Fiber counting and analysis in the diagnosis of asbestos-related disease. Hum Pathol 13:381, 1982.

342. Kuhn C III, Kuo TT: Cytoplasmic hyalin in asbestosis. A reaction of injured alveolar epithelium. Arch Pathol 95:190, 1973.

343. Warnock ML, Press M, Churg A: Further observations on cytoplasmic hyaline in the lung. Hum Pathol 11:59, 1980.

344. Davis JMG: The pathology of asbestos-related disease. Thorax 39:801, 1984.

345. Churg A, Wright JL: Small-airway lesions in patients exposed to non-asbestos mineral dusts. Hum Pathol 14:688, 1983.

346. Churg A: Asbestos fiber content of the lungs in patients with and without asbestos airways disease. Am Rev Respir Dis 127:470, 1983.

347. Churg A, Wright JL, Wiggs B, et al: Small airways disease and mineral dust exposure. Am Rev Respir Dis 131:139, 1985.

348. Cohen BM, Adasczik A, Cohen EM: Small airways changes in workers exposed to asbestos. Respiration 45:296, 1984.

349. Begin R, Cantin A, Berthiaume Y, et al: Airway function in lifetime-nonsmoking older asbestos population. Am J Med 75:631, 1983.

350. Rodrigues-Roisin R, Merchant JEM, Cochrane GM, et al: Maximal expiratory flow volume curves in workers exposed to asbestos. Respiration 39:158, 1980.

351. Secker-Walker RH, Ho JE: Regional lung function in asbestos workers: Observations and speculations. Respiration 43:8, 1982.

352. Bégin R, Masse S, Bureau MA: Morphologic features and function of the airways in early asbestosis in the sheep model. Am Rev Respir Dis 126:870, 1982.

353. Wright JL, Tron V, Filipenko D, et al: Pathophysiologic correlations in asbestos-induced airway disease in the guinea pig. Exp Lung Res 11:307, 1986.

354. Brody AR, Roe MW: Deposition pattern of inorganic particles at the alveolar level in the lungs of rats and mice. Am Rev Respir Dis 128:724, 1983.

355. Brody AR, Hill LH, Adkins B Jr, et al: Chrysotile asbestos inhalation in rats: Deposition pattern and reaction of alveolar epithelium and pulmonary macrophages. Am Rev Respir Dis 123:670, 1981.

356. Warheit DB, Chang LY, Hill LH, et al: Pulmonary macrophage accumulation and asbestos-induced lesions at sites of fiber deposition. Am Rev Respir Dis 129:301, 1984.

357. Warheit DB, George G, Hill LH, et al: Inhaled asbestos activates a complement-dependent chemoattractant for macrophages. Lab Invest 52:505, 1985.

358. Kagan E, Oghiso Y, Hartmann D-P: Enhanced release of a chemoattractant for alveolar macrophages after asbestos inhalation. Am Rev Respir Dis 128:680, 1983.

359. Lemaire I, Beaudoin H, Massé S, et al: Alveolar macrophage stimulation of lung fibroblast growth in asbestos-induced pulmonary fibrosis. Am J Pathol 122:205, 1986.

360. Adamson IYR, Bowden DH: Crocidolite-induced pulmonary fibrosis in mice. Cytokinetic and biochemical studies. Am J Pathol 122:261, 1986.

361. McLemore T, Corson M, Mace M, et al: Phagocytosis of asbestos fibers by human pulmonary alveolar macrophages. Cancer Lett 6:183, 1979.

362. Fasske E: Pathogenesis of pulmonary fibrosis induced by chrysotile asbestos. Longitudinal light and electron microscopic studies on the rat model. Virchows Arch 408:329, 1986.

363. Mossman BT, Kessler JB, Ley BW, et al: Interaction of crocidolite asbestos with hamster respiratory mucosa in organ culture. Lab Invest 36:131, 1977.

364. Samet JM, Epler GR, Gaensler EA, et al: Absence of synergism between exposure to asbestos and cigarette smoking in asbestosis. Am Rev Respir Dis 120:75, 1979.

365. Weiss W: Cigarette smoking, asbestos, and pulmonary fibrosis. Am Rev Respir Dis 104:223, 1971.

366. Rossiter CE, Harries PG: U.K. Naval Dockyards Asbestos Study: Survey of the sample population aged 50–59 years. Br J Ind Med 36:281, 1979.

367. Pearle J: Exercise performance and functional impairment in asbestos-exposed workers. Chest 80:701, 1981.

368. Kilburn KH, Lilis R, Anderson HA, et al: Interaction of asbestos, age, and cigarette smoking in producing radiographic evidence of diffuse pulmonary fibrosis. Am J Med 80:377, 1986.

369. Baker EL, Dagg T, Greene RE: Respiratory illness in the construction trades. I. The significance of asbestos-associated pleural disease among sheet metal workers. J Occup Med 27:483, 1985.

370. Finkelstein MM, Vingilis JJ: Radiographic abnormalities among asbestos-cement workers. An exposure-response study. Am Rev Respir Dis 129:17, 1984.

371. Lilis R, Selikoff IJ, Lerman Y, et al: Asbestosis: Interstitial pulmonary fibrosis and pleural fibrosis in a cohort of asbestos workers: Influence of cigarette smoking. Am J Ind Med 10:459, 1986.

372. McFadden D, Wright J, Wiggs B, et al: Cigarette smoke increases the penetration of asbestos fibers into airway walls. Am J Pathol 123:95, 1986.

373. Andrion A, Pira E, Mollo F: Pleural plaques at autopsy, smoking habits, and asbestos exposure. Eur J Respir Dis 65:125, 1984.

374. Turner-Warwick M, Parkes WR: Circulating rheumatoid and antinuclear factors in asbestos workers. Br Med J 1:886, 1965.

375. Doll NJ, Diem JE, Jones RN, et al: Humoral immunologic abnormalities in workers exposed to asbestos cement dust. J Allergy Clin Immunol 72:509, 1983.

376. deShazo RD, Hendrick DJ, Diem JE, et al: Immunologic aberrations in asbestos cement workers: Dissociation from asbestosis. J Allergy Clin Immunol 72:454, 1983.

377. Huuskonen MS, Rasanen JA, Juntunen J, et al: Immunological aspects of asbestosis: Patients' neurological signs and asbestosis progression. Am J Ind Med 5:461, 1984.

378. Haslam PL, Lukoszek A, Merchant JA, et al: Lymphocyte responses to phytohaemagglutinin in patients with asbestosis and pleural mesothelioma. Clin Exp Immunol 31:178, 1978.

379. Pierce R, Turner-Warwick M: Skin tests with tuberculin (PPD), Candida albicans and Trichophyton spp. in cryptogenic fibrosing alveolitis and asbestos related lung disease. Clin Allergy 10:229, 1980.

380. Lange A, Garncarek D, Tomeczako J, et al: Outcome of asbestos exposure (lung fibrosis and antinuclear antibodies) with respect to skin reactivity: An 8-year longitudinal study. Environ Res 41:1, 1986.

381. Toivanen A, Salmivalli M, Molnar G: Pulmonary asbestosis and autoimmunity. Br Med J 1:691, 1976.

382. Bégin R, Menard H, Decarie F, et al: Immunogenetic factors as determinants of asbestosis. Lung 165:159, 1987.

383. Gellert AR, Kitajewska JY, Uthayakumar S, et al: Asbestos fibres in bronchoalveolar lavage fluid from asbestos workers: Examination by electron microscopy. Br J Ind Med 43:170, 1986.

384. Xaubet A, Rodriguez-Roisin R, Bombi JA, et al: Correlation of bronchoalveolar lavage and clinical and functional findings in asbestosis. Am Rev Respir Dis 133:848, 1986.

385. Roggli VL, Piantadosi CA, Bell DY: Asbestos bodies in bronchoalveolar lavage fluid. A study of 20 asbestos-exposed individuals and comparison to patients with other chronic interstitial lung diseases. Acta Cytol 30:470, 1986.

386. De Vuyst P, Jedwab J, Dumortier P, et al: Asbestos bodies in bronchoalveolar lavage. Am Rev Respir Dis 126:972, 1982.

387. Bégin R, Drapeau G, Boileau R, et al: Enzyme activities of lung lavage in asbestosis. Clin Biochem 19:240, 1986.

388. Robinson BW, Rose AH, James A, et al: Alveolitis of pulmonary asbestosis. Bronchoalveolar lavage studies in crocidolite- and chrysotile-exposed individuals. Chest 90:396, 1986.

389. Costabel U, Bross KJ, Huck E, et al: Lung and blood lymphocyte subsets in asbestosis and in mixed dust pneumoconiosis. Chest 91:110, 1987.

390. Gellert AR, Macey MG, Uthayakumar S, et al: Lymphocyte subpopulations in bronchoalveolar lavage fluid in asbestos workers. Am Rev Respir Dis 132:824, 1985.

391. Gellert AR, Lewis CA, Langford JA, et al: Regional distribution of pulmonary epithelial permeability in normal subjects and patients with asbestosis. Thorax 40:734, 1985.

392. Gellert AR, Perry D, Langford JA, et al: Asbestosis. Bronchoalveolar lavage fluid proteins and their relationship to pulmonary epithelial permeability. Chest 88:730, 1985.

393. Bégin R, Cantin A, Drapeau G, et al: Pulmonary uptake of gallium-67 in asbestos-exposed humans and sheep. Am Rev Respir Dis 127:623, 1983.

394. Bégin R, Martel M, Desmarais Y, et al: Fibronectin and procollagen 3 levels in bronchoalveolar lavage of asbestos-exposed human subjects and sheep. Chest 89:237, 1986.

395. Churg AM, Warnock ML: Asbestos and other ferruginous bodies. Their formation and clinical significance. Am J Pathol 102:447, 1981.

396. Churg A, Warnock ML: Analysis of the cores of asbestos bodies from members of the general population: Patients with probable low-degree exposure to asbestos. Am Rev Respir Dis 120:781, 1979.

397. Kobayashi H, Okamura A, Ohnishi Y, et al: Generalized fibrosis associated with pulmonary asbestosis. Acta Pathol Jpn 33:1223, 1983.

398. Warnock ML, Churg AM: Asbestos bodies. Chest 77:129, 1980.

399. Kobayashi H, Ming ZW, Watanabe H, et al: A quantitative study on

12

the distribution of asbestos bodies in extrapulmonary organs. Acta Pathol Jpn 37:375, 1987.

400. Auerbach O, Conston AS, Garfinkel L, et al: Presence of asbestos bodies in organs other than the lung. Chest 77:133, 1980.

401. Roggli VL, Greenberg SD, McLarty JV, et al: Comparison of sputum and lung asbestos body counts in former asbestos workers. Am Rev Respir Dis 122:941, 1980.

402. Greenberg SD, Hurst GA, Christianson SC, et al: Pulmonary cytopathology of former asbestos workers. Am J Clin Pathol 66:815, 1976.

403. Roggli VL, Johnston WW, Kaminsky DB: Asbestos bodies in fine needle aspirates of the lung. Acta Cytol 28:493, 1984.

404. Suzuki Y, Churg J: Structure and development of the asbestos body. Am J Pathol 55:79, 1969.

405. Gross P, deTreville RTP, Cralley LJ, et al: Pulmonary ferruginous bodies. Development in response to filamentous dusts and a method of isolation and concentration. Arch Pathol 85:539, 1968.

406. Crouch E, Churg A: Ferruginous bodies and the histologic evaluation of dust exposure. Am J Surg Pathol 8:109, 1984.

407. Churg A, Warnock ML, Green M: Analysis of the cores of ferruginous (asbestos) bodies from the general population. Lab Invest 40:31, 1979.

408. Sebastien P, Gaudichet A, Bignon J, et al: Zeolite bodies in human lungs from Turkey. Lab Invest 44:420, 1981.

409. Dodson RF, O'Sullivan MF, Corn CJ, et al: Ferruginous body formation on a nonasbestos mineral. Arch Pathol Lab Med 109:849, 1985.

410. Steele RH, Thomson KJ: Asbestos bodies in the lung: Southampton (U.K.) and Wellington (New Zealand). Br J Ind Med 39:349, 1982.

411. Vollmer RT, Roggli VL: Asbestos body concentrations in human lung: Predictions from asbestos body counts in tissue sections with a mathematical model. Hum Pathol 16:713, 1985.

412. Roggli VL, Greenberg SD, Seitzman LW, et al: Pulmonary fibrosis, carcinoma, and ferruginous body counts in amosite asbestos workers. Am J Clin Pathol 73:496, 1980.

413. Roggli VL, Pratt PC: Numbers of asbestos bodies on iron-stained tissue sections in relation to asbestos body counts in lung tissue digests. Hum Pathol 14:355, 1983.

414. Dodson RF, Williams MG Jr, O'Sullivan MF, et al: A comparison of the ferruginous body and uncoated fiber content in the lungs of former asbestos workers. Am Rev Respir Dis 132:143, 1985.

415. Churg A, Warnock M: Asbestos fibers in the general population. Am Rev Respir Dis 122:669, 1980.

416. Case BW, Sebastien P: Environmental and occupational exposures to chrysotile asbestos: A comparative microanalytic study. Arch Environ Health 42:185, 1987.

417. Blesovsky A: The folded lung. Br J Dis Chest 60:19, 1966.

418. Menzies R, Fraser R: Round atelectasis. Pathologic and pathogenetic features. Am J Surg Pathol 11:674, 1987.

419. Dernevik L, Garzinsky P, Hultman E, et al: Shrinking pleuritis with atelectasis. Thorax 37:252, 1982.

420. Doyle TC, Lawler GA: CT features of rounded atelectasis of the lung. AJR 143:225, 1984.

421. Tallroth K, Kiviranta K: Round atelectasis. Respiration 45:71, 1984.

422. Mintzer RA, Gore RM, Vogelzang RL, et al: Rounded atelectasis and its association with asbestos-induced pleural disease. Radiology 139:567, 1981.

423. Hillerdal G, Hemmingsson A: Pulmonary pseudotumours and asbestos. Acta Radiol Diagn 21:615, 1980.

424. Mintzer RA, Cugell DW: The association of asbestos-induced pleural disease and rounded atelectasis. Chest 81:457, 1982.

425. Hurwitz M: Roentgenologic aspects of asbestosis. Am J Roentgenol 85:256, 1961.

426. Freundlich IM, Greening RR: Asbestosis and associated medical problems. Radiology 89:224, 1967.

427. Fletcher DE, Edge JR: The early radiological changes in pulmonary and pleural asbestosis. Clin Radiol 21:355, 1970.

428. Anton HC: Multiple pleural plaques, part II. Br J Radiol 41:341, 1968.

429. Zitting A, Huuskonen MS, Alanko K, et al: Radiographic and physiological findings in patients with asbestosis. Scand J Work Environ Health 4:275, 1978.

430. Sargent EN, Jacobson G, Gordonson JS: Pleural plaques: A signpost of asbestos dust inhalation. Semin Roentgenol 12:287, 1977.

431. Sargent EN, Gordonson J, Jacobson G, et al: Bilateral pleural thickening: A manifestation of asbestos dust exposure. Am J Roentgenol 131:579, 1978.

432. Sprince NL, Oliver LC, McLoud TC: Asbestos-related disease in plumbers and pipefitters employed in building construction. J Occup Med 27:771, 1985.

433. Lawson JP: Pleural calcification as a sign of asbestosis: A report of three cases. Clin Radiol 14:414, 1963.

434. Schneider L, Wimpfheimer F: Multiple progressive calcific pleural plaque formation: A sign of silicatosis. JAMA 189:328, 1964.

435. Oosthuizen SF, Theron CP, Sluis-Cremer GK: Calcified pleural plaques in asbestosis: An investigation into their significance. Med Proc (Johannesburg) 10:496, 1964.

436. MacKenzie FAF: The radiological investigation of the early manifestations of exposure to asbestos dust. Proc R Soc Med 64:834, 1971.

437. Begin R, Boctor M, Bergeron D, et al: Radiographic assessment of pleuropulmonary disease in asbestos workers: Posteroanterior, four view films, and computed tomograms of the thorax. Br J Ind Med 41:373, 1984.

438. Friedman AC, Fiel SB, Fisher MS, et al: Asbestos-related pleural disease and asbestosis: A comparison of CT and chest radiography. AJR 150:269, 1988.

439. Aberle DR, Gamsu G, Ray CS, et al: Asbestos-related pleural and parenchymal fibrosis: Detection with high-resolution CT. Radiology 166:729, 1988.

440. Rockoff SD, Kagan E, Schwartz A, et al: Visceral pleural thickening in asbestos exposure: The occurrence and implications of thickened interlobar fissures. J Thorac Imaging 2:58, 1987.

441. Fisher MS: Asymmetrical changes in asbestos-related disease. J Can Assoc Radiol 36:110, 1985.

442. Sargent EN, Boswell WD Jr, Ralls PW, et al: Subpleural fat pads in patients exposed to asbestos: Distinction from noncalcified pleural plaques. Radiology 152:273, 1984.

443. McLoud TC, Woods BO, Carrington CB, et al: Diffuse pleural thickening in an asbestos-exposed population: Prevalence and causes. AJR 144:9, 1985.

444. Sargent EN, Gordonson T, Jacobson G, et al: Bilateral pleural thickening: A manifestation of asbestos dust exposure. AJR 131:579, 1978.

445. Friedman AC, Fiel SB, Fisher MS, et al: Asbestos-related pleural disease and asbestosis: A comparison of CT and chest radiography. AJR 150:269, 1988.

446. Aberle DR, Gamsu G, Ray CS, et al: Asbestos-related pleural and parenchymal fibrosis: Detection with high-resolution CT. Radiology 166:729, 1988.

447. Rabinowitz JG, Efremidis SC, Cohen B, et al: A comparative study of mesothelioma and asbestosis using computed tomography and conventional chest radiography. Radiology 144:453, 1982.

448. Katz D, Kreel L: Computed tomography in pulmonary asbestosis. Clin Radiol 30:207, 1979.

449. Adams VI, Unni KK, Muhm JR, et al: Diffuse malignant mesothelioma of pleura. Diagnosis and survival in 92 cases. Cancer 58:1540, 1986.

450. Grant DC, Seltzer SE, Antman KH, et al: Computed tomography of malignant pleural mesothelioma. J Comput Assist Tomogr 7:626, 1983.

451. Goldstein B: Two malignant pleural mesotheliomas with unusual histological features. Thorax 34:375, 1979.

452. Nichols DM, Johnson MA: Calcification in a pleural mesothelioma. J Can Assoc Radiol 34:311, 1983.

453. Ashford RFU, Maher J, Drury A, et al: Radiation pneumonitis in a patient exposed to asbestos. Br J Radiol 54:74, 1981.

454. Smith AR: Pleural calcification resulting from exposure to certain dusts. Am J Roentgenol 67:375, 1952.

455. Kleinfeld M: Pleural calcification as a sign of silicatosis. Am J Med Sci 251:215, 1966.

456. Krige L: Asbestosis—with special reference to the radiological diagnosis. S Afr J Radiol 4:13, 1966.

457. Solomon A: Radiology of asbestosis. Environ Res 3:320, 1970.

458. Sargent EN, Jacobson G, Wilkinson EE: Diaphragmatic pleural calcification following short occupational exposure to asbestos. Am J Roentgenol 115:473, 1972.

459. Gaensler EA, Kaplan AI: Asbestos pleural effusion. Ann Intern Med 74:178, 1971.

460. Sluis-Cremer GK, Webster I: Acute pleurisy in asbestos exposed persons. Environ Res 5:380, 1972.

461. Epler GR, McLoud TC, Gaensler EA: Prevalence and incidence of benign asbestos pleural effusion in working population. JAMA 247:617, 1982.

462. Eisenstadt HB: Benign asbestos pleurisy. JAMA 192:419, 1965.

463. Smith KW: Pulmonary disability in asbestos workers. AMA Arch Ind Health 12:198, 1955.

464. Sperber M, Mohan KK: Computed tomography: A reliable diagnostic modality in pulmonary asbestosis. Comput Radiol 8:125, 1984.

465. Wollmer P, Jakobsson K, Albin M, et al: Measurement of lung density by x-ray computed tomography. Relation to lung mechanics in workers exposed to asbestos cement. Chest 91:865, 1987.

466. Yoshimura H, Hatakeyama M, Otsuji H, et al: Pulmonary asbestosis: CT study of subpleural curvillinear shadow. Work in progress. Radiology 158:653, 1986.

467. Hillerdal G: Asbestos exposure and upper lobe involvement. Am J Roentgenol 139:1163, 1982.

468. Solomon A, Goldstein B, Webster I, et al: Massive fibrosis in asbestosis. Environ Res 4:430, 1971.

469. Smyth MDP, Goodman NG, Basu AP, et al: Pulmonary asbestosis. Chest 60:270, 1971.
470. Eisenstadt HB: Asbestos pleurisy. Dis Chest 46:78, 1964.
471. Robinson BWS, Musk AW: Benign asbestos pleural effusion: Diagnosis and course. Thorax 36:896, 1981.
472. Hillerdal G: Non-malignant asbestos pleural disease. Thorax 36:669, 1981.
473. McGavin CR, Sheers G: Diffuse pleural thickening in asbestos workers: Disability and lung function abnormalities. Thorax 39:604, 1984.
474. Britton MG: Asbestos pleural disease. Br J Dis Chest 76:1, 1982.
475. Hilt B, Lien JT, Lund-Larsen PG: Lung function and respiratory symptoms in subjects with asbestos-related disorders: A cross-sectional study. Am J Ind Med 11:517, 1987.
476. Schüler P, Maturana V, Cruz E, et al: Pulmonary asbestosis. Rev Chil Enferm Torax 25:37, 1959.
477. Kleinfeld M, Messite J, Shapiro J: Clinical, radiological, and physiological findings in asbestosis. Arch Intern Med 117:813, 1966.
478. Murphy RLH Jr, Ferris BG Jr, Burgess WA, et al: Effects of low concentrations of asbestos: Clinical, environmental, radiologic and epidemiologic observations in shipyard pipe coverers and controls. N Engl J Med 285:1271, 1971.
479. Mitchell CA, Charney M, Schoenberg JB: Early lung disease in asbestos-product workers. Lung 154:261, 1978.
480. Shirai F, Kudoh S, Shibuya A, et al: Crackles in asbestos workers: Auscultation and lung sound analysis. Br J Dis Chest 75:386, 1981.
481. Begin R, Cantin A, Berthiaume Y, et al: Clinical features to stage alveolitis in asbestos workers. Am J Ind Med 8:521, 1985.
482. Berry G, Gilson JC, Holmes S, et al: Asbestosis: A study of dose-response relationships in an asbestos textile factory. Br J Ind Med 36:98, 1979.
483. Johnson WM, Lemen RA, Hurst GA, et al: Respiratory morbidity among workers in an amosite asbestos insulation plant. J Occup Med 24:994, 1982.
484. Huuskonen MS: Clinical features, mortality and survival of patients with asbestosis. Scand J Work Environ Health 4:265, 1978.
485. Picado C, Roisin RR, Sala H, et al: Diagnosis of asbestosis: Clinical, radiological and lung function data in 42 patients. Lung 162:325, 1984.
486. Coutts II, Gilson JC, Kerr IH, et al: Significance of finger clubbing in asbestosis. Thorax 42:117, 1987.
487. Barnhart S, Hudson LD, Mason SE, et al: Total lung capacity. An insensitive measure of impairment in patients with asbestosis and chronic obstructive pulmonary disease? Chest 93:299, 1988.
488. Bader ME, Bader RA, Selikoff IJ: Pulmonary function in asbestosis of the lung. An alveolar-capillary block syndrome. Am J Med 30:235, 1961.
489. Leathart GL: Clinical, bronchographic, radiological and physiological observations in ten cases of asbestosis. Br J Ind Med 17:213, 1960.
490. Wang ML, Lu PL: Lung function studies of asbestos workers. Scand J Work Environ Health 11(Suppl 4):34, 1985.
491. Divertie MB, Cassan SM, Brown AL Jr: Ultrastructural morphometry of the diffusion surface in a case of pulmonary asbestosis. Mayo Clin Proc 50:193, 1975.
492. Cookson WO, Musk AW, Glancy JJ: Asbestosis and cryptogenic fibrosing alveolitis: A radiological and functional comparison. Aust NZ J Med 14:626, 1984.
493. Wright PH, Hanson A, Kreel L, et al: Respiratory function changes after asbestos pleurisy. Thorax 35:31, 1980.
494. Cookson WO, Musk AW, Glancy JJ: Pleural thickening and gas transfer in asbestosis. Thorax 38:657, 1983.
495. Fournier-Massey G, Becklake MR: Pulmonary function profiles in Quebec asbestos workers. Bull Physiopathol Respir (Nancy) 11:429, 1975.
496. Agostoni P, Smith DD, Schoene RB, et al: Evaluation of breathlessness in asbestos workers: Results of exercise testing. Am Rev Respir Dis 135:812, 1987.
497. Selikoff IJ, Hammond EC, Churg J: Asbestos exposure, smoking, and neoplasia. JAMA 204:106, 1968.
498. Jodoin G, Gibbs GW, Macklem PT, et al: Early effects of asbestos exposure on lung function. Am Rev Respir Dis 104:525, 1971.
499. Becklake MR: Asbestos-related diseases of the lungs and pleura: Current clinical issues. Am Rev Respir Dis 126:187, 1982.
500. Stoeckle JD, Oliver LC, Hardy HL: Women with asbestosis in a medical clinic: Under reported women workers, delayed diagnosis and smoking. Women Health 7:31, 1982.
501. Oldham PD: Pneumoconiosis in Cornish china clay workers. Br J Ind Med 40:131, 1983.
502. Lerman Y, Ribak J, Selikoff IJ: Hazards of lung biopsy in asbestos workers. Br J Ind Med 43:165, 1986.
503. Payne CR, Jaques P, Kerr IH: Lung folding simulating peripheral pulmonary neoplasm (Blesovsky's syndrome). Thorax 35:936, 1980.
504. Inoshita T, Boyd WJ: Rounded atelectasis shown by computerized tomography. South Med J 79:764, 1986.
505. Segarra-Obiol F, Lopez-Ibanez P, Perez NJ: Asbestosis and tuberculosis. Am J Ind Med 4:755, 1983.
506. Armstrong BK, de Klerk NH, Musk AW, et al: Mortality in miners and millers of crocidolite in Western Australia. Br J Ind Med 45:5, 1988.
507. Williams R, Hugh-Jones P: The radiological diagnosis of asbestosis. Thorax 15:103, 1960.
508. Rossiter CE, Bristol LJ, Cartier PH, et al: Radiographic changes in chrysotile asbestos mine and mill workers of Quebec. Arch Environ Health 24:388, 1972.
509. McDonald JC: Asbestos and lung cancer: Has the case been proven? Chest 78(Suppl):374, 1980.
510. McDonald JC: Asbestos and lung cancer: Has the case been proven? Chest 78(Suppl):374, 1980.
511. Sluis-Cremer GK: The relationship between asbestosis and bronchial cancer. Chest 78(Suppl):380, 1980.
512. Selikoff IJ, Bader RA, Bader ME, et al: Asbestosis and neoplasia. Am J Med 42:487, 1967.
513. Weill H, Hughes J, Waggenspack C: Influence of dose and fiber type on respiratory malignancy risk in asbestos cement manufacturing. Am Rev Respir Dis 120:345, 1979.
514. Stovin PGI, Partridge P: Pulmonary asbestos and dust content in East Africa. Thorax 37:185, 1982.
515. Baba K: Indications of an increase of occupational pleural mesothelioma in Japan. Sangyo Ika Daigaku Zasshi 5:3, 1983.
516. McDonald AD, Fry JS, Woolley AJ, et al: Dust exposure and mortality in an American chrysotile textile plant. Br J Ind Med 40:361, 1983.
517. Wagner JC, Moncrieff CB, Coles R, et al: Correlation between fibre content of the lungs and disease in naval stockyard workers. Br J Ind Med 43:391, 1986.
518. Hughes JM, Weill H, Hammad YY: Mortality of workers employed in two asbestos cement manufacturing plants. Br J Ind Med 44:161, 1987.
519. Law MR, Ward FG, Hodson ME, et al: Evidence for longer survival of patients with pleural mesothelioma without asbestos exposure. Thorax 38:744, 1983.
520. Leading article: Asbestos pollution and pleural plaques. Med J Austral 1:444, 1981.
521. Selikoff IJ, Hammond EC: Asbestos and smoking (editorial). JAMA 242:458, 1979.
522. Berry G: Mortality of workers certified by pneumoconiosis medical panels as having asbestosis. Br J Ind Med 38:130, 1981.
523. Warnock M, Isenberg W: Asbestos burden and the pathology of lung cancer. Chest 89:20, 1986.
524. Kannerstein M, Churg J: Pathology of carcinoma of the lung associated with asbestos exposure. Cancer 30:14, 1972.
525. Wagner JC, Berry G, Pooley FD: Mesotheliomas and asbestos type in asbestos textile workers: A study of lung contents. Br Med J 285:603, 1982.
526. Baris YI, Sahin AA, Ozesmi M, et al: An outbreak of pleural mesothelioma and chronic fibrosing pleurisy in the village of Karain/Urgup in Anatolia. Thorax 33:181, 1978.
527. Auerbach O, Garfinkel L, Parks VR, et al: Histologic type of lung cancer and asbestos exposure. Cancer 54:3017, 1984.
528. Wagner JC: Current opinions on the asbestos cancer problem. Ann Occup Hyg 15:61, 1972.
529. Webster I: Malignancy in relation to crocidolite and amosite: Biological effects of asbestos. Lyon, IARC Scientific Publications, No. 8, 1973, p 195.
530. Asbestosis and malignant disease (Editorial). N Engl J Med 72:590, 1965.
531. Dement JM, Harris RL Jr, Symons MJ, et al: Exposures and mortality among chrysotile workers. Part II: Mortality. Am J Ind Med 4:421, 1983.
532. Elmes PC, Wade OL: Relationship between exposure to asbestos and pleural malignancy in Belfast. Ann NY Acad Sci 132:549, 1965.
533. Selikoff IJ, Hammond EC, Churg J: Mortality experiences of asbestos insulation workers: 1943–1968. In Shapiro HA (ed): International Conference on Pneumoconiosis, Johannesburg, 1969. London, Oxford University Press, 1970, p 180.
534. McDonald AD, Harper A, El-Attar OA, et al: Epidemiology of primary malignant mesothelial tumors in Canada. Cancer 26:914, 1970.
535. Churg A, Warnock ML, Bensch KG: Malignant mesothelioma arising after direct application of asbestos and fiber glass to the pericardium. Am Rev Respir Dis 118:419, 1978.
536. McConnochie K, Simonato L, Mavrides P, et al: Mesothelioma in Cyprus: The role of tremolite. Thorax 42:342, 1987.
537. Acheson ED, Bennett C, Gardner MJ, et al: Mesothelioma in a factory using amosite and chrysotile asbestos. Lancet 2:1403, 1981.
538. Thomas HF, Benjamin IT, Elwood PC, et al: Further follow-up study of workers from an asbestos cement factory. Br J Ind Med 39:273, 1982.

12

539. Glyseth B, Mowe G, Wannag A: Fibre type and concentration in the lungs of workers in an asbestos cement factory. Br J Ind Med 40:375, 1983.
540. Meurman LO, Kiviluoto R, Hakama M: Mortality and morbidity among the working population of anthophyllite asbestos miners in Finland. Br J Ind Med 31:105, 1974.
541. Armstrong BK, Musk AW, Baker JE, et al: Epidemiology of malignant mesothelioma in western Australia. Med J Aust 141:86, 1984.
542. Borow M, Couston A, Livornese L, et al: Mesothelioma following exposure to asbestos. A review of 72 cases. Chest 64:641, 1973.
543. Teta MJ, Lewinsohn HC, Meigs JW, et al: Mesothelioma in Connecticut, 1955–1977. Occupational and geographical associations. J Occup Med 25:749, 1983.
544. Solomons K: Malignant mesothelioma: Clinical and epidemiological features. A report of 80 cases. S Afr Med J 66:407, 1984.
545. Edge JR, Choudhury SL: Malignant mesothelioma of the pleura in Barrow-in-Furness. Thorax 33:26, 1978.
546. Martensson G, Larsson S, Zettergren L: Malignant mesothelioma in two pairs of siblings: Is there a hereditary predisposing factor? Eur J Respir Dis 65:179, 1984.
547. Hasan FM, Nash G, Kazemi H: The significance of asbestos exposure in the diagnosis of mesothelioma: A 28-year experience from a major urban hospital. Am Rev Respir Dis 115:761, 1977.
548. Antman KH, Corson JM, Li FP, et al: Malignant mesothelioma following radiation exposure. J Clin Oncol 1:695, 1983.
549. Antman KH, Ruxer RL Jr, Aisner J, et al: Mesothelioma following Wilms' tumor in childhood. Cancer 54:367, 1984.
550. Austin MB, Fechner RE, Roggli VL: Pleural malignant mesothelioma following Wilms' tumor. Am J Clin Pathol 86:227, 1986.
551. Berry G, Newhouse ML, Antonis P: Combined effect of asbestos and smoking on mortality from lung cancer and mesothelioma in factory workers. Br J Ind Med 42:12, 1985.
552. Gracey DR, Cugell DW, Bazley ES, et al: Pulmonary complications of asbestos exposure. Chest 59:77, 1971.
553. Finkelstein MM: Asbestosis in long-term employees of an Ontario asbestos-cement factory. Am Rev Respir Dis 125:496, 1982.
554. Jefferys DB, Vale JA: Malignant mesothelioma and gas-mask assemblers. Br Med J 2:607, 1978.
555. Scansetti G, Mollo F, Tiberi G, et al: Pleural mesothelioma after a short interval from first exposure in the wine filter industry. Am J Ind Med 5:335, 1984.
556. Hourihane DO: The pathology of mesotheliomata and an analysis of their association with asbestos exposure. Thorax 19:268, 1964.
557. Enticknap JB, Smither WJ: Peritoneal tumours in asbestosis. Br J Ind Med 21:20, 1964.
558. Selikoff IJ, Churg J, Hammond EC: Asbestos exposure and neoplasia. JAMA 188:22, 1964.
559. Snell PM, McGill P: Asbestos and laryngeal carcinoma. Lancet 2:416, 1973.
560. Newhouse ML, Berry G: Asbestos and laryngeal carcinoma. Lancet 2:615, 1973.
561. Libshitz HI, Wershba MS, Atkinson GW, et al: Asbestosis and carcinoma of the larynx. A possible association. JAMA 228:1571, 1974.
562. Gerber MA: Asbestosis and neoplastic disorders of the hematopoietic system. Am J Clin Pathol 53:204, 1970.
563. Hildick-Smith GY: The biology of talc. Br J Ind Med 33:217, 1976.
564. Messite J, Reddin G, Kleinfeld M: Pulmonary talcosis, a clinical and environmental study. AMA Arch Ind Health 20:408, 1959.
565. Wegman DH, Peters JM, Boundy MG, et al: Evaluation of respiratory effects in miners and millers exposed to talc free of asbestos and silica. Br J Ind Med 39:233, 1982.
566. Gamble JF, Fellner W, Dimeo MJ: An epidemiologic study of a group of talc workers. Am Rev Respir Dis 119:741, 1979.
567. Ahlmark A, Bruce T, Nyström Å: Pneumoconiosis (talcosis) in soapstone workers. Nord Med 59:287, 1958.
568. Berner A, Gylseth B, Levy F: Talc dust pneumoconiosis. Acta Pathol Microbiol Scand (A) 89:17, 1981.
569. Millman N: Pneumoconiosis due to talc in the cosmetic industry. Occup Med 4:391, 1947.
570. Moskowitz RL: Talc pneumoconiosis: A treated case. Chest 58:37, 1970.
571. Nam K, Gracey DR: Pulmonary talcosis from cosmetic talcum powder. JAMA 221:492, 1972.
572. Wells IP, Dubbins PA, Whimster WF: Pulmonary disease caused by the inhalation of cosmetic talcum powder. Br J Radiol 52:586, 1979.
573. Wells IP, Dubbins PA, Whimster WF: Pulmonary disease caused by the inhalation of cosmetic talcum powder. Br J Radiol 52:586, 1979.
574. Leading article: Accidental inhalation of talcum powder. Br Med J 4:5, 1969.
575. Gould SR, Barnardo DE: Respiratory distress after talc inhalation. Br J Dis Chest 66:230, 1970.
576. Bouchàma A, Chastre J, Gaudichet A, et al: Acute pneumonitis with bilateral pleural effusion after talc pleurodesis. Chest 86:795, 1984.
577. de Vuyst P, Dumortier P, Leophonte P, et al: Mineralogical analysis of bronchoalveolar lavage in talc pneumoconiosis. Eur J Respir Dis 70:150, 1987.
578. Vallyathan NV, Craighead JE: Pulmonary pathology in workers exposed to nonasbestiform talc. Hum Pathol 12:28, 1981.
579. Vallyathan NV, Green FHY, Craighead JE: Recent advances in the study of mineral pneumoconiosis. In Sommers SC, Rosen PP (eds): Pathology Annual, part II. New York, Appleton-Century-Crofts, 1980, p 15.
580. Lapenas DJ, Davis GS, Gale PN, et al: Mineral dusts as etiologic agents in pulmonary fibrosis: The diagnostic role of analytical scanning electron microscopy. Am J Clin Pathol 78:701, 1982.
581. Siegal W, Smith AR, Greenburg L: The dust inhaled in tremolite talc mining, including roentgenological findings in talc workers. Am J Roentgenol 49:11, 1943.
582. Kleinfeld M, Messite J, Tabershaw IR: Talc pneumoconiosis. AMA Arch Ind Health 12:66, 1955.
583. Gamble J, Greife A, Hancock J: An epidemiological-industrial hygiene study of talc workers. Ann Occup Hyg 26:841, 1982.
584. Seeler AO, Gryboski JS, MacMahon HE: Talc pneumoconiosis. AMA Arch Ind Health 19:392, 1959.
585. Porro FW, Patton JR, Hobbs AA Jr: Pneumoconiosis in the talc industry. Am J Roentgenol 47:507, 1942.
586. Alivisatos GP, Pontikakis AE, Terzis B: Talcosis of unusually rapid development. Br J Ind Med 12:43, 1955.
587. Kleinfeld M, Messite J, Shapiro J, et al: Effect of talc dust inhalation on lung function. Arch Environ Health 10:431, 1965.
588. Tukiainen P, Nickels J, Taskinen E, et al: Pulmonary granulomatous reaction: Talc pneumoconiosis or chronic sarcoidosis? Br J Ind Med 41:84, 1984.
589. Kleinfeld M, Messite J, Kooyman O, et al: Mortality among talc miners and millers in New York State. Arch Environ Health 14:663, 1967.
590. Kleinfeld M, Messite J, Shapiro J, et al: Effect of talc dust inhalation on lung function. Arch Environ Health 10:431, 1965.
591. Kleinfeld M, Messite J, Shapiro J, et al: Lung function in talc workers, a comparative physiologic study of workers exposed to fibrous and granular talc dust. Arch Environ Health 9:559, 1964.
592. Lockey JE, Brooks SM, Jarabek AM, et al: Pulmonary changes after exposure to vermiculite contaminated with fibrous tremolite. Am Rev Respir Dis 129:952, 1984.
593. Davies D, Cotton R: Mica pneumoconiosis. Br J Ind Med 40:22, 1983.
594. Dreesen WC, Dallavalle JM, Edwards TI, et al: Pneumoconiosis among mica and pegmatite workers. Public Health Bulletin No. 250, Washington, US Public Health Service, 1940, pp 1–74.
595. Vorwald AJ, MacEwen JD, Smith RG: Mineral content of lung in certain pneumoconioses. Arch Pathol 74:267, 1962.
596. Pimentel JC, Menezes AP: Pulmonary and hepatic granulomatous disorders due to the inhalation of cement and mica dusts. Thorax 33:219, 1978.
597. Skulberg KR, Gylseth B, Skaug V, et al: Mica pneumoconiosis: A literature review. Scand J Work Environ Health 11:65, 1985.
598. Campbell AH, Gloyne SR: A case of pneumoconiosis due to the inhalation of Fuller's earth. J Pathol Bacteriol 54:75, 1942.
599. Sakula A: Pneumoconiosis due to Fuller's earth. Thorax 16:176, 1961.
600. McNally WD, Trostler IS: Severe pneumoconiosis caused by inhalation of Fuller's earth. J Ind Hyg 23:118, 1941.
601. Sepulveda M-J, Vallyathan V, Attfield MO, et al: Pneumoconiosis and lung function in a group of kaolin workers. Am Rev Respir Dis 127:231, 1983.
602. Lapenas D, Gale P, Kennedy T, et al: Kaolin pneumoconiosis. Radiologic, pathologic, and mineralogic findings. Am Rev Respir Dis 130:282, 1984.
603. Lesser M, Zia M, Kilburn KH: Silicosis in kaolin workers and firebrick makers. South Med J 71:1242, 1978.
604. Altekruse EB, Chaudhary BA, Pearson MG, et al: Kaolin dust concentrations and pneumoconiosis at a kaolin mine. Thorax 39:436, 1984.
605. Lapenas DJ, Gale PN: Kaolin pneumoconiosis. A case report. Arch Pathol Lab Med 107:650, 1983.
606. Wagner JC, Pooley FD, Gibbs A, et al: Inhalation of china stone and china clay dusts: Relationship between the mineralogy of dust retained in the lungs and pathological changes. Thorax 41:190, 1986.
607. Edenfield RW: A clinical and roentgenological study of kaolin workers. Arch Environ Health 1:392, 1960.
608. Sheers G: Prevalence of pneumoconiosis in Cornish kaolin workers. Br J Ind Med 21:218, 1964.
609. Kennedy T, Rawlings W Jr, Baser M, et al: Pneumoconiosis in Georgia kaolin workers. Am Rev Respir Dis 127:215, 1983.
610. Hale LW: Pneumoconiosis in Cornwall. In King EJ, Fletcher CM (eds): Industrial Pulmonary Diseases: A Symposium held at the

Postgraduate Medical School of London, 18–20 September 1957 and 25–27 March 1958. London, J & A Churchill, 1960 pp 139–145.

611. Bristol LJ: Pneumoconioses caused by asbestos and by other siliceous and nonsiliceous dusts. Semin Roentgenol 2:283, 1967.

612. Hale LW, Gough J, King EJ, et al: Pneumoconiosis of kaolin workers. Br J Ind Med 13:251, 1956.

613. Herman SJ, Olscamp GC, Weisbrod GL: Pulmonary kaolin granulomas. J Can Assoc Radiol 33:279, 1982.

614. Barrie HJ, Gosselin L: Massive pneumoconiosis from a rock dust containing no free silica. Nepheline lung. Arch Environ Health 1:109, 1960.

615. Olscamp G, Herman SJ, Weisbrod GL: Nepheline rock dust pneumoconiosis. A report of 2 cases. Radiology 142:29, 1982.

616. Baris YI, Artvinli M, Sahin AA, et al: Diffuse lung fibrosis due to fibrous zeolite (erionite) exposure. Eur J Respir Dis 70:122, 1987.

617. Casey KR, Shigeoka JW, Rom WM, et al: Zeolite exposure and associated pneumoconiosis. Chest 87:837, 1985.

618. Baris YI, Sahin AA, Ozesmi M, et al: An outbreak of pleural mesothelioma and chronic fibrosing pleurisy in the village of Karain/Ürgüp in Anatolia. Thorax 33:181, 1978.

619. Baris YI, Saracci R, Simonato L, et al: Malignant mesothelioma and radiological chest abnormalities in two villages in Central Turkey. Lancet 1:984, 1981.

620. Artvinli M, Baris YI: Environmental fiber-induced pleuro-pulmonary diseases in an Anatolian village: An epidemiologic study. Arch Environ Health 37:177, 1982.

621. Attfield MD, Ross DS: Radiological abnormalities in electric-arc welders. Br J Ind Med 35:117, 1978.

622. Morgan WKC: Magnetite pneumoconiosis. J Occup Med 20:762, 1978.

623. Harding HE, McLaughlin AIG, Doig AT: Clinical, radiographic, and pathological studies of the lungs of electric-arc and oxacetylene welders. Lancet 2:394, 1958.

624. Stacy BD, King FJ, Harrison CV, et al: Tissue changes in rats' lungs caused by hydroxides, oxides and phosphates of aluminium and iron. J Pathol Bacteriol 77:417, 1959.

625. Harding HE, Grout JLA, Davies TAL: The experimental production of x-ray shadows in the lungs by inhalation of industrial dusts: I. Iron oxide. Br J Ind Med 4:223, 1947.

626. McLaughlin AIG: Iron and other radiopaque dusts. In King EJ, Fletcher CM (eds): Industrial Pulmonary Diseases: A Symposium held at the Postgraduate Medical School of London, 18–20 September 1957 and 25–27 March 1958, London, J & A Churchill, 1960, pp 146–167.

627. Hunnicutt TN Jr, Cracovaner DJ, Myles JT: Spirometric measurements in welders. Arch Environ Health 8:661, 1964.

628. Friede E, Rachow DO: Symptomatic pulmonary disease in arc welders. Ann Intern Med 54:121, 1961.

629. Enzer N, Sander OA: Chronic lung changes in electric arc welders. J Ind Hyg 20:333, 1938.

630. Harding HE, McLaughlin AIG, Doig AT: Clinical, radiographic and pathological studies of the lungs of electric arc and oxyacetylene welders. Lancet 2:394, 1958.

631. Angervall L, Hansson G, Rockert H: Pulmonary siderosis in electrical welders: A note on pathological appearance. Acta Pathol Microbiol Scand 49:373, 1960.

632. Johnson NF, Haslam PL, Dewar A, et al: Identification of inorganic dust particles in bronchoalveolar lavage macrophages by energy dispersive x-ray microanalysis. Arch Environ Health 41:133, 1986.

633. Guidotti TL, Abraham JL, DeNee PB, et al: Arc Welders' pneumoconiosis: Application of advanced scanning electron microscopy. Arch Environ Health 33:117, 1978.

634. Funahashi A, Schlueter DP, Pintar K, et al: Welders' pneumoconiosis: Tissue elemental microanalysis by energy dispersive x-ray analysis. Br J Ind Med 45:14, 1988.

635. Plamenac P, Nikulin A, Pikula B: Cytologic changes of the respiratory epithelium in iron foundry workers. Acta Cytol 18:34, 1974.

636. McLaughlin AIG, Grout JLA, Barrie HJ, et al: Iron oxide dust and the lungs of silver finishers. Lancet 1:337, 1945.

637. Sander OA: The nonfibrogenic (benign) pneumoconioses. Semin Roentgenol 2:312, 1967.

638. Antti-Poika M, Hassi J, Pyy L: Respiratory diseases in arc welders. Int Arch Occup Environ Health 40:225, 1977.

639. Low I, Mitchell C: Respiratory disease in foundry workers. Br J Ind Med 42:101, 1985.

640. Faulds JS: Haematite pneumoconiosis in Cumberland miners. J Clin Pathol 10:187, 1957.

641. McLaughlin AIG, Harding HE: The causes of death in iron and steel workers (non-foundry). Br J Ind Med 18:33, 1961.

642. Mun JM, Meyer-Bisch C, Pham QT, et al: Risk of lung cancer among iron ore miners: A proportional mortality study of 1,075 deceased miners in Lorraine, France. J Occup Med 29:762, 1987.

643. Smith GH, Williams FL, Lloyd OL: Respiratory cancer and air pollution from iron foundries in a Scottish town: An epidemiological and environmental study. Br J Ind Med 44:795, 1987.

644. Barrie HJ, Harding HE: Argyro-siderosis of the lungs in silver finishers. Br J Ind Med 4:225, 1947.

645. Robertson AJ, Whitaker PH: Radiological changes in pneumoconiosis due to tin oxide. J Fac Radiol 6:224, 1955.

646. Robertson AJ, Rivers D, Nagelschmidt G, et al: Benign pneumoconiosis due to tin dioxide. Lancet 1:1089, 1961.

647. Robertson AJ: Pneumoconiosis due to tin oxide. In King EJ, Fletcher CM (eds): Industrial Pulmonary Diseases: A Symposium held at the Postgraduate Medical School of London, September 18–20, 1957, and March 25–27, 1958. London, J & A Churchill, 1960, pp 168–184.

648. Arrigoni A: La pneumoconiosi da bario. Clin Med Ital 64:299, 1933.

649. Huppertz A: Barytlunge. (Baritosis.) Fortschr Röntgenstr 89:146, 1958.

650. Lévi-Valensi P, Drif M, Dat A, et al: A propos de 57 observations de barytose pulmonaire. Résultats d'une enquête systématique dans une usine de baryte. (Observations on 57 cases of barium sulfate pneumoconiosis: Results of a systematic investigation in a barium sulfate mill.) J Fr Med Chir Thorac 20:443, 1966.

651. Pendergrass EP, Greening RR: Baritosis. Report of a case. AMA Arch Ind Hyg 7:44, 1953.

652. Doig AT: Baritosis: A benign pneumoconiosis. Thorax 31:30, 1976.

653. McCallum RI: Detection of antimony in process workers' lungs by X-radiation. Trans Soc Occup Med 17:134, 1967.

654. Potkonjak V, Pavlovich M: Antimoniosis: A particular form of pneumoconiosis. I. Etiology, clinical and X-ray findings. Int Arch Occup Environ Health 51:199, 1983.

655. Cooper DA, Pendergrass EP, Vorwald AJ, et al: Pneumoconiosis among workers in an antimony industry. Am J Roentgenol 103:495, 1968.

656. Hoschek R: Röntgenologische lungenveränderungen durch seltene erden. Vorläufige mitteilung (Roentgenologic lung changes by rare earth elements. Preliminary communication.) Zentralbl Arbeitsmed 14:981, 1964.

657. Cain H, Egner E, Ruska J: Ablagerungen seltener erden in der menschlichen lunge und in tierexperiment. (Deposits of rare earth metals in the lungs of man, and in experimental animals). Virchows Arch 374:249, 1977.

658. Vocaturo G, Colombo F, Zanoni M, et al: Human exposure to heavy metals. Rare earth pneumoconiosis in occupational workers. Chest 83:780, 1983.

659. Sulotto F, Romano C, Berra A, et al: Rare-earth pneumoconiosis: A new case. Am J Ind Med 9:567, 1986.

660. Heuck F, Hoschek R: Cer-pneumoconiosis. Am J Roentgenol 104:777, 1968.

661. Hardy HL: Beryllium disease: A continuing diagnostic problem. Am J Med Sci 242:150, 1961.

662. American College of Chest Physicians Report of the Section on Nature and Prevalence Committee on Occupational Diseases of the Chest: Beryllium disease. Dis Chest 48:550, 1965.

663. Hardy H: Beryllium case registry progress report: 1962. Arch Environ Health 5:265, 1962.

664. Hasan FM, Kazemi H: Chronic beryllium disease: A continuing epidemiologic hazard. Chest 65:289, 1974.

665. Hasan FM, Kazemi H: Progress report, U.S. beryllium case registry, 1972. Am Rev Respir Dis 108:1252, 1973.

666. Beryllium disease among workers in a spacecraft-manufacturing plant—California. MMWR 32:419, 425, 1983.

667. Cullen MR, Kominsky JR, Rossman MD, et al: Chronic beryllium disease in a precious metal refinery. Clinical, epidemiologic, and immunologic evidence for continuing risk from exposure to low level beryllium fume. Am Rev Respir Dis 135:201, 1987.

668. Kanarek DJ, Wainer RA, Chamberlin RI, et al: Respiratory illness in a population exposed to beryllium. Am Rev Respir Dis 108:1295, 1973.

669. Constantinidis K: Acute and chronic beryllium disease. Br J Clin Pract 32:127, 1978.

670. Hazard JB: Pathologic changes of beryllium disease. The acute disease. AMA Arch Ind Health 19:179, 1959.

671. Frieman DG, Hardy HL: Beryllium disease. Hum Pathol 1:25, 1970.

672. DeNardi JM, Van Ordstrand HS, Curtis GH: Berylliosis. Summary and survey of all clinical types in ten year period. Cleve Clin Q 19:171, 1952.

673. Momose T, Koike S, Sakamoto A, et al: Impaired pulmonary function in acute beryllium poisoning. Nihon Rinsho 17:1229, 1959.

674. Shima M, Ohta K: Three cases of acute pneumonitis due to beryllium inhalation. Jpn J Chest Dis (Nippon Kyobu Rinsho), 19:707, 1960.

675. Hardy HL, Tabershaw IR: Delayed chemical pneumonitis occurring in workers exposed to beryllium compounds. J Ind Hyg Toxicol 28:197, 1946.

676. Deodhar SD, Barna B, Van Ordstrand HS: A study of the immunologic aspects of chronic berylliosis. Chest 63:309, 1973.

677. Hanifin JM, Epstein WI, Cline MJ: *In vitro* studies of granulomatous hypersensitivity to beryllium. J Invest Dermatol 55:284, 1970.
678. Henderson WR, Fukuyama K, Epstein WL, et al: *In vitro* demonstration of delayed hypersensitivity in patients with berylliosis. J Invest Dermatol 58:5, 1972.
679. Daniele RP: Cell-mediated immunity in pulmonary disease. Hum Pathol 17:154, 1986.
680. Williams WJ, Williams WR: Value of beryllium lymphocyte transformation tests in chronic beryllium disease and in potentially exposed workers. Thorax 38:41, 1983.
681. Aronchick JM, Rossman MD, Miller WT: Chronic beryllium disease: Diagnosis, radiographic findings, and correlation with pulmonary function tests. Radiology 163:677, 1987.
682. Rossman MD, Kern JA, Elias JA, et al: Proliferative response of bronchoalveolar lymphocytes to beryllium: A test for chronic beryllium disease. Ann Intern Med 108:687, 1988.
683. Prine JR, Brokeshoulder SF, McVean DE, et al: Demonstration of the presence of beryllium in pulmonary granulomas. Am J Clin Pathol 45:448, 1966.
684. Williams WJ, Kelland D: New aid for diagnosing chronic beryllium disease (CBD): Laser ion mass analysis (LIMA). J Clin Pathol 39:900, 1986.
685. Sprince ML, Kazemi H, Hardy HL: Current (1975) problem of differentiating between beryllium disease and sarcoidosis. Ann NY Acad Sci 278:654, 1976.
686. Gary JE, Schatzki R: Radiological abnormalities in chronic pulmonary disease due to beryllium. AMA Arch Ind Health 19:117, 1959.
687. Tebrock HE: Beryllium poisoning (berylliosis). X-ray manifestations and advances in treatment. Am J Surg 90:120, 1955.
688. Weber AL, Stoeckle JD, Hardy HL: Roentgenologic patterns in long-standing beryllium disease. Report of 8 cases. Am J Roentgenol 93:879, 1965.
689. Aronchick JM, Rossman MD, Miller WT: Chronic beryllium disease: Diagnosis, radiographic findings, and correlation with pulmonary function tests. Radiology 163:677, 1987.
690. Cotes JE, Gilson JC, McKerrow CB, et al: A long-term follow-up of workers exposed to beryllium. Br J Ind Med 40:13, 1983.
691. Hall TC, Wood CH, Stoeckle JD, et al: Case data from the beryllium registry. AMA Arch Ind Health 19:100, 1959.
692. Stockle JD, Hardy HL, Webber AL: Chronic beryllium disease: Long-term follow-up of sixty cases and selective review of the literature. Am J Med 46:545, 1969.
693. Resnick H, Roche M, Morgan WKC: Immunoglobulin concentrations in berylliosis. Am Rev Respir Dis 101:504, 1970.
694. Zimmer JG, Demis DJ: Associations between gout, psoriasis and sarcoidosis. Ann Intern Med 64:786, 1966.
695. Kelley WN, Goldfinger SE, Hardy HL: Hyperuricemia in chronic beryllium disease. Ann Intern Med 70:977, 1969.
696. Sprince NL, Kanarek DJ, Weber AL, et al: Reversible respiratory disease in beryllium workers. Am Rev Respir Dis 117:1011, 1978.
697. Gaensler EA, Verstraeten JM, Weil WB, et al: Respiratory pathophysiology in chronic beryllium disease. Review of thirty cases with some observations after long-term steroid therapy. AMA Arch Ind Health 19:32, 1959.
698. Andrews JI, Kazemi H, Hardy HL: Patterns of lung dysfunction in chronic beryllium disease. Am Rev Respir Dis 100:791, 1969.
699. Norris GF, Peard MC: Berylliosis: Report of two cases, with special reference to the patch test. Br Med J 1:378, 1963.
700. Curtis GH: The diagnosis of beryllium disease, with special reference to the patch tests. AMA Arch Ind Health 19:150, 1959.
701. Shaver CG, Riddell AR: Lung changes associated with the manufacture of alumina abrasives. J Ind Hyg Toxicol 29:145, 1947.
702. Bellot SM, Schade van Westrum JAFM, Wagenvoort CA, et al: Deposition of bauxite dust and pulmonary fibrosis. Pathol Res Pract 179:225, 1984.
703. Mitchell J: Pulmonary fibrosis in an aluminum worker. Br J Ind Med 16:123, 1959.
704. Mitchell J, Manning GB, Molyneux M, et al: Pulmonary fibrosis in workers exposed to finely powdered aluminum. Br J Ind Med 18:10, 1961.
705. Edling NPG: Aluminum pneumoconiosis. A roentgendiagnostic study of five cases. Acta Radiol 56:170, 1961.
706. McLaughlin AIG, Kazantzis G, King E, et al: Pulmonary fibrosis and encephalopathy associated with the inhalation of aluminum dust. Br J Ind Med 19:253, 1962.
707. De Vuyst P, DuMortier P, Schandene L, et al: Sarcoidlike lung granulomatosis induced by aluminum dusts. Am Rev Respir Dis 135:493, 1987.
708. Herbert A, Sterling G, Abraham J, et al: Desquamative interstitial pneumonia in an aluminum welder. Hum Pathol 13:694, 1982.
709. Vallyathan V, Bergeron WN, Robichaux PA, et al: Pulmonary fibrosis in an aluminum arc welder. Chest 81:372, 1982.
710. Chen W, Monnat RJ Jr, Chen M, et al: Aluminum induced pulmonary granulomatosis. Hum Pathol 9:705, 1978.
711. Miller R: Pulmonary alveolar proteinosis and aluminum dust exposure. Am Rev Respir Dis 130:312, 1984.
712. Denny JJ, Robson WD, Irwin DA: The prevention of silicosis by metallic aluminum. I. A preliminary report. Can Med Assoc J 37:1, 1937.
713. Campbell IK, Cass JS, Cholak J, et al: Aluminum in the environment of man. A review of its hygienic status. AMA Arch Ind Health 15:359, 1957.
714. Wyatt JP, Riddell ACR: The morphology of bauxite-fume pneumoconiosis. Am J Pathol 25:447, 1949.
715. Gilks R, Churg A: Aluminum-induced pulmonary fibrosis: Do fibers play a role? Am Rev Respir Dis 136:176, 1987.
716. Chan-Yeung M, Wong R, MacLean L, et al: Epidemiologic health study of workers in an aluminum smelter in British Columbia. Effects on the respiratory system. Am Rev Respir Dis 127:465, 1983.
717. Nilsen AM, Mylius EA, Gullvag BM: Alveolar macrophages from expectorates as indicators of pulmonary irritation in primary aluminum reduction plant workers. Am J Ind Med 12:101, 1987.
718. Davison AG, Haslam PL, Corrin B, et al: Interstitial lung disease and asthma in hard-metal workers: Bronchoalveolar lavage, ultrastructural, and analytical findings and results of bronchial provocation tests. Thorax 38:119, 1983.
719. Rizzato G, Lo Cicero S, Barberis M, et al: Trace of metal exposure in hard metal lung disease. Chest 90:101, 1986.
720. Coates EO Jr, Watson JHL: Diffuse interstitial lung disease in tungsten carbide workers. Ann Intern Med 75:709, 1971.
721. Demedts M: Cobalt lung in diamond polishers. Am Rev Respir Dis 130:130, 1984.
722. Kitamura H, Kitamura H, Tozawa T, et al: Cemented tungsten carbide pneumoconiosis. Acta Pathol Jpn 28:921, 1978.
723. Ruttner JR, Spycher MA, Stolkin I: Inorganic particulates in pneumoconiotic lungs of hard metal grinders. Br J Ind Med 44:657, 1987.
724. Sjogren I, Hillerdal G, Andersson A, et al: Hard metal lung disease: Importance of cobalt in coolants. Thorax 35:653, 1980.
725. Van Cutsem LJ, Ceuppens JL, Lacquet LM, et al: Combined asthma and alveolitis induced by cobalt in a diamond polisher. Eur J Respir Dis 70:54, 1987.
726. Anttila S, Sutinen S, Paananen M, et al: Hard metal lung disease: A clinical, histological, ultrastructural and X-ray microanalytical study. Eur J Respir Dis 69:83, 1986.
727. Tabatowski K, Roggli VL, Fulkerson WJ, et al: Giant cell interstitial pneumonia in a hard-metal worker. Cytologic, histologic and analytical electron microscopic investigation. Acta Cytol 32:240, 1988.
728. Forrest ME, Skerker LB, Nemirott MJ: Hard metal pneumoconiosis: Another cause of diffuse interstitial fibrosis. Radiology 128:609, 1978.
729. Bech AO, Kipling MD, Heather JC: Hard metal disease. Br J Ind Med 19:239, 1962.
730. Ratto D, Balmes J, Boylen T, et al: Pregnancy in a woman with severe pulmonary fibrosis secondary to hard metal disease. Chest 93:663, 1988.
731. Sprince NL, Chamberlin RI, Hales CA, et al: Respiratory disease in tungsten carbide production workers. Chest 86:549, 1984.
732. Funahashi A: Pneumoconiosis in workers exposed to silicon carbide. Am Rev Respir Dis 129:635, 1984.
733. Cordasco EM, Demeter SL, Kerkay J, et al: Pulmonary manifestations of vinyl and polyvinyl chloride (interstitial lung disease). Chest 78:6, 1980.
734. Mastrangelo G, Manno M, Marcer G, et al: Polyvinyl chloride pneumoconiosis: Epidemiological study of exposed workers. J Occup Med 21:540, 1979.
735. Antti-Poika M, Nordman H, Nickels J, et al: Lung disease after exposure to polyvinyl chloride dust. Thorax 41:566, 1986.
736. Arnaud A, De Santi PP, Garbe L, et al: Polyvinyl chloride pneumoconiosis. Thorax 33:19, 1978.
737. Prodan L, Suciu I, Pislaru V, et al: Experimental chronic poisoning with vinyl chloride (monochloroethylene). Ann NY Acad Sci 246:159, 1975.
738. Rode LE, Ophus EM, Gylseth B: Massive pulmonary deposition of rutile after titanium dioxide exposure. Acta Pathol Microbiol Scand (A) 89:455, 1981.
739. Elo R, Määttä K, Uksila E, et al: Pulmonary deposits of titanium dioxide in man. Arch Pathol 94:417, 1972.
740. Yamadori I, Ohsumi S, Taguchi K: Titanium dioxide deposition and adenocarcinoma of the lung. Acta Pathol Jpn 36:783, 1986.
741. Redline S, Barna BP, Tomashefski JF Jr, et al: Granulomatous disease associated with pulmonary deposition of titanium. Br J Ind Med 43:652, 1986.
742. Garabrant DH, Fine LJ, Oliver C, et al: Abnormalities of pulmonary function and pleural disease among titanium metal production workers. Scand J Work Environ Health 13:47, 1987.
743. Craighead JE, Adler KB, Butler GB, et al: Biology of disease. Health effects of Mount St. Helen's volcanic dust. Lab Invest 48:5, 1983.

744. Eisele JW, O'Halloran RL, Reay DT, et al: Deaths during the May 18, 1980 eruption of Mount St. Helens. Med Intelligence 305:931, 1981.
745. Merchant JA, Baxter P, Bernstein R, et al: Health implications of the Mount St. Helen's eruption: Epidemiological considerations. Ann Occup Hyg 26:911, 1982.
746. Baxter PJ, Ing R, Falk H, et al: Mount St. Helen's eruptions: The acute respiratory etiology of volcanic ash in a North American community. Arch Environ Health 38:138, 1983.
747. Hill JW: Health aspects of man-made mineral fibres. A review. Ann Occup Hyg 20:161, 1977.
748. Stanton MF, Layard M, Tegeris A, et al: Carcinogenicity of fibrous glass: Pleural response in the rat in relation to fiber dimension. J Natl Cancer Inst 58:587, 1977.
749. Gross P, Tuma J, deTreville RTP: Lungs of workers exposed to fiber glass. Arch Environ Health 23:67, 1971.
750. Gross P: Man-made vitreous fibers: An overview of studies on their biologic effects. Am Ind Hyg Assoc J 47:717, 1986.
751. Lee KP, Barras CE, Griffith FD, et al: Pulmonary response to glass fiber by inhalation exposure. Lab Invest 40:123, 1979.
752. Morgan RW, Kaplan SD, Bratsberg JA: Mortality study of fibrous glass production workers. Arch Environ Health 36:179, 1981.
753. Shannon HS, Hayes M, Julian JA, et al: Mortality experience of glass fibre workers. Br J Ind Med 41:35, 1984.
754. Enterline PE, Marsh GM, Esmen NA: Respiratory disease among workers exposed to man-made mineral fibers. Am Rev Respir Dis 128:1, 1983.
755. Bayliss DL, Dement JM, Wagoner JK, et al: Mortality patterns among fibrous glass production workers. Ann NY Acad Sci 271:324, 1976.
756. Goldsmith JR: Comparative epidemiology of men exposed to asbestos and man-made mineral fibers. Am J Ind Med 10:543, 1986.
757. Sixt R, Bake B, Abrahamsson G, et al: Lung function of sheet metal workers exposed to fiber glass. Scand J Work Environ Health 9:9, 1983.
758. Brody J, Miller A, Langer AM: Pneumoconiosis associated with exposure to glass and abrasive particles. Am J Ind Med 6:339, 1984.
759. Huuskonen MS, Tossavainen A, Koskinen H, et al: Wollastonite exposure and lung fibrosis. Environ Res 30:291, 1983.
760. Huuskonen MS, Jarvisalo J, Koskinen H, et al: Preliminary results from a cohort of workers exposed to wollastonite in a Finnish limestone quarry. Scand J Work Environ Health 9:169, 1983.
761. Hanke W, Sepulveda MJ, Watson A, et al: Respiratory morbidity in wollastonite workers. Br J Ind Med 41:474, 1984.
762. Clark TC, Harrington VA, Asta J, et al: Respiratory effects of exposure to dust in taconite mining and processing. Am Rev Respir Dis 121:959, 1980.
763. Gylseth B, Norseth T, Skaug V: Amphibole fibers in a taconite mine and in the lungs of the miners. Am J Ind Med 2:175, 1981.
764. Sander OA: Roentgen resurvey of cement workers. AMA Arch Ind Health 17:96, 1958.
765. McDowall ME: A mortality study of cement workers. Br J Ind Med 41:179, 1984.
766. Bohning DE, Atkins HL, Cohn SH: Long-term particle clearance in man: normal and impaired. Ann Occup Hyg 26:259, 1982.
767. Costello J, Graham WG: Vermont granite workers' mortality study. Am J Ind Med 13:483, 1988.
768. Struhar D, Harbeck RJ, Mason RJ: Lymphocyte populations in lung tissue, bronchoalveolar lavage fluid, and peripheral blood in rats at various times during the development of silicosis. Am Rev Respir Dis 139:28, 1989.
769. Vallyathan V, Shi X, Dalal NS, et al: Generation of free radicals from freshly fractured silica dust. Potential role in acute silica-induced lung injury. Am Rev Respir Dis 138:1213, 1988.
770. Craighead JE, Kleinerman J, Abraham JL, et al: Diseases associated with exposure to silica and nonfibrous silicate minerals. Arch Pathol Lab Med 112:673, 1988.
771. Bégin R, Ostiguy G, Cantin A, et al: Lung function in silica-exposed workers. A relationship to disease severity assessed by CT scan. Chest 94:539, 1988.
772. Hughes JM, Jones RN, Gilson JC, et al: Determinants of progression in sandblasters' silicosis. Ann Occup Hyg 26:701, 1982.
773. Nemery B, Veriter C, Brasseur L, et al: Impairment of ventilatory function and pulmonary gas exchange in non-smoking coalminers. Lancet 2:1427, 1987.
774. Susskind H, Acevedo JC, Iwai J, et al: Heterogeneous ventilation and perfusion: a sensitive indicator of lung impairment in non-smoking coalminers. Eur J Respir 1:232, 1988.
775. Sherson D, Maltbaek N, Olsen O: Small opacities among dental laboratory technicians in Copenhagen. Br J Ind Med 45:320, 1988.
776. Kern DG, Frumkin H: Asbestos-related disease in the jewelry industry: report of two cases. Am J Ind Med 13:407, 1988.
777. Cordier S, Lazar P, Brochard P, et al: Epidemiologic investigation of respiratory effects related to asbestos inside insulated buildings. Arch Environ Health 42:303, 1987.
778. Sison RF, Hruban RH, Moore GW, et al: Pulmonary disease associated with pleural "asbestos" plaques. Chest 95:831, 1989.
779. Antony VB, Owen CL, Hadley KJ: Pleural mesothelial cells stimulated by asbestos release chemotactic activity for neutrophils in vitro. Am Rev Respir Dis 139:199, 1989.
780. Bellis D, Andrion A, Delsedime L, et al: Minimal pathologic changes of the lung and asbestos exposure. Hum Pathol 20:102, 1989.
781. Hnizdo E, Sluis-Cremer GK: Effect of tobacco smoking on the presence of asbestosis at postmortem and on the reading of irregular opacities on roentgenograms in asbestos-exposed workers. Am Rev Respir Dis 138:1207, 1988.
782. Hayes AA, Rose AH, Musk AW, et al: Neutrophic chemotactic factor release and neutrophic alveolitis in asbestos-exposed individuals. Chest 94:521, 1988.
783. de Shazo RD, Morgan J, Bozelka B, et al: Natural killer cell activity in asbestos workers. Interactive effects of smoking and asbestos exposure. Chest 94:482, 1988.
784. Robinson BW, Rose AH, Hayes A, et al: Increased pulmonary gamma interferon production in asbestosis. Am Rev Respir Dis 138:278, 1988.
785. Warrock ML, Wolery G: Asbestos bodies and fibers and the diagnosis of asbestosis. Environ Res 44:29, 1987.
786. Hillerdal G: Rounded atelectasis. Clinical experience with 74 patients. Chest 95:836, 1989.
787. Rosenstock L, Barnhart S, Heyer NJ, et al: The relation among pulmonary function, chest roentgenographic abnormalities and smoking status in an asbestos-exposed cohort. Am Rev Respir Dis 138:272, 1988.
788. Enarson DA, Embree V, MacLean L, et al: Respiratory health in chrysotile asbestos miners in British Columbia: a longitudinal study. Br J Ind Med 45:459, 1988.
789. Fischbein L, Namade M, Sach RN, et al: Chronic constrictive pericarditis associated with asbestosis. Chest 94:646, 1988.
790. De Vuyst P, Dumortier P, Moulin E, et al: Asbestos bodies in bronchoalveolar lavage reflect lung asbestos body concentration. Eur Respir J 1:362, 1988.
791. Wheeler TM, Johnson EH, Coughlin D, et al: The sensitivity of detection of asbestos bodies in sputa and bronchial washings. Acta Cytol 32:647, 1988.
792. Wagner JC, Newhouse ML, Corrin B, et al: Correlation between fibre content of the lung and disease in East London asbestos factory workers. Br J Ind Med 45:305, 1988.
793. Alberts AS, Falkson G, Goedhals L, et al: Malignant pleural mesothelioma: a disease unaffected by current therapeutic maneuvers. J Clin Oncol 6:527, 1988.
794. Kishimoto T, Ono T, and Okada K: Acute myelocytic leukemia after exposure to asbestos. Cancer 62:787, 1988.
795. O'Brien AA, Moore DP, Keogh JA: Pulmonary berylliosis on corticosteroid therapy with cavitating lung lesions and aspergillomata: report on a fatal case. Postgrad Med J 63:797, 1987.
796. Musk AW, Beck BD, Greville HW, et al: Pulmonary disease from exposure to an artificial aluminum silicate: further observations. Br J Ind Med 45:246, 1988.
797. Shirakawa T, Kusaka Y, Fujimura N, et al: Occupational asthma from cobalt sensitivity in workers exposed to hard metal dust. Chest 95:29, 1989.
798. Bégin R, Dufresne A, Cantin A, et al: Carborundum pneumoconiosis. Fibers in the mineral activate macrophages to produce fibroblast growth factors and sustain the chronic inflammatory disease. Chest 95:842, 1989.
799. Hayashi H, Kajita A: Silicon carbide in lung tissue of a worker in the abrasive industry. Am J Ind Med 14:145, 1988.
800. Buist S: Personal communication, May, 1989.
801. Barrett TE, Pietra GG, Maycock RL, et al: Case report: Acrylic resin pneumoconiosis: report of a case in a dental student. Am Rev Respir Dis 139:841, 1989.
802. Loewen GM, Weiner D, McMahan J: Pneumoconiosis in an elderly dentist. Br J Ind Med 45:219, 1988.
803. Duma RJ: Particulate matter of particular interest. Ann Intern Med 78:146, 1973.

12

Pulmonary Disease Caused by Aspiration of Solid Foreign Material and Liquids

ASPIRATION OF SOLID FOREIGN BODIES

Aspiration of solid foreign bodies into the tracheobronchial tree occurs most often in small children. For example, more than 50 per cent of the 40 patients reported by Davis[1] were younger than 3 years of age and 79 per cent of the 66 patients documented by Weissberg and Schwarcz[2] were younger than 10 years of age; in one series of 33 children who survived aspiration, the mean age was 28 months,[3] and in another group of 23 infants and children who died, 78 per cent were between 2 months and 4 years of age.[4] However, although solid foreign body aspiration is most common in infants and children, it is important to remember that it does occur occasionally in older individuals.[184] In adults, aspiration of a solid foreign body is probably manifested most often as acute obstruction of the larynx or trachea, a clinical presentation commonly designated "café coronary" because of its frequent occurrence in restaurants and its resemblance to myocardial infarction (*see* later). In patients who have forgotten the original episode of aspiration or who recollect it only retrospectively, it can also cause repeated pneumonia, sometimes resulting in bronchiectasis.

Although the aspirated foreign bodies that have been described are of fascinating variety, including food, bone, pencils, rubber tubing, pins, needles, thermometers, metallic and plastic toys, and jewelry,[2, 5] the substance most commonly found is of vegetable origin. In a review of 160 patients, Brown and his colleagues[20] found that more than 85 per cent of aspirated bodies were of this type, the peanut being by far the most common. Vegetable material has also predominated in other series,[2, 3, 5, 7] the most common form varying with local dietary habits.[8]

Several specific solid foreign bodies deserve more comment. Inhalation of the flowering heads of various grasses has been reported by several investigators.[9–12] Although some of these—e.g., timothy grass—behave in a fashion similar to other bodies, others possess inflorescenses with well-developed terminal spikes (or awns) that project proximally towards the larger airways, causing the spikes to be inserted farther and farther into the lung periphery, much like a lobster entering a trap; this migration may be so extensive that the grass spike traverses the pleural space and is eventually extruded through the skin.[12, 13] Similar movement has been described in aspirated staples.[14] Any child who coughs and wheezes during the summer months should be suspected of having aspirated one of these grasses.[9] Broken fragments of teeth are occasionally aspirated following maxillofacial trauma, particularly in older children,[15] and roentgenograms of the chest should be obtained as a precautionary measure in all cases in which skull roentgenograms following trauma reveal absence or fracture of teeth. Mearns and England[16] have reported two incidents of young children who inhaled candies that dissolved in the tracheobronchial secretions and caused severe respiratory obstruction. The viscid fluid that formed as the candy dissolved was not expectorated, and bronchoscopy was necessary to remove it; the mucosal edema that resulted from the presence of the hyperosmolar sugar solution required 48 hours to resolve.

Pathologic Characteristics

In the early stages, the airway wall in immediate contact with the foreign body shows edema and a variable degree of inflammatory cellular infiltration or, if ulcerated, granulation tissue (Fig. 13–1); these reactions themselves contribute directly to airway narrowing. Foreign bodies, such as peanuts and other agents high in fatty acid content, are typically associated with an especially severe reaction. Vegetable material itself can absorb fluid and swell, increasing its effective size and resulting in an even greater degree of airway narrowing. Occasionally, the aspirated material becomes incorporated within granulation tissue in the bronchial wall and can appear grossly as a fungating tumor simulating carcinoma;[17] in such cases, the foreign material can usually be identified histologically in material obtained by endoscopic biopsy,[34] confirming the diagnosis (Fig. 13–1). Rare examples of true carcinoma associated with scarring and long-standing foreign body retention have been reported.[18] A more common result of such chronic retention is bronchial wall fibrosis and stenosis, usually accompanied by distal bronchiectasis and obstructive pneumonitis;[2, 19] in such circumstances, resection of the affected lung is often required.

Roentgenographic Manifestations

A wide variety of roentgenographic changes may be produced in the lungs. A nonreactive body, such as a tooth, may be discovered only incidentally on routine chest roentgenography.[20] In the majority of cases, however, changes in the lungs reflect the presence of partial or complete bronchial obstruction. The lower lobes are involved almost exclusively; contrary to common belief, left-sided aspiration is almost as common as right, a fact that has been attributed by Cleveland[21] to the equality of the right and left bronchial angles in the majority of children up to the age of 15 years. (According to this author, the more acute angle of the left bronchus usually seen in adults is caused by pressure from the contiguous aorta). The roentgenographic findings in the 160 patients reported by Brown and his associates[20] were as follows:

Obstructive overinflation	109	(68.1%)
Collapse	22	(13.8%)
"Infiltration"	17	(10.6%)
Radiopaque foreign body	15	(9.4%)
Bronchiectasis with recurrent local pneumonitis	3	
Pneumomediastinum	2	
Pneumothorax	1	

The number of patients with "obstructive overinflation" in this study is surprising. Because it can be very difficult to obtain roentgenograms of the chest in infants and young children at a point of maximal inspiration, particularly if there is respiratory distress and consequent tachypnea, we suspect that in the majority of cases the affected lung was *not* overinflated at a position of full inspiration and that instead the roentgenographic appearances reflected two effects: first, the ipsilateral lung *appeared* larger because roentgenograms were exposed at a position of slight expiration, thus exhibiting air trapping; and second, the ipsilateral lung exhibited increased radiolucency as a result of oligemia occasioned by hypoxic vasoconstriction (reflex reduction in perfusion in response to reduction in ventilation) (Fig. 13–2).

Because atelectasis was such an uncommon feature of the cases reported by Brown and associates,[1] it must be concluded that collateral air drift from adjacent normal lung parenchyma was an important factor in the majority. The low incidence of collapse or "infiltration" in this series differs from the findings of Davis,[1] who reported that 22 (55 per cent) of 40 patients who had aspirated solid foreign bodies showed roentgenographic evidence of basal collapse or consolidation.

In a patient in whom a foreign body impacts in a major bronchus, a roentgenogram exposed at inspiration may reveal no abnormality if insufficient time has elapsed for much air to be absorbed. In such circumstances, a roentgenogram exposed at full expiration will show air-trapping on the affected side and contralateral shift of the mediastinum. Because of the difficulty in communicating with infants and very young children and the resultant problems in obtaining good quality expiratory roentgenograms, Capitanio and Kirkpatrick[22] have adopted lateral decubitus roentgenography as a satisfactory alternative. They point out that when a child is placed on his or her side, the dependent hemithorax is splinted, restricting movement of the thoracic cage on that side. As a consequence, in normal children inflation of the dependent lung tends to be less than that of the upper lung. However, when air trapping is present in a dependent lung, the affected parenchyma tends to remain hyperlucent and of large volume. Thus, the presence of an obstructing endobronchial foreign body,

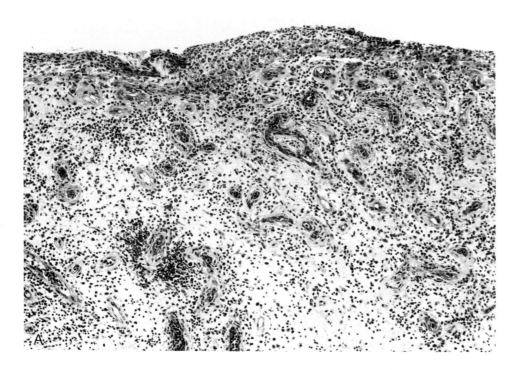

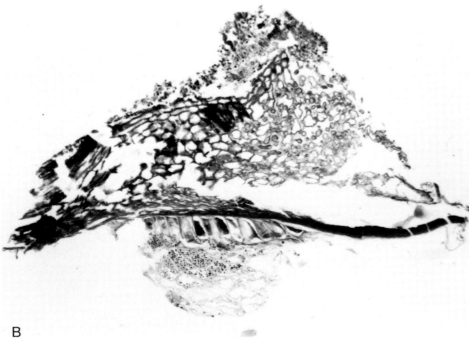

Figure 13–1. Foreign Body Aspiration: Bronchial Wall Ulceration. A histologic section of bronchial wall from a bronchoscopic biopsy specimen *(A)* shows complete loss of surface epithelium; the subepithelial layer consists only of granulation tissue. *B* is a histologic section of a fragment of vegetable material that was removed endoscopically from the same site at the time of biopsy. The patient was a 50-year-old man with partial atelectasis of the right upper lobe; there was no history of aspiration. *(A, × 100; B, × 90.)*

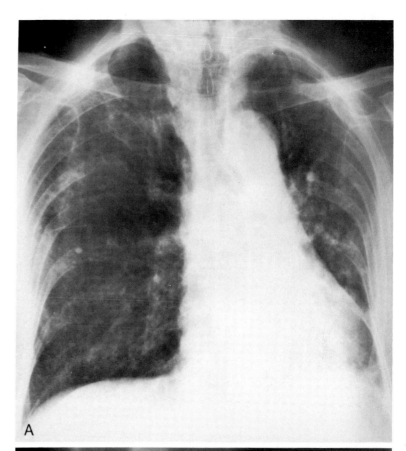

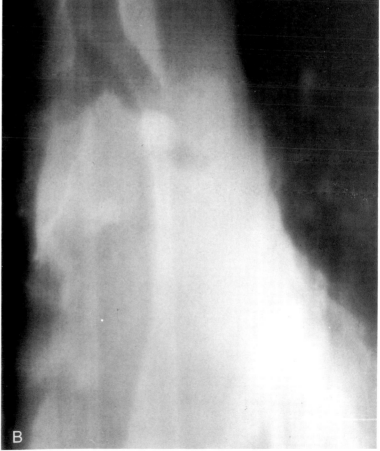

Figure 13–2. Aspiration of a Foreign Body with Impaction in a Main Bronchus. A posteroanterior roentgenogram *(A)* reveals moderate reduction in volume of the left lung accompanied by diffuse oligemia. A linear tomogram in anteroposterior projection *(B)* shows a circular opacity situated within and occupying the whole transverse diameter of the left main bronchus.

Illustration continued on following page

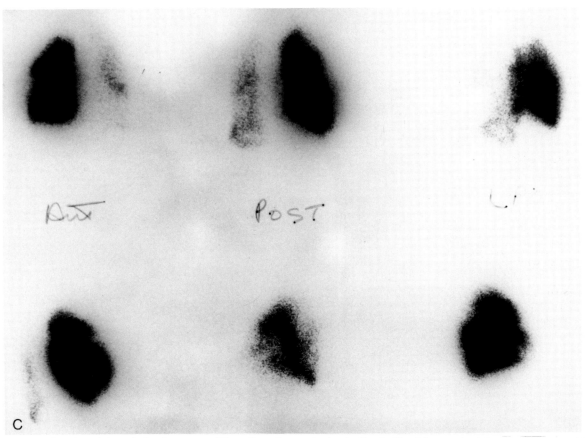

Figure 13–2. *Continued.* A perfusion lung scan *(C)* confirms the marked reduction in blood flow to the left lung, the result of hypoxic vasoconstriction. At bronchoscopy, a pill was successfully removed. The patient is an elderly man. (Courtesy of Dr. M. O'Donovan, Montreal General Hospital.)

as well as which lung is involved, usually will be easily established by bilateral lateral decubitus roentgenography, regardless of the degree of lung inflation at which the roentgenograms are exposed. Fluoroscopic examination will accomplish the same thing, revealing mediastinal "swing" and restricted diaphragmatic excursion on the affected side on deep respiration. In one series of 149 children who had aspirated foreign bodies, fluoroscopy revealed inspiratory mediastinal shift in 52 per cent.

Berger and his colleagues[23] have employed computed tomography (CT) to advantage in the identification of occult tracheobronchial foreign bodies in children; they emphasize that although this technique is not recommended as a routine in the diagnosis of foreign bodies, it can be of value in the more difficult cases. The value of lung scanning in the detection of endobronchial foreign bodies in infants and children also has been emphasized.[24] In five children subsequently shown to have aspirated radiolucent foreign bodies, who manifested normal physical findings and only minimal roentgenographic abnormalities, striking perfusion deficits were noted on lung scans. In all cases, the scans reverted to normal following removal of the foreign body. We believe that this procedure may be of value in selected cases, particularly when the clinical history is highly suggestive of aspiration and roentgenographic changes are equivocal (Fig. 13–2).

Four of five cases studied by Miller and colleagues,[25] in which there was delay between aspiration and roentgenography, showed only heavy markings or a nonspecific segmental opacity (probably constituting combined atelectasis and obstructive pneumonitis). It is assumed that this is the same change as that observed by Brown and colleagues[20] in approximately 10 per cent of their patients.

Bronchiectasis is an occasional complication of long-standing retention of a foreign body.[2] In one series of 500 patients with bronchiectasis,[26] long-retained and still present foreign bodies were identified in eight (four of the foreign bodies were vegetable and four mineral).

Clinical Manifestations

Although almost all adult patients remember choking at the time of aspiration,[20, 25] it may require much persistence to elicit the history, particularly when the episode occurred a long time before. In most instances, choking by children is recognized by nearby adults.[4, 185] As discussed previously, foreign bodies composed of vegetable matter, particularly peanuts and other material high in fatty acid, tend to cause an acute inflammatory response within a few hours or at most a few days, resulting in airway obstruction and consequent wheezing, rhonchi, and a localized decrease in breath sounds.[27] However, an asymptomatic interval may follow aspiration, especially when bronchi are not obstructed,[25] and such a latent period can extend to several months or even years if the aspirated material is bone or inorganic matter.[10, 11]

The "café coronary" syndrome[28] occurs in adults and is caused by lodgment of food in the upper airway, approximately a third being supraglottic.[29] Risk factors include old age, poor dentition, alcohol consumption, sedative drugs, chronic care institutionalization, and natural diseases, particularly parkinsonism, mental retardation, and psychiatric disorders.[29–31] Rarely, tracheal obstruction occurs as a result of impaction of a foreign body in the esophagus; such was the case in a 34-year-old mentally retarded patient who swallowed a 3 × 3-cm stone which came to rest in the upper esophagus and compressed the trachea from behind, resulting in death from asphyxiation.[32]

Acute upper airway obstruction results in air hunger, extreme cyanosis, venous distention, and coma; convulsions may be a manifestation of a risk factor itself (epilepsy) or the result of hypoxia occasioned by the airway obstruction.[33] The sudden onset of such a catastrophic episode can lead to a misdiagnosis of myocardial infarction; however, its development during a meal should suggest the true diagnosis. Current recommendations for the management of the choking victim[35] include the Heimlich maneuver, which consists of grasping the patient from behind and pressing the fist back and up in the epigastric area;[36] however, this maneuver is not without serious complications.[37–39]

ASPIRATION OF GASTRIC OR OROPHARYNGEAL SECRETIONS

The term aspiration pneumonia is employed by some to denote the inflammatory response in the lungs to infectious material aspirated from the mouth. This form of pneumonia is frequently caused by anaerobic organisms in patients with poor oral hygiene and is commonly associated with acute lung abscess; this type of aspiration is reviewed in Chapter 6 (see page 875). Although occasionally complicated by anaerobic bacterial infection, aspiration of oropharyngeal or gastric secretions, with or without admixed food particles, can also occur in a pure form and can cause significant pulmonary disease. This most often occurs as an isolated event:

1. In debilitated patients with chronic disease such as cancer.

2. In patients with oropharyngeal or airway intubation, such as those with a tracheostomy who have difficulty swallowing because of an overinflated cuff or those with a nasogastric tube in situ in the postoperative period[40–42] or with a feeding gastrotomy.[42, 43]

3. In unconscious patients in circumstances such as general anesthesia for emergency surgery or obstetric delivery,[44–46] pharyngeal-gastric colon interposition,[47] epileptic seizure, cardiopulmonary

resuscitation, electroconvulsive therapy, trauma, alcoholic stupor, or cerebrovascular accident.[48-52]

Such an event is not uncommon: in one series of 212 autopsies in which bronchopneumonia was identified, Fetterman and Moran[53] found food particles and associated inflammatory reaction in the lungs of 27 cases (12.7 per cent). In another study, Knoblich[54] identified 41 cases of "vegetable" aspiration pneumonia in approximately 1,500 autopsies. Because the presence of aspiration is usually determined pathologically by demonstrating food particles and because they are sometimes difficult to identify with certainty and may be sparse, the true incidence is undoubtedly higher.

In addition to these acute, often easily recognizable forms of aspiration, more chronic insidious disease can occur in association with various abnormalities of the upper gastrointestinal tract, including hypopharyngeal (Zenker's) diverticulum, benign or malignant esophageal stenosis or stricture, achalasia, congenital or acquired tracheoesophageal fistula, and neuromuscular disturbances in swallowing.[55-59, 186, 187] Probably of the same nature as aspiration associated with neuromuscular disturbances is the "fatigue" aspiration that sometimes occurs in otherwise normal infants toward the end of feeding, a potential cause of recurrent pneumonia. Patients with cystic fibrosis have been found to be subject to gastroesophageal reflux.[188] Chagas' disease, a parasitic disorder endemic to Brazil, causes myocardial and esophageal smooth muscle damage as a result of infestation with Trypanosoma cruzi, and has been reported to cause aspiration and recurrent pneumonia.[60] The incidence of both lipid pneumonia and pulmonary tuberculosis is higher in this form of esophageal dysfunction, the latter complication reflecting the tendency for mycobacterial organisms to proliferate in the fluid contents of a distended esophagus (see page 935).

Gastroesophageal reflux is a well-accepted cause of respiratory symptoms and repeated pneumonia, particularly in infants and children.[61-64] Evidence supporting this association derives from barium studies of the esophagus (particularly with cineradiography),[65] scintigraphic investigation employing various foods labeled with radionuclides,[43, 66, 67] esophageal pH recordings and manometry, and evidence of esophagitis on either esophagoscopy or biopsy.[68, 69] Some authors[64, 70, 71] recognize gastroesophageal reflux as a cause of asthma and have shown that bronchospasm can subside with antireflux therapy, including surgery when appropriate. It has also been postulated that gastroesophageal reflux can be responsible for diffuse interstitial fibrosis,[72-74] although support for this observation in published data is largely circumstantial and poorly controlled; Vraney and Pokorny[75] performed pulmonary function tests on 100 patients with gastroesophageal reflux and 100 matched controls and found no difference between the groups.

There is good evidence that aspiration of small amounts of oropharyngeal or gastric contents is common and may not be recognized by either patient or physician.[48] For example, of 300 unselected patients undergoing general anesthesia in whom Evans blue dye was injected into the stomach prior to anesthesia, 16 per cent showed bronchoscopic evidence of dye in the tracheobronchial tree postoperatively.[76] Similar findings have been noted in patients with neuromuscular disturbances in swallowing. In one study in which contrast material was instilled into the pharynx of normal control subjects and patients with myotonic dystrophy,[77] clearance time of the contrast material from the valleculae and pyriform sinuses was 1 to 3 seconds in the normal subjects and up to 1 hour in the patients; 12 of the patients were unaware of the aspiration of contrast material into their lungs. Aspiration of small amounts of oropharyngeal secretions is also probably common in patients with depressed consciousness and even in normal individuals during sleep.

Pathogenesis

Because of its highly irritating character, aspirated gastric fluid unaccompanied by a significant amount of admixed particulates is usually distributed more or less diffusely throughout both lungs in an explosive fashion as a result of violent coughing and the deep inspiration that such coughing engenders. Since the aspirate is liquid, it typically passes to the most peripheral airspaces, a process that can occur within seconds. The hydrochloric acid of the gastric juice is the chief offending agent and causes direct damage to the bronchiolar epithelium and alveolar wall with resulting increased alveolocapillary permeability.

Experimental studies suggest that pulmonary damage occurs predominantly when the pH of the aspirate is less than 2.5,[78] and it has been shown in rats[79] and in dogs[80] that prior neutralization of acid solutions instilled intratracheally reduces the severity of the pulmonary reaction. In humans it is generally assumed that the risk of pulmonary disease from gastric acid aspiration is also related to both the pH and the volume of aspirated stomach contents, being greatest when pH is less than 2.5 and the volume more than 25 ml. It should be noted, however, that there is considerable evidence that pulmonary damage also occurs when the pH of aspirated fluid is greater than 2.5; for example, several experimental and clinical studies have documented the development of pulmonary disease following the aspiration of neutralized gastric acid, distilled water, and isotonic saline (see later).[89-91] In addition, it has been shown repeatedly that antacids, modifiers of gastrointestinal tract motility, antiemetics, and H_2 receptor antagonists, singly or in combination, can increase pH and reduce gastric acid volume.[80–83] In theory, if such medication were to be administered at the appropriate time (1 to 1½ hours) before regurgitation and aspiration, it might be anticipated that a severe pulmonary reaction would be avoided, or at least diminished;[84] however, despite the widespread administration of antacids to women in labor, there has been little or no change in the incidence of maternal death from aspiration.[84] Furthermore, there are reports of fatal aspiration despite the use of antacids and the application of cricoid pressure.[85] (When considering the use of antacid therapy in such circumstances, it should be remembered that experimental inhalation of antacids can cause as much damage as gastric acid itself.[84])

During pregnancy, the morbidity resulting from aspiration of gastric contents appears to be particularly severe, and the mortality increased.[86] MacLennan[86] has suggested that underlying abnormal pulmonary water balance caused by either the pregnancy itself or therapeutic intervention may be responsible. It has also been postulated that incoordinate uterine contractions may be accompanied by failure of the stomach to empty, with resultant accumulation of a large volume of gastric contents.[85]

When aspirated gastric contents include an appreciable quantity of admixed particulates or when the aspirated material is derived from the oropharynx or esophagus, the pathogenesis of pulmonary damage appears to relate to both a nonspecific reaction to the liquid and a more specific inflammatory response to the various particulates.[87, 88] As noted previously, it has been shown in several clinical and experimental studies that pulmonary disease can develop as a result of aspiration of fluid with relatively high pH; for example, aspiration of neutralized gastric liquid (pH 5.9) that has been filtered to remove food particles results in significant but transient hypoxemia;[89] similarly, individual case reports have documented the development of severe pulmonary edema in patients who have aspirated fluid with a pH as high as 6.4.[90]

Pathologic studies have also shown evidence of lung damage caused by fluid of relatively neutral pH. Histologically, aspiration of gastric liquid at a pH higher than 4.0 has been shown to cause acute pneumonitis (characterized by edema, hemorrhage, and polymorphonuclear leukocyte infiltration) and bronchiolitis.[89, 91] In a study of the ultrastructure of pulmonary alveolar capillaries in Mendelson's syndrome, Alexander[92] examined the lungs of experimental animals into which solutions of varying pH and tonicity had been instilled. Pulmonary edema was present in all specimens, including those in which distilled water was utilized. Electron microscopy revealed fluid in the alveoli and separation of the vascular endothelium from the alveolar epithelium by interstitial fluid. The pH and tonicity were related to the reaction only in terms of degree and time.

Although these pathologic changes and the functional effects associated with them are less severe than when the pH of the aspirated fluid is less than 2.5,[89] they nevertheless imply that it is not acid alone that causes pulmonary damage. This has also been well illustrated in experimental studies in which pure solutions of ground-up meat and vegetable material have been aspirated, clearly resulting in a polymorphonuclear and granulomatous inflammatory response.[94] Gastrointestinal enzymes such as trypsin and pepsin are unlikely to have any pathogenetic effect by themselves.[88, 95]

Pathologic Characteristics

Pathologic changes depend on the nature and quantity of the aspirated material and on the frequency with which bouts of aspiration occur. Depending on the time after aspiration at which the lungs are examined, the gross appearance may be that of parenchymal edema and hemorrhage or an acute or organizing bronchopneumonia identical to that caused by bacteria. In occasional cases, foci of disease are relatively discrete and circumscribed and have been mistaken for miliary or endobronchial tuberculosis or bacterial abscesses.[87, 96] In the early stages, airway walls may be hyperemic and their lumens partly filled with a mucopurulent exudate.[53]

The histologic reaction to aspiration of relatively pure gastric liquid of low pH reflects the usually extensive acid-induced epithelial damage. In the airways, bronchitis and bronchiolitis are accompanied by focal ulceration and intraluminal exudate. In the early stages, the parenchyma shows only airspace edema and hemorrhage, followed rapidly by the appearance of necrotic debris and fibrin in the airspaces, and eventually by hyaline membrane formation. If the patient lives long enough, the exudate undergoes organization. This appearance is identical to diffuse alveolar damage of other etiologies (see Fig. 10–62, page 1936).

The pathologic appearance differs when there is a substantial amount of admixed particulate material in the aspirate. Edema, congestion, and hemorrhage followed by a polymorphonuclear influx are early findings in virtually all cases of both experimentally induced food aspiration[54, 88, 94] and in patients examined at autopsy (Fig. 13–3).[53] Food particles at first are found lying free within edema fluid in airway lumens and distal airspaces, but they rapidly develop a surrounding mantle of polymorphonuclear leukocytes (Fig. 13–3). Mononuclear phagocytic cells soon follow and increase in number thereafter. Foreign body giant cells, often of highly irregular shape and with numerous nuclei, can be found as early as 24 to 48 hours after the aspiration (Fig. 13–4). Well-organized granulomas often develop and surround identifiable fragments of meat or vegetable material or necrotic debris. At this stage, the disease foci may be relatively discrete and appear both grossly and histologically as multiple nodules resembling either hematogenous (miliary)

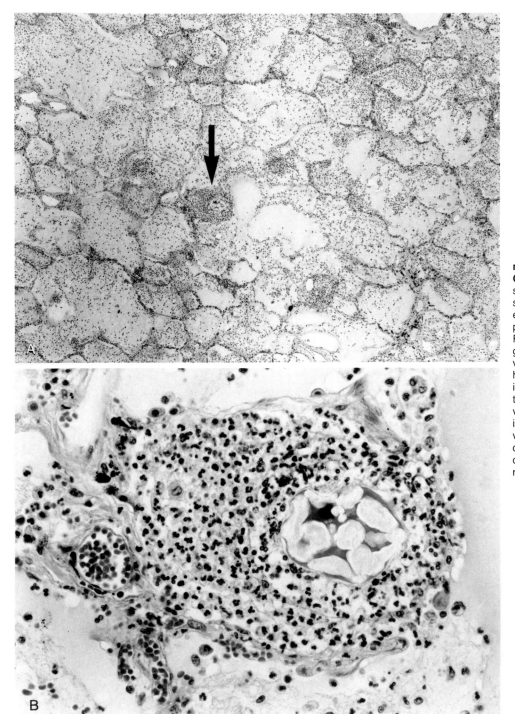

Figure 13–3. Acute Pneumonia Caused by Aspiration of Gastric Contents. A histologic section of lung parenchyma *(A)* shows airspaces consolidated by edema and numerous admixed polymorphonuclear leukocytes. Focally, leukocytes are aggregated around small particles of vegetable material *(arrow)*. A higher-power section of the area indicated by the arrow *(B)* reveals the foreign material to good advantage; its lobulated appearance is characteristic of leguminous vegetables. These sections were obtained at autopsy of a 65-year-old man with disseminated carcinoma. *(A,* × 40; *B,* × 300.)

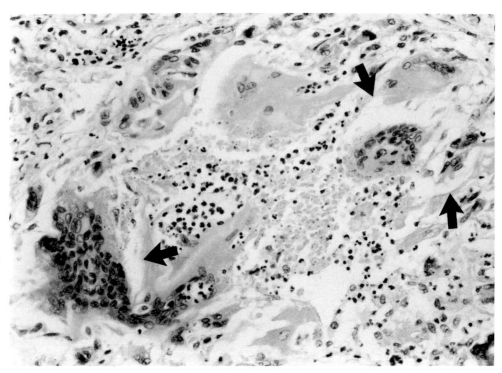

Figure 13–4. Foreign Body Giant Cell Reaction to Aspirated Gastric Contents. A histologic section through a focus of lower lobe pneumonia shows several mutinucleated giant cells surrounding necrotic material and multiple polymorphonuclear leukocytes. The giant cell at the lower left is quite irregular in shape and contains numerous nuclei, features characteristic of a reaction to aspirated foreign material, in this case vegetable. The vegetable fragments themselves are partly destroyed and are evident only as clear spaces within and adjacent to the giant cells *(arrows)*. (× 250.)

or endobronchial spread of tuberculosis (Fig. 13–5). A miliary pattern can sometimes be detected roentgenographically.[97]

With the exception of the reaction to lipid (*see* later), little difference has been shown in experimental studies between the reactions to different types of aspirated food,[94] although granulomas appear to develop more readily and persist longer in relation to leguminous vegetable material such as peas, beans, and lentils.[54, 88] In occasional cases, it may be difficult to identify food particles within the granulomas with conviction; examination of multiple sections and the use of polarization microscopy to identify the refractile cell walls found in many vegetables are necessary in these cases to arrive at the correct diagnosis.

Although the edema and hemorrhage of the early stage tend to be more or less diffuse throughout the parenchyma, the granulomatous inflammation is most severe in relation to membranous and respiratory bronchioles. Thus, some degree of bronchiolitis obliterans is not uncommon (Fig. 13–6); residual peribronchiolar fibrosis associated with distortion of the normal airway architecture and "bronchiolization" of the adjacent parenchyma may be the only evidence of prior aspiration (Fig. 13–6).

The development of secondary bacterial pneumonia in the areas of damaged lung or of lung abscess in the case of aspirates contaminated by anaerobic or other organisms can alter the typical histologic appearance.

Roentgenographic Manifestations

In the patient who has aspirated a large amount of relatively pure gastric secretion at a low pH (Mendelson's syndrome), the chest roentgenogram reveals general involvement of both lungs by typical patchy airspace consolidation similar in many ways to the pulmonary edema of cardiac origin or to the more diffuse permeability edema observed in the adult respiratory distress syndrome (ARDS). Discrete acinar shadows may be apparent, but most opacities are confluent (Fig. 13–7). The normal size of the heart and the absence of signs of pulmonary venous hypertension serve to differentiate the edema from that of cardiac origin.

In a review of the roentgenographic manifestations of aspiration of gastric contents in 60 patients, Landay and his colleagues[99] observed three basic patterns of disease: (1) extensive bilateral airspace consolidation (confluent acinar opacities), (2) widespread but fairly discrete acinar shadows, and (3) irregular opacities whose pattern did not fit into either of the other two categories (this last-named was the most common pattern, accounting for slightly over 40 per cent). Distribution was most commonly bilateral and multicentric but usually favored perihilar or basal regions. In uncomplicated cases, roentgenographic changes often worsened for several days but thereafter generally improved fairly rapidly. Worsening of the roentgenographic abnormalities after initial improvement was associ-

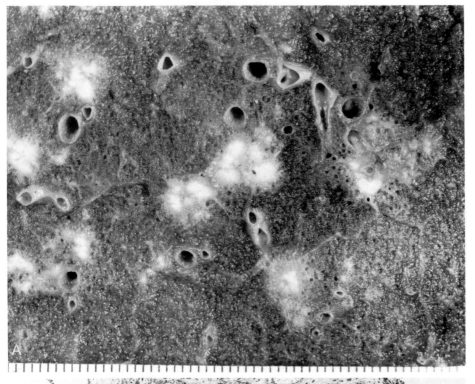

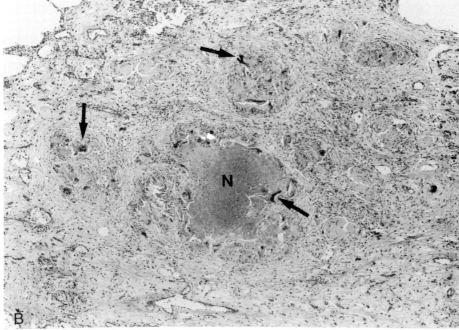

Figure 13–5. Aspiration of Gastric Contents Resembling Tuberculous Bronchopneumonia. A magnified view of lower lobe *(A)* shows multiple, fairly well-defined foci of white necrotic material surrounded by a thin rim of consolidated lung. The appearance resembles that seen in endobronchial spread of tuberculosis. A histologic section *(B)* reveals several fairly well-defined granulomas, one of which is related to necrotic material (N); these are surrounded by fibrous tissue containing scattered lymphocytes. Again, the appearance superficially resembles tuberculosis; however, the presence of numerous multinucleated giant cells, some with irregular shapes *(arrows)*, suggests that the etiology is food aspiration rather than infection *(B, × 40)*.

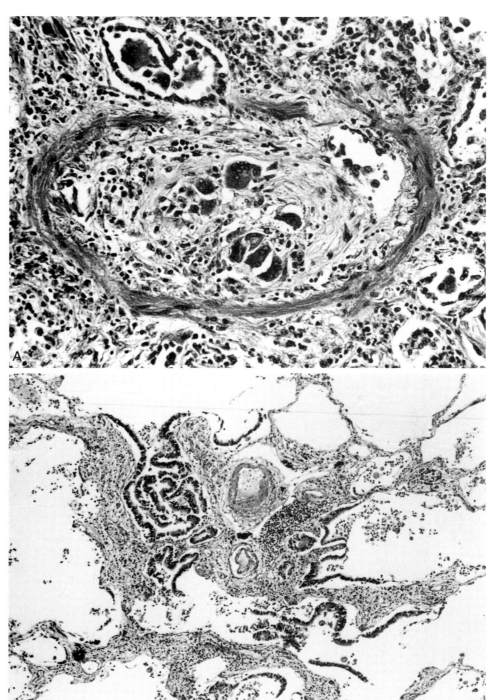

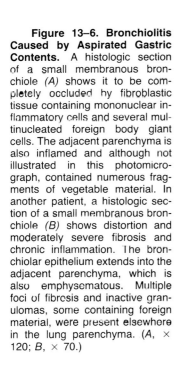

Figure 13–6. Bronchiolitis Caused by Aspirated Gastric Contents. A histologic section of a small membranous bronchiole (A) shows it to be completely occluded by fibroblastic tissue containing mononuclear inflammatory cells and several multinucleated foreign body giant cells. The adjacent parenchyma is also inflamed and although not illustrated in this photomicrograph, contained numerous fragments of vegetable material. In another patient, a histologic section of a small membranous bronchiole (B) shows distortion and moderately severe fibrosis and chronic inflammation. The bronchiolar epithelium extends into the adjacent parenchyma, which is also emphysematous. Multiple foci of fibrosis and inactive granulomas, some containing foreign material, were present elsewhere in the lung parenchyma. (A, × 120; B, × 70.)

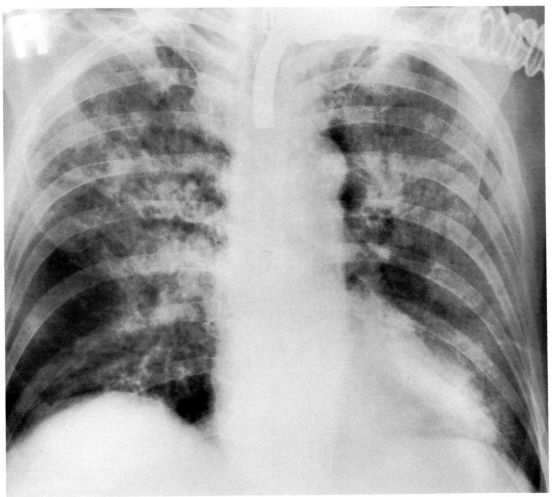

Figure 13–7. Acute Aspiration Pneumonia (Mendelson's Syndrome). While lying in a supine position following anesthesia, this 68-year-old man vomited and aspirated considerable quantities of vomitus. Anteroposterior roentgenography performed within 2 hours reveals extensive involvement of both lungs by patchy airspace consolidation typical of acute pulmonary edema. Although a few patchy shadows are present in the lower lung zones, the predominant involvement is in the upper zones, a distribution that can be explained, at least partly, by the position of the patient at the time of aspiration.

ated with the development of bacterial pneumonia, ARDS, or pulmonary embolism.

It is to be emphasized that this form of aspiration pneumonia may not show an anatomic distribution reflecting the influence of gravity. If the patient is lying in the prone or supine position at the time of aspiration, the highly irritative nature of the aspirate will result in widespread dissemination throughout the lungs; however, predominant changes may be unilateral if the patient is lying on his or her side. (Anyone who has employed the aspiration technique of bronchography described by Nordenstrom[100] and Priviteri[101] is familiar with the wide distribution of contrast material that occurs throughout the lung as a result of a single deep inspiration.) If the patient survives, resolution is

relatively rapid—averaging 7 to 10 days in our experience—about the same as for traumatic fat embolism but much slower than that for edema caused by acute cardiac decompensation.

In cases in which there is aspiration of oropharyngeal secretions or gastric contents with an appreciable amount of admixed food, the roentgenographic changes usually occur segmentally, involving one or more of the posterior segments of the upper or lower lobes (Fig. 13–8). The precise localization depends at least partly on the position of the patient at the time of aspiration.[102] Some degree of atelectasis is present in almost all cases, and the picture can be typical of bronchopneumonia (Fig. 13–9). With repeated aspiration, serial roentgenography over a period of months or years shows

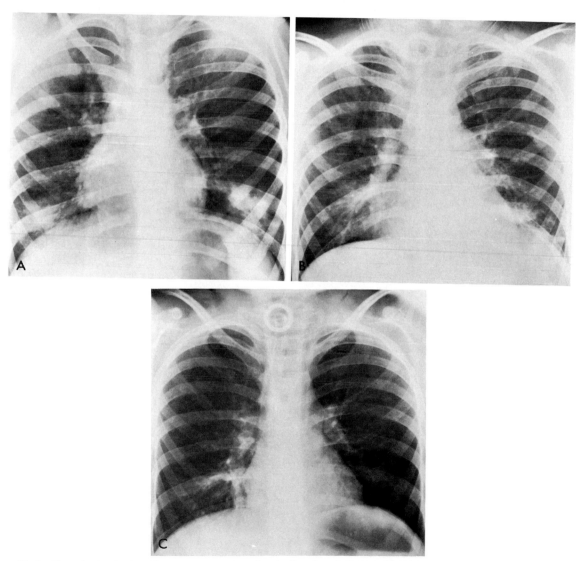

Figure 13–8. Chronic Aspiration Pneumonia in Myasthenia Gravis. A 9-year-old girl had had a history of frequent respiratory infections since infancy, complicated by bronchiolitis and bronchitis and by severe bronchiolar spasm. Positive skin tests suggested the presence of bronchial asthma. Epilepsy and myasthenia gravis were also part of the rather complicated clinical picture. The roentgenographic studies illustrated cover a period of almost 2 months. The first *(A)* reveals inhomogeneous segmental consolidation of both lower lobes and of the right middle lobe. Approximately 2 weeks later, the disease of the right lower lobe had resolved but the right middle lobe consolidation had extended; in addition there was new disease in the left lower lobe. Approximately 6 weeks later *(C)*, the pneumonia of both lower lobes had resolved completely, although there was still residual atelectasis and scarring in the middle lobe. This variation in the anatomic distribution of disease is typical of chronic recurrent aspiration pneumonia.

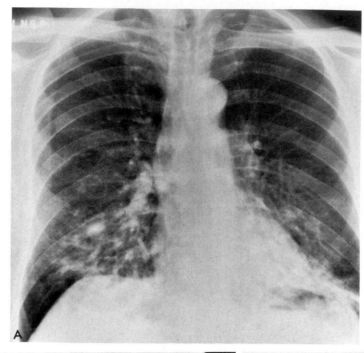

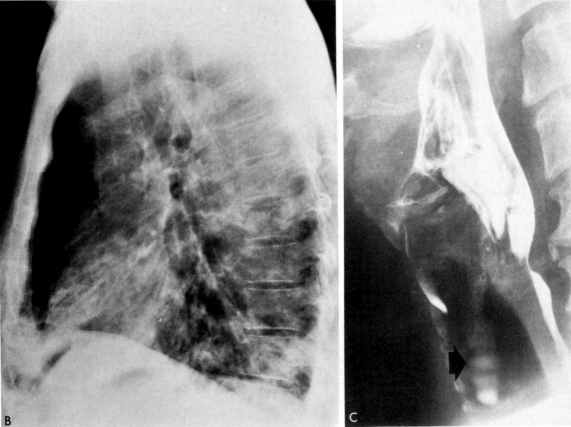

Figure 13–9. Aspiration Pneumonia (Carcinoma of the Pharynx).   A 54-year-old man was admitted to the hospital for investigation of an oropharyngeal mass that proved, on biopsy, to be primary carcinoma. Roentgenograms of the chest on admission were normal. During his hospitalization, he developed cough and low-grade fever. Chest roentgenograms in posteroanterior *(A)* and lateral *(B)* projections revealed extensive inhomogeneous, segmental consolidation of both lower lobes, the right middle lobe, and the lingula. The possibility that this was caused by aspiration was considered, and a barium swallow was performed. A view of the hypopharynx and upper trachea in lateral projection *(C)* shows barium in the upper trachea *(arrow)*. The fact that the pulmonary disease was largely confined to the lower lung zones suggests that the aspiration occurred when the patient was erect.

much variation in the anatomic distribution of segments involved, with disease clearing rather slowly in one segment and appearing anew in another (Fig. 13–10). A residuum of irregular accentuation

of linear markings may remain, probably representing peribronchial scarring. Two patients have been described whose chest roentgenograms revealed a reticulonodular pattern shown pathologi-

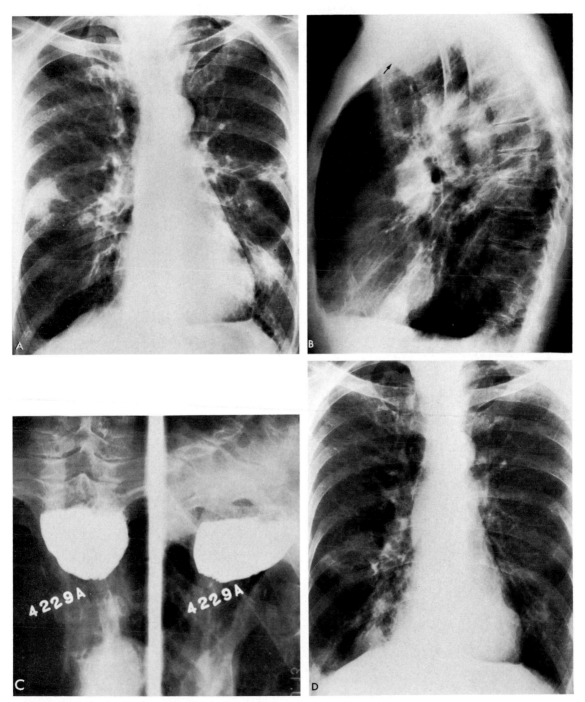

Figure 13–10. Chronic Aspiration Pneumonia Secondary to Zenker's Diverticulum. For approximately 2 years, a 48-year-old man had had recurrent episodes of acute lower respiratory infection associated with intermittent dysphagia. The roentgenograms illustrated extend over a period of 7 months. The first (A) reveals moderate pulmonary overinflation. Poorly defined homogeneous areas of consolidation are situated in the right midlung and in the left lower lobe, with irregular "streaking" in the axillary portion of the left lung. In lateral projection (B), the several areas of pneumonia are rather poorly visualized, but of greater significance is a homogeneous soft tissue density situated in the superior mediastinum and causing slight anterior displacement of the tracheal air column (arrow). The diagnosis of hypopharyngeal (Zenker's) diverticulum was confirmed by barium studies (C). Approximately 6 months after the first roentgenogram, a repeat study (D) shows almost complete clearing of the pneumonia of the left lung and of the axillary portion of the right lung. However, there is a new area of bronchopneumonia in the posterior basal segment of the right lower lobe. The episodes of recurrent aspiration pneumonia disappeared following surgical resection of the diverticulum.

cally to be related to a granulomatous reaction around food particles;[103] in another case of a mentally retarded adolescent with a defect in his swallowing mechanism, a miliary pattern was presumed to be caused by aspiration of lentils.[97]

Clinical Manifestations

The risk of acid aspiration pneumonia is present in all age groups, but because both gastric acidity and volume of secretion decrease as age increases,[104] the risk is theoretically greatest in children and least in the aged. Aspiration of gastric contents of low pH (Mendelson's syndrome) occurs most commonly in patients in a comatose state, often following induction of anesthesia. Intubation does not necessarily protect the lungs, because aspirated material situated within the airway above an inflated cuff can flood the lungs when the cuff is deflated; sometimes there is leakage around the cuff, a complication that has been described even with high-volume, low-pressure endotracheal cuffs.[105]

Respiratory distress may be noted before roentgenographic changes become manifest in the chest. In such situations, if clinical suspicion is high, fiberoptic bronchoscopy may reveal erythematous lesions of the tracheal mucosa and thus support the diagnosis.[106] In the early stages diffuse rales may be heard; once consolidation develops, patchy areas of bronchial breathing may be detected. Hypoxemia may be severe; in one series of 14 cases in which the arterial PO_2 was measured, the mean value was 49 mm Hg. If the patient survives the stage of acute pulmonary edema, cough, which is initially dry, may eventually become productive of copious purulent sputum; a variety of aerobic and anaerobic pathogens may be cultured from this material. Broad-spectrum antibiotics are indicated, but corticosteroids probably serve little or no purpose and can increase the risk of complicating gram-negative pneumonia.[49, 107]

In our experience patients who survive do not show clinical, physiologic, or roentgenographic sequelae. However, recovery may be prolonged: five adolescents who survived ARDS following gastric aspiration continued to show improvement in pulmonary function and gas transfer 18 months after the acute episode.[108] Despite these observations, long-term follow-up has revealed persistent respiratory insufficiency in some patients.[109]

The presence of chronic recurrent gastroesophageal reflux should be suspected in any patient with an unexplained cough or a history of repeated pneumonia. Although this applies mostly to infants and children,[61, 64, 68, 110] it is also applicable to adults who may also complain of choking, a symptom that is indicative of esophageal dysfunction. Even congenital tracheoesophageal fistula can escape diagnosis until adulthood (see page 727).[111, 112]

ASPIRATION OF LIPID

Lipid can accumulate in the lungs from either endogenous or exogenous sources. Accumulation of endogenous lipid is seen in such conditions as obstructive pneumonitis, pulmonary alveolar proteinosis, and lipid storage disease. These conditions are entirely different in nature from the exogenous forms[113, 114] and are considered elsewhere in this book. The term lipid (lipoid) pneumonia is restricted here to exogenous disease caused by the aspiration into the lungs of mineral oil or of the various vegetable or animal oils present in food or radiographic contrast media. This subject has been reviewed by Genereux,[115] and the interested reader is directed to this source for additional information, particularly with regard to radiologic-pathologic correlation.

Etiology and Pathogenesis

Mineral oil is probably the most common agent to cause lipid pneumonia, and a variety of medical, cultural, and occupational situations predispose to its aspiration. Disease occurs most frequently when the oil is used medically, particularly as a lubricant in infants with feeding difficulties, in old people who are constipated, and in patients with dysphagia caused by neurologic lesions, hypopharyngeal (Zenker's) diverticulum, esophageal carcinoma, or achalasia. Although oil-based nose drops are not used as widely now as formerly, cases of lipid pneumonia as a result of nasal medication containing liquid paraffin are still seen occasionally.[116, 117, 118] Experimental studies have shown that oil deposited in the nasal cavities of sleeping individuals can subsequently be identified in the lungs,[98] and it is presumably in this manner that pneumonia results in these individuals. Rarely, bronchopleural fistula formation and resultant lipid pneumonia have occurred secondary to oleothorax treatment of tuberculosis.[119]

Less common, nonmedical forms of lipid aspiration have also been described. For example, pneumonia has been attributed to the occupational inhalation of lipid in the form of an oil mist. Jones[120] based this diagnosis on the presence of a reticular pattern on the chest roentgenograms of 12 of 19 men exposed to mineral oil droplets that were produced during the cold reduction by water of mineral oil–coated, hot rolled strip steel. Cullen and coworkers[121] subsequently confirmed this association through examination of tissue obtained by transbronchial biopsy. The cleaning of airplane undercarriages with oil mists has also been reported to cause disease.[122] Although oil mist has been detected in piped air coming from oil-lubricated air compressors,[123] we are not aware of published reports of lung disease resulting from this source.

Diffuse interstitial lipid pneumonia has also been described in natives of Guyana who smoke tobacco known as "black-fat";[124] mineral oil and vaseline are added to the tobacco for flavoring and as humectants. The disease was identified in 56 individuals, who constituted 19.6 per cent of black-fat smokers in the area; there was no roentgenographic evidence of disease in a control group of nonsmokers. Lip gloss, a substance that contains a large amount of mineral oil, has been shown by biopsy to be the cause of a pulmonary mass.[125]

The pathogenesis of mineral oil–related fibrosis is not well understood. Chemically, mineral oil is a pure hydrocarbon and is believed to be inert, a feature that may explain the lack of airway-mediated cough reflex following aspiration.[126] It has been suggested that release of lysosomal enzymes by dead lipid-laden macrophages may be a factor in causing fibrosis.[126]

The principal *animal oils* associated with pneumonia are those in milk or milk products and in cod liver oil. Aspiration of these substances occurs predominantly in infants and young children during feeding. Pneumonia in a young infant has also been cited by Balakrishman[127] as being caused by the aspiration of ghee. One case of lipid pneumonia, verified by biopsy, has been reported in an engineer who tested the efficiency of fire extinguishers against simulated flash fires fueled with various commercial lards, shortenings, and rancid animal renderings.[128] In contrast to mineral oils, animal fats are hydrolyzed into fatty acids, presumably by lung lipases, and their presence in the lung can cause an acute hemorrhagic pneumonitis.[129]

Aspiration of *vegetable oils* occurs in a variety of circumstances and possesses great variability in its capacity to cause tissue damage.[129] It is probable that these substances most commonly are aspirated during eating or in association with vomiting of gastric contents, in which circumstances the oil is unlikely to be the sole offending agent; as a result, damage to the lung caused by the oil itself is difficult to assess. Occasionally, instances of pure vegetable oil aspiration have been documented; for example, an oily suspension of methenamine containing sesame and hydrogenated castor oil has been implicated as a cause of pneumonia in two senile patients.[130] Also, in a number of states in India, a local custom of smearing gingilli oil in babies' mouths is well recognized as a cause of pneumonia.[127] Finally, bronchographic contrast media such as Lipiodol (iodized ethyl esters of the fatty acids of poppy seed oil) and oily Dionosil (propyliodine in an arachis oil) have been associated with granulomatous and nonspecific pneumonitis.[131]

The pathogenesis of pulmonary disease resulting from vegetable oil aspiration is not completely understood. With some oils, there is virtually no pulmonary reaction, the oil remaining for prolonged periods in alveolar spaces without either fibrosis or significant inflammatory response.[129]

However, other vegetable oils cause tissue reactions similar to those associated with animal oils; as with the latter, hydrolysis can cause the release of fatty acids that can be important in pathogenesis.[129]

Pathologic Characteristics

As noted previously, the degree and quality of tissue reaction to aspirated oil are quite variable, being related to the quantity and frequency of aspiration, to the chemical characteristics of the oil itself, and to the complicating effects of other substances that may be aspirated at the same time. The initial reaction to many animal oils and some vegetable oils is an acute bronchopneumonia characterized by edema, intra-alveolar hemorrhage, and a mixed polymorphonuclear and mononuclear infiltrate. Macrophages become finely vacuolated as they ingest the lipid; although most macrophages remain within alveolar airspaces or are transported up the mucociliary escalator, some enter the lymphatics and can cause hyperplasia of lymphoid tissue in the lung and mediastinum.[132] Giant cell and granuloma formation can be absent or quite extensive. In the early stages of milk aspiration, amorphous, eosinophilic material resembling fibrin can sometimes be identified within alveoli and terminal airways, representing collections of unaltered milk itself.[132]

The reaction to aspirated mineral oil is characterized in the early stage by an intra-alveolar infiltrate of macrophages, accompanied by minimal, if any, acute inflammatory reaction. The oil is rapidly emulsified and phagocytosed, resulting in fine vacuolation of macrophages that may fill the alveoli (Fig. 13–11). With time, these macrophages become predominantly interstitial in location and decrease in number; the small oil droplets in turn coalesce to form relatively large, round or oval droplets situated within multinucleated giant cells (Fig. 13–11). Typically, the nuclei of these cells are compressed into a flattened rim at the edge of the oil droplet. True granulomas do not develop. Fibrous tissue containing scattered collections of lymphocytes surrounds the giant cells (Fig. 13–12). In the early stages, droplets can also be identified apparently lying free within interstitial tissues and the media of small arteries; endarteritis obliterans can be seen in later stages. Grossly, the area of fibrosis can form a fairly well-circumscribed, stellate tumor (sometimes termed "paraffinoma"; Fig. 13–13), or can be more diffuse and patchy in appearance, resembling an area of nonspecific, organized pneumonitis.

The precise characterization of an oily substance within the lung can be difficult without a clinical history. The staining reactions of the various oils have been described by Wagner and colleagues.[133] Thin-layer chromatography, chemical analysis, and infrared spectroscopy have been used for definitive identification.[118, 134–136]

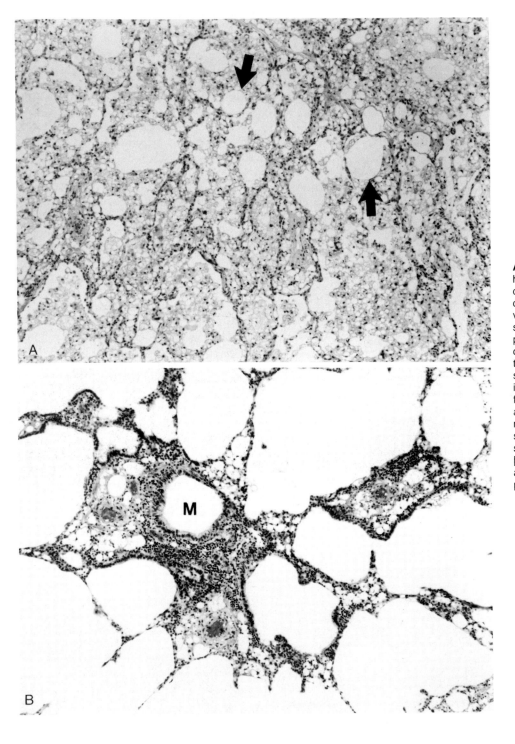

Figure 13–11. Mineral Oil Aspiration: Early Stages. A histologic section of lung parenchyma *(A)* shows complete filling of alveolar airspaces by finely vacuolated macrophages; occasional oval clear spaces *(arrows)* probably represent free mineral oil. Note that the parenchymal interstitium is virtually normal. A somewhat later stage is revealed in a histologic section from a different patient *(B)*, in which the airspaces are largely devoid of macrophages; instead, the interstitium (especially adjacent to a small membranous bronchiole [M]) shows a lymphocytic infiltrate and numerous lipid-laden macrophages. *(A,* × 80; *B,* × 80.)

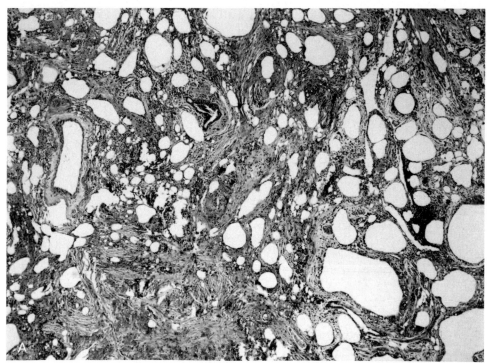

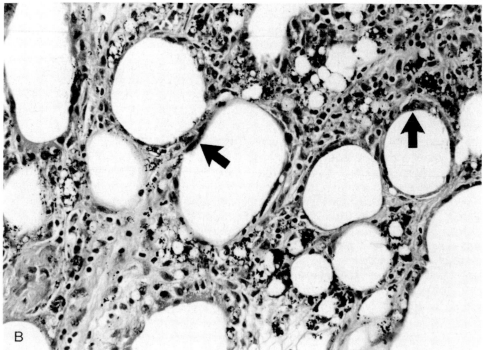

Figure 13–12. Mineral Oil Aspiration: Chronic Stage. A histologic section from a well-circumscribed parenchymal nodule *(A)* shows fibrous tissue with admixed lymphocytes and numerous clear spaces of variable size and shape. At higher magnification *(B)*, many of the clear spaces can be seen to be surrounded by a thin rim of cytoplasm containing multiple, somewhat flattened nuclei *(arrows)*. The clear spaces represent foci of mineral oil within multinucleated giant cells. (*A*, × 40; *B*, × 250.)

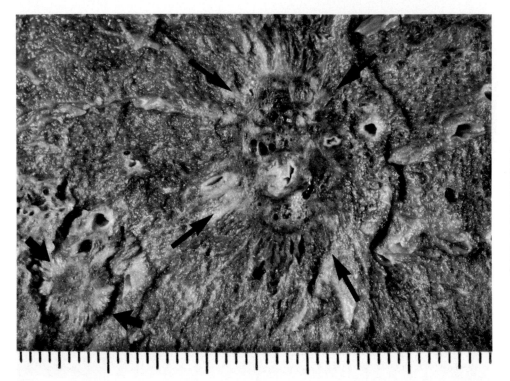

Figure 13–13. Mineral Oil Aspiration: "Paraffinoma." A magnified view of a lower lobe (resected for a presumptive diagnosis of carcinoma) shows two fairly well defined nodules, one round *(short arrows)* and the other oval with a somewhat spiculated appearance *(long arrows)*. Multiple small cystic spaces within the nodules represent foci of mineral oil accumulation.

Roentgenographic Manifestations

In the early stages, the typical pattern of disease caused by mineral oil aspiration is alveolar consolidation. Depending on the quantity of oil aspirated, the resultant airspace shadows can be confluent or discrete—in fact, isolated acinar shadows may form a distinctive feature during the early stages. Although the roentgenographic pattern varies, its most common form is relatively homogeneous consolidation of one or more segments, often in precise segmental distribution (Fig. 13–14). In most cases, the lower lobes are predominantly affected, although in debilitated patients, because of their recumbent position, involvement is likely to occur in the superior segment of a lower lobe or the posterior segment of an upper lobe.[113, 137–139] The consolidated area may be several centimeters in diameter, with poorly defined or fairly sharply defined margins (Fig. 13–15). Another, almost as common manifestation is a peripheral mass, sometimes with fairly well circumscribed margins simulating peripheral pulmonary carcinoma (Fig. 13–16).[140] This lesion also develops chiefly in the dependent portions of the lung, although sometimes in the middle lobe or lingula. Linear shadows radiating from the periphery of such a localized mass result from the interlobular septal thickening caused by infiltration of lipid-laden macrophages and secondary chronic inflammation. In one instance, necropsy revealed ossification of multiple deposits of lipid material.[141] Rarely, the acute phase of the process can be associated with cavitation, probably related to concomitant anaerobic infection.[115, 116] Because the oil is carried from the alveoli into the interstitial space by macrophages, a predominantly interstitial pattern can develop in the later stages. Withdrawal of the medication may be followed by slow but progressive roentgenographic resolution (Fig. 13–17). By dint of its low attenuation, the lipid nature of a pulmonary mass can sometimes be confirmed by computed tomography (CT).[142]

Clinical Manifestations

In most cases of mineral oil aspiration, the patient is asymptomatic and the abnormality is discovered on a screening chest roentgenogram; in fact, it is probable that the diagnosis is made most frequently by pathologists through histologic examination of tissue removed at thoracotomy performed on the basis of an erroneous diagnosis of pulmonary carcinoma.[139] Some patients complain of chronic cough and pleuritic pain.[139] If sufficient oil is aspirated over a long period, diffuse pulmonary fibrosis and eventually cor pulmonale may develop.[143, 144] The diagnosis may be suspected from a history of exposure to oily substances, particularly if obstructive esophageal disease is present. The finding of fat droplets in macrophages in the sputum[113] or BAL fluid[117] adds weight to the diagnosis, although fat can sometimes be identified in the sputum of normal subjects and its presence is not incontrovertible evidence of pulmonary disease. Two groups of workers[145, 146] have stressed the diagnostic value of the quantification of lipid-laden alveolar macrophages in fluid obtained by BAL. TTNA[142] or transbronchial biopsy will generally

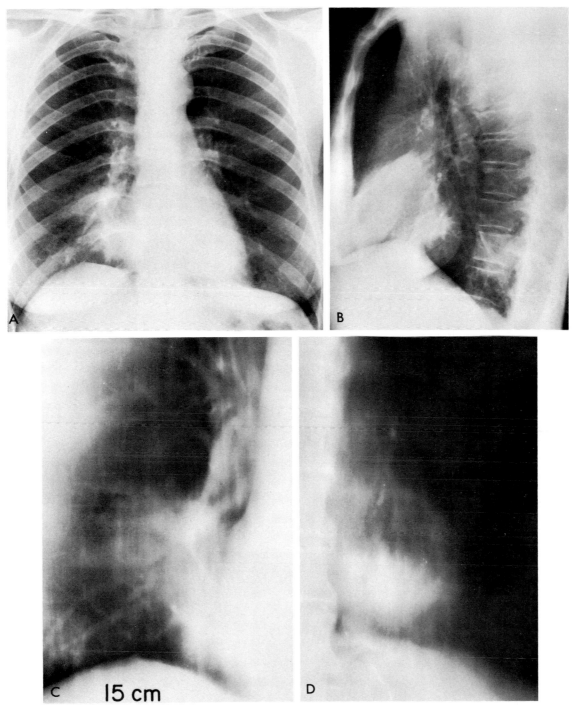

Figure 13–14. Exogenous Lipid Pneumonia. Posteroanterior *(A)* and lateral *(B)* roentgenograms of a 53-year-old asymptomatic woman reveal rather poorly defined shadows of homogeneous density situated in the right middle lobe, the anterior segment of the right lower lobe, and the posterior basal segment of the left lower lobe. Tomographic sections of the right and left lungs *(C and D)* in anteroposterior projection show the consolidations to better advantage. An air bronchogram can be identified in the left lesion. Thorough clinical and laboratory investigations failed to reveal the cause of these shadows. Ten years later, the patient died following rupture of a congenital berry aneurysm of the anterior cerebral artery. Necropsy revealed chronic lipid pneumonitis of both lower lobes and the right middle lobe.

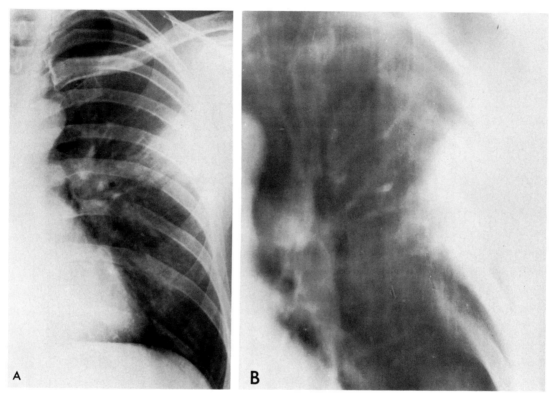

Figure 13–15. Exogenous Lipid Pneumonia. A 39-year-old aircraft mechanic whose main occupation involved the cleaning of aircraft engines with vaporized mineral oil was admitted to the hospital with a 3-week history of chest pain. The pain was sharp, steady, and severe and was located in the region of the apex of the heart; it was accentuated by coughing and deep breathing. There was no associated shortness of breath, cough, sputum, or hemoptysis. A view of the left hemithorax from a posteroanterior roentgenogram (A) (the right lung was clear) reveals a triangular shadow of homogeneous density lying in the axillary zone, possessing a rather indistinctly defined margin. A few line shadows extend from the mass toward the left hilum. An anteroposterior tomogram (B) shows the shadow to be somewhat better defined than was thought on the standard roentgenogram. The mass is homogeneous in density and shows neither cavitation nor calcification. All clinical and laboratory investigations proved negative, and the lobe was resected. Histologically, the appearance was typical of lipid pneumonitis. (Courtesy of St. Mary's Hospital, Montreal.)

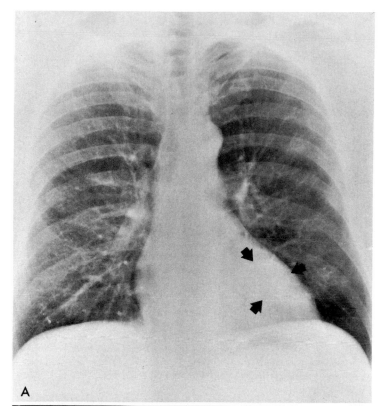

Figure 13–16. Exogenous Lipid Pneumonia Simulating Carcinoma. Posteroanterior *(A)* and lateral *(B)* roentgenograms reveal a poorly defined homogeneous opacity in the posterior portion of the left lower lobe *(arrows).*

Illustration continued on following page

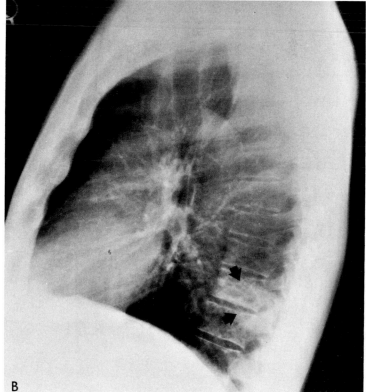

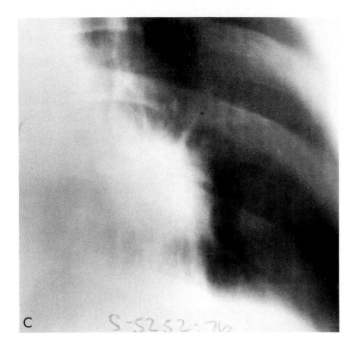

Figure 13–16 *Continued* A tomogram in anteroposterior projection *(C)* shows a multitude of linear strands extending outward into contiguous lung, creating an appearance usually identified with pulmonary carcinoma. The resected lobe revealed lipid pneumonia. The patient was an asymptomatic 42-year-old man who had used oily nose drops for many years.

establish the diagnosis with reasonable certainty; the latter procedure may be preferable, in that endoscopy will exclude the possibility of an obstructing neoplasm. A patient has been described[147] in whom lipid pneumonia caused by chronic aspiration of a "vaporizing ointment" was associated with hypercalcemia and with suppressed levels of parathyroid hormone and elevated levels of calcitriol in the serum; following surgical excision of the lesion, serum calcium and calcitriol levels rapidly returned to normal.

There is some evidence that the presence of mineral oil in the lungs is associated with an increased risk for the development of pulmonary carcinoma (*see* page 1337); however, in a study of a cohort of 792 men exposed to cutting fluids that contained mineral oil, the incidence of death from pulmonary carcinoma was not higher than in a nonexposed control population.[145]

There is a paucity of studies of pulmonary function in patients who have aspirated mineral oil. In one of the five patients described by Cullen and coworkers,[121] lung volumes were reduced and PaO_2 fell on exercise. Improvement in pulmonary function has been shown to correlate with the measured quantity of oil expectorated.[148]

ASPIRATION OF LIQUIDS

ASPIRATION OF WATER (NEAR-DROWNING)

Drowning can be defined as death caused by asphyxia as a result of submersion in liquid, providing the victim succumbs within 24 hours of the submersion episode. By contrast, near-drowning is defined as survival (at least temporarily) following a submersion episode; the term still applies if the victim dies more than 24 hours after the submersion episode. The term secondary near-drowning has been applied in those patients who die from complications of the initial submersion accident (e.g., superimposed infection). Orlowski[149] has suggested that this term be abandoned because it only adds confusion to an already confusing terminology. He suggests that the specific cause of death should be stated as a complication of a near-drowning incident.

Drowning is the third leading cause of death in children in the United States, following motor vehicle accidents and cancer. However, mortality rates fail to reflect the large morbidity from anoxic brain damage in near-drowning accidents: one-third of survivors of near-drowning are moderately to severely neurologically impaired. Near-drowning accidents are estimated to be 500 to 600 times more common than drowning, indicating the magnitude of the problem.[149]

Of the 1,587 drownings that occurred in Los Angeles County during the 9-year period 1976 to 1984, 44.5 per cent were in private swimming pools; the highest incidence of these was in children and toddlers between the ages of 1 and 3 years.[150] Near-drowning in the Australian surf is not uncommon, a high survival rate being attributable to the National Surf Life-Saving Association of Australia; the peak age range for drowning and near-drowning in Australia is 14 to 25 years rather than childhood.[151] A male predominance in near-drowning episodes is very strong, being 12:1 for boat-related submersions and 5:1 for those by other means.[152]

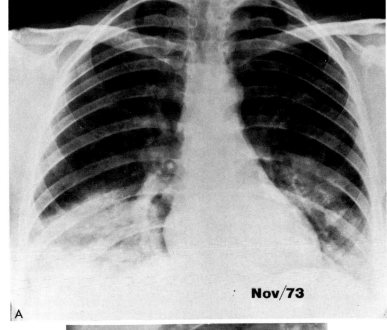

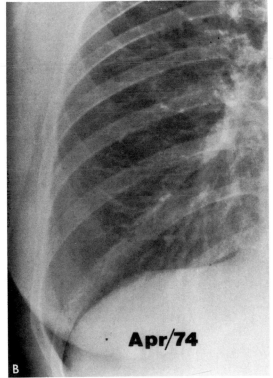

Figure 13–17. Exogenous Lipid Pneumonia with Complete Roentgenographic Resolution. For several years prior to the roentgenogram illustrated in (A), a asymptomatic middle-aged woman had been using oily nose drops many times a day for a stuffy nose. The roentgenogram reveals massive consolidation of both lower lung zones, the right more than the left. The consolidation is homogeneous except for a well-defined air bronchogram. Although the diagnosis of exogenous lipid pneumonia must be regarded as presumptive because a biopsy was not performed, the facts that the patient was asymptomatic and that oil droplets were identified in the sputum constitute reasonably convincing evidence. No treatment was given other than a change in the nose drops to a nonoily mixture. Six months later (B), all signs of pulmonary disease had disappeared. (Courtesy of Queen Elizabeth Hospital, Montreal, and Montreal Chest Hospital Center.)

Pathogenesis

In experimental animals the effects of inhaling sea water (which has about three times the tonicity of human extracellular fluid) differ from those of inhaling fresh water (whose salt content is negligible). By contrast, in humans there is little difference between the consequences of salt water and fresh water inhalation, both causing severe hypoxemia and acidosis. There is no convincing evidence that other factors such as hemodilution (secondary to fresh water inhalation) and hemoconcentration (secondary to salt water inhalation) have a significant modulating effect. The importance of the tonicity of the aspirated fluid in animals was dramatically illustrated by Klystra,[153] who showed that mice submerged in suitably oxygenated physiologic saline solution could survive for 18 hours, whereas if this medium was replaced by sea water or tap water the mice succumbed in less than 12 minutes. A practical application of this observation is that in Denmark some swimming pools are reported to be filled with isotonic saline solution rather than fresh water! However, Klystra[154] has theorized that whereas oxygenation of blood by human lungs breathing suitably oxygenated saline would be adequate, it is almost certain that carbon dioxide could not be eliminated at the necessary rate, even in the total absence of physical effort.

DRY DROWNING

In an individual whose laryngeal reflexes are brisk, spasm may prevent inhalation of water. If the spasm is maintained until the resulting cerebral anoxia causes paralysis of the respiratory center, the individual can lose consciousness without entrance of water into the lung. Because persons in whom this occurs are the group that has the highest recovery rate and is undoubtedly the one containing many cases that are not reported, it is difficult to estimate the number of victims who experience dry drowning; the incidence has been reported to range from 20 to 40 per cent[155] and from 10 to 15 per cent.[156] Clinically, patients present a picture of simple asphyxia.

So-called dry drowning may be related to the presence in humans of a "diving reflex." The full-blown diving reflex occurs in certain birds and mammals that customarily dive for their food; they develop marked bradycardia and a redistribution of cardiac output away from hypoxia-resistant organs. The human diving reflex is probably most active in the young, which may explain their higher incidence of complete neurologic recovery following near-drowning, especially in cold water.[157]

NEAR-DROWNING IN SEA WATER

In near-drowning in either sea or fresh water, there is usually a period of apnea and struggling, which may be followed by violent inspiratory effort.

Water enters the mouth and at first is swallowed in large quantities and then is inhaled. Both tonicity and volume have considerable bearing on the outcome, at least in the experimental animal. Modell and Moya[158] showed in dogs that the chance of survival was very small if the volume of sea water inhaled exceeded 10 ml/pound body weight, the critical volume of fresh water being 20 ml/pound. These figures correspond to about 1.5 and 3 liters, respectively, for 70 kg humans.[159] Because its tonicity is greater than that of blood, when sea water enters the alveoli of an experimental animal, water is drawn out of the blood into the alveoli, and ions of sodium, magnesium, calcium, and chloride pass into the blood.[155] At the same time there is a transfer of protein into the alveoli. All of these movements result in rapid hemoconcentration and hypovolemia. There follows a slowing of the pulse, a fall in blood pressure, and death in 4 to 5 minutes from hypoxemia and metabolic acidosis. In humans, pulmonary edema is almost invariable, being observed roentgenographically in 27 of 32 patients studied by Hasan and colleagues.[160] In the latter group of sea water victims, serum electrolyte changes were minimal, including slight hypokalemia in 17 patients and minimal elevation of serum sodium in approximately 25 per cent of patients.

NEAR-DROWNING IN FRESH WATER

In experimental animals, when fresh water enters the alveoli the situation is reversed. Because of the blood's greater tonicity, inhaled water is immediately absorbed into the circulation, producing marked hemodilution and hemolysis of red cells. In the experiments on dogs carried out by Modell and Moya,[158] inhalation of 20 ml of fresh water per pound body weight raised the free hemoglobin in the plasma to about 1.5 gm/dl, which represents about 10 per cent of total blood hemoglobin; blood volume rose by approximately 50 per cent. In experimental near-drowning in fresh water, serum potassium levels rise considerably and serum sodium levels fall; both changes may be factors in causing ventricular fibrillation. However, changes in plasma sodium and potassium levels tend to be transient and maximal at 3 to 5 minutes after immersion.[159]

As pointed out by Miles,[155] the theoretical and experimental differences between the effects of inhalation of salt and fresh water have tended to confuse the issue as far as humans are concerned, because complete investigations are seldom made during recovery. Where it has been possible to carry out such examinations, no evidence of significant electrolyte transfer, hemoconcentration, or hemodilution has been found.[161] Similarly, no clinical differences are seen between fresh water and salt water drowning victims.[162]

Although there is no conclusive evidence regarding the exact sequence of events that occurs in humans when water is inhaled, it is not the same as that observed in experimental animals. It is clear that water entering the alveoli must act as an irritant, whatever its tonicity and whichever way electrolytes flow, and such irritation could quite possibly cause increased permeability of pulmonary capillaries. In both fresh and salt water drowning, there is considerable loss of protein from the blood, manifested pathologically in fatal cases by hyaline membrane formation in the alveoli and clinically by the characteristic foam found in the airways. In a study of ultrastructure of pulmonary alveolar capillaries in Mendelson's syndrome, Alexander[163] examined the lungs of experimental animals into which solutions of varying pH and tonicity had been instilled. Pulmonary edema was present in all specimens, including those in which distilled water was the aspirated fluid. The pH and tonicity increased the reaction only in terms of degree and time, suggesting to Sladen and Zauder[164] that the pathologic process caused by fresh water aspiration is similar to that produced by acid aspiration and that the major mechanism must be increased capillary permeability. In the cases studied by Fuller,[161] morphologic evidence of pulmonary parenchymal damage was seen in all victims whether they survived for a few minutes or for several days; hemorrhagic, desquamative, and exudative reactions developed even in those patients who survived only a few minutes. A polymorphonuclear inflammatory response may occur with extreme rapidity, as in the case described by Heitzman.[165]

In many cases, the water inhaled contains debris such as small marine organisms, sand, mud, fuel oil, sewage, and other pollutants, all of which increase the hazard to the lungs. These substances can directly cause pulmonary injury and an inflammatory cellular reaction;[166] as a result, deterioration in clinical status may follow initial improvement. For example, a patient who has recovered consciousness and seems to be progressing favorably may, within a few hours, show increasing respiratory distress with progressive restlessness, breathlessness, pain in the chest, cyanosis, and cough. It is probable that the major causes of this deterioration are progressive pulmonary edema, ARDS, and pneumonia resulting from toxic debris. Sand that is aspirated along with water can be radiopaque as a result of its calcium carbonate content, and can cause a "sand bronchogram";[167] bronchoscopic removal of the sand can result in prompt clinical improvement.

Roentgenographic Manifestations

The roentgenographic changes in near-drowning have been reviewed extensively by Rosenbaum and colleagues[168] and more recently by Hunter and Whitehouse[169] and Putman and colleagues.[170] Hunter and Whitehouse[169] addressed the roentgenographic aspects of fresh water near-drowning only,

but the report of 36 patients by Hasan and colleagues[160] revealed no significant differences in the roentgenographic picture between fresh and sea water aspiration. The basic roentgenographic finding is one of pulmonary edema (Fig. 13–18), the severity presumably depending upon the amount of water inhaled; in the most severe cases there is almost complete opacification of both lungs. Airspace edema is generally bilateral and symmetric but in less severe cases can be predominantly parahilar and midzonal. Three of the 16 patients studied by Hunter and Whitehouse[169] showed no roentgenographic abnormality and presumably represented examples of "dry near-drowning"; the remaining 13 patients showed pulmonary edema that improved rather quickly over 3 to 5 days and resolved completely in 7 to 10 days. These authors noted that once resolution had begun, the radiographic findings often disappeared in as little as 12 to 24 hours. In four of the 36 patients described by Hasan and colleagues,[160] the roentgenographic changes persisted or worsened, findings that were consistent with the clinical diagnosis of bacterial pneumonia, with or without ARDS (Fig. 13–19). Putman and colleagues[170] emphasized the delay observed in some patients before there is roentgenographic evidence of pulmonary edema, sometimes as long as 24 to 48 hours.

Clinical Manifestations

According to Miles,[155] the period between the onset of respiratory failure and cardiac arrest rarely exceeds 3 to 4 minutes. The resulting cerebral hypoxia results in cerebral edema that can have prolonged after-effects. It is apparent that when prolonged submersion occurs in cold water, chances of survival are improved, possibly because the hypothermia serves to protect the brain from hypoxic injury. For example, at least 28 cases of recovery with intact neurologic faculties have been reported after submersion in ice-cold water for 15 minutes or more. In all these cases, water temperature was below 10° C and often below 5° C, and the patients were hypothermic. One report documents a 2½-year-old girl who had complete neurologic recovery after submersion in ice cold water for approximately 66 minutes.[152]

The most important clinical consequence of near-drowning is severe hypoxemia caused by shunting of blood through airless lung parenchyma. Whether the shunt is related to diffuse alveolar damage caused by hypertonic salt water or to diffuse atelectasis resulting from surfactant disruption from fresh water, the consequences are similar.[171]

Hasan and colleagues[160] reviewed in detail the clinical manifestations in 36 patients with near-drowning, 32 in salt water and four in chlorinated pools. Ages ranged from 3 to 89 years, and 33 of the 36 survived. Only nine of the 36 patients were unconscious on arrival at the hospital. Respiratory

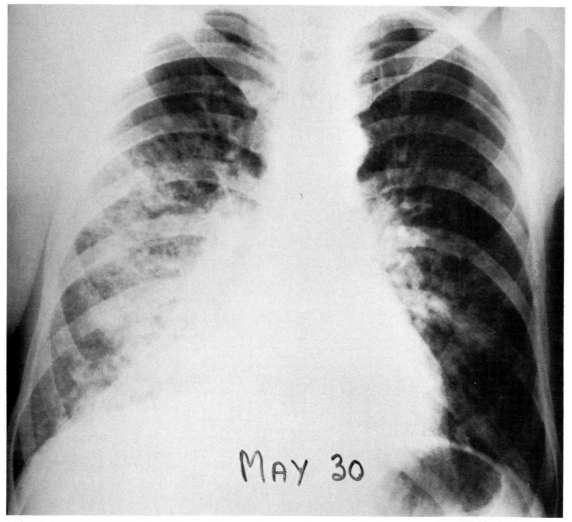

Figure 13–18. Near-Drowning in Sea Water.   The man whose roentgenogram is shown was immersed for an indeterminate time in sea water. There is evidence of extensive bilateral airspace edema, more marked in the right than the left lung. The edema cleared in 3 days. (Courtesy of Yale University, New Haven, Connecticut.)

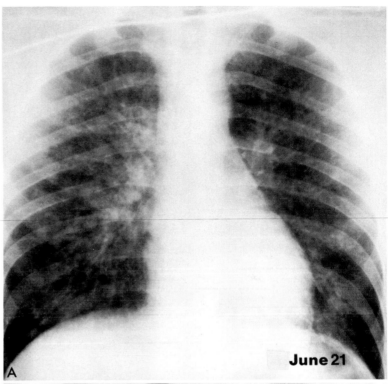

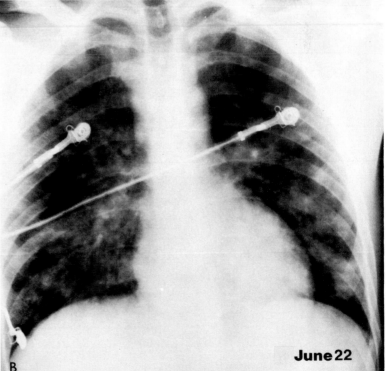

Figure 13–19. Near-Drowning in Fresh Water. A 19-year-old man was immersed in a dirty, badly polluted, fresh-water lake for a period of about 4 minutes before being rescued; he was under the influence of drugs at the time. The roentgenogram obtained shortly after his arrival in the emergency department *(A)* reveals widespread patchy airspace consolidation evenly distributed throughout both lungs. Heart size and configuration are normal. Twenty-four hours later *(B),* the upper zones of both lungs had cleared considerably, although moderate edema persists in the lower zones.

Illustration continued on following page

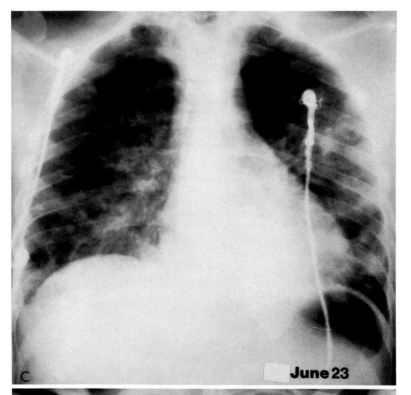

June 23

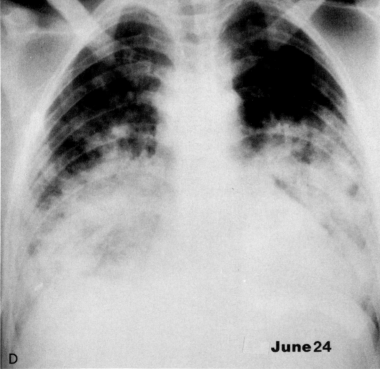

June 24

Figure 13–19. *Continued.* Forty-eight hours later *(C)*, the edema appeared to have worsened somewhat in the lower zones. Three days after the acute episode *(D)*, massive airspace consolidation had developed throughout the lower two-thirds of both lungs, and the patient's clinical status had deteriorated markedly. This represents the characteristic sequence of events following near-drowning in badly polluted water and the development of acute pneumonia caused by chemicals and debris.

frequency was generally increased to between 30 and 40 breaths per minute during the initial 24 hours, and thereafter it returned to normal levels. Only one patient had hemoptysis. Fine inspiratory crackles were heard in all patients, and wheezing was noted in a few. In 11 patients, the electrocardiogram showed nonspecific S-T segment and T-wave changes, abnormal patterns that reverted to normal within 36 hours. Severe hypoxemia was a constant finding, mean PaO_2 being 55 mm Hg (SD ± 0.17), and base excess − 10 mEq/liter (SD ± 9). Of the three patients who died, one developed pneumonia 2 days after admission, one showed refractory pulmonary edema 2 hours after admission, and the third patient was dead on arrival, the cause of death being unknown. The metabolic acidosis is presumably caused by the formation of lactic acid in the hypoxic tissues of a person struggling to survive. Respiratory acidosis is usually not observed in near-drowning patients, probably because victims are artificially ventilated before initial arterial blood gas samples are drawn in the hospital.[160] Although most patients recover completely, a few manifest roentgenographic evidence of persistent fibrosis and linear opacities months after recovery.[172]

Serum electrolyte abnormalities have been reported in near-drowning victims from the Dead Sea, in which electrolyte concentration is extremely high;[173] sodium content is some three times higher than ordinary sea water, whereas the potassium, calcium, and magnesium concentrations are 15, 36, and 26 times higher than Mediterranean sea water. Yagil and associates[173] have reported eight cases of men drowning in the Dead Sea in whom significant hypernatremia, hypercalcemia, and hypermagnesemia were thought to have contributed to death, perhaps as a result of cardiac arrhythmias. Hypoglycemia has also been reported in near-drowning victims.[174]

The prognosis in patients with near-drowning has been reviewed by Modell and associates on the basis of a retrospective study of 91 victims, 81 of whom survived.[175] Patients who were alert on arrival in the emergency room survived, but those who were comatose and whose pupils were fixed and dilated invariably died. All patients with normal chest roentgenograms survived, although several had significant hypoxemia. Only two of the survivors manifested residual neurologic damage.

Few patients have had pulmonary function testing following near-drowning; in one study of two individuals, an initial restrictive ventilatory pattern and abnormal gas exchange resolved completely over a 16-week follow-up period.[176] In another study, ten asymptomatic children were examined a mean of 3.3 years after submersion accidents: only mild abnormalities of peripheral airway dysfunction were detected; however, seven of the ten demonstrated bronchial hyper-responsiveness to inhaled methacholine.[177]

Finally, it is important to remember that individuals with near-drowning following a dive into shallow water must be suspected of having head or cervical spine injuries.[178]

ASPIRATION OF HYPERTONIC CONTRAST MEDIA

A number of reports have appeared in the literature describing the development of acute pulmonary edema following aspiration of water-soluble contrast media,[179–181] commonly in patients with chronic pulmonary disease. This fact should alert radiologists to exercise caution in employing water-soluble media in circumstances in which there is danger of aspiration. This subject is dealt with in detail in Chapter 14.

ASPIRATION OF MISCELLANEOUS LIQUIDS

Aspiration of *alcohol* in various concentrations has been studied experimentally by Moran and Hellstrom:[182] in the early stages, they found parenchymal edema, hemorrhage, and hyaline membranes consistent with diffuse alveolar damage; in animals that survived for 1 to 4 weeks there was a prominent bronchiolitis obliterans. Pure *carbohydrate solutions*, if administered to rabbits in sufficient quantity and concentration, have been shown to cause edema, acute pneumonia, and fibrosis.[183] Experimental aspiration of *kerosene* causes pulmonary congestion and focal bronchopneumonia accompanied by a shift to the left of the static pressure-volume curve and an increase in total lung capacity.[93]

REFERENCES

1. Davis CM: Inhaled foreign bodies in children. An analysis of 40 cases. Arch Dis Child 41:402, 1966.
2. Weissberg D, Schwartz I: Foreign bodies in the tracheobronchial tree. Chest 91:730, 1987.
3. Keith FM, Charrette EJP, Lynn RB, et al: Inhalation of foreign bodies by children: A continuing challenge in management. Can Med Assoc J 122:52, 1980.
4. Mittleman RE: Fatal choking in infants and children. Am J Forensic Med Pathol 5:201, 1984.
5. Jackson C: Observations on the pathology of foreign bodies in the air and food passages. Based on the analysis of 628 cases. Surg Gynecol Obstet 28:201, 1919.
6. Henry WJ, Miscall L: Rapidly reversible atelectasis due to change in position. J Thorac Cardiovasc Surg 41:686, 1961.
7. Blazer S, Naveh Y, Friedman A: Foreign body in the airway. A review of 200 cases. Am J Dis Child 134:68, 1980.
8. Abdulmajid OA, Ebeid AM, Motaweh MM, et al: Aspirated foreign bodies in the tracheobronchial tree: Report of 250 cases. Thorax 31:635, 1976.
9. Jewett TC Jr, Butsch WL: Trials with treacherous timothy grass. J Thorac Cardiovasc Surg 50:124, 1965.
10. Merriam JC Jr, Storrs RC, Hoefnagel D: Lung disease caused by aspirated timothy-grass heads. Am Rev Respir Dis 90:947, 1964.
11. Godfrey RC: The behaviour of inhaled grass inflorescences. Lancet 2:273, 1957.
12. Pneumocutaneous fistula secondary to aspiration of grass (letter). J Pediatr 82:737, 1973.
13. Hilman BC, Kurzweg FT, McCook WW Jr, et al: Foreign body aspiration of grass inflorescences as a cause of hemoptysis. Chest 78:306, 1980.
14. Jackson C, Jackson CL: Staples and double-pointed tacks as foreign bodies: Mechanical problems of bronchoscopic extraction. Arch Otolaryngol 22:603, 1935.
15. Pochaczevsky R, Leonidas JC, Feldman F, et al: Aspirated and ingested teeth in children. Clin Radiol 24:349, 1973.
16. Mearns AJ, England RM: Dissolving foreign bodies in the trachea and bronchus. Thorax 30:461, 1975.
17. Chopra S, Simmons DH, Cassan SM, et al: Case reports. Bronchial obstruction by incorporation of aspirated vegetable material in the bronchial wall. Am Rev Respir Dis 112:717, 1975.
18. Weiss E, Krusen FH: Foreign body in the lung for thirty-five years complicated by abscess and tumor formation. JAMA, Feb. 18, 1922, p 506 (Vol 78).
19. Tarkka M, Anttila S, Sutinen S: Bronchial stenosis after aspiration of an iron tablet. Chest 93:439, 1988.
20. Brown BS, Ma H, Dunbar JS, et al: Foreign bodies in the tracheobronchial tree in childhood. J Can Assoc Radiol 14:158, 1963.
21. Cleveland RH: Symmetry of bronchial angles in children. Radiology 133:89, 1979.
22. Capitanio MA, Kirkpatrick JA: The lateral decubitus film: An aid in determining air-trapping in children. Radiology 103:460, 1972.
23. Berger PE, Kuhn JP, Kuhns LR: Computed tomography and the occult tracheobronchial foreign body. Radiology 134:133, 1980.
24. Rudavsky AZ, Leonidas JC, Abramson AL: Lung scanning for the detection of endobronchial foreign bodies in infants and children: Clinical and experimental studies. Radiology 108:629, 1973.
25. Miller GA, Gianturco C, Neucks HG: The asymptomatic period in retained foreign bodies of the bronchus. AMA J Dis Child 95:282, 1958.
26. Kürklü EU, Williams MA, le Roux BT: Bronchiectasis consequent upon foreign body retention. Thorax 28:601, 1973.
27. Leading article: Inhaled foreign bodies. Br Med J 282:1649, 1981.
28. Berkmen YM: Aspiration and inhalation pneumonias. Semin Roentgenol 15:73, 1980.
29. Mittleman RE: The fatal café coronary. JAMA 247:1285, 1982.
30. Irwin RS, Ashba JK, Braman SS, et al: Food asphyxiation in hospitalized patients. JAMA 237:2744, 1977.
31. Hsieh HH, Bhatia SC, Andersen JM, et al: Psychotropic medication and nonfatal cafe coronary. J Clin Psychopharmacol 6:101, 1986.
32. Mittleman M, Perek J, Kolkov Z, et al: Fatal aspiration pneumonia caused by an esophageal foreign body. Ann Emerg Med 14:365, 1985.
33. Northcote RJ: Pulmonary aspiration presenting with generalized convulsions. Scott Med J 28:368, 1983.
34. Ristagno RL, Kornstein MJ, Hansen-Flaschen JH: Diagnosis of occult meat aspiration by fiberoptic bronchoscopy. Am J Med 80:154, 1986.
35. Montoya D: Management of the choking victim. Can Med Assoc J 135:305, 1986.
36. Heimlich HJ, Uhley MH, Netter FH: The Heimlich maneuver. Clin Symp 31:1, 1979.
37. Roehm EF, Twiest MW, Williams RC Jr: Abdominal aortic thrombosis in association with an attempted Heimlich maneuver. JAMA 249:1186, 1983.
38. Croom DW: Rupture of stomach after attempted Heimlich maneuver (Letter). JAMA 250:2602, 1983.
39. Feldman T, Mallon SM, Bolooki H, et al: Fatal acute aortic regurgitation in a person performing the Heimlich maneuver (Letter). N Engl J Med 315:1613, 1986.
40. Alessi DM, Berci G: Aspiration and nasogastric intubation. Otolaryngol Head Neck Surg 94:486, 1986.
41. Miller KS, Tomlinson JR, Sahn SA: Pleuropulmonary complications of enteral tube feedings. Two reports, review of the literature, and recommendations. Chest 88:230, 1985.
42. Burtch GD, Shatney CH: Feeding gastrostomy. Assistant or assassin? Am Surg 51:204, 1985.
43. Cole MJ, Smith JT, Molnar C, et al: Aspiration after percutaneous gastrostomy. Assessment by Tc-99m labeling of the enteral feed. J Clin Gastroenterol 9:90, 1987.
44. Rutishauser M: Die maligne lungencaverne. (The malignant pulmonary cavity.) Schweiz Med Wochenschr 95:349, 1965.
45. McCormick PW, Hay RG, Griffin RW: Pulmonary aspiration of gastric contents in obstetric patients. A report of two patients treated by artificial ventilation. Lancet 1:1127, 1966.
46. Berris B, Kasler D: Pulmonary aspiration of gastric acid: Mendelson's syndrome. Can Med Assoc J 92:905, 1965.
47. Gallagher JD, Smith DS, Meranze J, et al: Aspiration during induction of anaesthesia in patients with colon interposition. Can Anaesth Soc J 32:56, 1985.
48. Cameron JL, Zuidema GD: Aspiration pneumonia. Magnitude and frequency of the problem. JAMA 219:1194, 1972.
49. Dines DE, Titus JL, Sessler AD: Aspiration pneumonitis. Mayo Clin Proc 45:347, 1970.
50. Aspiration pneumonitis (Editorial). (Massachusetts Medical Society, Committee on Maternal Welfare.) N Engl J Med 286:487, 1972.
51. Nicholl RM, Holland EL, Brown SS: Mendelson's syndrome: Its treatment by tracheostomy and hydrocortisone. Br Med J 2:745, 1967.
52. Lawes EG, Baskett PJ: Pulmonary aspiration during unsuccessful cardiopulmonary resuscitation. Intensive Care Med 13:379, 1987.
53. Fetterman GH, Moran TJ: Food aspiration pneumonia. Penn Med J 45:810, 1942.
54. Knoblich R: Pulmonary granulomatosis caused by vegetable particles. So-called lentil pulse pneumonia. Am Rev Respir Dis 99:380, 1969.
55. Hughes RL, Freilich RA, Bytell DE, et al: Aspiration and occult esophageal disorders: Clinical conference in pulmonary disease from Northwestern University Medical School; Chicago. Chest 80:489, 1981.
56. Christie DL, O'Grady LR, Mack DV: Incompetent lower esophageal sphincter and gastroesophageal reflux in recurrent acute pulmonary disease of infancy and childhood. J Pediatr 93:23, 1978.
57. Hillemeir C, Buchin PJ, Gryboski J: Esophageal dysfunction in Down's syndrome. J Pediatr Gastroenterol Nutr 1:101, 1982.
58. McArthur MS: Pulmonary complications of benign esophageal disease. Am J Surg 151:296, 1986.
59. Donald IP, Gear MW, Wilkinson SP: A life-threatening respiratory complication of gastro-oesophageal reflux in a patient with tetraplegia. Postgrad Med J 63:397, 1987.
60. Camara EJ, Lima JAC, Oliveira GB, et al: Pulmonary findings in patients with chagasic megaesophagus. Study of autopsied cases. Chest 83:87, 1983.
61. Hrabovsky EE, Mullett MD: Patterns of pediatric gastroesophageal reflux. Am Surg 51:212, 1985.
62. Olson NR: The problem of gastroesophageal reflux. Otolaryngol Clin North Am 19:119, 1986.
63. Barish CF, Wu WC, Castell DO: Respiratory complications of gastroesophageal reflux. Arch Intern Med 145:1882, 1985.
64. Hoyoux C, Forget P, Lambrechts L, et al: Chronic bronchopulmonary disease and gastroesophageal reflux in children. Pediatr Pulmonol 1:149, 1985.

65. Ekberg O, Hilderfors H: Defective closure of the laryngeal vestibule: Frequency of pulmonary complications. AJR 145:1159, 1985.
66. McVeagh P, Howman-Giles R, Kemp A: Pulmonary aspiration studied by radionuclide milk scanning and barium swallow roentgenography. Am J Dis Child 141:917, 1987.
67. Crausaz FM, Favez G: Aspiration of solid food particles into lungs of patients with gastroesophageal reflux and chronic bronchial disease. Chest 93:376, 1988.
68. Euler AR, Byrne WJ, Ament ME, et al: Recurrent pulmonary disease in children: A complication of gastroesophageal reflux. Pediatrics 63:47, 1979.
69. Hoyoux C, Forget P, Garzaniti N, et al: Is the macroscopic aspect of the esophagus at endoscopy indicative of reflux esophagitis? Endoscopy 18:4, 1986.
70. Orringer MB: Respiratory symptoms and esophageal reflux. Chest 76:618, 1979.
71. Harper PC, Bergner A, Kaye MD: Antireflux treatment for asthma. Improvement in patients with associated gastroesophageal reflux. Arch Intern Med 147:56, 1987.
72. Davis MV: Evolving concepts regarding hiatus hernia and gastroesophageal reflux. Ann Thorac Surg 7:120, 1969.
73. Pearson JEG, Wilson RSE: Diffuse pulmonary fibrosis and hiatus hernia. Thorax 26:300, 1971.
74. Mays EE, Dubois JJ, Hamilton GB: Pulmonary fibrosis associated with tracheobronchial aspiration. A study of the frequency of hiatal hernia and gastroesophageal reflux in interstitial pulmonary fibrosis of obscure etiology. Chest 69:512, 1976.
75. Vraney GA, Pokorny C: Pulmonary function in patients with gastroesophageal reflux. Chest 76:678, 1979.
76. Culver GA, Makel HP, Beecher HK: Frequency of aspiration of gastric contents by lungs during anesthesia and surgery. Ann Surg 133:289, 1951.
77. Pruzanski W, Profis A: Pulmonary disease and myotonic dystrophy. Am Rev Respir Dis 91:874, 1965.
78. Baker GL, Heublein GW: Postoperative aspiration pneumonitis. Am J Roentgenol 80:42, 1958.
79. Taylor G, Pryse-Davies J: The prophylactic use of antacids in the prevention of the acid-pulmonary-aspiration syndrome (Mendelson's syndrome). Lancet 1:288, 1966.
80. Chen CT, Toung TJ, Haupt HM, et al: Evaluation of the efficacy of Alka-Seltzer Effervescent in gastric acid neutralization. Anesth Analg 63:325, 1984.
81. Gipson SL, Stovall TG, Elkins TE, et al: Pharmacologic reduction of the risk of aspiration. South Med J 79:1356, 1986.
82. Harris PW, Morison DH, Dunn GL, et al: Intramuscular cimetidine and ranitidine as prophylaxis against gastric aspiration syndrome: A randomized double-blind study. Can Anaesth Soc J 31:599, 1984.
83. Manchikanti L, Grow JB, Colliver JA, et al: Bicitra (sodium citrate) and metoclopramide in outpatient anesthesia for prophylaxis against aspiration pneumonitis. Anesthesiology 63:378, 1985.
84. Cimetidine and the acid-aspiration syndrome (Editorial). Lancet 1:465, 1980.
85. Robinson JS, Thompson JM: Fatal aspiration (Mendelson's) syndrome despite antacids and cricoid pressure. Lancet 2:228, 1979.
86. MacLennan FM: Maternal mortality from Mendelson's syndrome: An explanation? Lancet 1:587, 1986.
87. Vidyarthi SC: Diffuse miliary granulomatosis of the lungs due to aspirated vegetable cells. Arch Pathol 83:215, 1967.
88. Teabeaut JR II: Aspiration of gastric contents: An experimental study. Am J Pathol 28:51, 1952.
89. Schwartz DJ, Wynne JW, Gibbs CP, et al: The pulmonary consequences of aspiration of gastric contents at pH values greater than 2.5. Am Rev Respir Dis 121:119, 1980.
90. Bond VK, Stoelting RK, Gupta CD: Pulmonary aspiration syndrome after inhalation of gastric fluid containing antacids. Anesthesiology 51:452, 1979.
91. Wynne JW, Reynolds JC, Hood I, et al: Steroid therapy for pneumonitis induced in rabbits by aspiration of foodstuff. Anesthesiology 51:11, 1979.
92. Alexander IGS: The ultrastructure of the pulmonary alveolar vessels in Mendelson's (acid pulmonary aspiration) syndrome. Br J Anaesth 40:408, 1968.
93. Scharf SM, Heimer D, Goldstein J: Pathologic and physiologic effects of aspiration of hydrocarbons in the rat. Am Rev Respir Dis 124:625, 1981.
94. Moran TJ: Experimental food-aspiration pneumonia. AMA Arch Pathol 52:350, 1951.
95. Moran TJ: Experimental aspiration pneumonia: IV. Inflammatory and reparative changes produced by intratracheal injections of autologous gastric juice and hydrochloric acid. AMA Arch Pathol 60:122, 1955.
96. Crome L, Valentine JC: Pulmonary nodular granulomatosis caused by inhaled vegetable particles. J Clin Pathol 15:21, 1962.
97. Ros PR: Lentil aspiration pneumonia (Letter). JAMA 251:1277, 1984.
98. Quinn LH, Meyer OO: The relationship of sinusitis and bronchiectasis. Arch Otolaryngol 10:152, 1929.
99. Landay MJ, Christensen EE, Bynum LJ: Pulmonary manifestations of acute aspiration of gastric contents. Am J Roentgenol 131:587, 1978.
100. Nördenstrom B: Bronchography by aspiration of contrast media. Acta Radiol 44:281, 1955.
101. Priviteri CA: Physiological bronchography. Am J Roentgenol 73:958, 1955.
102. Brock RC, Hodgkiss F, Jones HO: Bronchial embolism and posture in relation to lung abscess. Guy's Hosp Rep 91:131, 1948.
103. Coriat P, Labrousse J, Vilde F, et al: Diffuse interstitial pneumonitis due to aspiration of gastric contents. Anaesthesia 39:703, 1984.
104. Manchikanti L, Colliver JA, Marrero TC, et al: Assessment of age-related acid aspiration risk factors in pediatric, adult, and geriatric patients. Anesth Analg 64:11, 1985.
105. MacRae W, Wallace P: Aspiration around high-volume, low-pressure endotracheal cuff. Br Med J 283:1220, 1981.
106. Campinos L, Duval G, Couturier M, et al: The value of early fibreoptic bronchoscopy after aspiration of gastric contents. Br J Anaesth 55:1103, 1983.
107. Wolfe JE, Bone RC, Ruth WE: Effects of corticosteroids in the treatment of patients with gastric aspiration. Am J Med 63:719, 1977.
108. Brandstetter RD, Conetta R, Sander NW, et al: Adult respiratory distress syndrome in adolescents due to aspiration of gastric contents. NY State J Med 86:513, 1986.
109. Sladen A, Zanca P, Hadnott WH: Aspiration pneumonitis: The sequelae. Chest 59:448, 1971.
110. Baer M, Maki M, Nurminen J, et al: Esophagitis and findings of long-term esophageal pH recording in children with repeated lower respiratory tract symptoms. J Pediatr Gastroenterol Nutr 5:187, 1986.
111. Baimbridge MV, Keith HI: Oesophago-bronchial fistula in the adult. Thorax 20:226, 1965.
112. Sacks RP, Du Bois JJ, Geiger JP, et al: The esophagobronchial fistula. Case report and review of the literature. Am J Roentgenol 99:204, 1967.
113. Sundberg RH, Kirschner KE, Brown MJ: Evaluation of lipid pneumonia. Dis Chest 36:594, 1959.
114. Robbins LL, Sniffen RC: Correlation between the roentgenologic and pathologic findings in chronic pneumonitis of the cholesterol type. Radiology 53:187, 1949.
115. Genereux GP: Lipids in the lungs: Radiologic-pathologic correlation. J Can Assoc Radiol 21:2, 1970.
116. Borrie J, Gwynne JF: Paraffinoma of lung: Lipoid pneumonia. Report of two cases. Thorax 28:214, 1973.
117. Spatafora M, Bellia V, Ferrara G, et al: Diagnosis of a case of lipoid pneumonia by bronchoalveolar lavage. Respiration 52:154, 1987.
118. Blondal T, Hartvig P, Bengtsson A, et al: An unnecessary case of paraffin oil pneumonia. Acta Med Scand 213:227, 1983.
119. McBurney RP, Jamplis RW, Hedberg G: Oil granuloma and lipoid pneumonitis: A complication of oleothorax. J Thorac Surg 29:271, 1955.
120. Jones JG: An investigation into the effects of exposure to an oil mist in workers in a mill for the cold reduction of steel strip. Ann Occup Hyg 3:264, 1961.
121. Cullen MR, Balmes JR, Robins JM, et al: Lipoid pneumonia caused by oil mist from a steel rolling tandem mill. Am J Ind Med 2:51, 1981.
122. Foe RB, Bigham RS Jr: Lipid pneumonia following occupational exposure to oil spray. JAMA 155:33, 1954.
123. Bushman JA, Clark PA: Oil mist hazard in piped air supplies. Br Med J 3:588, 1967.
124. Miller GJ, Ashcroft MT, Beadnell HMSG, et al: The lipoid pneumonia of blackfat tobacco smokers in Guyana. Q J Med 40:457, 1971.
125. Becton DL, Lowe JE, Falletta JM: Lipoid pneumonia in an adolescent girl secondary to use of lip gloss. J Pediatr 105:421, 1984.
126. Scully RE, Galdabini JJ, McNeely BU: Case 19–1977. Lipoid pneumonia. N Eng J Med 296:1105, 1977.
127. Balakrishman S: Lipoid pneumonia in infants and children in South India. Br Med J 4:329, 1973.
128. Oldenberger D, Maurer WJ, Beltaos E, et al: Inhalation lipoid pneumonia from burning fats. A newly recognized industrial hazard. JAMA 222:1288, 1972.
129. Pinkerton H: The reaction to oils and fats in the lung. Arch Pathol 5:380, 1928.
130. Timmerman RJ, Schroe JA: Lipoid pneumonia caused by methenamide mandelate suspension. JAMA 225:1524, 1973.
131. Felton WL II: The reaction of pulmonary tissue to lipiodol. J Thorac Surg 25:530, 1953.
132. Moran TJ: Milk-aspiration pneumonia in human and animal subjects. AMA Arch Pathol 55:286, 1953.

13

133. Wagner JC, Adler DI, Fuller DN: Foreign body granulomata of the lungs due to liquid paraffin. Thorax 10:157, 1955.
134. Fox B: Liquid paraffin pneumonia—with chemical analysis and electronmicroscopy. Virchows Arch 382:339, 1979.
135. Heckers H, Melcher F-W, Dittmar K, et al: Paraffin oil pneumonia. Analysis of saturated hydrocarbons in different human tissue. J Chromatogr 146:91, 1978.
136. Levade T, Salvayre R, Dongay G, et al: Chemical analysis of the bronchoalveolar washing fluid in the diagnosis of liquid paraffin pneumonia. J Clin Chem Clin Biochem 25:45, 1987.
137. Forbes G, Bradley A: Liquid paraffin as a cause of oil aspiration pneumonia. Br Med J 2:1566, 1958.
138. Eyal Z, Borman JB, Milwidsky H: Solitary oil granuloma of the lung. A report of three cases. Br J Dis Chest 55:43, 1961.
139. Guidry LD, Clagett OT, McDonald JR, et al: Pulmonary resection for mineral oil granulomas. Ann Surg 150:67, 1959.
140. Kennedy JD, Costello P, Balikian JP, et al: Exogenous lipoid pneumonia. AJR 136:1145, 1981.
141. Salm R, Hughes EW: A case of chronic paraffin pneumonitis. Thorax 25:762, 1970.
142. Wheeler PS, Stitik FP, Hutchins GM, et al: Diagnosis of lipoid pneumonia by computed tomography. JAMA 245:65, 1981.
143. Steinberg I, Finby N: Lipoid (mineral oil) pneumonia and cor pulmonale due to cardiospasm. Report of a case. Am J Roentgenol 76:108, 1956.
144. Casey JF: Chronic cor pulmonale associated with lipoid pneumonia. JAMA 177:896, 1961.
145. Corwin RW, Irwin RS: The lipid-laden alveolar macrophage as a marker of aspiration in parenchymal lung disease. Am Rev Respir Dis 132:576, 1985.
146. Colombo JL, Hallberg TK: Recurrent aspiration in children: Lipid-laden alveolar macrophage quantitation. Pediatr Pulmonol 3:86, 1987.
147. Rolla AR, Granfone A, Balogh K, et al: Granuloma-related hypercalcemia in lipoid pneumonia. Am J Med Sci 292:313, 1986.
148. Heckers H, Melcher F-W, Dittmar K, et al: Long-term course of mineral oil pneumonia. Lung 155:101, 1978.
149. Orlowski JP: Drowning, near drowning and ice water drowning. JAMA 260:390, 1988.
150. O'Carroll PW, Alkon E, Weiss B: Drowning mortality in Los Angeles County, 1977 to 1984. JAMA 260:380, 1988.
151. Manolios N, Mackie I: Drowning and near-drowning on Australian beaches patrolled by life-savers: A 10-year study, 1973–1983. Med J Aust 148:165, 1988.
152. Bolte RG, Black PG, Bowers CCP, et al: The use of extracorporeal rewarming in a child submerged for 66 minutes. JAMA 260:377, 1988.
153. Kylstra JA: Survival of submerged mammals. N Engl J Med 272:198, 1965.
154. Kylstra JA: Experiments in water-breathing. Sci Am 219:1123, 1968.
155. Miles S: Drowning. Br Med J 3:597, 1968.
156. Orlowski JP: Drowning, near-drowning, and ice-water submersions. Pediatr Clin North Am 34:75, 1987.
157. Sarnaik AP, Vohra MP: Near-drowning: Fresh, salt, and cold water immersion. Clin Sports Med 5:33, 1986.
158. Modell JH, Moya F: Effects of volume of aspirated fluid during chlorinated fresh water drowning. Anesthesiology 27:662, 1966.
159. Leading Article: Drowning. Lancet 2:441, 1968.
160. Hasan S, Avery WG, Fabian C, et al: Near drowning in humans: A report of 36 patients. Chest 59:191, 1971.
161. Fuller RH: The 1962 Wellcome Prize Essay: "Drowning and the postimmersion syndrome. A clinicopathologic study." Milit Med 128:22, 1963.

162. Bradley ME: Near-drowning: CPR is just the beginning. J Respir Dis 2:37, 1981.
163. Alexander IGS: The ultrastructure of the pulmonary alveolar vessels in Mendelson's (acid pulmonary aspiration) syndrome. Br J Anaesth 40:408, 1968.
164. Sladen A, Zauder HL: Methylprednisolone therapy for pulmonary edema following near drowning. JAMA 215:1793, 1971.
165. Heitzman ER: The Lung: Radiologic-Pathologic Correlations. St. Louis, The CV Mosby Co, 1973, pp 127, 137.
166. Noguchi M, Kimula Y, Ogata T: Muddy lung. Am J Clin Pathol 83:240, 1985.
167. Bonilla-Santiago Capt. J, Fill Capt. WL: Sand aspiration in drowning and near drowning. Radiology 128:301, 1978.
168. Rosenbaum HT, Thompson WL, Fuller RH: Radiographic pulmonary changes in near drowning. Radiology 83:306, 1964.
169. Hunter TB, Whitehouse WM: Freshwater near-drowning: Radiological aspects. Radiology 112:51, 1974.
170. Putman CE, Tummillo AM, Myerson DA, et al: Drowning: Another plunge. Am J Roentgenol 125:543, 1975.
171. Gonzalez-Rothi RJ: Near drowning: Consensus and controversies in pulmonary and cerebral resuscitation. Heart Lung 16:474, 1987.
172. Glauser FL, Smith WR: Pulmonary interstitial fibrosis following near-drowning and exposure to short-term high oxygen concentrations. Chest 68(Suppl):373, 1975.
173. Yagil Y, Stalnikowicz R, Michaeli J, et al: Near drowning in the Dead Sea: Electrolyte imbalances and therapeutic implications. Arch Intern Med 145:50, 1985.
174. Boles JM, Mabille S, Scheydecker JL, et al: Hypoglycaemia in salt water near-drowning victims. Intensive Care Med 14:80, 1988.
175. Modell JH, Graves SA, Ketover A: Clinical course of 91 consecutive near-drowning victims. Chest 70:231, 1976.
176. Jenkinson SG, George RB: Serial pulmonary function studies in survivors of near drowning. Chest 77:6, 1980.
177. Laughlin JJ, Eigen H: Pulmonary function abnormalities in survivors of near drowning. J Pediatr 100:26, 1982.
178. Modell JH: Near drowning. Circulation 74(Suppl IV):27, 1986.
179. Ansell G: A national survey of radiological complications: Interim report. Clin Radiol 19:175, 1968.
180. Reich SB: Production of pulmonary edema by aspiration of water-soluble nonabsorbable contrast media. Radiology 92:367, 1969.
181. Chiu CL, Gambach RR: Hypaque pulmonary edema: A case report. Radiology 111:91, 1974.
182. Moran TJ, Hellstrom HR: Experimental aspiration pneumonia. V. Acute pulmonary edema, pneumonia, and bronchiolitis obliterans produced by injection of ethyl alcohol. Am J Clin Pathol 27:300, 1957.
183. Smith RH, Moran TJ: Experimental aspiration pneumonia. III. Pneumonia produced by intratracheal injection of carbohydrate solutions. AMA Arch Pathol 57:194, 1954.
184. McGuirt WF, Holmes KD, Feehs R, et al: Tracheobronchial foreign bodies. Laryngoscope 98:615, 1988.
185. Laks Y, Barzilay Z: Foreign body aspiration in childhood. Pediatr Emerg Care 4:102, 1988.
186. Diehl JT, Thomas L, Bloom MB, et al: Tracheoesophageal fistula associated with Barrett's ulcer: the importance of reflex control. Ann Thorac Surg 45:449, 1988.
187. Coelho CA, Ferrante R: Dysphagia in postpolio sequelae: report of three cases. Arch Phys Med Rehabil 69:634, 1988.
188. Stringer DA, Sprigg A, Juodis E, et al: The association of cystic fibrosis, gastroesophageal reflux, and reduced pulmonary function. J Can Assoc Radiol 39:100, 1988.

NAME INDEX

Reference numbers are in **bold face**
and are followed by the numbers of the pages
on which they are cited.

SUBJECT INDEX

Note: Page numbers in *italics* refer to illustrations;
page numbers followed by t refer to tables.